Inflammatory Diseases of Blood Vessels

Inflammatory Diseases of Blood Vessels

edited by

Gary S. Hoffman
Cleveland Clinic Foundation
Cleveland, Ohio

Cornelia M. Weyand
Mayo Clinic and Mayo Foundation
Rochester, Minnesota

MARCEL DEKKER, INC.   NEW YORK • BASEL

ISBN: 0-8247-0269-7

This book is printed on acid-free paper.

Headquarters
Marcel Dekker, Inc.
270 Madison Avenue, New York, NY 10016
tel: 212-696-9000; fax: 212-685-4540

Eastern Hemisphere Distribution
Marcel Dekker AG
Hutgasse 4, Postfach 812, CH-4001 Basel, Switzerland
tel: 41-61-261-8482; fax: 41-61-261-8896

World Wide Web
http://www.dekker.com

The publisher offers discounts on this book when ordered in bulk quantities. For more information, write to Special Sales/Professional Marketing at the headquarters address above.

To our spouses and children
without whose support and love
our accomplishments and joys would be incomplete:
Jörg, Dominic, and Isabel Goronzy
Diane, Matthew, and Timothy Hoffman

Preface

Inflammatory Diseases of Blood Vessels is a comprehensive overview of the science and clinical consequences of vascular inflammation in health and disease. Chapters cover basic topics that would be of interest to scientists and clinicians from a broad range of disciplines.

Vascular inflammation has become of interest in atherosclerosis and myocardial infarction, as well as many different forms of primary and secondary idiopathic systemic vasculitis. Diagnostic methods and tools, as well as new developments in treatment, challenge practicing clinicians in rheumatology, nephrology, pulmonology, clinical immunology, cardiology, vascular medicine, cardiovascular surgery, and pathology.

We have tried to serve all of these constituencies by reviewing accepted principles in the science of vascular diseases and clinical medicine, as well as including new information about the most promising areas of discovery that we hope will change the understanding and practice of medicine in the future.

To achieve our goals, we have selected contributors who are leading worldwide authorities in their fields. We have admired their work over the years and are very grateful for their help in making this volume comprehensive. We believe that this book will be a valuable and frequently used reference.

The authors are indebted to our patients and colleagues who have helped to educate and nurture our appreciation of the mechanisms and clinical consequences of vascular inflammation.

Anthony S. Fauci, M.D., Director of the National Institute of Allergy and Infectious Diseases, has played a major role in delineating mechanisms whereby immunosuppressive agents modulate immune responses and become effective therapies for formerly fatal inflammatory vascular diseases. It was in his program that one of us (GSH) was first exposed to an extraordinary spectrum of systemic vasculitides and provided with unique opportunities to study patients with a team of talented scientists.

We are grateful to our students and fellows, who have trusted in our mentorship and have joined us in the pursuit of knowledge. Their work in the laboratory, where they explored with endless enthusiasm the immunopathology of vascular inflammation, has critically shaped our concepts and ideas. Their help will be needed in bringing molecular biology, genomics, and proteonomics to our patients.

Gary S. Hoffman
Cornelia M. Weyand

Contents

III. Secondary Vasculitides

Contributors

Dwomoa Adu, M.D., F.R.C.P. Consultant Nephrologist, Queen Elizabeth Hospital, Edgbaston, Birmingham, England

Paul A. Bacon, M.D., F.R.C.P. (UK) Chairman, Department of Rheumatology, University of Birmingham Medical School, Birmingham, England

Karyl S. Barron, M.D. Deputy Director, Division of Intramural Research, National Institute of Allergy and Infectious Diseases, National Institutes of Health, Bethesda, Maryland

Luigi M. Biasucci, M.D. Catholic University of Sacred Heart, Rome, Italy

Isabel Bielsa Hospital Germans Trias i Pujol, Badalona, Spain

Johannes Björnsson, M.D. Consultant, Department of Laboratory Medicine and Pathology; Professor of Pathology, Mayo Medical School; Mayo Clinic and Mayo Foundation, Rochester, Minnesota

Peter C. Brooks, Ph.D. University of Southern California School of Medicine, Los Angeles, California

Leonard H. Calabrese, M.D. Professor of Medicine and Vice Chairman, Rheumatic and Immunological Diseases, Cleveland Clinic Foundation, Cleveland, Ohio

Kenneth T. Calamia, M.D. Department of Rheumatology, Mayo Clinic Jacksonville, Jacksonville, Florida

Jeffrey P. Callen, M.D. Professor of Medicine and Chief, Division of Dermatology, University of Louisville, Louisville, Kentucky

Edwin S.L. Chan, M.D., F.R.C.P.C. Department of Medicine/Rheumatology, New York University School of Medicine, New York, New York

Maria Cinta-Cid, M.D. Department of Internal Medicine, Hospital Clinic i Provincial, Barcelona, Spain

Paul Cockwell, Ph.D., M.R.C.P. Department of Nephrology, Queen Elizabeth Hospital, Birmingham, England

Blanca Coll-Vinent   Hospital Clinic i Provincial, Barcelona, Spain

Pascal Cohen, M.D.   Hôpital Avicenne, Bobigny, France

Jan W. Cohen Tervaert, M.D., Ph.D.   Professor, Clinical Immunology, University Hospital, Maastricht, The Netherlands

Mary Frances Cotch, Ph.D.   Program Director, Collaborative Clinical Research, National Eye Institute, National Institutes of Health, Bethesda, Maryland

Bruce N. Cronstein, M.D.   Professor of Medicine, Department of Medicine/Rheumatology, New York University School of Medicine, New York, New York

Elena Csernok, Ph.D.   Rheumaklinik Bad Bramstedt GmbH, University of Lübeck, Bad Bramstedt, Germany

Rossana Danese, M.D., F.A.C.E.   Department of Endocrinology, Cleveland Clinic Foundation, Cleveland, Ohio

David D'Cruz, M.D., F.R.C.P.   Consultant Rheumatologist, The Lupus Research Unit, St. Thomas' Hospital, London, England

Paul DeMarco, M.D.   Balboa Naval Medical Center, San Diego, California

Michael J. Dillon, M.D., F.R.C.P.   Professor of Medicine, Cardiothoracic Unit, Special Pediatric Unit, Hospital for Sick Children, London, England

George F. Duna, M.D., F.A.C.P.   Clinical Assistant Professor, Baylor College of Medicine, Houston, Texas

Ronald J. Falk, M.D.   Professor of Medicine and Chief, Division of Nephrology, Department of Medicine, University of North Carolina, Chapel Hill, North Carolina

Scott D. Flamm, M.D.   The Texas Medical Center, Houston, Texas

Paul R. Fortin, M.D., M.P.H., F.R.C.P. (C)   Director of Clinical Research, Arthritis Center of Excellence, and Associate Professor of Medicine, University Health Network, University of Toronto, Toronto, Ontario, Canada

Robert I. Fox, M.D., Ph.D.   Division of Allergy and Rheumatology, Scripps Memorial Hospital and Research Foundation, La Jolla, California

Joseph M. Giordano, M.D.   Professor and Chairman, Department of Surgery, George Washington University Medical Center, Washington, D.C.

Jörg J. Goronzy, M.D., Ph.D.   Professor, Departments of Medicine and Immunology, Mayo Clinic and Mayo Foundation, Rochester, Minnesota

Wolfgang L. Gross, M.D., Ph.D.   Professor of Medicine, Rheumaklinik Bad Bramstedt GmbH, University of Lübeck, Bad Bramstedt, Germany

Loïc Guillevin, M.D. Professor of Medicine and Chairman, Department of Internal Medicine, Hôpital Avicenne, Université Paris–Nord, Bobigny, France

Göran K. Hansson, M.D., Ph.D. Professor, Center for Molecular Medicine and Department of Medicine, Karolinska Institutet and Karolinska Hospital, Stockholm, Sweden

Edward D. Harris, Jr., M.D. George DeForest Barnett Professor of Medicine, Department of Medicine/Rheumatology, Stanford University School of Medicine, Stanford, California

Loubna Hassanieh University of Southern California School of Medicine, Los Angeles, California

Joichiro Hayashi, Ph.D. The Scripps Research Institute, La Jolla, California

Barton F. Haynes, M.D. Frederic M. Hanes Professor and Chair, Department of Medicine, Duke University Medical Center, Durham, North Carolina

Peter Heeringa, Ph.D. Department of Pathology and Laboratory Medicine, University of North Carolina, Chapel Hill, North Carolina

Gary S. Hoffman, M.D. Professor of Medicine, Harold C. Schott Chair, and Chairman, Department of Rheumatic and Immunologic Diseases, and Director, Center for Vasculitis Care and Research, Cleveland Clinic Foundation, Cleveland, Ohio

Byron J. Hoogwerf, M.D., F.A.C.P., F.A.C.E. Department of Endocrinology, and Director, Internal Medicine Residency Program, Cleveland Clinic Foundation, Cleveland, Ohio

Graham R.V. Hughes, M.D., F.R.C.P. Professor of Medicine, Lupus Unit, St. Thomas' Hospital, London, England

Gene G. Hunder, M.D. Professor of Medicine, Department of Internal Medicine/Rheumatology, Mayo Clinic and Mayo Foundation, Rochester, Minnesota

David Jayne Consultant in Nephrology and Vasculitis, Department of Medicine, Addenbrooke's Hospital, Cambridge, England

J. Charles Jennette, M.D. Brinkhous Distinguished Professor and Chair, Department of Pathology and Laboratory Medicine, University of North Carolina, Chapel Hill, North Carolina

Jukka Juvonen, M.D., Ph.D. Chief, Department of Internal Medicine, Central Hospital of Kainuu, Kajaani, Finland

Tatu Juvonen, M.D., Ph.D. Professor and Chairman, Department of Surgery, University of Oulu, Oulu, Finland

Cees G.M. Kallenberg, M.D., Ph.D. Professor, Clinical Immunology, University Hospital, Groningen, The Netherlands

M. Bashar Kahaleh, M.D. Professor of Rheumatology, Department of Medicine, Medical College of Ohio, Toledo, Ohio

Munther A. Khamashta, M.D., Ph.D., M.R.C.P.   Deputy Director, Lupus Unit, St. Thomas' Hospital, London, England

Robert P. Kimberly, M.D.   Professor, Department of Medicine/Clinical Immunology and Rheumatology, University of Alabama at Birmingham, Birmingham, Alabama

Hynda K. Kleinman, Ph.D.   Research Chemist and Chief, Cell Biology, National Institute of Dental & Craniofacial Research, National Institutes of Health, Bethesda, Maryland

E. Carwile LeRoy, M.D.   Professor, Department of Microbiology and Immunology, Medical University of South Carolina, Charleston, South Carolina

François Lhote, M.D.   Hôpital Avicenne, Bobigny, France

Giovanna Liuzzo, M.D.   Institute of Cardiology, Catholic University of Sacred Heart, Rome, Italy

Katherine M. Malinda, Ph.D.   National Institute of Dental & Craniofacial Research, National Institutes of Health, Bethesda, Maryland

Brian F. Mandell, M.D., Ph.D.   Education Program Director, Rheumatic and Immunologic Diseases, Cleveland Clinic Foundation, Cleveland, Ohio

Gopal K. Marathe, Ph.D.   Human Molecular Biology and Genetics, University of Utah, Salt Lake City, Utah

Tashiaki Maruyama, M.D., Ph.D.   The Scripps Research Institute, La Jolla, California

Attilio Maseri, M.D., Ph.D.   Professor, Institute of Cardiology, Catholic University of Sacred Heart, Rome, Italy

Eric L. Matteson, M.D., M.P.H.   Associate Professor, Division of Rheumatology, Department of Medicine, Mayo Clinic and Mayo Foundation, Rochester, Minnesota

Rex M. McCallum, M.D.   Associate Clinical Professor, Department of Medicine, Duke University Medical Center, Durham, North Carolina

Thomas M. McIntyre, Ph.D.   Human Molecular Biology and Genetics, University of Utah, Salt Lake City, Utah

Peter A. Merkel, M.D., M.P.H.   Assistant Professor of Medicine, Rheumatology Section, Boston University School of Medicine, Boston, Massachusetts

Paul Michelson, M.D.   Scripps Memorial Hospital and Research Foundation, La Jolla, California

Rocco Misiani, M.D.   Director, Unità Operativa di Medicina Interna, Ospedali Riuniti di Bergamo, Bergamo, Italy

Fujio Numano, M.D., Ph.D.   Professor, Third Department of Internal Medicine, Tokyo Medical and Dental University, Tokyo, Japan

J. Desmond O'Duffy, M.D., F.R.C.P.   Private Practice, Sarasota, Florida

Chester V. Oddis, M.D.   Associate Professor, Department of Medicine, University of Pittsburgh School of Medicine, Pittsburgh, Pennsylvania

Jeffrey W. Olin, D.O.   Director, The Heart and Vascular Institute, Morristown, New Jersey

M. Lourdes Ponce, Ph.D.   National Institute of Dental & Craniofacial Research, National Institutes of Health, Bethesda, Maryland

Stephen M. Prescott, M.D.   Director, Huntsman Cancer Institute, University of Utah, Salt Lake City, Utah

Jaya K. Rao, M.D., M.H.S.   Assistant Professor, Department of Medicine, Duke University, Durham, North Carolina

Karen E. Rendt, M.D.   Education Program Co-Director, Department of Rheumatic and Immunologic Diseases, Center for Vasculitis Care and Research, Cleveland Clinic Foundation, Cleveland, Ohio

Caroline O.S. Savage, M.D., Ph.D., F.R.C.P.   Professor, Department of Medical Sciences, University of Birmingham Medical School, Birmingham, England

Markku J. Savolainen, M.D., Ph.D.   Professor of Medicine, Department of Internal Medicine, University of Oulu, Oulu, Finland

Yoshinori Seko, M.D., Ph.D.   Research Associate, Department of Cardiovascular Medicine, University of Tokyo, Tokyo, Japan

Prediman K. Shah, M.D.   Shapell and Webb Chair and Director, Cardiology and Atherosclerosis Research Center, Cedars Sinai Medical Center, and Professor of Medicine, University of California, Los Angeles, California

Michael C. Sneller, M.D.   Chief, Immunologic Diseases Section, Laboratory of Immunoregulation, National Institute of Allergy and Infectious Diseases, National Institutes of Health, Bethesda, Maryland

Ulrich Specks, M.D.   Associate Professor, Division of Pulmonary and Critical Care Medicine, Mayo Clinic and Mayo Foundation, Rochester, Minnesota

Sudhakar Sridharan, M.D.   Department of Rheumatic and Immunologic Diseases, Cleveland Clinic Foundation, Cleveland, Ohio

E. William St. Clair, M.D.   Associate Professor, Department of Medicine, Duke University Medical Center, Durham, North Carolina

Anthony W. Stanson, M.D.   Department of Radiology, Mayo Clinic and Mayo Foundation, Rochester, Minnesota

Ilona S. Szer, M.D., F.A.A.P., F.A.C.R.   Director, Division of Pediatric Rheumatology, Children's Hospital of San Diego, and Professor of Pediatrics, University of California School of Medicine, San Diego, La Jolla, California

Arthur Topoulos, M.D.   Department of Vascular Medicine, Cleveland Clinic Foundation, Cleveland, Ohio

Robert M. Valente, M.D.   Arthritis Center of Nebraska, Lincoln, Nebraska

Dimitrios Vassilopoulos, M.D.   Department of Rheumatic and Immunologic Diseases, Cleveland Clinic Foundation, Cleveland, Ohio

Alexandra Villa-Forte, M.D.   Department of Rheumatic and Immunologic Diseases, Cleveland Clinic Foundation, Cleveland, Ohio

Cornelia M. Weyand, M.D., Ph.D.   Barbara Woodward Lips Professor of Medicine and Immunology, Departments of Medicine and Immunology, Mayo Clinic and Mayo Foundation, Rochester, Minnesota

Richard D. White, M.D., F.A.C.C.   Head, Cardiovascular Imaging, Department of Radiology, Cleveland Clinic Foundation, Cleveland, Ohio

Guy A. Zimmerman, M.D.   Human Molecular Biology and Genetics, University of Utah, Salt Lake City, Utah

1

Vasculitis: A Dialogue Between the Artery and the Immune System

Cornelia M. Weyand

Mayo Clinic and Foundation, Rochester, Minnesota

I. INTRODUCTION

Vasculitides are chronic inflammatory diseases in which blood vessel walls are targeted by an immune insult. For the last decades, necrosis of the vessel wall as well as thrombotic occlusion of the vascular lumen have been considered to be the major pathological pathways. The standard paradigm for the immunopathogenesis of inflammatory vasculopathies has centered around the assumption that endothelial injury is the leading event followed by the formation of inflammatory cell infiltrates within and around the vessel wall. It is now clear that this paradigm is oversimplified. From advances in cell and molecular biology, immunology, and molecular genetics, several new key concepts have emerged that, when integrated with the clinical syndromes of vasculitis, will facilitate an explosion of new knowledge and improved patient care.

One of the major revelations in vascular diseases is that the traditional separation of noninflammatory and inflammatory vasculopathies is incorrect. Atherosclerotic vascular disease, the underlying pathology for ischemic heart disease and stroke, is the leading cause of death and disability in the Western world. There is plentiful evidence that immune cells and inflammatory pathways participate in atherogenesis, particularly in the events leading to plaque rupture and acute ischemia. It has been proposed that inflammation is a critical component of atherosclerosis, bringing it in alignment with the classic vasculitides.

Conceptually, the most important developments stem from the realization that the vascular pathology caused by inflammation results from contributions of both the attacking immune cells and the responding blood vessel wall. The vascular tissue is not merely an innocent bystander being insulted by immune-mediated effector mechanisms. Rather, the vessel wall serves as a "partner in crime" with an injury response program, providing protection and regeneration, but most importantly, also maladaptive responses. Both the immune insult and the blood vessel have significant effects on each other and have to be understood as an interactive unit. While the injury initiated by the immune reaction in and around the blood vessel wall is influential on the initiation of the disease, the reaction pattern of the attacked blood vessel is equally important in determining whether the interaction between the immune system and the vasculature will be beneficially or detrimentally resolved. The importance of this concept is best exemplified by the hyperproliferative reaction of the intima, originally intended to repair tissue injury, but which leads to lumen occlusion and ischemia.

Most chapters in this book highlight individual components of the inflammatory infiltrates and blood vessel wall and their possible involvement in disease. The purpose of this chapter is to focus on arteries, clinically the most relevant targets of vascular disease, and to draw attention to the key concept that the artery's perspective is critical in modulating and controlling the disease process. Having accepted that the blood vessel contributes to pathology, it is evident that particular features of this tissue will impact the outcome of vascular inflammation. Variations in the composition of different territories of the vascular tree should be reflected by heterogeneity of disease and could provide an explanation for the fascinating clinical observation that consequences of vasculitis differ with the site, the size, and the number of affected vessels. The clinical relevance of this conceptually new view of inflammatory blood vessel disease will be the ability to therapeutically target not only the immune system but also its "partner in crime."

II. STRUCTURAL SPECIFICS OF THE ARTERIAL WALL

To fulfill its role in transport, exchange, and vasomotor control, the arterial wall contains several cell types, arranged in defined wall layers, and a complex array of extracellular matrix (Fig. 1). In normal vessels, the lining of the lumen is formed by a single-cell layer of endothelium, forming a nonadhesive and nonthrombogenic luminal surface. Lateral interactions between endothelial cells control transendothelial permeability and the extravasation of leukocytes from the blood into the surrounding tissue space. Extensive studies have demonstrated that the endothelial lining is an interface that is dynamic in nature and rapidly responds to stimuli received from the circulation and from neighboring cells and tissues (1). Besides its unique anatomical position between the circulation and the tissues, the cellular constituents of the endothelium have been found to possess an impressive repertoire of functions. In response to stimuli, they are capable of produc-

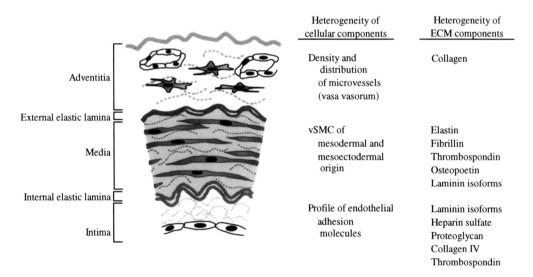

Figure 1 Structure of the arterial wall. The vessel wall of small to large arteries consists of three layers: intima, media, and adventitia. While this structural organization is universal, arteries of different sizes and localizations differ in the cellular and the matrix components that form these layers. Therefore, inflammatory cells infiltrating into the arterial wall will encounter quite distinct microenvironments with implications for the immune interactions defining the vascular disease process. Also, molecular heterogeneity among vascular beds should translate into differences of response patterns to the inflammatory attack.

ing effector molecules, such as nitric oxide, cytokines, growth factors, vasoactive peptides, fibrinolytic factors, and procoagulant and anticoagulant substances (1,2). Stimuli have been identified that increase the expression of adhesion molecules on the endothelial lining, regulating the process of leukocyte recruitment under physiological and pathological conditions (3,4).

It is important to realize that endothelial cells are not limited to the arterial lumen but also line the vasa vasorum. The vascular wall is a relatively avascular tissue, comparable to cartilage that completely lacks vascularization. Oxygen and nutrients are delivered to the wall layers by diffusion from the lumen. Arteries reaching a critical wall thickness form a capillary network in the adventitia. Whether macroendothelial and microendothelial cells play different roles in vasculitis has not been firmly demonstrated, but it is very likely that they are involved in different aspects of the disease process and have different contributions in distinct vascular territories.

Contractility of the vascular wall is a function of the medial layer, composed of vascular smooth muscle cells (vSMCs). A central premise of modern vascular biology is that vSMCs have the unique ability to switch from a contractile to a synthetic phenotype (5). Associated with this phenotypic switch, vSMCs acquire migratory capability and begin to proliferate. Vascular smooth muscle cell migration, proliferation, and extracellular matrix production have been implicated as the critical steps in the formation of hyperplastic intima. The origin of the intimal SMCs remains a matter of debate and the former paradigm that they derive from the medial layer has been challenged (6). With enormous flexibility in phenotype and function, vSMCs could also serve as partners in immune reactions. This concept has not been explored in vasculitic lesions.

Information is least available about the adventitia, a layer of soft tissue surrounding the artery. This soft tissue has only been regarded as a passive structural support component of the vascular wall, but recent data suggest a possible active, if not central, role of the adventitial layer in atherogenesis and in vasculitis (7,8). Specifically, the adventitia contains the capillary network of vasa vasorum, thus providing access to the arterial wall not only for macromolecular particles but also for immune cells. Accelerated growth and redistribution of microcapillaries in the adventitia has been implicated as an early event in atherogenesis.

Functional aspects of the vascular wall in physiological and pathological situations cannot be separated from extracellular matrix proteins (9). Different compartments of the wall contain various matrix types. The basement membrane matrix manufactured by endothelial cells is composed of laminin, type IV collagen, and heparin sulfate proteoglycan. Different sets of isoforms of these basic components are used to assemble basement membranes surrounding the SMCs of the media. The media is characterized by sheets of collagenous and elastic tissues with particular concentration of elastin and fibrillin in the elastic laminae, and the matrix of the adventitia is enriched for collagens (10). Cell matrix interactions have been studied in the maintenance of the vascular structure and angiogenesis (11,12), but their involvement in vascular pathologies is not well understood. It can be expected that the molecular composition of the vascular wall has important influence on how immune reactions evolve.

III. TARGET-TISSUE SUSCEPTIBILITY: NOT ALL ARTERIES ARE EQUAL

A characteristic feature of vasculitides is their preference for defined vascular beds. The selectivity of individual syndromes is clinically used, particularly when imaging techniques or sites for tissue biopsies are chosen. As an example, Takayasu's arteritis targets the aorta and its primary branches. Giant cell arteritis (GCA), a closely related entity, can cause aortitis but consistently spares the primary branches and is essentially not found in the common carotid, innominate, proximal subclavian, visceral, or common iliac arteries. Giant cell arteritis classically manifests in the second- to fifth-order branches of the aorta with a strong preference for upper extremity and cranial arteries. Once extracranial arteries penetrate into the skull, they no longer serve as a target for GCA but appear to be protected from the disease. One obvious conclusion is that the ability of the host to generate an immune response is not sufficient for disease initiation or progression. But, how is the inflammation targeted? Specific features of the local environment must determine whether a particular vessel serves as a site for vasculitis. The factors predisposing arteries for inflammatory attack are incompletely known but variations in the cellular and molecular composition of the vasculature cannot be without relevance (Table 1 and Fig. 1).

Blood vessels in different territories are specialized and are able to adapt to unique conditions and requirements of the organs they supply (13,14). Differences in endothelial cell function in different regions are indicated by tissue-specific homing of lymphocytes (15). Proof for biochemical differences of vascular beds has recently be provided by in vivo targeting experiments (16,17). In these experiments, peptide libraries expressed on the surface of a bacteriophage were used for in vivo targeting studies. The phages homed to organs, and different peptide motifs were recovered from each tissue. These data show that vasculature expresses organ- and tissue-specific heterogeneity and that molecular differences of blood vessels can serve as molecular addresses. It has also been suggested that the composition of matrix proteins varies in arterial territories (10).

The functional relevance of vasa vasorum in providing access to the arterial wall for inflammatory cells raises the possibility that the arrangement of these microcapillary vessels is a defining factor in arterial vulnerability. Studies on the structure and distribution of vasa vasorum are an emerging field of investigation and technologies are being developed that will allow for the construction of three-dimensional maps of adventitial vasa vasorum (18).

Additional variability in arterial wall components is introduced by the vSMCs (14). Smooth muscle cells of the blood vessel and gut arise from the mesenchyme (19). However, differences in lineage exist. In the head and neck, the mesenchyme derives from the ectoderm, suggesting that SMCs in these regions are genetically distinct. Support for this model has come from the demonstration that cultured mesoectodermal SMCs have unique properties, such as increased production of elastin (20). Smooth muscle cells of mesoectodermal origin may react differently from those of mesodermal origin, providing a clue for the targeting of GCA to head and neck arteries.

Data have now accumulated that in at least some of the arteritides antigen-specific immune responses occur in the arterial wall (21). In this disease concept, availability of eliciting antigen could contribute to target-tissue susceptibility in arteritis (see Table 1). Differences in the composition of the arterial wall could alter the spectrum of autoantigens. Alternatively, exogenous antigens could specifically infect tissue-residing cells represented in restricted areas. No experimental data are available that this is the case. Even for vasculitides associated with infectious diseases, such as hepatitis C, it has not been unequivocally documented that antigen is recognized at the site of vascular inflammation.

Table 1   Possible Mechanisms of Target-Tissue Susceptibility in Vasculitis

---

Variable spectrum of autoantigens expressed by vessels in different territories
Diversity in the vascular wall microenvironment
   Heterogeneity of endothelial cells represented in different vascular territories
   Variations in the extracellular matrix proteins expressed by different vascular beds
   Differences in the distribution of vasa vasorum
   Variability in vascular smooth muscle cells
Heterogeneity in the susceptibility of vascular wall cells toward infections
   Targeting of different cell populations
   Variations in the expression of cellular receptors
   Diverse reaction pattern of infected cells

Differential vulnerability of arterial territories is not limited to the primary vasculitides but also holds for atherosclerotic disease. Atherosclerosis is now considered an inflammatory disorder (22), and a purely mechanical view of obstructive arterial disease due to atheroma formation is being abandoned. Arterial occlusive disease in patients with atherosclerosis can be widespread, involving the coronary, cerebral, and peripheral circulation. However, it is not unusual that clinically significant disease, particularly acute clinical complication, occurs in patients with disease limited to a certain territory. It is also notable that the mammary and gastroepiploic arteries remain free of disease, even in hosts with severe atherosclerosis, allowing them to be used in coronary bypass surgery.

IV. CELLULAR INTERACTIONS IN THE INFLAMED ARTERIAL WALL

Pathological events in the blood vessel wall not only display selectivity for a vascular bed but they also acquire a distinct topography within the different regions of the wall. Lesions of atherosclerosis are strictly limited to the intima. Other parts of the arterial wall participate, but it is now clear that different tissue structures serve different functions. A detailed picture of the involvement of different layers of the arterial wall in vasculitis has been gathered for GCA (Fig. 2) (23). The underlying principle implies that arterial cells have means of communicating to invading cells where they are, where to go, and what to do, thereby inducing specific response patterns in the resident cells.

Inflammatory lesions in GCA are composed of T cells, most of which are CD4 T cells, and macrophages. B cells are rare, if not absent, from the vascular infiltrates (24). Activated forms of macrophages give rise to granulomas; macrophage polykaryons, multinucleated giant cells, are often found. Histomorphological hallmarks of GCA include granuloma formation, predominantly in the media, and fragmentation of the elastic laminae at the adventitial–medial and medial–intimal borders (25). Multinucleated giant cells are known to have a tendency to lie at the media–intima junction, often in vicinity to degraded internal elastic lamina. This arrangement could suggest that this vasculitis emerges as a response to an inert instigator, such as destroyed elastic tissue, and that the center of the immunological events coincides with the granulomas.

Experimental data support a more complex disease model. Evidence suggests that the critical events of T-cell activation and possibly antigen recognition originate in the adventitia (7, 21,24). The key cytokine in GCA, interferon-γ (IFN-γ) (26), derives from CD4 T cells in the adventitia, distant from the site of granuloma formation and elastic membrane destruction (7). The specific cellular and noncellular components of the adventitia that direct and regulate CD4+ IFN-γ–producing cells have not been identified, but obvious candidates include the vasa vasorum modulating cell adhesion and migration, specialized antigen presenting cells such as interdigitating dendritic cells, and the restricted expression of endogenous or exogenous antigen. The adventitia is also the residence for interleukin (IL)-1β– and IL-6–producing macrophages, cells equipped to support T-cell activation (23).

The complexity of cell–cell interactions in arteritis is exemplified by the finding that IFN-γ produced by adventitial T cells has regulatory functions for events occurring in proximal wall layers of the artery. How can cellular interactions occur distally and how do anatomical and biochemical characteristics of the arterial wall contribute to cell–cell interactions between the adventitia and the intima? Evidence for signal exchange between cells in distinct anatomical locations comes from studies demonstrating that macrophage effector functions in the media and intima are closely correlated with IFN-γ production in the adventitia. It is conceivable that extracellular matrix components of the vascular wall participate in the transport of such signals. Inflammatory cells in the media are functionally distinct from those in the adventitia. Medial

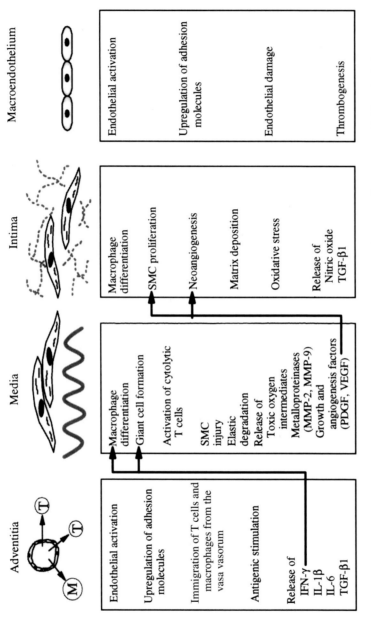

Figure 2 Compartmentalization of immune events in the arterial wall environment. In most vasculitides, the inflammatory response involves all layers of the arterial wall. Nevertheless, the immune response is compartmentalized with immune cells exerting different functions in different layers, suggesting that cellular and matrix components of the vessel wall regulate the differentiation of immune cells and their gene expression profile upon stimulation. Vessel wall components may also be important in facilitating communication among immune cells in different layers, e.g., cytokine-producing cells in the adventitia and metalloproteinase-secreting macrophages in the media. The schematic diagram has been modeled on giant cell arteritis, for which most data are available, but the model can be extended to other vasculitides.

macrophages specialize in the synthesis of matrix metalloproteinases (MMPs) (27) and growth factors (28). A critical cellular element is multinucleated giant cells, which have various secretory functions. They represent the major cellular source of platelet-derived growth factor (PDGF) and vascular endothelial growth factor (VEGF) in addition to producing MMP-2. Production of a variety of growth factors indicates that giant cells are not just a calamity of vascular damage with a role in removing debris. Instead, they appear to have a regulatory function for cells residing in the arterial wall, such as vSMCs and endothelial cells (29). Mechanisms of giant cell formation in the media are not understood and the nature of the stimuli controlling their activity also remains to be elucidated. Giant cells express IFN-γ receptors and could thus receive signals from IFN-γ–producing T cells located distant from them. The contribution of various other signals relevant in giant cell formation has to be inferred from the lack of polykaryons among macrophages directly intermingling with IFN-γ–producing T cells and from the specialized functional profile of macrophages accumulated in the arterial media.

The intima provides the proper environment for other molecular events. Macrophages recruited to the intima are characterized by their ability to produce nitric oxide synthase (NOS-2) (23). Nitric oxide is a paracrine signaling molecule in the vascular wall. In addition to its role in regulating vasomotor functions, it also has destructive potential. Recent observations indicate that NOS-2 production by intimal macrophages directly reflects specific features of the microenvironment. Hyperplastic intima is rich in laminin, which is known to interact with molecules of the integrin family (30). We have found that the laminin α-chain can induce transcription of NOS-2 in human macrophages. Interaction of macrophages with laminin results in the translocation of the transcription factors STAT-1 and NFκB into the nucleus, where they regulate gene function by binding to DNA motifs in the NOS-2 promoter region. Taking these experimental data into account, it can be proposed that matrix proteins in the intimal layer communicate with invading macrophages and regulate their functional differentiation. This is an excellent example of vascular wall components altering the function of immune cells, indicating that cross-talk between invading cells and arterial wall cells is a dialogue. Differences in microenvironment and compartmentalization of immune reactions should lead to a spectrum of structural lesions in inflammatory blood vessel diseases. In holding with this concept, blood vessels targeted by inflammatory attack display several different abnormalities. This is best visualized in small, medium-sized, and large arteries where different compartments are created due to the formation of the vessel wall. A listing of lesions typically found in arteritis is given in Table 2, including the pathomechanisms underlying the pathological findings. Due to the multitude of cell types and the definition of wall layers, more than one immunopathway has relevance in arteritis (see Table 2).

Table 2 Morphological Changes in Arteritis

Structural lesion in arteritis	Pathomechanism
Adventitial scarring	Extracellular matrix deposition
Fragmentation of elastic membranes	Tissue-degrading enzymes
Patchy disappearance of smooth muscle cells (SMCs)	SMC necrosis (SMC apoptosis) Membrane damage mediated by reactive oxygen species
Formation of new microvessels	Neoangiogenesis
Intimal hyperplasia	Myofibroblast migration and proliferation
Thrombotic occlusion	Prothrombogenic state of endothelial lining

V. RESPONSE-TO-INJURY PROGRAM OF THE ARTERY: PROTECTIVE AND MALADAPTIVE REACTION PATTERNS

The traditional paradigm assumes that the immune insult directed toward the vascular wall leads to tissue damage, wall rupture, and hemorrhage. However, hemorrhage is an infrequent complication of vasculitis. Inflammation of capillaries and small arteries can cause bleeding, but in the vasculitides targeting medium-sized and large vessels, aneurysm formation is only expected in patients with polyarteritis nodosa. In all other entities, vascular stenosis with tissue infarct is the typical pattern of vascular morbidity. How does vessel occlusion develop and why do intramural inflammatory infiltrates induce vascular wall rupture so infrequently? The arterial wall, like other organs, does not remain passive when injured. Rather, a response-to-injury program is initiated with the goal to protect and repair. Unfortunately, this response is often maladaptive, exacerbating the injury, delaying healing, and inducing structural changes that are detrimental to the patient, such as the formation of hyperplastic intima. The fibroproliferative response of the intimal layer is associated with an increase in smooth muscle cells and excessive deposition of matrix proteins (Table 3).

Intimal hyperplasia is a complex process that has been best examined in atherosclerotic plaques and in models of restenosis following arterial injury set by dilatation (Fig. 3) (31). It is possible that the molecular pathways involved in regulation of this injury response are similar in different vascular diseases. However, factors initiating the process and elements controlling disease progression are likely different in the multiple forms of vasculitis, atherogenesis, and allograft vasculopathy.

Myofibroblasts that form the thickened intima may derive from the media or the adventitia. Whether the originating cell is a smooth muscle cell that undergoes phenotypic changes or a fibroblast that acquires new functional capabilities is unsolved. Injury response starts with directed cell migration of myofibroblasts across the medial elastic lamina, a metalloproteinase-dependent process. Myofibroblast mobility and proliferation are modulated by polypeptide growth factors and cytokines provided in the milieu of the arterial wall. Such growth factors are present in very low abundance in the uninjured arterial wall and their overexpression is a typical feature of the injury response program. Synthesis of extracellular matrix proteins is probably regulated by similar mediators. Additional regulatory events have not yet been defined at the molecular level, but

Table 3 Injury Response of the Arterial Wall

Protective
  Heat shock proteins
  Aldose reductase in smooth muscle cells
Regenerative
  Matrix production
  Repair of media injury
Maladaptive
  Cytokine-mediated endothelial activation
    Recruitment of inflammatory cells
  Formation of microcapillaries
    Accessibility of media and intima to inflammatory cells
  Mobilization, migration, and proliferation of smooth muscle cells
    Intimal hyperplasia
  Aldose reductase in T cells and macrophages
    Protection of inflammatory cells from oxidative damage

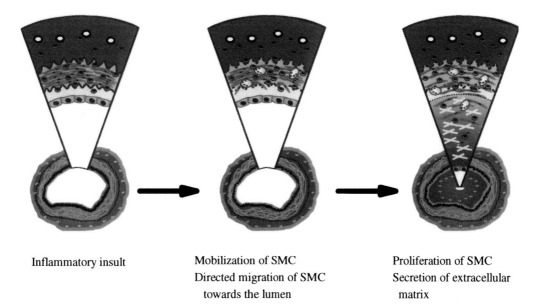

| Inflammatory insult | Mobilization of SMC
Directed migration of SMC
towards the lumen | Proliferation of SMC
Secretion of extracellular
matrix |

Figure 3 Intimal hyperplasia—the major maladaptive response of inflamed arteries. In response to the inflammatory insult, smooth muscle cells are mobilized, proliferate, and migrate to the intima. These smooth muscle cells switch from a contractile to a secretory phenotype enabling them to produce matrix molecules. Smooth muscle cell mobilization and proliferation are under the control of metalloproteinases and growth factors secreted mainly by tissue-infiltrating macrophages and by giant cells in the media. The end result is a concentric hyperplastic intima that occludes the lumen.

cell–cell interactions with inflammatory cells, other non-SMCs, and matrix components could potentially influence the response to arterial injury.

Some aspects of the interplay between growth-regulatory molecules, immune cells recruited to the lesions, and cellular components of the vessel wall have been studied. In GCA, PDGF-A and PDGF-B are abundantly produced in affected arteries (28). The majority of the PDGF-producing cells are mononuclear cells, specifically macrophages. The supply of PDGF in the lesions has been associated not only with the degree of luminal obstruction but also with clinical signs of ischemia, lending support to the concept that the response-to-injury program of the arterial wall has clinical relevance in vasculitis.

Only a specialized subset of intramural macrophages, multinucleated giant cells, can provide PDGF in GCA. The production of growth factors by invading inflammatory cells suggests that the arterial repair mechanisms causing clinical complications are ultimately under the control of the infiltrating immune cells. Hyperplastic intima in inflamed temporal arteries can be distinguished from that in allograft vasculopathy. In the latter model, intimal myofibroblasts themselves were found to release PDGF, suggesting an autocrine amplification of cellular hyperproliferation (32). Neointimal cells do not contribute to PDGF synthesis in GCA, but instead inflammatory cells, particularly multinucleated giant cells, are the major regulators of growth factor production.

Multinucleated giant cells have been implicated in other aspects of the response-to-injury program in GCA. Besides their ability to secrete MMPs and PDGF, they also transcribe and synthesize VEGF (29). Vascular endothelial growth factor is a polypeptide growth factor with a critical role in the formation of new blood vessels. Neoangiogenesis is one of the structural changes typical of the chronically inflamed arterial wall. Microvessels are normally restricted to the adventitia and are only found in the media and in the hyperplastic intima under pathological conditions. Careful regulation of neoangiogenesis is suggested by a distinct topography of newly formed capillaries, which are arranged in the outer one-third of the intimal layer. Growth of new blood vessels in the arterial wall is not a random process but has been associated with the presence of multinucleated giant cells and the degree of internal elastic lamina fragmentation. Molecular studies have indicated that tissue production of VEGF is correlated with the transcription of IFN-γ, raising the possibility that T lymphocytes influence the availability of angiogenic factors. Tissue IFN-γ has been shown to be highest in arteries with giant cell formation. Because giant cells are the source of VEGF, IFN-γ could act in regulating giant cell activity.

The response-to-injury program accompanying vascular inflammation is not completely detrimental. The array of genes upregulated in inflamed arteries includes molecules that are protective and regenerative. An example is the overexpression of aldose reductase (AR) in affected temporal arteries of GCA patients (33). Aldose reductase is a member of the aldo–keto reductase superfamily and is a monomeric NADPH (reduced form of nicotinamide adenine dinucleotide phosphate) dependent oxidoreductase with broad substrate specificity for carbonyl compounds (34,35). Colocalization of AR with lipid peroxidation products in the vascular lesions led to the hypothesis that the toxic aldehyde 4-hydroxynoneal could be a substrate for the enzyme (33). Blocking of AR in vivo with specific enzyme inhibitors led to increased production of toxic aldehydes and an increase in the number of apoptotic cells in the arterial wall. The model holds that inflammatory injury upregulates AR, an oxidative defense mechanism that functions by detoxifying toxic products of lipid peroxidation. An intriguing aspect of this model is which cells are the beneficiaries of this tissue-protective mechanism. Preventing smooth muscle cell apoptosis would clearly limit vascular wall damage; thus, AR could function by preserving medial thickness. However, it is also possible that AR protects tissue-infiltrating lymphocytes and macrophages. Mononuclear cells in the vascular lesions produced high concentrations of AR in their cytoplasm. By upregulating AR, macrophages, the producers of reactive oxygen species, could protect themselves from the cytopathic effects of toxic oxygen metabolites. Therefore, induction of AR could prevent suicide of the attacker, but would ultimately be to the disadvantage of the patient because it would amplify the immune insult. Careful studies will be necessary to understand the negative and positive effects mediated by the genetic program of the arterial wall in response to the immune attack. These studies promise to identify novel targets for immunosuppression in vasculitis, and to open up entirely new areas of therapeutic interventions by focusing on the artery's maladaptive contribution to disease.

REFERENCES

1. Cines DB, Pollak ES, Buck CA, Loscalzo J, Zimmerman GA, McEver RP, Pober JS, Wick TM, Konkle BA, Schwartz BS, Barnathan ES, McCrae KR, Hug BA, Schmidt AM, Stern DM. Endothelial cells in physiology and in the pathophysiology of vascular disorders. Blood 1998; 91:3527–3561.
2. Krishnaswamy G, Kelley J, Yerra L, Smith JK, Chi DS. Human endothelium as a source of multifunctional cytokines: molecular regulation and possible role in human disease. J Interferon Cytokine Res 1999; 19:91–104.
3. Butcher EC, Picker LJ. Lymphocyte homing and homeostasis. Science 1996; 272:60–66.
4. Wang J, Springer TA. Structural specializations of immunoglobulin superfamily members for adhesion to integrins and viruses. Immunol Rev 1998; 163:197–215.
5. Andres V. Control of vascular smooth muscle cell growth and its implication in atherosclerosis and restenosis (review). Int J Mol Med 1998; 2:81–89.
6. Wilcox JN, Scott NA. Potential role of the adventitia in arteritis and atherosclerosis. Int J Cardiol 1996; 54(suppl):S21–S35.

7. Wagner AD, Bjornsson J, Bartley GB, Goronzy JJ, Weyand CM. Interferon-gamma-producing T cells in giant cell vasculitis represent a minority of tissue-infiltrating cells and are located distant from the site of pathology. Am J Pathol 1996; 148:1925–1933.

8. Kwon HM, Sangiorgi G, Ritman EL, McKenna C, Holmes DRJ, Schwartz RS, Lerman A. Enhanced coronary vasa vasorum neovascularization in experimental hypercholesterolemia. J Clin Invest 1998; 101:1551–1556.

9. Coats WD, Jr., Faxon DP. The role of the extracellular matrix in arterial remodelling. Semin Interv Cardiol 1997; 2:167–176.

10. Ruoslahti E, Engvall E. Integrins and vascular extracellular matrix assembly. J Clin Invest 1997; 100: S53–S56.

11. Ruoslahti E, Vaheri A. Cell-to-cell contact and extracellular matrix. Curr Opin Cell Biol 1997; 9:605–607.

12. Hynes RO, Wagner DD. Genetic manipulation of vascular adhesion molecules in mice. J Clin Invest 1997; 100:S11–3.

13. Garlanda C, Dejana E. Heterogeneity of endothelial cells. Specific markers. Arterioscler Thromb Vasc Biol 1997; 17:1193–1202.

14. Shanahan CM, Weissberg PL. Smooth muscle cell heterogeneity: Patterns of gene expression in vascular smooth muscle cells in vitro and in vivo. Arterioscler Thromb Vasc Biol 1998; 18:333–338.

15. Butcher EC. Leukocyte-endothelial cell recognition: Three (or more) steps to specificity and diversity. Cell 1991; 67:1033–1036.

16. Pasqualini R, Ruoslahti E. Organ targeting in vivo using phage display peptide libraries. Nature 1996; 380:364–366.

17. Rajotte D, Arap W, Hagedorn M, Koivunen E, Pasqualini R, Ruoslahti E. Molecular heterogeneity of the vascular endothelium revealed by in vivo phage display. J Clin Invest 1998; 102:430–437.

18. Kwon HM, Sangiorgi G, Ritman EL, Lerman A, McKenna C, Virmani R, Edwards WD, Holmes DR, Schwartz RS. Adventitial vasa vasorum in balloon-injured coronary arteries: Visualization and quantitation by a microscopic three-dimensional computed tomography technique. J Am Coll Cardiol 1998; 32:2072–2079.

19. Archer SL. Diversity of phenotype and function of vascular smooth muscle cells. J Lab Clin Med 1996; 127:524–529.

20. Majesky MW, Schwartz SM. An origin for smooth muscle cells from endothelium? Circ Res 1997; 80:601–603.

21. Weyand CM, Goronzy JJ. Giant cell arteritis as an antigen-driven disease. Rheum Dis Clin North Am 1995; 21:1027–1039.

22. Ross R. Atherosclerosis—An inflammatory disease. N Engl J Med 1999; 340:115–126.

23. Weyand CM, Wagner AD, Bjornsson J, Goronzy JJ. Correlation of the topographical arrangement and the functional pattern of tissue-infiltrating macrophages in giant cell arteritis. J Clin Invest 1996; 98:1642–1649.

24. Martinez-Taboada V, Brack A, Hunder GG, Goronzy JJ, Weyand CM. The inflammatory infiltrate in giant cell arteritis selects against B lymphocytes. J Rheumatol 1996; 23:1011–1014.

25. Lie JT. Illustrated histopathologic classification criteria for selected vasculitis syndromes. American College of Rheumatology Subcommittee on Classification of Vasculitis. Arthritis Rheum 1990; 33: 1074–1087.

26. Weyand CM, Tetzlaff N, Bjornsson J, Brack A, Younge B, Goronzy JJ. Disease patterns and tissue cytokine profiles in giant cell arteritis. Arthritis Rheum 1997; 40:19–26.

27. Nikkari ST, Hoyhtya M, Isola J, Nikkari T. Macrophages contain 92-kD gelatinase (MMP-9) at the site of degenerated internal elastic lamina in temporal arteritis. Am J Pathol 1996; 149:1427–1433.

28. Kaiser M, Weyand CM, Bjornsson J, Goronzy JJ. Platelet-derived growth factor, intimal hyperplasia, and ischemic complications in giant cell arteritis. Arthritis Rheum 1998; 41:623–633.

29. Kaiser M, Younge B, Bjornsson J, Weyand CM, Goronzy JJ. Formation of new vasa vasorum in vasculitis: Production of angiogenic cytokines by multinucleated giant cells. Am J Pathol 1999; in press.

30. Quaranta V, Plopper GE. Integrins and laminins in tissue remodeling. Kidney Int 1997; 51:1441–1446.

31. Faxon DP, Coats W, Currier J. Remodeling of the coronary artery after vascular injury. Prog Cardiovasc Dis 1997; 40:129–140.

32. Alpers CE, Davis CL, Barr D, Marsh CL, Hudkins KL. Identification of platelet-derived growth factor A and B chains in human renal vascular rejection. Am J Pathol 1996; 148:439–451.
33. Rittner HL, Hafner V, Klimiuk PA, Szweda LI, Goronzy JJ, Weyand CM. Aldose reductase functions as a detoxification system for lipid peroxidation products in vasculitis. J Clin Invest 1999; 103:1007–1013.
34. Bohren KM, Bullock B, Wermuth B, Gabbay KH. The aldo-keto reductase superfamily. cDNAs and deduced amino acid sequences of human aldehyde and aldose reductases. J Biol Chem 1989; 264:9547–9551.
35. Flynn TG, Green NC. The aldo-keto reductases: An overview. Adv Exp Med Biol 1993; 328:251–257.

2
Endothelial Cell Adhesion Molecules

Maria Cinta-Cid and Blanca Coll-Vinent
Hospital Clinic í Provincial

Isabel Bielsa
Hospital Germans Trias i Pujol, Badalona, Spain

I. INTRODUCTION

Tissue infiltration by leukocytes is the pathological substrate of many chronic inflammatory and autoimmune diseases, including vasculitis. The development of inflammatory infiltrates in tissues requires dynamic and precisely regulated interactions among leukocytes, endothelial cells, and the underlying basement membrane and interstitial matrix (1). Such interactions are mediated by a complex array of leukocyte surface receptors and their ligands on the endothelial cell membrane. On the leukocyte surface, carbohydrates closely related to sialylated forms of Lewis[x] and Lewis[a] antigens, selectins, and integrins interact in a sequential and precisely regulated manner with specific counterreceptors on the endothelial cell surface. Again, these include carbohydrate-bearing mucins, selectins, and immunoglobulin superfamily members. The main molecules involved in the interactions among leukocytes, endothelial cells, and extracellular matrix proteins are summarized in Table 1. Descriptions of their structural as well as functional properties have been addressed in detail in recent, comprehensive reviews (1–6).

The transition from a circulating leukocyte to a tissue-infiltrating leukocyte requires a series of coordinated events. First, when an appropriate stimulus induces the endothelium to express selectins and to display ligands for leukocyte selectins, circulating leukocytes slow down and roll over the endothelial surface. This phenomenon is mediated mainly by labile interplays between carbohydrates and selectins, which accumulate in philopodia allowing interactions between relatively distant cells. Subsequently, leukocyte integrins, which are usually in a nonadherent conformation status, become activated. The intracellular mechanisms underlying integrin activation are not completely understood. Integrin activation may follow interactions mediated by selectins and can be triggered by soluble factors (chemokines) or by leukocyte homotypic interactions mediated by costimulatory molecules (7).

Chemokines include a growing family of small polypeptides with chemotactic activity on leukocytes (1,8,9). Four major families of chemokines have been described according to the relative location of characteristic cystein residues: C, C-C (β chemokines), C-X-C (α chemokines), and C-X3-C chemokines (8,9). With a few exceptions, α chemokines attract neutrophils, β chemokines attract monocytes, eosinophils, and basophils, and the members of both families can attract different subsets of lymphocytes. Chemokines are usually immobilized by interactions

Table 1 Adhesion Molecules Involved in Interactions Between Leukocytes and
Endothelial Cells

Leukocytes	Endothelium
Selectins/carbohydrates	Selectins/carbohydrates
L-selectin (CD62L)	Glycam-1[a]
	CD34[a]
	MadCAM (mucin-like domain)[a]
PSGL-1[a]	P-selectin (CD62P)
?	E-selectin
CLA[a]	
Integrins	Immunoglobulins
αLβ2 (CD11a/CD18) LFA-1	ICAM-1 (CD54)
	ICAM-2 (CD102)
αMβ2 (CD11b/CD18) Mac-1	ICAM-1 (CD54)
αXβ2 (CD11c/CD18) gp 150,95	ICAM-1 (CD54)
α4β1 (CD49d/Cd29) VLA-4	VCAM-1 (CD106)
α4β7 (CD49d/CD?) LPAM-1	MadCAM-1
	VCAM-1 (CD106)
αvβ3 (CD51/CD61)	PECAM-1 (CD31)

[a]Selectins interact with carbohydrates related to sialyl Lewis^x and sialyl Lewis^a carried by these
mucin-like glycoproteins.

with proteoglycans, which are crucial components of the glycocalix of endothelial cells and extracellular matrix proteins. Recently, a chemokine coupled to a mucinlike membrane protein expressed on activated endothelial cells has been demonstrated to serve both as a chemotactic factor and as an adhesion molecule for monocytes and for activated T lymphocytes. This molecule, named fractalkine, is the first member of the C-X3-C class of chemokines (8). Together with adhesion molecules, chemokines and chemokine receptors account for a high number of combinatorial possibilities determining the diversity and the specificity of the components of the inflammatory infiltrates, as well as, according to recent contributions, the specificity of tissue targeting (1,8,10,11).

Leukocyte integrins interacting with endothelial cells belong mainly to the β2, β1, β3, and β7 families (see Table 1). Counterreceptors for leukocyte integrins are constitutively expressed by endothelial cells (intercellular adhesion molecule-1 [ICAM-1], ICAM-2, and platelet–endothelial cell adhesion molecule-1 [PECAM-1]) or can be induced (vascular cell adhesion molecule-1 [VCAM-1]) or upregulated (ICAM-1) upon cytokine stimulation (1). Cytokines involved in endothelial adhesion molecule regulation are mainly interleukin-1 (IL-1), tumor necrosis factor-α (TNF-α), interleukin-4 (IL-4), and interferon-γ (IFN-γ) (12).

Interactions between integrins and immunoglobulin superfamily members account for the strong adhesion and spreading of leukocytes over the endothelium and for subsequent transmigration through the endothelial cell junctions. In this process, homotypic interactions between PECAM-1 on leukocytes and on endothelial cells may function as a molecular zipper allowing leukocyte transmigration with minimal disruption of the endothelial cell monolayer (6). The role of cadherins in leukocyte transmigration is also being investigated (13,14).

Besides their chemotactic activity, chemokines induce cell polarization. In a polarized migrating leukocyte, chemokine receptors and activated integrins accumulate at the leading edge whereas ICAMs are redistributed at the trailing part of the cell in an elongated, pseudopod-like formation named uropod (13,14). Interactions between uropod-located ICAMs and β2 integrins

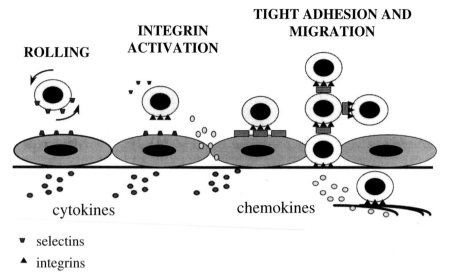

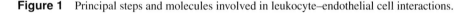

▼ selectins

▲ integrins

▭ immunoglobulin-like molecules

Figure 1 Principal steps and molecules involved in leukocyte–endothelial cell interactions.

in surrounding leukocytes may drag additional cells during the transmigration process (13,14) (Fig. 1). On the other hand, signals driven by ICAM-3 engagement by β2 integrins on surrounding cells activate both β1 and β2 integrin function in transmigrating leukocytes, enhancing their adhesion to endothelial cells and underlying matrix (7). Together, these mechanisms constitute a migratory amplifying cascade.

Leukocytes, then, interact with extracellular matrix proteins, mainly through β1, β3, and β5 integrins. Integrin-mediated interactions with endothelial cells and extracellular matrix proteins trigger matrix-metalloproteinase production by leukocytes which allows basement membrane disruption and progression through the interstitial matrix (15).

Interactions mediated by adhesion molecules are part of the physiological inflammatory response to injury. Persistent expression of inducible endothelial adhesion molecules as well as excessive activation of leukocyte integrins have been observed in a variety of inflammatory diseases, including vasculitis (2,16). Along with functional studies and experimental animal models, these observations suggest that adhesion molecules have a crucial role in the development, amplification, and perpetuation of inflammatory infiltrates and subsequent tissue damage in many chronic inflammatory diseases (2,16).

II. ADHESION MOLECULES IN INFLAMMATORY DISEASES OF BLOOD VESSELS

The systemic vasculitides include a highly heterogeneous group of clinicopathological entities (17). Although the potential etiological role of some infectious agents, particularly viruses, and other environmental factors is increasingly being considered, the triggering agents remain unknown for the majority of primary vasculitides (16,19).

Several immunopathogenic mechanisms able to produce blood vessel inflammation have been identified. These include immune complex deposition and complement activation, antineu-

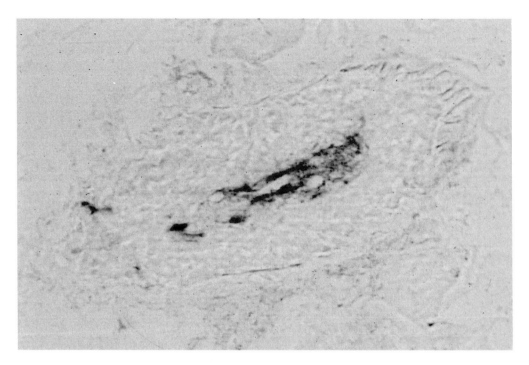

Figure 2 Muscle biopsy from a patient with classical polyarteritis nodosa showing E-selectin expression by the luminal endothelium of a minimally involved vessel. Immunohistochemical staining with the mAb 1.2 B6. Alkaline phosphatase antialkaline phosphatase (APAAP) method (100×).

trophil cytoplasmic antibody enhancement of neutrophil-mediated vessel damage, generation of antiendothelial cell antibodies, and a delayed-type hypersensitivity reaction driven by specific recognition of a putative antigen residing in the vessel wall (17–21). These mechanisms are not mutually exclusive and they may act simultaneously or sequentially with a variable predominance depending on the specific vasculitis syndrome or along the evolving course of each disease.

Irrespective of the primary immunopathogenic events leading to blood vessel inflammation, leukocytes are recruited into inflammatory foci by complex interplays with the endothelium and underlying matrix mediated by adhesion molecules.

A. Immunopathogenic Mechanisms of Vessel Damage and Adhesion Molecules

Most of the primary immunopathogenic mechanisms that are thought to play a role in the pathogenesis of blood vessel inflammation in vasculitis have been shown to include among their main effects altered modulation of adhesion molecule expression or function (18). In vitro studies have shown that complement activation products such as C1q induce E-selectin, ICAM-1, and VCAM-1 in cultured endothelial cells (22). Adhesion molecule expression and function are required for immune complex and complement-mediated vessel damage in vivo (23–25). Recent studies have shown that antineutrophil cytoplasmic antibodies (ANCAs) binding to membrane-associated proteinase 3 on endothelial cells may induce E-selectin and VCAM-1 expression by endothelial cells (26,27). The ANCA binding to neutrophils increases integrin expression and integrin-mediated adhesion, partially through Fc-mediated mechanisms (28,29). Studies with monoclonal blocking

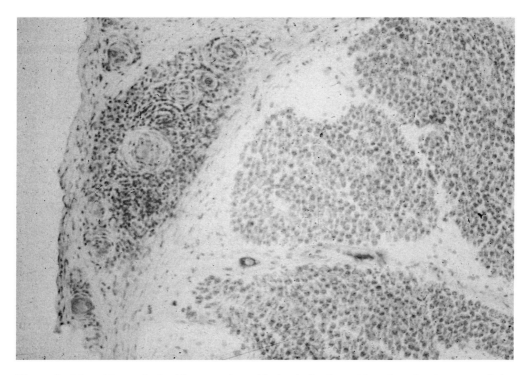

Figure 3 Nerve biopsy obtained from a patient with classical polyarteritis nodosa showing a strongly inflamed perineural artery. ICAM-1 expression by the luminal endothelium is slight. By contrast, strong expression of ICAM-1 can be observed in surrounding microvessels. Immunostaining with the mAb RR 1/1 (APAAP technique) (100×).

antibodies have shown that enhancement of TNF-induced neutrophil activation by ANCAs is, at least, partially dependent on homotypic interactions mediated by neutrophil integrins (30).

Anti–endothelial cell antibodies have been detected in a variety of vasculitides, particularly in patients with active disease (31,32). Although their specific role in the development of vascular inflammation has not been fully characterized, in vitro studies have shown that anti–endothelial cell antibody binding to endothelial cells induces endothelial adhesion molecule expression (33). Whether this phenomenon results from in vitro manipulation of endothelial cells or is a pathophysiologically relevant effect remains to be elucidated.

It has been also shown that, in vasculitis, activated lymphocytes and macrophages actively produce IL-1, TNF-α, and IFN-γ (34,35), the main inducers of endothelial adhesion molecules (12). A topographical relationship between inducer cytokines and endothelial adhesion molecule expression has been demonstrated in tissue samples from patients with microscopic polyangiitis (36). In addition, endothelial adhesion molecules may be modulated by steroid hormones. In this regard, estrogen has been shown to increase TNF-induced adhesion molecules E-selectin, ICAM-1, and VCAM-1 by endothelial cells (37). This fact may contribute to female predominance in many chronic inflammatory diseases.

Most of our current appreciation of the role that adhesion molecules might play in the development of inflammatory infiltrates in vasculitis comes from: studies performed on circulating leukocytes, studying adhesion molecule expression in tissue samples, and the detection of soluble circulating forms of adhesion molecules in sera from patients with various vasculitis syndromes.

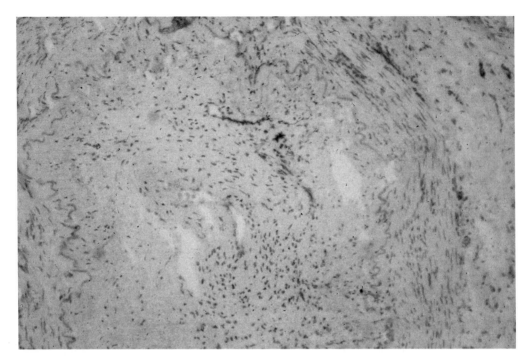

Figure 4   Neovessels within inflammatory infiltrates strongly express VCAM-1 in giant cell arteritis lesions. Temporal artery biopsy section stained with the mAb BBIG-VI (APAAP method) (100×).

B.   Expression of Adhesion Molecules by Circulating Leukocytes from Patients with Vasculitis

Several authors have studied the expression and function of β1 and β2 integrins in circulating leukocytes from patients with active vasculitis. The CD4+ T lymphocytes from patients with systemic lupus erythematosus and vasculitis express higher density of surface integrins of the β1 and β2 families and show a higher adherence to cultured TNF-stimulated endothelial cells and to extracellular matrix proteins than lymphocytes from systemic lupus erythematosus patients without vasculitis or than lymphocytes from healthy donors (38). Lymphocytes and monocytes from patients with Wegener's granulomatosis also express higher density of β1 and β2 integrins than leukocytes from healthy people (39,40). However, leukocyte adherence depends not only on the amount of surface integrins but mainly on their avidity status. Moreover, leukocyte adhesion and transmigration are tightly regulated by the microenvironment at the inflammatory foci. Consequently, the biological significance of the increased integrin expression by circulating leukocytes in patients with vasculitis is unclear and probably reflects an increased number of activated leukocytes in the bloodstream.

C.   Tissue Expression of Endothelial Adhesion Molecules

Expression of endothelial adhesion molecules and their leukocyte receptors in involved tissues may probably reflect the type of leukocyte–endothelial cell interactions participating in the development of blood vessel inflammation. Expression of adhesion molecules in lesions has been investigated in sizable and homogeneous series of patients with cutaneous leukocytoclastic vasculitis, Kawasaki disease, classical polyarteritis nodosa, and giant cell arteritis (41–44). In all of

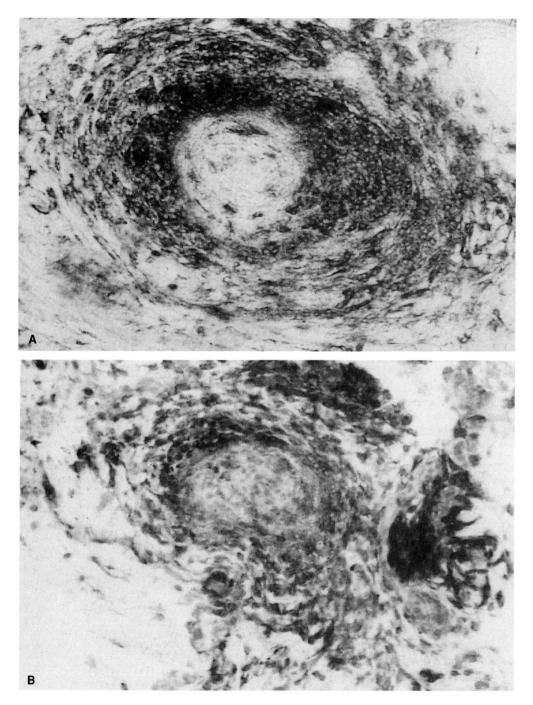

Figure 5   (A) The common β chain of β2 integrins is strongly expressed by leukocytes infiltrating the arterial wall in classical polyarteritis nodosa, whereas (B) ICAM-3 expression is mainly observed in leukocytes surrounding adventitial microvessels. Serial sections stained with the mAb MEM-48 (A) and 152-1D2 (B), respectively (APAAP technique) (100×).

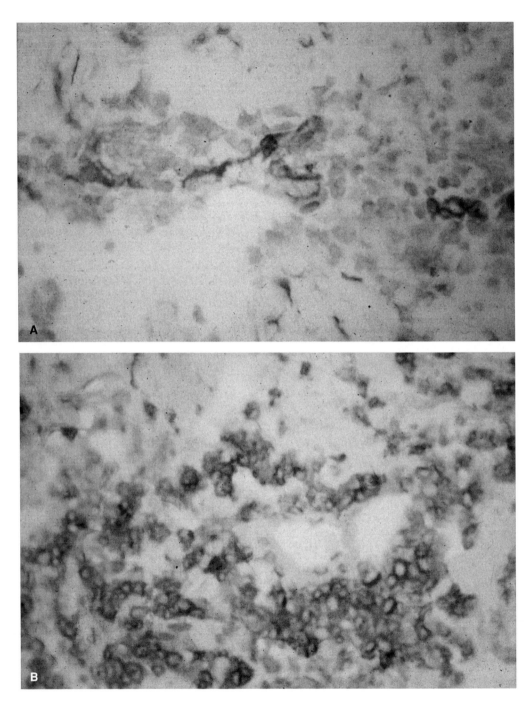

Figure 6   (A) Endothelial E-selectin expression in a skin biopsy from a patient with cutaneous leukocy-toclastic vasculitis. (B) In early lesions, inflammatory infiltrates include a high percentage of CLA-express-ing leukocytes. Immunostaining with the mAbs 1.2 B6 (A) and HECA 472 (B) (peroxidase antiperoxidase technique) (250×).

them, expression of inducible adhesion molecules E-selectin and VCAM-1 by endothelial cells can be detected at some point. Constitutive expression of ICAM-1 is usually upregulated. In glomerular lesions of Wegener's granulomatosis and microscopic polyangiitis, as well as in ANCA-associated necrotic and crescentic glomerulonephritis, VCAM-1 and ICAM-1 expression can be observed at the glomerular tuft as well as in tubular epithelial cells (45,46).

In small-vessel vasculitis, endothelial adhesion molecule expression occurs in the luminal endothelium (41). However, in medium-sized vasculitis, such as classical polyarteritis nodosa, the luminal endothelium only expresses constitutive or inducible adhesion molecules at early stages. As the inflammatory process proceeds, the luminal endothelium is damaged and the vascular lumen is occluded. Endothelial adhesion molecules are then strongly expressed by adventitial neovessels (43). Extensive neovascularization also occurs in giant cell (temporal) arteritis lesions, particularly in the adventitia and at the intima–media junction where the granulomatous reaction takes place (44). This observation suggests that, in large and medium-sized vessels, infiltrating leukocytes do not come from the vascular lumen. Rather, inflammatory cells penetrate the vessel wall through the adventitial vasa vasorum and neovessels. Inflammation-induced angiogenesis has, therefore an important role in amplifying and perpetuating the inflammatory response in large- and medium-sized-vessel vasculitis.

D. Dynamic Pattern of Endothelial Cell Adhesion Molecule Expression

Endothelial cell adhesion molecule expression varies along the subsequent stages of the inflammatory process in vasculitis. This variation has been studied in cutaneous leukocytoclastic vasculitis and in polyarteritis nodosa where the simultaneous occurrence of lesions at various histological stages is a common finding. In both processes, E-selectin expression is preferentially detected in early infiltrates, whereas in fully developed inflammatory lesions, E-selectin expression decreases and endothelial expression of ICAM-1 and VCAM-1 predominates (42,44). These observations are concordant with in vitro studies where, in cytokine-stimulated cultured endothelial cells, E-selectin expression is early and transient whereas ICAM-1 and VCAM-1 expression appears later and is more persistent (1–3). E-selectin expression correlates with the presence of abundant neutrophils (41,43) whereas mononuclear cells are the main cell population in later stages when ICAM-1 and VCAM-1 expression predominates (41). In healing lesions, endothelial adhesion molecule expression decreases along with a reduction in the number of infiltrating leukocytes. In renal lesions of ANCA-associated glomerulonephritis, glomerular expression of ICAM-1 and VCAM-1 also decreases when glomeruli become obliterated by crescent formation (45,46).

E. Adhesion Receptor Expression by Infiltrating Leukocytes

Leukocyte selectins play an important role in the initial interactions with endothelial cells but, subsequently, when the strong adhesion mediated by integrins begins, leukocyte selectins are shed from the cell surface (3,12). Consistently, infiltrating leukocytes in vasculitis do not disclose a substantial expression of L-selectin (43,44). By contrast, an intense expression of leukocyte integrins is detected, as it is observed in leukocytes that have migrated to specific compartments in other diseases (16). In addition, a topographical relationship is observed between integrin expression by infiltrating leukocytes and their respective ligands of the immunoglobulin superfamily by endothelial cells (43,44). Among them, LFA-1/ICAM-1–and VLA-4/VCAM-1–mediated interactions seem to play an important role in the development of vascular infiltrates in vasculitis. In medium-sized and large vessels, leukocytes surrounding small neovessels have phenotypic characteristics of activated and transmigrating leukocytes, specifically, strong expression of lymphocyte-function-associated molecule-1 (LFA-1) and very-late-activation antigen-4 (VLA-4)

(1,2,12). Adventitial leukocytes surrounding neovessels also show strong expression of ICAM-3. As mentioned above, ICAM-3 is a signaling molecule with a crucial role in the transmigration process (7,13,14). By contrast, ICAM-3 expression is less intense in leukocytes that have invaded the vessel wall and are located at the media. These show, instead, an intense expression of the common chain of β2 integrins (43,44).

F. Tissue-Specific Targeting

Vasculitis syndromes tend to target specific organs or specific vessels. Several factors potentially contributing to tissue specificity in vasculitis have been considered. Hemodynamic factors have been thought to play a role in the location of immune-complex–mediated vasculitis. In this regard, turbulence may favor immune complex deposition and may facilitate the development of polyarteritis nodosa lesions at branch points (17,19). Hydrostatic pressure may contribute to the predominance of cutaneous leukocytoclastic vasculitis in lower extremities. A specialized, complex microvasculature such as the renal glomerulus may favor the deposition of immune complexes in the kidney (17,19). The potential site of antigen encounter may address inflammatory response to the upper and lower airways in Wegener's granulomatosis and to large vessels in granulomatous arteritis (21,47).

Adhesion molecules mediating leukocyte–endothelial cell interactions may contribute to the specificity of tissue targeting. To date, most of the adhesion molecules mediating leukocyte–endothelial cell interactions identified seem to play a crucial but general role in the development of inflammatory infiltrates. A few molecular interactions mediating tissue specificity have been identified. The recognition of these interactions comes from studies investigating the pattern of lymphocyte recirculation and homing to different lymphoid organs. In this regard, the carbohydrate determinant CLA (cutaneous lymphocyte antigen) confers skin homing capability to lymphocytes. While neutrophils are able to interact with E-selectin, only skin-homing lymphocytes displaying CLA can interact with E-selectin. The CLA–E-selectin interactions appear to mediate cutaneous tropism in several inflammatory disorders, including graft-versus-host disease (17) and dermatomyositis (48). Interestingly, in the latter case, E-selectin expression can be detected in the skin but not in muscle vessels (49). Recently, concomitant expression of CLA-bearing lymphocytes and endothelial E-selectin has been demonstrated in early stages of cutaneous vasculitis (50).

Interactions mediated by lymphocyte α4β7 and endothelial mucosal-addressing cell adhesion molecule-1 (MadCAM-1) recruit lymphocytes into mucosa-associated lymphoid tissue of the gut (1). Lymphocytes infiltrating the gastrointestinal tract in several conditions, such as lymphoma or inflammatory bowel disease, exhibit, indeed, α4β7 expression (51). According to recent contributions, interactions mediated by tissue-specific endothelial chemokines and highly versatile specific chemokine receptors expressed by different lymphocyte subsets seem to be the major determinant of tissue targeting (8–11). These interactions have not yet been studied in vasculitis.

G. Adhesion Molecules in Animal Models

The functional relevance of interactions mediated by adhesion molecules in the pathogenesis of vasculitis has been investigated in animal models. In a murine model of systemic vasculitis induced by immunization against *Mycobacterium butyricum,* the administration of monoclonal blocking antibodies and the application of vital microscopy have demonstrated the important participation of interactions mediated by selectins and by α4 integrins in leukocyte adhesion and transmigration through postcapillary venules (52). Similarly, ICAM-1 deficiency considerably reduces the development of vasculitis in MRL/lpr mice, and VCAM-1 deficiency or blocking α4 integrins prevents the development of β-glucan–induced granulomatous vasculitis (40,52). Although none of these models satisfactorily represents specific human vasculitic syndromes, these findings underline the functional importance of interactions mediated by adhesion molecules in the development of vascular inflammation.

H. Effect of Corticosteroid Treatment on Adhesion Molecule Expression

In vitro studies have shown that corticosteroids may suppress endothelial cell adhesion molecule expression induced by endotoxins or by cytokines (54). In addition, corticosteroids inhibit the production of proinflammatory cytokines which are the main inducers of adhesion molecule expression (55).

The effect of treatment on adhesion molecule expression in patients with vasculitis is not well defined. Immunoglobulin therapy decreases endothelial cell adhesion molecule expression in skin samples from patients with Kawasaki disease (42). Preliminary cross-sectional studies show a substantial decrease in E-selectin and VCAM-1 expression in lesions from patients with giant cell arteritis treated with corticosteroids for up to one month but some expression still persists (44). A decrease in endothelial adhesion molecule expression in synovial biopsies from patients with polymyalgia rheumatica treated with corticosteroids has also been observed (56). However, corticosteroid and immunosuppressive treatment of patients with polyarteritis nodosa for a few days does not modify substantially adhesion molecule expression (43).

I. Circulating Soluble Adhesion Molecules

Soluble selectins and immunoglobulin superfamily members can be detected in human plasma and other body fluids, and increased levels have been detected in a variety of disorders, including infections, malignant tumors, and chronic inflammatory diseases (57). Soluble adhesion molecule fragments are shed from the cell surface by proteolytic cleavage or are directly generated as splice variants lacking the transmembrane and cytoplasmic domains (57). Circulating adhesion molecules probably have some regulatory role but their biological significance is still unclear. Since soluble forms of adhesion molecules are released by endothelial cells stimulated by cytokines, elevated circulating adhesion molecule concentrations have been considered a consequence of endothelial cell activation in response to inflammatory stimuli. Some adhesion molecules such as ICAM-1 and VCAM-1 are also expressed and released by activated lymphocytes and macrophages. Consequently, their increase may reflect immune activation and does not necessarily indicate endothelial cell exposure to proinflammatory cytokines.

Studies in large and homogeneous series of patients have demonstrated that circulating soluble E-selectin (sE-selectin), ICAM-1 (sICAM-1), and VCAM-1 (sVCAM-1) concentrations are elevated in patients with systemic vasculitis, such as polyarteritis nodosa, Kawasaki disease, Wegener's granulomatosis, and microscopic polyangiitis (40,58–61). In general, there is some correlation with the extent of the disease, particularly in Kawasaki disease (59,60) and in Wegener's granulomatosis (40,61). Circulating adhesion molecule levels usually correlate with levels of circulating proinflammatory cytokines such as TNF-α (59) or IL-6 (60) and with acute-phase proteins such as C-reactive protein (CPR); however, such correlations are appropriate or variable (40, 61). A decrease in the concentration of soluble adhesion molecules is usually observed with treatment (40,58,62), particularly in acute, monophasic disorders such as Kawasaki disease (40,59, 60). In chronic, relapsing vasculitis, correlation between adhesion molecule levels and disease activity is not satisfactory enough to use levels as a guide for therapeutic decisions (G. S. Hoffman, unpublished) (40,58,63). Moreover, circulating adhesion molecules usually increase during concurrent diseases, such as infections (40,61). Persistent elevated levels of adhesion molecules despite clinically apparent remission induced by treatment have been detected in polyarteritis nodosa and in Wegener's granulomatosis (40,62). This observation may indicate persistent exposure of endothelial cells to a remaining inflammatory microenvironment, which may predispose to the high relapse rates observed among many vasculitides.

Interestingly, in cutaneous leukocytoclastic vasculitis and in Schönlein–Henoch purpura, sICAM-1 levels are similar to normal controls (40). In the latter, only sE-selectin appears to be increased (61). In large-vessel vasculitis such as giant cell (temporal) arteritis, only sICAM-1 has been found to be significantly elevated compared with age- and sex-matched controls (62). Although endothelial VCAM-1 and E-selectin expression are both observed in temporal arteritis lesions, the endothelial surface contributing to the release of adhesion molecules is much less in large-vessel vasculitis compared with widespread small-vessel vasculitis. Elevated sICAM-1 with normal levels of other, more specific endothelial adhesion molecules can be also found in other granulomatous nonvasculitic diseases, such as sarcoidosis (64). This observation suggests that activated monocytes or macrophages could also contribute to the release of sICAM-1.

Other leukocyte and endothelial adhesion molecules, such as sP-selectin, sL-selectin, and sICAM-3, have been much less investigated in vasculitis. No significant changes in P-selectin concentrations have been found in polyarteritis nodosa or in giant cell arteritis (58,62). Elevated levels of sICAM-3 have been found in rheumatoid vasculitis (40) but not in giant cell arteritis (62). By contrast, sL-selectin levels are decreased in polyarteritis nodosa patients and in patients with other autoimmune diseases (58,65). Low levels of sL-selectin have also been observed in conditions characterized by widespread endothelial activation, such as adult respiratory distress syndrome (66). Low concentrations of sL-selectin might be due to a reduction in its release or sequestration in diseased tissue.

III. SUMMARY

An increasing number of contributions provide evidence supporting a crucial role for adhesion molecules in the development of vascular inflammation in vasculitis. Interactions mediated by adhesion molecules are complex and dynamic and their participation in the pathogenesis of vessel inflammation is just beginning to be appreciated. Preferential adhesion pathways involved in different vasculitides and the type of interactions participating in tissue-specific targeting are exciting aspects that await further investigation. Emerging concepts suggest that new therapeutic approaches targeting adhesion molecules might complement the therapeutic effects of corticosteroid and immunosuppressive agents in vasculitis (16,67).

ACKNOWLEDGMENTS

The data generated by the authors have been supported by grants from Fondo de Investigación Sanitaria (FIS 95/0860 and FIS 98/0443).

REFERENCES

1. Springer TA. Traffic signals on endothelium for lymphocyte recirculation and leukocyte emigration. Annu Rev Physiol 1995; 57:827–872.
2. Mojcik CF, Shevach EM. Adhesion molecules: A rheumatologic perspective. Arthritis Rheum 1997; 40:991–1004.
3. Tedder TF, Steeber DA, Chen A, Engel P. The selectins: Vascular adhesion molecules. FASEB J 1995; 9:866–873.
4. Hynes RO. Integrins: Versatility, modulation, and signaling in cell adhesion. Cell 1992; 69:11–25.

5. Gahmberg CG. Leukocyte adhesion: CD11/CD18 integrins and intercellular adhesion molecules. Curr Opin Cell Biol 1997; 9:643–650.

6. Bianchi E, Bender JR, Blasi F, Pardi R: Through and beyond the way: Late steps in leukocyte transendothelial migration. Immunol Today 1997; 18:586–591.

7. Adams DH, Lloyd. Chemokines: Leukocyte recruitment and activation cytokines. Lancet 1997; 349: 490–495.

8. Nelson PJ, Krensky AM. Chemokines, lymphocytes and viruses: What goes around, comes around. Curr Opin Immunol 1998; 10:265–270.

9. Cid MC, Esparza J, Juan M, Miralles A, Ordi J, Vilella R, Urbano-Márquez A, Gayà A, Vives J, Yagüe J: Signaling through CD50 (ICAM-3) stimulates T lymphocyte binding to human umbilical vein endothelial cells and extracellular matrix proteins via an increase in $\beta 1$ and $\beta 2$ integrin function. Eur J Immunol 1994; 24:1377–1382.

10. Foxman EF, Campbell JJ, Butcher EC. Multistep navigation and the combinatorial control of leukocyte chemotaxis. J Cell Biol 1997; 139:1349–1360.

11. Gunn MD, Tangemann K, Tam C, Cyster JG, Rosen SD, Williams LT. A chemokine expressed in lymphoid high endothelial venules promotes the adhesion and chemotaxis of naive T lymphocytes. Proc Natl Acad Sci USA 1998; 98:258–263.

12. Springer TA. Traffic signals for lymphocyte recirculation and leukocyte emigration: The multistep paradigm. Cell 1994; 76:301–314.

13. del Pozo MA, Cabañas C, Montoya MC, Ager A, Sánchez-Mateos P, Sánchez-Madrid F. ICAMs redistributed by chemokines to cellular uropods as a mechanism for recruitment of T lymphocytes. J Cell Biol 1997; 137:493–508.

14. del Pozo MA, Sánchez-Mateos P, Sánchez-Madrid F. Cellular polarization induced by chemokines: A mechanism for leukocyte recruitment? Immunol Today 1996; 17:127–31.

15. Esparza J, Vilardell C, Calvo J, Juan M, Yagüe J, Cid MC. Fibronectin up-regulates gelatinase B (MMP-9) and induces coordinated expression of gelatinase A (MMP-2) and its activator MT1-MMP (MMP-14) by human T lymphocyte cell lines. A process repressed through RAS/MAP kinase signaling pathways. Blood 1991; 94:2754–2766.

16. Cid MC, Coll-Vinent B, Grau JM. Cell adhesion molecules in leukocyte/endothelial cell/extracellular matrix interactions. Clinical relevance and potential therapeutic implications. Med Clin (Barc) 1997; 108:503–511.

17. Fauci AS, Haynes BF, Katz P. The spectrum of vasculitis: Clinical, pathologic, immunologic and therapeutic considerations. Ann Intern Med 1978; 89:660–676.

18. Cid MC. New developments in the pathogenesis of systemic vasculitis. Curr Opin Rheumatol 1996; 8: 1–11.

19. Cid MC, Fauci AS, Hoffman GS. The vasculitides: Classification, diagnosis and pathogenesis. In: Khamashta M, Font J, Hughes GRV, eds. Autoimmune Connective Tissue Diseases. Barcelona: Doyma, 1993:149–162.

20. Sundy JS, Haynes BF. Pathogenic mechanisms of vessel damage in vasculitis syndromes. Rheum Dis Clin North Am 1995; 21:861–881.

21. Weyand, CM, Goronzy JJ. Giant-cell arteritis as an antigen-driven disease. Rheum Dis Clin North Am 1995; 21:1027–1039.

22. Lozada CJ, Levin IR, Hirschhorn R, Naime D, Whitlow MS, Recht PA, et al. Identification of C1q as the heat-labile serum cofactor required for immune complexes to stimulate endothelial expression of the adhesion molecules E-selectin and intercellular and vascular cell adhesion molecules 1. Proc Natl Acad Sci USA 1995; 92:8378–8382.

23. Argenbright LW, Barton RW. Interactions of leukocyte integrins with intercellular adhesion molecule 1 in the production of inflammatory vascular injury in vivo: The Schwartzman reaction revisited. J Clin Invest 1992; 89:259–272.

24. Brady HR. Leukocyte adhesion molecule and kidney diseases. Kidney Int 1994; 45:1285–1300.

25. Mulligan MS, Varani J, Warren JS, Till GO, Smith CW, Anderson DC, et al. Roles of $\beta 2$ integrins of rat neutrophils in complement and oxygen radical-mediated acute inflammatory injury. J Immunol 1992; 148:1847–1857.

26. Mayet WJ, Meyer zum Buschenfelde KH. Antibodies to proteinase 3 increase adhesion of neutrophils to human endothelial cells. Clin Exp Immunol 1993; 94:440–446.

27. Mayet WJ, Schwarting A, Orth T, Duchman R, Meyer zum Buschenfelde KH. Antibodies to proteinase 3 mediate expression of vascular cell adhesion molecule-1 (VCAM-1). Clin Exp Immunol 1996; 103:259–267.

28. Mulder AHL, Heeringa P, Brower E, Limburg PC, Kallenberg CGM. Activation of granulocytes by anti-neutrophil cytoplasmic antibodies (ANCA): A FcγRII-dependent process. Clin Exp Immunol 1994; 98:270–278.

29. Keogan MR, Rifkin I, Ronda N, Lockwood CM, Brown DL. Anti-neutrophil cytoplasmic antibodies increase neutrophil adhesion to cultured human endothelium. Adv Exp Med Biol 1993; 336:115–119.

30. Reumaux D, Vossebeld PJ, Roos D, Verhoeven AJ. Effect of tumor necrosis factor-induced integrin activation on Fcγ receptor II-mediated signal transduction: Relevance for activation of neutrophils by anti-proteinase 3 or anti-myeloperoxidase antibodies. Blood 1995; 86:3189–3195.

31. Cervera R, Navarro M, López-Soto A, Cid MC, Font J, Esparza J, Ingelmo M, Urbano-Márquez A. Anti-endothelial cell antibodies in Behçet disease. Cell binding specificity and correlation with clinical activity. Ann Rheum Dis 1994; 53:265–267.

32. Ferraro G, Meroni PL, Tincani A, Sinicio A, Barcellini W, Radice A, et al. Anti-endothelial cell antibodies in patients with Wegener's granulomatosis and microscopic polyarteritis. Clin Exp Immunol 1990; 79:47–53.

33. Del Papa N, Guidalhi L, Sironi M, Shoenfeld Y, Mantovani A, Tincani A, et al. Anti-endothelial cell IgG antibodies from Wegener's granulomatosis bind to human endothelial cells in vitro and induce adhesion molecule expression and cytokine secretion. Arthritis Rheum 1996; 39:758–766.

34. Weyand CM, Hicok KC, Hunder GG, Goronzy JJ. Tisue cytokine patterns in patients with polymyalgia rheumatica and giant-cell arteritis. Ann Intern Med 1994; 121:484–491.

35. Noronha IL, Kruger C, Andrassy K, Ritz E, Waldherr R. In situ production of TNF-α, IL-1β and IL-2R in ANCA-positive glomerulonephritis. Kidney Int 1993; 43:682–692.

36. Bradley JR, Lockwood CM, Thiru S. Endothelial cell activation in patients with systemic vasculitis. Q J Med 1994; 87:741–745.

37. Cid MC, Kleinman HK, Grant DS, Schnaper HW, Fauci AS, Hoffman GS. Estradiol enhances leukocyte binding to tumor necrosis factor (TNF)-stimulated endothelial cells vian an increase in TNF-induced adhesion molecules E-selectin, intercellular adhesion molecule type 1, and vascular cell adhesion molecule type 1. J Clin Invest 1994; 93:17–25.

38. Takeuchi T, Amano K, Sekine H, Koide J, Abe T. Up-regulated expression and function of integrin receptors in systemic lupus erythematosus patients with vasculitis. J Clin Invest 1993; 92:3008–3016.

39. Haller H, Eichhorn J, Pieper K, Göbel U, Luft FC. Circulating leukocyte integrin expression in Wegener's granulomatosis. J Am Soc Nephrol 1996; 7:40–48.

40. Cohen Tervaert JW, Kallenberg CGM. Cell adhesion molecules in vasculitis. Curr Opin Rheumatol 1997; 9:16–25.

41. Sais G, Vidaller A, Jugcla A, Condom E, Peyri J. Adhesion molecule expression and endothelial cell activation in cutaneous leukocytoclastic vasculitis: An immunohistologic and clinical study in 42 patients. Arch Dermatol 1997; 133:443–450.

42. Leung DYM, Kurt-Jones E, Newburger JW, Cotran RS, Burns JC, Pober JS. Endothelial cell activation and increased interleukin-1 secretion in the pathogenesis of acute Kawasaki disease. Lancet 1990; 339:1298–1302.

43. Coll-Vinent B, Cebrián M, Cid MC, Font C, Esparza J, Juan M, et al. Dynamic pattern of endothelial cell adhesion molecule expression in muscle and perineural vessels from patients with classical polyarteritis nodosa. Arthritis Rheum 1998; 41:435–444.

44. Cid MC, Cebrián M, Font C, Coll-Vinent B, Hernández-Rodríguez J, Esparza J, Urbano-Márquez A, Grau JM. Cell adhesion molecules in the development of inflammatory infiltrates in giant-cell arteritis. Arthritis Rheum 2000; 43:184–196.

45. Pall AA, Howie AJ, Adu D, Richards GM, Inward CD, Milford DV, et al. Glomerular vascular cell adhesion molecule-1 expression in renal vasculitis. J Clin Pathol 1996; 49:238–242.

46. Rastaldi MP, Ferrario F, Tunesi S, Yang L, d'Amico G. Intraglomerular and interstitial leukocyte infiltration, adhesion molecules, and interleukin-1α expression in 15 cases of antineutrophil cytoplasmic autoantibody-associated renal vasculitis. Am J Kidney Dis 1996; 27:48–57.

47. Nikkari S, Relman DA. Molecular approaches for identification of infectious agents in Wegener's granulomatosis and other vasculitides. Curr Opin Rheumatol 1999; 11:11–16.

48. Hausmann G, Mascaró JM Jr, Herrero C, Cid MC, Palou J, Mascaró J. Immunohistochemical study of endothelial cell adhesion molecules in cutaneous lesions of dermatomyositis. Acta Dermatol Venereol (Stockh) 1996; 76:222–225.

49. Cid MC, Grau JM, Casademont J, Tobías E, Picazo A, Pedrol E, Coll-Vinent B, Esparza J, Urbano-Márquez A. Leukocyte/endothelial cell adhesion receptors in muscle biopsies from patients with idiopathic inflammatory myopathies. Clin Exp Immunol 1996; 104:467–473.

50. Bielsa I, Carrascosa JM, Hausmann G, Ferrandiz C. An immunohistopathologic study in cutaneous necrotizing vasculitis. J Cutan Pathol 2000; 27:130–135.

51. Drillenburg P, van der Voort R, Koopman G, Dragosics B, van Krieken JH, Kluin P, et al. Preferential expression of the mucosal homing receptor integrin α4β7 in gastrointestinal non-Hodgkin lymphomas. Am J Pathol 1997; 150:919–927.

52. Johnston B, Issekutz TB, Kubes P. The α4 integrin supports leukocyte rolling and adhesion in chronically inflamed postcapillary venules in vivo. J Exp Med 1996; 183: 1995–2006.

53. Bullard DC, King PD, Hicks MJ, Dupont B, Beaudet AL, Elkon KB. Intercellular adhesion molecule-1 deficiency protects MRL Mpj-Fas (lpr) mice from early lethality. J Immunol 1997; 159:2058–2067.

54. Cronstein BN, Kimmel SC, Levin IR, Martiniuk F, Weissman G. A mechanism for the antiinflammatory effects of corticosteroids: The glucocorticoid receptor regulates leukocyte adhesion to endothelial cells and expression of endothelial leukocyte adhesion molecule 1 and intercellular adhesion molecule 1. Proc Natl Acad Sci USA 1992; 89:9991–9995.

55. Brack A, Rittner HL, Younge BR, Kaltschmidt C, Weyand CM, Goronzy JJ. Glucocorticoid-mediated repression of cytokine gene transcription in human arteritis-SCID chimeras. J Clin Invest 1997; 99: 2842–50.

56. Meliconi R, Pulsatelli L, Melchiorri C, Frizziero L, Salvarani C, Macchioni P, et al. Synovial expression of cell adhesion molecules in polymyalgia rheumatica. Clin Exp Immunol 1997; 107:494–500.

57. Gearing AJH, Newman W. Circulating adhesion molecules in disease. Immunol Today 1993; 14:506–512.

58. Coll-Vinent B, Grau JM, López-Soto A, Oristrell J, Font C, Bosch X, Mirapeix E, Urbano-Márquez A, Cid MC. Circulating soluble adhesion molecules in patients with classical polyarteritis nodosa. Br J Rheumatol 1997; 36:1178–1183.

59. Furukawa S, Imai K, Matsubara T, Yone K, Yachi A, Okumura K, et al. Increased levels of circulating intercellular adhesion molecule 1 in Kawasaki disease. Arthritis Rheum 1992; 35:672–677.

60. Kim DS, Lee KY. Serum soluble E-selectin levels in Kawasaki disease. Scand J Rheumatol 1994; 23: 283–286.

61. Stegeman CA, Cohen Tervaert JW, Huitema MG, de Jong PE, Kallenberg CGM. Serum levels of soluble adhesion molecules intercellular adhesion molecule 1, vascular cell adhesion molecule 1, vascular cell adhesion molecule 1, and E-selectin in patients with Wegener's granulomatosis: Relationship to disease activity and relevance during follow-up. Arthritis Rheum 1994; 37:1228–1235.

62. Coll-Vinent B, Vilardell C, Font C, Oristrell J, Hernández-Rodríguez J, Yagüe J, Urbano-Márquez A, Grau JM, Cid MC. Circulating soluble adhesion molecules in patients with giant-cell arteritis. Correlation between soluble intercellular adhesion molecule-1 (sICAM-1) levels and disease activity. Ann Rheum Dis 1999; 58:189–192.

63. John S, Neumayer HH, Weber M. Serum circulating ICAM-1 levels are not useful to indicate active vasculitis or early renal allograft rejection. Clin Nephrol 1994; 42:369–275.

64. Shijubo N, Imai K, Shigehara K, Hinoda Y, Abe S. Circulating soluble intercellular adhesion molecule-1 (sICAM-1) in patients with sarcoidosis. Clin Exp Immunol 1996; 106:549–554.

65. Blann AD, Sanders PA, Herrick A, Jayson MI. Soluble L-selectin in the connective tissue diseases. Br J Haematol 1996; 95:192–194.

66. Donnelly SC, Haslett C, Dransfield I, Robertson CE, Carter DC, Ross JA, et al. Role of selectins in de-
     velopment of adult respiratory distress syndrome. Lancet 1994; 344:215–219.
67. Rothlein R, Jaeger JR. Clinical applications of antileukocyte adhesion molecule monoclonal anti-
     bodies. In: Austen KF, Burakoff SJ, Rosen FS, Strom TS, eds. Therapeutic Immunology. Cambridge:
     Blackwell, 1996:347–353.

3

Extracellular Matrix

Hynda K. Kleinman, Katherine M. Malinda, and M. Lourdes Ponce
National Institute of Dental & Craniofacial Research, National Institutes of Health, Bethesda, Maryland

I. INTRODUCTION

Most cells in multicellular organisms contact, on at least one of their surfaces, an intricate meshwork of interacting extracellular molecules that constitutes the extracellular matrix. The amount and type of extracellular matrix is highly variable, especially during development, and is tissue dependent (1). There is considerable evidence that the extracellular matrix has many structural and biological functions in tissues (Table 1). Much of the information on the biological activity of the extracellular matrix has come from in vitro studies with cells grown on purified matrices and on isolated components, and from the elucidation of the role of matrix molecules in diseases (2–4). The importance of the extracellular matix in development is further confirmed with the identification of various genetic diseases. Also, the biochemistry of these molecules is beginning to be understood at the structural level and active sites have been identified using fragments, antibodies, and synthetic peptides. Because of their important biological activities, some of these extracellular matrix molecules have the potential to be used therapeutically for tissue repair and possibly to control disease progression.

The extracellular matrix varies considerably in its functions (see Table 1) and tissue-specific components (1,5). It was initially thought to form the major structural support of tissues and to connect various organ systems, but it is now clear that other functions exist. During embryonic development and in wound healing, the matrix provides a substructure on which the cells migrate. Growth factors/cytokines are present in the extracellular matrix which serves as a storage depot for these bioactive molecules. Resident cells adhere to the extracellular matrix which provides signals for the cells to grow and/or differentiate. Extracellular matrix components are used in vitro to stimulate cell survival and differentiation. In vivo, matrix components have been used to promote tissue repair. This chapter focuses on the extracellular matrix underlying endothelial cells, which is termed the basement membrane (6).

II. BASEMENT MEMBRANE

The basal surfaces of endothelial cells are in contact with a basement membrane, the thin extracellular matrix that separates the endothelium from the underlying stroma (1,2). This matrix serves as a selective barrier to cells and to macromolecules and also is a storage depot for cytokines, growth factors, and proteases (7). The major components of this matrix are collagen IV,

Table 1 Functions of the Extracellular Matrix

Forms the supporting structures between cells
Provides a substructure for cell movement
Is a major storage site for soluble and insoluble substances
Provides signals and induces cells to differentiate
Connects organ systems
Absorbs shock/compression

which does not form fibers, a heparan sulfate proteoglycan, perlecan, and two glycoproteins, laminin and entactin. It should be noted that not all basement membranes contain the same amounts or types of components. The actual amount of each component in the endothelial cell basement membrane has not been defined due to its relative low abundance.

Degradation of the basement membrane is the first step in angiogenesis (8,9). The endothelial cells then migrate from the vessel into the tissue. The cells proliferate in the region of the vessel where the basement membrane was degraded, and these new cells form the migrating column of cells. The migrating cells then undergo tube formation. Finally, there is a resynthesis and deposition of the basement membrane, which provides structural integrity to the mature vessel.

The basement membrane maintains the endothelial cell phenotype and integrity of the endothelium (9). The biological interaction of basement membrane with endothelial cells has been defined using a substrate of reconstituted basement membrane termed matrigel (Table 2) (10,11). Matrigel is isolated from an epithelial tumor and contains all of the known basement membrane components. At 4°C, matrigel at 10 mg/ml is a liquid, and at 24°C it forms a gel in about 30 min. Matrigel that has been allowed to gel on a culture dish forms an active biomatrix substratum for many cell types. Endothelial cells plated on gelled basement membrane cease growth and form capillary-like structures with a lumen in 18 h (Fig. 1). This morphological differentiation mimics many of the steps in angiogenesis and has been used as a relatively quick in vitro screen to assay for angiogenic and antiangiogenic compounds (Table 3) (12,13). For the most part, known proan-

Table 2 Components of the Basement Membrane Matrigel

Abundant components
  Laminin
  Type IV collagen
  Perlecan (heparan sulfate proteoglycan)
  Nidogen/entactin
Growth factors
  TGF-βs (transforming growth factor)
  FGF (fibroblast growth factor)
  EGF (epidermal growth factor)
  PDGF (platelet derived growth factor)
  IGF (insulin-like growth factor)
Proteases
  72 KDa MMP-2
  92 KDa MMP-9
  Urokinase
  Tissue-type plasminogen activator
  Amylase

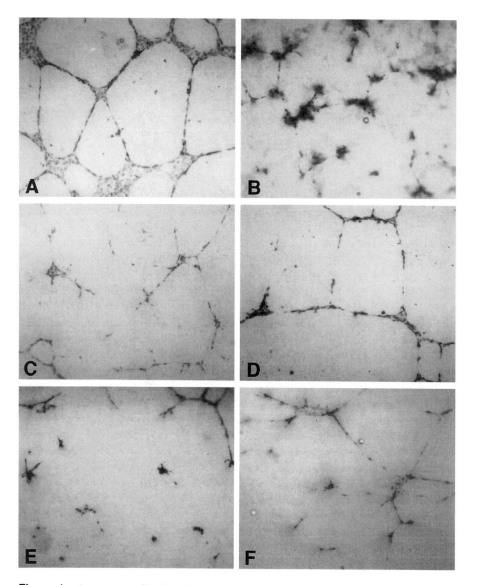

Figure 1   Appearance of endothelial cells on basement membrane matrigel after 18 h in the presence of various laminin peptides. The upper left panel shows the cell morphology in the absence of added peptides. Here tubelike structures with a lumen are observed. In the presence of various active peptides from the laminin γ chain, tube formation is disrupted indicating an active peptide for either angiogenesis or antiangiogenesis. (From Ref. 32.)

giogenic factors, such as estradiol, fibroblast growth factor (FGF), haptoglobin, scatter factor/hepatocyte growth factor (HGF), etc., promote tube formation. Antiangiogenic factors, such as tissue inhibitor of metalloproteinase (TIMP), interferon-inducible protein (IP-10), etc., block endothelial cell tube formation on matrigel. Many substances block/disrupt tube formation and need to be further tested before conclusions can be made about their angiogenic or antiangiogenic activity. For example, the laminin peptide SIKVAV (ser-ile-lys-val-ala-val) causes the tubes to "submerge" into the matrigel and appear fragmented (14). When tested in additional assays, such as

Table 3 Factors That Promote or Inhibit Tube Formation on Matrigel and Angiogenesis in Other Assays

Factor	Tube assay	Other angiogenesis assays
bFGF	Promotes	Promotes in all assays
TGF-β	Promotes	Promotes in ear model
Scatter factor	Promotes	Promotes in eye model
Haptoglobin	Promotes	Promotes in sponge implant
IP-10	Inhibits	Inhibits in many assays
Estrogen	Promotes	Promotes in many assays
TIMP	Inhibits	Inhibits in many assays
Thymosin β$_4$	Promotes	Promotes wound healing
Thymosin α$_1$	Promotes	Promotes wound healing

the sponge implant and chick chorioallantoic membrane assay (CAM), this peptide was found to be proangiogenic, and to be able to increase protease activity and tumor growth (15,16). Thus, any material that affects tube formation on matrigel should be further analyzed in different assays to determine if it actually inhibits or stimulates angiogenesis.

Interestingly, basement membrane can also promote tumor cell growth in vivo in part through its angiogenic activity (17). When basement membrane is coinjected with tumor cells, growth can be accelerated some three- to eightfold. Approximately twice as many vessels per area are observed in the matrigel growth-stimulated tumors versus tumors grown in the absence of matrigel (18). Many human tumors are difficult to grow in mice either as minced pieces or single cells. When coinjected with basement membrane, the incidence of tumor take is nearly 100% for many different types of tumors. There are many angiogenic factors in matrigel but when it is injected alone little angiogenesis occurs. When coinjected with tumor cells, considerable angiogenesis is observed which helps the tumor to grow. Since more angiogenesis is observed with the tumor cells in matrigel than with the tumor cells alone, it is likely that factors released by the tumor cells either activate, work in synergy, and/or release the angiogenic activity in the matrigel (19). The exact mechanism is not known.

A. Laminin

Laminin is the first extracellular matrix protein to be synthesized in the developing embryo and is thought to be a major contributor to early embryonic differentiation because of its diverse biological activities (20). One of the chains of laminin is observed at the two-cell stage. Laminin interacts with itself, collagen IV, perlecan, and entactin, and is also thought to be important in the assembly of the basement membrane. Laminin is composed of three chains designated α, β, and γ, which are held together by disulfide bonds (Fig. 2). At least five α, three β, and two γ chains have been described. Although genetically distinct, the chains are homologous in structure. The α chain, Mr = 400,000, contains three globular domains at the amino terminus that are separated by EGF-like (epidermal growth factor) repeats. Another EGF-like repeat is adjacent to a coiled-coil domain that has a large terminal globule at the carboxyl end. The β and γ chains contain the three amino terminal globules separated by EGF-like repeats and the coiled-coil domain but lack the carboxyl terminal globule. These chains assemble into different laminin isoforms such that 12 have been described to date but others likely exist (21). Laminins display tissue- and temporal-specific locations and presumably tissue-specific functions. The laminin produced by endothelial cells has not yet been definitely identified but is probably laminin-8 (α4β1γ1) (22).

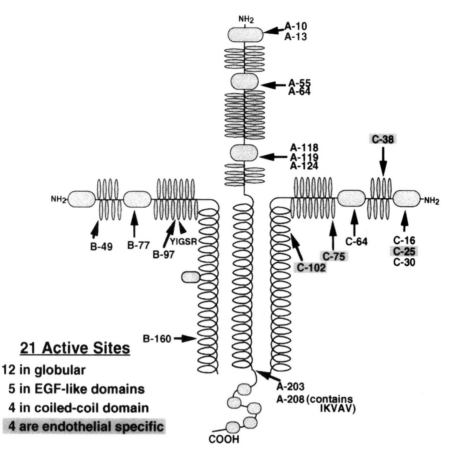

Figure 2 Schematic model of laminin-1 showing locations of some active peptides. The amino terminal globules are separated by EGF-like repeats while the carboxyl region, where the three chains are associated, is a coiled-coil structure.

B.   Laminin Peptides Active with Endothelial Cells

There is considerable interest in laminin because of its potent and diverse biological activities both in vitro and in vivo. It promotes cell adhesion, migration, growth, differentiation, neurite outgrowth, tumor growth, and metastases. It is active with endothelial cells as well. A number of active sites on laminin have been identified using fragments, recombinant proteins, and synthetic peptides (23). Several synthetic peptides duplicating laminin sequences have been found to affect angiogenesis. For example, YIGSR (tyr-ile-gly-ser-arg) blocks lung colonization, tumor growth, and angiogenesis in the rabbit eye model and in the chick CAM assay (24–27). It also blocks endothelial cell tube formation on matrigel. The laminin peptide SIKVAV is proangiogenic as discussed above (14). The physiological role of these and other sites on laminin is not known. It is possible that some but not all are active in the intact molecule. It is also possible that during angiogenesis and tumor invasion, when the basement membrane is degraded by the invading endothelial and tumor cells, fragments of laminin could become active for angiogenesis. Laminin is very protease sensitive and thus would be expected to be degraded.

The entire laminin molecule has been duplicated by synthetic peptides of approximately 12 amino acids and tested with various cell types, including endothelial cells (28–32). Endothelial cells were tested for cell adhesion and tube formation in the presence of the peptides. Many of the active peptides did not directly stimulate tube formation but rather disrupted it as expected (see Fig. 1). This assay revealed that certain laminin peptides in solution could affect tubes but did not indicate if the peptide was a stimulator or an inhibitor. Interestingly, many of the peptides disrupted the tubes resulting in differing morphologies, which suggests different mechanisms of action. The active peptides that disrupted tube formation and/or promoted endothelial cell adhesion were then tested for endothelial cell migration, ability to compete with laminin and other matrix substrates for attachment, aortic ring outgrowth, and sprouting from chick chorioallantoic membranes (i.e., in vivo angiogenesis). Some 21 active peptides were identified, four of which were not active with any other cell type tested, including tumor cells, neural cells, and salivary gland cells (Table 4).

The identification of 21 laminin-derived peptides active for endothelial cells suggests that there are a large number of active sites. It is possible that some are false positives due to charge but this number is likely to be small. It should be noted that more than 12 different receptors have been identified for laminin (33). Also, given the number and diversity of biological activities, one would expect multiple active sites. Since the laminin chains are so highly homologous, it is also possible that some of the active peptides are from homologous regions. This is expected given that 12 of the active peptides are localized in the highly homologous amino terminal globular domains. The evidence for the actual biological relevance of these sites awaits identification of the cellular receptors and functional studies using blocking antibodies.

III. SUMMARY

The extracellular matrix is comprised of highly diverse interacting molecules that regulate the structure and function of organs and tissues. The basement membrane, in particular, has been shown to promote endothelial cell differentiation in vitro confirming its biological role. The impressive biological response of cells to matrix components, such as laminin, can be duplicated by small synthetic peptides comprising the active sites. Some 21 active sites on laminin have been described for endothelial cells. These sites may be active on the intact molecules or, alternatively, they become available during the breakdown of the basement membrane matrix during angiogenesis and tumor metastasis.

Table 4 Laminin Peptides Active with Endothelial Cells

Chain	Tested	Active	Specificity	Location
α1	323	9	All cell types[a]	7 in N terminal globules 2 in coiled-coil domain
β1	187	5	All cell types	2 in EGF repeats 1 in coiled-coil domain 1 in signal region 1 in N terminal globule
γ1	154	7	3 with all cell types 4 only with endothelial cells	4 in N terminal globules 2 in EGF repeats 1 in coiled-coil domain

[a]The cell types that were tested include B16F10 melanoma, HT1080 fibrosarcoma, PC12 pheochromocytoma, HSG salivary gland cells, NG108 neuroblastoma × glioma, and primary cerebellar granule neurons.

REFERENCES

1. Hay ED. Cell Biology of Extracellular Matrix. New York: Plenum, 1991.
2. Klett CC, Diegelmann RF. Hereditary disorders of connective tissue: A review. Wound Rep Reg 1997; 3:3–11.
3. Mundlos S, Olsen BR. Heritable diseases of the skeleton. FASEB J 1997; 11:125–132, 227–233.
4. Ryan MC, Christiano AM, Engvall E, Wewer UM, Miner JH, Sanes JR, Burgeson RE. The functions of laminins: Lessons from in vivo studies. Matrix Biol 1996; 15369–15381.
5. Ninomiya Y, Olsen BR, Ooyama T. Extracellular Matrix-Cell Interaction. Basel: Karger, 1998.
6. Rohrbach DH, Timpl R. Molecular and Cellular Aspects of Basement Membranes. San Diego: Academic, 1993.
7. Vukicevic S, Kleinman HK, Luyten FP, Roberts AB, Roche NS, Reddi AH. Identification of multiple active growth factors in basement membrane Matrigel suggests caution in interpretation of cellular activity related to extracellular matrix components. Exp Cell Res 1992; 202:1–8.
8. Thorgeirsson UP, Linday CK, Cottam DW, Gomez DE. Tumor invasion, proteolysis and angiogenesis. J Neurooncol 1993; 18:89–103.
9. Grant DS, Kleinman HK. Regulation of capillary formation by laminin and other components of the extracellular matrix. In: Goldberg ID, Rosen EM, eds. Regulation of Angiogenesis. Basel: Birkhauser Verlag, 1997:317–333.
10. Kubota Y, Kleinman HK, Martin GR, Lawley TJ. Role of laminin and basement membrane in the morphological differentiation of human endothelial cells into capillary-like structures. J Cell Biol 1988; 107:1589–1598.
12. Grant DS, Morales D, Cid MC, Kleinman HK. Angiogenesis models identify factors which regulate endothelial cell differentiation. In: Maragoudakis ME, ed. Angiogenesis, Molecular Biology, Clinical Aspects. New York: Plenum, 1994:51–60.
13. Cid MC, Grant GS, Hoffman GS, Auerbach R, Fauci AS, Kleinman HK. Identification of haptoglobin as an angiogenic factor in sera from patients with systemic vasculitis. J Clin Invest 1993; 91:977–985.
14. Grant DS, Kinsella JL, Fridman R, Auerbach R, Piasecki BA, Yamada Y, Zain M, Kleinman HK. Interaction of endothelial cells with a laminin A chain peptide (SIKVAV) in vitro and induction of angiogenic behaviour in vivo. J Cellul Physiol 1992; 153:614–625.
15. Kanemoto T, Reich R, Royce L, Greatorex D, Adler SH, Shiraishi N, Martin GR, Yamada Y, Kleinman HK. Identification of an amino acid sequence from laminin A chain that stimulates metastasis and collagenase IV production. Proc Natl Acad Sci USA 1990; 87:2279–2283.
16. Sweeney TM, Kibbey MC, Zain M, Fridman R, Kleinman HK. Basement membrane and the SIKVAV laminin-derived peptide promote tumor growth and metastases. Cancer Met Rev 1991; 10:245–254.
17. Fridman R, Kibbey MC, Royce LS, Zain M, Sweeney TM, Jicha DL, Yannelli JR, Martin GR, Kleinman HK. Basement membrane (matrigel) enhances both the incidence and growth of subcutaneously injected human and murine tumors. J Natl Cancer Inst 199; 83:769–774.
18. Kibbey MC, Grant DS, Kleinman HK. Role of the SIKVAV site of laminin in promotion of angiogenesis and tumor growth: An in vivo model. J Natl Cancer Inst 1992; 84:1633–1638.
19. Martin, GR, Liotta, LA, Kleinman, HK. Interactions of tumor cells with basement membrane and laminin-1. In: Eckblom P, Timpl R, eds. The Laminins. Reading, UK: Harwood, 1996:277–290.
20. Timpl R, Brown JC. The laminins. Matrix Biol 1994; 4:275–286.
21. Burgeson RE, Chiquet M, Deutzmann R, Ekblom P, Engel J, Kleinman HK, Martin GR, Meneguzzi G, Paulsson M, Sanes J, Timpl R, Trygvasson K, Yamada Y, Yurchenco PS. A new nomenclature for the laminins. Matrix Biol 1994; 14:209–211.
22. Frieser M, Nockel H, Pausch F, Roder C, Hanh A, Deutzmann R, Sorokin LM Cloning of the mouse laminin α4 cDNA. Expression in a subset of endothelium. Eur J Biochem 1997; 246:727–735.
23. Kleinman HK, Weeks BS, Schnaper HW, Kibbey MC, Yamamura K, Grant DS. The laminins: A family of basement membrane glycoproteins important in cell differentiation and tumor metastasis. Vitamins Horm 1993; 47:161–186.
24. Graf J, Iwamoto Y, Sasaki M, Martin GR, Kleinman HK, Robey FA, Yamada Y. Identification of an

amino acid sequence in laminin mediating cell attachment, chemotaxis and receptor binding. Cell 1987; 48:989–996.

25. Iwamoto Y, Robey FA, Graf J, Sasaki M, Kleinman HK, Yamada Y, Martin GR. YIGSR, a synthetic laminin peptide, inhibits experimental metastasis formation. Science 1987; 238:1132–1134.

26. Sakamoto N, Iwahana M, Tanaka NG, Osada Y. Inhibition of angiogenesis and tumor growth by a synthetic laminin peptide, CDPGYIGSR. Cancer Res 1991; 51:903–906.

27. Kim WH, Schnaper WH, Nomizu M, Yamada Y, Kleinman HK. Apoptosis in human fibrosarcoma cells is induced by a multimeric synthetic tyr-ile-gly-ser-arg (YIGSR)-containing polypeptide from laminin. Cancer Res 1994; 54:5005–5010.

28. Nomizu M, Kim WH, Yamaura K, Utani A, Song SY, Otaka A, Roller PP, Kleinman HK, Yamada Y. Identification of cell binding sites in the laminin α1 chain carboxyterminal globular domain by systematic screening of synthetic peptides. J Biol Chem 1996; 270:20583–20590.

29. Nomizu M, Kuratomi Y, Song SY, Ponce ML, Hoffman MP, Powell SK, Miyoshi K, Otaka A, Kleinman HK, Yamada Y. Identification of cell binding sequences in mouse laminin γ1 chain by systematic peptide screening. J Biol Chem 1997; 272:32198–32205.

30. Nomizu M, Kuratomi Y, Malinda KM, Song SY, Miyoshi K, Otaka A, Powell SK, Hoffman MP, Kleinman HK, Yamada Y. Cell binding sequences in mouse laminin α1 chain. J Biol Chem 1998; 273: 32491–32499.

31. Malinda KM, Nomizu M, Chung M, Delgado M, Kuratomi Y, Yamada Y, Kleinman HK, Ponce ML. Identification of laminin α1 and β1 chain peptides active for endothelial cells adhesion, tube formation, and aortic sprouting. FASEB J 1999; 13:53–62.

32. Ponce ML, Nomizu M, Delgado MC, Kuratomi Y, Hoffman MP, Powell S, Yamada Y, Kleinman HK, Malinda KM. Identification of endothelial cell binding sites on the laminin γ1 chain. Circ 1999; 84: 688–694.

33. Powell SK, Kleinman HK. Neuronal laminins and their cellular receptors. Int J Biochem Cell Biol 1997; 29:401–414.

4
Autoantibodies in Vasculitis

Cees G.M. Kallenberg
University Hospital, Groningen, The Netherlands

Jan W. Cohen Tervaert
University Hospital, Maastricht, The Netherlands

I. INTRODUCTION

Vasculitis is a condition characterized by inflammation of blood vessels. Its clinical manifestations are dependent on the localization and size of the involved vessels as well as on the nature of the inflammatory process. Vasculitis can be secondary to other conditions or can constitute a primary, in most of the cases, idiopathic disorder (1). Underlying conditions in the secondary vasculitides are infectious diseases, connective tissue diseases, and hypersensitivity disorders. Immune complexes, either deposited from the circulation or formed in situ, are involved, in many cases, in the pathophysiology of the secondary vasculitides. These complexes are supposedly composed of microbial antigens in the case of underlying infectious diseases, autoantigens in the connective tissue diseases, and nonmicrobial exogenous antigens in the hypersensitivity disorders. Although immune deposits can be demonstrated in the involved vessel wall by direct immunofluorescence in biopsy material, the specificities of the antibodies and their corresponding antigens have not been demonstrated in most of the cases.

The primary vasculitides are, with the exception of Schönlein–Henoch purpura and cryoglobulinemia-associated vasculitis, characterized by paucity of immune deposits. The pathophysiology of vessel wall inflammation in these conditions is far from clarified. In the 1980s, autoantibodies to cytoplasmic constituents of myeloid cells were detected in patients with idiopathic necrotizing small-vessel vasculitides. These antineutrophil cytoplasmic antibodies (ANCAs), particularly those reacting with proteinase 3 (Pr3) and myeloperoxidase (MPO), were shown to be sensitive and specific for Wegener's granulomatosis, microscopic polyangiitis, and necrotizing crescentic glomerulonephritis, with absent or scant immune complex deposits. This suggests that the autoantibodies are involved in the pathogenesis of the associated diseases and positions these diseases within the spectrum of autoimmune disorders. Besides ANCA, antiendothelial cell antibodies (AECAs) have been described in patients with idiopathic systemic vasculitis. Such AECAs, could possibly play a role in the pathophysiology of vasculitis. There are, however, many uncertainties regarding the antigenic specificities of AECAs and their clinical and pathophysiological significance in systemic vasculitis.

This chapter primarily focuses on the significance of ANCAs in systemic vasculitis. Additionally, the possible role of AECAs in the idiopathic vasculitides is discussed.

II. ANTINEUTROPHIL CYTOPLASMIC ANTIBODIES IN SYSTEMIC VASCULITIS

A. Antigenic Specificities and Disease Associations

1. c-ANCAs and Proteinase 3

Antineutrophil cytoplasmic antibodies were first described by Davies et al. (2) in 1982 in a few patients with segmental necrotizing glomerulonephritis. In 1985, van der Woude et al. (3) reported the presence of autoantibodies reacting with cytoplasmic components of neutrophils and monocytes in patients with Wegener's granulomatosis (WG). The antibodies produced a cytoplasmic fluorescence pattern with accentuation of the area within the nuclear lobes when tested by indirect immunofluorescence (IIF) on ethanol-fixed neutrophils (Fig. 1), and were later designated c-ANCAs. Goldschmeding et al. (4) demonstrated that the target antigen of c-ANCAs was a 29-kDa serine protease contained within the azurophilic or α-granules of neutrophils that was different from elastase and cathepsin G, the other serine proteases in these granules. Further studies (5–7) confirmed that this 29-kDa serine protease was identical to proteinase 3, which had already been described by Kao et al. (8). Proteinase 3 has been cloned and shown to be a 29-kDa glycoprotein of 228 amino acids (9). It is synthesized as a preproenzyme. A signal peptide at the N terminus is first proteolytically cleaved. Cleavage of the propeptide results in proteolytic activity of the enzyme. Finally, a peptide of seven residues is cleaved from the carboxy terminus which does not seem to influence enzymatic activity of Pr3 (10). Proteinase 3 is present both in monocytes and granulocytes and appears early in mono-myeloid differentiation. It is thought to be present in only myeloid cells (11), although Mayet et al. have described the occurrence of Pr3, both at the RNA and protein level, in a number of other cell types including endothelial cells (12,13). In endothelial cells, cytokine stimulation induces surface expression of Pr3, which would make Pr3 accessible for the autoantibodies and might, thus, be relevant for the pathogenesis of vasculitis as will be discussed later. Whether or not Pr3 is present in endothelial cells is controversial. Proteinase 3, as recognized by human autoantibodies, has been found in humans and baboons only. Recently, a homologue of Pr3 not recognized by human antibodies has been described in mice and shows 69% homology with human Pr3 (14).

Proteinase 3 is a serine protease that is slightly cationic (pI 7.6–9.0), has proteolytic activity and is physiologically inhibited by α_1-antitrypsin (15). The Pr3-α_1-antitrypsin complexes can be detected in inflammatory fluids (15) and in sera, as shown in a study of patients with WG (16). Deficiency of α_1-antitrypsin occurs more frequently than expected in patients with anti-Pr3 autoantibodies and WG. However, patients with α_1-antitrypsin deficiency do not appear to have an increased prevalence of c-ANCAs (17). Thus, a causal relationship between α_1-antitrypsin deficiency and the development of c-ANCA/anti-Pr3 and WG has not been substantiated.

Upon full activation of myeloid cells, degranulation occurs and Pr3, together with other granule constituents, is released. In vitro stimulation of neutrophils with low doses of proinflammatory cytokines, such as tumor necrosis factor-α (TNF-α), interleukin-1 or interleukin-8, results in membrane expression of Pr3 (and other granule constituents, such as MPO and lactoferrin) (18). These so-called primed neutrophils expressing Pr3 and MPO can be further stimulated by ANCAs as will be discussed later. Surface expression of Pr3 occurs in some individuals in a low percentage of resting neutrophils (19) and, also in apoptotic neutrophils (20).

Detection of autoantibodies to Pr3 is classically done by IIF on ethanol-fixed neutrophils (21), in which they, generally, produce a cytoplasmic pattern (see Fig. 1). The c-ANCA pattern is, however, not always identical with anti-Pr3 and antigen-specific assays such as Pr 3-specific ELISAs (enzyme-linked immunosorbent assays) are required for as final test specificity. Those assays either use purified Pr3 (22) in a directly coated system or use a Pr3-specific monoclonal antibody to capture Pr3 from an α-granule extract (4,23). It should be realized that purification of

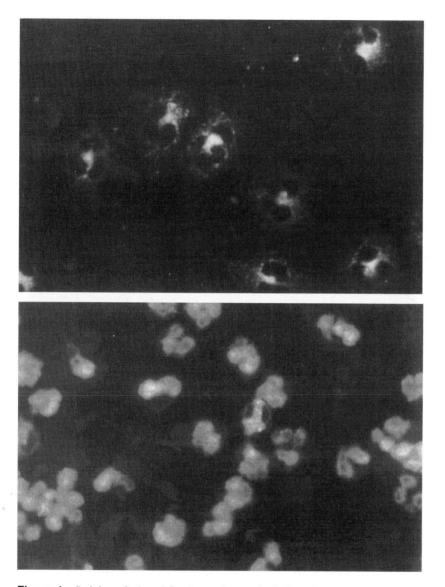

Figure 1 Staining of ethanol-fixed granulocytes by indirect immunofluorescence. Upper panel: characteristic cytoplasmic staining pattern with accentuation of the fluorescence intensity in the area within the nuclear lobes (c-ANCAs). Lower panel: perinuclear staining pattern (p-ANCAs).

Pr3 from buffy coats, as done by ion-exchange chromatography, is very laborious and requires large amounts of donor leukocytes. Furthermore, the capture ELISA has the advantage of having Pr3 presented in its native configuration, which is important since the human autoantibodies primarily react with conformational epitopes. This probably explains why recombinant proteins are, as yet, unsatisfactory for use in ELISA with the exception of Pr3 expressed in a human mast cell line (24) and, possibly, recombinant Pr3 from a baculo-virus expression system (unpublished observation). As shown in a collaborative European study, standardization of the assays is of utmost importance (22).

2. p-ANCAs and Myeloperoxidase

Following the description of c-ANCA as a marker for WG, several groups observed that a number of sera, from patients suspected of having vasculitis, produced a perinuclear fluorescence pattern on ethanol-fixed neutrophils. Falk and Jennette (25) and our group (26) described MPO as a major antigen for p-ANCA–positive sera in patients with crescentic glomerulonephritis and/or necrotizing vasculitis. Myeloperoxidase is a highly cationic protein (pI 11.0) with a molecular weight of 146 kDa, and consists of two chains. By immunoprecipitation at least two bands of approximately 60 and 42 kDa, representing a complete and a partly degraded single chain, are recognized by monoclonal and human polyclonal antibodies (4).

Myeloperoxidase is present, like Pr3, in the azurophilic or α-granules of myeloid cells, but not in other cells. Human MPO shows considerable homology with mouse and rat MPO. Immunization of rats with human MPO results in the generation of antihuman MPO antibodies that cross-react with rat MPO (27), generating anti-MPO autoantibodies. The latter is relevant for the development of experimental models of anti-MPO–associated vasculitis/glomerulonephritis (28).

MPO plays a critical role in the generation of reactive oxygen species. It catalyzes the generation of hypochlorite from hydrogen peroxide and chloride anion. Ceruloplasmin is its natural inhibitor (29). Comparable to Pr3, full activation of neutrophils results in the release of MPO whereas priming of neutrophils with low concentrations of proinflammatory cytokines results in surface expression of MPO relevant for anti-MPO (ANCA)–induced neutrophil activation (18).

Detection of anti-MPO can be screened for IIF on ethanol-fixed neutrophils (21) (see Fig. 1), where anti-MPO produces a perinuclear fluorescence pattern. This perinuclear pattern is an artifact of ethanol fixation. When neutrophils are fixed with a cross-linking fixative such as paraformaldehyde, anti-MPO–positive sera produce a cytoplasmic staining pattern. It has become clear that ANCAs of diverse specificities, such as lactoferrin, glucuronidase, elastase, cathepsin G, and others, also produce a p-ANCA pattern (30,31). The latter autoantibodies occur in a wide variety of idiopathic inflammatory disorders other than vasculitis (30,31). Many p-ANCA–positive sera in those conditions have not yet been characterized with respect to their antigenic specificities. Thus, for the detection of anti-MPO, antigen-specific assays are required.

3. Other Target Antigens of ANCAs in Systemic Vasculitis

As discussed below, Pr3 and MPO are the major target antigens of ANCAs in the systemic vasculitides. Two other antigens are recognized by ANCAs in these diseases. One is human leukocyte elastase (HLE), a 30-kDa serine protease from azurophilic granules. Autoantibodies to HLE as tested by capture ELISA have been detected in a few sera from patients with symptoms suggesting WG (32). The highly infrequent occurrence of anti-HLE does not warrant inclusion of testing for anti-HLE in the routine laboratory work-up for patients with vasculitis. Bactericidal permeability-increasing protein (BPI) is another antigen recognized by autoantibodies in systemic vasculitis. Bactericidal permeability-increasing protein, a 54-kDa protein localized in the azurophilic granules, is cytotoxic for gram-negative bacteria. It interacts with both the bacterial envelope and cell-free lipopolysaccharide, leading to bacterial killing and neutralization of free endotoxin. Zhao et al. (33) reported that ANCAs directed to BPI were found in sera from patients with small-vessel vasculitides who were negative for anti-Pr3 or anti-MPO. Anti-BPI occur also in chronic infectious diseases, particularly in patients with cystic fibrosis who are carriers of *Pseudomonas aeruginosa* (34), and in idiopathic inflammatory diseases such as primary sclerosing cholangitis (35).

4. Associations of Anti-Pr3 and Anti-MPO with Clinical Disease Entities in Systemic Vasculitis

Following the original description of c-ANCAs in WG (3), three major studies on more than 200 patients have found a sensitivity of c-ANCA/anti-Pr3 of 90% for extended WG characterized by the triad of granulomatous inflammation of the respiratory tract, systemic vasculitis, and necrotizing crescentic glomerulonephritis (36–38). The sensitivity of anti-Pr3 for limited WG, i.e., disease manifestations without obvious renal involvement, was 75% (37). Specificity of anti-Pr3 for WG or related small-vessel vasculitides was 98% when selected groups of patients with idiopathic inflammatory or infectious diseases were tested (36,37). The aforementioned studies were performed by groups highly experienced in ANCA testing. The high sensitivity and specificity of c-ANCAs for WG have, however, been questioned (39). Rao et al. (40) performed a meta-analysis on the role of c-ANCA testing in the diagnosis of WG. Summarizing current literature, they found a sensitivity of 66% and a specificity of 98% of c-ANCAs for a diagnosis of WG. Sensitivity rose to 91% when patients with active disease only were considered. Anti-Pr3 also occurs in primary vasculitides other than WG: 25–40% of patients with microscopic polyangiitis (MPA), 20–30% of patients with idiopathic necrotizing and crescentic glomerulonephritis (NCGN), and a minority of patients with Churg–Strauss syndrome test positive for anti-Pr3 (42). Anti-Pr3 has only very infrequently been reported in other disorders (41).

Whereas anti-Pr3 is primarily associated with WG, anti-MPO is found in primary vasculitis patients with a more diverse presentations (26,42). In WG, most of the patients who test negative for anti-Pr3, are positive for anti-MPO. Also, some 60% of patients with MPA, 65% of those with idiopathic NCGN, and 60% of those with Churg–Strauss syndrome are positive for anti-MPO (26,41,42). Anti-MPO has also been detected in 30–40% of patients with anti-GBM disease (43). These patients are considerably older than patients with anti-GBM only, may have clinical signs suggesting associated vasculitis, and, possibly, have a better renal outcome. Furthermore, anti-MPO has been reported in connective tissue diseases, such as systemic lupus erythematosus (SLE) (44), and in various drug-induced disease states, such as hydralazine-induced glomerulonephritis and vasculitis-like syndromes associated with propylthiouracil, other antithyroid medications, minocycline, and penicillamine (45). It is clear from the previous data that there is a clinical overlap between patients with anti-Pr3 and anti-MPO. To further define the clinical characteristics of anti-Pr3– versus anti-MPO–associated vasculitis/glomerulonephritis, Franssen et al. (46) analyzed the clinical course of consecutive patients with anti-Pr3– and anti-MPO–associated vasculitis/glomerulonephritis. They observed that patients with anti-Pr3 had a more fulminant course prior to diagnosis, with more severe inflammation in their renal biopsies. In addition, anti-Pr3–positive patients had more extra-renal disease manifestations, granuloma formation, and relapsed more frequently compared with anti-MPO–positive patients. These differences may, at least in part, be explained by a higher neutrophil-activating capacity of anti-Pr3 compared with anti-MPO as shown by in vitro studies (47). Testing for ANCAs in patients suspected of vasculitis should include tests for both anti-Pr3 and anti-MPO. A large, prospective European collaborative study has analyzed the sensitivity and specificity of anti-Pr3/anti-MPO for the idiopathic *small-to-medium-sized*-vessel vasculitides (48). This study found that the combination of cANCA by IIF and anti-Pr3 by ELISA or pANCA by IIF and anti-MPO by ELISA had a specificity of 98.4% in a group of 153 patients with either WG, MPA, or idiopathic NCGN compared with 184 disease controls and 740 healthy subjects. In that multicenter study, the sensitivity of cANCA + anti-Pr3 or pANCA + anti-MPO for WG, MPA, or idiopathic NCGN was 73, 67, and 82%, respectively. These numbers are somewhat lower than in other studies, possibly since patients with minor disease activity were included as well. In conclusion, anti-Pr3/anti-MPO, but not p-ANCA alone, are highly specific and reasonably sensitive markers for the idiopathic necrotizing small-vessel vasculitides.

B. Induction of Antineutrophil Cytoplasmic Antibodies

Antineutrophil cytoplasmic antibodies are primarily of the immunoglobulin G (IgG) class (49) although IgM-class antibodies have also been described (50). Analysis of the IgG-subclass distribution of anti-Pr3 and anti-MPO shows that antigen binding is primarily mediated by the IgG1 and IgG4 subclasses (49). Immunoglobulin G3 subclasses of ANCAs as studied for anti-Pr3 are present as well, particularly in patients with WG and renal involvement (49). These data suggest that the antibodies arise during an antigen-driven, T-cell–dependent immune response. Several groups have, therefore, analyzed the in vitro proliferative capacity of peripheral blood T cells on stimulation with Pr3 and MPO (51). Generally, patients with WG positive for anti-Pr3 responded more frequently and more strongly to Pr3 than controls, although lymphocytes from a substantial number of controls also proliferated in response to Pr3. In contrast, most patients with anti-MPO did not show in vitro lymphocyte proliferation to MPO, nor did most of the controls. Until now, no dominant T-cell epitopes have been identified for Pr3 or MPO. Identifying these epitopes may give a clue to a possible inducing agent that underlies development of anti-Pr3 or anti-MPO.

What do we know about the induction or regulation of autoantibody production in relation to disease expression? Unfortunately, no consistent observations are available showing that the development of anti-Pr3 or anti-MPO precedes the clinical expression of the associated diseases. Some data, however, suggest that exogenous factors are involved. First, certain drug therapies, particularly propylthiouracil and hydralazine, are associated with the development of anti-MPO, sometimes in conjunction with vasculitis-like diseases or glomerulonephritis (45). Second, mercuric chloride–induced autoimmune disease in rats involves the development of anti-MPO and, under certain circumstances, the occurrence of vasculitis, particularly in the gut (52). The mechanisms underlying drug- and mercuric chloride–induced anti-MPO production are, however, far from clarified.

It has been noted that reappearance or rises in anti-Pr3 levels are associated with or followed by reactivation of the disease in many patients (36,53,54). These findings have, however, been questioned in other studies (55). A meta-analysis of the available literature showed that 94 out of 197 rises in ANCA levels were followed by a relapse of WG, whereas 81 out of 157 relapses were preceded by a rise in ANCA titer (56). Differences in methodologies, however, do not allow a firm conclusion as to the diagnostic sensitivity and specificity of a rise in ANCA titer for an ensuing relapse of the associated disease. Although a rise in titer should alert the physician to the possibility of an ensuing relapse, treatment based on rises in ANCA levels cannot be recommended based on the data presently available. Nevertheless, the question remains what induces reappearance or rise in titer of anti-Pr3? In this respect, studies by Stegeman et al. (57,58) may be relevant. They observed that chronic nasal carriage of *Staphylococcus aureus* was a significant risk factor for the occurrence of relapses in patients with WG (57). Also, persistence of c-ANCA after induction of remission in these patients was a significant risk factor for relapse. Persistence of c-ANCA during remission was not independent of chronic nasal carriage of *S. aureus*, which might suggest that both factors are related. Furthermore, Stegeman et al. (58) demonstrated that maintenance treatment with co-trimoxazole in patients with WG resulted in a 60% reduction of relapses. How *S. aureus* may induce disease relapses is, presently, not clear but several hypotheses have been formulated including a role of *S. aureus*–derived superantigens stimulating the (auto)immune response (59).

C. Pathogenic Potential of Antineutrophil Cytoplasmic Antibodies in Systemic Vasculitides: In Vitro Experimental Findings

1. Interaction of ANCAs with Polymorphonuclear Granulocytes

Falk et al. (60) were the first to demonstrate that polymorphonuclear granulocytes (PMNs) can be activated by ANCAs, resulting in their production of reactive oxygen species and release of lysosomal enzymes. Polymorphonuclear granulocytes need, however, to be primed before they can be activated. Priming is a process of preactivation that can be accomplished in vitro with low doses of proinflammatory cytokines, such as tumor necrosis factor-α (TNF-α), interleukin-1 (IL-1), or IL-8, and results in surface expression of the target antigens of ANCAs, such as Pr3 and MPO. In this way, the antigens are available for interaction with the antibodies.

How activation of primed PMNs occurs after interaction with ANCAs has not been fully analyzed. Kettritz et al. (61) showed that ANCA-induced PMN activation is dependent on crosslinking of surface molecules, as ANCA IgG and F(ab')$_2$ fragments, but not Fab fragments, were capable of stimulating the production of oxygen radicals by primed PMNs. Others, however, have not been able to find activation of primed PMNs by using F(ab')$_2$ fragments of ANCAs (62, 63) and suggest that activation occurs via interaction of the autoantibodies with Fc$_\gamma$ receptors (Fc$_\gamma$R). The ANCA-induced PMN activation was strongly inhibited when blocking monoclonal antibodies against Fc$_\gamma$RII were used. The Fc$_\gamma$RIIa is the only Fc$_\gamma$ receptor that interacts with IgG2 and also has a particular affinity for the IgG3 subclass. Interestingly, in patients with WG experiencing relapses, it was observed that increases in in vitro PMN-activating capacity of serum IgG correlated with increases in levels of the IgG3 subclass of anti-Pr3, and not with that of the other subclasses (64). This, also, suggests that Fc$_\gamma$R-interaction is involved in ANCA-induced PMN activation. Reumaux et al. (65) demonstrated that, besides priming of PMNs and binding of ANCAs, a third factor is needed for in vitro PMN activation, and that is adherence of PMNs to a surface. Blocking antibodies to β_2 integrins, particularly CD18, inhibited PMN activation, suggesting that ANCA-induced PMN activation only occurs when primed PMNs are bound to a surface, e.g., endothelial cells, a process dependent on adhesion molecules, especially the β_2 integrins.

What are the in vitro effects of ANCA-induced PMN activation? As mentioned before, activated PMNs produce and secrete reactive oxygen species, they degranulate lysosomal enzymes, including Pr3, MPO and elastase, and they produce inflammatory mediators, such as TNF-α, IL-1, IL-8, and leukotriene B$_4$ (18). As a consequence, other cells are attracted, primed, and activated, which results in a strong amplification of inflammation. The process is markedly enhanced in the presence of extracellular arachidonic acid (66), which also contributes to an increase in inflammation. Finally, upon activation by ANCAs, PMNs express increased levels of adhesion molecules, including β_2 integrins, that facilitate binding to and transmigration through the endothelial monolayer (18). In vitro studies have shown that interaction among (primed) PMNs, ANCAs, and activated endothelial cells can result in damage to the endothelial cells by toxic products released from the activated PMNs (67). In addition, lysosomal constituents, including Pr3 and MPO, may bind to the endothelial cell surface, serving as "planted" antigens and targets for ANCAs. Indeed, endothelial cells can be coated in vitro with these antigens (68). Furthermore, in vitro incubation of endothelial cells with Pr3 induces production of IL-8 (69), endothelial cell apoptosis (70), and endothelial cell detachment and lysis (71). These effects were independent of the serine protease activity of Pr3. Taken together, although the exact mechanisms involved are not fully elucidated, there is evidence that ANCAs, in vitro, are able to augment and sustain a PMN-mediated inflammatory reaction, particularly affecting endothelial cells.

2.   Interaction of ANCAs with Monocytes

Since Pr3 and MPO are also constituents of granules from monocytes, these cells are likely to be targets for ANCAs as well. The ANCAs stimulate monocytes to produce and release reactive oxygen species, IL-8, and monocyte chemoattractant protein-1 (MCP-1) (72,73). In vivo, ANCA-induced MCP-1 secretion may play an important role in the formation of granulomas by amplification of local monocyte recruitment. Fluorescence-activated cell sorter (FACS) analysis of circulating monocytes of patients with WG showed the presence of MPO and Pr3 on the cell surface during active disease and relapses, and monocytes do express FcγRIIa (74). This suggests that the mechanisms underlying ANCA-induced monocyte activation are similar to those observed for PMNs.

3.   Interaction of ANCAs with Endothelial Cells

As discussed previously, Mayet et al. (12,13) described Pr3 expression by endothelial cells that was not confirmed by others (11). Expression of Pr3, as demonstrated by Mayet et al. (12), was increased and translocation of the enzyme to the cell membrane was observed after stimulation of endothelial cells with either TNF-α, interferon (IFN), or IL-1, making Pr3 available for interaction with circulating ANCAs. It should, however, be noted that within vascular lesions in ANCA-associated vasculitis, deposits of immunoglobulins are absent or scant. Therefore, direct or indirect binding of ANCAs to endothelial cells as a pathophysiological mechanism in the development of ANCA-associated vasculitis has been disputed. Further in vitro studies have demonstrated some other potentially pathogenic effects of anti-Pr3 on endothelial cells. De Bandt et al. (75) showed that anti-Pr3 are able to induce upregulation of adhesion molecules and expression of IL-1 and tissue factor by endothelial cells. Sibelius et al. (13) observed that incubation of endothelial cells with anti-Pr3 resulted in phosphoinositide hydrolysis–related signal transduction followed by the synthesis of prostacyclin and platelet-activating factor and by increased endothelial protein leakage. Thus, anti-Pr3 may potentially affect endothelial cells in ANCA-associated vasculitis. However, the expression of Pr3 by endothelial cells is not uniformly accepted.

A schematic representation of the immune mechanisms supposedly involved in the pathophysiology of ANCA-associated vasculitis is given in Figure 2 (18).

4.   Interaction of ANCAs with Their Target Antigens

Antineutrophil cytoplasmic antibodies may also affect the enzymatic properties of their target antigens. Binding of anti-Pr3 to Pr3 can inhibit the irreversible inactivation of Pr3 by α_1-antitrypsin although most anti-Pr3–positive sera also inhibit the enzymatic activity of Pr3. Binding of anti-Pr3 to Pr3 may interfere with the clearance of Pr3 released from neutrophils. Dissociation of active Pr3 from these complexes may contribute to tissue injury. A longitudinal study of WG patients showed that disease activity correlated better with the amount of inhibitory activity of anti-Pr3 on the inactivation of Pr3 by α_1-antitrypsin than with the anti-Pr3 titer itself (76).

Anti-MPO may likewise interfere with the enzymatic activity of its target enzyme. In addition, anti-MPO may interfere with binding of MPO to its natural inhibitor ceruloplasmin (29). Correlations between clinical disease activity of anti-MPO–associated vasculitis and such in vitro effects of anti-MPO have not been described.

D.   Pathogenic Potential of Antineutrophil Cytoplasmic Antibodies in Systemic Vasculitides: In Vivo Experimental Findings

Although the aforementioned findings suggest that ANCAs are potentially pathogenic, in vivo experimental models are clearly needed to further analyze how these autoantibodies can induce spe-

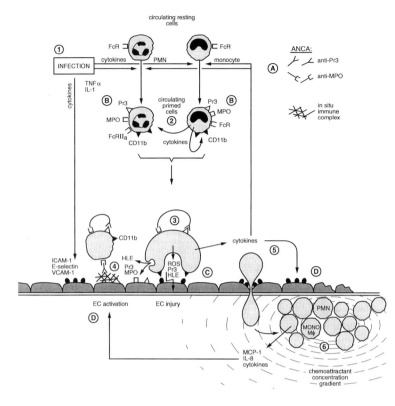

Figure 2 Schematic representation of the immune mechanisms supposedly involved in the pathophysiology of ANCA-associated vasculitides. (1) Cytokines released due to (local) infection cause upregulation of adhesion molecules on the endothelium and priming of neutrophils and/or monocytes. (2) Circulating primed neutrophils and/or monocytes express the ANCA antigens on the cell surface. (3) Adherence of primed neutrophils and/or monocytes to the endothelium, followed by activation of these cells by ANCAs. Activated neutrophils and/or monocytes release reactive oxygen species (ROS) and lysosomal enzymes, which leads to endothelial cell injury and eventually to necrotizing inflammation. (4) Degranulation of proteinase 3 (Pr3) and myeloperoxidase (MPO) by these ANCA-activated neutrophils and/or monocytes results in endothelial cell activation, endothelial cell injury, or even endothelial cell apoptosis. Furthermore, bound Pr3 and MPO serve as planted antigens, resulting in in situ immune complexes, which in turn attract other neutrophils. (5) ANCA-induced monocyte activation leads to production of monocyte chemoattractant protein-1 (MCP-1) and interleukin 8 (IL-8) production by these cells. The release of chemoattractants by these cells amplifies monocyte and neutrophil recruitment possibly leading to granuloma formation. (6) (A) to (D) represent the four prerequisites for endothelial cell damage by ANCA: (A) the presence of ANCAs, (B) expression of the target antigens for ANCAs on primed neutrophils and monocytes, (C) the necessity of an interaction between primed neutrophils and endothelium via β_2 integrins, and finally, (D) activation of endothelial cells. (From Ref. 18.)

cific lesions in intact animals. To date, several animal models have been described but none of them seems fully equivalent to the human situation.

Development of anti-MPO antibodies has been described in Brown Norway (BN) rats exposed to mercuric chloride (52). These anti-MPO antibodies are generated as part of a polyclonal response that includes antinuclear antibodies, antibodies to DNA, collagen, thyroglobulin, and components of the glomerular basement membrane. The animals develop inflammatory lesions in many organs, especially in the duodenum and cecum, where necrotizing leukocytoclastic vasculitis of submucosal vessels is apparent and is accompanied by a neutrophilic and mononuclear infiltrate. Pretreatment of the animals with antibiotics markedly reduces the vasculitic lesions suggesting that microbial factors are involved in the expression of the lesions. Although anti-MPO antibodies are present in mercuric chloride–treated BN rats, their pathogenic potential is not apparent from this model.

In 1993, Kinjoh et al. (77) described an inbred strain of mice, derived from (BXSBx MRL/Mp-lpr/lpr)F1 hybrid mice, that spontaneously developed rapidly progressive crescentic glomerulonephritis and necrotizing vasculitis. These mice develop antibodies to MPO, again as part of a polyclonal response including other autoantibodies as well. Another recombinant congenic strain of mice, designated McH5-lpr/lpr, spontaneously develop granulomatous arteritis, particularly in the kidneys, but, in most cases, without glomerulonephritis (78). Anti-MPO and anti-DNA titers are low in these mice, particularly compared with titers in the "Kinjoh" mice. The impact of these findings for our understanding of human ANCA-associated vasculitis/glomerulonephritis is not clear.

In order to develop a model for anti-MPO–associated glomerulonephritis, Brouwer et al. (79) immunized BN rats with human MPO in complete Freund's adjuvant. MPO-immunized rats developed antibodies to human MPO cross-reacting with rat MPO. Immunized rats subsequently had perfused into the renal artery products of activated neutrophils, including proteolytic enzymes, MPO, and its substrate hydrogen peroxide (H_2O_2). In contrast to control immunized rats, MPO-immunized rats developed severe necrotizing crescentic glomerulonephritis with interstitial infiltrates and vasculitis but without immune deposits. Immune deposits were present in the very initial phase but later disappeared, perhaps because of neutrophil activation by anti-MPO antibodies, inducing necrotizing inflammation with breakdown of immune deposits. Since ANCA-associated vasculitis is a systemic disease, Heeringa et al. (80) injected MPO-immunized BN rats in the jugular vein with a neutrophil lysosomal extract and H_2O_2. These rats developed severe necrotizing vasculitis in the lungs and gut. To further prove the phlogistic potential of anti-MPO antibodies, they also injected MPO-immunized BN rats with a subnephritogenic dose of rabbit anti–glomerular basement membrane (GBM) antibodies. In control immunized rats only minor lesions developed. The MPO-immunized rats, which had developed anti–rat MPO antibodies, showed severe renal lesions with fibrinoid necrosis of glomerular capillaries and crescent formation (28). This demonstrates that the anti-MPO immune response was able to severely aggravate the anti-GBM disease in this model.

The aforementioned models all relate to anti-MPO–associated vasculitides. Induction of autoimmunity to Pr3 in experimental models is hampered by the fact that the equivalent of human Pr3 in rats and mice shows only a restricted homology to human Pr3 (14). Human Pr3-ANCAs do not recognize rat or mouse Pr3 as tested by IIF, and immunization of rats with human Pr3 does not result in the formation of antibodies that react with cytoplasmic components of rat myeloid cells. Therefore, at present, the role of autoimmunity to Pr3 cannot be studied in in vivo experimental models. Induction of autoantibodies to Pr3 has, however, been described in mice by the group of Shoenfeld using idiotypic manipulation (81). In this model affinity purified human anti-Pr3 antibodies are injected into mice. These mice develop Pr3-specific anti-idiotypic antibodies after 2 weeks, and anti–anti-idiotypic antibodies that react with Pr3 after 4 months. Surprisingly, sera from these mice also reacted with human MPO and endothelial surface proteins. After 8 months, some mice developed inflammatory lesions in their lungs. Reactivity of the antibodies to mouse Pr3 was, however, not demonstrated, which questions the autoimmune basis of this model.

Taken together, a fully satisfying animal model for anti-Pr3– or anti-MPO–associated vasculitis/glomerulonephritis is presently not available. Some data from experimental studies do, however, support a pathophysiological role for ANCAs.

E. Conclusion

Both Pr3-ANCAs and MPO-ANCAs, but not ANCAs alone as tested by IIF, are important diagnostic markers for Wegener's granulomatosis, microscopic polyangiitis, Churg–Strauss syndrome and idiopathic necrotizing crescentic glomerulonephritis. Changes in levels of Pr3-ANCAs and possibly MPO-ANCAs are related to changes in disease activity although this correlation is far from absolute. In vitro studies clearly demonstrate the potential of the antibodies to interact with myeloid cells resulting in their activation and enhanced destructive activity toward endothelial cells. In vivo experimental models, although not perfect imitators of the human situation, support a pathophysiological role for MPO-ANCAs.

III. ANTIENDOTHELIAL CELL ANTIBODIES

Antiendothelial cell antibodies (AECAs) represent a heterogeneous group of antibodies found in various inflammatory diseases. Nearly three decades ago, these antibodies were reported by Lindquist and Osterland (82), who detected specific staining of the vascular endothelium by several serum samples during testing for antinuclear antibodies on mouse kidney sections as tissue substrate. Later, cultured human endothelial cells (ECs) were used as a substrate to detect AECAs and it was found that AECAs react with different endothelial antigens ranging in molecular weight from 25–200 kDa as demonstrated by immunoprecipitation of crude extracts from ECs (83).

In vitro, it has been demonstrated that AECAs may directly cause EC injury and/or apoptosis of ECs or interfere with several EC functions (84). Therefore, AECAs have been postulated to be of pathophysiological relevance. Their pathophysiological role, however, is uncertain. It is not known if these antibodies are generated before or after vascular damage or if they actually cause vascular dysfunction in vivo. Here, we discuss the possible role of AECAs in the pathophysiology of vasculitis and the value of AECAs as markers of disease activity.

A. Methods of Detection

Antiendothelial cell antibodies are usually detected by enzyme-linked immunosorbent assays (ELISAs) using as a substrate cultured human umbilical vein endothelial cells (HUVEC) that are passaged three to four times (83–87). Confluent cells are usually fixed with gluturaldehyde or paraformaldehyde to avoid nonspecific IgG binding. Fixation, however, induces increased permeability of EC membranes. Reactivity of patient sera in an AECA-ELISA in which fixed ECs are used may therefore be partially attributed to reaction with intracellular constituents. In addition, fixation induces EC membrane alterations that facilitate binding of antibodies to negatively charged phospholipids (88). To avoid these artifacts, several groups have used ELISAs with unfixed ECs to detect AECAs (86,87). Unfortunately, very few reports have compared detection of AECAs on fixed ECs with that on unfixed ECs. Antiendothelial cell antibodies also can be detected by methods such as immunofluorescence assays, radioimmunoassays, FACS analysis, immunoblotting, and immunoprecipitation, and by cell-mediated functional assays such as complement-dependent cytotoxicity (CDC) and antibody-dependent cytotoxicity (ADCC) (83). Results obtained in these tests may differ. Substrates other than HUVEC have been used, e.g., cell membrane extracts, cells from renal or adipose microvasculature, an endothelial–epithelial cell line (i.e., EAhy 926), or a spontaneously transformed EC line, ECV 304 (83). Each of these substrates has its own advantages and disadvantages. Despite these differences, concentrated efforts are currently being made to standardize tests for the detection of AECAs.

B. Endothelial Antigens

Antiendothelial cell antibodies are a group of autoantibodies directed against a variety of endothelial autoantigens. The antigens recognized by AECAs are, generally, not specific for ECs (83). Endothelial cell–specific AECAs are only found in a few instances, e.g., in sera from patients with Kawasaki disease (KD). In most other cases, AECAs react not only with ECs, but also with other cells such as fibroblasts and/or peripheral blood mononuclear cells, as demonstrated by absorption studies (83).

The EC antigens either show a constitutive and stable expression or can be modulated by cytokines (83). Cryptic antigens have been described as well (89). In some cases, activation of EC by cytokines may be a prerequisite for the detection of AECAs (83). Finally, antigenic determinants for AECA may in fact be molecules that adhere to ECs, e.g., deoxyribonucleic acid (DNA), β_2-glycoprotein I (β_2-GPI), and/or MPO (83). These so-called "planted" antigens adhere to the endothelium either directly, through charge-mediated mechanisms (MPO, β_2-GPI), or indirectly, via a DNA/histone bridge (DNA). Serum samples have been shown to contain MPO, DNA, and/or β_2-GPI (83). Myeloperoxidase, β_2-GPI, and/or DNA present in these samples may adhere to ECs during incubation of ECs with sera. Thus, anti-DNA, anti-β_2-GPI and/or anti-MPO, when present in the sera, may falsely be detected as AECAs. This phenomenon that occurs in vitro may also occur in vivo although no data are available that prove in vivo binding. Many AECA antigens are still not well characterized.

1. Constitutive Endothelial Antigens

Human leukocyte antigen (HLA) class I antigens, normally present on ECs, are not a major antigenic determinant for AECAs as, for most AECA-positive sera, no significant loss of AECA activity is observed after absorption with other cells expressing HLA class I antigens (83). Furthermore, AECA-positive sera are usually negative for the presence of anti–HLA class I antibodies as detected in a cytotoxicity assay against a large panel of human lymphocyte donors (90), and react with ECs from donors with different HLA phenotypes to the same extent. Many constitutive endothelial antigens for AECAs are not yet characterized. When proteins are extracted from lysed endothelial cells, transferred to nitrocellulose membranes, and subsequently incubated with serum samples from patients, IgG antibodies to several protein bands can be detected by immunoblotting. When cell surface membrane proteins are selectively radiolabeled and subsequently used in immunoprecipitation assays, some disease-specific endothelial antigens can be immunoprecipitated, such as a 125-kDa band in WG and a 200-kDa band in SLE (86). Antiendothelial cell antibodies distinct from those that react with cell surface membrane proteins have also been described. These AECA may react with extracellular matrix (ECM) components. By testing serum samples from patients with various systemic vasculitides, Direskeneli et al. (91) found a 25% reduction of AECA binding after incubation of the sera with a crude extract of ECM components. Different extracellular matrix components may be target antigens of AECAs such as collagen types II, IV, and VII, vimentin, and/or laminin (84,91,92). Antibodies to collagen II and IV have been described in a large variety of diseases, including vasculitis (91,93), antibodies to laminin in a high proportion of patients with primary Raynaud's phenomenon and/or systemic sclerosis (92), and antivimentin antibodies in patients with SLE (94).

2. Cryptic Antigens

Human leukocyte antigen class II determinants are present on activated ECs only, and could represent target antigens for AECAs. Antibodies to HLA class II antigens are implicated in the pathogenesis of rejection of transplanted organs (83). Proteinase 3 may be another cryptic target antigen for AECAs.

3. "Planted" Antigens

Cationic proteins from leukocytes may be target antigens both for ANCAs and, as planted antigens, for AECAs. Cationic ANCA antigens, in particular MPO, may bind to ECs after being released by activated neutrophils and/or monocytes. Binding to ECs occurs, probably, via a charge-mediated mechanism (68). Another example of a "planted" antigen for AECAs is β_2-GPI. Anti–β_2-GPI antibodies have been described in diseases such as SLE, primary antiphospholipid syndrome, and Sneddon's syndrome (83). The β_2-GPI adheres to EC membranes (84) and may be present in sera. Furthermore, EC-bound β_2-GPI is recognized by anti–β_2-GPI antibodies (95). Deoxyribonucleic acid is another example of a "planted antigen" (96). During testing for AECAs on fixed ECs, some groups found a strong association between AECAs and anti-DNA antibodies in SLE patients (83). In addition, monoclonal anti-DNA antibodies also bind to EC membranes (96). This binding was, at least partially, caused by binding of DNA/anti-DNA immune complexes to ECs and was enhanced by the addition of histones. Furthermore, treatment of HUVEC with DNase reduced the binding of monoclonal DNA antibodies to HUVEC by 20%, suggesting that DNA may indeed be present on the surface of HUVEC (96).

C. Disease Associations

Antiendothelial cell antibodies are described in a variety of diseases, such as connective tissue diseases, systemic vasculitides, and others (83). Their associations with the vasculitides are discussed here.

1. Large-Vessel Vasculitis

In 1967, Nakao et al. (97) reported antiaortic antibodies in patients with Takayasu's arteritis (TA). However, these findings could not be reproduced (98). Brasile et al. (99) later described AECAs in three patients with temporal arteritis and one with TA. One of the serum samples was also tested for reactivity with frozen cadaveric vessel sections from different anatomical sites and reacted with the iliac artery, the inferior mesenteric artery and veins, but not with the aorta. Others have reported high titers of AECAs in almost all patients with TA, confirmed by ELISA, FACS analysis, and confocal microscopy (100). Salojin et al. (101), however, found AECAs in only 7 of 21 (33%) patients with TA and 8 of 26 (31%) patients with temporal arteritis.

2. Medium-Sized-Vessel Vasculitis

Brasile et al. (99) reported AECAs in four patients with polyarteritis nodosa (PAN), whereas only 10 of 32 (31%) patients with PAN gave a positive reaction in the study of Salojin et al. (101). In Kawasaki disease, IgM AECAs were observed in 53% of patients, whereas IgG AECAs were only infrequently seen (102). The antigens involved are still not well characterized, but cytokine-inducible epitopes may be important (103). Complement-dependent cytotoxicity has been found in the majority of KD sera (102,103), particularly when cytokine-stimulated ECs were used as a substrate (103). By ELISA, however, AECA binding can be detected on both nonstimulated and TNF-α–stimulated ECs (102). Antiendothelial cell antibodies may be a marker of disease activity in KD, insofar as the antibodies disappear in convalescent patients (103).

3. Small-Vessel Vasculitis

In WG, MPA, and Churg–Strauss syndrome, AECAs are frequently found (prevalence 40–100%) (85,87,90,104,105). About 40% of AECA in the small-vessel vasculitides are, however, only borderline positive (85,87). Antiendothelial cell antibodies are more frequently found in patients with MPO-ANCAs than in those with Pr3-ANCAs (85). The endothelial antigens recognized by AECAs in these diseases are not well characterized. Some Pr3-ANCAs may bind to ECs (12), but cross-absorption studies show that most serum samples bind to ECs independent of their binding to ANCA antigens (106). Protein bands of 25, 68, 125, 155, and 180 kDa were detected by immunoblotting. The 68- and 125-kDa bands were characteristic for WG patients (86). Immunoglobulin G binding to EC was enhanced by pretreatment of ECs with TNF-α or IL-1 (85). Antiendothelial cell antibodies from patients with WG activated ECs resulting in increased expression of adhesion molecules and secretion of IL-6, IL-8, and MCP-1 (87,106). These effects were more prominent in patients with high AECA titers than in those with borderline titers (87). The AECA levels correlate with disease activity (90,104) and increasing AECA titers may be used as a marker of relapse, especially in ANCA-negative cases (107). In a prospective study on 10 patients followed during a mean period of 36 weeks, a rise of AECA titers was seen in 8 of 11 relapses and patients persistently positive for AECAs were at risk of a subsequent relapse (107).

D. Pathogenetic Role

The correlation between changes in AECA titers and disease activity suggests a role for AECAs in the induction of vessel wall damage, although it does not exclude the possibility that AECAs are a result of vascular injury. Several mechanisms have been proposed by which AECAs may play a role in the pathophysiology of vasculitis. Binding of AECAs to ECs may result in activation of ECs. Upregulated expression of endothelial adhesion molecules such as E-selectin, intercellular adhesion molecule-1 (ICAM-1), and/or vascular cell adhesion molecule-1 (VCAM-1) was found after incubation of ECs with IgG AECAs (106). Similar findings were reported for anti-Pr3, anti–β_2-GPI, and anti–HLA class I antibodies (84,108,109). Activation by AECAs may also result in the secretion of chemoattractants and/or cytokines (87,106). In addition, binding of AECAs to ECs may cause inhibition of prostacyclin production by ECs (110). More recently, it has been shown that AECAs from patients with vasculitis and/or systemic sclerosis may induce apoptosis of ECs (88). During this process, anionic phospholipids (most notably phosphatidylserine) are exposed on the surface of the cells providing binding sites for β_2-GPI and, subsequently, antiphospholipid antibodies (111). This may result in proinflammatory clearance of apoptotic cells (112). Alternative mechanisms by which AECAs could be a trigger in the pathogenesis of associated diseases are CDC and/or ADCC. Complement-dependent cytotoxicity toward cytokine-activated ECs has been reported in Kawasaki's disease (102,103) but not in other forms of vasculitis, and ADCC has occasionally been demonstrated using serum samples from patients with WG or MPA (85).

A definite animal model supporting a pathophysiological role of AECAs has not yet been developed, but several models are suggestive in this respect. Injection of antibodies to EC antigens, such as angiotensin-converting enzyme (ACE) or factor VIII von Willebrand, induces lung injury and/or glomerulonephritis in rabbits and rats (83). Furthermore, AECAs can be detected in serum samples from lupus-prone (MRL 1pr/1pr) mice (84). In an anti-idiotypic animal model, AECAs were induced in mice immunized with human IgG having AECA activity. The appearance of AECAs in these animals was associated with glomerular vascular inflammation (113).

E. Conclusion

Antiendothelial cell antibodies are detected in a variety of vasculitic and other inflammatory disorders. They are of limited value in the differential diagnosis of these diseases. Several studies support a role for AECAs in the pathophysiology of certain vasculitides. The antibodies may activate ECs, induce apoptosis, and induce complement-mediated and/or antibody-dependent vascular damage. Further characterization of putative target antigens would be helpful in the search for a possible pathophysiological role of these antibodies.

REFERENCES

1. Jennette JC, Falk RJ, Andrassy K, et al. Nomenclature of systemic vasculitides. Proposal of an international consensus conference. Arthritis Rheum 1994; 37:187–192.
2. Davies DJ, Moran JE, Niall JF, Ryan G. Segmental necrotizing glomerulonephritis with antineutrophil antibody: Possible arbovirus aetiology. Br Med J 1982; 285:606.
3. van der Woude FJ, Rasmussen N, Lobatto S, Wiik A, Permin H, van Es LA, van der Giessen M, van der Hem GK, The TH. Autoantibodies to neutrophils and monocytes: A new tool for diagnosis and a marker of disease activity in Wegener's granulomatosis. Lancet ii:425–429, 1985.
4. Goldschmeding R, van der Schoot CE, ten Bokkel Huinink D, Hack CE, van den Ende ME, Kallenberg CGM, von dem Borne AEGKr. Wegener's granulomatosis autoantibodies identify a novel diisopropylfluorophosphate-binding protein in the lysosomes of normal human neutrophils. J Clin Invest 1989; 84:1577–1587.
5. Niles JL, McCluskey RT, Ahmad MF, Arnaout MA. Wegener's granulomatosis autoantigen is a novel serine proteinase. Blood 1989; 74:1888–1893.
6. Jennette JC, Hoidal JR, Falk RJ. Specificity of anti-neutrophil cytoplasmic autoantibodies for proteinase 3. Blood 1990; 75:2263–2264.
7. Lüdemann J, Utecht B, Gross WL. Anti-neutrophil cytoplasm antibodies in Wegener's granulomatosis recognize an elastinolytic enzyme. J Exp Med 1990; 171:357–362.
8. Kao RC, Wehner MG, Skubitz KM, Gray BH, Hoidal JR. Proteinase 3: A distinct human polymorphonuclear leucocyte proteinase that produces emphysema in hamsters. J Clin Invest 1988; 82:1963–1973.
9. Campanelli D, Melchior M, Fu Y, Nakata N, Shuman H, Nathan C, Gabay JE. Cloning of cDNA for proteinase 3: A serine protease, antibiotic, and autoantigen from human neutrophils. J Exp Med 1990; 172:1709–1715.
10. Jenne DE. Gene structure of ANCA target antigens: Implications for the pathogenesis of vasculitis. Sarcoidosis Vasculitis and Diffuse Lung Diseases 1996; 13:209–213.
11. King WJ, Adu D, Daha MR, et al. Endothelial cells and renal epithelial cells do not express the Wegener's autoantigen, proteinase 3. Clin Exp Immunol 1995; 102:98–105.
12. Mayet WJ, Csernok E, Szymkowiak C, Gross WL, Meyer zum Büschenfelde KH. Human endothelial cells express proteinase 3, the target antigen of anti-cytoplasmic antibodies in Wegener's granulomatosis. Blood 1993; 82:1221–1229.
13. Sibelius U, Hattar K, Schenkel A et al. Wegener's granulomatosis: Anti-proteinase 3 antibodies are potent inductors of human endothelial cell signaling and leakage response. J Exp Med 1998; 187:497–503.
14. Jenne DE, Fröhlich L, Hummel AM, Specks U. Cloning and functional expression of the murine homologue of proteinase 3: Implications for the design of murine models of vasculitis. FEBS Lett 1997; 408:187–190.
15. Dolman KM, van de Wiel BA, Kam CM, Abbink JJ, Hack CE, Sonnenberg A, Powers JC, von dem Borne AEGKr, Goldschmeding R. Determination of proteinase 3/alpha$_1$-antitrypsin complexes in inflammatory fluids. FEBS Lett 1992; 314:117–121.
16. Henshaw TJ, Malone CC, Gabay JE, Williams RC Jr. Elevations of neutrophil proteinase 3 in serum of patients with Wegener's granulomatosis and polyarteritis nodosa. Arthritis Rheum 1994; 37:104–112.
17. Esnault VLM, Testa A, Audrain M, Rogé C, Hamidou M, Barrier JH, et al. Alpha 1-antitrypsin genetic polymorphism in ANCA-positive systemic vasculitis. Kidney Int 1993; 43:1329–1332.
18. Muller Kobold AC, van der Geld YM, Limburg PC, Cohen Tervaert JW, Kallenberg CGM. Pathophysiology of ANCA-associated glomerulonephritis. Nephrol Dial Transplant 1999; 14:1366–1375.

19. Halbwachs Mecarelli L, Bessou G, Lesavre P, Lopez S, Witko Sarsat V. Bimodal distribution of proteinase 3 (Pr3) surface expression reflects a constitutive heterogeneity in the polymorphonuclear neutrophil pool. FEBS Lett 1995; 374:29–33.

20. Gilligan HM, Bredy B, Brady HR, et al. Antineutrophil cytoplasmic autoantibodies interact with primary granule constituents on the surface of apoptotic neutrophils in the absence of neutrophil priming. J Exp Med 1996; 184: 2231–2241.

21. Wiik A. Delineation for a standard procedure for indirect immunofluorescence detection of ANCA. APMIS 1989; 97:S12–S13.

22. Hagen EC, Andrassy K, Csernok E, Daha MR, Gaskin G, Gross WL, et al. Development and standardization of solid phase assays for the detection of antineutrophil cytoplasmic antibodies (ANCA): A report on the second phase of an international cooperative study on the standardization of ANCA assays. J Immunol Meth 1996; 196:1–15.

23. Westman KW, Selga D, Bygren P, Segelmark M, Baslund B, Wiik A, Wieslander J. Clinical evaluation of a capture ELISA for detection of proteinase-3 antineutrophil cytoplasmic antibody. Kidney Int 1998; 53:1230–1236.

24. Sun J, Fass DN, Hudson JA, Viss MA, Homburger HA, Specks U. Capture-ELISA based on recombinant proteinase 3 (Pr3) is sensitive for Pr3-ANCA testing and allows detection of Pr3 and Pr3-ANCA/Pr3 immune complexes. J Immunol Meth 1998; 221:111–123.

25. Falk RJ, Jennette JC. Anti-neutrophil cytoplasmic autoantibodies with specificity for myeloperoxidase in patients with systemic vasculitis and idiopathic necrotizing and crescentic glomerulonephritis. N Engl J Med 1988; 318:1651–1657.

26. Cohen Tervaert JW, Goldschmeding R, Elema JD, Limburg PC, van der Giessen M, Huitema MG, Koolen MI, Hené RJ, The TH, van der Hem GK, von dem Borne AEGKr, Kallenberg CGM. Association of autoantibodies to myeloperoxidase with different forms of vasculitis. Arthritis Rheum 1990; 33:1264–1272.

27. Heeringa P, Brouwer E, Klok PA, Huitema MG, van den Born J, Weening JJ, Kallenberg CGM. Autoantibodies to myeloperoxidase aggravate mild anti-glomerular-basement-membrane-mediated glomerular injury in the rat. Am J Pathol 1996; 149:1695–1706.

28. Heeringa P, Brouwer E, Cohen Tervaert JW, Weening JJ, Kallenberg CGM. Animal models of antineutrophil cytoplasmic antibody associated vasculitis. Kidney Int 1998; 53:253–263.

29. Griffin SV, Chapman PT, Lianos EA, Lockwood CM. The inhibition of myeloperoxidase by ceruloplasmin can be reversed by anti-myeloperoxidase antibodies. Kidney Int 1999; 55:917–925.

30. Kallenberg CGM, Mulder AHL, Cohen Tervaert JW. Antineutrophil cytoplasmic antibodies: A still growing class of autoantibodies in inflammatory disorders. Am J Med 1992; 93: 675–682.

31. Hoffman GS, Specks U. Antineutrophil cytoplasmic antibodies. Arthritis Rheum 1998; 41:1521–1537.

32. Cohen Tervaert JW, Mulder AHL, Stegeman CA, Elema JD, Huitema MG, The TH, Kallenberg CGM. The occurrence of autoantibodies to human leukocyte elastase in Wegener's granulomatosis and other inflammatory disorders. Ann Rheum Dis 1993; 52:115–120.

33. Zhao MH, Jones SJ, Lockwood CM. Bactericidal/permeability-increasing protein (BPI) is an important antigen for anti-neutrophil cytoplasmic autoantibodies (ANCA) in vasculitis. Clin Exp Immunol 1995; 99:49–56.

34. Zhao MH, Jayne DRW, Ardiles L et al. Autoantibodies against bactericidal/permeability-increasing protein (BPI) in cystic fibrosis. Q J Med 1996; 89:259–265.

35. Roozendaal C, van Milligen de Wit AWM, Haagsma EB, Horst G, Schwarze C, Peter HH, Kleibeuker JH, Cohen Tervaert JW, Limburg PC, Kallenberg CGM. Anti-neutrophil cytoplasmic antibodies (ANCA) in primary sclerosing cholangitis: Defined specificities may be associated with distinct clinical features. Am J Med 1998; 105:393–399.

36. Cohen Tervaert JW, van der Woude FJ, Fauci AS, Ambrus JL, Velosa J, Keane WF, Meijer S, van der Giessen M, The TH, van der Hem GK, Kallenberg CGM: Association between active Wegener's granulomatosis and anticytoplasmic antibodies. Arch Intern Med 1989; 149:2461–2465.

37. Nölle B, Specks V, Lüdemann J, Rohrbach MS, De Remee DA, Gross WL: Anticytoplasmic autoantibodies: Their immunodiagnostic value in Wegener's granulomatosis. Ann Int Med 1989; 111:28–40.

38. Weber MFA, Andrassy K, Pullig O, Koderisch J, Netzer K. Antineutrophil cytoplasmic antibodies and

antiglomerular basement membrane antibodies in Goodpasture's syndrome and Wegener's granulomatosis. J Am Soc Nephrol 1992; 2:1227–1234.

39. Rao JK, Allen NB, Feussner JR, Weinberger M. A prospective study of antineutrophil cytoplasmic antibody (c-ANCA) and clinical criteria in diagnosing Wegener's granulomatosis. Lancet 1995; 346: 926–931.

40. Rao JK, Weinberger M, Oddone EZ, et al. The role of antineutrophil cytoplasmic antibody testing in the diagnosis of Wegener granulomatosis. Ann Intern Med 1995; 123:925–932.

41. Kallenberg CGM, Brouwer E, Weening JJ, Cohen Tervaert JW. Anti-neutrophil cytoplasmic antibodies: Current diagnostic and pathophysiological potential. Kidney Int 1994; 46:1–15.

42. Cohen Tervaert JW, Limburg PC, Elema JD, Huitema MG, Horst G, The TH, Kallenberg CGM. Detection of autoantibodies against myeloid lysosomal enzymes: A useful adjunct to classification of patients with biopsy-proven necrotizing arteritis. Am J Med 1991; 91:59–66.

43. Jayne DRW, Marshall PD, Jones SJ, Lockwood CM. Autoantibodies to GBM and neutrophil cytoplasm in rapidly progressive glomerulonephritis. Kidney Int 1990; 37:965–970.

44. Merkel PA, Polisson RP, Chang Y, Skates SJ, Niles JL. Prevalence of antineutrophil cytoplasmic antibodies in a large inception cohort of patients with connective tissue disease. Ann Intern Med 1997; 126:866–873.

45. Merkel PA. Drugs associated with vasculitis. Curr Opinion Rheumatol 1998; 10:45–50.

46. Franssen CFM, Gans ROB, Arends B, Hageluken C, ter Wee PM, Gerlag PGG, Hoorntje SJ. Differences between anti-myeloperoxidase and anti-proteinase 3 associated renal disease. Kidney Int 1995; 47:193–199.

47. Franssen CFM, Huitema MG, Muller Kobold AC, Oost-Kort W, Limburg PC, Tiebosch A, et al. In vitro neutrophil activation by antibodies to proteinase 3 and myeloperoxidase from patients with crescentic glomerulonephritis. J Am Soc Nephrol 1999; 10:1506–1515.

48. Hagen EC, Daha MR, Hermans J, Andrassy K, Csernok E, et al. Diagnostic value of standardized assays for anti-neutrophil cytoplasmic antibodies in idiopathic systemic vasculitis. EC/BCR project for ANCA assay standardization. Kidney Int 1998; 53:743–753.

49. Brouwer E, Cohen Tervaert JW, Horst G, Huitema MG, van der Giessen M, Limburg PC, Kallenberg CGM. Predominance of IgG4 subclass of anti-neutrophil cytoplasmic autoantibodies in patients with Wegener's granulomatosis and clinically related disorders. Clin Exp Immunol 1991; 83:379–386.

50. Esnault VL, Soleimani B, Keogan MT, Brownlee AA, Jayne DR, Lockwood CM. Association of IgM with IgG ANCA in patients presenting with pulmonary hemorrhage. Kidney Int 1992; 41:1304–1310.

51. Mathieson PW, Oliviera DBG. The role of cellular immunity in systemic vasculitis. Clin Exp Immunol 1995; 100:183–185.

52. Mathieson PW, Thiru S, Oliveira DBG: Mercuric chloride-treated Brown Norway rats develop widespread tissue injury including necrotizing vasculitis. Lab Invest 1992; 67:121–129.

53. Egner W, Chapel HM. Titration of antibodies against neutrophil cytoplasmic antigens is useful in monitoring disease activity in systemic vasculitides. Clin Exp Immunol 1990; 82:244–249.

54. Jayne DRW, Gaskin G, Pusey CD, Lockwood CM. ANCA and predicting relapse in systemic vasculitis. Q J Med 1995; 88:127–133.

55. Kerr GR, Fleischer THA, Hallahan CD, et al. Limited prognostic value of changes in antineutrophil cytoplasmic antibody titer in patients with Wegener's granulomatosis. Arthritis Rheum 1993; 36:365–371.

56. Cohen Tervaert JW, Stegeman CA, Kallenberg CGM. Serial ANCA testing is useful in monitoring disease activity of patients with ANCA-associated vasculitides. Sarcoidosis 1996; 13:241–245.

57. Stegeman CA, Cohen Tervaert JW, Sluiter WJ, Manson W, Jong de PE, Kallenberg CGM. Association of chronic nasal carriage of Staphylococcus aureus and higher relapse rates in Wegener's granulomatosis. Ann Intern Med 1994; 113:12–17.

58. Stegeman CA, Cohen Tervaert JW, de Jong PE, Kallenberg CGM. Trimethoprim-sulfamethoxazole for the prevention of relapses of Wegener's granulomatosis. N Engl J Med 1996; 335:16–20.

59. Cohen Tervaert JW, Popa ER, Bos NA. The role of superantigens in vasculitis. Curr Opinion Rheumatol 1999; 11:24–33.

60. Falk RJ, Terrell RS, Charles LA, Jennette JC. Anti-neutrophil cytoplasmic autoantibodies induce neu-

trophils to degranulate and produce oxygen radicals in vitro. Proc Natl Acad Sci USA. 1990; 87: 4115–4119.

61. Kettritz R, Jennette JC, Falk RJ. Crosslinking of ANCA antigens stimulates superoxide release by human neutrophils. J Am Soc Nephrol 1997; 8:386–394.

62. Porges AJ, Redecha PB, Kimberly WT, Csernok E, Gross WL, Kimberly RP. Anti-neutrophil cytoplasmic antibodies engage and activate human neutrophils via Fcgg RIIa. J Immunol 1994; 153: 1271–1280.

63. Mulder AH, Heeringa P, Brouwer E, Limburg PC, Kallenberg CGM. Activation of granulocytes by anti-neutrophil cytoplasmic antibodies (ANCA): A Fcgg RII-dependent process. Clin Exp Immunol 1994; 98:270–278.

64. Mulder AH, Stegeman CA, Kallenberg CGM. Activation of granulocytes by anti-neutrophil cytoplasmic antibodies (ANCA) in Wegener's granulomatosis: A predominant role for the IgG3 subclass of ANCA. Clin Exp Immunol 1995; 101:227–232.

65. Reumaux D, Vossebeld PJ, Roos D, Verhoeven AJ. Effect of tumor necrosis factor-induced integrin activation on Fcgg receptor II-mediated signal transduction: Relevance for activation of neutrophils by anti-proteinase 3 or anti-myeloperoxidase antibodies. Blood 1995; 86:3189–3195.

66. Grimminger F, Hattar K, Papavassilis C, Temmesfeld B, Csernok E, Gross WL. Neutrophil activation by anti-proteinase 3 antibodies in Wegener's granulomatosis: Role of arachidonic acid and leukotriene B4 generation. J Exp Med 1996; 184:1567–1572.

67. Savage CO, Pottinger BE, Gaskin G, Pusey CD, Pearson JD. Autoantibodies developing to myeloperoxidase and proteinase 3 in systemic vasculitis stimulate neutrophil cytotoxicity toward cultured endothelial cells. Am J Pathol 1992; 141:335–342.

68. Ballieux BE, Zondervan KT, Kievit P, et al. Binding of proteinase 3 and myeloperoxidase to endothelial cells: ANCA-mediated endothelial damage through ADCC? Clin Exp Immunol 1994; 97: 52–60.

69. Berger SP, Seelen MA, Hiemstra PS, et al. Proteinase 3, the major autoantigen of Wegener's granulomatosis, enhances IL-8 production by endothelial cells in vitro. J Am Soc Nephrol 1996; 7:694–701.

70. Yang JJ, Kettritz R, Falk RJ, Jennette JC, Gaibo ML. Apoptosis of endothelial cells induced by neutrophil serine proteases proteinase 3 and elastase. Am J Pathol 1996; 149:1617–1626.

71. Ballieux BE, Hiemstra PS, Klar Mohamad N, et al. Detachment and cytolysis of human endothelial cells by proteinase 3. Eur J Immunol 1994; 24:3211–3215.

72. Ralston DR, Marsh CB, Lowe MP, Wewers MD. Antineutrophil cytoplasmic antibodies induce monocyte IL-8 release. Role of surface proteinase 3, alpha1-antitrypsin, and Fcγ receptors. J Clin Invest 1997; 100:1416–1424.

73. Casselman BL, Kilgore KS, Miller BF, Warren JS: Antibodies to neutrophil cytoplasmic antigens induce monocyte chemoattractant protein-1 secretion from human monocytes. J Lab Clin Med 1995; 126:495–502.

74. Muller Kobold AC, Kallenberg CGM, Cohen Tervaert JW. Monocyte activation in patients with Wegener's granulomatosis. Ann Rheum Dis 1999; 58:237–245.

75. de Brandt M, Olliviec V, Meyer O, Babin-Chevaye C, Kherhai F, Prost D de, Hakim J, Pasquier C. Induction of interleukin-1 and subsequent tissue factor expression by anti-proteinase 3 antibodies in human umbilical vein endothelial cells. Arthritis Rheum 1997; 40:2030–2038.

76. Dolman KM, Stegeman CA, van de Wiel BA, Hack CE, von dem Borne AEGKr, Kallenberg CGM, Goldschmeding R. Relevance of classic anti-neutrophil cytoplasmic autoantibody (cANCA)-mediated inhibition of proteinase 3–α1-antitrypsin complexation to disease activity in Wegener's granulomatosis. Clin Exp Immunol 1993; 93:405–410.

77. Kinjoh K, Kyoguko M, Good RA. Genetic selection for crescent formation yields mouse strain with rapidly progressive glomerulonephritis and small vessel vasculitis. Proc Natl Acad Sci USA 1993; 90: 3413–3417.

78. Nose M, Nishimura M, Ito MR, Itoh J, Shibata T, Sugisaki T. Arteritis in a novel congenic strain of mice derived from MRL/*lpr* lupus mice. Am J Pathol 1996; 149:1763–1796.

79. Brouwer E, Huitema MG, Klok PA, Cohen Tervaert JW, Weening JJ, Kallenberg CGM. Anti-myelo-

peroxidase associated proliferative glomerulonephritis: An animal model. J Exp Med 1993; 177:905–914.

80. Heeringa P, Foucher P, Klok PA, Huitema MG, Cohen Tervaert JW, Weening JJ, Kallenberg CGM. Systemic injection of products of activated neutrophils and H_2O_2 in myeloperoxidase-immunized rats leads to necrotizing vasculitis in the lungs and gut. Am J Pathol 1997; 151:131–140.

81. Blank M, Tomer Y, Stein M, Kopolovic J, Wiik A, Meroni PL, Conforti G, Shoenfeld Y. Immunization with anti-neutrophil cytoplasmic antibody (ANCA) induces the production of mouse ANCA and perivascular lymphocyte infiltration. Clin Exp Immunol 1995; 102:120–130.

82. Lindqvist KJ, Oosterland CK. Human antibodies to vascular endothelium. Clin Exp Immunol 1971; 9:753–762.

83. Belizna C, Cohen Tervaert JW. Specificity, pathogenicity, and clinical value of antiendothelial cell antibodies. Seminars Arthritis Rheum 1997; 27:98–109.

84. Meroni PL, Del Papa N, Raschi E, Tincani A, Balestrieri G, Youinou P. Antiendothelial cell antibodies (AECA): From a laboratory curiosity to another useful autoantibody. In: Shoenfeld Y, ed. The Decade of Autoimmunity. Amsterdam: Elsevier, 1999:285–294.

85. Savage COS, Pottinger BE, Gaskin G, Lockwood CM, Pusey CD, Pearson JD. Vascular damage in Wegener's granulomatosis and microscopic polyarteritis: Presence of AECA and their relation to ANCA. Clin Exp Immunol 1991; 85:14–19.

86. Del Papa N, Conforti G, Gambini D, La Rosa L, Tincani A, D'Cruz D, Khamashta M, Hughes GRV, Balestrieri G, Meroni LP. Characterisation of the endothelial surface proteins recognized by AECA in primary and secondary autoimmune vasculitis. Clin Immunol Immunopathol 1994; 70(3):211–216.

87. Muller Kobold AC, van Wijk RT, Franssen CFM, Molema G, Kallenberg CGM, Cohen Tervaert JW. In vitro upregulation of E-selectin and induction of interleukin-6 in endothelial cells by autoantibodies in Wegener's granulomatosis and microscopic polyangiitis. Clin Exp Rheumatol 1999; 17:433–440.

88. Bordron A, Dueymes M, Levy Y, Jamin C, Leroy JP, Piette JC, Shoenfeld Y, Youinou PY. The binding of some human antiendothelial cell antibodies induces endothelial cell apoptosis. J Clin Invest 1998; 101:2029–2035.

89. Koenig DW, Barley-Maloney L, Daniel TO. A western blot assay detects autoantibodies to cryptic endothelial antigens in thrombotic microangiopathies. J Clin Immunol 1993; 13:204–210.

90. Ferraro G, Meroni PL, Tincani A, Sinico A, Barcellini W, Radice A, Gregorini G, Froldi M, Borghi MO, Balestrieri G. AECA in patients with Wegener granulomatosis and micropolyarteritis. Clin Exp Immunol 1990; 79:47–53.

91. Direskeneli H, D'Cruz D, Khamashta AM, Hughes RV. Autoantibodies against EC, ECM, and human collagen IV in patients with systemic vasculitis. Clin Immunol Immunopathol 1994; 70:206–210.

92. Gabrielli A, Montroni M, Rupoli S, Caniglia ML, De Lustro F, Danieli G. A retrospective study of antibodies against basement membrane antigens (type IV collagen and laminin) in patients with primary and secondary Raynaud's phenomenon. Arthritis Rheum 1988; 31:1433–1436.

93. Moreland LW, Gay RE, Gay S. Collagen antibodies in patients with vasculitis and systemic lupus erythematosus. Clin Immunol Immunopathol 1991; 60:412–418.

94. Blaschek MA, Boehmen M, Jouquan J, Simitizis AM, Fifas S, Le Goff P, Youinou P. Relation of antivimentin antibodies to anticardiolipin antibodies in systemic lupus erythematosus. Ann Rheum Dis 1988; 47:708–716.

95. Del-Papa N, Guidali L, Spatola L, Bonara P, Borghi MO, Tincani A, Balestrieri G, Meroni PL. Relationship between anti-phospholipid and anti-endothelial cell antibodies III: Beta 2 glycoprotein I mediates the antibody binding to endothelial membranes and induces the expression of adhesion molecules. Clin Exp Rheumatol 1995; 13:179–186.

96. Chan TM, Frampton G, Staines NA, Hobby P, Perry GJ, Cameron JS. Different mechanisms by which anti-DNA MoAbs bind to human EC and glomerular mesangial cells. Clin Exp Immunol 1992; 88:68–74.

97. Nakao K, Ikeda K, Kimata M. Takayasu's arteritis: Clinical report of 84 cases and immunological studies of 7 cases. Circulation 1967; 53:1141–1144.

98. Chopra P, Datta RK, Dasgupta A, Bhargava S. Nonspecific aortaarteritis (Takayasu's disease): An immunologic and autopsy study. Jpn Heart J 1983; 24:549–556.

99. Brasile L, Kremer J, Clarke J, Cerrili J. Identification of an autoantibody to vascular endothelial cell-specific antigen in patients with systemic vasculitis. Am J Med 1987; 87:74–80.

100. Eichhorn J, Sima D, Thiele B, Lindschau C, Turowski A, Schmidt H, Schneider W, Haller H, Luft FC. Anti-endothelial cell antibodies in Takayasu arteritis. Circulation 1996; 94:2396–2401.

101. Salojin KV, Le-Tonqueze M, Nassovov EL, Blouch MT, Baranov AA, Saraux A, Guillevin L, Fiessinger JN, Piette JC, Youinou P. Anti-endothelial cell antibodies in patients with various forms of vasculitis. Clin Exp Rheumatol 1996; 14:163–169.

102. Kaneko K, Savage COS, Pottinger BE, Shah V, Pearson JD, Dillon MJ. AECA can be cytotoxic to EC without cytokine prestimulation and correlate with ELISA antibody measurement in Kawasaki disease. Clin Exp Immunol 1994; 8:264–269.

103. Leung DYM, Geha RS, Newburger JW, Burns JC, Fiers W, Lapierre LA, Pober JS. Two monokines, IL-1 and TNF, render cultured vascular EC susceptible to lysis by antibodies circulating during Kawasaki syndrome. J Exp Med 1986; 164:1958–1972.

104. Gobel U, Eichhorn J, Kettritz R, Briedigkeit L, Sima D, Lindschau C, Haller H, Luft FC. Disease activity and autoantibodies to endothelial cells in patients with Wegener's granulomatosis. Am J Kidney Dis 1996; 28:186–194.

105. Schmitt WH, Csernok E, Kobayashi S, Klinkenborg A, Reinhold-Keller E, Gross WL. Churg-Strauss syndrome: Serum markers of lymphocyte activation and endothelial damage. Arthritis Rheum 1998; 41:445–452.

106. Del-Papa N, Guidali L, Sironi M, Shoenfeld Y, Mantovani A, Tincani A, Balestrieri G, Radice A, Sinico RA, Meroni PL. Anti-endothelial cell IgG antibodies from patients with Wegener's granulomatosis bind to human endothelial cells in vitro and induce adhesion molecule expression and cytokine secretion. Arthritis Rheum 1996; 39:758–766.

107. Chan TM, Frampton G, Jayne DR, Perry GJ, Lockwood CM, Cameron JS. Clinical signifiance of AECA in systemic vasculitis: A longitudinal study comparing AECA and ANCA. Am J Kidney Dis 1993; 22:387–392.

108. Mayet WJ, Meyer-zum-Büschenfelde KH. Antibodies to proteinase 3 increase adhesion of neutrophils to human endothelial cells. Clin Exp Immunol 1993; 94:440–446.

109. Bian H, Harris PE, Mulder A, Reed EF. Anti-HLA antibody ligation to HLA class I molecules expressed by endothelial cells stimulates tyrosine phosphorylation, inositol phosphate generation, and proliferation. Hum Immunol 1997; 53:90–97.

110. Lindsey NJ, Henderson FI, Malia R, Milford-Ward MA, Greaves M, Hughes P. Inhibition of prostacyclin release by endothelial binding anticardiolipin antibodies in thrombosis-prone patients with SLE and the anti-phospholipid syndrome. Br J Rheumatol 1994; 33:20–26.

111. Bordron A, Dueymes M, Levy Y, Jamin C, Ziporen L, Piette JC, Shoenfeld Y, Youinou P. Anti-endothelial cell antibody binding makes negatively charged phospholipids accessible to antiphospholipid antibodies. Arthritis Rheum 1998; 41:1738–1747.

112. Manfredi AA, Rovere P, Heltai S, Galati G, Nebbia G, Tincani A, et al. Apoptotic cell clearance in systemic lupus erythematosus. II. Role of β2-glycoprotein I. Arthritis Rheum 1998; 41:215–223.

113. Damianovich M, Gilburd B, George J, Del-Papa N, Afek A, Goldberg I, Kopolovic Y, Roth D, Barkai G, Meroni PL, Shoenfeld Y. Pathogenic role of anti-endothelial cell antibodies in vasculitis. An idiotypic experimental model. J Immunol 1996; 156:4946–4951.

5
T Cells in Vascular Disease

Jörg J. Goronzy

Mayo Clinic and Foundation, Rochester, Minnesota

I. INTRODUCTION

The host immune response is an integrated system of natural (innate) and specific immune mechanisms. By recognizing antigen with exquisite specificity, the specific immune responses direct and focus inflammatory processes to the site of antigen where they orchestrate and amplify the natural immune reactions. In contrast to the innate immune response, the specific immune system memorizes antigenic encounters. In subsequent encounters, as is the case with antigen reexposure or chronic antigen persistence, specific immune responses become increasingly effective and, therefore, more difficult to interrupt by immunosuppressive therapy. Like physiological immune responses, the inflammation in vasculitic syndromes has components of specific and of natural immunity. The spectrum varies from dominant T-cell involvement in large-vessel vasculitides to the predominance of innate immune mechanisms in small-vessel inflammation. Even within a vasculitic entity, the relative contribution of the different immune mechanisms can vary, possibly as a function of disease duration as exemplified in polyarteritis nodosa.

T cells are the principal mediators of specific immunity. They recognize antigen in the form of antigenic peptides complexed to major histocompatibility complex (MHC) molecules on the surface of antigen-presenting cells (1). Principally, two classes of MHC molecules can be distinguished. The MHC class I molecules are expressed on all somatic cells, predominantly present endogenous peptides derived from cytoplasmic proteins, and are recognized by CD8 T cells. The MHC class II molecules have a very restricted tissue distribution. They bind antigens that are endocytosed by specialized antigen-presenting cells, such as dendritic cells, macrophages, and B cells, and they present the antigenic peptides to CD4 T cells. T-cell receptor stimulation by the appropriate MHC-peptide complex initiates a cascade of events that culminates in the clonal expansion of the antigen-specific T cell, the release of cytokines, and the differentiation of the T cell into an effector cell.

II. MOLECULAR BASIS OF T-CELL ACTIVATION

T cells express a clonally distributed T-cell receptor (TCR) to recognize peptide MHC complexes (2). In the majority of T cells, the receptor consists of a α and β chains, covalently linked by disulfide bonds. A less common subset of T cells is composed of γ and δ chains (3). Both types of T-cell receptors signal through the CD3 molecule, which consists of four chains (γ, δ, and 2ε) non-

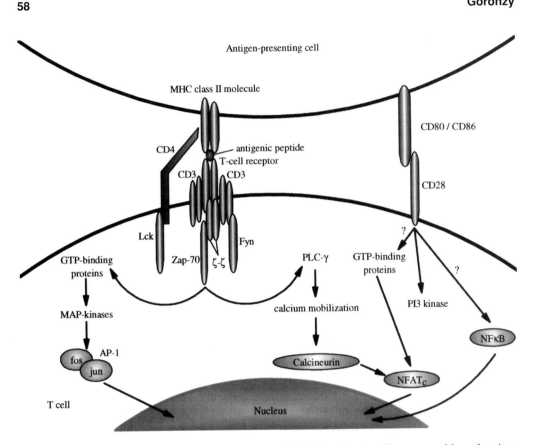

Figure 1   Schematic diagram of molecular pathways in T-cell activation. Upon recognition of antigen complexed with MHC class II (or class I) molecules, CD4 (or CD8 in case of CD8 T cells) is clustered with the T-cell receptor complex and induces the phosphorylization of domains on the invariant chains of the CD3 molecule as well as on the ζ–ζ dimer. Phosphorylization of these sites allows for the docking and subsequent phosphorylization of a number of proteins, among them ZAP-70 and PLC-γ. PLC-γ activation initiates a cascade of events that results in the intracellular mobilization of calcium and the activation of calcineurin and the nuclear transcription factor NFAT. ZAP-70 docking, over a series of intermediary steps, leads to the activation of a cascade of serine-threonine kinases (MAP kinases) that activate or induce the transcription of several transcription factors, including AP-1. These signaling events do not induce complete T-cell activation unless the CD28 costimulatory pathway is activated. CD28-induced signaling is less well defined but may preferentially influence the activation of the transcription factors NFAT and NFκB. Activated transcription factors are translocated into the nucleus and initiate the transcription of multiple genes, including the cytokine genes IFN-γ and IL-2.

covalently associated with the T-cell receptor and the ζ-chain homodimer (4). Upon antigenic triggering of the T-cell receptor, the CD3/ζ complex transduces signals that lead to T-cell activation (Fig. 1). However, T-cell receptor–transduced signals are usually not sufficient to activate a T cell. The coordinate stimulation of two independent signaling pathways is required for T-cell activation. This "two-signal hypothesis" provides a possible explanation of how self- and nonself-antigens are distinguished and how tolerance to self is achieved (5). T cells that receive signals from the TCR in the absence of costimulatory signals are rendered incapable of responding to an antigen, even if that antigen is later presented again in the context of costimulatory molecules. This form of T-cell activation has been termed "clonal anergy." Also, T cells solely stimulated through the TCR in the absence of costimulatory signals fail to induce antiapoptotic proteins and tend to undergo apoptosis.

Several costimulatory molecules on T cells have been described, the most important of which is the CD28 molecule (6,7). The ligands for the CD28 molecule, CD80 and CD86, are only expressed on professional antigen-presenting cells under normal circumstances. Costimulation through the CD28 molecules is essential to induce the transcription of interleukin-2 (IL-2) and the antiapoptotic protein bcl-xL. Lack of costimulation via CD28 has been postulated as the major mechanism of maintaining peripheral tolerance of CD4 T cells to self-antigens. Obviously, CD4 T cells should be tolerized when somatic cells aberrantly express MHC class II molecules and present self-antigens in the absence of CD80 and CD86 expression. If antigen-presenting cells express the ligand for the CD28 molecule, incorporate exogenous antigen, and process and present it to CD4 T cells, T cell activation is initiated. Tolerance mechanisms for CD8 T cells are slightly different because activated CD4 T cells may substitute for the costimulatory signals. Accordingly, CD8 T cells are inactivated if they recognize MHC class I–associated antigens in the absence of T-cell help.

III. HLA AND DISEASE ASSOCIATION

The MHC region encompasses a cluster of several genes, many of which are involved in T-cell regulation, that display allelic polymorphisms within the human population. The MHC class I region includes at least six genes, HLA-A, -B, -C, -E, -F, and -G; at least HLA-A, -B, and -C are polymorphic. The MHC class II region encodes for the α and β chains of the HLA-DR, HLA-DQ, and HLA-DP molecules. HLA polymorphisms, in particular allelic variants of MHC class II molecules, have been found to function as predisposing factors for chronic inflammatory diseases, particularly those with autoimmune characteristics (8). Because HLA polymorphisms determine the specific binding of antigenic peptides and directly interact with T-cell receptor molecules, the HLA association of these autoimmune syndromes implies that antigen recognition by T cells is a critical step in the pathogenesis (Table 1).

The large-vessel vasculitides, Takayasu's arteritis and giant cell arteritis (GCA), are both associated with MHC polymorphisms. In Takayasu's arteritis, MHC class I molecules encoded at the HLA-B locus are enriched in different ethnic populations, indicating that stimulation of CD8 T cells by antigenic peptides may be critically involved in this inflammatory disease (9). In Japanese patients with Takayasu's disease, associations with HLA-B52 and with HLA-B39 have been reported (10). An association with HLA-B52 is also present in the Native American population, whereas HLA-B39 appears to be the disease-associated allele in the Mexican population (11). Associations with MHC class II antigens are less pronounced in patients with Takayasu's arteritis. Increased frequencies of HLA-DRB1*1502 allele in the Japanese population and HLA-DRB1*1301 in the Mexican population may be in linkage disequilibrium with HLA-B52 and HLA-B39, respectively. Only in Caucasians has an association with HLA-DR4 alleles has been described (12). In summary, the HLA association studies suggest that stimulation of CD8 T cells is a primary event in Takayasu's arteritis.

In contrast, GCA is associated with HLA-DRB1 polymorphisms, implicating CD4 T cells as the major immune regulators in this vasculitis. In patients with GCA, HLA-DRB1*04 alleles are highly enriched. Sequence comparison of disease-associated alleles in GCA have supported the hypothesis that the association reflects a polymorphic configuration within the peptide binding site of the HLA molecule (13). The peptide binding site consists of a floor of β pleated sheets bordered by two α helices. Polymorphic residues are clustered in pockets that represent the sites of peptide binding. Polymorphisms in the α helices directly contribute to MHC-T cell receptor

Table 1 T Cells and MHC Disease Association: Implications for the Pathogenesis of Vasculitides

Clinical example:	Takayasu's arteritis	Giant cell arteritis	Rheumatoid vasculitis	Wegener's granulomatosis
Disease-associated MHC genes:	MHC class I polymorphism	MHC class II polymorphism	Homozygosity of MHC class II polymorphism	No discernible HLA association
Pathomechanism:	Binding of selected antigenic peptide → Stimulation of cytotoxic CD8 T cells → Blood vessel wall damage Inflammation	Binding of selected antigenic peptides → Stimulation of CD4 T cells → Activation of effector macrophages Induction of arterial wall injury-response program → Arterial damage Luminal occlusion	Positive thymic selection of CD4 T cells → Autoreactive T cell repertoire → Anti-self-immune response → Endothelial damage Vascular wall damage	Multiple peptide-MHC combinations → Stimulation of T cells → Production of ANCA antibodies Activation of neutrophils Intravascular and extravascular inflammation

interaction (14). The finding that polymorphic residues associated with GCA map to the floor suggests that the binding of selected peptides is a crucial initial step. These MHC-peptide complexes then could activate CD4 T cells to sustain the inflammation in GCA. Patients with GCA share the HLA-DRB1*04 association with patients with polymyalgia rheumatica (PMR), a minor variant of GCA, with predominantly systemic manifestations but no clinical evidence of vascular inflammation (15). This implies that the activation of CD4 T cells by specific MHC-peptide complexes precedes the vasculitic inflammation and, by itself, is not sufficient to induce vasculitis.

In rheumatoid vasculitis, a different mechanism also implicating HLA-DR4 and CD4 T cells appears to be functional (see Table 1). Rheumatoid arthritis (RA) itself is associated with selected HLA-DRB1*04 alleles that share a peptide stretch encompassing amino acid positions 67–74 (16). These residues are located on the α helix of the β chain and form a peptide binding pocket, and they are also able to directly interact with residues on the juxtaposed TCR molecule. The risk of developing extraarticular complications of RA (i.e., rheumatoid vasculitis) is correlated with expression of disease-associated HLA-DRB1*04 genes on both haplotypes, either in the form of HLA-DRB1*04 homozygosity or HLA-DRB1*0401/0404/0408 heterozygosity (17). This gene–dose effect predisposing for rheumatoid vasculitis raises the question whether MHC-dependent functions other than selective binding of peptides have a role in pathogenesis (18). Inheritance of a single copy of an HLA-DR molecule should be sufficient to initiate antigen-specific T-cell responses (8). Alternatively, it has been suggested that the direct interaction between MHC and TCR molecules is of immediate importance in the extraarticular spreading of RA and vascular complications. Dosing of an HLA-DR polymorphism has been demonstrated to skew the repertoire of T cells selected in the thymus. Indeed, patients with RA and two disease-associated alleles have been shown to select a unique set of T-cell receptors in CD4 T cells (19). How differences in the available T-cell pool translate into vascular damage and inflammation remains to be elucidated.

For the majority of vasculitic syndromes, no definitive MHC association has been established, making it unlikely that the trimolecular interaction among TCR, peptide, and MHC represents a primary risk factor for disease. However, the absence of an HLA-association does not imply that T cells are not involved in regulating and amplifying vascular inflammation. To the contrary, immune responses to many common antigens are characteristically not associated with HLA alleles because each protein antigen can harbor many different antigenic peptides that can bind to different allelic MHC variants. The presence of an HLA association is evidence in favor of T-cell involvement while its absence does not allow for any conclusions on the possible relevance of selected antigens or MHC molecules.

IV. T-CELL HOMING TO VASCULAR TISSUES AND LOCAL T-CELL ACTIVATION

T cells are generally primed by a specific antigen in primary lymphoid tissues where they recognize antigen on professional antigen-presenting cells, such as dendritic cells. To fulfill the tasks of tissue surveillance, the primed lymphocytes circulate and then adhere to and migrate through the blood vessel endothelial layer. In principle, there are two possible ports of entry into the vascular tissue, macroendothelium and, at least in medium-sized to large blood vessels, via the microendothelium of the vasa vasorum. In noninflamed arteries, vasa vasorum are usually confined to the adventitia; however, during inflammation, new blood vessels can be found in the media and even in the intima, making these tissues accessible to the influx of lymphocytes (20). Lymphocyte immigration is governed by a complex cascade of events that include adhesion and leukocyte extraversation directed by adhesion molecules and locally produced chemokines (21,22).

Most adhesion molecules are absent on endothelial cells under physiological conditions. Cytokines, such as interleukin-1 (IL-1) and tumor necrosis factor-α (TNF-α), are produced by the innate immune system and have a rather broad effect on endothelial cells to induce the expression of a variety of adhesion molecules. Thus, mechanisms to facilitate lymphocyte extravasation are in place in primarily T-cell–induced vasculitides, such as Takayasu's arteritis and GCA, and also in vasculitides with a predominant component of natural immunity, such as polyarteritis nodosa and Wegener's granulomatosis. Not surprisingly, lymphomononuclear infiltrates can be found in all vasculitides involving small to large arteries.

Upon tissue entry, lymphocytes need to reencounter antigen in restriction to the appropriate MHC molecule to be locally activated and to exert effector functions. The MHC class I molecules are expressed on all somatic cells where they can be recognized by CD8 T cells. The MHC class II molecules can be aberrantly expressed on endothelial cells and on some tissue-resident cells. More importantly, the vasculitic inflammation contains numerous professional antigen-presenting cells, such as macrophages and dendritic cells, that can take up soluble antigens by phagocytosis or pinocytosis and present the antigenic peptide to the tissue-infiltrating CD4 T cells.

The function of T cells in vasculitic lesions has best been studied in GCA (23). In this arteritis, lymphomononuclear infiltrates are present in all three layers of the artery. However, activated T cells are only found in the adventitia (24). Therefore, these T cells are likely to have entered the arterial tissue through the vasa vasorum in the adventitia. They express several activation markers, including IL-2 receptor on their cell surface and interferon-γ (IFN-γ) in their cytoplasm. They have reorganized their cytoskeletal structure, as is the case in T cells that are in the process of antigen recognition. In the adventitia, they are intermingled with IL-1– and IL-6–producing macrophages that likely represent the antigen-presenting cells. Formal proof for the hypothesis that the inflammation in GCA depends on the recognition of antigen by selected CD4 T cells has been developed in adoptive transfer experiments using a human tissue–SCID (severe combined immunodeficiency) mouse chimera model (25). In these experiments, inflamed temporal artery biopsy specimens were engrafted into SCID mice. Antibody-mediated depletion of T cells abrogated the production of the macrophage-derived cytokines IL-1 and IL-6 in the engrafted tissue, demonstrating that their production is T-cell dependent. Conversely, adoptive transfer of tissue-derived CD4 T-cell clones, but not of blood-derived control clones, into SCID mouse chimeras engrafted with autologous inflamed temporal arteries induced increased expression of the T-cell–derived cytokine IFN-γ, as well as IL-1 and IL-6. These experiments demonstrated that adoptively transferred T cells home to the tissue via the microendothelium, are locally activated to produce IFN-γ, and stimulate macrophages to produce monokines.

The nature of the antigen presumably recognized on tissue-infiltrating macrophages is unknown. However, indirect conclusions can be drawn from TCR studies of tissue-infiltrating T cells. Studies in GCA have shown that a small percentage of tissue-infiltrating T cells is clonally expanded. T cells with identical TCR sequences have been detected at different sites of the biopsy specimens or even in the left and right temporal arteries from the same patient (26). These data suggest that T cells are first primed in extravascular tissue and are then seeded to different arteries via the vasa vasorum where they recognize the identical antigen.

V.   FUNCTIONAL HETEROGENEITY OF T LYMPHOCYTES:
THE TH1–TH2 PARADIGM AND VASCULITIS

Upon initial antigenic contact, naive CD4 T cells start to differentiate into cytokine-producing effector cells (Fig. 2). The functional extremes of this differentiation are TH1 and TH2 cells. TH1 cells mainly produce high concentrations of IFN-γ and lymphotoxin-α, whereas TH2 cells are

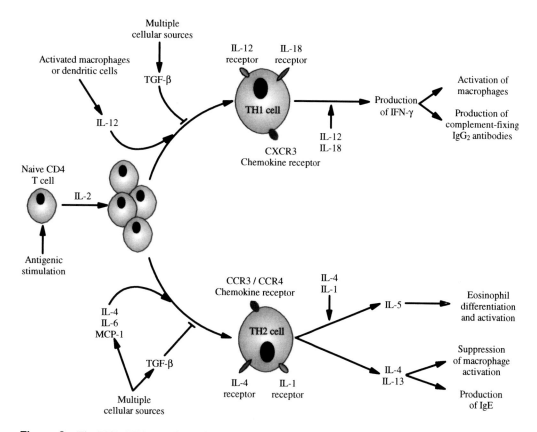

Figure 2 The TH1–TH2 paradigm of T-cell differentiation. In the early stages of T-cell activation, naive T cells are susceptible to the local environment, in particular cytokines locally produced by cells of the innate immune system. Depending on this environment, T cells differentiate into TH1 and TH2 effector cells that differ in the expression of chemokine and cytokine receptors and in their ability to produce cytokines. TH1 and TH2 cells show different homing patterns, their activation is amplified by different cytokines (IL-12 and IL-18 versus IL-1 and IL-4, respectively), and they produce different profiles of lymphokines.

specialized to produce IL-4 and IL-5. Other cytokines, such as IL-10, can be produced by both cell types. The commitment to either pathway depends on the environment during the initial T-cell priming (27,28). Priming in the presence of IL-12 initiates the differentiation into TH1 cells while initial stimulation in the presence of IL-4 and IL-6 shuts off the expression of the IL-12 receptor and promotes differentiation into TH2 cells. It has to be emphasized that human T cells cannot be as clearly subsetted as murine T cells based upon their cytokine profile. However, there seems to be preferential production of either TH1- or TH2-associated cytokines. There is also evidence that TH1 and TH2 cells express different chemokine receptors, supporting the notion that they are functionally distinct subsets. Both TH1 and TH2 cells express CD40 ligand upon stimulation that binds to CD40 on B cells; both cell types can, therefore, provide B-cell help. However, TH1 cells preferentially induce a switch to IgG2 antibodies while IL-4 produced by TH2 cells supports the production of IgE. Interferon-γ and IL-4 have partial antagonistic functions on macrophages and monocytes. Interferon-γ is the most potent cytokine to activate macrophages while IL-4 has mainly macrophage-downregulating properties.

Based on the observation that TH1 and TH2 cells cross-regulate and control each other's effector functions, the TH1–TH2 paradigm has been used to develop a hypothetical model of autoimmune disease (29). In this model, an acute inflammatory response does not resolve, but turns into a chronic inflammation if T cells commit to a pathway that is biologically and immunologically unfavorable. Subsequent studies have shown that most autoimmune responses are associated with commitment to the TH1 pathway. Preferential activation of TH2 cells is a typical feature of allergic diseases. Although this model is attractive, it remains unproven that the commitment to either pathway is causative and favors the generation of a chronic vasculitic response.

Even if the TH1–TH2 model does not provide a valid model for the pathogenesis of vasculitides, pathological events in the vasculitic lesion are dependent on the profile and amount of cytokines produced. Analysis of tissue cytokines in temporal artery specimens from patients with GCA by immunohistochemistry as well as by semiquantitative polymerase chain reaction (PCR) identified IFN-γ as the major T-cell–derived cytokine (30). In the majority of tissues, IL-4 and IL-5 were not present, supporting the notion that tissue-infiltrating T cells have a TH1 phenotype. This cytokine profile is consistent with the representation of cell types in the infiltrates. Eosinophils are completely absent, as one would expect, if T cells do not produce IL-5. Macrophages, many of which are highly activated and form granulomata, are the dominant cell type in the lesions. Giant cells that derive from the fusion of activated macrophages are another histological hallmark. Both of these phenomena are IFN-γ-dependent. Further support for the central role of IFN-γ comes from semiquantification of IFN-γ messenger ribonucleic acid (mRNA) in tissues from PMR patients that do not have obvious mononuclear infiltrates and no structural damage to the arterial wall. Typically, in these tissues, IL-2, a T-cell–derived cytokine, is detectable but IFN-γ cannot be found (30). In contrast, temporal arteries characterized by a high number of giant cells and extensive intimal hyperplasia have the highest in situ production of IFN-γ (31). Specimens with intermediate IFN-γ production show no or minimal intimal hyperplasia and no or few giant cells. None of the tissues contained significant amounts of IL-4. Also, there was no evidence that the inflammatory response and the vascular damage were inversely correlated with the presence of other antiinflammatory cytokines such as IL-10 and transforming growth factor- β (TGF-β). These data indicate that the tissue-destructive changes correlate with the quantity of a TH1 response in the tissue, but not with a variable imbalance between TH1 and TH2 responses.

Granulomatous lesions are characteristic not only for GCA but also for other vasculitides such as Wegener's granulomatosis and Churg–Strauss vasculitis. Patients with Wegener's granulomatosis appear to have a bias to produce TH1-type cytokines even in the periphery (32). This is particularly evident in the granulomatous lesion, where exclusively IFN-γ and no IL-4 or IL-5 is found (33). In contrast, Churg–Strauss vasculitis develops on the background of a chronic asthmatic condition that is generally characterized by a TH2 response, IgE overproduction, and eosinophilia. One would therefore expect that the vasculitic lesions show typical features of a TH2 response. Results reported so far, however, are not unequivocal. A predominant production of IL-6 and IL-10 has been described (34). These cytokines can be produced by a variety of cells, including macrophages, and do not allow for the conclusion of there being a predominant TH2 response in the tissue.

VI. FUNCTIONAL HETEROGENEITY OF T CELLS: THE NATURAL KILLER T CELL IN VASCULITIS

Studies in several vasculitides have recently identified a T-cell type in the circulation that appears to be of functional relevance for the development of vasculitis (Table 2). This T-cell type is char-

Table 2 Properties of CD4$^+$ NK T Cells in Vasculitis

Form large clonal populations	→	Hyperresponsiveness to stimulatory antigens
Express homologous T-cell receptor sequences in different patients	→	Recognize the same antigen
Lack CD28 expression	→	Have escaped regulation by CD80 and CD86
Exhibit resistance to apoptosis (bcl-2 overexpression)	→	Increased longevity
Express MHC class I-recognizing KIR and KAR receptors	→	Are regulated by MHC class I molecules
Are cytotoxic	→	Direct damage of targeted cells—Effector function in vasculitis?
Produce large amounts of IFN-γ	→	Activate effector macrophages—Tissue damage and granuloma formation in vasculitis?

acterized by the lack of expression of the costimulatory molecule CD28 and is, therefore, not controlled by the classical tolerance mechanisms involving CD28 and CD80/86. CD28^{null} CD8 T cells commonly occur in the elderly with increasing age and have also been found in several chronic infections including HIV. CD28^{null} CD4 T cells are very infrequent in normal healthy individuals. CD4 CD28^{null} T cells are found in patients with rheumatoid vasculitis (35), and CD4 CD28^{null}, as well as CD8 CD28^{null}, T cells are expanded in Wegener's granulomatosis (36). One typical feature of CD28-deficient T cells is their potential to form large clonal populations in the circulation (37). Studies in RA, as well as polyarteritis nodosa, have shown that TCRs expressed by large clonal populations share sequence homologies in different patients (38,39). Four out of eight patients with polyarteritis nodosa had clonally expanded CD4 T cells in the peripheral blood that expressed TCR with conserved β chains. These four patients also had the same HLA-DR allele, HLA-DRB1*0401, suggesting that the T-cell clones from these patients recognized the same antigenic peptide in the context of HLA-DR4.

In addition to the loss of CD28 expression, CD4 CD28^{null} T-cell clones have several features that distinguish them from normal T cells (see Table 2): first, they produce large amounts of IFN-γ upon stimulation; second, they express several markers of natural killer (NK) cells, in particular, MHC-recognizing receptors of the immunoglobulin superfamily (40); and third, they have lost their ability to provide B-cell help but express granzyme B and perforin, enabling them to be cytotoxic. These three features, cytotoxic activity, high production of IFN-γ, and expression of cell surface molecules that are generally found on NK cells, emphasize the close relationship of CD28^{null} CD4 T cells with NK cells. However, in contrast to NK cells, these T cells express TCR α and β chains as the cell surface molecules that control antigen recognition and cell activation.

The ability of these T cells to recognize self-MHC and to exert cytotoxic activity may be important functionally in the development of vascular damage. Additional support for the concept that these cells are relevant for vascular inflammation has come from studies describing increased frequencies of these cells in patients with unstable angina (41). The current model proposes that unstable angina occurs when inflammation of a minimally obstructive plaque leads to plaque rupture and superimposed thrombosis. Patients with unstable angina frequently have highly elevated acute phase responses and carry increased frequencies of IFN-γ–producing cells. Studies in these patients have shown that IFN-γ mainly derives from the CD28^{null} population and that the frequencies of CD4 CD28^{null} T cells are significantly increased compared with patients with stable angina. Clonally expanded CD4 CD28^{null} cells have been demonstrated to infiltrate into unstable, but not stable, plaques, supporting the model that they contribute directly to plaque instability

(42). Thus, this cell population may be an important effector T-cell population capable of inflicting endothelial and vascular damage in a variety of inflammatory vessel diseases, ranging from classical vasculitic conditions such as Wegener's granulomatosis, rheumatoid vasculitis, and polyarteritis nodosa to a subset of patients with atherosclerotic disease.

VII. EFFECTOR FUNCTIONS OF T CELLS IN VASCULITIS

In principal, T cells exert effector functions by one of three mechanisms. First, CD8 T cells and CD4 NK T cells, but not normal CD4 T cells, express perforin and granzyme B and can induce apoptosis in target cells that they recognize via the T-cell receptor. Second, all T cells can produce cytokines upon stimulation, albeit in different combinations as described for TH1 and TH2 cells. Third, following triggering of the T-cell receptor, T cells transiently express cell surface molecules and thereby interact with and activate resident cells and other immune cells. A classical example is CD40 ligand expressed on activated CD4 T cells. The receptor for CD40 ligand, CD40 is present on a variety of cells including CD8 T cells and B cells. Binding of CD40 ligand to CD40 provides a signal that is crucial for the activation and proliferation of CD40-expressing cells.

Evidence has been provided that all three T-cell effector mechanisms are relevant in vascular inflammation, with preference for certain pathways dominating T-cell involvement in certain vasculitic syndromes. In theory, cytotoxic activity could be directed against endothelial cells as well as other resident cells, such as smooth muscle cells. Induction of endothelial cell apoptosis by T cells in vivo has not been demonstrated, but it is possible that CD4 NK T cells exert such an activity in rheumatoid vasculitis and Wegener's granulomatosis. Activated endothelial cells express MHC class II molecules and can be recognized by these cells as long as they also express the relevant antigenic peptide. One possible antigen is the antineutrophil cytoplasmic antibody (ANCA) antigen in Wegener's granulomatosis that has been shown to be present on endothelial cells. In unstable angina, CD4 NK T cells may function by inducing apoptosis in the endothelial and smooth muscle cells overlying the atherosclerotic plaque, thereby causing the disruption of the endothelial layer, providing the bed for superimposed thrombosis.

Conclusive evidence for cytotoxic activity has been shown for Takayasu's arteritis (43). From the MHC class I association of the disease, a primary role of CD8 T cells could be predicted. Indeed, the inflammatory infiltrate predominantly consists of CD8 T cells and classical NK cells. Perforin release by these cells has been demonstrated, documenting their in vivo activity. The target cells appears to be smooth muscle cells in the media and certainly not endothelial cells, suggesting a role of effector T cells in smooth muscle cell apoptosis and in the destruction of the medial layer.

The CD4 effector T cells exert their function via indirect mechanisms by interacting with CD8 T cells, B cells, or cells of the innate immune system. They control the production of autoantibodies, in particular, the isotype switch and affinity maturation that leads to high-affinity pathogenic antibodies. Therefore, it is not surprising that T-cell reactivity to myeloperoxidase and proteinase 3 can be found in ANCA-associated vasculitides (44).

Interaction of CD4 T cells with tissue-infiltrating macrophages frequently results in granuloma formation, a histological hallmark of several vasculitides, including GCA and Wegener's granulomatosis. Experiments in animal models have shown that granuloma formation is a strictly T-cell–dependent process. Although both TH1 and TH2 cytokines have been reported to facilitate granuloma formation (45), IFN-γ is the strongest macrophage activator and is the key cytokine in granulomatous vasculitides. Granulomatous lesions are tissue injurious, most notably by their ability to produce reactive oxygen species (46). Again, the preferred targets of these tissue injurious pathways are smooth muscle cells in the media, as is also the case for the CD8 T cell-mediated cytotoxicity in Takayasu's disease. The formation of granulomatous lesions exemplifies how the T-cell system and the innate immune system cooperate to produce destructive inflammation in the vessel wall.

REFERENCES

1. Germain RN, Margulies DH. The biochemistry and cell biology of antigen processing and presentation. Ann Rev Immunol 1993; 11:403–450.
2. Jorgensen JL, Reay PA, Ehrich EW, Davis MM. Molecular components of T-cell recognition. Annu Rev Immunol 1992; 10:835–873.
3. Haas WP, Pereira P, Tonegawa S. Gamma/delta cells. Nature 1995; 375:155–158.
4. Chan AC, Desai DM, Weiss A. The role of protein tyrosine kinases and protein tyrosine phosphatases in T cell antigen receptor signal transduction. Annu Rev Immunol 1994; 12:555–592.
5. Miller JFAP, Morahan G. Peripheral T cell tolerance. Annu Rev Immunol 1992; 10:51–69.
6. Linsley PS, Ledbetter JA. The role of the CD28 receptor during T cell responses to antigens. Annu Rev Immunol 1993; 11:191–212.
7. Lenschow DJ, Walunas TL, Bluestone JA. CD28/B7 system of T cell costimulation. Annu Rev Immunol 1996; 14:233–258.
8. Nepom GT, Erlich H. MHC class-II molecules and autoimmunity. Annu Rev Immunol 1991; 9: 493–525.
9. Weyand CM, Goronzy JJ. Molecular approaches toward pathological mechanisms in giant cell arteritis and Takayasu's arteritis. Curr Opin Rheumatol 1995; 7:30–36.
10. Kitamura HY, Kobayashi, Kimura A, Numano F. Association of clinical manifestations with HLA-B alleles in Takayasu arteritis. Int J Cardiol 1998; 66(suppl 1):S121–126.
11. Rodriguez-Reyna TS, Zuniga-Ramos J, Salgado N, Hernandez-Martinez B, Vargas-Alarcon G, Reyes-Lopez PA, Granados J. Intron 2 and exon 3 sequences may be involved in the susceptibility to develop takayasu arteritis. Int J Cardiol 1998; 66(Suppl 1):S135–138.
12. Volkman DJ, Mann DL, Fauci AS. Association between Takayasu's arteritis and a B-cell alloantigen ·in North Americans. N Engl J Med 1982; 306:464–465.
13. Weyand CM, Hicok KC, Hunder GG, Goronzy JJ. The HLA-DRB1 locus as a genetic component in giant cell arteritis. Mapping of a disease-linked sequence motif to the antigen binding site of the HLA-DR molecule. J Clin Invest 1992; 90:2355–2361.
14. Madden DR. The three-dimensional structure of peptide-MHC complexes. Annu Rev Immunol 1995; 13:587–622.
15. Weyand CM, Hunder NNH, Hicok KC, Hunder GG, Goronzy JJ. HLA-DRB1 alleles in polymyalgia rheumatica, giant cell arteritis, and rheumatoid arthritis. Arthritis Rheum 1994; 37:514–520.
16. Winchester R. The molecular basis of susceptibility to rheumatoid arthritis. Adv Immunol 1994; 56: 389–466.
17. Weyand CM, Xie C, Goronzy JJ. Homozygosity for the HLA-DRB1 allele selects for extraarticular manifestations in rheumatoid arthritis. J Clin Invest 1992; 89:2033–2039.
18. Weyand CM, Goronzy JJ. Functional domains on HLA-DR molecules. Implications for the linkage of HLA-DR genes to different autoimmune diseases. Clin Immunol Immunopath 1994; 70:91–98.
19. Walser-Kuntz DR, Weyand CM, Weaver AJ, O'Fallon WM, Goronzy JJ. Mechanisms underlying the formation of the T cell receptor repertoire in rheumatoid arthritis. Immunity 1995; 2:597–605.
20. Kaiser M, Young BR, Bjornsson J, Weyand CM, Goronzy JJ. Formation of new vasa vasorum in vasculitis: production of angiogenic cytokines by multinucleated giant cells. Am J Pathol 1999; 155:765–774.
21. Springer TA. Traffic signals for lymphocyte recirculation and leukocyte emigration: the multistep paradigm. Cell 1994; 76:301–314.
22. Salmi M, Jalkanen S. How do lymphocytes know where to go: Current concepts and enigmas of lymphocyte homing. Adv Immunol 1997; 64:139–218.
23. Weyand CM, Goronzy JJ. Arterial wall injury in giant cell arteritis. Arthritis Rheum 1999; 42: 844–853.
24. Wagner AD, Bjornsson J, Bartley GB, Goronzy JJ, Weyand CM. Interferon-gamma-producing T cells

in giant cell vasculitis represent a minority of tissue-infiltrating cells and are located distant from the site of pathology. Am J Pathol 1996; 148:1925–1933.

25. Brack A, Geisler A, Martinez-Taboada VM, Young BR, Goronzy JJ, Weyand CM. Giant cell vasculitis is a T cell-dependent disease. Mol Med 1997; 3:530–543.

26. Weyand CM, Schonberger J, Oppitz U, Hunder NN, Hicok KC, Goronzy JJ. Distinct vascular lesions in giant cell arteritis share identical T cell clonotypes. J Exp Med 1994; 179:951–960.

27. Seder RA, Paul WE. Acquisition of lymphokine-producing phenotype by CD4+ T cells. Annu Rev Immunol. 1994; 12:635.

28. O'Garra A. Cytokines induce the development of functionally heterogeneous T helper cell subsets. Immunity 1998; 8:275.

29. Romagnani S. Lymphokine production by human T cells in disease states. Annu Rev Immunol 1994; 12:227–257.

30. Weyand CM, Hicok KC, Hunder GG, Goronzy JJ. Tissue cytokine patterns in patients with polymyalgia rheumatica and giant cell arteritis. Ann Intern Med 1994; 121:484–491.

31. Weyand CM, Tetzlaff N, Bjornsson J, Brack A, Younge B, Goronzy JJ. Disease patterns and tissue cytokine profiles in giant cell arteritis. Arthritis Rheum 1997; 40:19–26.

32. Ludviksson BR, Sneller MC, Chua KS, Talar-Williams C, Langford CA, Ehrhardt RO, Fauci AS, Strober W. Active Wegener's granulomatosis is associated with HLA-DR+ CD4+ T cells exhibiting an unbalanced Th1-type T cell cytokine pattern: Reversal with IL-10. J Immunol 1998; 160:3602–3609.

33. Csernok E, Trabandt A, Muller A, Wang GC, Moosig F, Paulsen J, Schnabel A, Gross WL. Cytokine profiles in Wegener's granulomatosis: Predominance of type 1 (Th1) in granulomatous inflammation. Arthritis Rheum 1999; 42:742–750.

34. Fujioka A, Yamamoto T, Takasu H, Kawano K, Masuzawa M, Katsuoka K, Jinno S. The analysis of mRNA expression of cytokines from skin lesions in Churg-Strauss syndrome. J Dermatol 1998; 25:171–177.

35. Martens PB, Goronzy JJ, Schaid D, Weyand CM. Expansion of unusual CD4+ T cells in severe rheumatoid arthritis. Arthritis Rheum 1997; 40:1106–1114.

36. Moosig F, Csernok E, Wang GC, Gross WL. Costimulatory molecules in Wegener's granulomatosis (WG): Lack of expression of CD28 and preferential up-regulation of its ligands B7-1 (CD80) and B7-2 (CD86) on T cells. Clin Exp Immunol 1998; 114:113–118.

37. Schmidt D, Goronzy JJ, Weyand CM. CD4+ CD7– CD28– T cells are expanded in rheumatoid arthritis and are characterized by autoreactivity. J Clin Invest 1996; 97:2027–2037.

38. Schmidt D, Martens PB, Weyand CM, Goronzy JJ. The repertoire of CD4+ CD28– T cells in rheumatoid arthritis. Mol Med 1996; 2:608–618.

39. Grunewald J, Halapi E, Wahlstrom J, Giscombe R, Nityanand S, Sanjeevi C, Lefvert AK. T-cell expansions with conserved T-cell receptor beta chain motifs in the peripheral blood of HLA-DRB1*0401 positive patients with necrotizing vasculitis. Blood 1998; 92:3737–3744.

40. Lanier LL. NK cell receptors. Annu Rev Immunol 1998; 16:359–393.

41. Liuzzo G, Kopecky SL, Frye RL, O'Fallon WM, Maseri A, Goronzy JJ, Weyand CM. Perturbation of the T cell repertoire in patients with unstable angina. Circulation 1999; 100:2135–2190.

42. Liuzzo G, Goronzy JJ, Yang H, Kopecky SL, Holmes DR, Frye RL, Weyand CM. Monoclonal T cell proliferation and plaque instability in acute coronary syndromes. Circulation 2000; 101:2883–2888.

43. Seko Y, Minota S, Kawasaki A, Shinkai Y, Maeda K, Yagita H, Okumura K, Sato O, Takagi A, Tada Y, Yazaki Y. Perforin-secreting killer cell infiltration and expression of a 65-kD heat-shock protein in aortic tissue of patients with Takayasu's arteritis. J Clin Invest 1994; 93:750–758.

44. Griffiths M, Coulthart A, Pusey C. T cell responses to myeloperoxidase and proteinase 3 in patients with systemic vasculitis. Clin Exp Immunol 1996; 103:253–258.

45. Chensue SW, Warmington K, Ruth J, Lincoln P, Kuo MC, Kunkel SL. Cytokine responses during mycobacterial and schistosomal antigen-induced pulmonary granuloma formation: Production of Th1 and Th2 cytokines and relative contribution of tumor necrosis factor. Am J Pathol 1994; 145:1105–1113.

46. Rittner HL, Hafner V, Klimiuk PA, Szweda LI, Goronzy JJ, Weyand CM. Aldose reductase functions as a detoxification system for lipid peroxidation products in vasculities. J Clin Invest 1999; 103:1007–1013.

6
Neutrophils in Vasculitis

Edwin S. L. Chan and Bruce N. Cronstein
New York University School of Medicine, New York, New York

I. INTRODUCTION

The neutrophil plays a central role in the pathogenesis of many inflammatory disorders of the vasculature. The presence of neutrophils in vasculitic lesions, including those of Wegener's granulomatosis, leukocytoclastic vasculitis, etc., bears witness to this (Fig. 1). Cochrane's classic demonstration that neutrophils are required for tissue injury in Arthus vasculitis, which does not develop in rabbits depleted of neutrophils, lends further support to the hypothesis that neutrophils are not passive bystanders in these lesions (1,2). In the human, counterparts to the Arthus reaction include immune complex–mediated vasculitides such as cryoglobulinemia, Schönlein–Henoch purpura, and vasculitis associated with hepatitis B and C infections. The neutrophil is also featured prominently in many antibody-associated diseases, for instance, Goodpasture's syndrome, the ANCA-associated vasculitides (e.g., polyarteritis nodosa, Wegener's granulomatosis, microscopic polyarteritis), as well as vasculitides putatively associated with antiendothelial antibodies (e.g., Kawasaki disease). Regardless of the etiology, the neutrophil clearly contributes to vessel injury in many different types of vasculitides.

II. NEUTROPHIL RECRUITMENT AT INFLAMMATORY SITE

Although the effector functions of neutrophils are central to the vascular injury associated with vasculitis, neutrophils must be present at the site in order to contribute to the vasculitic lesion. Neutrophil recruitment is therefore no less critical an event than what happens afterward in the tissue. Of essence to this is the neutrophil's ability to respond to the various environmental signals generated to enlist its participation.

The binding of the neutrophil to the vascular endothelium and its subsequent transmigration is orchestrated by the cellular adhesion molecules present on both cell types. The expression of these adhesion molecules is modulated by the presence of inflammatory mediators, immune reactants, and complement components (3–5). In this multistep process, neutrophils first adhere to the endothelium by virtue of their surface L-selectin, which preferentially binds to the sialyl Lewis X antigen present on glycoproteins and glycolipids on both neutrophilic and endothelial surfaces (3,6). Concurrently, the influence of local inflammatory mediators, such as histamine, thrombin, tumor necrosis factor-α (TNF-α) and interleukin-1 (IL-1) promote both endothelial expression of E-selectin and the translocation of P-selectin from Weibel-Palade bodies to the cell

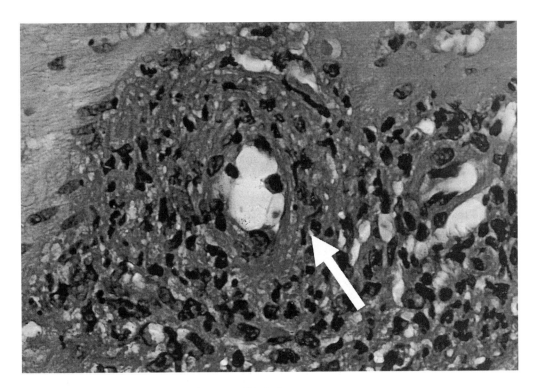

Figure 1   Infiltration of neutrophils in a vasculitic lesion.

surface, allowing further interaction with neutrophilic surface oligosaccharides (3,5,7–9). Subsequent rolling and adhesion are accompanied by activation of the integrin CD11b/CD18, which interacts primarily with intercellular adhesion molecule-1 (ICAM-1) on the endothelial surface, a member of the immunoglobulin family of adhesion molecules (10–14). The adhesive process is downregulated by nitric oxide (11,15).

The cellular expression of adhesive molecules is, however, by no means a static process and the sequential activation and inactivation of molecules such as CD11b/CD18 and the resultant fluctuations in the degree of adhesive interaction contribute to the transmigration of neutrophils across the endothelium, a process that requires the participation of platelet endothelial cell adhesion molecule-1 (PECAM-1) (10,16,17). Transmigration is felt to take place via intercellular junctions for the most part, but transmigration directly through intact endothelial cells may also occur (18–20). To accomplish this, digestion of the basement membrane and matrix components is a necessity. The neutrophil possesses both receptors for matrix molecules (e.g., laminin) and a large armament of digestive enzymes, some of which are expressed on the cell surface following stimulation, including gelatinase, elastase, and cathepsin G, which help to achieve this goal (21–26). Chemotaxins generated in the inflammatory milieu further augment this recruitment process. These include complement proteins (e.g., C5a), arachidonic acid metabolites (leukotriene B_4 [LTB_4]), lipids (platelet-activating factor), cytokines and growth factors (interleukin-8, transforming growth factor-β) as well as the N-formulated oligopeptides generated by bacteria that have invaded the tissues (f-Met-Leu-Phe) (27–31). The neutrophil responds to these molecular signals by following the chemical gradient from low to high concentration. The functional importance of some of these chemotaxins may be related to their ability to activate as well as attract neutrophils, particularly at the higher concentrations found after the neutrophil has homed to the inflammatory site (32–35).

Neutrophils are able to produce some of these chemotaxins themselves (e.g., IL-8) and, in turn, propagate the further recruitment of their own kind (36).

III. RESPIRATORY BURST AND GENERATION OF REACTIVE OXYGEN METABOLITES

Reactive oxidants generated by neutrophils possess enormous destructive powers, a line of defense primarily devised to protect against invading microorganisms. Defects in the molecular pathways in the generation of oxygen radicals result in recurrent and life-threatening infections, as seen in the genetic disorder, chronic granulomatous disease (CGD) (37,38). These pathways can be initiated not only by microbial infections, but also a variety of inflammatory stimuli capable of activating neutrophils through G-protein–linked receptors and the subsequent activation of various protein kinases and phospholipases (39–41), which may result in the destruction of host tissues, including the human vasculature (42,43). This function, known as the "respiratory burst," requires the reducing activity of reduced nicotinamide-adenine dinucleotide phosphate (NADPH) by an oxidase unique to neutrophils and other phagocytes (44).

Latent NADPH oxidase in the membrane of resting neutrophils is activated rapidly at the site of the forming phagosome (45). Active NADPH oxidase is assembled from various proteins found in the plasma membrane and cytosol of the neutrophil. The first component of the multi-molecular complex was identified in studies of patients with the X-linked form of CGD (46), whose neutrophils lack a membrane-bound b-type cytochrome known as flavocytochrome b_{558}, so named because of its characteristic α-band absorbance at 558 nm. This cytochrome is a heteromeric glycoprotein consisting, in the membrane, of an α subunit, p22^{phox} (a 22-kDa phagocyte oxidase), and a β subunit, gp91^{phox} (47–49). The cytosolic fraction is comprised of at least three different factors, p47^{phox}, p67^{phox}, and the small guanine triphosphatase protein, p21^{rac} (50–55). The assembly of the NADPH oxidase complex requires the translocation of the cytosolic proteins to the membrane surface where they associate with the subunits already there (56–61).

Neutrophils, once stimulated, utilize oxygen in vastly increased amounts. While oxygen is a relatively inert molecule under the physiological conditions of the resting cell, its reactivity increases dramatically in the presence of the reducing conditions conferred upon it by the oxidase system. Reduction involves the acceptance of electrons and, ultimately, the generation of water. In a series of reactions directed toward this final goal, three intermediates are formed that are highly reactive and the resultant activity of these molecules may culminate in tissue destruction (42,43,62).

The acceptance of the first electron gives rise to the first reactive product, the superoxide anion (O_2^-) (63). When two superoxide anions react together in a dismutation reaction, either spontaneously or catalyzed by the enzyme superoxide dismutase, hydrogen peroxide (H_2O_2) is formed (64–66). In the presence of ferrous ions, further reduction of H_2O_2 leads to the production of the hydroxyl radical ($\cdot$OH) through a series of reactions originally described by Fenton and Haber-Weiss (67–72). Activation of the neutrophil also releases the enzyme myeloperoxidase from the azurophilic granules. The interaction of myeloperoxidase with H_2O_2 results in the oxidation of halide ions and the production of hypohalous acids—in particular, hypochlorous acid (72–76). The powerful oxidant activity of hypochlorous acid is capable of destroying living tissues, particularly in concert with the chloramines derived from its reaction with nitrogen-containing compounds (43,77–79). Oxygen radicals and their derivatives may deplete the main energy resource, adenosine triphosphate, in target-tissue cells causing cellular dysfunction, and the continuation of this process may lead to cell death (80,81). These oxygen radicals also inactivate α_1-antitrypsin, an enzyme that normally inhibits neutrophilic granular elastase, thus allowing the elastase to exert widespread, uncontrolled proteolytic activity (82–87). Another protease inhibitor capable of inhibiting collagenase activity, α_2-macroglobulin, is similarly inactivated (43,88–91). Furthermore, the many toxins generated by the activated neutrophil may act synergistically in their mediation of tissue injury (92–94).

IV. DEGRANULATION

Neutrophils have a variety of granules in their cytoplasm containing a diversity of macromolecules, some of which are listed in Table 1. Of particular interest are the enzymic contents, which include elastase, myeloperoxidase, proteinase 3, collagenase, and gelatinase. While the antimicrobial role of some of these enzymes is clear, the same enzymes can be destructive to host tissues when released. The granular contents can be discharged into the immediate surroundings in at least three different ways. First, a host of chemical mediators can activate neutrophils to degranulate. These stimuli include activated complement components (e.g., C1q, C5a), immunoglobulins and immune complexes, cytokines (e.g., TNF-α), and arachidonic acid metabolites (e.g., LTB$_4$) (95–100). The neutrophil displays specific receptors on its surface for some of these immune reactants, the ligation of which leads to intracellular signaling events. These receptors include the IL-8 receptor, receptors for the constant region of immunoglobulin molecules, FcγRII and FcγRIII, the C5a receptor, and complement receptors CR1 and CR3, which are capable of interacting with complement components C3b and C4b, and iC3b, respectively, enhancing the phagocytic function of neutrophils for opsonized particles (101–103). Receptors for C3a are also important triggers for the respiratory burst (104). Granular contents can also be released from the dying neutrophils seen in the leukocytoclastic vasculitides. Last, the neutrophil may secrete its granular contents during a process described as "regurgitation upon eating"; granules fuse with the forming phagosome before it has been completely internalized and the granule contents can escape to the extracellular space (105). Neutrophils can secrete their specific and azurophilic granules independently (106–107). Regardless of how the degranulation process is activated, the discharge of granular enzymes contributes to the digestion that culminates in widespread tissue destruction (42). In addition to classical enzymatic digestion, execution of tissue destruction may assume many shapes or forms. Neutrophil defensins, for instance, alter membrane permeability in the target tissue in a charge- or voltage-dependent manner (108–110). The inflammatory environment is particularly conducive to the destructive activity as a result of the protective milieu generated that allows the enzymes to be sheltered from inactivation by protease inhibitors such as α_1-antitrypsin and β_2-macroglobulin, as described above. The same matrix or vessel wall component can be degraded by different enzymes released in the degranulation process, for instance, collagen, an important constituent of the vessel wall, can be degraded by collagenase, elastin, cathepsin G, and gelatinase; and individual enzymes, in turn, usually have multiple functions (111–118).

V. ROLE OF NEUTROPHILS IN ANTINEUTROPHIL CYTOPLASMIC ANTIBODY–MEDIATED VASCULITIDES

We have already mentioned the existence of the proteases, proteinase 3 and myeloperoxidase, in the neutrophil, the principal ligands for c-ANCA and p-ANCA, respectively. The nature and diagnostic utility of these antineutrophil cytoplasmic antibodies (ANCAs) are covered elsewhere in this volume. Surface expression of the target molecules for ANCAs on activated neutrophils, however, has been implicated in the pathogenesis of ANCA-associated diseases (119–124). Inflammatory cytokines, such as TNF-α and IL-8, prevalent in the inflammatory environment, help to stimulate their surface expression, which by interacting with ANCAs may stimulate neutrophil

Table 1 Contents of Neutrophilic Granules

	Azurophilic granules	Secondary granules	Tertiary granules	Secretory vesicle
Enzymes	5′-Nucleotidase α-Fucosidase α-Manosidase Acid phosphatase Arylsulfatase Azurocidin β-Glucosaminadase β-Glucuronidase Cathepsins Elastase Lysozyme Myeloperoxidase Phospholipase A Proteinase 3 Sialidase	Collagenase Heparanase Histaminase Lysozyme Plasminogen activator Sialidase	Acetyltransferase Gelatinase	
Nonenzymic proteins/peptides	Bacterial/permeability-inducing protein Defensins Ubiquitin	HCap 18 Lactoferrin Vitamin B_{12}-binding protein		
Other macromolecules	Chondroitin sulfate Glycosaminoglycans Heparin-binding protein Heparin sulfate	β_2-Microglobulin		
Endocytosis-derived plasma proteins				Albumin Immunoglobulins Transferrin
Membrane-associated proteins	CD63 CD68	CD11b/CD18 CD66 CD67 Fibronectin receptor Flavocytochrome b_{558} Formyl peptide receptor G protein α-subunit Laminin receptor Rap 1/2 Thrombospondin receptor TNF receptor Vitronectin receptor	CD11b/CD18 DAG-deacylating enzyme Formyl peptide receptor	Alkaline phosphatase CD11b/CD18 Complement receptor 1 Flavocytochrome b_{558} Formyl peptide receptor Uroplasminogen-activating receptor

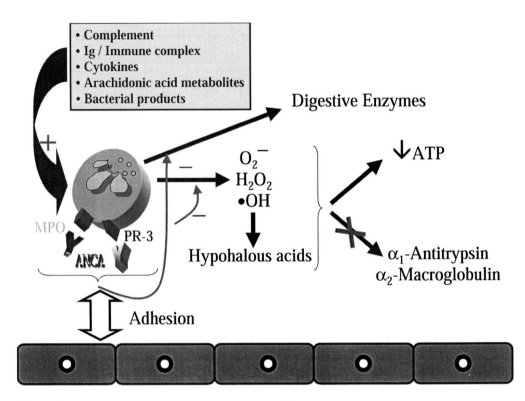

Figure 2   Mechanisms of tissue destruction by neutrophils.

degranulation or generate toxic oxygen radicals resulting in vessel injury (124,125). The necessity for cytokine priming may also account for the increased incidence of upper respiratory infections occurring shortly before the onset of the vasculitic manifestations in some ANCA-associated diseases (126). Alternatively, ANCAs may activate the neutrophil through ligation with FcγRII or FcγRIII on the neutrophil surface with similar consequences (127–129). The potential for disengagement of the surface myeloperoxidase and proteinase 3 from the neutrophil exists and the subsequent formation of immune complexes with ANCAs may result in tissue damage through complement fixation (119). Interaction with ANCAs may also have a shielding effect on the secreted proteases themselves, which may escape from inactivation by circulating protease inhibitors (119). Cross-linkage of ANCA antigens also induces tissue damage by releasing superoxide anions from neutrophils (130). These mechanisms, although speculative, all highlight the important part the neutrophil plays in the pathogenesis of the ANCA-associated diseases.

VI.   THERAPEUTIC MODIFICATION OF NEUTROPHILIC ACTIVITY

Some of the most commonly used drugs in the therapy of vasculitis exert their antiinflammatory actions partly through influencing the neutrophil's activities in the generation of vascular damage. Salicylates inhibit the adhesion of activated neutrophils to the endothelium, a process mediated in part by the release of adenosine (131). Neutrophil transmigration across the endothelium is also decreased by nonsteroidal antiinflammatory drugs (NSAIDs) (132). By affecting arachidonic metabolism in the endothelium, chemorepellents for neutrophils may be produced after treatment with NSAIDs (133). Corticosteroids, known to downregulate endothelial expression of ELAM-1 and ICAM-1, share this capacity to reduce neutrophil adhesion (134). Shedding of L-selectin from the neutrophil surface is another mechanism deployed by some NSAIDs which may limit neutrophil recruitment (135). Neutrophils are incapable of regenerating L-selectin once it has been shed, unlike the vascular endothelium (136,137). Conversely, an increase in adhesion molecules like ICAM-1 and P-selectin in the gastric mucosal vasculature, induced by NSAIDs such as indomethacin, may explain the frequently observed side effect of NSAID-induced gastropathy (138). Decrease in endothelial adhesiveness for neutrophils is also seen with colchicine therapy, and the microtubular disruptive properties of colchicine have been linked to selectin shedding in neutrophils, thereby decreasing their accumulation at the inflamed site (139,140). The NSAIDs have the ability to inhibit neutrophil degranulation, aggregation, and superoxide anion generation, properties that vary among different NSAIDs (141–144). Corticosteroids are also capable of limiting oxidant production in the neutrophil by inhibiting respiratory burst oxidase, but only at extreme concentrations (145). They may modify neutrophilic lysosomal enzyme release and accumulation, and may also inhibit apoptosis in neutrophils (146,147). The formation of superoxide anions is inhibited by adenosine, and endogenous antiinflammatory agent released by methotrexate-treated cells and tissues (148–152). Finally, neutrophilic inactivation of protease inhibitors may also be modulated by NSAIDs (153,154).

VII. SUMMARY

In summary, the neutrophil possesses a large array of destructive powers that it deploys inappropriately against host vascular tissue in the course of various vasculitic disorders (Fig. 2). Current therapy of these disorders may function, in part, by ameliorating some of the neutrophil's deleterious activities. As we learn more about the mechanisms of action of some of these therapeutic agents, it is likely that previous unnoticed antineutrophilic properties will be further uncovered. This knowledge complements the growing understanding of the pathophysiological role of the neutrophil in vascular diseases and may provide suitable targets for future therapy.

REFERENCES

1. Cochrane, CG, WO Weigle, and FJ Dixon. The role of polymorphonuclear leukocytes in the initiation and cessation of the Arthus vasculitis. J Exp Med 1959; 110:481–494.
2. Cochrane, CG. Immunologic tissue injury mediated by neutrophilic leukocytes. Adv Immunol 1968; 9:97–162.
3. Cronstein, BN, and G Weissmann. The adhesion molecules of inflammation. Arthritis Rheum 1993; 36:147–157.
4. Lozada, C, RI Levin, M Huie, R Hirschhorn, D Naime, M Whitlow, PA Recht, B Golden, and BN Cronstein. Identification of C1q as the heat-labile serum cofactor required for immune complexes to stimulate endothelial expression of the adhesion molecules E-selectin and intercellular and vascular cell adhesion molecules 1. Proc Natl Acad Sci USA 1995; 92:8378–8382.
5. Bevilacqua, MP, and RM Nelson. Endothelial-leukocyte adhesion molecules in inflammation and metastasis. Thromb Haemost 1993; 70:152–154.
6. Osborn, L. Leukocyte adhesion to endothelium in inflammation. Cell 1990; 62:3–6.
7. Lorant, DE, KD Patel, TM McIntyre, RP McEver, SM Prescott, and GA Zimmerman. Coexpression of GMP-140 and PAF by endothelium stimulated by histamine or thrombin: A juxtacrine system for adhesion and activation of neutrophils. J Cell Biol 1991; 115:223–234.
8. Burns, AR, RA Bowden, Y Abe, DC Walker, SI Simon, ML Entman, and CW Smith. P-selectin mediates neutrophil adhesion to endothelial cell borders. J Leukoc Biol 1999; 65:299–306.

9. Essani, NA, MA Fisher, CA Simmons, JL Hoover, A Farhood, and H Jaeschke. Increased P-selectin gene expression in the liver vasculature and its role in the pathophysiology of neutrophil-induced liver injury in murine endotoxin shock. J Leukocyte Biol 1998; 63:288–296.

10. Smith, CW, SD Marlin, R Rothlein, C Toman, and DC Anderson. Cooperative interactions of LFA-1 and Mac-1 with intercellular adhesion molecule-1 in facilitating adherence and transendothelial migration of human neutrophils in vitro. J Clin Invest 1989; 83:2008–2017.

11. Albelda, SM, CW Smith, and PA Ward. Adhesion molecules and inflammatory injury. FASEB J 1994; 8:504–512.

12. Smith, CW. Leukocyte-endothelial cell interactions. Semin Hematol 1993; 30:45–53; discussion 54–55.

13. Smith, CW. Endothelial adhesion molecules and their role in inflammation. Can J Physiol Pharmacol 1993; 71:76–87.

14. Rainger, GE, C. Buckley, DL Simmons, and GB Nash. Cross-talk between cell adhesion molecules regulates the migration velocity of neutrophils. Curr Biol 1997; 7:316–325.

15. Kubes, P, M Suzuki, and DN Granger. Nitric oxide: An endogenous modulator of leukocyte adhesion. Proc Natl Acad Sci USA 1991; 88:4651–4655.

16. Muller, WA, SA Weigl, X Deng, and DM Phillips. PECAM-1 is required for transendothelial migration of leukocytes. J Exp Med 1993; 178:449–460.

17. Michiels, C, T Arnould, and J Remacle. Role of PECAM-1 in the adherence of PMN to hypoxic endothelial cells. Cell Adhes Commun 1998; 5:367–374.

18. Feng, D, JA Nagy, K Pyne, HF Dvorak, and AM Dvorak. Neutrophils emigrate from venules by a transendothelial cell pathway in response to FMLP. J Exp Med 1998; 187:903–915.

19. Del Maschio, A, A Zanetti, M Corada, Y Rival, L Ruco, MG, Lampugnani, and E. Dejana. Polymorphonuclear leukocyte adhesion triggers the disorganization of endothelial cell-to-cell adherens junctions. J Cell Biol 1996; 135:497–510.

20. Allport, JR, H Ding, T Collins, ME Gerritsen, and FW Luscinskas. Endothelial-dependent mechanisms regulate leukocyte transmigration: A process involving the proteasome and disruption of the vascular endothelial-cadherin complex at endothelial cell-to-cell junctions. J Exp Med 1997; 186:517–527.

21. Bohnsack, JF, SK Akiyama, CH Damsky, WA Knape, and GA Zimmerman. Human neutrophil adherence to laminin in vitro. Evidence for a distinct neutrophil integrin receptor for laminin. J Exp Med 1990; 171:1221–1237.

22. Owen, CA, MA Campbell, SS Boukedes, and EJ Campbell. Inducible binding of bioactive cathepsin G to the cell surface of neutrophils. A novel mechanism for mediating extracellular catalytic activity of cathepsin G. J Immunol 1995; 155:5803–5810.

23. Owen, CA, MA Campbell, PL Sannes, SS Boukedes, and EJ Campbell. Cell surface-bound elastase and cathepsin G on human neutrophils: A novel, non-oxidative mechanism by which neutrophils focus and preserve catalytic activity of serine proteinases. J Cell Biol 1995; 131:775–789.

24. Owen, CA, and EJ Campbell. Neutrophil proteinases and matrix degradation. The cell biology of pericellular proteolysis. Semin Cell Biol 1995; 6:367–376.

25. Delclaux, C, C Delacourt, MP D'Ortho, V Boyer, C Lafuma, and A Harf. Role of gelatinase B and elastase in human polymorphonuclear neutrophil migration across basement membrane. Am J Respir Cell Mol Biol 1996; 14:288–295.

26. Hayashi, M, RR Schellenberg, S Tsang, and CR Roberts. Matrix metalloproteinase-9 in myeloid cells: Implications for allergic inflammation. Int Arch Allergy Immunol 1999; 118:429–432.

27. Chenoweth, DE, and TE Hugli. Demonstration of specific C5a receptor on intact human polymorphonuclear leukocytes. Proc Natl Acad Sci USA 1978; 75:3943–3947.

28. Dos Santos, C, and D Davidson. Neutrophil chemotaxis to leukotriene B4 in vitro is decreased for the human neonate. Pediatr Res 1993; 33:242–246.

29. Damerau, B, E Grunefeld, and W Vogt. Chemotactic effects of the complement-derived peptides C3a, C3ai and C5a (classical anaphylatoxin) on rabbit and guinea-pig polymorphonuclear leukocytes. Naunyn Schmiedebergs Arch Pharmacol 1978; 305:181–184.

30. Mulder, K, and IG Colditz. Migratory responses of ovine neutrophils to inflammatory mediators in vitro and in vivo. J Leukoc Biol 1993; 53:273–278.

31. Reibman, J, S Meixler, TC Lee, LI Gold, BN Cronstein, KA Haines, SL Kolasinski, and G Weissmann. Transforming growth factor beta 1, a potent chemoattractant for human neutrophils, bypasses classic signal-transduction pathways. Proc Natl Acad Sci USA 1991; 88:6805–6809.

32. Ehrengruber, MU, T Geiser, and DA Deranleau. Activation of human neutrophils by C3a and C5A. Comparison of the effects on shape changes, chemotaxis, secretion, and respiratory burst. FEBS Lett 1994; 346:181–184.

33. Huang, R, JP Lian, D Robinson, and JA Badwey. Neutrophils stimulated with a variety of chemoattractants exhibit rapid activation of p21-activated kinases (paks): Separate signals are required for activation and inactivation of paks. Mol Cell Biol 1998; 18:7130–7138.

34. McPhail, LC, and R Snyderman. Activation of the respiratory burst enzyme in human polymorphonuclear leukocytes by chemoattractants and other soluble stimuli. Evidence that the same oxidase is activated by different transductional mechanisms. J Clin Invest 1983; 72:192–200.

35. English, D, JS Roloff, and JN Lukens. Chemotactic factor enhancement of superoxide release from fluoride and phorbol myristate acetate stimulated neutrophils. Blood 1981; 58:129–134.

36. Cassatella, MA, F Bazzoni, M Ceska, I Ferro, M Baggiolini, and G Berton. IL-8 production by human polymorphonuclear leukocytes. The chemoattractant formyl-methionyl-leucyl-phenylalanine induces the gene expression and release of IL-8 through a pertussis toxin-sensitive pathway. J Immunol 1992; 148:3216–3220.

37. Holmes, B, AR Page, and RA Good. Studies of the metabolic activity of leukocytes from patients with a genetic abnormality of phagocytic function. J Clin Invest 1967; 46:1422–1432.

38. Quie, PG, JG White, B Holmes, and RA Good. In vitro bactericidal capacity of human polymorphonuclear leukocytes: Diminished in chronic granulomatous diseases of childhood. J Clin Invest 1967; 46:668–679.

39. Henderson, LM, JB Chappell, and OT Jones. Superoxide generation is inhibited by phospholipase A2 inhibitors. Role for phospholipase A2 in the activation of the NADPH oxidase. Biochem J 1989; 264: 249–255.

40. Dana, R, HL Malech, and R Levy. The requirement for phospholipase A2 for activation of the assembled NADPH oxidase in human neutrophils [published erratum appears in Biochem J 1994 (Mar 15); 298(Pt 3):759]. Biochem J 1994; 297:217–223.

41. Klebanoff, SJ, MA Vadas, JM Harlan, LH Sparks, JR Gamble, JM Agosti, and AM Waltersdorph. Stimulation of neutrophils by tumor necrosis factor. J Immunol 1986; 136:4220–4225.

42. Dallegri, F, and L Ottonello. Tissue injury in neutrophilic inflammation. Inflamm Res 1997; 46:382–391.

43. Weiss, SJ. Tissue destruction by neutrophils [see comments]. N Engl J Med 1989; 320:365–376.

44. Sbarra, AJ, and ML Karnovsky. The biochemical basis of phagocytosis. 1. Metabolic changes during the ingestion of particles by polymorphonuclear leukocytes. J Biol Chem 1959; 234:1355–1362.

45. Morel, F, J Doussiere, and PV Vignais. The superoxide-generating oxidase of phagocytic cells. Physiological, molecular and pathological aspects. Eur J Biochem 1991; 201:523–546.

46. Segal, AW, OT Jones, D Webster, and AC Allison. Absence of a newly described cytochrome b from neutrophils of patients with chronic granulomatous disease. Lancet 1978; 2:446–449.

47. Rotrosen, D, CL Yeung, TL Leto, HL Malech, and CH Kwong. Cytochrome b558: the flavin-binding component of the phagocyte NADPH oxidase. Science 1992; 256:1459–1462.

48. Parkos, CA, RA Allen, CG Cochrane, and AJ Jesaitis. Purified cytochrome b from human granulocyte plasma membrane is comprised of two polypeptides with relative molecular weights of 91,000 and 22,000. J Clin Invest 1987; 80:732–742.

49. Parkos, CA, RA Allen, CG Cochrane, and AJ Jesaitis. The quaternary structure of the plasma membrane b-type cytochrome of human granulocytes. Biochim Biophys Acta 1988; 932:71–83.

50. Rotrosen, D, CL Yeung, and JP Katkin. Production of recombinant cytochrome b558 allows reconstitution of the phagocyte NADPH oxidase solely from recombinant proteins. J Biol Chem 1993; 268: 14256–14260.

51. Lomax, KJ, TL Leto, H Nunoi, JI Gallin, and HL Malech. Recombinant 47-kilodalton cytosol factor restores NADPH oxidase in chronic granulomatous disease [published erratum appears in Science 1989 (Nov 24); 246(4933):987]. Science 1989; 245:409–412.

52. Leto, TL, KJ Lomax, BD Volpp, H Nunoi, JM Sechler, WM Nauseef, RA Clark, JI Gallin, and HL

Malech. Cloning of a 67-kD neutrophil oxidase factor with similarity to a noncatalytic region of p60c-src. Science 1990; 248:727–730.

53. Volpp, BD, WM Nauseef, JE Donelson, DR Moser, and RA Clark. Cloning of the cDNA and functional expression of the 47-kilodalton cytosolic component of human neutrophil respiratory burst oxidase [published erratum appears in Proc Natl Acad Sci USA 1989 (Dec); 86(23):9563]. Proc Natl Acad Sci USA 1989; 86:7195–7199.

54. Leto, TL, MC Garrett, H Fujii, and H Nunoi. Characterization of neutrophil NADPH oxidase factors p47-phox and p67-phox from recombinant baculoviruses. J Biol Chem 1991; 266:19812–19818.

55. Abo A, E Pick, A Hall, N Totty, CG Teahan, and AW Segal. Activation of the NADPH oxidase involves the small GTP-binding protein p21rac1. Nature 1991; 353:668–670.

56. Nauseef, WM, BD Volpp, S McCormick, KG Leidal, and RA Clark. Assembly of the neutrophil respiratory burst oxidase. Protein kinase C promotes cytoskeletal and membrane association of cytosolic oxidase components. J Biol Chem 1991; 266:5911–5917.

57. Clark, RA, BD Volpp, KG Leidal, and WM Nauseef. Two cytosolic components of the human neutrophil respiratory burst oxidase translocate to the plasma membrane during cell activation. J Clin Invest 1990; 85:714–721.

58. Clark, RA, BD Volpp, KG Leidal, and WM Nauseef. Translocation of cytosolic components of neutrophil NADPH oxidase. Trans Assoc Am Physicians 1989; 102:224–230.

59. Heyworth, PG, JT Curnutte, WM Nauseef, BD Volpp, DW Pearson, H Rosen, and RA Clark. Neutrophil nicotinamide adenine dinucleotide phosphate oxidase assembly. Translocation of p47-phox and p67-phox requires interaction between p47-phox and cytochrome b558. J Clin Invest 1991; 87:352–356.

60. Heyworth, PG, BP Bohl, GM Bokoch, and JT Curnutte. Rac translocates independently of the neutrophil NADPH oxidase components p47phox and p67phox. Evidence for its interaction with flavocytochrome b558. J Biol Chem. 1994; 269:30749–30752.

61. Quinn, MT, T Evans, LR Loetterle, AJ Jesaitis, and GM Bokoch. Translocation of Rac correlates with NADPH oxidase activation. Evidence for equimolar translocation of oxidase components. J Biol Chem 1993; 268:20983–20987.

62. Aust, SD, CE Thomas, LA Morehouse, M Saito, and JR Bucher. Active oxygen and toxicity. Adv Exp Med Biol 1986; 197:513–526.

63. Babior, BM, RS Kipnes, and JT Curnutte. Biological defense mechanisms. The production by leukocytes of superoxide, a potential bactericidal agent. J Clin Invest 1973; 52:741–744.

64. Weiss, SJ, J Young, AF LoBuglio, A Slivka, and NF Nimeh. Role of hydrogen peroxide in neutrophil-mediated destruction of cultured endothelial cells. J Clin Invest 1981; 68:714–721.

65. Iyer, GYN, DMF Islam, and JH Quastel. Biochemical aspects of phagocytosis. Nature 1961; 192:535–541.

66. Weening, RS, R Wever, and D Roos. Quantitative aspects of the production of superoxide radicals by phagocytizing human granulocytes. J Lab Clin Med 1975; 85:245–252.

67. Fenton, HJH. Oxidation of tartaric acid in the presence of iron. J Chem Soc 1894; 65:899–910.

68. Haber, F, and J Weiss. The catalytic decomposition of hydrogen peroxide by iron salts. Proc R Soc Lond 1934; 147:332–351.

69. Halliwell, B, and JM Gutteridge. Oxygen free radicals and iron in relation to biology and medicine: Some problems and concepts. Arch Biochem Biophys 1986; 246:501–514.

70. Aust, SD, LA Morehouse, and CE Thomas. Role of metals in oxygen radical reactions. J Free Radic Biol Med 1985; 1:3–25.

71. Winterbourn, CC. Toxicity of iron and hydrogen peroxide: The Fenton reaction. Toxicol Lett 1995; 82–83:969–974.

72. Kettle, AJ, and CC Winterbourn. Superoxide enhances hypochlorous acid production by stimulated human neutrophils. Biochim Biophys Acta 1990; 1052:379–385.

73. Weiss, SJ, R Klein, A Slivka, and M Wei. Chlorination of taurine by human neutrophils. Evidence for hypochlorous acid generation. J Clin Invest 1982; 70:598–607.

74. Winterbourn, CC. Myeloperoxidase as an effective inhibitor of hydroxyl radical production. Implications for the oxidative reactions of neutrophils. J Clin Invest 1986; 78:545–550.

75. Winterbourn, CC, and AJ Kettle. Reactions of myeloperoxidase with superoxide and hydrogen peroxide: significance for its function in the neutrophil. Basic Life Sci 1988; 49:823–827.

76. Hampton, MB, AJ Kettle, and CC Winterbourn. Inside the neutrophil phagosome: Oxidants, myeloperoxidase, and bacterial killing. Blood 1998; 92:3007–3017.

77. Test ST, and SJ Weiss. The generation and utilization of chlorinated oxidants by human neutrophils. Adv Free Rad Biol Med 1986; 2:91–116.

78. Grisham, MB, MM Jefferson, DF Melton, and EL Thomas. Chlorination of endogenous amines by isolated neutrophils. Ammonia-dependent bactericidal, cytotoxic, and cytolytic activities of the chloramines. J Biol Chem 1984; 259:10404–10413.

79. Halliwell, B, JR Hoult, and DR Blake. Oxidants, inflammation, and anti-inflammatory drugs. FASEB J 1988; 2:2867–2873.

80. Dallegri, F, R Goretti, A Ballestrero, L Ottonello, and F Patrone. Neutrophil-induced depletion of adenosine triphosphate in target cells: Evidence for a hypochlorous acid-mediated process. J Lab Clin Med 1988; 112:765–772.

81. Johnson, RJ, SJ Guggenheim, SJ Klebanoff, RF Ochi, A Wass, P Baker, M Schulze, and WG Couser. Morphologic correlates of glomerular oxidant injury induced by the myeloperoxidase-hydrogen peroxide-halide system of the neutrophil. Lab Invest 1988; 58:294–301.

82. Smedly, LA, MG Tonnesen, RA Sandhaus, C Haslett, LA Guthrie, RB Johnston, Jr, PM Henson, and GS Worthen. Neutrophil-mediated injury to endothelial cells. Enhancement by endotoxin and essential role of neutrophil elastase. J Clin Invest 1986; 77:1233–1243.

83. Zaslow, MC, RA Clark, PJ Stone, JD Calore, GL Snider, and C Franzblau. Human neutrophil elastase does not bind to alpha 1-protease inhibitor that has been exposed to activated human neutrophils. Am Rev Respir Dis 1983; 128:434–439.

84. Zaslow, MC, RA Clark, PJ Stone, J Calore, GL Snider, and C Franzblau. Myeloperoxidase-induced inactivation of alpha 1-antiprotease in hamsters. J Lab Clin Med 1985; 105:178–184.

85. Stone, PJ, EC Lucey, R Breuer, TG Christensen, MC Zaslow, RA Clark, C Franzblau, and GL Snider. Oxidants from neutrophil myeloperoxidase do not enhance elastase-induced emphysema in the hamster. Respiration 1993; 60:137–143.

86. Ossanna, PJ, ST Test, NR Matheson, S Regiani, and SJ Weiss. Oxidative regulation of neutrophil elastase-alpha-1-proteinase inhibitor interactions. J Clin Invest 1986; 77:1939–1951.

87. Carrell, RW. Alpha 1-antitrypsin: Molecular pathology, leukocytes, and tissue damage. J Clin Invest 1986; 78:1427–1431.

88. Ohlsson, K. Alpha1-antitrypsin and alpha2-macroglobulin. Interactions with human neutrophil collagenase and elastase. Ann NY Acad Sci 1975; 256:409–419.

89. Ohlsson, K, and H Tegner. Granulocyte collagenase, elastase and plasma protease inhibitors in purulent sputum. Eur J Clin Invest 1975; 5:221–227.

90. Ohlsson, K. Granulocyte collagenase and elastase and their interactions with alpha1-antitrypsin and alpha2-macroglobulin. In: Reich E, et al., eds. Proteases and Biological Control. Cold Spring Harbor: Cold Spring Harbor Laboratory, 1975:591–602.

91. Ohlsson, K, and I Olsson. Neutral proteases of human granulocytes. IV. Interaction between human granulocyte collagenase and plasma protease inhibitors. J Lab Clin Med 1977; 89:269–277.

92. Ginsburg, I, RS Mitra, DF Gibbs, J Varani, and R Kohen. Killing of endothelial cells and release of arachidonic acid. Synergistic effects among hydrogen peroxide, membrane-damaging agents, cationic substances, and proteinases and their modulation by inhibitors. Inflammation 1993; 17:295–319.

93. Varani, J, I Ginsburg, L Schuger, DF Gibbs, J Bromberg, KJ Johnson, US Ryan, and PA Ward. Endothelial cell killing by neutrophils. Synergistic interaction of oxygen products and proteases. Am J Pathol 1989; 135:435–438.

94. Ginsburg, I, R Misgav, A Pinson, J Varani, PA Ward, and R Kohen. Synergism among oxidants, proteinases, phospholipases, microbial hemolysins, cationic proteins, and cytokines. Inflammation 1992; 16:519–538.

95. Borregaard, N, L Christensen, OW Bejerrum, HS Birgens, and I Clemmensen. Identification of a highly mobilizable subset of human neutrophil intracellular vesicles that contains tetranectin and latent alkaline phosphatase. J Clin Invest 1990; 85:408–416.

96. Solomkin, JS, LA Cotta, PS Satoh, JM Hurst, and RD Nelson. Complement activation and clearance in acute illness and injury: Evidence for C5a as a cell-directed mediator of the adult respiratory distress syndrome in man. Surgery 1985; 97:668–678.

97. Zhou, HL, M Chabot-Fletcher, JJ Foley, HM Sarau, MN Tzimas, JD Winkler, and TJ Torphy. Association between leukotriene B4-induced phospholipase D activation and degranulation of human neutrophils. Biochem Pharmacol 1993; 46:139–148.

98. Richter, J, J Ng-Sikorski, I Olsson, and T Andersson. Tumor necrosis factor-induced degranulation in adherent human neutrophils is dependent on CD11b/CD18-integrin-triggered oscillations of cytosolic free Ca^{2+}. Proc Natl Acad Sci USA 1990; 87:9472–9476.

99. Tenner, AJ, and NR Cooper. Identification of types of cells in human peripheral blood that bind C1q. J Immunol 1981; 126:1174–1179.

100. Tenner, AJ. C1q receptors: Regulating specific functions of phagocytic cells. Immunobiology 1998; 199:250–264.

101. Unkeless, JC. Function and heterogeneity of human Fc receptors for immunoglobulin G. J Clin Invest 1989; 83:355–361.

102. Samanta, AK, S Dutta, and E Ali. Modification of sulfhydryl groups of interleukin-8 (IL-8) receptor impairs binding of IL-8 and IL-8-mediated chemotactic response of human polymorphonuclear neutrophils. J Biol Chem 1993; 268:6147–6153.

103. Richard, S, CA Farrell, AS Shaw, HJ Showell, and PA Connelly. C5a as a model for chemotactic factor-stimulated tyrosine phosphorylation in the human neutrophil. J Immunol 1994; 152:2479–2487.

104. Elsner, J, M Oppermann, W Czech, and A Kapp. C3a activates the respiratory burst in human polymorphonuclear neutrophilic leukocytes via pertussis toxin-sensitive G-proteins. Blood 1994; 83: 3324–3331.

105. Zurier, RB, S Hoffstein, and G Weissmann. Mechanisms of lysosomal enzyme release from human leukocytes. I. Effect of cyclic nucleotides and colchicine. J Cell Biol 1973; 58:27–41.

106. Wright, DG, DA Bralove, and JI Gallin. The differential mobilization of human neutrophil granules. Effects of phorbol myristate acetate and ionophore A23187. Am J Pathol 1977; 87:237–284.

107. Pryzwansky, KB, EK MacRae, JK Spitznagel, and MH Cooney. Early degranulation of human neutrophils: Immunocytochemical studies of surface and intracellular phagocytic events. Cell 1979; 18:1025–1033.

108. Fujii, G, ME Selsted, and D Eisenberg. Defensins promote fusion and lysis of negatively charged membranes. Protein Sci 1993; 2:1301–1312.

109. Cociancich, S, A Ghazi, C Hetru, JA Hoffmann, and L Letellier. Insect defensin, an inducible antibacterial peptide, forms voltage-dependent channels in Micrococcus luteus. J Biol Chem 1993; 268: 19239–19245.

110. Ganz, T, and RI Lehrer. Defensins. Curr Opin Immunol 1994; 6:584–589.

111. Virca, GD, G Metz, and HP Schnebli. Similarities between human and rat leukocyte elastase and cathepsin G. Eur J Biochem 1984; 144:1–9.

112. Hasty, KA, MS Hibbs, AH Kang, and CL Mainardi. Secreted forms of human neutrophil collagenase. J Biol Chem 1986; 261:5645–5650.

113. Mainardi, CL, KA Hasty, and MS Hibbs. Collagen degradation by inflammatory phagocytes. J Rheumatol 1987; 14(spec no):59–60.

114. Murphy, G, U Bretz, M Baggiolini, and JJ Reynolds. The latent collagenase and gelatinase of human polymorphonuclear neutrophil leucocytes. Biochem J 1980; 192:517–525.

115. Murphy, G, JJ Reynolds, U Bretz, and M Baggiolini. Partial purification of collagenase and gelatinase from human polymorphonuclear leucocytes. Analysis of their actions on soluble and insoluble collagens. Biochem J 1982; 203:209–2021.

116. Travis, J. Structure, function, and control of neutrophil proteinases. Am J Med 1988; 84:37–42.

117. Travis, J, A Dubin, J Potempa, W Watorek, and A Kurdowska. Neutrophil proteinases. Caution signs in designing inhibitors against enzymes with possible multiple functions. Ann NY Acad Sci 1991; 624:81–86.

118. Travis, J, and H Fritz. Potential problems in designing elastase inhibitors for therapy. Am Rev Respir Dis 1991; 143:1412–1415.

119. Sundy, JS, and BF Haynes. Vasculitis: Pathogenic mechanisms of vessel damage. In: Gallin, JI, Snyderman, R, eds. Inflammation: Basic Principles and Clinical Correlates. 3d ed. Philadelphia: Lippincott Williams & Wilkins, 1999:995–1016.

120. Brouwer, E, JJ Weening, PA Klok, MG Huitema, JW Tervaert, and CG Kallenberg. Induction of an humoral and cellular (auto)immune response to human and rat myeloperoxidase (MPO) in Brown-Norway (BN), Lewis and Wistar Kyoto (WKY) rat strains. Adv Exp Med Biol 1993; 336:139–142.

121. Kallenberg, CG, E Brouwer, JJ Weening, and JW Tervaert. Anti-neutrophil cytoplasmic antibodies: Current diagnostic and pathophysiological potential. Kidney Int 1994; 46:1–15.

122. Kallenberg, CG, E Brouwer, AH Mulder, CA Stegeman, JJ Weening, and JW Tervaert. ANCA—Pathophysiology revisited. Clin Exp Immunol 1995; 100:1–3.

123. Csernok, E, J Ludemann, WL Gross, and DF Bainton. Ultrastructural localization of proteinase 3, the target antigen of anti-cytoplasmic antibodies circulating in Wegener's granulomatosis. Am J Pathol 1990; 137:1113–1120.

124. Csernok, E, M Ernst, W Schmitt, DF Bainton, and WL Gross. Activated neutrophils express proteinase 3 on their plasma membrane in vitro and in vivo. Clin Exp Immunol 1994; 95:244–250.

125. Falk, RJ, RS Terrell, LA Charles, and JC Jennette. Anti-neutrophil cytoplasmic autoantibodies induce neutrophils to degranulate and produce oxygen radicals in vitro. Proc Natl Acad Sci USA 1990; 87: 4115–4119.

126. Fauci, AS, BF Haynes, P Katz, and SM Wolff. Wegener's granulomatosis: Prospective clinical and therapeutic experience with 85 patients for 21 years. Ann Intern Med 1983; 98:76–85.

127. Kocher, M, JC Edberg, HB Fleit, and RP Kimberly. Antineutrophil cytoplasmic antibodies preferentially engage FcγRIIIb on human neutrophils. J Immunol 1998; 161:6909–6914.

128. Porges, AJ, PB Redecha, WT Kimberly, E Csernok, WL Gross, and RP Kimberly. Anti-neutrophil cytoplasmic antibodies engage and activate human neutrophils via FcγRIIa. J Immunol 1994; 153:1271–1280.

129. Mulder, AH, P Heeringa, E Brouwer, PC Limburg, and CG Kallenberg. Activation of granulocytes by anti-neutrophil cytoplasmic antibodies (ANCA): a FcγRII-dependent process. Clin Exp Immunol 1994; 98:270–278.

130. Kettritz, R, JC Jennette, and RJ Falk. Crosslinking of ANCA-antigens stimulates superoxide release by human neutrophils. J Am Soc Nephrol 1997; 8:386–394.

131. Cronstein, BN, M Van de Stouwe, L Druska, RI Levin, and G Weissmann. Nonsteroidal antiinflammatory agents inhibit stimulated neutrophil adhesion to endothelium: Adenosine dependent and independent mechanisms. Inflammation 1994; 18:323–335.

132. Dapino, P, L Ottonello, and F Dallegri. The anti-inflammatory drug nimesulide inhibits neutrophil adherence to and migration across monolayers of cytokine-activated endothelial cells. Respiration 1994; 61:336–341.

133. Buchanan, MR, TA Haas, M Lagarde, and M Guichardant. 13-Hydroxyoctadecadienoic acid is the vessel wall chemorepellant factor, LOX. J Biol Chem 1985; 260:16056–16059.

134. Cronstein, BN, SC Kimmel, RI Levin, F Martiniuk, and G Weissmann. A mechanism for the antiinflammatory effects of corticosteroids: The glucocorticoid receptor regulates leukocyte adhesion to endothelial cells and expression of endothelial-leukocyte adhesion molecule 1 and intercellular adhesion molecule 1. Proc Natl Acad Sci USA 1992; 89:9991–9995.

135. Diaz-Gonzalez, F, I Gonzalez-Alvaro, MR Campanero, F Mollinedo, MA del Pozo, C Munoz, JP Pivel, and F Sanchez-Madrid. Prevention of in vitro neutrophil-endothelial attachment through shedding of L-selectin by nonsteroidal antiinflammatory drugs. J Clin Invest 1995; 95:1756–1765.

136. Gonzalez-Alvaro, I, L Carmona, F Diaz-Gonzalez, R Gonzalez-Amaro, F Mollinedo, F Sanchez-Madrid, A Laffon, and R Garcia-Vicuna. Aceclofenac, a new nonsteroidal antiinflammatory drug, decreases the expression and function of some adhesion molecules on human neutrophils. J Rheumatol 1996; 23:723–729.

137. Crowell, RE, and DE Van Epps. Nonsteroidal antiinflammatory agents inhibit upregulation of CD11b, CD11c, and CD35 in neutrophils stimulated by formyl-methionine-leucine-phenylalanine. Inflammation 1990; 14:163–171.

138. Morise, Z, S Komatsu, JW Fuseler, DN Granger, M Perry, AC Issekutz, and MB Grisham. ICAM-1

and P-selectin expression in a model of NSAID-induced gastropathy. Am J Physiol 1998; 274:G246–G252.

139. Cronstein, BN, Y Molad, J Reibman, E Balakhane, RI Levin, and G Weissmann. Colchicine alters the quantitative and qualitative display of selectins on endothelial cells and neutrophils. J Clin Invest 1995; 96:994–1002.

140. Asako, H, P Kubes, BA Baethge, RE Wolf, and DN Granger. Colchicine and methotrexate reduce leukocyte adherence and emigration in rat mesenteric venules. Inflammation 1992; 16:45–56.

141. Kaplan, HB, HS Edelson, HM Korchak, WP Given, S. Abramson, and G Weissmann. Effects of non-steroidal anti-inflammatory agents on human neutrophil functions in vitro and in vivo. Biochem Pharmacol 1984; 33:371–378.

142. Abramson S, H Edelson, H Kaplan, W Given, and G Weissmann. The inactivation of the polymor-phonuclear leukocyte by non-steroidal anti-inflammatory drugs. Inflammation 1984; 8(suppl):S103–S108.

143. Neal, TM, MC Vissers, and CC Winterbourn. Inhibition by nonsteroidal anti-inflammatory drugs of superoxide production and granule enzyme release by polymorphonuclear leukocytes stimulated with immune complexes or formyl-methionyl-leucyl-phenylalanine. Biochem Pharmacol 1987; 36:2511–2517.

144. Neal, TM, MC Vissers, and CC Winterbourn. Inhibition of neutrophil-mediated degradation of iso-lated basement membrane collagen by nonsteroidal antiinflammatory drugs that inhibit degranula-tion. Arthritis Rheum 1987; 30:908–913.

145. Umeki, S, and R Soejima. Hydrocortisone inhibits the respiratory burst oxidase from human neu-trophils in whole-cell and cell-free systems. Biochim Biophys Acta 1990; 1052:211–215.

146. Schleimer, RP, HS Freeland, SP Peters, KE Brown, and CP Derse. An assessment of the effects of glucocorticoids on degranulation, chemotaxis, binding to vascular endothelium and formation of leukotriene B4 by purified human neutrophils. J Pharmacol Exp Ther 1989; 250:598–605.

147. Weyts, FA, G Flik, and BM Verburg-van Kemenade. Cortisol inhibits apoptosis in carp neutrophilic granulocytes. Dev Comp Immunol 1998; 22:563–572.

148. Cronstein, BN, ED Rosenstein, SB Kramer, G Weissmann, and R Hirschhorn. Adenosine; a physio-logic modulator of superoxide anion generation by human neutrophils. Adenosine acts via an A2 re-ceptor on human neutrophils. J Immunol 1985; 135:1366–1371.

149. Cronstein, BN, RI Levin, J Belanoff, G Weissmann, and R Hirschhorn. Adenosine: an endogenous in-hibitor of neutrophil-mediated injury to endothelial cells. J Clin Invest 1986; 78:760–770.

150. Cronstein, BN, SM Kubersky, G Weissmann, and R Hirschhorn. Engagement of adenosine receptors inhibits hydrogen peroxide (H_2O_2) release by activated human neutrophils. Clin Immunol Immuno-pathol 1987; 42:76–85.

151. Cronstein, BN, SB Kramer, G Weissmann, and R Hirschhorn. Adenosine: A physiological modulator of superoxide anion generation by human neutrophils. J Exp Med 1983; 158:1160–1177.

152. Cronstein, BN, D Naime, and E Ostad. The antiinflammatory mechanism of methotrexate. Increased adenosine release at inflamed sites diminishes leukocyte accumulation in an in vivo model of inflam-mation. J Clin Invest 1993; 92:2675–2682.

153. Dallegri, F, L Ottonello, P Dapino, and C Sacchetti. Effect of nonsteroidal antiinflammatory drugs on the neutrophil promoted inactivation of alpha-1-proteinase inhibitor. J Rheumatol 1992; 19:419–423.

154. Dallegri, F, L Ottonello, P Dapino, and M Bevilacqua. The anti-inflammatory drug nimesulide res-cues alpha-1-proteinase inhibitor from oxidative inactivation by phagocytosing neutrophils. Respira-tion 1992; 59:1–4.

7
Oxygen Metabolites and Vascular Damage

Thomas M. McIntyre, Gopal K. Marathe, Guy A. Zimmerman, and Stephen M. Prescott
University of Utah, Salt Lake City, Utah

I. INTRODUCTION: FREE RADICALS AND REACTIVE OXYGEN SPECIES

Free radicals are atoms or molecules with an unpaired electron in the outer shell, and in complex molecules these may be centered on carbon, nitrogen, or oxygen. The definition of free radicals from a biologist's point of view is extended by defining a new category, reactive oxygen species (ROS), to include peroxides that are not radicals. However, peroxides can easily form them and play a central role in metabolism and inflammation. Thus this definition of ROS encompasses peroxides, which are radical precursors. The reason this chemistry is of interest to biologists is that the reactivity of radicals is high as they seek to pair with another atom and complete its own unfilled orbital. The free energy to be gained by this reaction means that many normally stable chemical bonds are susceptible to attack. The result is the facile addition of atoms and molecules to other molecules, or the rearrangement of the molecule that is exploited, for example, in the generation of the many leukotrienes, prostanoids, and thromboxanes that coordinate cellular actions in complex organisms. Radicals and reactive oxygen species are also used by the inflammatory cells of higher organisms to aid in the destruction of invading organisms, a mission that becomes apparent in chronic granulomatous disease where the ability of inflammatory cells to generate reactive oxygen species on demand is lost. Oxidants (in a currently undefined fashion) also regulate gene transcription through modulation of intracellular signal pathways leading to the activation of the transcription factors NF-kB (1) and AP-1 (2). Oxidants also alter vascular tone, acting both as vasoconstrictors and vasodilators, so their final effect is variable (3). Free radicals, oxidants, and reactive oxygen species play diverse roles in metabolism, but by their very nature are able to cause inappropriate responses and widespread destruction. This capacity for mayhem is checked by mobile antioxidants, as well as dedicated intracellular and extracellular catabolic pathways. It is when this suppressive ability is overcome, even when the loss of control is only local, that a number of unintended events relevant to vascular biology become manifest. One of these consequences we know the most about is reviewed here: mimicry of physiological inflammatory processes.

II. PHYSIOLOGICAL INFLAMMATION

Inflammation is a regulated physiological process so relevant to human history that the written literature reaches back two millenia. The modern era in understanding the cellular and molecular basis for these early observations began in the nineteenth century with the microscopic observation of the microcirculatory system immediately after application of a noxious stimulus. These early microscopists found that leukocytes (white corpuscles of unknown function then) interacted with the wall of vessels traversing the stimulus. Initially this was visualized as rolling along the vessel wall, followed by a sudden transition to a stationary cell, and then appearance outside of intact vessels (4). A detailed understanding of the mechanisms that accomplished this rapid transition had to wait until it became possible to study the key cell type in this first step of inflammation, endothelial cells, in isolation, a process that only became facile in the early 1970s (5). With the culture of human endothelial cells, in a way that maintained their highly differentiated phenotype, came a clear distinction of the various activation states of endothelial cells. More complex systems such as the Stamper–Woodruff assay using tissue sections and organ culture (6), and now transgenic and gene-targeted mice (7) all have defined the individual components that allow the rapid recruitment of specific inflammatory cells to localized tissue beds in a transient, regulated fashion.

Quiescent endothelial cells, except at specialized sites that allow continuous monitoring by the immune system, do not display a surface that favors interaction with inflammatory cells. Rather, quiescent endothelium is actively nonthrombotic through continuous production of prostacyclin and nitric oxide, a short-lived radical that raises cAMP levels in target cells that dampens its own program of activation, adhesion, and migration. In addition to a basal production of prostacyclin and nitric oxide that prevents platelet activation, adhesion, and release of platelet-derived growth factors, the production of these two molecules can be increased by stimulated transcription and translation of isoforms of the synthetic enzymes, inducible nitric oxide synthase and cyclooxygenase-2 (8). These two compounds also have a role in endothelial cell-dependent vasorelaxation that encourages blood flow and decreases endothelial cell interaction with circulating cells. These two agents do not, however, fully explain the endothelial cell–dependent vasorelaxation. At least one unidentified endothelial cell–hyperpolarizing factor relaxes vascular smooth muscle (9).

Activation of endothelial cells changes this antithrombotic state to one that results in the rapid adhesion of inflammatory cells described by Cohnheim in the nineteenth century (4). This is not an all-or-nothing change from one state to another, but rather the resulting activated endothelial cells reflect the nature of the stimulatory agent (10). We divide the activation state of endothelial cells into those responses that occur almost immediately and those early responses that take an hour or more to develop. In general, division of the activation state in a temporal fashion correlates with the molecular changes that define the state, although at least one agonist can induce elements of both the immediate and the early activation states (11). The changes induced by agonists of either class are twofold: expression of an adhesion molecule by the activated endothelial cells that binds specific circulating cells and sequesters them against the vascular wall, and the expression by the activated endothelial cells of molecules that specifically activate the sequestered inflammatory cells (12). This two-step model (13) of adhesion or tethering of leukocytes followed by activation underlies both the rapid (14) and early (15) types of endothelial cell activation.

The activation state of endothelial cells after exposure to, for example, thrombin or histamine defines the immediate phenotype that promotes the binding and activation of resting leukocytes. For the rapid activation of endothelial cells, the tethering molecule is P-selectin, a Ca^{2+}-dependent molecule that binds sialyl Lewis-X–modified proteins expressed by leukocytes (16). The molecule expressed by leukocytes is P-selectin glycoprotein ligand-1 (17), and the interaction between endothelial cell P-selectin and this ligand is rapid. A rapid ligand–receptor interaction allows the first, fleeting interaction of the two cell types, but it is the additional rapidity of the reverse interaction between these two molecules (18) that is responsible for the rolling of leukocytes along the microvasculature in response to the flow still experienced by the leukocyte. A rapid on-and-off binding of the P-selectin ligand has the advantage of slowing the leukocyte and localizing it to the vascular wall, but in a way that allows the leukocyte the mobility that it will need to complete its journey across the vascular wall.

The trip across the endothelial cell barrier is initiated by the second change in the phenotype of endothelial cells after activation, the localized expression of an activation molecule that initiates the leukocyte's own motility and activation program. In the immediate-type of endothelial cell response, this leukocyte agonist is platelet-activating factor (PAF). This leukocyte agonist was originally named after its first known biological function as it was being identified as the component in blood isolated from anaphylactic rabbits that was responsible for platelet activation and hypotension (19). It was separately identified as a antihypotensive agent (20) and its structure defined as a phosphatidylcholine with two modifications; it contained an ether bond at the first position of the glycerol backbone, and an acetate esterifed at the second (21). Leukocytes possess a receptor that specifically recognizes this molecule, even in a virtual sea of other phosphatidylcholine molecules that comprise mammalian cellular membranes. This receptor, and there currently is only one known, has been cloned (22) and been found to be a member of the abundant class of receptors that span the extracellular membrane seven times and functionally couple to intracellular G proteins. Platelet-activating factor, like the lipid mediators derived from arachidonate, is not normally present in endothelial cells, but is rapidly synthesized and expressed on the outer surface of endothelial cells activated with, among other stimuli, thrombin and histamine (21). Endothelial cells are activated by leukotriene C_4 and D_4 with a similar surface expression of PAF and P-selectin, although the kinetics lag somewhat behind those of thrombin (23). The key point here is that PAF, a highly potent leukocyte agonist, is not released from the activated endothelial cells, but rather remains on the outer surface. The mechanism by which this occurs is not known, but it is presented by the endothelial cells in such a way that the leukocytes juxtaposed with the activated endothelial cells by P-selectin are able to respond to it through their PAF receptors (Fig. 1). The result of this is that only those leukocytes interacting with the endothelium are activated by the PAF expressed by activated endothelial cells, a form of juxtacrine signaling (14) that actually was the phenomenon that led the early biologists to conclude that changes in the vascular wall accounted for leukocyte adhesion—a deduction that explained why leukocytes adhered only to the side of the vessel exposed to trauma and why leukocytes released from this localized site never were seen to reattach downstream.

The importance of PAF and P-selectin in the early steps of inflammation suggests that their presence must be carefully controlled, and, in fact, this is the case. P-selectin is constitutively present in endothelial cells, but resides in specialized intracellular granules, Weibel-Palade bodies, that additionally contain von Willebrand factor. Activation of endothelial cells in ways that increase the levels of intracellular Ca^{2+} result in the fusion of these vesicles with the plasma membrane, release of the soluble von Willebrand factor, and deposition of P-selectin on the surface of the activated endothelial cells (24). Activated endothelial cells rapidly initiate the synthesis of PAF in a process controlled by intracellular Ca^{2+} (25) and phosphorylation of the synthetic enzyme (26). The physiological inflammatory response is marked by its transient nature with the peak change in endothelial cell properties occurring by 30 min after stimulation with agonists that induce an immediate response, and by 8 h for those that induce the early response. For P-selectin expressed on the surface of activated endothelial cells, this reversal occurs through rapid reinternalization with some contribution by proteolysis, especially of platelet-expressed P-selectin, to generate circulating soluble P-selectin (27). Abnormally prolonged expression of P-selectin is correlated with vascular damage. P-selectin is expressed for weeks at aortic branch points of rabbits destined to develop atherosclerosis at this site, and this expression precedes early macrophage infiltration that drives atherogenesis (28). The effects of surface-bound PAF are controlled by its

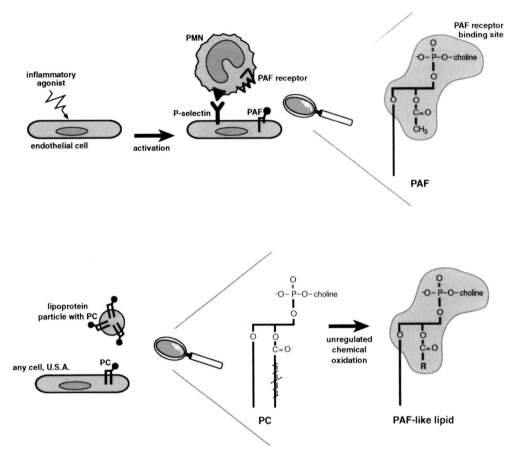

Figure 1   Regulated cellular synthesis and chemical oxidation of cellular or lipoprotein phosphatidyl-choline generates PAF-receptor agonists. Activated endothelial cells, as opposed to quiescent cells, translocate the leukocyte-binding protein P-selectin from intracellular granules to their plasma membrane that then sequesters circulating polymorphonuclear leukocytes (PMN) against the activated endothelial cell. Simultaneously, platelet-activating factor (PAF), synthesized only in activated cells in a two-step enzymatic process, is expressed on the plasma membrane of activated cells. Activation of the leukocyte PAF receptor induces its own program of shape change, adhesion, and migration. The regulated and localized expression of these two molecules localizes the inflammatory reaction. In contrast, oxidative fragmentation of phosphatidyl-choline (PC) also generates ligands and activators of the PAF receptor. This, however, occurs through un-regulated chemical reactions and results in unregulated inflammatory responses.

rapid hydrolysis and inactivation by PAF acetylhydrolase that circulates in a fully active state in association with specific lipoprotein particles (29). This enzyme is able to circulate in an active state, rather than as an inactive zymogen, without deleterious effects subsequent to hydrolysis of lipoprotein and membrane phosphatidylcholines because of its specificity for PAF. This issue becomes important below when we discuss the effect oxidants have on this carefully controlled system of inflammation.

There is one other issue to be discussed before we consider how oxidants disturb physiological inflammation, and that is an additional function of P-selectin. Activated platelets express P-selectin (and hence the P in the name) and this causes leukocytes to adhere to them (30), an event that underlies the formation of leukocyte–platelet clusters in vivo (31). Formation of these clusters will alter the function of the incorporated monocyte by priming them for an enhanced response to soluble agonists (32,33). In addition, activation of platelets and their expression of P-selectin underlie a puzzling paradox in in vivo models of inflammation where leukocyte rolling and adhesion occurs both in arterioles and venules (34). Yet, immunolocalization studies place P-selectin just in postcapillary venules (35). It now appears that platelets line the vascular wall, an event that is not easily visualized, and it is platelet-(P)-selectin that localizes leukocytes to regions of the microcirculation that lack endogenous P-selectin.

III. OXIDANTS AND THE INFLAMMATORY SYSTEM

Physiological inflammation is a regulated, reversible homeostatic process. In contrast, some components of the inflammatory cascade can be recruited in an uncoordinated, unregulated manner. The culprits here are oxidizing radicals and ROS produced in quantities that overcome local antioxidants to damage macromolecules. Lipid oxidation products are of particular importance as these have an abundance of easily oxidized double bonds. As now has become apparent, the effect of oxidizing radicals can be disproportionate to their amount as some of these activate inflammatory responses in an uncontrolled way. Over the past decade robust markers of in vivo oxidative reactions have been developed, some of the oxidatively generated biological mimetics have been identified, some of the biological events they induce have been discovered, and a correlation of oxidatively generated mediators with disease states has been established. This chapter focuses on two classes of oxidatively generated lipid mediators, oxidized arachidonate and phosphatidylcholines.

IV. MARKERS OF OXIDATION

Free radicals by their very nature are transient and quite difficult to quantitate in vivo, so a definition of the types and amounts of ROS and radicals in any given event is not possible. One advance that has had a significant effect on the field in this regard is the development of isoprostanes (36,37), and now isoleukotrienes (38) and isolevuglandins (39), as markers (and effectors) of in vivo oxidative stress and nonenzymatic oxidative reactions. Arachidonate, as a consequence of its four double bonds, is susceptible to oxidation, and this is the basis for the enzymatic control of oxidative attack to generate the potent and varied eicosanoid arachidonate metabolites. Similar reactions occur without the aid of an enzymatic reaction mechanism to direct the reaction curve, with the result that numerous positional and stereochemical homologues of these enzymatic products are produced in an uncontrolled way. Some of these are biologically active. The best characterized of these are the isoprostanes first identified (40) as arachidonate oxidation products whose generation did not depend on cyclooxygenase activity (41). Isoprostanes are produced in abundance as arachidonate is oxidized and many of these are chemically stable, two attributes that underlie the use of isoprostane levels as surrogate markers of oxidation. Whether these compounds would accurately reflect endogenous oxidative reactions was questioned when it was determined that platelets form some isoprostane through a cyclooxygenase-dependent oxidation (42). However this reaction is a minor source (43), and except perhaps for urine where renal cyclooxygenase may contribute to the excreted isoprostanes, quantification of several isoprostanes (44,45) has correlated well with oxidation states in vitro (46) and in vivo (47–49). The confidence gained through the correlation of isoprostane generation in smokers (49,50), a habit that introduces an immense radical load into the lungs (51) and the circulation (52), validates the use of this approach in other disease states where oxidant involvement is suspected but not proved (53,54). Quantitation of isoprostanes also provides a convenient method to quantitate the progression of vascular damage in conditions where oxidants have been shown to play a major part in disease progression (47,48,55). Other lipid oxidation products, generated in vitro from oxidative attack on phosphatidylcholine (56,57), are found in atherosclerotic plaques (58) and likely mark nonenzymatic oxidative processes. However, quantitation and identification of these lipid oxidation products is more laborious and difficult than gas chromatography–mass spectrometry with an internal standards protocol that has made isoprostane quantitation so accurate and facile.

V. MIMETICS OF ARACHIDONATE METABOLITES

Arachidonate is oxidized by cytochromes, lipoxygenases, and cyclooxygenases to a host of mediators including hydroperoxyeicosanoic acids, thromboxanes, leukotrienes, and prostaglandins that regulate processes ranging from parturition to apoptotic cell death. Nonenzymatic oxidation produces an even wider variety of homologues, and some of these are biologically active. The initial description of the prostaglandin-like compounds (40) showed that infusion of one of the isoprostanes either into a peripheral vein or intrarenally caused a marked parallel reduction in renal blood flow and glomerular filtration rate. One of the isoprostanes with this activity, 8-epi-PGF$_{2\alpha}$, acts at least partially through the thromboxane A$_2$ receptor (59). Vasoconstriction is also apparent in other vascular beds, such as those of the retina (60) and the coronary arteries (61). Some isoprostanes bind the prostaglandin F$_{2\alpha}$ (PGF$_{2\alpha}$) receptor and both an isoprostane and prostaglandin F$_{2\alpha}$ induce cardiac cell hypertrophy, although other unidentified events come into play as the signaling pathways leading to this functional response are different (62). Now after a second type of cyclooxygenase has been identified with particular relevance to regulated inflammatory processes (63), whose specific inhibition is actively being sought by the pharmaceutical industry, we find an alternative, uncontrolled route to prostaglandin-like arachidonate metabolites that may be just as important.

VI. OXIDIZED PHOSPHOLIPIDS

The main target of oxidizing species and radicals are bonds adjacent to olefinic bonds. Enzymatic and chemical oxidation of free arachidonate generates important intercellular mediators as well as reactive chemical products (e.g., reactive aldehydes and conjugated aldehydes). A recent example is modification of apolipoprotein B100 of low-density lipoprotein (LDL) by arachidonate oxidation products that created protein adducts that stimulated macrophage growth (64). However, the bulk of cellular fatty acids are not free but are esterified in complex lipids (phospholipids, triglycerides, and cholesterol esters). Oxidation of these acyl residues creates reactive phospholipids that, like the reactive fragments generated from fatty acid oxidation, modify protein lysyl residues (65,66). For example, ectopic expression of the lipase PAF acetylhydrolase (67,68), which specifically hydrolyzes PAF and oxidatively fragmented phospholipids, protects cells from oxidant-induced apoptosis (69). This shows that the intact phospholipid, rather than water-soluble products from fatty acid oxidation, is deleterious in peroxide-stressed cells.

VII. PAF-LIKE PHOSPHOLIPIDS

Other products of oxidative attack on phospholipids may produce problems by mimicking the structure of endogenous agonists, and so activate receptors for physiological ligands like the PAF receptor (69a). The first of these to be identified (70) were the PAF-like agonists generated by the oxidation of phosphatidylcholine containing a polyunsaturated fatty acyl residue in the 2 position of the glycerol backbone. Recent data from our research group define a new class of oxidatively generated phospholipid mediators that activate a member of the nuclear hormone receptor family, peroxisomal proliferator–activated receptor gamma (PPARγ). PPARγ activates at least one inflammatory gene through a novel responsive element (Davies et al., unpublished).

The bulk of cellular and lipoprotein phosphatidylcholines contain an esterified fatty acyl residue at the first position of the glycerol backbone (the *sn*-1 position) as well as the second position. However, some phosphatidylcholines contain a fatty alcohol residue in an ether bond at the *sn*-1 position, and these are the precursors for biologically active PAF [1-fatty alcohol 2-acetyl]phosphocholine. A homologue of PAF with an *sn*-1 esterified fatty acyl residue is also made by activated cells (71), but this is a poor activator of the PAF receptor, so only PAF is relevant to the inflammatory process. Cellular synthesis of PAF is a tightly regulated process where a cytosolic, calcium-dependent phospholipase A$_2$ cleaves the long-chain *sn*-2 fatty acyl residue to generate a lysoPAF backbone and a free fatty acid. Intriguingly, ether phosphatidylcholines are highly enriched with arachidonoyl residues at the *sn*-2 position, so this phospholipase A$_2$ activity generates precursors for two classes of lipid mediators, PAF, and eicosanoids. Next, an acetyltransferase, which is regulated by phosphorylation (26), transfers an acetyl group from acetyl coenzyme A to the free hydroxyl of the lysoPAF. The product of this cellular synthetic pathway is PAF (1-O-alkyl-2-acetyl-*sn*-glycero-3-phosphocholine). This activates inflammatory cells expressing the PAF receptor that specifically recognizes the bond at the 1 position, the short acetyl residue at the 2 position, and the choline head group. This receptor can activate leukocytes and platelets that express it when confronted with PAF concentrations as low as 10^{-15} M.

In contrast to the regulated synthesis of PAF, unregulated chemical oxidation fragments phospholipids into species that also bind to and activate the PAF receptor. Initially a series of vasopressor lipids were found in the extracts of bovine brain (72), and the structure of these vasopressor lipids was found to be a complex group of phosphatidylcholines with a series of a short, and often derivatized *sn*-2 residues. We found such phospholipids could be generated from the oxidative fragmentation of biological (73,74) or synthetic (70) phosphatidylcholines. Thus, the activities extracted from brains, as well as those found in atherosclerotic lesions (58), appeared to be oxidatively fragmented phospholipids. Importantly, we find many of these phospholipids are capable of activating the receptor for PAF, even though they lack the acetyl function of authentic PAF. That is, oxidation of synthetic or biological phosphatidylcholines generates PAF mimetics by fragmentation of the *sn*-2 fatty acyl residue to short residues recognized by the PAF receptor. The formation of these compounds is the result of a series of competing chemical reactions, some of which can be exponential, and therefore are not subjected to enzymatic or biological control. We have ectopically expressed the PAF receptor in a cell line that normally does not possess this receptor and found that, like PAF, certain oxidatively fragmented phospholipids activated just those cells that expressed the PAF receptor (74). We also have purified membranes from cells expressing the PAF receptor, and found that purified PAF receptors also directly bind certain oxidatively fragmented phospholipids (Marathe et al., unpublished). Thus, oxidative fragmentation of cellular and lipoprotein phosphatidylcholines creates fragmented phospholipids that are potent ligands and activators of the PAF receptor. This, in turn, would suggest that this unregulated, oxidative process could induce an inflammatory reaction in a local environment or systemically when endogenous antioxidant defenses are overwhelmed. Clearly this response can be created ex vivo when we provide a robust burst of oxidizing radicals. The question that remains is whether a sufficient suppression of endogenous antioxidant defenses can be attained in vivo to allow the inappropriate and rampant formation of inflammatory PAF-like compounds.

VIII. PAF-LIKE LIPIDS IN VIVO

To answer the question posed above, we exposed hamsters to second-hand cigarette smoke by drawing the smoke of one cigarette into a chamber over a period of 10 min. Cigarette smoke is a rich source of oxidizing species, and it has been estimated (75) that a single puff of cigarette smoke contains 5 nmol of oxidizing radicals. This is an immense radical load: while it may be difficult to accurately quantitate extracellular lung water, dissolving this amount of long-lived and reactive radicals in even 1 ml would produce micromolar amounts of radicals continuously delivered over the time it takes to smoke a cigarette. Thus, if we are to find a condition where the load of oxidizing radicals could overwhelm antioxidant defenses and generate PAF-like lipids, cigarette smoking should be a premier candidate. This cigarette smoke exposure protocol has been shown to induce a rapid, and, more importantly, systemic inflammatory response. Typically, few leukocytes interact with the vessel wall in the microcirculation of normal animals, but by 10 min after exposure to cigarette smoke both leukocytes and leukocyte-platelet aggregates are clearly seen rolling, tumbling, and stationary in both the arterioles and venules of the skin (76). This pronounced inflammatory response extends well away from the initial oxidant stress of the lungs, but clearly is the result of oxidant stress and not the myriad of inhaled chemicals to be found in cigarette smoke. The evidence for this is that either the antioxidant vitamin C (77), or injection of superoxide dismutase (78) blocks these telltale signs of smoke-induced inflammation. The systemic inflammation, then, precedes from the inhalation of oxidants.

We determined whether the inhaled oxidants generate PAF-like mimetics and whether these would be essential for the systemic inflammatory response by isolating blood from control hamsters and animals exposed to cigarette smoke. The lipids in these blood samples were extracted, purified, and assayed for PAF-like bioactivity. We found (79) activity in the blood of cigarette smoke–exposed animals that activates leukocytes in an in vitro adhesion assay that detects PAF activity. The bulk of this inflammatory activity, purified by high-performance liquid chromatography (HPLC), migrated as oxidatively fragmented phospholipids, while the plasma obtained from control animals did not contain any proinflammatory lipids. These data show that cigarette smoke results in the rapid accumulation of inflammatory compounds in the circulation. Examination of the level of this activity in control animals, those exposed to cigarette smoke, or animals exposed to cigarette smoke after a course of dietary vitamin C was conducted to determine if the accumulation of these compounds was sensitive to antioxidant therapy. We found that most animals exposed to cigarette smoke had proinflammatory PAF-like phospholipids in their blood, but that dietary vitamin C suppressed the accumulation of these compounds such that there was no difference between these animals and control animals. This is evidence that the proinflammatory phospholipids were derived from an oxidative reaction. Since vitamin C prevented the formation of these compounds and the systemic inflammation, we conclude that biologically active oxidized phospholipids account for the systemic inflammation that occurs immediately after cigarette smoking. It is instructive that a similar rapid systemic inflammatory response is observed when hamsters are injected with LDL oxidized outside the animal (80). Similarly, humans rapidly express PAF or PAF-like lipids in their circulation just after smoking (81). In addition, cigarette smoking causes a very marked retention of leukocytes in the lungs of humans (82) and animals (83) during their first pass through this bed. We take this as strong evidence that pathologically relevant levels of oxidant stresses occur in vivo, that these oxidants are capable of generating PAF-like phospholipid mediators, and these mediators can induce an inflammatory response.

Recent data demonstrate that oxidatively fragmented phospholipids also accumulate in atherosclerotic lesions (58), so it appears that oxidants can generate inflammatory phospholipids at appropriate sites and times to also have a role in the early events of atherogenesis. Additionally ionizing radiation is a well characterized source of radicals, and endothelial cells exposed to this source of radicals also generate oxidatively fragmented phospholipids with PAF-like activity (84). Although smoking and radiation can generate large amounts of oxidizing radicals, it is possible that other sources, while less prolific in their generation of reactive oxygen species, may produce a similar inappropriate stimuli to inflammation. One source of radicals that is often overlooked is diet. This is particularly true for fried foods where, for instance, french fries may contain up to 8% oxidized materials (85). This radical source is detrimental because feeding rabbits a diet enriched in oxidized oil increased the amount of lipid peroxides in circulating lipoprotein particles (86), which are the immediate precursors for oxidatively fragmented phospholipids. This increase in circulating oxidized lipids increased the rate of atherogenesis two- to fourfold (87). This occurred when animals were fed oxidized oils well below that found in just a medium-sized order of french fries. Moreover, humans who ingest oxidized lipid show increased levels of oxidized lipids in their circulating lipoprotein particles (85,88), suggesting this as another important source of oxidizing radicals and inflammatory compounds that may exacerbate atherosclerotic and diabetic vascular disease (88).

IX. EXTENSION OF THE INFLAMMATORY REACTION

Reactive oxygen species may directly generate inflammatory responses by creating inflammatory mimetics of PAF, but they also can induce the inappropriate synthesis of authentic PAF. Endothelial cells stimulated with hydrogen peroxide, in contrast to organic peroxides that generate oxidatively fragmented phospholipids with PAF-like activity (73), enzymatically synthesize PAF (89). A similar event is found in epithelial cells exposed to a peroxide load (90), where extension of the original insult through the synthesis of PAF may attract leukocytes into oxidatively damaged dermis.

An additional effect of oxidants on the inflammatory process is through their effect on endothelial cell proteins that tether leukocytes to activated endothelium. Leukocyte extravasation is a two-step process (13) where P-selectin brings passing leukocytes into the proximity of the PAF synthesized and localized on activated endothelial cells (11,12). Oxidants cause endothelial cells to express P-selectin not in the regulated and transient way induced by physiological agonists, but rather for quite prolonged periods of time (91). P-selectin is stored in endothelial-cell Weibel-Palade bodies that also contain von Willebrand factor; accordingly, endothelial cells release von Willebrand factor when exposed to the reactive oxygen species and superoxide (92). There may be a small additional effect of oxidants on the transcription of P-selectin, even though this is not the major form of its regulated expression on the surface of endothelial cells, as antioxidants interfere with its induction (93). The net result is prolonged P-selectin expression on endothelial cells that will bind slowly passing leukocytes where oxidant-induced PAF synthesis and the formation of PAF-like agonists is occurring. This suggests that the inflammatory response may be quite susceptible to inappropriate regulation.

REFERENCES

1. Collins, T. Endothelial nuclear factor-kB and the initiation of the atherosclerotic lesion. Lab Invest 1995; 68:499–508.
2. Sen, CK, and L Packer. Antioxidant and redox regulation of gene transcription. FASEB J 1996; 10: 709–720.
3. Gurtner, GH, and T Burke-Wolin. Interactions of oxidant stress and vascular reactivity. Am J Physiol 1991; 260:L207–211.
4. Cohnheim, J. Lectures on General Pathology: A Handbook for Practitioners and students. London: The New Sydenham Society, 1889.
5. Jaffe, EA, RL Nachman, CG Becker, and CR Minick. Culture of human endothelial cells derived from umbilical veins. J Clin Invest 1973; 52:2745–2756.
6. Zimmerman, GA, RE Whatley, TM McIntyre, DM Benson, and SM Prescott. Endothelial cells for studies of platelet-activating factor and arachidonate metabolites. Methods Enzymol 1990; 187:520–535.
7. Ley, K. Gene-targeted mice in leukocyte adhesion research. Microcirculation 1995; 2:141–150.

8. Wu, KK. Injury-coupled induction of endothelial eNOS and COX-2 genes: A paradigm for thromboresistant gene therapy. Proc Assoc Am Physicians 1998; 110:163–170.

9. Feletou, M, and PM Vanhoutte. The alternative: EDHF. J Mol Cell Cardiol 1999; 31:15–22.

10. Cines, DB, ES Pollak, CA Buck, J Loscalzo, GA Zimmerman, RP McEver, JS Pober, TM Wick, BA Konkle, BS Schwartz, ES Barnathan, KR McCrae, BA Hug, AM Schmidt, and DM Stern. Endothelial cells in physiology and in the pathophysiology of vascular disorders. Blood 1998; 91:3527–3561.

11. McIntyre, TM, V Modur, SM Prescott, and GA Zimmerman. Molecular mechanisms of early inflammation. Thromb Haemost 1997; 78:302–305.

12. Zimmerman, GA, TM McIntyre, and SM Prescott. Adhesion and signaling in vascular cell-cell interactions. J Clin Invest 1997; 100:S3–5.

13. Zimmerman, GA, SM Prescott, and TM McIntyre. Endothelial cell interactions with granulocytes: Tethering and signaling molecules. Immunol Today 1992; 13:93–100.

14. Lorant, DE, KD Patel, TM McIntyre, RP McEver, SM Prescott, and GA Zimmerman. Coexpression of GMP-140 and PAF by endothelium stimulated by histamine or thrombin: A juxtacrine system for adhesion and activation of neutrophils. J Cell Biol 1991; 115:223–234.

15. Springer, TA. Traffic signals for lymphocyte recirculation and leukocyte emigration: The multistep paradigm. Cell 1994; 76:301–314.

16. Powell, LD, and A Varki. I-type lectins. J Biol Chem 1995; 270:14243–14246.

17. Moore, KL, KD Patel, RE Bruehl, L Fugang, DA Johnson, HS Lichenstein, RD Cummings, DF Bainton, and RP McEver. P-selectin glycoprotein ligand-1 mediates rolling of human neutrophils on P-selectin. J Cell Biol 1995; 128:661–671.

18. Mehta, P, RD Cummings, and RP McEver. Affinity and kinetic analysis of P-selectin binding to P-selectin glycoprotein ligand-1. J Biol Chem 1998; 273:32506–32513.

19. Benveniste, J, PM Henson, and C Cochrane. Leukocyte-dependent histamine release from rabbit platelets: The role for IgE, basophils and a platelet-activating factor. J Exp Med 1972; 136:1356–1375.

20. Blank, ML, F Snyder, LW Byers, B Brooks, and EE Muirhead. Antihypertensive activity of an alkyl ether analog of phosphatidylcholine. Bioch Biophys Res Comm 1979; 90:1194–1200.

21. Prescott, SM, TM McIntyre, and GA Zimmerman. Platelet-activating factor: A phospholipid mediator of inflammation. In: JI Gallin, and R Snyderman, eds. Inflammation: Basic Principles and Clinical Correlates. Philadelphia: Lippincott Williams & Wilkins, 1999:387–396.

22. Honda Z, M Nakamura, I Miki, M Minami, T Watanabe, Y Seyama, H Okado, H Toh, K Ito, T Miyamoto, and T Shimizu. Cloning by functional expression of platelet-activating factor receptor from guinea-pig lung. Nature 1991; 349:342–346.

23. McIntyre, TM, GA Zimmerman, and SM Prescott. Leukotrienes C_4 and D_4 stimulate human endothelial cells to synthesize platelet-activating factor and bind neutrophils. Proc Natl Acad Sci USA 1986; 83:2204–2208.

24. McEver, RP. Regulation of function and expression of P-selectin. Agents Actions [Suppl] 1995; 47:117–119.

25. Whatley, RE, P Nelson, GA Zimmerman, DL Stevens, CJ Parker, TM McIntyre, and SM Prescott. The regulation of platelet-activating factor production in endothelial cells. J Biol Chem 1989; 264:6325–6333.

26. Holland, MR, ME Venable, RE Whatley, GA Zimmerman, TM McIntyre, and SM Prescott. Activation of the acetyl-coenzyme A: Lysoplatelet-activating factor acetyltransferase regulates platelet-activating factor synthesis in human endothelial cells. J Biol Chem 1992; 267:22883–22890.

27. Fijnheer, R, CJ Frijns, J Korteweg, H Rommes, JH Peters, JJ Sixma, and HK Nieuwenhuis. The origin of P-selectin as a circulating plasma protein. Thromb Haemost 1997; 77:1081–1085.

28. Sakai, A, N Kume, E Nishi, K Tanoue, M Miyasaka, and T Kita. P-selectin and vascular cell adhesion molecule-1 are focally expressed in aortas of hypercholesterolemic rabbits before intimal accumulation of macrophages and T lymphocytes. Arterioscler Thromb Vasc Biol 1997; 17:310–316.

29. Stafforini, DM, TM McIntyre, GA Zimmerman, and SM Prescott. Platelet-activating factor acetylhydrolases. J Biol Chem 1997; 272:17895–17898.

30. Ostrovsky, L, AJ King, S Bond, D Mitchell, DE Lorant, GA Zimmerman, R Larsen, XF Niu, and P Kubes. A juxtacrine mechanism for neutrophil adhesion on platelets involves platelet-activating factor and a selectin-dependent activation process. Blood 1998; 91:3028–3036.

31. Lehr, HA, AM Olofsson, TE Carew, P Vajkoczy, UH von Andrian, C Hubner, MC Berndt, D Steinberg, K Messmer, and KE Arfors. P-selectin mediates the interaction of circulating leukocytes with platelets and microvascular endothelium in response to oxidized lipoprotein in vivo. Lab Invest 1994; 71:380–386.

32. Weyrich, AS, TM McIntyre, RP McEver, SM Prescott, and GA Zimmerman. Monocyte tethering by P-selectin regulates monocyte chemotactic protein-1 and tumor necrosis factor-α secretion: Signal integration and NF-kB translocation. J Clin Invest 1995; 95:2297–2303.

33. Weyrich, AS, MR Elstad, RP McEver, TM McIntyre, KL Moore, JH Morrissey, SM Prescott, and GA Zimmerman. Activated platelets signal chemokine synthesis by human monocytes. J Clin Invest 1996; 97:1525–1534.

34. Lehr, HA, C Hubner, B Finckh, S Angermuller, D Nolte, U Beisiegel, A Kohlschutter, and K Messmer. Role of leukotrienes in leukocyte adhesion after systemic administration of oxidatively modified human low density lipoprotein in hamsters. J Clin Invest 1991; 88:9–14.

35. Davenpeck, KL, TW Gauthier, KH Albertine, and AM Lefer. Role of P-selectin in microvascular leukocyte-endothelial interaction in splanchnic ischemia-reperfusion. Am J Physiol 1994; 267:H622–630.

36. Morrow, JD, Y Chen, CJ Brame, J Yang, SC Sanchez, J Xu, WE Zackert, JA Awad, and LJ Roberts. The isoprostanes: Unique prostaglandin-like products of free-radical-initiated lipid peroxidation. Drug Metab Rev 1999; 31:117–139.

37. Morrow, JD, and LJ Roberts. The isoprostanes: Unique bioactive products of lipid peroxidation. Prog Lipid Res 1997; 36:1–21.

38. Harrison, KA, and RC Murphy. Isoleukotrienes are biologically active free radical products of lipid peroxidation. J Biol Chem 1995; 270:17273–17278.

39. Brame, CJ, RG Salomon, JD Morrow, and LJ Roberts II. Identification of extremely reactive gamma-ketoaldehydes (isolevuglandins) as products of the isoprostane pathway and characterization of their lysyl protein adducts. J Biol Chem 1999; 274:13139–13146.

40. Morrow, JD, KE Hill, RF Burk, TM Nammour, KF Badr, and LJ Roberts. A series of prostaglandin F2-like compounds are produced in vivo in humans by a non-cyclooxygenase, free radical-catalyzed mechanism. Proc Natl Acad Sci USA 1990; 87:9383–9387.

41. Morrow, JD, KE Hill, RF Burk, TM Nammour, KF Badr, and LJD Roberts. Formation of unique biologically active prostaglandins in vivo by a non-cyclooxygenase free radical catalyzed mechanism. Adv Prostaglandin Thromboxane Leukotriene Res 1991; 21A:125–128.

42. Pratico, D, JA Lawson, and GA FitzGerald. Cyclooxygenase-dependent formation of the isoprostane, 8-epi prostaglandin F2 alpha. J Biol Chem 1995; 270:9800–9808.

43. Catella, F, MP Reilly, N Delanty, JA Lawson, N Moran, E Meagher, and GA FitzGerald. Physiological formation of 8-epi-PGF2 alpha in vivo is not affected by cyclooxygenase inhibition. Adv Prostaglandin Thromboxane Leukotriene Res 1995; 23:233–236.

44. Morrow, JD, and LJ Roberts II. Mass spectrometric quantification of F2-isoprostanes in biological fluids and tissues as measure of oxidant stress. Methods Enzymol 1999; 300:3–12.

45. Morrow, JD, WE Zackert, JP Yang, EH Kurhts, D Callewaert, R Dworski, K Kanai, D Taber, K Moore, JA Oates, and LJ Roberts. Quantification of the major urinary metabolite of 15-F2t-isoprostane (8- iso-PGF2alpha) by a stable isotope dilution mass spectrometric assay. Anal Biochem 1999; 269:326–331.

46. Lynch, SM, JD Morrow, LJ Roberts II, and B Frei. Formation of non-cyclooxygenase-derived prostanoids (F_2-isoprostanes) in plasma and low density lipoprotein exposed to oxidative stress in vitro. J Clin Invest 1994; 93:998–1004.

47. Pratico, D, RK Tangirala, DJ Rader, J Rokach, and GA FitzGerald. Vitamin E suppresses isoprostane generation in vivo and reduces atherosclerosis in ApoE-deficient mice. Nat Med 1998; 4:1189–1192.

48. Delanty, N, MP Reilly, D Pratico, JA Lawson, JF McCarthy, AE Wood, ST Ohnishi, DJ Fitzgerald, and GA FitzGerald. 8-epi PGF2 alpha generation during coronary reperfusion. A potential quantitative marker of oxidant stress in vivo. Circulation 1997; 95:2492–2499.

49. Morrow, JD, B Frei, AW Longmire, JM Gaziano, SM Lynch, Y Shyr, WE Strauss, JA Oates, and LJ Roberts. Increase in circulating products of lipid peroxidation (F_2-isoprostanes) in smokers. N Engl J Med 1995; 332:1198–1203.

50. Reilly, M, N Delanty, JA Lawson, and GA FitzGerald. Modulation of oxidant stress in vivo in chronic cigarette smokers. Circulation 1996; 94:19–25.
51. Pryor, WA, and K Stone. Oxidants in cigarette smoke. Ann NY Acad Sci 1993; 686:12–28.
52. Miller, ER III, LJ Appel, L Jiang, and TH Risby. Association between cigarette smoking and lipid peroxidation in a controlled feeding study. Circulation 1997; 96:1097–1101.
53. Markesbery, WR, and JM Carney. Oxidative alterations in Alzheimer's disease. Brain Pathol 1999; 9:133–146.
54. Montine, TJ, MF Beal, D Robertson, ME Cudkowicz, I Biaggioni, H O'Donnell, WE Zackert, LJ Roberts, and JD Morrow. Cerebrospinal fluid F2-isoprostanes are elevated in Huntington's disease. Neurology 1999; 52:1104–1105.
55. Gniwotta, C, JD Morrow, LJ Roberts, 2nd, and H Kuhn. Prostaglandin F2-like compounds, F2-isoprostanes, are present in increased amounts in human atherosclerotic lesions. Arterioscler Thromb Vasc Biol 1997; 17:3236–3241.
56. Stremler, KE, DM Stafforini, SM Prescott, GA Zimmerman, and TM McIntyre. An oxidized derivative of phosphatidylcholine is a substrate for the platelet-activating factor acetylhydrolase from human plasma. J Biol Chem 1989; 264:5331–5334.
57. Stremler, KE, DM Stafforini, SM Prescott, and TM McIntyre. Human plasma platelet-activating factor acetylhydrolase: Oxidatively-fragmented phospholipids as substrates. J Biol Chem 1991; 266:11095–11103.
58. Watson, AD, N Leitinger, M Navab, KF Faull, S Horkko, JL Witztum, W Palinski, D Schwenke, RG Salomon, W Sha, G Subbanagounder, AM Fogelman, and JA Berliner. Structural identification by mass spectrometry of oxidized phospholipids in minimally oxidized low density lipoprotein that induce monocyte/endothelial interactions and evidence for their presence in vivo. J Biol Chem 1997; 272:13597–135607.
59. Takahashi, K, TM Nammour, M Fukunaga, J Ebert, JD Morrow, LJD Roberts, RL Hoover, and KF Badr. Glomerular actions of a free radical-generated novel prostaglandin, 8-epi-prostaglandin F2 alpha, in the rat. Evidence for interaction with thromboxane A2 receptors. J Clin Invest 1992; 90:136–141.
60. Lahaie, I, P Hardy, X Hou, H Hassessian, P Asselin, P Lachapelle, G Almazan, DR Varma, JD Morrow, LJ Roberts, 2nd, and S Chemtob. A novel mechanism for vasoconstrictor action of 8-isoprostaglandin F2 alpha on retinal vessels. Am J Physiol 1998; 274:R1406–1416.
61. Kromer, BM, and JR Tippins. Coronary artery constriction by the isoprostane 8-epi prostaglandin F2 alpha. Br J Pharmacol 1996; 119:1276–1280.
62. Kunapuli, P, JA Lawson, JA Rokach, JL Meinkoth, and GA FitzGerald. Prostaglandin F2alpha (PGF2alpha) and the isoprostane, 8,12-iso-isoprostane F2alpha-III, induce cardiomyocyte hypertrophy. Differential activation of downstream signaling pathways. J Biol Chem 1998; 273:22442–22452.
63. Jones, DA, DP Carlton, TM McIntyre, GA Zimmerman, and SM Prescott. Molecular cloning of human prostaglandin endoperoxide synthase type II and demonstration of expression in response to cytokines. J Biol Chem 1993; 268:9049–9054.
64. Martens, JS, M Lougheed, A Gomez-Munoz, and UP Steinbrecher. A modification of apolipoprotein B accounts for most of the induction of macrophage growth by oxidized low density lipoprotein. J Biol Chem 1999; 274:10903–10910.
65. Steinbrecher, UP, S Parthasarathy, DS Leake, JL Witztum, and D Steinberg. Modification of low density lipoprotein by endothelial cells involves lipid peroxidation and degradation of LDL phospholipids. Proc Natl Acad Sci USA 1984; 81:3883–3887.
66. Horkko, S, E Miller, DW Branch, W Palinski, and JL Witztum. The epitopes for some antiphospholipid antibodies are adducts of oxidized phospholipid and beta2 glycoprotein 1 (and other proteins). Proc Natl Acad Sci USA 1997; 94:10356–103561.
67. Stafforini, DM, SM Prescott, and TM McIntyre. Human plasma platelet-activating factor acetylhydrolase: Purification and properties. J Biol Chem 1987; 262:4223–4230.
68. Tjoelker, LW, C Wilder, C Eberhardt, DM Stafforini, G Dietsch, B Schimpf, S Hooper, H Le Trong, LS Cousens, GA Zimmerman, Y Yamada, TM McIntyre, SM Prescott, and PW Gray. Anti-inflammatory properties of a PAF acetylhydrolase. Nature 1995; 374:549–553.

69. Matsuzawa, A, K Hattori, J Aoki, H Arai, and K Inoue. Protection against oxidative stress-induced cell death by intracellular PAF-acetylhydrolase II. J Biol Chem 1997; 272:32315–32320.

69a. Marathe, GK, S Davies, KA Harrison, et al. Inflammatory platelet-activating factor-like phospholipids in oxidized low-density liporoteins are fragmented alkyl phosphatidyl cholines. J Biol Chem 1999; 247:28395–28404.

70. Smiley, PL, KE Stremler, SM Prescott, GA Zimmerman, and TM McInytre. Oxidatively fragmented phosphatidylcholines activate human neutrophils through the receptor for platelet-activating factor. J Biol Chem 1991; 266:11104–11110.

71. Whatley, RE, KL Clay, FH Chilton, M Triggiani, GA Zimmerman, TM McIntyre, and SM Prescott. Relative amounts of 1-O-alkyl- and 1-acyl-2-acetyl-sn-glycero-3-phosphocholine in stimulated endothelial cells. Prostaglandins 1992; 43:21–29.

72. Tokumura, A, K Kamiyasu, K Takauchi, and H Tsukatani. Evidence for existence of various homologues and analogues of platelet activating factor in a lipid extract of bovine brain. Biochem Biophys Res Comm 1987; 145:415–425.

73. Patel, KD, GA Zimmerman, SM Prescott, and TM McIntyre. Novel leukocyte agonists are released by endothelial cells exposed to peroxide. J Biol Chem 1992; 267:15168–15175.

74. Heery, JM, M Kozak, DM Stafforini, DA Jones, GA Zimmerman, TM McIntyre, and SM Prescott. Oxidatively modified LDL contains phospholipids with PAF-like activity and stimulates the growth of smooth muscle cells. J Clin Invest 1995; 96:2322–2330.

75. Church, DF, and WA Pryor. Free-radical chemistry of cigarette smoke and its toxicological implications. Environ Health Perspect 1985; 64:111–126.

76. Lehr, H-A. Adhesion-promoting effects of cigarette smoke on leukocytes and endothelial cells. Ann NY Acad Sci 1993; 686:112–119.

77. Lehr, HA, B Frei, and KE Arfors. Vitamin C prevents cigarette smoke-induced leukocyte aggregation and adhesion to endothelium in vivo. Proc Natl Acad Sci USA 1994; 91:7688–7692.

78. Lehr, HA, E Kress, MD Menger, HP Friedl, C Hubner, KE Arfors, and K Messmer. Cigarette smoke elicits leukocyte adhesion to endothelium in hamsters: Inhibition by CuZn-SOD. Free Radic Biol Med 1993; 14:573–581.

79. Lehr, HS, AS Weyrich, RK Saetzler, A Jurek, KE Arfors, GA Zimmerman, SM Prescott, and TM McIntyre. Vitamin C blocks inflammatory PAF mimetics created by cigarette smoking. J Clin Invest 1997; 99:2358–2364.

80. Lehr, HA, C Hubner, D Nolte, B Finckh, U Beisiegel, A Kohlschutter, and K Mebmer. Oxidatively modified human low-density lipoprotein stimulates leukocyte adherence to the microvascular endothelium in vivo. Res Exp Med 1991; 191:85–90.

81. Imaizumi, T, K Satoh, H Yoshida, H Kawamura, M Hiramoto, and S Takamatsu. Effect of cigarette smoking on the levels of platelet-activating factor-like lipid(s) in plasma lipoproteins. Atherosclerosis 1991; 87:47–55.

82. MacNee, W, B Wiggs, AS Belzberg, and JC Hogg. The effect of cigarette smoking on neutrophil kinetics in human lungs. N Engl J Med 1989; 321:924–928.

83. Terashima, T, ME Klut, D English, J Hards, JC Hogg, and SF van Eeden. Cigarette smoking causes sequestration of polymorphonuclear leukocytes released from the bone marrow in lung microvessels. Am J Respir Cell Mol Biol 1999; 20:171–177.

84. Kimura, H, NZ Wu, R Dodge, DP Spencer, BM Klitzman, TM McIntyre, and MW Dewhirst. Inhibition of radiation-induced up-regulation of leukocyte adhesion to endothelial cells with the PAF inhibitor, BN52021. Int J Radiat Oncol Biol Phys 1995; 33:627–633.

85. Staprans, I, JH Rapp, X-M Pan, KY Kim, and KR Feingold. Oxidized lipids in the diet are a source of oxidized lipid in chylomicrons of human serum. Arterioscler Thromb 1994; 14:1900–1905.

86. Staprans, I, JH Rapp, X-M Pan, and KR Feingold. The effect of oxidized lipids in the diet on serum lipoprotein peroxides in control and diabetic rats. J Clin Invest 1994; 92:638–643.

87. Staprans, I, JH Rapp, X-M Pan, DA Hardman, and KR Feingold. Oxidized lipids in the diet accelerate the development of fatty streaks in cholesterol-fed rabbits. Arterioscler Thromb Vasc Biol 1996; 16: 533–538.

88. Staprans, I, DA Hardman, X-M Pan, and KR Feingold. Effect of oxidized lipids in the diet on oxidized lipid levels in postprandial serum chylomicrons of diabetic patients. Diabetes Care 1999; 22:300–306.

89. Lewis, MS, RE Whatley, P Cain, TM McIntyre, SM Prescott, and GA Zimmerman. Hydrogen peroxide stimulates the synthesis of platelet-activating factor by endothelium and induces endothelial cell-dependent neutrophil adhesion. J Clin Invest 1988; 82:2045–2055.

90. Travers, JB. Oxidative stress can activate the epidermal platelet-activating factor receptor. J Invest Dermatol 1999; 112:279–283.

91. Patel, KD, GA Zimmerman, SM Prescott, RP McEver, and TM McIntyre. Oxygen radicals induce human endothelial cells to express GMP-140 and bind neutrophils. J Cell Biol 1991; 112:749–759.

92. Vischer, UM, L Jornot, CB Wollheim, and JM Theler. Reactive oxygen intermediates induce regulated secretion of von Willebrand factor from cultured human vascular endothelial cells. Blood 1995; 85: 3164–3172.

93. Xia, L, J Pan, L Yao, and RP McEver. A proteasome inhibitor, an antioxidant, or a salicylate, but not a glucocorticoid, blocks constitutive and cytokine-inducible expression of P-selectin in human endothelial cells. Blood 1998; 91:1625–1632.

8

Cytokines and Vascular Inflammation

Elena Csernok and Wolfgang L. Gross
University of Lübeck, Bad Bramstedt, Germany

I. INTRODUCTION

Since the term cytokines was first introduced in 1974, an enormous amount of work has been done to identify and characterize the cytokines and to describe their functions and roles in varied circumstances. Cytokines are proteins or glycoproteins produced by various cell types, but most frequently by lymphocytes, monocytes/macrophages, mast cells, and fibroblasts. They are powerful local mediators that influence important biological processes, including cell survival, proliferation, repair, and fibrosis. Also, these proteins mediate the initiation and maintenance of immune responses and inflammation. Their importance to physiological and pathological processes is undoubted and the clinical application of both the molecules and their antagonists is assuming increasing importance.

Cytokines include proteins described in the literature as interleukins (1–18 at present), interferons (α, β, γ), growth factors or mitogenic cytokines (G-CSF, GM-CSF, VEGF, PDGF), tumor necrosis factors (TNFs), transforming growth factor-β (TGF-β), and chemotactic cytokines (chemokines). To date, at least 90 cytokines have been identified and characterized and every month more novel cytokine molecules are identified, each with a perplexing multiplicity and redundancy of action.

Cytokines mediate their biological effects by binding to their cognate cell–associated receptors. This interaction initiates intracellular signaling pathways that mediate the effector function by activating gene transcription. Cytokines are rarely released as a single species. An individual cytokine is able to stimulate the production of many others generating a network response. Generally, these molecules are produced in small amounts (picomolar to nanomolar concentrations) and act nonenzymatically in a paracrine or autocrine fashion in the local milieu in which they are produced. A minority of cytokines circulate in a bioactive form to be distributed to various tissues via the circulation. The production of cytokines is transient and subject to complex and strict controls and interactions with other cell regulators, such as hormones and neuropeptides.

The goal of this chapter is to provide a survey of cytokines potentially operative in the pathogenesis of vasculitis. Since cytokines are pleiotropic (they exert diverse functions on varied type of cells and tissues), and mediate overlapping activities, the role of specific cytokines that are active in the vascular inflammation requires careful dissection. What needs to be established is which cytokines have the most influence on pathological mechanisms responsible for vessel damage in a given syndrome. This information is not easy to obtain, as the importance of cytokines in pathogenesis may not strongly correlate with their abundance.

II. VASCULAR INFLAMMATION

Over the past few years, novel pathogenic mechanisms leading to vascular inflammation and injury have been discovered. Inflammation is normally a localized, protective response to tissue injury. This process is associated with production of cytokines and chemokines that recruit and activate inflammatory cells. Cytokines such as IL-1β and TNF-α are released early and alter blood flow, increase vascular permeability, increase leukocyte adhesion, promote migration of leukocytes to the inflammatory site, and stimulate these cells to destroy inciting agents. Infiltrating inflammatory cells produce cytokines that amplify an ongoing response. The inflammatory response is typically self-limiting. Changes in the regulatory mechanisms lead to chronic inflammation. Vasculitis, as a clinicopathological process, may occur as a primary process or as a component of another, underlying disease. The clinical spectrum of vasculitides is wide and varied. The vasculitic syndromes share a common histopathological substrate—inflammation and necrosis of the vessel walls—and are generally thought to be mediated by immunopathological mechanisms. Irrespective of the primary immunopathogenic events leading to vasculitis, activation of vascular endothelium by several cytokines plays a pivotal role in the localization and propagation of vascular injury. Cytokine-induced accumulation of inflammatory infiltrates in the blood vessel wall is the common phenomenon shared by all vasculitides, and advances have been made in understanding the interactions between leukocytes recruited into inflammatory site and vascular endothelial cells. The spectrum of cytokines produced simultaneously within the blood vessels encompasses both proinflammatory and antiinflammatory activities, and it seems that in vasculitic lesions the balance is in favor of proinflammatory molecules.

A.   Analysis of Cytokines in Vasculitic Syndromes

Analysis of cytokine action in vasculitic disorders has been limited to some clinical experiments and is confined mainly to the analysis of blood (serum/plasma and cells) and the in situ expression of cytokines in vasculitic lesions.

It is now well established that the development of inflammatory infiltrates in vessel walls relies on dynamic interactions among leukocytes, endothelial cells, and extracellular matrix proteins. Adhesion molecules and cytokines released by endothelial cells and activated inflammatory cells recruited in blood vessels represent key factors in this process. It is evident from our current understanding that vasculitic disorders are associated with abnormal cytokine and cytokine receptor expression. Not surprisingly, both quantitative and qualitative abnormalities of cytokine production have been described in patients with systemic vasculitis. Because cytokines act in autocrine, paracrine, or endocrine manner, their detection in vasculitic lesions has significant pathophysiological relevance. It is likely that these mediators actively participate in the pathogenesis of vessel occlusion and repair of vasculitis. The main cytokines particular relevant for the pathogenesis of various vasculitides are summarized in Table 1.

The findings concerning serum or plasma levels of cytokines in vasculitic syndromes are difficult to interpret since these may be affected by soluble cytokine receptors, inhibitors, and natural antibodies to cytokines. The increase of serum levels of proinflammatory cytokines in vasculitis patients could explain, at least in part, the presence of systemic manifestations (fever, weight loss, malaise) that are common in vasculitic disease. Several studies have provided evidence that in the context of vasculitis, constitutional symptoms are linked closely to the presence of elevated levels of circulating cytokines and soluble cytokine receptors that are shed from the cell surface, such as sIL-2R, sTNFR or sIL-6R (11,21,29).

Table 1 Principal Cytokines Known to Be Involved in the Pathogenesis of Various Vasculitis Syndromes

Cytokine	Cellular source	Function/potential role in vessel damage
Proinflammatory cytokines		
IL-1α, β	Monocytes, macrophages, EC, T cells, NK cells, etc.	Induces ELAM-1 and ICAM-1 on endothelial cells; induces procoagulant activity in EC; decreases fibrinolytic activity of EC; activates T cells
TNF-α	Monocytes, tissue macrophages, T, B cells, EC, NK cells, etc.	Similar to IL-1; enhances ANCA antigen expression
Lymphotoxin	Monocytes, tissue macrophages, T cells	Induces MHC class II, ELAM-1, and ICAM-1 on endothelial cells
Interferon-γ	T cells, NK cells	Induces MHC class II, ELAM-1, and ICAM-1 on endothelial cells
IL-2	T cells, B cells	Activates T-cells
IL-6	Monocytes/macrophages, EC, smooth muscle cells, T cells	Stimulates T-cell proliferation; stimulates B-cell immunoglobulin production; stimulates fibroblast proliferation
IL-12	B cells, monocytes, macrophages	Increases cytokine production (IFN-γ), proliferation and cytotoxicity on T and K cells
Immune regulatory cytokines		
IL-4	T cells, mast cells	Activates T- and B-cells
IL-10	T, B cells, macrophages, keratinocytes	Inhibits proinflammatory cytokine synthesis, APC function cell inhibited immunity
IL-13	T cells, mast cells, etc.	Regulates B cells and monocyte activity
TGF-β	Monocytes, macrophages, lymphocytes, dendritic cells	Stimulates angiogenesis; increases collagen synthesis; induces TNF-α and IL-1; downregulates growth of EC
Chemotactic cytokines		
IL-8/NAP-1	Endothelial cells, monocytes, tissue macrophages, fibroblasts	Chemoattractant for neutrophils; downregulates ELAM-1-CD15 interactions, induces ANCA antigen expression
Eotaxin	Epithelial cells and phagocytic cells	Chemoattractant for eosinophils and basophils
Mitogenic cytokines		
Platelet-activating factor (PAF)	Platelets, EC, monocyte/ macrophages, eosinophils, neutrophils	Primes neutrophils to release lysosomal enzymes when binding IC; directly stimulates neutrophils to produce superoxidase radicals and release proteolytic enzymes
VEGF	EC	EC mitogen in vitro and a potent angiogenic factor in vivo

III. PROINFLAMMATORY CYTOKINES

Tumor necrosis factors (TNFs) have well-documented proinflammatory effects in endotoxic shock, tissue inflammation, and autoimmunity. These cytokines are mediators of both specific and nonspecific biological responses and represent a link between immune responses and inflammatory reactions. Tumor necrosis factor-α represents a two-edged sword, in which catabolic effects (cachexia), tissue damage, and death can result from excessive uncontrolled production. Tumor necrosis factor-α is a pleiotropic cytokine produced by macrophages, activated T lymphocytes, and smooth muscle cells. Both mature TNF (often called TNF-α) and lymphotoxin (often called TNF-β) have the same molecular weight (17 kDa) and, similar to interleukin-1, have a precursor form that can remain intracellular. The two forms, TNF-α and TNF-β, represent two distinct but related gene products. Tumor necrosis factor-α exerts its action through two cell surface receptors (p55 and p75 TNFR).

Interleukin-1 is the term for two polypeptides (IL-1α and IL-1β) that possess a wide spectrum of inflammatory, metabolic, physiological, hematopoietic, and immunological properties. Although both forms of IL-1 are distinct gene products, they recognize the same cell surface receptors and share various biological activities. The biological properties of TNF-α are remarkably similar to those of IL-1, particularly the nonimmunological effects of IL-1. Both TNF-α and IL-1 induce the expression of a wide variety of genes (i.e., cytokines IL-1–8, TNF-α, IFN-γ, adhesion molecules, etc.) or suppress the expression of other genes (e.g., albumin, cytochrome P450, etc.).

Interleukin-6 (IL-6) is a 26-kDa cytokine that shares most inflammatory effects with IL-1 or TNF-α, and synergizes with these cytokines to amplify the immune response. In some models, the production of IL-6 appears to be under control of IL-1. Like IL-1 and TNF-α, IL-6 is an endogenous pyrogen and an inducer of acute-phase proteins.

Generally, activation of monocytes/macrophages by different stimuli rapidly induces a group of proinflammatory cytokines, including TNF-α, IL-1α and β, and IL-6. These proinflammatory cytokines are produced by cells participating in the development of vascular lesions. A variety of cell types, including macrophages, T lymphocytes, fibroblasts, endothelial cells, and smooth muscle cells, all of which are present in the inflamed vessel wall, can express the receptors for TNF and are therefore capable of responding to TNF if it is produced during inflammation. Interleukin-1 and TNF-α induce accumulation of leukocytes at local sites of inflammation (probably the physiologically most important local effects of TNF) and stimulate endothelial cell adhesiveness for leukocytes. The biological effects of these cytokines also include activation and migration of leukocytes (T cells, B cells, macrophages, and neutrophils) and procoagulant activities, including the stimulation of tissue factor–like activity and the downregulation of the antithrombotic protein C/protein S pathway.

Several lines of evidence indicate that TNF-α plays a significant role in the development of vascular lesions in human vasculitic syndromes. Elevated levels of TNF-α have been detected in both sera and tissue from patients with different forms of vasculitis. Many studies have demonstrated that TNF (as protein or messenger ribonucleic acid [mRNA]) and its receptors can be detected in almost all vasculitic disorders. Enhanced TNF-α gene expression in mononuclear cells in patients with systemic vasculitis (8), as well as elevated serum levels of TNF-α (12) and soluble TNF receptors (sTNF-55R) and sTNF-75R), have been detected (10,21,27). The effects mediated by TNF-α in vasculitic disorders are presented in Figure 1.

Several studies have focused on the in situ expression of proinflammatory cytokines in vasculitic lesions. In 1993, Noronha et al. (22), in their pioneering work, demonstrated by using different methods [reverse transcriptase-polymerase chain reaction (RT-PCR), in situ hybridization, and immunohistochemical techniques] the production of IL-1 and TNF-α in renal glomeruli from

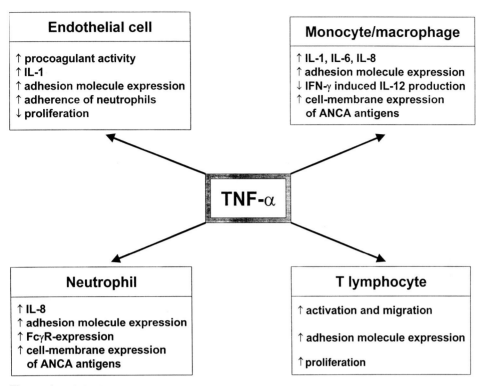

Figure 1 Biological activities of TNF-α in vasculitis.

patients with Wegener's granulomatosis (WG) and microscopic polyangiitis (MPA). Weyand et al. (36) detected by the same technique a number of proinflammatory, angiogenic, and fibrogenic cytokines (IL-1, IL-2, IL-6, TNF-α, interferon-γ [IFN-γ], TGF-β and granulocyte-macrophage colony-stimulating factor [GM-CSF]) in giant cell arteritis (GCA) and polymyalgia rheumatica (PMR) lesions. Patients with PMR and GCA share in situ production of mRNA specific for macrophage-derived cytokines. T cells recruited to vasculitic lesions in patients with GCA predominantly produce IL-2 and IFN-γ. Patients with PMR do not show interferon production, suggesting that IFN-γ may be involved in the progression to overt arteritis (36). Evidence has accumulated that local production of IFN-γ by CD4+ T cells is critical for the formation of inflammatory infiltrates in GCA. Wagner et al. (35) demonstrated that the putatively disease-relevant CD4+ T cells, which are secreting IFN-γ and express IL-2R, represent a very small population of tissue-infiltrating T cells. Interferon-γ–producing T cells in vasculitic lesions of GCA express several markers that identify them as T cells that have been recently stimulated by an antigen-specific receptor. The regulatory function of IFN-γ–producing T cells appears to extend into the inner media and intima where pathological changes in GCA are most pronounced (35).

A. Effects of Proinflammatory Cytokines on Cells Active in Vascular Inflammation

Abnormal production of proinflammatory cytokines is a key element in the immunopathology of systemic vasculitis (26). In vitro experiments indicate that TNF-α in interplay with other cytokines plays a pivotal role in neutrophil-mediated vascular injury. Recently, Bratt and Palmblad (4) analyzed how cytokine stimulation of endothelial cells (ECs) in vitro activates the cytotoxic capacity of polymorphonuclear neutrophil leukocytes (PMN). In this in vitro model of vasculitis, the authors demonstrated that IL-1β, TNF-α, and IFN-γ, act as powerful promoters of cytokine-mediated neutrophil-dependent injury to endothelial cells. Many previous studies have documented that stimulated PMN can cause injury to EC. Chemotactic peptide FMLP or the physiologically occurring lipid product of arachidonic acid, LXA_4, directly stimulate PMN to confer a consistent cytotoxicity. The effect of these two stimuli is dependent on release of proteases, oxygen radicals, and expression of PMN adhesion molecules, and requires Ca^{2+} and Mg^{2+} ions. However, the cytokine-mediated process presented in that work is an example of endothelial injury mediated by neutrophils in the absence of neutrophil agonists. The cytotoxic process of vascular inflammation is dependent on expression of adhesion molecules and may be associated with stimulated nitric oxide (NO) production (4).

Defective apoptosis regulation might lead to a persistent presence of inflammatory cells causing damage to vessel walls. Recently, Tanigushi et al. (32) have demonstrated that mice defective in Fas-mediated apoptotic mechanisms develop a granulomatous arteritis through macrophage activation that might be amplified by macrophage colony-stimulating factor (M-CSF). Both MRL/gld and MRL/lpr strains can develop spontaneous granulomatous arteritis, with infiltration by Mac-2 macrophages and CD4+ T cells, due to defective apoptotic mechanisms. The M-CSF was shown to enhance Fas antigen and Mac-2 expression on spleen cells from MRL/+ mice, as well as granuloma formation. This model clearly demonstrated how the cytokine stimulation and interaction between T cells and macrophages can generate and potentiate permanent damage to vessel walls (32).

The experimental evidence summarized above indicates that cytokines activate endothelial cells in ways that lead to leukocyte accumulation and activation into the blood vessel wall. Recruited inflammatory cells release a variety of cytokines and growth factors. Their effects on endothelial cells and smooth muscle cells account for systemic clinical symptoms and vasculitis. Endothelial cells undergo morphological and functional changes at the sites of cell-mediated immune and inflammatory reactions. Endothelial cells are now known to contribute directly to the control of many aspects of vascular homeostasis, including the process of blood coagulation and fibrinolysis, platelet activation, vasomotor tone and vascular permeability, vessel growth and remodeling, and leukocyte trafficking in normal and pathological conditions. Until recently, vascular endothelium was regarded as an "innocent bystander" or as a victim of the vasculitic processes. A growing body of evidence indicates that endothelial injury is a fundamental step in the development of all types of vasculitis. Recent data have demonstrated that ECs may play an initiating role in vascular disease. Recently, Johnson et al. (15) have demonstrated that adult vascular ECs (venous and arterial endothelial cells) costimulate production of IL-2 and IFN-γ, but not IL-4, by mature T cells. This finding may be important in understanding vasculitis or atherosclerosis.

B. Proinflammatory Cytokines and Antineutrophil Cytoplasmic Antibody–Mediated Vasculitis

Advances have been made in understanding the pathogenesis of WG and MPA by discovery of the presence of antineutrophil cytoplasmic antibodies (ANCAs) in these diseases. The ANCAs have been postulated to play a pathogenic role in vessel injury in these vasculitic syndromes. In vitro data indicate that these autoantibodies enhance the effector pathway of immune responses relevant to vascular inflammation. Accessibility of ANCA antigens appears to be a prerequisite for such an interaction. Tumor necrosis factor-α (and other cytokines such as IL-1 and IL8-8) induces expression of ANCA target antigens on the surface of human neutrophils and monocytes and also induces neutrophils and endothelial cells to increase their expression of adhesion molecules, leading to adhesion of activated neutrophils to the vascular endothelium. Circulating ANCAs bind to membrane-associated antigens and influence neutrophil and monocyte function. This interaction leads to enhanced production of reactive oxygen species and degranulation (ANCA cytokine sequence theory), which damage the vessel walls and the surrounding tissues (13). Furthermore, the release of proteolytic enzymes may subsequently induce shedding of sTNF receptors (TNFRs) from the cell surface or release of sTNF-55R to the intracellular pool (24). While sTNFRs may potentially protect cells for further activation by TNF-α, it has been demonstrated that TNFRs stabilize the bioactivity of TNF-α (1), and hence may contribute to TNF-mediated neutrophil/monocyte activation.

Very recently, Cockwell et al. (5) have studied the role of IL-8 in ANCA-associated glomerulonephritis (GN). They analyzed the intraglomerular expression of IL8 in ANCA-associated GN by in situ hybridization and immunohistochemistry. In vitro, they investigated ANCA-stimulated neutrophil IL-8 production by ELISA (enzyme-linked immunosorbent assay), and the effect of IL-8 on ANCA-stimulated neutrophil supernatants by chemotactic and transendothelial assays. They proposed that the production of IL-8 by ANCA-stimulated neutrophils within the intravascular compartment may frustrate neutrophil transmigration, encourage intravascular stasis, and contribute to bystander damage of glomerular endothelial cells (5).

In summary, proinflammatory cytokines are the orchestrators of neutrophil migration and function in ANCA-associated vasculitis. These cytokines mediate a complex series of endothelial/leukocyte interactions.

C. Proinflammatory Cytokines and Mechanisms of Pathogenic Immune Complex Formation

Among proposed mechanisms of endothelial injury, the most important and best studied is immune complex (IC)–mediated injury. However, the mechanism of IC targeting to specific areas of blood vessels is largely unknown. Elevated circulating levels of cytokines such as TNF-α and INF-γ have been reported in IC-associated vasculitis (12,20). Tumor necrosis factor-α and IFN-γ regulate EC gene expression and cause morphological change. The role of leukocyte FcγR in the pathogenesis of IC-associated vasculitis has been recognized (31). Recently, Pan et al. (23) reported for the first time that TNF-α and IFN-γ enhanced low-affinity FcγR expression on human aortic ECs in vitro. The authors suggested that FcγR expressed on inflammatory cytokine-stimulated ECs may contribute to the specific localization of circulating IC in blood vessel endothelium and thereby contribute to vasculitis (23).

Taken together, the data presented above indicate that proinflammatory cytokines TNF-α, IL-β, and IL-6 are key cytokines in human vasculitic syndromes. Whatever the initial antigenic stimuli may be, these cytokines play a pivotal part and might be appropriate therapeutic targets. However, the consequences of anticytokine therapy on the immune system (host defense, Th1/Th2 balance, leukocyte and endothelial cell activities) are still unexplored.

IV. MITOGENIC CYTOKINES

Vascular endothelial growth factor (VEGF) is an endothelial cell mitogen in vitro and a potent angiogenic factor in vivo (9). The main inducer of VEGF is hypoxia, but its expression is regulated by a variety of hormones, growth factors, and cytokines (Il-6, TGF-β). It is detected in areas where ECs are proliferating and also around microvessels in areas were ECs are normally quiescent. In mice deficient for VEGF expression, the formation of blood vessels is severely impaired, whereas overexpression of VEGF in quail results in hypervascularity and hyperpermeability (9). Concerning the function of VEGF, Li et al. (17) hypothesized that it may be important in pathobiology of vasculitis and they measured levels of VEGF in the serum from patients with active WG. The VEGF levels are raised in WG compared with controls and may be a marker of disease activity. However, VEGF does not seem to be specific for a particular disease. It is probably a nonspecific marker for vascular disorders in which EC damage/repair occurs (17).

To elucidate the involvement of VEGF in the pathogenesis of Kawasaki disease (KD), Terai et al. (33) investigated 30 patients with acute KD, comparing the time course of plasma VEGF levels with clinical symptoms and laboratory findings. They also measured the plasma levels of TGF-β and TNF-α, both of which can upregulate VEGF in vitro. They found markedly elevated VEGF levels in plasma from patients with acute KD. The VEGF levels at the appearance of rash and/or edema of hands and feet were also elevated and in 23% patients, plasma levels remained increased after the resolution of these symptoms. Furthermore, the authors found that the plasma levels of VEGF were highly correlated with those of TGF-β. Vascular endothelial growth factor may be involved in the hyperpermeability of local blood vessels in acute KD (33).

Platelet-derived growth factor (PDGF) is produced locally in the blood vessel wall and regulates mobilization, migration, and proliferation of vascular smooth muscle cells (VSMC). In a recent study, Kaiser et al. (16) explored the hypothesis that GCA is associated with vaso-occlusion resulting from a growth factor–dependent fibroproliferative process. They demonstrated that PDGF, a prototypic growth factor implicated in driving intimal hyperplasia in nonvasculitic arterial diseases, is upregulated in tissue-infiltrating and stromal cells in arteries affected by GCA. CD68+ macrophages, smooth muscle cells, and multinucleated giant cells produced PDGF, whereas hyperplastic intimal tissue did not. Correlation of tissue expression of PDGF and ischemic complications suggested that PDGF has a role in arterial occlusion in GCA. The excessive fibroproliferative response, leading to luminal narrowing could be distinguished from the stenosing process in atherosclerosis and postangioplasty restenosis, suggesting that there are different response patterns to arterial injury. In GCA, macrophages at the media–intima border were the dominant source of PDGF. The authors concluded that inhibition of intimal proliferation should be a major goal of treatment in GCA, and therapeutic measures targeting the action of PDGF could complement steroid therapy, which causes a high rate of side effects in the elderly population affected by GCA (16).

V.   IMMUNOREGULATORY CYTOKINES

A.   T Lymphocyte–Derived Cytokines in Vasculitic Syndromes

The characterization of different subsets of T helper (Th) cells is directly related to their cytokine profiles and several disorders may now be classified according to the predominance of a particular T helper cell subset. We will briefly summarize the Th1/Th2 hypothesis and how it relates to vasculitides, and highlight recent studies that question this hypothesis.

1.   The Th1/Th2 Model

The discovery of T helper lymphocyte subsets (Th1 and Th2) that differ in their cytokine secretion patterns and effector functions has provided a model for understanding how cytokines regulate pathological immune and inflammatory responses.

Figure 2 summarizes the cell types and cytokines involved in the polarization of T cells and the major differences between Th1 and Th2 cells in terms of cytokine profile and function. Th1 lymphocytes secrete interleukin 2 (IL-2), IFN-γ, and tumor necrosis factor-β (TNF-β or lymphotoxin). Th2 cells, on the other hand, secrete IL-4, IL-5, IL-6, IL-9, IL-10, and IL-13. Both cell types

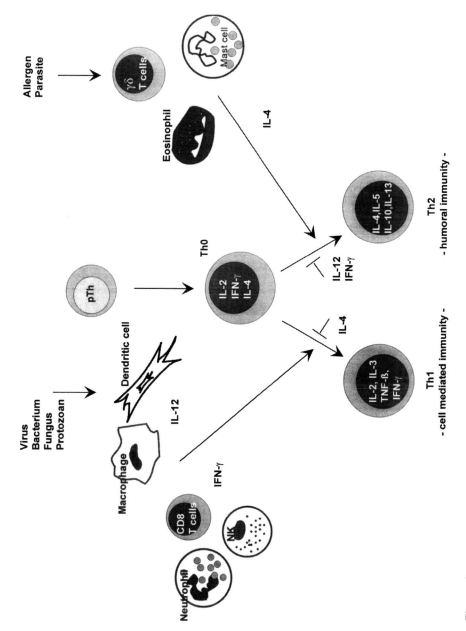

Figure 2 Cell types and cytokines.

originate from the same precursor lymphocyte (Th0) and their differentiation is partially determined by cytokines present at time of antigen recognition. The presence of IFN-γ and IL-12 favors the Th1 phenotype, while IL-4 and IL-10 promote generation of Th2 cells. Thus, cytokines themselves can alter the subsequent cytokine profile produced by T cells. Th1 cells support cell-mediated immunity, while Th2 cells provide B-cell help and also suppress cell-mediated immunity.

The balance between cytokines from Th1 and those from Th2 cells is thus critical in determining the outcome of the immune and inflammatory response and any disturbance could have profound pathological effects.

2. The Th1/Th2 Concept and Vasculitic Disorders

There is now considerable interest in evaluating whether development of vascular lesions are due to abnormalities of the Th1/Th2 balance. Few studies have directly addressed the predominance of a particular T-helper-cell subset in vasculitic syndromes.

Analysis of tissue cytokine patterns in patients with PMR and GCA (see above) indicated that the granulomatous reaction in GCA is associated with a localized immune response of exclusively the Th1 pathway. The pattern of T cell–derived cytokines found in inflamed tissue indicated that a selected type of helper T cells, the IFN-γ–producing T cells, are crucially involved in the formation of the granulomatous infiltrate (36).

Recently, our group has investigated the cytokine pattern (Th1 and Th2) in WG by analyzing the profile of cytokine secretion by T cells derived from tissue with granulomatous inflammation (nasal mucosal biopsy specimens) or from an area close to the site of granulomatous inflammation (bronchoalveoler lavage [BAL]) and, for comparison, from peripheral blood (PB). In this study we used different experimental approaches, and cytokines were detected by ELISA and a competitive RT-PCR. Our results demonstrate that the Th1 pattern is the main cytokine profile exhibited by T-cell clones (TCCs) isolated from nasal biopsy specimens displaying granulomatous inflammation and, to a lesser extent, by TCCs and T cell lines (TCLs) generated from BAL cells. In addition, both polyclonal CD4+ and CD8+ T cells from PB and BAL produced predominantly IFN-γ. These findings fit well with the concept that T cells play a triggering role in the pathogenesis of WG (7). Lúdvíksson et al. (18) addressed the question if WG falls in the same or different category as GCA by examining the profile of cytokine secretion of circulating T-cell populations from patients with WG. They found that active WG is associated with HLA-DR+ CD4+ T cells exhibiting an unbalanced Th1-type T-cell cytokine pattern.

The mechanisms responsible for the preferential development of Th1 cells in granuloma have not yet been investigated. Th1-dominant responses are very effective in eradicating infectious agents, including those hidden within the cells; however, if the Th1 response is not effective or is excessively prolonged, it may become dangerous for the host due to both the activity of cytotoxic cytokines and the strong activation of phagocytic cells. The local secretion of high levels of IFN-γ may represent an important amplification loop leading to a tissue-destructive inflammatory response in patients. The IFN-γ activates local macrophages and granulocytes to produce proinflammatory cytokines and toxic metabolites, which cause damage to the tissue and maintain the inflammation.

Interleukin-12 produced by macrophages in response to various stimuli is a potent inducer of IFN-γ production. Interferon-γ, in turn, markedly enhances IL-12 production. Recently, Hodge-Dudour et al. (14) demonstrated that TNF can inhibit IFN-γ priming for enhanced IL-12 production and thereby interrupt the amplification loop involving IFN-γ and IL-12. To determine whether TNF inhibition of IFN-γ–induced IL-12 production contributed to the resolution of an inflammatory response in vivo, the responses of TNF+/+ and TNF–/– mice injected with *Corynebacterium parvum* were compared. TNF–/– mice developed a delayed, but vigorous, inflammatory response leading to death, whereas TNF+/+ mice exhibited a prompt response that resolved. Serum IL-12 levels were elevated threefold in *C. parvum*-treated TNF–/– mice compared with TNF+/+ mice. Treatment with anti–IL-12 antibody led to resolution of the response to *C. parvum* in TNF–/– mice. The authors conclude that the role of TNF in limiting the extent and duration of inflammatory responses in vivo involves its capacity to regulate macrophage IL-12 production (14).

Fujioka et al. (38) recently investigated the mRNA expression of cytokines from skin lesions in Churg–Strauss syndrome. Cytokine mRNA expression differed according to the degree of cellular infiltration. In the presence of marked infiltration, counteracting Th1 and Th2 cytokines were simultaneously detected; the former included IL-12 and IFN-γ, and the latter IL-6 and IL-10. The concurrence of both types of cytokines could be attributed to different factors. For example, IL-6 is involved in the formation of immune complexes by IgG, and IL-12 and IFN-γ appeared to participate in the development of granuloma. It is also inferred that the dominance of one of the two types of cytokines depends on the clinical phase of the disease.

Sugi-Ikai et al. (30) analyzed the Th1 (IL-12 and IFN-γ) and Th2 (IL-4) cytokine profile of CD4+ and CD8+ cells in peripheral blood in patients with active and inactive Behçet's disease (BD) and the effect of immunosuppressive drugs on the profile of cytokine-producing cells was evaluated. The frequencies of Th1 cytokine-producing CD4+ and CD8+ cells increased in patients with active BD. Effective immunosuppressive treatment decreased the population of Th1-producing cells. These results suggest a possible role for Th1 cytokine–producing cells in the immunopathogenesis of BD (30).

Taken together, there is some clinical and experimental evidence that the dysregulation of the Th1/Th2 cytokine balance may play a key role in orchestrating the immune response in vasculitic diseases. However, cytokines, predicted by the Th1/Th2 hypothesis to either promote or prevent injury, may have dual functions in the immunopathogenesis of vasculitis disorders. IFN-γ, which activates macrophages, may play a critical role in downregulating activated T cells. Conversely, IL-4, which has important antiinflammatory properties, also induces polyclonal B cell activation. The Th1/Th2 concept is a useful paradigm for understanding T cell differentiation and regulation, but the immune responses and disease manifestations in vasculitic syndromes are more complex and may not be so highly polarized as to depend on only one effector population.

B. Transforming Growth Factor-β

Transforming growth factor-β is a small family of multifunctional cytokines (TGF-β1, 2, and 3) that display both growth-promoting and growth-inhibitory properties on a wide range of cell types. In animal models of human autoimmune disease, local or systemic administration of TGF-β can modulate the onset and course of inflammatory processes (2,3). Transforming growth factor is produced by every hematopoietic cell lineage, including dendritic cells, macrophages, lymphocytes, and natural killer (NK) cells. Although a number of different experimental systems have produced conflicting results regarding the influence of TGF-β on T helper differentiation, the production of this cytokine by antigen-specific T cells may define a unique Th subset, referred to as TGF-β–producing Th cells, or Th3. This cytokine has received recent attention in vasculitic disorders. Transforming growth factor-β stimulates angiogenesis and increases collagen synthesis. In temporal artery biopsies from patients with GCA and PMR, TGF-β levels were elevated and promoted migration of inflammatory cells to the vessel wall. Furthermore, it was demonstrated that this cytokine diminished growth of endothelial cells and induced expression of other cytokines, such as TNF-α and IL-1 (37). Our own laboratory (6) has investigated the expression of TGF-β and possible interactions of this cytokine with ANCA autoantigen (proteinase 3 [PR3]) in WG. Specifically, we examined the effects of TGF-β on translocation of the lysosomal enzymes to the cell surface of PMNs and possible activation of nonbioactive, latent TGF-β by these enzymes. The TGF-β1 isoform was found to be overexpressed in WG and to correlate with disease activity, while TGF-β2 levels were not elevated. Flow cytometry analysis of TGF-β1 function showed TGF-β1 to be a potent translocation factor for PR3 comparable with other neutrophil activating factors such as IL-8. The membrane expression of PR3 on primed PMNs increased by up to 51% after incubation with TGF-β1. Moreover, PR3 itself was revealed as a potent activator of latent TGF-β, and thus was able to mediate the biological effects of this cytokine. These surprising findings, together with other TGF-β capabilities, such as induction of angiogenesis and its strong chemotactic capacity, indicate that TGF-β might serve as a proinflammatory factor involved in the cascade of immunological events and resulting in inflammation and tissue destruction in WG (6). Thus, further investigation and prospective studies are necessary to clarify the clinical and pathophysiological role of these phenomena in the pathogenesis of vasculitic disease.

VI. CYTOKINES: CLUES TO THE PATHOLOGY OF VASCULITIC SYNDROMES?

Most of the vasculitic syndromes are mediated by immunopathogenic mechanisms that have been traditionally classified into four types (I–IV) analogous to those described by Coombs and Gell for the various forms of hypersensitivity reactions (13). Accordingly, clinicopathological and immunohistochemical studies led to the terms allergic angiitis (type I reaction), autoantibody-associated vasculitis (type II reaction), immune complex vasculitis (type III reaction) and vasculitis associated with T cell–mediated hypersensitivity (type IV reaction). We have attempted to apply this simplistic approach to what is now known about the role of cytokines in the pathogenesis of vasculitic syndromes. A simplified scheme is depicted in Figure 3.

A. Type I: Vasculitides Strongly Associated with Atopic Disorders (Allergic Vasculitis)

Urticarial vasculitis (UV) and, more characteristically, Churg–Strauss syndrome (CSS) are vasculitides strongly associated with atopic disorders, or type I reactions, in the classification of Gell and Coombs. In these disease entities, activated Th2 lymphocytes play a central role through their production of cytokines, such as IL-4, IL-5, IL-13, mediating the accumulation of mast cells, basophils, and eosinophils and the hyperproduction of IgE. Bridging of IgE-receptors on these cells leads to secretion of inflammatory and toxic mediators. While UV is predominantly induced by degranulation of mast cells, in CSS activation of eosinophils is a central feature, where eosinophil cationic protein, eosinophil-derived neurotoxin, and lipid mediators (LTC4, platelet activation factor [PAF]) seem to play a major role in induction of eosinophilic vasculitis. Interleukin-5 and to a lesser extent GM-CSF or IL-3 act as specific growth and differentiation factors for eosinophils and are selective chemoattractants in tissue. Furthermore, IL-5 induces the expression of adhesion molecules CD18/11b, promoting enhanced adhesion of eosinophils on human microvascular endothelial cells in vitro. Interleukin-5, and also IL-3 and GM-CSF, activate eosinophils in vitro, leading to degranulation (34). Moreover, eotaxin is a selective and highly potent chemotaxin for eosinophils, which specifically binds to the chemokine receptor CCR3, expressed on eosinophils, and activates these cells. In this regard, PAF and eotaxin can act synergistically. More recently, the treatment with interferon-α has shown to counterbalance the Th2 predominance in CSS (38).

B. Type II: Vasculitides Strongly Associated with Autoantibodies

The ANCA-associated vasculitides (WG, MPA) and Goodpasture's syndrome (antiglomerular basement membrane antibody disease [GBM]) belong to type II immune reactions, or vasculi-

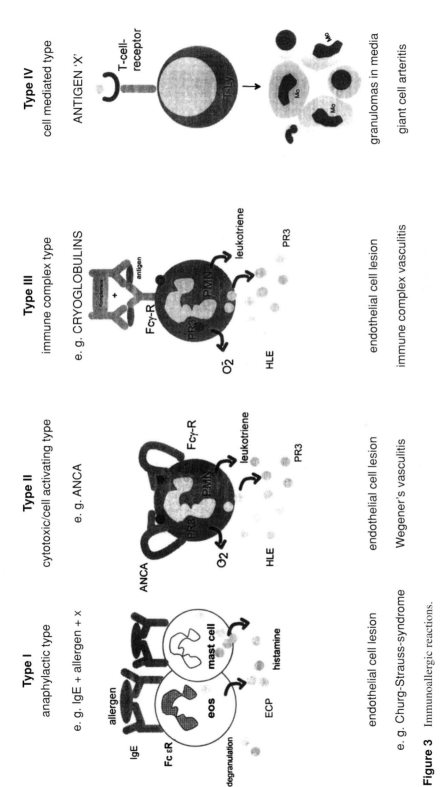

Figure 3 Immunoallergic reactions.

tides strongly associated with autoantibodies. As described above, autoantibodies (ANCAs) are involved in the immunopathogenic mechanisms of these vasculitides, resulting in necrotizing inflammation of blood vessel walls (ANCA cytokine sequence theory) and pauci-immune vasculitis. In pauci-immune vasculitides no (or only few) immune deposits will be found in contrast to the linear deposition of GBM-antibodies seen in Goodpasture's syndrome. The severity of the initial injury is influenced by the amount of antibody bound, the rate of binding, and the extent of priming of leukocytes. For example, injury is increased by the proinflammatory cytokines TNF-α and IL-1. Mouse strains that are predisposed to a Th1-type immune response develop crescentic glomerulonephritis (rapidly progressive renal vasculitis) after receiving a subnephritogenic dose of heterologous anti-GBM antiserum, whereas mice predisposed to a Th2-type response do not (19). In addition, a combination of two Th2-type cytokines (IL-4 and IL-10) suppress crescent formation (25).

C. Type III: Vasculitides Strongly Associated with Immune Complexes

Circulating immune complexes or in situ immune complex formation are widely accepted as inducers for vasculitis. The pathogenic mechanisms leading to Schönlein–Henoch purpura, essential cryoglobulinemic vasculitis, cutaneous leukocytoclastic angiitis, and classic polyarteritis nodosa can therefore be characterized as vasculitides strongly associated with immune complexes (type III reaction). Immunohistochemical demonstration of humoral immune components (immunoglobulins, complement factors) in situ in blood vessel walls, often combined with polyclonal hypergammaglobulinemia and autoantibody production (antinuclear antibodies, rheumatoid factor), are hallmarks of these conditions. Th2-type cytokines, such as IL-10 and IL-6, seem to play a central role by promoting B-cell activation. In MRL/lpr mice deficient in IL-4 and in the mercuric chloride ($HgCl_2$)–induced autoimmune syndrome, Th2-type cytokines exaggerate immune complex nephritis (25).

D. Type IV: Vasculitides Strongly Associated with T Cell–Mediated Hypersensitivity

The type IV immune reaction summarizes vasculitides strongly associated with T cell–mediated hypersensitivity and includes large-vessel vasculitides (giant cell arteritis and Takayasu's arteritis). These are often described as granulomatous vasculitides, however without deposition of immune complexes in situ or ANCA association. Characteristically, accumulation of lymphocytes and monocytes can be seen in blood vessel walls, with a preponderance of IFN-γ producing CD4+ T cells (Th1-type cells).

Although this scheme allows a simple classification according to central pathogenic mechanisms, more than one type of immune reaction may be involved during the course of a single disease entity, and overlap syndromes may occur.

VII. SUMMARY

This chapter summarized the work of several laboratories investigating cytokine expression in vasculitic disorders over the last 10 years. From the data presented it is apparent that while many studies have been performed to investigate cytokines, both in peripheral blood and in the local vasculitic lesions, their role in the pathophysiology of the vasculitic disorders is not yet completely clear. Cytokines play a role in all forms of inflammation. It is no surprise that the increased presence of these mediators in vasculitis has been convincingly demonstrated. Our knowledge of the precise role of cytokines and the extent to which they are relevant in different phases of disease processes is still very limited. Based on current understanding of the pathogenesis of sytemic vasculitis, it can be postulated that cytokine-mediated changes in the expression and function of adhesion molecules coupled with inappropiate activation of inflammatory cells and endothelial cells are the primary factors influencing the degree and location of vessel damage in the vasculitic syndromes. Progress in the study of cytokines in vessel injury will provide new concepts regarding the pathogenesis of vasculitic syndromes and will probably reveal new therapeutic opportunities.

REFERENCES

1. Aderka D, Engelmann H, Maor Y, Brakebusch C, Wallach D. Stabilization of the bioactivity of tumor necrosis factor by its soluble receptors. J Exp Med 1992; 175:323–329.
2. Allen JB, Manthey CL, Hand AR, O'Hura K, Ellingworth L, Wahl SM. Rapid onset synovial inflammation and hyperplasia induced by transforming growth factor β. J Exp Med 1990; 171:231–247.
3. Brandes ME, Allen JB, Ogawa Y, Wahl SM. TGFβ1 suppresses leucocyte recruitment and synovial inflammation in experimental arthritis. J Clin Invest 1991; 87:1108–1113.
4. Bratt J, Palmblad J. Cytokine-induced neutrophil-mediated injury of human endothelial cells. J Immunol 1997; 159:912–918.
5. Cockwell P, Brooks CJ, Adu D, Savage COS. Interleukin-8: A pathogenetic role in antineutrophil cytoplasmic autoantibody-associated glomerulonephritis. Kidney Int 1999; 55:852–863.
6. Csernok E, Szymkowiak C, Mistry N, Daha MR, Gross WL, Kekow J. TGF-beta expression and interactions with proteinase 3 in ANCA-associated vasculitis. Clin Exp Immunol 1996; 105:104–111.
7. Csernok E, Trabandt A, Müller A, Wang G, Moosig F, Paulsen J, Schnabel A, Gross WL. Cytokine profiles in Wegener's granulomatosis: Predominance of type 1 (Th1) in the granulomatous inflammation. Arthritis Rheum 1999; 42:742–750.
8. Deguchi Y, Shibata N, Kishimoto S. Enhanced expression of the tumour necrosis factor/cachectin gene in peripheral blood mononuclear cells from patients with systemic vasculitis. Clin Exp Immunol 1990; 81:311–314.
9. Ferrara N. The role of vascular endothelial growth factor in the regulation of blood vessel growth. In: Bicknell R, Levis CE, Ferrara N, eds. Tumor Angiogenesis. Oxford: Oxford University Press, 1997: 185–199.
10. Field M, Cook A, Gallagher G. Immuno-localisation of tumour-necrosis factor and its receptors in temporal arteritis. Rheumatol Int 1997; 17:113–118.
11. Gattorno M, Picco P, Barbano G, Stalla F, Sormani MP, Buoncompagni A, Gusmano R, Borrone C, Pistoia V. Differences in tumor necrisis factor-a soluble receptor serum concentrations between patients with Henoch-Schönlein purpura and pediatric systemic lupus erythematosus: Pathogenetic implications. J Rheumatol 1998; 25:361–365.
12. Grau G, Lomband P, Gysler C. Serum cytokine changes in systemic vasculitis. Immunology 1989; 68: 196–198.
13. Gross WL. Immunopathogenesis of vasculitis. In: Klippel JH, Dieppe PA, eds. Rheumatology. 2d ed. London: Mosby, 1997:1–8.
14. Hodge-Dufour J, Marino MW, Horton MR, Jungbluth A, Burdick MD, Strieter RM, Noble PW, Hunter CA, Puré E. Inhibition of interferon-γ induced interleukin-12 production: A potential mechanism for the anti-inflammatory activities of tumor necrosis factor. Proc Natl Acad Sci USA 1998; 95:13806–13811.
15. Johnson DR, Hauser IA, Voll RE, Emmrich F. Arterial and venular endothelial cell costimulation of cytokine secretion by human T cell clones. J Leukocyte Biol 1998; 63:612–619.
16. Kaiser M, Weyand CM, Björnsson J, Goronzy JJ. Platelet-derived growth factor, intimal hyperplasia, and ischemic complications in giant cell arteritis. Arthritis Rheum 1998; 41:623–633.
17. Li CG, Reynolds I, Ponting JM, Holt PJL, Hillarby MC, Kumar S. Serum levels of vascular endothe-

lial growth factor (VEGF) are markedly elevated in patients with Wegener's granulomatosis. Brit J Rheumatol 1998; 37:1303–1306.

18. Lúdvíksson BR, Sneller M, Chua KS, Talar-Williams C, Langford CA, Ehrhardt RO, Fauci AS, Strober W. Active Wegener's granulomatosis is associated with HLA-DR+ CD4+ T cells exhibiting an unbalanced Th1-type T cell cytokine pattern: Reversal with IL-10. J Immunol 1998; 160:3602–3609.

19. Mathieson PW. The ins and outs of glomerular crescent formation. Clin Exp Immunol 1997; 110:155–157.

20. Matsubara T, Furukawa S, Yabuta K. Serum levels of TNF, IL-2 receptor, and IFN-γ in Kawasaki disease involved coronary-artery lesions. Clin Immunol Immunopathol 1990; 56:29–36.

21. Nassonov EL, Samsonov MY, Tilz GP, Beketova T, Semenkova EN, Baranov A, Wachter H, Fuchs D. Serum concentrations of neopterin, soluble interleukin-2 receptor, and soluble tumor necrosis factor receptor in Wegener's granulomatosis. J Rheumatol 1997; 24:666–670.

22. Noronha IL, Kruger C, Andrassy K, Ritz E, Waldherr R. In situ production of TNF-α, IL-1-β and IL-2R in ANCA-positive glomerulonephritis. Kidney Int 1993; 43:682–692.

23. Pan L-F, Kreisle RA, Shi Y-D. Dectection of Fcγ receptors on human endothelial cells stimulated with cytokines tumour necrosis factor-alpha (TNF-α) and interferon-gamma (IFN-γ). Clin Exp Imunol 1998; 112:533–538.

24. Porteu F, Nathan C. Mobilizable intracellular pool of p55 (type I) tumor necrosis factor receptors in human neutrophils. J Leukoc Biol 1992; 52:122–124.

25. Ring GH, Lakkis FG. T lymphocyte-derived cytokines in experimental glomerulonephritis: Testing the Th1/Th2 hypothesis. Nephrol Dial Transplant 1998; 13:1101–1103.

26. Robertson CR, McCallum RM. Changing concepts in pathophysiology of the vasculitides. Curr Opinion Rheumatol 1994; 6:3–10.

27. Roux-Lombard P, Lin HC, Peter JB, Dayer JM. Elevated serum levels of TNF soluble receptors in patients with positive antineutrophil cytoplasmic antibodies. Br J Rheumatol 1994; 33:428–431.

28. Roux-Lombard P. The interleukin-1 family. Eur Cytokine Netw 1998; 9:565–576.

29. Schmitt WH, Heesen C, Csernok E, Rautmann A, Gross WL. Elevated serum levels of soluble interleukin-2 receptor in patients with Wegener's granulomatosis. Arthritis Rheum 1992:35(9): 1088–1096.

30. Sugi-Ikai N, Nakazawa M, Nakamura S, Ohno S, Minami M. Increased frequencies of interleukin-2- and interferon-gamma-producing T cells in patients with active Behcet's disease. Invest Ophthalmol Vis Sci 1998; 39(6):996–1004.

31. Sylvestre DL, Ravetch JV. Fc receptors initiate the Arthus reaction: Redefining the inflammatory cascade. Science 1994; 265:1095–1098.

32. Tanigushi Y, Ito MR, Mori S, Yonehara S, Nose M. Role of macrophages in the development of arteritis in MRL strains of mice with a deficit in Fas-mediated apoptosis. Clin Exp Immunol 1996; 106: 26–34.

33. Terai M, Yasukawa K, Narumoto S, Tateno S, Oana S, Kohno Y. Vascular endothelial growth factor in acute Kawasaki disease. Am J Cardiol 1999; 83:337–339.

34. Tsukadaira A, Okubo Y, Kitano K, Horie S, Momose T, Takashi S, Suzuki J, Isobe M, Sekiguchi M. Eosinophil active cytokines and surface analysis of eosinophils in Churg-Strauss syndrome. Allergy Asthma Proc 1999;20(1):39–44.

35. Wagner AD, Björnsson J, Bartley GB, Goronzy JJ, Weyand CM. Interferon-γ-producing T cells in giant cell vasculitis represent a minority of tissue-infiltrating cells and are located distant from the site of pathology. Am J Pathol 1996; 148:1925–1933.

36. Weyand CM, Hicok KC, Hunder GG, Goronzy JJ. Tissue cytokine patterns in patients with polymyalgia rheumatica and giant cell arteritis. Ann Intern Med 1994; 121:484–491.

37. Weyand CM, Goronzy JJ. Giant cell arteritis as an antigen-driven disease. Rheum Dis Clin North Am 1995; 21: 1027–1039.

38. Fujioka A, Yamamoto T, Takasu H, Kawano K, Maruzawa M, Katsuoka K, Jinno S. The analysis of mRNA expression of cytokines from skin lesions in Churg-Strauss syndrome. J Dermatol 1998; 25: 171–177.

9

Fc Receptors in Vascular Diseases

Robert P. Kimberly

University of Alabama at Birmingham, Birmingham, Alabama

I. INTRODUCTION

IgGs are the most abundant immunoglobulins, and perhaps for that reason, the term "Fc receptors" typically refers to the three families of IgG binding proteins encoded in the human genome and expressed constitutively by one or more specific cell types. These three families, $Fc_\gamma RI$, $Fc_\gamma RII$, and $Fc_\gamma RIII$, contain eight distinct genes and generate even more protein products by alternative splicing within several of the genes. However, the human genome also encodes for receptors for other immunoglobulin classes (IgA, IgD, IgE, and IgM) as well as for Fc receptors with specialized functions in immunoglobulin transport (the neonatal Fc receptor, FcRn; and the polymeric Ig receptor). Although our level of knowledge about each of these other receptors varies, it is certainly likely that at least several of them play an important role in vascular diseases. Intuitively, the IgA receptor ($Fc_\alpha R$, CD89) probably plays an important role in the vasculitis of Schönlein–Henoch purpura, and the IgE receptor ($Fc_\varepsilon R$, CD23) clearly plays a role in the vascular permeability of some urticarias and possibly urticarial vasculitis. In addition to all of these endogenously encoded receptors, it is also important to remember that cells infected with certain herpes viruses can express virally encoded proteins that have Fc receptor–like binding capacity (Fig. 1). These proteins, whose true functions are unknown, raise interesting possibilities for the role of antibodies and immunologically relevant cells in virally induced vascular injury.

From an immunologist's perspective, vascular disease implies "vasculitis"—that is, clear evidence of substantial inflammation leading to vascular damage and a repertoire of clinical diseases, including cutaneous and systemic vasculitides. Of course, vascular diseases encompass a much broader spectrum of pathology than just overt and predominant inflammation with vessel destruction. The interface between classical vasculitis and vasculopathies, including atherosclerosis, has been blurred by new pathophysiological insights. Indeed, immune system cells and low levels of chronic inflammation may play an important part in the development of lesions in atherosclerosis.

Recognizing that the context can be large, the focus of this chapter will be primarily receptors that bind IgG. These receptors may also have other ligands (1–4), and the principles and directions established may pertain to other Fc receptors and Ig binding proteins.

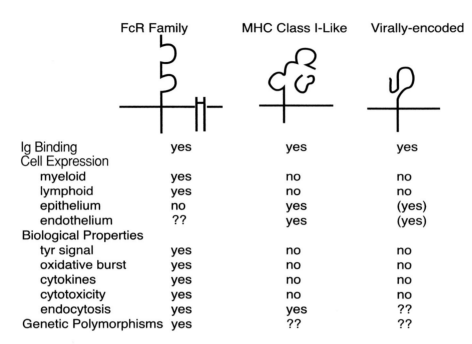

	FcR Family	MHC Class I-Like	Virally-encoded
Ig Binding	yes	yes	yes
Cell Expression			
myeloid	yes	no	no
lymphoid	yes	no	no
epithelium	no	yes	(yes)
endothelium	??	yes	(yes)
Biological Properties			
tyr signal	yes	no	no
oxidative burst	yes	no	no
cytokines	yes	no	no
cytotoxicity	yes	no	no
endocytosis	yes	yes	??
Genetic Polymorphisms	yes	??	??

Figure 1 Types of Fc receptor–like proteins. Each of the immunoglobulin classes binds to distinct endogenous human Fc receptors. Among receptors for IgG, there are three families, each with multiple genes. Differences in Ig binding and signal transduction properties, as well as cell type–specific expression and unique genetic polymorphisms characterize these receptors. Unrelated is the MHC Class I–like receptor involved in Ig transport and catabolism. Virally encoded proteins bear no structural similarities to the endogenous human receptors.

II. SPECTRUM OF Fc RECEPTORS AND Ig BINDING PROTEINS

A. Fc$_\gamma$RI Family

The Fc$_\gamma$RI (CD64) family contains three genes, but only the full-length A gene product (Fc$_\gamma$RIa) has been identified unequivocally as a mature protein on the cell surface (5). Unlike the other human Fc$_\gamma$ receptors, Fc$_\gamma$RIa has three Ig-like extracellular domains and is a high-affinity receptor ($K_a \sim 10^9$ M^{-1}) that binds monomeric IgG. Fc$_\gamma$RIa binds immune complexes or clustered arrays of IgG with a higher net avidity than monomer, but other Fc$_\gamma$ receptors may be more likely to mediate first binding contact with soluble immune complexes since Fc$_\gamma$RIa is typically saturated with monomer. Two different Fc$_\gamma$RIB transcripts, one with a stop codon in EC3 and one splice variant with EC3 deleted (6), can be identified by polymerase chain reaction (PCR), but the human EC3 deletion variant has been difficult to demonstrate as an expressed protein. The cytoplasmic domain of Fc$_\gamma$RIa does not contain a tyrosine activation motif (ITAM) or recognized docking sites for SH2 and/or SH3 domain-containing molecules. Tyrosine phosphorylation events, which are essential for Fc$_\gamma$RIa function, are mediated through the associated Fc$_\varepsilon$RI γ chain that contains an ITAM and is also found in association with Fc$_\gamma$RIII, Fc$_\alpha$RI, and Fc$_\varepsilon$RI (7,8). As with other ITAMs, tyrosine phosphorylation of Fc$_\varepsilon$RI γ chain involves both src kinases (e.g., hck) and syk kinase (9). Fc$_\gamma$RIa mediates phagocytosis, degranulation, generation of a respiratory burst, cytokine production [tumor necrosis factors-α (TNF-α) interleukin 1 (IL-1), interleukin 6 (IL-6), antibody-dependent cell-mediated cytotoxicity (ADCC), and antigen presentation. Interestingly, it also binds C-reactive protein (CRP) and provides one pathway through which CRP modulates the immune response (2).

The Fc$_\gamma$RIa gene has several nonsynonymous, missense single nucleotide polymorphisms (SNPs) that change coding sequence. A rare mutation at codon 92 in EC1 leads to a "stop" codon. Several individuals with this mutation appear clinically well (10). The biology of other coding region SNPs has not been established.

B. Fc$_\gamma$RII Family

The three genes in the Fc$_\gamma$RII family encode glycoproteins of about 40 kDa (11–15). While the extracellular domains of each of these gene products are highly homologous, the cytoplasmic domain of the B gene, which contains a distinctive inhibitory signaling motif, diverges significantly from the A and C genes. All three Fc$_\gamma$RII family gene products are low-affinity receptors ($K_a <$ 10^7 M^{-1}) that do not bind IgG monomer and preferentially bind arrays of IgG as found in immune complexes, opsonized microorganisms, and IgG-coated particles. Three different isoforms are derived from the B gene. Fc$_\gamma$RIIb1 and Fc$_\gamma$RIIb2 differ by a 19 amino acid cytoplasmic domain insert in Fc$_\gamma$RIIb1. Fc$_\gamma$RIIb3 lacks part of the signal peptide. Fc$_\gamma$RIIb1 is expressed in lymphocytes while Fc$_\gamma$RIIb2 is expressed by some myeloid cells. The C gene, the result of an unequal crossover between the IIA and IIB gene, has an Fc$_\gamma$RIIb-like extracellular domain and an Fc$_\gamma$RIIa-like cytoplasmic domain.

The cytoplasmic domain of Fc$_\gamma$RIIa contains an ITAM, which is necessary for a wide variety of receptor-mediated functions, including the respiratory burst, degranulation, phagocytosis, cytokine production and release, and antibody-dependent cellular cytotoxicity. Fc$_\gamma$RIIa signaling involves tyrosine phosphorylation and engages members of the src family of kinases (e.g., fgr) as well as syk kinase (16). Although pertussis toxin, a classical G-protein inhibitor, alters some net signaling functions, G-proteins do not appear to play a primary role in Fc$_\gamma$RIIa signal transduction. Other pathways, such as sphingomyelin-sphingomyelinase, are not yet clearly defined. Because the Fc$_\gamma$RIIb isoform has a tyrosine inhibition motif (ITIM) in the cytoplasmic domain, it has the potential to play an important downregulatory role in cell activation. Fc$_\gamma$RIIb recruits tyrosine phosphatases including SHP-1 and SHIP to signaling complexes (17).

The coding regions of both Fc$_\gamma$RIIa and Fc$_\gamma$RIIb have several missense SNPs that lead to structural polymorphisms (18,19). The two predominant alleles of Fc$_\gamma$RIIa differ by two amino acids, the first at residue 27 in the first extracellular Ig-like domain (EC1) [glutamine (Q) to tryptophan (W)] and the second at residue 131 in EC2 [arginine (R) to histidine (H)]. The change from R to H at residue 131 dramatically affects the binding of human IgG2. The R131 allele, which binds human IgG2 poorly, is associated with certain bacterial infections and with autoimmune disease in some ethnic groups. Conversely, the H131 allele, which binds human IgG2 efficiently, may be associated with an increased risk of heparin-induced thrombocytopenia and of thrombosis in patients with autoimmune antiphospholipid syndrome. The H131 allele may have an increased affinity for human IgG3. A rare substitution in codon 127, changing glutamine (Q) to lysine (K), restores moderate IgG2 binding in the context of the low-binding R131 allele (20). Interestingly, Fc$_\gamma$RIIa has recently been identified as the second receptor for CRP (3,4). This binding is allele sensitive with relative avidities reciprocal to those for IgG2. The impact of the Q127K polymorphism on CRP binding has not been studied.

C. Fc$_\gamma$RIII Family

The Fc$_\gamma$RIII family contains two genes that yield two distinct gene products (11–15). Fc$_\gamma$RIIIa (CD16a) has an intermediate affinity for ligand ($K_a \sim 1$–2×10^7 M^{-1}) and binds monomeric IgG in solution (21). Because multipoint binding leads to a net gain in avidity, Fc$_\gamma$RIIIa preferentially binds immune complexes and clustered arrays of IgG just like other FcR. Fc$_\gamma$RIIIa is a transmembrane protein that associates with Fc$_\varepsilon$RI γ chain in the plasma membrane and requires γ chain both for expression and for signal transduction (22–25). In mast cells, FcRIIIa associates with the β subunit of the high-affinity IgE receptor to form a receptor complex composed of an α chain (Fc$_\gamma$RIIIa), a β chain, and two γ chains (26). This complex does not occur in natural killer cells or mononuclear phagocytes and β chain probably serves to amplify signal transduction. Like other Fc$_\gamma$ receptors, signal transduction depends on tyrosine phosphorylation events which are mediated through the ITAM of the Fc$_\varepsilon$RI γ chain.

Like Fc$_\gamma$RIa and Fc$_\gamma$RII, Fc$_\gamma$RIIIa is structurally polymorphic and these polymorphisms impact on receptor function. Initial evidence suggested that SNPs located in the third exon encoding EC1 and predicting an amino acid change from leucine (L) to arginine (R) or from leucine (L) to histidine (H), might alter binding of human IgG. However, with exploration of the membrane-proximal EC2 domain, a nonconservative T to G substitution that predicts a change of phenylalanine (F) into valine (V) at amino acid 176 (27,28) was found. Multiple studies have demonstrated that EC2 strongly influences ligand binding, and crystal structure now confirms that EC2 contains the ligand binding surface for IgG (29,30). Thus, Fc$_\gamma$RIIIa in V176 homozygotes binds substantially more monomeric IgG1 and IgG3 relative to F176 homozygotes despite identical levels of receptor expression.

Fc$_\gamma$RIIIb (CD16b), the second member of the Fc$_\gamma$RIII family, is a low-affinity receptor ($K_a <$ 10^7 M^{-1}) with expression restricted to neutrophils and eosinophils. Like Fc$_\gamma$RIIa, Fc$_\gamma$RIIIb does not bind monomeric IgG in solution but does bind IgG aggregates. Fc$_\gamma$RIIIb is unique in its linkage to the plasma membrane through a glycosylphosphatidyl inositol (GPI) anchor (31,32). With cell activation, Fc$_\gamma$RIIIb may be released from the cell surface through cleavage by serine protease(s). Fc$_\gamma$RIIIb is rapidly reexpressed by translocation of pre-formed receptor from intracellular stores in secretory vesicles. Fc$_\gamma$RIIIb binds human IgG1 and IgG3 with minimal binding of IgG2 and IgG4. Some evidence suggests suggests that Fc$_\gamma$RIIIb is responsible for IgG3-triggered neutrophil responses (33). Despite the lack of transmembrane and cytoplasmic domains, Fc$_\gamma$RIIIb does initiate tyrosine phosphorylation–dependent signal transduction and cell activation, although the range of cell programs elicited differs in some aspects from that initiated by Fc$_\gamma$RIIa (34). Clustering of Fc$_\gamma$RIIIb can initiate an oxidative burst, degranulation, augmentation of Fc$_\gamma$RIIa-mediated phagocytosis, capacitation of CR3 for phagocytosis, and ADCC for some cell targets.

The Fc$_\gamma$FIIIb has two commonly recognized allelic forms, originally defined serologically as the NA1 and NA2 alloantigens (35). The Fc$_\gamma$RIIIB gene has five SNPs, and the Fc$_\gamma$RIIIb protein product has four polymorphic amino acid residues. These SNPs are grouped into two predominant genotypes; combinatorial grouping of these sites to yield a larger number of alleles does not occur. The "SH" polymorphism, found in <5% of the NA2 Caucasian donors, reflects an uncommon mutation from C to A at nt 266 in codon 78 [alanine (A) to aspartic acid (D)] (36). The NA1 and NA2 alleles have different quantitative levels of function despite comparable binding of IgG-opsonized erythrocytes (37,38). In normal donors, the NA1 isoform mediates a larger Fc$_\gamma$R-mediated phagocytic response and a quantitatively larger oxidative burst and/or degranulation response relative to the NA2 allele. The NA1 and NA2 alleles do have different numbers of N-linked glycosylation sites and are differentially glycosylated in vivo. These posttranslational modifications may mediate interactions with the β2 integrin, CD11b/18 (CR3), in the neutrophil plasma membrane and alter net receptor function (39).

D. Fc Receptors for Other Ig Classes

Fc$_\alpha$RI consists of a single family of molecules most probably derived by alternative splicing from a single gene (40–44). The dominant protein product, Fc$_\alpha$RIa (CD89), is a heavily and variably glycosylated transmembrane protein. Like Fc$_\gamma$RIa and Fc$_\gamma$RIIIa, Fc$_\alpha$RIa lacks recognized signaling motifs in its cytoplasmic domain and associates with Fc$_\varepsilon$RI γ chain which has an ITAM (45);

but unlike $Fc_\gamma RIIIa$, $Fc_\alpha RIa$ does not require the $Fc_\epsilon RI \gamma$ chain for expression. Similar to $Fc_\gamma RIa$ and $Fc_\gamma RIIIa$, $Fc_\alpha RIa$ can initiate degranulation, a respiratory burst, and phagocytosis at least in some experimental systems (46–48). Despite these parallels, $Fc_\alpha RI$ has several distinctive features that suggests it may have some unique functions. It is not encoded on chromosome 1 in the $Fc_\gamma R$ gene cluster but rather on chromosome 19 near the KIR inhibitory receptors. Structurally, it is also distinct in having its ligand interaction site in EC1 rather than EC2.

In many ways, $Fc_\epsilon RI$, the high-affinity receptor for IgE, has served as the prototypic Ig receptor for studies of signal transduction and activation of cell programs (49,50). It forms a multichain signaling complex with the ligand binding $Fc_\epsilon RI \alpha$ chain, the $Fc_\epsilon RI \gamma$ chain and the β chain from the tetraspan family of molecules. In contrast, the IgD receptor bears no structural homology to other FcRs and is a member of the scavenger receptor superfamily. Neither its function, nor the function of the IgM receptor which has not yet been cloned, is well understood.

E. The "Brambell" Fc Receptor, FcRn

The MHC class I-related Fc receptor, FcRn, mediates the intestinal absorption of maternal IgG in neonatal rodents and the transplacental transport of maternal IgG in humans by receptor-mediated transcytosis. FcRn is also expressed by endothelial cells where it modulates the catabolism of serum IgG (51–53). Beta 2 microglobulin knockout mice, which lack a functional FcRn, have altered clearance of IgG and this appears to impact on the pathophysiology of some antibody mediated diseases (54,55). Unlike other FcRs, however, FcRn does not directly activate or modulate cell injury programs and inflammatory responses.

F. Viral Proteins with Fc Receptor Binding Activity

Herpes simplex virus (HSV), varicella-zoster virus (VZV), and cytomegalovirus (CMV) each have endogenous viral genes encoding Fc binding proteins (56–61). The HSV glycoprotein, gE, binds IgG and together with a second glycoprotein, gI, the complex can bind with high avidity. Similar to the glycoproteins encoded by VZV and CMV, neither gE nor gI have any homology with the endogenous human Fc receptors. Although their function is not known, ligation of the viral Fc receptors expressed by infected cells does not activate cells. Perhaps they serve as decoy receptors to prevent ADCC, but perhaps they also capture circulating immune complexes and promote an adhesion cascade for circulating Fc receptor bearing cells.

III. SPECTRUM OF CELLS EXPRESSING Fc RECEPTORS

In the development of vascular disease, Fc receptors might play a role if they are expressed by endothelial cells, if they activate circulating cells, or if they activate cells adherent to endothelium or present in vascular lesions. Fc receptors might also modulate resident vascular dendritic cells or, indirectly through activation of myeloid cells, modulate infiltrating lymphoid cells. An understanding, therefore, of the spectrum of cells expressing Fc receptors becomes important in considering models of pathogenesis.

$Fc_\gamma RIa$ is expressed on myeloid cells (monocytes, macrophages, and CD34+ myeloid progenitor cells) and can be induced on neutrophils by interferon-γ (IFN-γ), IL-10, and granulocyte colony-stimulating factor (G-CSF). $Fc_\gamma RIIa$ is widely found on myeloid cells, platelets, dendritic cells, and perhaps dermal microvascular endothelial cells. $Fc_\gamma RIIb$ is expressed on B lymphocytes and on some myeloid cells while $Fc_\gamma RIIc$ is expressed on some natural killer (NK) cells. $Fc_\gamma RIIIa$ is expressed on NK cells and, depending on the stage of differentiation, on mononuclear phagocytes and renal mesangial cells. Its expression by monocytes is markedly enhanced by IFN-α and by transforming growth factor-β (TGF-β) and decreased by IL-4. Interferon-γ and IL-10, two cytokines that significantly affect Fc$_\gamma$RI expression, have little effect on Fc$_\gamma$RIIIa. Fc$_\gamma$RIIIb is mostly restricted to high-density expression on neutrophils although there is some expression on eosinophils.

Fc$_\alpha$RIa is constitutively expressed on human neutrophils and monocytes with about 6000 to 7000 copies per cell. Its expression is upregulated on activated neutrophils. Among cytokines, TNF-α, IL-8, and GM-CSF increase surface expression of Fc$_\alpha$RIa while IFN-γ and TGF-β downregulate it. Fc$_\epsilon$RI α chain is found on effector cells—mast cells, basophils, and eosinophils—typically associated with an allergic diathesis, but it is also present on antigen presenting cells such as mononuclear phagocytes and dendritic cells. The IgD receptor is expressed in the lymphoid compartment during T cell development and does not appear to be related to the inflammatory response in the periphery.

Of course, the HSV, VZV and CMV Fc receptors are expressed by virally infected cells. The location and density of expression will vary according to the infection, but endothelial cells are often a target.

IV. MODELS OF PATHOPHYSIOLOGY: ADHESION AND ACTIVATION

Although the ITAM-containing Fc receptors are typically conceptualized as receptors that activate cell programs, in the context of vascular disease one can think of Fc receptors both as adhesion and activation receptors (Figs. 2–4). Depending of the degree of activation, one may have

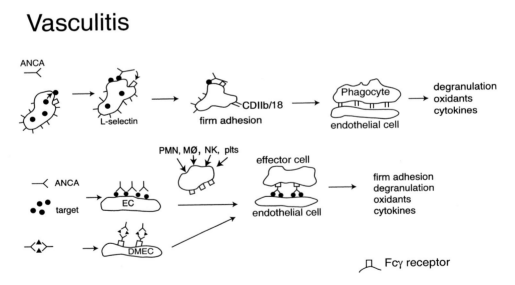

Figure 2   Models of Fc receptors in vasculitis. Specific antibody may target antigens on the surface of circulating cells, subsequently engage Fc receptors on the same cells and trigger them for a variety of cell programs. Alternatively, antibody may target non–Fc receptor bearing cells and then serve simultaneously as "adhesion" and "triggering" molecules for recruited Fc bearing cells. These latter cells might include neutrophils, monocytes, platelets, and NK cells. Immune complexes could serve the same role for both circulating and fixed tissue cells bearing Fc receptors.

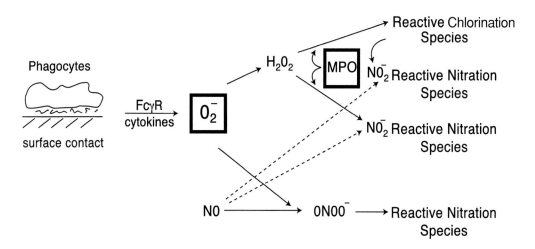

Figure 3   Fc receptors and oxidant-dependent reactions. Phagocytes, especially in the context of surface contact, produce a vigorous respiratory burst in response to cytokines and Fc receptor ligation. In addition, Fc receptors deliver potent signals for degranulation. Superoxide (O_2^-) and myeloperoxidase from azurophilic granules are essential elements for generating reactive chlorination and nitration species.

Vasculopathy

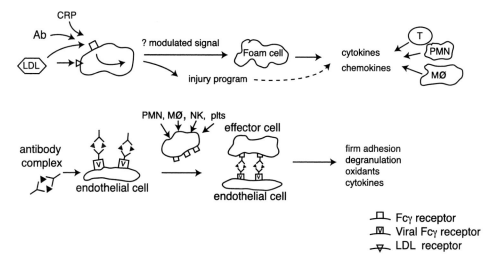

Figure 4   Models of Fc receptors in vasculopathy. Modified LDL may be internalized both by Fc receptors and scavenger receptors, perhaps leading to a modified repertoire of cell programs promoting low-grade inflammation and foam cell formation. Alternatively, virally infected endothelial cells can express IgG binding proteins, which could focus immune complexes on the endothelial surface and recruit Fc-receptor-bearing inflammatory cells.

frank inflammation with "vasculitis" or, perhaps, a much more subtle activation and tissue injury program that over time appears more compatible with less inflammatory "vasculopathy." Atherosclerosis is a compelling example of such subtle activation involving inflammatory cells.

A.   Inflammation with Histological Vasculitis

Vasculitis most probably represents an interplay between an activated endothelium and activated, infiltrating inflammatory cells. However, the nature of the cell injury programs elicited may vary with the properties of the activating stimuli and the types of inflammatory cells recruited. Several different models of antibody-mediated engagement and recruitment of effector cells are possible (see Fig. 2): (1) following antigen-specific binding of antibody to circulating cells, Fc receptor–mediated activation of these cells promotes a proadhesive phenotype, firm adhesion to the endothelium and triggering of a tissue injury program, (2) antibody bound to endothelial cells in an antigen-specific fashion facilitates adhesion of circulating cells or of cells rolling on the endothelium and at the same time triggers a tissue injury program in the effector cell, and (3) antibody bound to endothelial cells in a "nonspecific" fashion, perhaps by immune complexes interacting with endogenously expressed Fc receptors, facilitates adhesion of effector cells and triggers tissue injury programs. The first model has been proposed as a framework for understanding the pathophysiological role of antineutrophil cytoplasmic antibodies (ANCAs) in Wegener's granulomatosis (WG) (62–64), and as such there are several stated elements of the hypothesis that need to be examined. In WG, attention has focused on neutrophils because they are the primary source of proteinase 3, the distinctive ANCA target antigen characteristic of WG.

Element #1: Can Fc_γ Receptors Activate Neutrophils and Promote a
Proadhesive Phenotype?

Neutrophils constitutively express $Fc_\gamma RIIa$ and $Fc_\gamma RIIIb$, and $Fc_\gamma RIa$ can be induced by cytokines such as interferon-γ and GM-CSF. These receptors initiate a wide variety of functions in neutrophils, including the upregulation of CD11b/CD18 necessary for firm adhesion, the respiratory burst, and exocytosis of $1°$, $2°$ and secretory granules (see Figs. 2 and 3). These effector mechanisms can lead to chemical modification of proteins and lipids; targets range from microbial invaders to bystander tissues including endothelial cells. The signaling pathways engaged by $Fc_\gamma RIa$, $Fc_\gamma RIIa$ and $Fc_\gamma RIIIb$ each have some distinctive properties (63,65), and therefore the nature of the neutrophil cell programs elicited by Fc_γ receptor ligation and clustering may vary according to the type of receptor engaged, the stoichiometry of clustering, and the recruitment of other molecules to the signaling cluster capable of modulating the net signaling event. Notably, $Fc_\gamma RIIIb$ has the interesting property of upregulating the CD11b/CD18 adhesion molecule before promoting L-selectin shedding (63). This sequence of events suggests that $Fc_\gamma RIIIb$-mediated activation of neutrophils in the circulation could promote both the rolling and the firm adhesion interactions of neutrophils with endothelial cells.

Element #2: Do ANCAs Activate Neutrophils in an Fc_γ Receptor–Dependent Fashion?

The ANCAs clearly activate neutrophils displaying ANCA targets in an Fc_γ receptor–dependent fashion that favors $Fc_\gamma RIIIb$ (62,65–68). Some ANCAs may be able to fix complement and, perhaps, (co)engage complement receptors; and whether Fc_γ receptors constitute the only pathway for ANCA-mediated activation remains a fruitful area for investigation (69). However, the experimental precedent for an "ANCA-$Fc_\gamma R$" model of pathogenesis in the ANCA(+) vasculitides is clearly established. Intrinsic to this model is the importance of understanding the qualitative and quantitative nature of Fc_γ receptor signaling, especially as induced by ANCAs. The ANCAs preferentially engage Fc_γRIIIb and its unique signaling program (64). This program may have important consequences for neutrophil apoptosis as well as for effector functions.

Element #3: Do In Vitro Experiments Translate to the In Vivo Setting of the ANCA(+) Vasculitides?

The ANCA target antigens are found on the plasma membrane of circulating neutrophils from WG patients. Circulating neutrophils also show other signs of submaximal activation (70). Neutrophils are found in vasculitic lesions; and in some settings, some correlations between ANCA titer, ANCA IgG subclass distribution, and disease activity have been found. The ANCA target display by neutrophils probably results from fusion of intracellular azurophilic granules with the plasma membrane induced by activation stimuli. However, display of ANCA target on cell surfaces can, most probably, also be passively acquired. Exocytosis due to activation with degranulation or to spontaneous apoptosis leads to discharge of granule contents. Passive adsorption of these contents, perhaps as a small vesicle or "ectosome" (71), provides a mechanism for recruiting additional effector cells as well as for targeting other cells (e.g., endothelial cells).

Genetics provides an interesting window on the Fc_γR model in the ANCA(+) vasculitides. One might anticipate that Fc_γR genetic polymorphisms might influence disease phenotype. Fc_γRIIa SNPs do not seem to be important (72,73), a finding which is not surprising since IgG2 ANCAs are not prominent in disease. However, Fc_γRIIIb SNPs may influence disease severity (74,75). Such observations, based on naturally occurring functional point mutants, strongly support a role for Fc_γ receptors in pathogenesis.

Element #4: Do All ANCA Targets Have the Same Biology and Same Disease Phenotype?

Each ANCA target has a characteristic biology. They may reside in different granule compartments, have different resident times on the surface of the neutrophils, have different access to ectosomes, and be handled differently once released from cellular structures. Accordingly, it is not surprising that different ANCAs may not be equivalent (76). The roles of Fc_γRIa, Fc_γRIIb, and Fc_γRIIc, and the factors that affect their expression will be important modifiers in different clinical settings. However, the different signaling pathways may present important opportunities for selective intervention. The relationship of ANCA target type, ANCA class and subclass, specific Fc_γ receptor expression, and corresponding genetic variants all need to be examined in relationship to clinical phenotype.

Of course, none of the three different models of antibody-mediated engagement and recruitment of effector cells are mutually exclusive. Indeed, the recognition that proteinase 3 and myeloperoxidase are characteristically "sticky" suggests that both direct target display on neutrophils and passive adsorption may play a role in pathogenesis of ANCA(+) vasculitides. Similarly, in immune complex vasculitis, circulating complexes might bind to circulating cells or to fixed tissue cells expressing Fc receptors. And, of course, antibodies to endothelial cells or to vascular wall constituents can bind directly to their target antigens and present their respective Fc pieces to Fc receptor bearing cells.

B. Noninflammatory Vasculopathy

Thorough analysis of the pathogenesis of atherosclerosis is beyond the scope of this chapter. Nonetheless, several elements suggest that Fc receptor bearing inflammatory cells may play an important role (see Figs. 3 and 4). Mononuclear phagocytes are the precursors to foam cells, and the footprints of an inflammatory response can be found in atherosclerotic plaques: chlorinated and nitrated proteins indicate degranulation and a respiratory burst, and various chemokines suggest an orchestrated recruitment of immune cells (77,78). Cytokines modulate the athersclerotic response (79).

Generation of reactive chlorination species requires both an oxidative burst and the availability of myeloperoxidase from azurophilic granules. Interestingly, although reactive nitration species may be formed by several different pathways, those derived from the myeloperoxidase (MPO)-catalyzed reaction of H_2O_2 with NO_2^- are highly effective in modifying low-density lipoprotein (LDL) for receptor-mediated uptake by macrophages (77). Fc receptors are among the most potent stimuli for both the oxidative burst and neutrophil degranulation. Blockade of this pathway may be one explanation for the effectiveness of IVIg in retarding the development of athersclerosis in the ApoE knockout model of atherogenesis (80). Of course, postulating a role for Fc receptors in atherosclerosis focuses the search on the appropriate ligand—perhaps antibodies to modified LDL (81) or perhaps C-reactive protein. Quantitatively, the activation response must be modest compared with inflammatory vasculitis, but qualitatively many of the same mechanisms may apply. Thus receptors that recognize opsonins of the innate immune system as well as opsonins reflecting adaptive, acquired immunity may play an equally broad role in the spectrum of vascular disease.

REFERENCES

1. Salmon JE, Kapur S, Kimberly RP. Opsonin-independent ligation of Fc_γ receptors. The 3G8-bearing receptors on neutrophils mediate the phagocytosis of concanavalin A-treated erythrocytes and nonopsonized Escherichia coli. J Exp Med 1987; 166:1798–813.
2. Crowell RE, Du Clos TW, Montoya G, Heaphy E, Mold C. C reactive protein receptors on the human monocytic cell line U937. Evidence for additional binding to $Fc_\gamma RI$. J Immunol 1991; 147:3445–3451.
3. Bharadwaj D, Stein MP, Volzer M, Mold C, Du Clos TW. The major receptor for C-reactive protein on leukocytes is Fc_γ receptor II. J Exp Med 1999; 190:585–590.
4. Stein MP, Edberg JC, Kimberly RP, Mangan EK, Bharadwaj D, Mold C, Du Clos TW. C-reactive protein binding to $Fc_\gamma RIIa$ on human monocytes and neutrophils is allele specific. J Clin Invest. In press.
5. Ernst LK, van de Winkel JGJ, Chiu IM, Anderson CL. Three genes for the human high affinity Fc receptor for IgG (FcgRI) encode four distinct transcription products. J Biol Chem 1992; 267:15692–15700.
6. Porges AJ, Redecha PB, Doebele R, Pan LC, Salmon JE, Kimberly RP. Novel Fc_γ receptor I family gene products in human mononuclear cells. J Clin Invest 1992; 90:2102–2109.
7. Ernst LK, Duchemin AM, Anderson CL. Association of the high-affinity receptor for IgG (FcgRI) with the γ subunit of the IgE receptor. Proc Natl Acad Sci USA 1993; 90:6023–6027.
8. Scholl PR, Geha RS. Physical association between the high-affinity IgG receptor (FcgRI) and the γ subunit of the high-affinity IgE receptor ($Fc_\varepsilon RI_\gamma$). Proc Natl Acad Sci USA 1993; 90:8847–8850.
9. Wang AV, Scholl PR, Geha RS. Physical and functional association of the high affinity immunoglobulin G receptor ($Fc_\gamma RI$) with the kinases Hck and Lyn. J Exp Med 1994; 180:1165–1170.
10. Van de Winkel JGJ, de Wit TP, Ernst LK, Capel PJA, Ceuppens JL. Molecular basis for a familial defect in phagocyte expression of IgG receptor I (CD64). J Immunol 1995; 154:2896–2903.
11. Unkeless JC, Scigliano E, Freedman VH. Structure and function of human and murine receptors for IgG. Annu Rev Immunol 1988; 6:251–281.
12. Ravetch JV, Kinet JP. Fc receptors. Annu Rev Immunol 1991; 9:457–492.
13. Hulett MD and Hogarth PM. Molecular basis of Fc receptor function. Adv Immunol 1994; 57:1–127.
14. Kimberly RP, Salmon JE, Edberg JC. Receptors for immunoglobulin G. Molecular diversity and implications for disease. Arthritis Rheum 1995; 38:306–314.

15. Daeron M. Fc receptor biology. Annu Rev Immunol 1997; 15:203–234.
16. Hamada F, Aoki M, Akiyama T, Toyoshima K. Association of immunoglobulin G Fc receptor II with Src-like protein-tyrosine kinase Fgr in neutrophils. Proc Natl Acad Sci USA 1993; 90:6305–6309.
17. Malbec O, Fridman WH, Daeron M. Negative regulation of hematopoietic cell activation and proliferation by Fc_γ RIIB. Curr Topics Microbiol Immunol 1999; 244:13–27.
18. Warmerdam PAM, van de Winkel JGJ, Vlug A, Westerdal NAC, Capel PJA. A single amino acid in the second Ig-like domain of the human Fc_γ receptor II is critical in human IgG2 binding. J Immunol 1991; 147:1338–1343.
19. Clark MR, Stuart SG, Kimberly RP, Ory PA, Goldstein IM. A single amino acid distinguishes the high-responder from low-responder form of Fc receptor II on human monocytes. Eur J Immunol 1991; 21: 1911–1916.
20. Norris CF, Pricop L, Millard SS, Taylor SM, Surrey S, Schwartz E, Salmon JE, McKenzie SE. A naturally occurring mutation in Fc_γRIIA: a Q to K 127 change confers unique binding properties to the R131 allelic form of the receptor. Blood 1997; 91:656–662, 1998.
21. Edberg JC, Kimberly RP. Cell-type specific glycoforms of Fc_γRIIIa (CD16): Differential ligand binding. J Immunol 1997; 159:3849–3857.
22. Bonnerot C, Amigorena S, Choquet D, Pavlovich R, Choudroun V, Fridman WH. Role of associated γ chain in tyrosine kinase activation via murine Fc_γRIII. EMBO J 1992; 11:2747–2757.
23. Wirthmueller U, Kurosaki T, Murakami MS, Ravetch JV. Signal transduction by Fc_γRIII (CD16) is mediated through the γ chain. J Exp Med 1992; 175:1381–1390.
24. Park JG, Murray RK, Chien P, Darby C, Schreiber AD. Conserved tyrosine residues of the γ subunit are required for a phagocytic signal mediated by Fc_γRIIIA. Blood 1993; 92:2073–2079.
25. Greenberg S, Chang P, Silverstein SC. Tyrosine phosphorylation of the γ subunit of Fc_γ receptors, p72syk and paxillin during Fc receptor mediated phagocytosis in macrophages. J Biol Chem 1994; 269:3897–3902.
26. Kurosaki T, Gander I, Wirthmueller U, Ravetch JV. The β subunit of the FcεRI is associated with the Fc_γRIII on mast cells. J Exp Med 1992; 175:447–451.
27. Wu J, Edberg JC, Redecha PB, Bansal V, Guyre PM, Coleman K, Salmon JE, Kimberly RP. A novel polymorphism of Fc_γRIIIa (CD16) alters receptor function and predisposes to autoimmune disease. J Clin Invest 1997; 100:1059–1070.
28. Koene HR, Kleijer M, Algra J, Roos D, von dem Borne AE, de Haas M. Fc_γRIIIa-158V/F polymorphism influences the binding of IgG by natural killer cell Fc_γRIIIa, independently of the Fc_γRIIIa-48L/R/H phenotype. Blood 1997; 90:1109–1114.
29. Powell MS, Barton PA, Emmanouilidis D, Wines BD, Neumann GM, Peitersz GA, Maxwell KF, Garrett TP, Hogarth PM. Biochemical analysis and crystallisation of Fc gamma RIIa, the low affinity receptor for IgG. Immunol Lett 1999; 68:17–23.
30. Sondermann P, Jacob U, Kutscher C, Frey J. Characterization and crystallization of soluble human Fc_γ receptor II (CD32) isoforms produced in insect cells. Biochemistry 1999; 38:8469–8477.
31. Edberg JC, Kimberly RP. Modulation of Fcγ and complement receptor function by the glycosyl-phosphatidylinositol-anchored form of Fc_γRIII. J Immunol 1994; 152:5826–5835.
32. Edberg JC, Salmon JE, Kimberly RP. Functional capacity of Fcγ receptor III (CD16) on human neutrophils. Immunol Res 1992; 11:239–251.
33. Voice JK, Lachmann PJ. Interactions of defined soluble IgG immune complexes with Fc and complement receptors on human neutrophils (PMN). Proc Int Cong Immunol 1995; 9:4626.
34. Edberg JC, Moon JJ, Chang DJ, Kimberly RP. Differential regulation of human neutrophil Fc_γRIIa (CD32) and Fc_γRIIIb (CD16)-induced Ca2+ transients. J Biol Chem 1998; 273:8071–8079.
35. Huizinga TW, Kleijer M, Tetteroo PA, Roos D, von dem Borne AEG Kr. Biallelic neutrophil Na-antigen system is associated with a polymorphism on the phosphoinositol-linked Fcγ receptor III (CD16). Blood 1990; 75:213–217.
36. Bux J, Stein EL, Bierling P, Fromont P, Clay M, Stroncek D, Santoso S. Characterization of a new alloantigen (SH) on the human neutrophil Fcγ receptor IIIb. Blood 1997; 89:1027–1034.
37. Salmon JE, Edberg JC, Kimberly RP. Fcγ receptor III on human neutrophils. Allelic variants have functionally distinct capacities. J Clin Invest 1990; 85:1287–1295.

38. Salmon JE, Millard SS, Brogle NL, Kimberly RP. Fcγ receptor IIIb enhances Fcγ receptor IIa function in an oxidant-dependent and allele-sensitive manner. J Clin Invest 1995; 95:2877–2885.

39. Zhou MJ, Brown EJ. CR3 (Mac-1, aM b2, CD11b/CD18) and FcγRIII cooperate in generation of a neutrophil respiratory burst: Requirement for FcγRIII and tyrosine phosphorylation. J Cell Biol 1994; 125:1407–1416.

40. Morton HC, Schiel AE, Janssen SWJ, van de Winkel JGJ. Alternatively spliced forms of the human myeloid Fcα receptor (CD89) in neutrophils. Immunogenetics 1996; 43:246–247.

41. Patry C, Sibille Y, Lehuen A, Monteiro RC. Identification of Fcα receptor (CD89) isoforms generated by alternative splicing that are differentially expressed between blood monocytes and alveolar macrophages. J Immunol 1996; 156:4442–4448.

42. Pleass RJ, Andrews PD, Kerr MA, Woof JM. Alternative splicing of the human IgA Fc receptor CD89 in neutrophils and eosinophils. Biochem J 1996; 318:771–777.

43. Reterink TJF, Verweij CL, van Es LA, Daha MR. Alternative splicing of IgA Fc receptor (CD89) transcripts. Gene 1996; 175:279–280.

44. van Dijk TB, Bracke M, Caldenhoven E, Raaijmakers JAM, Lammers JWJ, Koenderman L, de Groot RP. Cloning and characterization of $Fc_\alpha Rb$, a novel Fc_α receptor (CD89) isoform expressed in eosinophils and neutrophils. Blood 1996; 88:4229–4238.

45. Morton HC, Van den Herik-Oudijk IE, Vossebeld P, Snijders A, Verhoeven AJ, Capel PJA, Van de Winkel JGJ. Functional association between the human myeloid immunoglobulin A Fc receptor (CD89) and FcR γ chain: Molecular basis for CD89/FcR γ chain association. J Biol Chem 1995; 270:29781–29787.

46. Stewart WW, Mazengera RL, Shen L, Kerr MA. Unaggregated serum IgA binds to neutrophil FcaR at physiological concentrations and is endocytosed but cross-linking is necessary to elicit a respiratory burst. J Leukocyte Biol 1994; 56:481–487.

47. Mackenzie SJ, Kerr MA. IgM monoclonal antibodies recognizing FcαR but not FcγRIII trigger a respiratory burst in neutrophils although both trigger an increase in intracellular calcium levels and degranulation. Biochem J 1995; 306:519–523.

48. Patry C, Herbelin A, Lehuen A, Bach JF, Monteiro RC. Fcα receptors mediate release of tumour necrosis factor-α and interleukin-6 by human monocytes following receptor aggregation. Immunology 1995; 86:1–5.

49. Kinet JP. 1999. The high-affinity IgE receptor (Fc epsilon RI): From physiology to pathology. Annu Rev Immunol 1999; 17:931–972.

50. Garman SC, Kinet JP, Jardetzky TS. Crystal structure of the human high-affinity IgE receptor. Cell 1998; 95:951–961.

51. Simister NE, Ahouse JC. The structure and evolution of FcRn. Res Immunol 1996; 147:333–337.

52. Ghetie V, Ward ES. FcRn: The MHC class I-related receptor that is more than an IgG transporter. Immunol Today 1997; 18:592–598.

53. Dickinson BL, Badizadegan K, Wu Z, Ahouse JC, Zhu X, Simister NE, Blumberg RS, Lencer WI. Bidirectional FcRn-dependent IgG transport in a polarized human intestinal epithelial cell line. J Clin Invest 1999; 104:903–911.

54. Israel EJ, Wilsker DF, Hayes KC, Schoenfeld D, Simister NE. Increased clearance of IgG in mice that lack β 2-microglobulin: Possible protective role of FcRn. Immunol 1996; 89:573–578.

55. Liu Z, Roopenian DC, Zhou X, Christianson GJ, Diaz LA, Sedmak DD, Anderson CL. Beta₂-microglobulin-deficient mice are resistant to bullous pemphigoid. J Exp Med 1997; 186:777–783.

56. Litwin V, Grose C. Herpesviral Fc receptors and their relationship to the human Fc receptors. Immunol Res 1992; 11:226–238.

57. Weeks BS, Sundaresan P, Nagashunmugam T, Kang E, Friedman HM. The herpes simplex virus-1 glycoprotein E (gE) mediates IgG binding and cell-to-cell spread through distinct gE domains. Biochem Biophys Res Comm 1997; 235:31–35.

58. Litwin V, Jackson W, Grose C. Receptor properties of two varicella-zoster virus glycoproteins, gpI and gpIV, homologous to herpes simplex virus gE and gI. J Virol 1992; 66:3643–3651.

59. MacCormac LP, Grundy JE. Human cytomegalovirus induces an Fc γ receptor (Fc γR) in endothelial

cells and fibroblasts that is distinct from the human cellular Fc gammaRs. J Infect Dis 1996; 174:1151–1161.

60. Thale R, Lucin P, Schneider K, Eggers M, Koszinowski UH. Identification and expression of a murine cytomegalovirus early gene coding for an Fc receptor. J Virol 1994; 68:7757–7765.

61. Stannard LM, Hardie DR. An Fc receptor for human immunoglobulin G is located within the tegument of human cytomegalovirus. J Virol 1991; 65:3411–5.

62. Porges AJ, Redecha PB, Kimberly WT, Csernok E, Gross WL, Kimberly RP. Anti-neutrophil cytoplasmic antibodies engage and activate human neutrophils via Fc$_\gamma$RIIa. J Immunol 1994; 153:1271–1280.

63. Kocher M, Siegel ME, Edberg JC, Kimberly RP. Cross-linking of Fc$_\gamma$ receptor IIa and Fc$_\gamma$ receptor IIIb induces different proadhesive phenotypes on human neutrophils. J Immunol 1997; 159:3940–3948.

64. Kocher M, Edberg JC, Fleit HB, Kimberly RP. Antineutrophil cytoplasmic antibodies preferentially engage Fc$_\gamma$RIIIb on human neutrophils. J Immunol 1998; 161:6909–6914.

65. Edberg JC, Lin CT, Lau D, Unkeless JC, Kimberly RP. The Ca2+ dependence of human Fc$_\gamma$ receptor-initiated phagocytosis. J Biol Chem 1995; 270:22301–22307.

66. Falk RJ, Terrell RS, Charles LA, Jennette JC. Anti-neutrophil cytoplasmic autoantibodies induce neutrophils to degranulate and produce oxygen radicals in vitro. Proc Natl Acad Sci USA 1990; 87:4115–4119.

67. Mulder AH, Stegeman CA, Kallenberg CG. Activation of granulocytes by anti-neutrophil cytoplasmic antibodies (ANCA) in Wegener's granulomatosis: A predominant role for the IgG3 subclass of ANCA. Clin Exp Immunol 1995; 101:227–232.

68. Cockwell P, Brooks CJ, Adu D, Savage CO. Interleukin-8: A pathogenetic role in antineutrophil cytoplasmic autoantibody-associated glomerulonephritis. Kid Int 1999; 55:852–863.

69. Kettritz R, Jennette JC, Falk RJ. Crosslinking of ANCA-antigens stimulates superoxide release by human neutrophils. J Am Soc Nephrol 1997; 8:386–394.

70. Muller Kobold AC, Mesander G, Stegeman CA, Kallenberg CG, Cohen Tervaert JW. Are circulating neutrophils intravascularly activated in patients with anti-neutrophil cytoplasmic antibody (ANCA)-associated vasculitides? Clin Exp Immunol 1998; 114:491–499.

71. Hess C, Sadallah S, Hefti A, Landmann R, Schifferli JA. Ectosomes released by human neutrophils are specialized functional units. J Immunol 1999; 163:4564–4573.

72. Edberg JC, Wainstein E, Wu J, Csernok E, Sneller MC, Hoffman GS, Keystone EC, Gross WL, Kimberly RP. Analysis of Fc$_\gamma$RII gene polymorphisms in Wegener's granulomatosis. Exp Clin Immunogenet 1997; 14:183–195.

73. Tse WY, Abadeh S, McTiernan A, Jefferis R, Savage CO, Adu D. No association between neutrophil FcγRIIa allelic polymorphism and anti-neutrophil cytoplasmic antibody (ANCA)-positive systemic vasculitis. Clin Exp Immunol 1999; 117:198–205.

74. Wainstein E, Edberg J, Csernok E, Sneller M, Hoffman G, Keystone E, Gross W, Salmon J, Kimberly R. FcγRIIIB alleles predict renal dysfunction in Wegener's granulomatosis. Arthritis Rheum 1996; 39:S210.

75. Dijstelbloem HM, Scheepers RH, Oost WW, Stegeman CA, van der Pol WL, Sluiter WJ, Kallenberg CG, van de Winkel JG, Tervaert JW. Fc γ receptor polymorphisms in Wegener's granulomatosis: Risk factors for disease relapse. Arthritis Rheum 1999; 42:1823–1827.

76. Franssen CF, Huitema MG, Muller Kobold AC, Oost-Kort WW, Limburg PC, Tiebosch A, Stegeman CA, Kallenberg CG, Tervaert JW. In vitro neutrophil activation by antibodies to proteinase 3 and myeloperoxidase from patients with crescentic glomerulonephritis. J Am Soc Nephrol 1999; 10:1506–1515.

77. Podrez EA, Schmitt D, Hoff HF, Hazen SL. Myeloperoxidase-generated reactive nitrogen species convert LDL into an atherogenic form in vitro. J Clin Invest 1999; 103:1547–1560.

78. Frostegard J, Ulfgren AK, Nyberg P, Hedin U, Swedenborg J, Andersson U, Hansson GK. Cytokine expression in advanced human atherosclerotic plaques: Dominance of pro-inflammatory (Th1) and macrophage-stimulating cytokines. Atherosclerosis 1999; 145:33–43.

79. Gu L, Okada Y, Clinton SK, Gerard C, Sukhova GK, Libby P, Rollins BJ. Absence of monocyte chemo-

attractant protein-1 reduces atherosclerosis in low density lipoprotein receptor-deficient mice. Molec Cell 1998; 2:275–281.

80. Nicoletti A, Kaveri S, Caligiuri G, Bariety J, Hansson GK. Immunoglobulin treatment reduces atherosclerosis in apo E knockout mice. J Clin Invest 1998; 102:910–918.
81. Huang Y, Jaffa A, Koskinen S, Takei A, Lopes-Virella MF. Oxidized LDL-containing immune complexes induce Fc γ receptor I-mediated mitogen-activated protein kinase activation in THP-1 macrophages. Arterioscler Thromb Vasc Biol 1999; 19:1600–1607.

10
Pathophysiology of Atherothrombosis: Role of Inflammation

Prediman K. Shah

Cedars Sinai Medical Center and University of California, Los Angeles, California

I. INTRODUCTION

Arterial occlusive disorders include atherosclerosis of native arteries, accelerated atherosclerosis involving vein grafts and arteries of transplanted organs, and restenosis following angioplasty and stenting. Atherosclerotic vascular disease is a leading cause of death and disability throughout the United States and other industrialized nations and consumes enormous fiscal resources. An improved understanding of the pathophysiology of atherosclerosis and thrombosis is likely to lead to improved prevention, diagnosis, and treatment of this common disorder.

Atherosclerosis involves the development of a plaque composed of variable amounts of lipids, lipoproteins, extracellular matrix (collagen, proteoglycans, glycosaminoglycans), calcium, vascular smooth muscle cells, inflammatory cells (chiefly monocyte-derived macrophages, T lymphocytes, and mast cells), and new blood vessels (angiogenesis). A body of evidence now suggests that atherosclerosis represents a chronic inflammatory response to vascular injury caused by a variety of agents that activate or injure endothelium and promote lipoprotein infiltration, retention, and modification, combined with leukocyte retention and activation (1).

II. SHEAR STRESS AND ENDOTHELIAL INFLAMMATORY GENE ACTIVATION AT SITES OF PREDILECTION

The sites of predilection for atherosclerosis are characterized by low shear stress, evidence of endothelial activation with expression of leukocyte adhesion molecules, and increased influx and/or prolonged retention of lipoproteins (2,3) (Table 1). Specific arterial sites, such as branches, bifurcations, and curvatures, cause characteristic alterations in the flow of blood, including decreased shear stress and increased turbulence. Changes in flow alter the expression of genes that have elements in their promoter regions that respond to shear stress. For example, the genes for intercellular adhesion molecule 1, platelet-derived growth factor B chain, and tissue factor in endothelial cells have these elements, and their expression is increased by reduced shear stress (4–11). Rolling and adherence of inflammatory cells (monocytes and T cells) occur at these sites as a result of the upregulation of adhesion molecules on both the endothelium and the leukocytes.

Table 1   Key Steps in Atherogenesis Highlighting Role of Inflammation at Various Steps

1. Endothelial activation with increased infiltration of atherogenic lipoproteins at sites of low or oscillating shear stress (branch points and flow dividers)
2. Subendothelial retention and modification of atherogenic lipoproteins (LDL/VLDL)
3. Endothelial activation with increased mononuclear leukocyte (inflammatory cell) adhesion, chemotaxis, and subendothelial recruitment
4. Subendothelial inflammatory cell activation with lipid ingestion through monocyte scavenger receptor expression resulting in foam cell formation
5. Intimal migration and proliferation of medial/adventitial smooth muscle cells/myofibroblasts in response to growth factors released by activated monocytes with matrix production and formation of fibrous cap and fibrous plaque
6. Abluminal plaque growth with positive (outward) arterial adventitial remodeling preserving lumen size in early stages; later plaque growth or negative remodeling results in luminal narrowing
7. Neoangiogenesis due to angiogenic stimuli produced by inflammatory cells (macrophages) and other arterial wall cells (VEGF, IL-8)
8. Death of foam cells by necrosis/apoptosis leading to necrotic lipid-core formation
9. Plaque disruption (rupture of fibrous cap or endothelial erosion) due to inflammatory cell–mediated matrix degradation and death of matrix-synthesizing smooth muscle cells.
10. Exposure of thrombogenic substrate (lipid-core containing tissue factor derived from inflammatory cells) following plaque disruption with arterial thrombosis

At these sites, specific molecules form on the endothelium that are responsible for the adherence, migration, and accumulation of monocytes and T cells. Such adhesion molecules, which act as receptors for glycoconjugates and integrins present on monocytes and T cells, include several selectins, intercellular adhesion molecules, and vascular-cell adhesion molecules (4–11). Molecules associated with the migration of leukocytes across the endothelium, such as platelet-endothelial-cell adhesion molecules act in conjunction with chemoattractant molecules generated by the endothelium, smooth muscle, and monocytes—such as monocyte chemotactic protein-1 (MCP-1), osteopontin, and modified low-density lipoprotein (LDL)—to attract monocytes and T cells into the artery (2–11). Chemokines may be involved in the chemotaxis and accumulation of macrophages in fatty streaks (12). Activation of monocytes and T cells leads to upregulation of receptors on their surfaces, such as the mucinlike molecules that bind selectins, integrins that bind adhesion molecules of the immunoglobulin superfamily, and receptors that bind chemoattractant molecules. These ligand–receptor interactions further activate mononuclear cells, induce cell proliferation, and help define and localize the inflammatory response at the sites of lesions.

In genetically modified mice that are deficient in apolipoprotein E (and have hypercholesterolemia), intercellular adhesion molecule-1 (ICAM-1) is constitutively increased at lesion-prone sites long before the lesions develop (8). In contrast, vascular cell adhesion molecule 1 (VCAM-1) is absent in normal mice but is present at the same sites as ICAM-1 in mice with apolipoprotein E deficiency (8). Mice that are completely deficient in ICAM-1, P-selectin, CD18, or combinations of these molecules, have reduced atherosclerosis in response to lipid feeding. Proteolytic enzymes may cleave adhesion molecules such that in situations of chronic inflammation it may be possible to measure the "shed" molecules in plasma as markers of a sustained inflammatory response to help identify patients at risk for atherosclerosis or other inflammatory diseases (13–17).

III. KEY ROLE OF ENDOTHELIAL ACTIVATION/DYSFUNCTION AND INFLAMMATION IN ATHEROGENESIS

Several studies have suggested that one of the earliest steps in atherogenesis is endothelial activation or injury/dysfunction with infiltration and retention and modification of atherogenic lipoproteins (predominantly the apo B containing lipoproteins) in the subendothelial space of the vessel wall (18–26) (Table 2).

Various factors that may contribute to endothelial activation or the development of endothelial injury/dysfunction predisposing to atherosclerosis, including risk factors such as elevated and modified LDL/VLDL cholesterol; reduced HDL cholesterol; oxidant stress caused by cigarette smoking, hypertension, and diabetes mellitus; genetic alterations; elevated plasma homocysteine concentrations; infectious microorganisms such as herpes viruses or *Chlamydia pneumoniae;* estrogen deficiency; and advancing age (21,22). Endothelial activation and injury/dysfunction may manifest in (1) increased adhesiveness of the endothelium to inflammatory cells (leukocytes) or platelets, (2) increased vascular permeability, (3) change from an anticoagulant to a procoagulant phenotype, (4) change from a vasodilator to a vasoconstrictor phenotype or, (5) change from a growth-inhibiting to a growth-promoting phenotype through elaboration of cytokines. Abnormal vasomotor function has been one of the most well-studied manifestations of endothelial dysfunction in subjects with either established atherosclerosis or in those with risk factors for atherosclerosis. Normal healthy endothelium produces nitric oxide from arginine through the action of a family of enzymes known as nitric oxide synthases (21,22). Nitric oxide acts as a local vasodilator by increasing smooth muscle cell cyclic guanosine monophosphate (GMP) levels while at the same time inhibiting platelet aggregation and smooth muscle cell proliferation (21,22). In the presence of risk factors, a reduced vasodilator response to endothelium-

Table 2   Endothelial Activation/Dysfunction in Atherosclerosis

Phenotypic features
1. Reduced vasodilator and increased vasoconstrictor capacity
    —enhanced oxidant stress with increased inactivation of nitric oxide
    —increased expression of endothelin
2. Enhanced leukocyte (inflammatory cell) adhesion and recruitment
    —increased adhesion molecule expression (ICAM, VCAM)
    —increased chemotactic molecule expression (MCP-1, IL-8)
3. Increased prothrombotic and reduced fibrinolytic phenotype
4. Increased growth-promoting phenotype

Factors contributing to endothelial activation/dysfunction
1. Dyslipidemia and atherogenic lipoprotein modification
    —elevated LDL, VLDL, LP(a)
    —LDL modification (oxidation, glycation)
    —Reduced HDL
2. Increased angiotensin II and hypertension
3. Insulin resistance and diabetes
4. Estrogen deficiency
5. Smoking
6. Hyperhomocysteinemia
7. Advancing age
8. Infection?

dependent vasodilator stimuli or even paradoxical vasoconstrictor response to such stimuli have been observed in large vessels as well as in the microcirculation, even in absence of structural abnormalities in the vessel wall (21,22). These abnormal vasomotor responses have been attributed to reduced bioavailability of endothelium-derived relaxing factor(s), specifically nitric oxide, due to rapid inactivation of nitric oxide by oxidant stress or excess generation of asymmetric dimethylarginine and/or increased production of vasoconstrictors such as endothelin (21,22).

One of the major contributors to endothelial injury is LDL cholesterol modified by processes such as oxidation, glycation (in diabetes), aggregation, association with proteoglycans, or incorporation into immune complexes (21–23,26,27). Oxidized LDL has been shown to be present in the atheroscleroitic lesions of both experimental animals as well as in humans (28). Subendothelial retention of LDL particles results in progressive oxidation and its subsequent internalization by macrophages through the scavenger receptors (26). The internalization leads to the formation of lipid peroxides and facilitates the accumulation of cholesterol esters, even finally resulting in the formation of foam cells. Once modified and taken up by macrophages, LDL activates the foam cells. In addition to its ability to injure these cells, modified LDL is chemotactic for other monocytes and can upregulate the expression of genes for macrophage colony-stimulating factor (M-CSF) and monocyte chemotactic protein derived from endothelial cells (29–32). Thus, it may help expand the inflammatory response by stimulating the replication of monocyte-derived macrophages and the entry of new monocytes into lesions. Continued inflammatory response stimulates migration and proliferation of smooth muscle cells that accumulate within the areas of inflammation to form an intermediate fibroproliferative lesion resulting in thickening of the artery wall.

The inflammatory and immune response in atherosclerosis consists of accumulation of monocyte-derived macrophages and specific subtypes of T lymphocytes at every stage of the disease (33–39). The fatty streak, the earliest type of lesion, common in infants and young children, consists of monocyte-derived macrophages, macrophage-derived foam cells and T lymphocytes. The critical role of the macrophage in atherogenesis is supported by the virtual absence (or drastic reduction) of atherosclerosis when M-CSF null genotype is introduced in murine models of severe dyslipidemia induced by diet or genetic manipulation (40–41).

Continued inflammation results in increased numbers of macrophages and lymphocytes, which both emigrate from the blood and multiply within the lesion. Activation of these cells leads to the release of proteolytic enzymes, cytokines, chemokines, and growth factors, which can induce further damage and eventually lead to focal necrosis. Necrosis and/or apoptosis of foam cells results in the formation of the necrotic lipid core in the plaque. Thus, cycles of accumulation of mononuclear cells, migration and proliferation of smooth muscle cells, and formation of fibrous tissue lead to further enlargement and restructuring of the lesion, so that it becomes covered by a fibrous cap that overlies a core of lipid and necrotic tissue resulting in the formation of an advanced and complicated atherosclerotic plaque.

The inflammatory response itself can influence lipoprotein transfer within the vessel wall. Proinflammatory cytokines, such as tumor necrosis factor-α (TNF-α), interleukin-1 (IL-1), and M-CSF increase binding of LDL to endothelium and smooth muscle and increase the transcription of the LDL-receptor gene (1). After binding to scavenger receptors in vitro, modified LDL initiates a series of intracellular events that include the induction of proteases and inflammatory cytokines (1). Thus, a vicious circle of inflammation, modification of lipoproteins, and further inflammation can be maintained in the artery by the presence of these modified lipoproteins.

Monocyte-derived macrophages are present in various stages of atherogenesis and act as scavenging and antigen-presenting cells. They produce cytokines, chemokines, growth-regulating molecules, tissue factor, metalloproteinases, and other hydrolytic enzymes. The continuing entry, survival, and replication of monocytes/macrophages in lesions depend in part on growth factors, such as M-CSF and granulocyte-macrophage colony-stimulating factor (GM-CSF), whereas IL-2 is involved in a similar manner for T lymphocytes.

Activated macrophages as well as lesional smooth muscle cells express class II histocompatibility antigens such as HLA-DR that allow them to present antigens to T lymphocytes (1,33–39). Atherosclerotic lesions contain both CD4 and CD8 T cells implicating the immune system in atherogenesis (33–39). T cell activation, following antigen processing, results in production of various cytokines, such as interferon-γ (IFN-γ) and TNF-α and β, which can further enhance the inflammatory response (1). Antigens presented include oxidized LDL and heat shock protein 60 which may participate in the immune response in atherosclerosis (2,33–39).

Macrophages, T cells, endothelial and smooth muscle cells in the atherosclerotic lesions express CD40 ligand and its receptor, which may play a role in atherogenesis by regulating the function of inflammatory cells (42–45). The antiatherogenic effect of CD40 blocking antibodies in the murine model of atherosclerosis suggests that CD40-mediated signaling may play an important role in atherogenesis (46).

Platelet adhesion and mural thrombosis are ubiquitous in the initiation and generation of the lesions of atherosclerosis in animals and humans (1). Platelets can adhere to dysfunctional endothelium, exposed collagen, and macrophages. When activated, platelets release their granules, which contain cytokines and growth factors that, together with thrombin, may contribute to the migration and proliferation of smooth muscle cells and monocytes. Activation of platelets leads to the formation of free arachidonic acid, which can be transformed into prostaglandins such as thromboxane A2, one of the most potent vasoconstricting and platelet-aggregating substances known, or into leukotrienes, which can amplify the inflammatory response.

Angiotensin II, a potent vasoconstrictor, may also contribute to atherogenesis by stimulating the growth of smooth muscle, increasing oxidant stress, inducing LDL oxidation, and promoting an inflammatory response (1,46–50).

Elevated plasma homocysteine concentrations, resulting from enzymatic defects or vitamin deficiency, may facilitate atherothrombosis by inducing endothelial dysfunction with a reduction in vasodilator capacity and enhanced prothrombotic phenotype and smooth muscle cell replication (51–55). Hyperhomocysteinemia is associated with an increased risk of atherosclerosis of the coronary, peripheral, and cerebral arteries (51–55). Trials are underway to determine whether reduction of plasma homocysteine levels by vitamins such as folic acid, B_6, and B_{12}, can reduce atherothrombotic events in humans (55).

IV. POTENTIAL ROLE OF INFECTION IN ATHEROTHROMBOSIS

It is likely that a number of stimuli are responsible for provoking and sustaining a chronic inflammatory response in the vessel wall in atherosclerosis. Among the key potential culprits are the modified lipoproteins and infectious agents. Oxidatively modified lipoproteins can induce a variety of proinflammatory genes in the vessel wall that are responsible for recruiting and activating inflammatory cells such as ICAM- and VCAM-type adhesion molecules, chemotactic cytokines such as MCP-1, IL-8, and colony-stimulating factors such as M-CSF. In addition to modified lipoproteins, there is now a body of evidence suggesting that arterial wall infections with organisms such as *Chlamydia pneumoniae*, CMV/herpes virus, as well as remote infections such as chronic bronchitis, gingivitis, and *Helicobacter pylori* infection may affect inflammation, thereby contributing to atherogenesis and/or plaque disruption and thrombosis in the presence of preexisting atherosclerosis (56–68) (Table 3). Increased titers of antibodies to these organisms have been used as a predictor of further adverse events in patients who have had a myocardial infarction. Organisms, particularly *Chlamydia pneumoniae,* have been identified in atheromatous

Table 3 Potential Role of Infection in Atherosclerosis and Thrombosis

Infectious organisms implicated
1. Viruses
    —herpes virus
    —CMV
2. Bacteria
    —*Chlamydia pneumoniae*
    —*Helicobacter pylori*
    —*Porphyromonas gingivalis?*

Mechanisms(s) by which infections may contribute to atherothrombosis
1. Direct infection of the vascular wall with endothelial injury, inflammatory cell recruitment, and activation (*Chlamydia pneumoniae*, herpes virus, CMV)
2. Immune-mediated vascular injury through molecular mimicry (*Chlamydia pneumoniae*)
3. Remote infections with systemic activation of the inflammatory response (*Helicobacter pylori*, *Porphyromonas gingivalis*)

lesions in coronary arteries and in other organs obtained at autopsy. The case for *Chlamydia pneumoniae* is of particular interest since both in the hypercholesterolemic rabbit as well as in genetically hyperlipidemic mice, acceleration of atherosclerosis with *C. pneumoniae* infection has been demonstrated (64,65). In addition, pilot clinical trials of antichlamydial macrolide antibiotics have raised the possibility that such therapy may reduce the risk of recurrent coronary events (66,67). In vitro studies have suggested that *C. pneumoniae* can trigger proatherogenic events, such as foam cell formation, procoagulant activity, and metalloproteinase activity in monocytes, probably mediated by its heat shock protein 60 (HSP60) (56). Molecular antigenic mimicry between certain chlamydia antigens and myosin have also raised the additional possibility that such antigenic mimicry could be involved in an immune-mediated vascular and myocardial injury (68). Large-scale clinical trials are currently underway to more clearly define the role of chlamydia infection in atherothrombosis. Although there is no direct evidence that these organisms can cause the lesions of atherosclerosis, it is nevertheless possible that infection, combined with other risk factors, may contribute to atherogenesis or destabilization of preexisting atherosclerotic lesions in some patients.

V. ANGIOGENESIS IN ATHEROSCLEROSIS

Angiogenesis or neovascularization is an essential process that supports chronic inflammation and fibroproliferation, processes that are involved in atherogenesis. Several studies have demonstrated increased neoangiogenesis in atherosclerotic lesions and hypercholesterolemia has been shown to increase adventitial neovascularity in porcine arteries before the development of an atherosclerotic lesion (69–72). Proinflammatory chemokines such as IL-8 and other angiogenic growth factors such as vascular endothelial growth factor (VEGF) have been demonstrated in atherosclerotic lesions where they could contribute to angiogenesis (73). Recent preliminary data demonstrating an inhibitory effect of angiostatin in murine model of atherosclerosis suggests the potential proatherogenic role for angiogenesis (74).

VI. ROLE OF INFLAMMATION IN PLAQUE RUPTURE, PLAQUE EROSION, AND THROMBOSIS

Thrombosis complicating atherosclerosis is the mechanism by which atherosclerosis leads to acute ischemic syndromes of unstable angina, non–Q- and Q-wave myocardial infarction and many cases of sudden cardiac death (75–78). In most cases, coronary thrombosis occurs as a result of uneven thinning and rupture of the fibrous cap, often at the shoulders of a lipid-rich lesion where macrophages and T cells enter, accumulate, and are activated, and where apoptosis may occur (75–78) (Fig. 1). Thinning of the fibrous cap may result from elaboration of matrix-degrading metalloproteinases (MMPs) such as collagenases (MMP-1, MMP-13), gelatinases (MMP-2, MMP-9), elastases (MMP-12), and stromelysins (MMP-3), and/or other proteases such as cathepsins, by inflammatory cells, chiefly macrophages (75–80). These proteases may be induced or activated by oxidized LDL, cell-to-cell interaction between macrophages and activated T cells, CD40 ligation, mast cell–derived proteases, oxidant radicals, matrix proteins such as Tenascin-C, and infectious agents (75–81). Thinning may also result from increased smooth muscle cell death by apoptosis/necrosis and consequent reduced matrix production (82,83).

Inflammatory cells, specifically the macrophages, are also the main source of tissue factor in the atherosclerotic plaque (84–86). Tissue factor, when exposed to circulating blood, interacts with activated factor VII to generate activated factor X; activated factor X in turn cleaves thrombin from prothrombin. Thrombin is involved in recruiting and activating platelets as well as the clotting cascade, thereby initiating thrombus formation. Tissue factor expression is increased in atherosclerotic plaques, particularly in unstable coronary syndromes (85,86). The lipid core of the atheromatous lesion is heavily impregnated with tissue factor derived from dead (possibly apoptotic) macrophages and foam cells, accounting for its high thrombogenicity (87). Macrophage tissue factor expression may be induced by a variety of signals in the atherosclerotic plaque, including various cytokines, infectious agents, and oxidized lipoproteins. Thrombosis may also occur on a proteoglycan-rich matrix without a large lipid core, and in such cases, evidence of superficial endothelial erosion is found (88). This plaque erosion may account for thrombosis in a relatively higher proportion of young victims of sudden death, particularly in women and smokers (88). The precise molecular basis for these plaque erosions is not clear although endothelial desquamation through activation of basement membrane–degrading MMP may be involved (80).

Plaques with a large lipid core, active inflammatory infiltration, and a thinned fibrous cap are therefore considered vulnerable or unstable plaques. Their identification may be particularly difficult because they may not produce symptoms because of lack of flow-limiting stenoses and may thus escape detection by stress testing and even angiography. Inflammation in atherosclerosis may be accompanied by elevation of circulating proinflammatory markers such as C-reactive protein (CRP), interleukin-6, serum amyloid A, and a variety of soluble leukocyte adhesion molecules (89–93). Elevated CRP levels have been shown to predict an increased risk of adverse cardiac events in patients with symptomatic vascular disease as well as in asymptomatic subjects at risk for vascular disease (89).

VII. CONCLUSIONS

Atherosclerosis is a complex disease process that involves lipoprotein influx, lipoprotein modification, increased pro-oxidant stress, and inflammatory, angiogenic, and fibroproliferative responses intermingled with extracellular matrix and lipid accumulation, resulting in the formation of an atherosclerotic plaque. Endothelial activation/dysfunction is common in atherosclerosis and

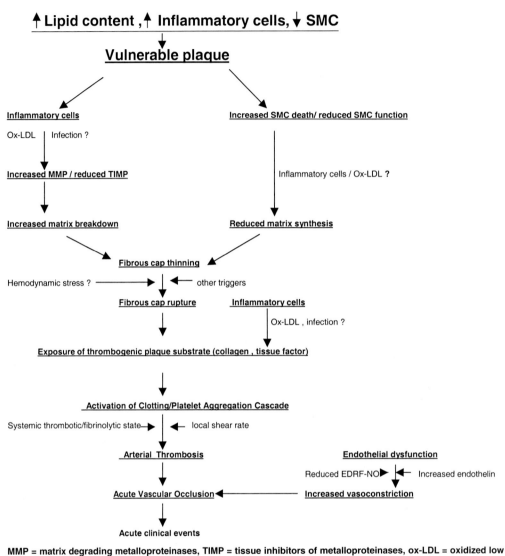

↑ Lipid content , ↑ Inflammatory cells, ↓ SMC

Vulnerable plaque

Inflammatory cells   Increased SMC death/ reduced SMC function

Ox-LDL | Infection ?

Increased MMP / reduced TIMP   Inflammatory cells / Ox-LDL ?

Increased matrix breakdown   Reduced matrix synthesis

Fibrous cap thinning

Hemodynamic stress ? ———————→ ←— other triggers

Fibrous cap rupture   Inflammatory cells

Ox-LDL , infection ?

Exposure of thrombogenic plaque substrate (collagen , tissue factor)

Activation of Clotting/Platelet Aggregation Cascade

Systemic thrombotic/fibrinolytic state→ ←— local shear rate

Arterial Thrombosis   Endothelial dysfunction

Reduced EDRF-NO▶ ◀— Increased endothelin

Acute Vascular Occlusion◀———————— Increased vasoconstriction

Acute clinical events

MMP = matrix degrading metalloproteinases, TIMP = tissue inhibitors of metalloproteinases, ox-LDL = oxidized low
density lipoprotein, EDRF-NO = endothelium derived relaxation factor-Nitric Oxide

Figure 1 Schematic describing the pathways and steps involved in disruption of atherosclerotic plaques
with consequent thrombosis.

often manifests as a reduced vasodilator or enhanced vasoconstrictor phenotype that contributes
to luminal compromise. Thrombosis resulting from plaque rupture or superficial erosion complicates atherosclerosis, often resulting in abrupt luminal occlusion with resultant acute ischemic
syndromes. Infectious agents may contribute to the inflammatory response and thus to destabilization of lesions. An improved understanding of the pathophysiology of atherosclerosis is providing novel directions for its prevention and treatment. In particular, the recognition of the important role of inflammation could lead to novel therapeutic interventions directed at selective
inhibition of inflammatory cascade in the vessel wall. Targeting inflammatory triggers such as

lipoproteins, angiotensin II, possible infectious agents, and others is likely to lead to improved outcomes in patients with atherosclerosis.

REFERENCES

1. Ross R. Atherosclerosis: An inflammatory disease. N Engl J Med 1999; 340:115–126.
2. McMillan DE. Blood flow and the localization of atherosclerotic plaques. Stroke 1985; 16:582–587.
3. Gotlieb AI, Langille BL. The role of rheology in atherosclerotic coronary artery disease. In: Fuster V, Ross R, Topol EJ, eds. Atherosclerosis and Coronary Artery Disease. Vol. 1. Philadelphia: Lippincott-Raven, 1996:595–606.
4. Nagel T, Resnick N, Atkinson WJ, Dewey CF Jr, Gimbrone MA Jr. Shear stress selectively upregulates intercellular adhesion molecule-1 expression in cultured human vascular endothelial cells. J Clin Invest 1994; 94:885–891.
5. Resnick N, Collins T, Atkinson W, Bonthron DT, Dewey CF Jr, Gimbrone MA Jr. Platelet-derived growth factor B chain promoter contains a cis-acting fluid shear-stress-responsive element. Proc Natl Acad Sci USA 1993; 90:4591–4595.
6. Lin MC, Almus-Jacobs F, Chen HH, et al. Shear stress induction of the tissue factor gene. J Clin Invest 1997; 99:737–744.
7. Mondy JS, Lindner V, Miyashiro JK, Berk BC, Dean RH, Geary RL. Platelet-derived growth factor ligand and receptor expression in response to altered blood flow in vivo. Circ Res 1997; 81:320.
8. Nakashima Y, Raines EW, Plump AS, Breslow JL, Ross R. Upregulation of VCAM-1 and ICAM-1 at atherosclerosis-prone sites on the endothelium in the ApoE-deficient mouse. Arterioscler Thromb Vasc Biol 1998; 18:842–851.
9. Springer TA, Cybulsky MI. Traffic signals on endothelium for leukocytes in health, inflammation, and atherosclerosis. In: Fuster V, Ross R, Topol EJ, eds. Atherosclerosis and Coronary Artery Disease. Vol. 1. Philadelphia: Lippincott-Raven, 1996:511–538.
10. Muller WA, Weigl SA, Deng X, Phillips DM. PECAM-1 is required for transendothelial migration of leukocytes. J Exp Med 1993; 178:449–460.
11. Giachelli CM, Lombardi D, Johnson RJ, Murry CE, Almeida M. Evidence for a role of osteopontin in macrophage infiltration in response to pathological stimuli in vivo. Am J Pathol 1998; 152:353–358.
12. Boisvert WA, Santiago R, Curtiss LK, Terkeltaub RA. A leukocyte homologue of the IL-8 receptor CXCR-2 mediates the accumulation of macrophages in atherosclerotic lesions of LDL receptor-deficient mice. J Clin Invest 1998; 101:353–363.
13. Herren B, Raines EW, Ross R. Expression of a disintegrin-like protein in cultured human vascular cells and in vivo. FASEB J 1997; 11:173–180.
14. Black RA, Rauch CT, Kozlosky CJ, et al. A metalloproteinase disintegrin that releases tumor-necrosis factor-(alpha) from cells. Nature 1997; 385:729–733.
15. Moss ML, Jin S-LC, Milla ME, et al. Cloning of a disintegrin metalloproteinase that processes precursor tumour necrosis factor-(alpha). Nature 1997; 385:733–736.
16. De Caterina R, Basta G, Lazzerini G, et al. Soluble vascular cell adhesion molecule-1 as a biohumoral correlate of atherosclerosis. Arterioscler Thromb Vasc Biol 1997; 17:2646–2654.
17. Hwang S-J, Ballantyne CM, Sharrett AR, et al. Circulating adhesion molecules VCAM-1, ICAM-1, and E-selectin in carotid atherosclerosis and incident coronary heart disease cases: the Atherosclerosis Risk in Communities (ARIC) study. Circulation 1997; 96:4219–4225.
18. Napoli C, D'Armiento FP, Mancini FP, et al. Fatty streak formation occurs in human fetal aortas and is greatly enhanced by maternal hypercholesterolemia: intimal accumulation of low density lipoprotein and its oxidation precede monocyte recruitment into early atherosclerotic lesions. J Clin Invest 1997; 100:2680–2690.
19. Stary HC, Chandler AB, Glagov S, et al. A definition of initial, fatty streak, and intermediate lesions of atherosclerosis: A report from the Committee on Vascular Lesions of the Council on Arteriosclerosis, American Heart Association. Circulation 1994; 89:2462–2478.

20. Simionescu N, Vasile E, Lupu F, Popescu G, Simionescu M. Prelesional events in atherogenesis: Accumulation of extracellular cholesterol-rich liposomes in the arterial intima and cardiac valves of the hyperlipidemic rabbit. Am J Pathol 1986; 123:109–125.

21. Kinlay S, Ganz P. Role of endothelial dysfunction in coronary artery disease and implications for therapy. Am J Cardiol 1997; 80:111–161.

22. Lerman A, Edwards BS, Hallett JW, Heublein DM, Sandberg SM, Burnett JC Jr: Circulating and tissue endothelin immunoreactivity in advanced atherocslerosis. N Engl J Med 1991; 325:997–1001.

23. Steinberg D. Low density lipoprotein oxidation and its pathobiological significance. J Biol Chem 1997; 272:20963–20966.

24. Khoo JC, Miller E, McLoughlin P, Steinberg D. Enhanced macrophage uptake of low density lipoprotein after self-aggregation. Arteriosclerosis 1988; 8:348–358.

25. Khoo JC, Miller E, Pio F, Steinberg D, Witztum JL. Monoclonal antibodies against LDL further enhance macrophage uptake of LDL aggregates. Arterioscler Thromb 1992; 12:1258–1266.

26. Navab M, Berliner JA, Watson AD, et al. The Yin and Yang of oxidation in the development of the fatty streak: A review based on the 1994 George Lyman Duff Memorial Lecture. Arterioscler Thromb Vasc Biol 1996; 16:831–834.

27. Griendling KK, Alexander RW. Oxidative stress and cardiovascular disease. Circulation 1997; 96: 3264–3265.

28. YIa-Herttuala S, Palinski W, Rosenfeld ME, et al. Evidence for the presence of oxidatively modified low density lipoprotein in atherosclerotic lesions of rabbit and man. J Clin Invest 1989; 84:1086–1095.

29. Han J, Hajjar DP, Febbraio M, Nicholson AC. Native and modified low density lipoproteins increase the functional expression of the macrophage class B scavenger receptor, CD36. J Biol Chem 1997; 272:21654–1659.

30. Rajavashisth TB, Andalibi A, Territo MC, et al. Induction of endothelial cell expression of granulocyte and macrophage colony-stimulating factors by modified low-density lipoproteins. Nature 1990; 344: 254–257.

31. Quinn MT, Parthasarathy S, Fong LG, Steinberg D. Oxidatively modified low density lipoproteins: A potential role in recruitment and retention of monocyte/macrophages during atherogenesis. Proc Natl Acad Sci USA 1987; 84:2995–2998.

32. Leonard EJ, Yoshimura T. Human monocyte chemoattractant protein-1 (MCP-1). Immunol Today 1990; 11:97–101.

33. Jonasson L, Holm J, Skalli O, Bondjers G, Hansson GK. Regional accumulations of T cells, macrophages, and smooth muscle cells in the human atherosclerotic plaque. Arteriosclerosis 1986; 6:131–138.

34. van der Wal AC, Das PK, Bentz van de Berg D, van der Loos CM, Becker AE. Atherosclerotic lesions in humans: In situ immunophenotypic analysis suggesting an immune mediated response. Lab Invest 1989; 61:166–170.

35. Libby P, Ross R. Cytokines and growth regulatory molecules. In: Fuster V, Ross R, Topol EJ, eds. Atherosclerosis and Coronary Artery Disease. Vol. 1. Philadelphia: Lippincott-Raven, 1996:585–594.

36. Raines EW, Rosenfeld ME, Ross R. The role of macrophages. In: Fuster V, Ross R, Topol EJ, eds. Atherosclerosis and Coronary Artery Disease. Vol. 1. Philadelphia: Lippincott-Raven, 1996:539–555.

37. Hansson GK, Libby P. The role of the lymphocyte. In: Fuster V, Ross R, Topol EJ, eds. Atherosclerosis and Coronary Artery Disease. Vol. 1. Philadelphia: Lippincott-Raven, 1996:557–568.

38. Hansson GK, Jonasson L, Seifert PS, Stemme S. Immune mechanisms in atherosclerosis. Arteriosclerosis 1989; 9:567–578.

39. Stemme S, Faber B, Holm J, Wiklund O, Witztum JL, Hansson GK. T lymphocytes from human atherosclerotic plaques recognize oxidized low density lipoprotein. Proc Natl Acad Sci USA 1995; 92:3893–3897.

40. Qiao J-H, Tripathi J, Mishra NK, et al. Role of macrophage colony-stimulating factor in atherosclerosis: studies of osteopetrotic mice. Am J Pathol 1997; 150:1687–1699.

41. Rajavashisth, T, Qiao JH, Tripathi S, Tripathi J, Mishra N, Hua M, Wang XP, Loussararian A, Clinton S, Libby P, Lusis A. Heterozygous osteopetrotic (op) mutation reduces atherosclerosis in LDL receptor-deficient mice. J Clin Invest 1998; 101:2702–2710.

42. Hollenbaugh D, Mischel-Petty N, Edwards CP, et al. Expression of functional CD40 by vascular endothelial cells. J Exp Med 1995; 182:33–40.

43. Mach F, Schonbeck U, Bonnefoy J-Y, Pober JS, Libby P. Activation of monocyte/macrophage functions related to acute atheroma complication by ligation of CD40: induction of collagenase, stromelysin, and tissue factor. Circulation 1997; 96:396–399.

44. Schonbeck U, Mach F, Sukhova GK, et al. Regulation of matrix metalloproteinase expression in human vascular smooth muscle cells by T lymphocytes: A role for CD40 signaling in plaque rupture? Circ Res 1997; 81:448–454.

45. Schonbeck U, Mach F, Bonnefoy J-Y, Loppnow H, Flad H-D, Libby P. Ligation of CD40 activates interleukin 1(beta)-converting enzyme (caspase-1) activity in vascular smooth muscle and endothelial cells and promotes elaboration of active interleukin 1(beta). J Biol Chem 1997; 272:19569–19574.

46. Mach F, Schonbeck U, Sukhova GK, Atkinson E, Libby P. Reduction of atherosclerosis in mice by inhibition of CD40 signalling. Nature 1998; 394:200–203.

47. Chobanian AV, Dzau VJ. Renin angiotensin system and atherosclerotic vascular disease. In: Fuster V, Ross R, Topol EJ, eds. Atherosclerosis and Coronary Artery Disease. Vol. 1. Philadelphia: Lippincott-Raven, 1996:237–242.

48. Gibbons GH, Pratt RE, Dzau VJ. Vascular smooth muscle cell hypertrophy vs. hyperplasia: Autocrine transforming growth factor-beta 1 expression determines growth response to angiotensin II. J Clin Invest 1992; 90:456–461.

49. Lacy F, O'Connor DT, Schmid-Schonbein GW. Plasma hydrogen peroxide production in hypertensives and normotensive subjects at genetic risk of hypertension. J Hypertens 1998; 16:291–303.

50. Swei A, Lacy F, DeLano FA, Schmid-Schonbein GW. Oxidative stress in the Dahl hypertensive rat. Hypertension 1997; 30:1628–1633.

51. Nehler MR, Taylor LM Jr, Porter JM. Homocysteinemia as a risk factor for atherosclerosis: A review. Cardiovasc Surg 1997; 6:559–567.

52. Nygard O, Nordrehaug JE, Refsum H, Ueland PM, Farstad M, Vollset SE. Plasma homocysteine levels and mortality in patients with coronary artery disease. N Engl J Med 1997; 337:230–236.

53. Malinow MR. Plasma homocyst(e)ine and arterial occlusive disease diseases: A mini-review. Clin Chem 1995; 41:173–176.

54. Verhoef P, Stampfer MJ. Prospective studies of homocysteine and cardiovascular disease. Nutr Rev 1995; 53:283–288.

55. Omenn GS, Beresford SAA, Motulsky AG. Preventing coronary heart disease: B vitamins and homocysteine. Circulation 1998; 97:421–424.

56. Libby P, Egan D, Skarlatos S. Roles of infectious agents in atherosclerosis and restenosis: An assessment of the evidence and need for future research. Circulation 1997; 96:4095–4103.

57. Hendrix MG, Salimans MM, van Boven CP, Bruggeman CA. High prevalence of latently present cytomegalovirus in arterial walls of patients suffering from grade III atherosclerosis. Am J Pathol 1990; 136:23–28.

58. Jackson LA, Campbell LA, Schmidt RA, et al. Specificity of detection of Chlamydia pneumoniae in cardiovascular atheroma: Evaluation of the innocent bystander hypothesis. Am J Pathol 1997; 150:1785–1790.

59. Thom DH, Wang SP, Grayston JT, et al. Chlamydia pneumoniae strain TWAR antibody and angiographically demonstrated coronary artery disease. Arterioscler Thromb 1991; 11:547–551.

60. Melnick JL, Adam E, Debakey ME. Cytomegalovirus and atherosclerosis. Eur Heart J 1993; 14(suppl K):30–38.

61. Hajjar DP, Fabricant CG, Minick CR, Fabricant J. Virus-induced atherosclerosis: Herpesvirus infection alters aortic cholesterol metabolism and accumulation. Am J Pathol 1986; 122:62–70.

62. Nicholson AC, Hajjar DP. Herpesviruses in atherosclerosis and thrombosis: etiologic agents or ubiquitous bystanders? Arterioscler Thromb Vasc Biol 1998; 18:339–348.

63. Shah PK. Plaque disruption and coronary thrombosis: new insight into pathogenesis and prevention. Clin Cardiol 1997; 20(II):38–44.

64. Muhlestein JB, Anderson JL, Hammond EH, Zhao L, Trehan S, Schwobe EP, Carlquist JF. Infection with Chlamydia pneumoniae accelerates the development of atherosclerosis and treatment with azithromycin prevents it in a rabbit model. Circulation 1998; 97:633–636.

65. Hu H, Pierce GN, Zhong G. The atherogenic effects of chlamydia are dependent on serum cholesterol and specific to Chlamydia pneumoniae. J Clin Invest 1999; 103:747–753.

66. Gurfinkel E, Bozovich G, Daroca A, Beck E, Mautner B. Randomised trial of roxithromycin in non-Q-wave coronary syndromes: ROXIS Pilot Study. ROXIS Study Group [see comments]. Lancet 1997; 350:404–407.

67. Gupta S, Leatham EW, Carrington D, Mendall MA, Kaski JC, Camm AJ. Elevated Chlamydia pneumoniae antibodies, cardiovascular events, and azithromycin in male survivors of myocardial infarction. Circulation 1997; 96:404–407.

68. Bachmaier K, Neu N, de la Maza LM, Pal S, Hessel A, Penninger JM. Chlamydia infections and heart disease linked through antigenic mimicry. Science 1999; 283:1335–1339.

69. Folkman J. Angiogenesis in cancer, vascular, rheumatoid and other diseases. Nature Med 1995; 1: 27–31.

70. Barger AC, Beeuwkes R, Iainey LL, Siverman KJ. Hypothesis: Vasa vasorum and neovascularization of human coronary arteries. N Engl J Med 1984; 310:175–177.

71. O'Brien ER, Garvin MR, Dev R, Stewart DK, Hiniohara T, Simpson JB, Schwartz SM. Angiogenesis in human atherosclerotic plaques. Am J Pathology 1994; 145:883–894.

72. Kwon HM, Sangiorgi G, Ritman EL, McKenna C, Holmes DL, Schwartz RS, Lerman A: Enhanced coronary vasa vasorum neovascularization in experimental hypercholesterolemia. J Clin Invest 1998; 101:1551–1556.

73. Wang N, Tabas I, Winchester R, Ravalli S, Rabbani L, Tall A. Interleukin-8 is induced by cholesterol loading of macrophages and expressed by macrophage foam-cells in human atheroma. J Biol Chem 1996; 271:8837–8842.

74. Moulton KS, Heller E, Konerding MA, Flynn E, Palinski W, Folkman J. Angiogenesis inhibitor endostatin or TNP-470 reduces intimal neovascularization and plaque growth in apolipoprotein E deficient mice. Circulation 1999; 99:1726–1732.

75. Falk E, Shah PK, Fuster V. Pathogenesis of plaque disruption. In: Fuster V, Ross R, Topol EJ, eds. Atherosclerosis and Coronary Artery Disease. Vol. 2. Philadelphia: Lippincott-Raven, 1996:492–510.

76. Lee RT, Libby P. The unstable atheroma. Arterioscler Thromb Vasc Biol 1997; 17:1859–1867.

77. Shah PK. Role of inflammation and metalloproteinases in plaque disruption and thrombosis. Vasc Med 1998; 3:199–206.

78. Shah PK. Plaque disruption and thrombosis. Potential role of inflammation and infection. Cardiol Clin 1999; 17:271–281.

79. Xu XP, Meisel SR, Ong JM, Kaul S, Cercek B, Rajavashisth TB, Sharifi B, Shah PK. Oxidized low-density lipoprotein regulates matrix metalloproteinase-9 and its tissue inhibitor in human monocyte-derived macrophages. Circulation 1999; 99:993–998.

80. Rajavashisth TB; Xu XP; Jovinge S, Meisel S, MD;, Xu XO, Chai NN, Fishbein MC, Kaul S, Cercek B, Sharifi B, Shah PK: Membrane type 1 matrix metalloproteinase expression in human atherosclerotic plaques: Evidence for activation by proinflammatory mediators. Circulation 1999; 99:3103–3109.

81. Wallner K, Shah PK, Fishbein MC, Forrester JS, Kaul S, Sharifi BG. Tenascin-C Is expressed in macrophage-rich human coronary atherosclerotic plaque. Circulation 1999; 16:1284–1289.

82. Geng Y-J, Libby P. Evidence for apoptosis in advanced human atheroma: Colocalization with interleukin-1 beta-converting enzyme. Am J Pathol 1995; 147:251–266.

83. Wallner K, Li Chen, Shah PK, Sharifi, BG: The EGF-L domain of tenascin-c induces apoptosis of smooth muscle celss in a caspase independent manner. Circulation (abstr) 1999; 100:1–485.

84. Wilcox JN, Smith KM, Schwartz SM, Gordon D. Localization of tissue factor in the normal vessel wall and in the atherosclerotic plaque. Proc Natl Acad Sci USA 1989; 86:2839–2843.

85. Moreno PR, Bernardi VH, López-Cuéllar J, Murcia AM, Palacios IF, Gold HK, Mehran R, Sharma SK, Nemerson Y, Fuster V, Fallon JT. Macrophages, smooth muscle cells, and tissue factor in unstable angina. Implications for cell-mediated thrombogenicity in acute coronary syndromes. Circulation 1996; 94:3090–3097.

86. Toschi V, Gallo R, Lettino M, et al. Tissue factor modulates the thrombogenicity of human atherosclerotic plaque. Circulation 1997; 95:594–599.

87. Fernandez-Ortiz A, Badimon JJ, Falk E, Fuster V, Meyer B, Mailhac A, Weng D, Shah PK, Badimon L. Characterization of the relative thrombogenicity of atherosclerotic plaque components: Implications for consequences of plaque rupture. J Am Coll Cardiol 1994; 23:1562–1569.

88. Burke AP, Farb A, Malcom GT, Liang Y, Smialek J, Virmani R: Effect of risk factors on the mechanism of acute thrombosis and sudden coronary death in women. Circulation 1998; 97(21):2110–2116.

89. Ridker PM, Cushman M, Stampfer MJ, Tracy RP, Hennekens CH. Inflammation, aspirin, and the risk of cardiovascular disease in apparently healthy men. N Engl J Med 1997; 336:973–979.

90. Haverkate F, Thompson SG, Pyke SD, Gallimore JR, Pepys MB. Production of C-reactive protein and risk of coronary events in stable and unstable angina: European Concerted Action on Thrombosis and Disabilities Angina Pectoris Study Group. Lancet 1997; 349:462–466.

91. Toss H, Lindahl B, Siegbahn A, Wallentin L. Prognostic influence of increased fibrinogen and C-reactive protein levels in unstable coronary artery disease. Circulation 1997; 96:4204–4210.

92. Berk BC, Weintraub WS, Alexander RW. Elevation of C-reactive protein in 'active' coronary artery disease. Am J Cardiol 1990; 65:168–172.

93. Levenson J, Giral P, Razavian M, Gariepy J, Simon A. Fibrinogen and silent atherosclerosis in subjects with cardiovascular risk factors. Arterioscler Thromb Vasc Biol 1995; 15:1263–1268.

11
Infectious Aspects of Atherosclerosis

Markku J. Savolainen
University of Oulu, Oulu, Finland

Jukka Juvonen
Kainuu Central Hospital, Kajaani, Finland

Tatu Juvonen
Oulu University Hospital, Oulu, Finland

I. INTRODUCTION

The possibility of an association between atherosclerosis and infectious diseases was proposed as early as the beginning of this century (1,2). During the last two decades, there has been a renewed interest in this hypothesis, especially since 1978, when Fabricant et al. found that chickens infected with a herpes-type virus developed vascular lesions resembling human atherosclerosis (3). Another burst of research interest followed after the study by Saikku et al. (4) associating *Chlamydia pneumoniae* with atherosclerosis.

II. INFECTION AS A RISK FACTOR FOR ATHEROSCLEROSIS

The association between atherosclerosis and infections is based mainly on seroepidemiological data, which are to some extent supported by animal studies. In addition, some studies have demonstrated the presence of infectious agents in atherosclerotic lesions, and pathogens have occasionally been isolated from the diseased vessel wall. A number of infectious agents and conditions have been associated with atherosclerosis, and there are many potential mechanisms that could be initiated by infections and eventually lead to atherothrombogenesis. However, prospective studies and interventions have not been able to give final proof on this matter. On the contrary, some recent studies tend to reject this hypothesis.

In this chapter, we review the current evidence for the role of infections in the development of atherosclerosis and its complications. The postulates originally set out by Robert Koch in 1890 are used as a basis of approving or rejecting the hypothesis that proposes that infectious agents are a causative factor in atherosclerotic diseases (Table 1). Moreover, it is reasonable to expect that eradication of the pathogen will reduce the probability of an individual acquiring the disease or its complications.

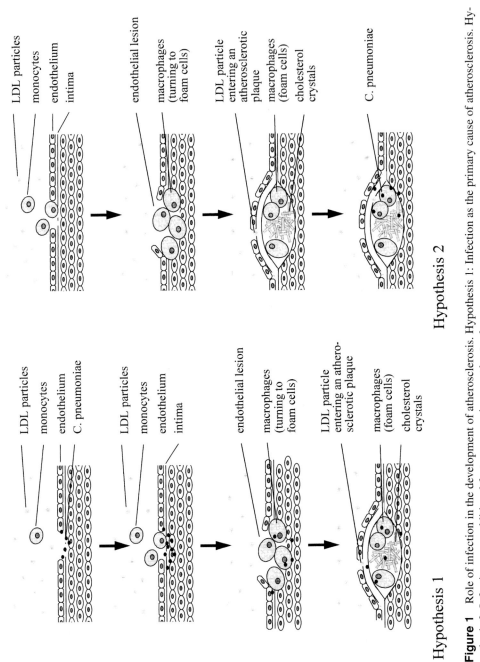

Figure 1 Role of infection in the development of atherosclerosis. Hypothesis 1: Infection as the primary cause of atherosclerosis. Hypothesis 2: Infection as an additional factor or as an innocent bystander.

Table 1   Infectious Agents Implicated in the Development of Atherosclerosis

Viruses
   Herpes (HSV-1, HSV-2)
   Cytomegalovirus
Other microbes
   Chlamydia pneumoniae
   Helicobacter pylori

Table 2   Koch's Postulates in Relation to the Pathogenesis of Atherosclerosis

Original postulates	Postulates applied to atherosclerosis as an infectious disease caused by *C. pneumoniae*
1. The pathogen must be present in every case of the disease.	1. Antigen or DNA found in atherosclerotic lesions (36–40)
2. The pathogen must be isolated from the host and grown in vitro.	2. Chlamydia grown from lesions (44–46)
3. The specific disease must be reproduced when a pure culture of the pathogen is inoculated into a healthy susceptible host.	3. Experimental studies in rabbits have given positive results (47–50)
4. The same pathogen must be recovered again from the experimentally infected host.	4. Not proven.

A.   Seroepidemiological Evidence (Cross-Sectional Studies)

1.   Herpes Viruses

Results from experimental studies (3) raised considerable interest in attempting to link viral infections to atherosclerosis. Out of the seven herpes viruses known to infect humans, herpes simplex virus type 1 (HSV-1) and type 2 (HSV-2), in addition to cytomegalovirus, have been implicated in the genesis, progression, and complications of atherosclerosis. Serological evidence of HSV-1 and HSV-2 is so far lacking. By contrast, research has been focused on the human cytomegalovirus, a third member of the herpes virus family.

2.   Cytomegalovirus

High antibody titers against cytomegalovirus (CMV) (one of the herpes viruses) are found more frequently in patients undergoing surgery for atherosclerosis than in matched controls (5). This finding has also been made in diabetics (6). A significant correlation between CMV antibodies and carotid-intimal-medial thickness has been found in a case–control study (7) and in a prospective study (8). Seroepidemiological data also link CMV infection to atherosclerosis in transplanted hearts (9). Recently, however, two studies failed to demonstrate any association between CMV serology and atherosclerosis (10,11).

3.   *C. pneumoniae*

Seroconversion against an epitope of chlamydial lipopolysaccharide (LPS) has been observed during acute myocardial infarction (4). Further studies with microimmunofluorescence demonstrated the presence of constantly elevated IgG and IgA titers against *C. pneumoniae* in two-thirds of men with acute myocardial infarction and in half of men with chronic coronary heart disease.

By contrast, only one out of six was seropositive among the controls. In hindsight, it is interesting to note that a similar observation was already made in the 1940s but remained unrecognized for decades (12).

The possibility that coronary heart disease makes a patient more vulnerable to *C. pneumoniae* infection or that acute myocardial infection reactivates infection was excluded by the results of the Helsinki Heart Study, where elevated IgG or IgA antibody titers and/or the presence of immunocomplexes, 3 to 6 months earlier, were associated with acute myocardial infection or sudden cardiac death (13).

Elevated *C. pneumoniae* antibody titers were associated with angiographically demonstrated coronary heart disease, while in another study by the same group the association was limited solely to smokers (14). A comparison between 67 healthy men and 103 consecutive age-matched males with angiographically verified coronary heart disease showed that 22% of the coronary heart disease cases but only 5% of the controls had high antibody titers against *C. pneumoniae.* Other studies have also reported that high antibody titers are an independent risk factor for coronary heart disease (15,16).

Patients with coronary heart disease have immune complexes containing chlamydial LPS or *C. pneumoniae*–specific proteins more often than control subjects (17,18).

4. Other Infections

The magnitude of coronary artery intimal thickening is associated with acute systemic infections in children (19). *Helicobacter pylori* antibodies have also been described as a risk factor for coronary heart disease and myocardial infarction (20). The more virulent (CagA-positive) of the two inflammatory *H. pylori* strains seems to correlate with an increased risk of coronary heart disease (21). In a case–control study (22), dental infections have been associated with increased prevalence of coronary heart disease and myocardial infarction. In a prospective study, dental infections were associated with a higher incidence of recurrent coronary events (23).

B. Seroepidemiological Evidence (Prospective Studies)

1. Cytomegalovirus

Major interest in restenosis (a major problem after coronary angioplasty) and CMV has emerged in recent years. Restenosis occurred in 43% of CMV-antibody-positive but only in 8% of CMV-negative patients (24). More evidence for the possible role of CMV has been gathered by studies showing that the risk of restenosis correlates with high anti-CMV titers (25) and with IgG antibodies rather than IgM (24). Moreover, stable IgG levels during follow-up point to a prior infection rather than an acute one as the risk factor for restenosis.

In contrast to restenosis, no relationship between CMV seropositivity and development of myocardial infarction could be found in a 10-year follow-up of the Caerphilly prospective heart disease study (26,27).

2. *C. pneumoniae*

Although retrospective and cross-sectional studies in most cases have shown a positive association between *C. pneumoniae* and the presence of coronary heart disease, prospective data are sparse. Recently, two large studies revealed no evidence of association between *C. pneumoniae* IgG seropositivity and the risk of future myocardial infarction (28,29). By contrast, IgA antibodies, a marker for active or chronic infection with *C. pneumoniae,* were significantly associated with prevalent coronary disease, fatal myocardial infarction, and all-cause mortality (28).

3. Other Infections

In a prospective study, dental infection increased the incidence of recurrent coronary events (23). In another prospective study, seropositivity for *H. pylori* was not associated with increased mean intima–media thickness of the carotid artery, a measure of subclinical atherosclerosis (30).

C. Demonstration of Pathogens in Atherosclerotic Lesions

1. Viruses

Cytomegalovirus or herpes virus DNA or antigen has been demonstrated in atherosclerotic lesions (31–33). Viral DNA or antigen has been found in atherosclerotic lesions in patients undergoing cardiovascular surgery, in the coronary arteries of young trauma victims, in the carotid arteries of patients scheduled for vascular surgery and in transplant-associated atherosclerosis (31). However, a review of published studies revealed only a small difference in the proportion of atheromatous and nonatheromatous blood vessels positive for CMV (34). The presence of virus did not correlate with serum antibody titers (35).

2. *C. pneumoniae*

The presence of *C. pneumoniae* in atherosclerotic lesions has been demonstrated with many different techniques, including electron microscopy (EM), immunohistochemistry and DNA amplification. Using EM of coronary atheromas, structures similar to pear-shaped electron-dense bodies (EBs) with the descriptive characteristics of *C. pneumoniae* were found in the lipid-rich core material of fibrolipid plaques and intimal smooth muscle cells (36). Tissue sections from 5 out of 7 patients stained positively with chlamydial genus-specific and *C. pneumoniae* species-specific antibodies.

In another study, including autopsy cases, *C. pneumoniae* was detected by immunohistochemistry (IHC) or the polymerase chain reaction (PCR) in atherosclerotic lesions at different stages from 20 out of 36 cadavers studied, and EM revealed organisms resembling *C. pneumoniae* EBs in 6 of the 21 plaques studied. *C. pneumoniae* was found only in the diseased vessel wall (intimal smooth muscle cells, foam cells, and central necrotic area of the plaque) (37). The presence of *C. pneumoniae* was also shown by IHC and PCR in early atheromatous lesions (6 out of 7 atheromas and 2 out of 11 intimal thickenings) of young people (ages 15 to 34) who died of sudden trauma, but not in histologically normal arterial tissues from the same cadavers (38). *C. pneumoniae* has also been found by PCR and IHC in carotid arteries removed from patients suffering from advanced, symptomatic arteriosclerosis (39). Whether *C. pneumoniae* can be detected in coronary atherectomy tissue is still not clear. An early study (40) showed a high prevalence of chlamydia only in coronary arteries diseased by atherosclerosis whereas a recent study (41) demonstrated a low prevalence. Additional evidence against *C. pneumoniae* as a causative factor in atherosclerosis has been reported in a recent study (42) showing no correlation between the distribution of *C. pneumoniae* and the severity or extent of atherosclerosis.

If chlamydia were only an "innocent bystander," it should also be found in arteries diseased by processes other than atherosclerosis. With direct immunofluorescence, chlamydial antigen was present in 71 out of 90 coronary artery specimens from symptomatic patients undergoing coronary atherectomy, but only in 1 out of 24 nonatherosclerotic coronary specimens (39).

3. *Helicobacter pylori*

In a recent report (43), *H. pylori* was not detected by PCR in atherosclerotic plaques from carotid endarterectomy samples.

D. Isolation and Culture of Pathogens from Atherosclerotic Lesions

1. Viruses

Thus far, it has not been possible to culture viruses from human atherosclerotic lesions.

2. *C. pneumoniae*

C. pneumoniae has recently been isolated both from the coronary artery of a patient with advanced arteriosclerosis and from cases of carotid atherosclerosis (44,45). Viable *C. pneumoniae* was found in 11 (16%) out of 70 atherosclerotic specimens taken by endarterectomy from coronary arteries (46).

E. Inoculation of Pathogens into Experimental Animals

1. Viruses

In 1978, Fabricant et al. (3) established an animal model for atherosclerosis by infecting normocholesterolemic pathogen-free chickens with a herpes virus that caused malignant lymphomas of T-cell origin in chickens (Marek's disease virus). Atherosclerotic lesions developed in the aorta and its major branches as well as in the coronary arteries. Such lesions could be prevented by vaccination.

2. *C. pneumoniae*

Both mouse and rabbit models have been used for studying *C. pneumoniae* infection and atherosclerosis (47,48). After intranasal infection of mice with *C. pneumoniae*, the organism was much more frequently detected in the atheromatous aortas of atherosclerosis-suspectible apolipoprotein E–deficient mice than in the aortas of the wild-type strain (48). Intranasal infection of New Zealand White rabbits with *C. pneumoniae* maintained on normal diet and reinfected 3 weeks later produced aortic inflammatory changes, intimal thickening, or fibroid plaques resembling atherosclerosis in 6 of 9 animals. Three of the rabbits with atherosclerotic lesions were *C. pneumoniae*–positive by immunohistochemistry. Atherosclerotic lesions were not detected in controls (49). Repeated intranasal inoculation of rabbits with *C. pneumoniae*, fed a modestly cholesterol-enriched diet, significantly increased the maximal intimal thickness compared with uninfected controls and infected rabbits that received the antichlamydial agent azithromycin (50).

III. POTENTIAL PATHOPHYSIOLOGICAL MECHANISMS

Some of the most important pathological events in the development of atherosclerotic plaque include: endothelial damage, inflammatory cell infiltration with accumulation of lipids and extracellular matrix, platelet aggregation, and smooth muscle cell proliferation. Infection may be linked to these events in several ways (1). We will consider mechanisms by which *C. pneumoniae* may influence atherosclerosis.

A. Lipopolysaccharide

Circulating or local deposition of bacterial LPS can damage the endothelium, possibly by stimulating the production of inflammatory cytokines and growth factors (51). The activation of macrophages by LPS or LPS-induced cytokines leads to increased formation of immunogenic and atherogenic oxidized low-density lipoproteins (LDL) (52). There are also remarkable changes in the hemostatic system related to infections. Bacterial LPS may induce the release of tissue factor (the initiator of the extrinsic coagulation pathway) and activate Hageman factor (a participant in the intrinsic pathway). It induces monocytes to aggregate platelets, to produce factor VII activity, and to generate plasminogen activator inhibitors. Infections are also known to increase blood viscosity by increasing the concentrations of plasma fibrinogen, factor VIII, β-thromboglobulin, and thromboxane, whereas levels of antithrombin III are reduced (1,53,54). Recently it has been demonstrated that *C. pneumoniae* infection activates NF-κB and induces tissue factor and plasminogen activator inhibitor-1 expression in vascular smooth muscle cells and endothelial cells (55).

B. Heat Shock Proteins

Heat shock proteins (HSPs) are highly conserved proteins with notable homology among different species ranging from bacteria to humans. Autoantibodies to mycobacterial HSP65 have been demonstrated in atherosclerotic patients (56). Because atherosclerotic lesions show many features of autoimmune reactions and express human HSPs, it has been postulated that a cross-reaction between bacterial and host HSPs may contribute to immune activation. *C. pneumoniae* and periodontal pathogens have marked homology to human and mycobacterial HSPs. Immunological cross-reactions may hence occur (56–58). Chlamydial HSP60 frequently colocalizes with human HSPs in plaque macrophages of human atherosclerotic lesions. Both human and chlamydial HSPs induce tumor-necrosis factor-α (TNF-α) and matrix metalloproteinase production by macrophages (60). Anti-HSP65 titers correlate with both the severity and the extent of coronary atherosclerosis (60) and are associated with carotid atherosclerosis (61). Successful eradication of *H. pylori* leads to a significant fall in the titers of anti-HSP65 (60).

C. Persistent Infection

Both *C. pneumoniae* and CMV can infect human macrophages, endothelial cells, and smooth muscle cells (62–64). Chlamydia can cause persistent infections, thereby providing an opportunity for a chronic low-grade inflammation. In the setting of persistent chlamydial infections, the host response seems to be a major contributor to the development of the disease (58,65,66). Persistent infection and chronic stimulation of the host with chlamydial antigens is associated with poor clinical outcomes. Primary *C. trachomatis* ocular infection in humans and monkeys resolves with little or no residual tissue damage. However, recurrent infections produce an intense inflammatory reaction and cause scarring trachoma (67). On the other hand, trauma or changes in immunological circumstances may reactivate quiescent chlamydial infection (58,65,67). By analogy with trachoma, it is tempting to speculate that in some immunologically vulnerable subjects *C. pneumoniae* may persist in the arterial wall after the primary infection. The trauma activating the infection could be caused by mechanical stress. Multiple *C. pneumoniae* reinfections during one's lifetime might activate an immunological response to *C. pneumoniae* antigens in the arterial wall. The LPS of *C. pneumoniae* may cause endothelial damage in spite of the fact that its endotoxin activity is much lower than that of gram-negative enterobacteria (68,69). The persistence of *C. pneumoniae* or its antigens in the arterial wall may lead to release of inflammatory cytokines or adhesion molecules and ultimately to an inflammatory reaction (65).

This hypothesis is supported by recent studies focusing on degenerative aortic valves (70). *C. pneumoniae* species-specific antigen was present in 53% of the aortic valves in a cross-sectional autopsy study. Positive staining with the *C. pneumoniae* species-specific antibody was found in 44% of normal valve specimens and in 83% of the valves with signs of "early lesions" of aortic valve stenosis. In younger subjects, 60% of the valves were positive for the species-specific antibody, although their valves were macroscopically normal. Among subjects over age 60, the prevalence of "early lesions" was significantly greater if the person was positive for *C. pneumoniae* (87% vs. 14%). The finding that *C. pneumoniae* persists in aortic valves and is more common after the macroscopically normal valve evolves to having an "early lesion" provides additional evidence for the participation of *C. pneumoniae* in the pathogenesis of vascular diseases.

D. Conventional Risk Factors

Infections may also modify conventional risk factors. The release of cytokines may induce the synthesis of acute phase proteins, such as fibrinogen or lipoprotein(a), in liver and influence lipid metabolism (15,65). In unstable angina, high fibrinogen levels seems to be associated with persistent *C. pneumoniae* infection (72). During infection, lipid metabolism and glucose tolerance may become impaired. Subjects with chronic *C. pneumoniae* infection, defined by persistent IgG and IgA antibodies, have higher cholesterol and triglyceride and lower HDL cholesterol concentrations than subjects without detectable antibodies (73).

IV. PREVENTION OF ATHEROSCLEROSIS BY ANTIMICROBIAL TREATMENT

If infection plays a role in the pathogenesis of atherosclerosis, vaccination or intervention with antibiotics should prevent vascular lesions. This issue has obvious clinical implications and is the focus of several recent studies.

A. Vaccination Against Viruses

In a prototype prevention study, Fabricant et al. (3) reported in 1983 that atherosclerotic lesions induced by herpes virus could be prevented by preimmunizing chickens with a turkey herpes virus vaccine.

B. Intervention Studies Targeting *C. pneumoniae*

In the first human intervention study of treatment for *Chlamydia* (74), 213 survivors of myocardial infarctions were followed up for 18 months. Significant cardiac ischemic events occurred among 7% of patients who had undetectable IgG against *C. pneumoniae,* 15% who had moderate IgG titers, and 28% who had high IgG (>64) titers. By contrast, primary cardiac end points only occurred in 8% of patients with high IgG titers who were treated with azithromycin (74).

In another randomized study, doxycyclin or placebo was given for 4 months to 34 patients with chronic coronary artery disease and mild hypertension or moderate hypercholesterolemia and previous bypass operation. After a follow-up of 6 months, the treatment groups were similar with regard to *C. pneumoniae* antibodies or coronary heart disease risk factors (75).

A more recent addition to the list of intervention studies is the ACADEMIC study (76), which showed no benefit of azithromycin treatment in 150 coronary heart disease patients positive for *C. pneumoniae* antibodies as compared with placebo with regard to clinical events or antibody titers. However, the global score of inflammation markers was improved by the antibiotic therapy.

The authors of the ROXIS study first reported positive results based on preliminary analysis of 202 patients with unstable angina or non-Q wave infarction randomized to receive roxithromycin 150 mg orally twice a day or placebo for 30 days. After a follow-up of 6 months, the primary composite triple end point (cardiac ischemic death, acute myocardial infarction, severe recurrent ischemia) rate was significantly reduced in the roxithromycin group (77). In the final report, however, no beneficial effect was observed (78). It is noteworthy that the preliminary positive results were reported in one of the leading medical journals with a high impact factor, whereas the final report with negative results was published in a journal read by a much smaller group of specialists. The publication bias has recently been emphasized (79).

V. HOW STRONG IS THE EVIDENCE SO FAR?

There are limitations in the studies concerning the associations between atheroclerosis and infections. First, many seroepidemiological studies have had methodological limitations with the size of the study populations or with the influence of confounding factors. Second, the presence of an antigen, DNA, RNA, or even a viable pathogen does not prove a causal relationship since the pathogen can also be an innocent bystander harbored in damaged tissue.

As pointed out recently (80) with regard to *C. pneumoniae,* if the pathogen plays a role in the etiology of atherosclerosis and its complications, the role could be related to the initiation of the disease, the progression of the disease, or the complicating events. The evidence gathered so far suggests that infectious agents, such as *C. pneumoniae,* may be involved in the genesis of atherosclerotic lesions at least in some patients. The results from prospective studies are still contradictory and large interventional studies are definitely needed in order to demonstrate the antiatherosclerotic effect of macrolide antibiotics in subjects with *C. pneumoniae* infection.

Table 3 Studies of Infectious Agents in the Development of Atherosclerosis

	Evidence (reference numbers)	
	FOR	*AGAINST*
Epidemiological association (cross-sectional studies)		
Herpes viruses (HSV-1, HSV-2)	—	—
Cytomegalovirus	5–9	10–11
Chlamydia pneumoniae	4,13–18	—
Helicobacter pylori	20,21	—
Other infections (dental infections)	22	—
Epidemiological association (prospective studies)		
Cytomegalovirus	24,25	26,27
Chlamydia pneumoniae	28	28,29
Helicobacter pylori	—	30
Other infections (dental infections)	23	—
Evidence of antigen or DNA of pathogen in lesions		
Herpes/cytomegalovirus	31,32	34,35
Chlamydia pneumoniae	36–40	41,42
Helicobacter pylori	—	43
Growth of pathogen from atherosclerotic lesions		
Chlamydia pneumoniae	44–46	—
Inoculation of pathogens into experimental animals		
Herpes	3	—
Chlamydia pneumoniae	47–50	—

Table 4 Randomized Prospective Prevention Trials

Reference	Drug	Treatment	Follow-up	Patients	End points
74	Azithromycin	3–6 days	18 months	213	reduced
75	Doxycyclin	4 months	6 months	34	no effect
76	Azithromycin	3 months	6 months	150	no effect
78	Roxithromycin	30 days	6 months	202	no effect

VI. FUTURE PERSPECTIVES

Our understanding of the roles microorganisms may play in the development and progression of atherosclerotic diseases is rapidly changing. The implications of infection enhancing atherogenesis are profound in regard to treatment with antimicrobials or vaccination. At present, the results of clinical trials with antibiotics are inconclusive (81). We feel such approaches deserve further exploration and should include larger numbers of patients and more clearly defined subsets.

We must also be mindful of the possibility that eradication of microorganisms that are found in atherosclerotic lesions may have yet to be considered deleterious effects.

REFERENCES

1. Mattila KJ, Valtonen VV, Nieminen MS, Asikainen S. Role of infection as a risk factor for atherosclerosis, myocardial infarction, and stroke. Clin Infect Dis 1998; 26:719–734.
2. Kuvin JT, Kimmelstiel CD. Infectious causes of atherosclerosis. Am Heart J 1999; 137:216–226.
3. Fabricant CG, Fabricant J, Minick CR, Litrenta MM. Herpesvirus-induced atherosclerosis in chickens. Fed Proc 1983; 42:2476–2479.
4. Saikku P, Leinonen M, Mattila K, Ekman MR, Nieminen MS, Mäkelä PH, Huttunen JK, Valtonen V. Serological evidence of an association of a novel Chlamydia, TWAR, with chronic coronary heart disease and acute myocardial infarction. Lancet 1988; 2(8618):983–986.
5. Adam E, Melnick JL, Probtsfield JL, Petrie BL, Burek J, Bailey KR, McCollum CH, DeBakey ME. High levels of cytomegalovirus antibody in patients requiring vascular surgery for atherosclerosis. Lancet 1987; 2(8554):291–293.
6. Visseren FL, Bouter KP, Pon MJ, Hoekstra JB, Erkelens DW, Diepersloot RJ. Patients with diabetes mellitus and atherosclerosis: A role for cytomegalovirus? Diabetes Res Clin Pract 1997; 36:49–55.
7. Sorlie PD, Adam E, Melnick SL, Folsom A, Skelton T, Chambless LE, Barnes R, Melnick JL. Cytomegalovirus/herpesvirus and carotid atherosclerosis: The ARIC Study. J Med Virol 1994; 42:33–37.
8. Nieto FJ, Adam E, Sorlie P, Farzadegan H, Melnick JL, Comstock GW, Szklo M. Cohort study of cytomegalovirus infection as a risk factor for carotid intimal-medial thickening, a measure of subclinical atherosclerosis. Circulation 1996; 94:922–927.
9. Grattan MT, Moreno-Cabral CE, Starnes VA, Oyer PE, Stinson EB, Shumway NE. Cytomegalovirus infection is associated with cardiac allograft rejection and atherosclerosis. JAMA 1989; 261:3561–3566.
10. Ossewaarde JM, Feskens EJ, De Vries A, Vallinga CE, Kromhout D. Chlamydia pneumoniae is a risk factor for coronary heart disease in symptom-free elderly men, but Helicobacter pylori and cytomegalovirus are not. Epidemiol Infect 1998; 120:93–99.
11. Adler SP, Hur JK, Wang JB, Vetrovec GW. Prior infection with cytomegalovirus is not a major risk factor for angiographically demonstrated coronary artery atherosclerosis. J Infect Dis 1998; 177:209–212.

12. Coutts WE, Davila M. Lymphogranuloma venereum as a possible cause of arteriosclerosis and other arterial conditions. J Trop Med Hyg 1945; 48:46–51.
13. Saikku P, Leinonen M, Tenkanen L, Linnanmäki E, Ekman MR, Manninen V, Mänttäri M, Frick MH, Huttunen JK. Chronic Chlamydia pneumoniae infection as a risk factor for coronary heart disease in the Helsinki Heart Study. Ann Intern Med 1992; 116:273–278.
14. Thom DH, Grayston JT, Siscovick DS, Wang SP, Weiss NS, Daling JR. Association of prior infection with Chlamydia pneumoniae and angiographically demonstrated coronary artery disease. JAMA 1992; 268:68–72.
15. Mendall MA, Carrington D, Strachan D, Patel P, Molineaux N, Levi J, Toosey T, Camm AJ, Northfield TC. Chlamydia pneumoniae: Risk factors for seropositivity and association with coronary heart. J Infect 1995; 30:121–128.
16. Miettinen H, Lehto S, Saikku P, Haffner SM, Rönnemaa T, Pyörälä K, Laakso M. Association of Chlamydia pneumoniae and acute coronary heart disease events in non–insulin dependent diabetic and nondiabetic subjects in Finland. Eur Heart J 1996; 17:682–688.
17. Leinonen M, Linnanmäki E, Mattila K, Nieminen MS, Valtonen V, Leirisalo-Repo M, Saikku P. Circulating immune complexes containing chlamydial lipopolysaccharide in acute myocardial infarction. Microb Pathog 1990; 9:67–73.
18. Linnanmäki E, Leinonen M, Mattila K, Nieminen M, Valtonen V, Saikku P. Chlamydia pneumoniae-specific circulating immune complexes in patients with chronic coronary heart disease. Circulation 1993; 87:1130–1134.
19. Pesonen E. Infection and intimal thickening: Evidence from coronary arteries in children. Eur Heart J 1994; 15(suppl C):57–61.
20. Mendall MA, Goggin PM, Molineaux N, Levy J, Toosy T, Strachan D, Camm AJ, Northfield TC. Relation of Helicobacter pylori infection and coronary heart disease. Br Heart J 1994; 71:437–439.
21. Pasceri V, Cammarota G, Patti G, Cuoco L, Gasbarrini A, Grillo RL, Fedeli G, Gasbarrini G, Maseri A. Association of virulent Helicobacter pylori strains with ischemic heart disease. Circulation 1998; 97:1675–1679.
22. Mattila KJ, Nieminen MS, Valtonen VV, Rasi VP, Kesäniemi YA, Syrjälä SL, Jungel PS, Isoluoma M, Hietaniemi K, Jokinen MJ. Association between dental health and acute myocardial infarction. Br Med J 1989; 298:779–781.
23. Mattila K, Valtonen VV, Nieminen M, Huttunen J. Dental infection and the risk of new coronary events: Prospective study of patients with documented coronary artery disease. Clin Infect Dis 1995; 20:588–592.
24. Zhou YF, Leon MB, Waclawiw MA, Popma JJ, Yu ZX, Finkel T, Epstein SE. Association between prior cytomegalovirus infection and the risk of restenosis after coronary atherectomy. N Engl J Med 1996; 335:624–630.
25. Blum A, Giladi M, Weinberg M, Kaplan G, Pasternack H, Laniado S, Miller H. High anti-cytomegalovirus (CMV) IgG antibody titer is associated with coronary artery disease and may predict post-coronary balloon angioplasty restenosis. Am J Cardiol 1998; 81:866–868.
26. Strachan DP, Carrington D, Mendall MA, Butland BK, Sweetnam PM, Elwood PC. Cytomegalovirus seropositivity and incident ischaemic heart disease in the Caerphilly prospective heart disease study. Heart 1999; 81:248–251.
27. Ridker PM, Hennekens CH, Stampfer MJ, Wang F. Prospective study of Herpes simplex virus, cytomegalovirus, and the risk of future myocardial infarction and stroke. Circulation 1999; 98:2796–2799.
28. Strachan DP, Carrington D, Mendall MA, Ballam L, Morris J, Butland BK, Sweetnam PM, Elwood PC. Relation of Chlamydia pneumoniae serology to mortality and incidence of ischaemic heart disease over 13 years in the Caerphilly prospective heart disease study. Br Med J 1999; 318:1035–1039.
29. Ridker PM, Kundsin RB, Stampfer MJ, Poulin S, Hennekens CH. Prospective study of Chlamydia pneumoniae IgG seropositivity and risks of future myocardial infarction. Circulation 1999; 99:1161–1164.
30. Folsom AR, Nieto FJ, Sorlie P, Chambless L, and Graham DY. Helicobacter pylori seropositivity and coronary heart disease incidence. Circulation 1998; 98:845–850.

31. Benditt EP, Barrett T, McDougall JK. Viruses in the etiology of atherosclerosis. Proc Natl Acad Sci USA 1983; 80:6386–6389.

32. Melnick JL, Adam E, Debakey ME. Cytomegalovirus and atherosclerosis. Eur Heart J 1993; 14(suppl K):30–38.

33. Taylor-Robinson D, Thomas BJ. Chlamydia pneumoniae in arteries: The facts, their interpretation, and future studies. J Clin Pathol 1998; 51:793–797.

34. Danesh J, Collins R, Peto R. Chronic infections and coronary heart disease: Is there a link? Lancet 1997; 350(9075):430–436.

35. Chiu B, Viira E, Tucker W, Fong IW. Chlamydia pneumoniae, cytomegalovirus, and herpes simplex virus in atherosclerosis of the carotid artery. Circulation 1997; 96:2144–2148.

36. Shor A, Kuo CC, Patton DL. Detection of Chlamydia pneumoniae in coronary arterial fatty streaks and atheromatous plaques. S Afr Med J 1992; 82:158–161.

37. Kuo CC, Shor A, Campbell LA, Fukushi H, Patton DL, Grayston JT. Demonstration of Chlamydia pneumoniae in atherosclerotic lesions of coronary arteries. J Infect Dis 1993; 167:841–849.

38. Kuo CC, Grayston JT, Campbell LA, Goo YA, Wissler RW, Benditt EP. Chlamydia pneumoniae (TWAR) in coronary arteries of young adults (15–34 years old). Proc Natl Acad Sci USA 1995; 92:6911–6914.

39. Grayston JT, Kuo CC, Coulson AS, Campbell LA, Lawrence RD, Lee MJ, Strandness ED, Wang SP. Chlamydia pneumoniae (TWAR) in atherosclerosis of the carotid artery. Circulation 1995; 92:3397–3400.

40. Muhlestein JB, Hammond EH, Carlquist JF, Radicke E, Thomson MJ, Karagounis LA, Woods ML, Anderson JL. Increased incidence of Chlamydia species within the coronary arteries of patients with symptomatic atherosclerotic versus other forms of cardiovascular disease. J Am Coll Cardiol 1996; 27:1555–1561.

41. Jantos CA, Nesseler A, Waas W, Baumgartner W, Tillmanns H, Haberbosch W. Low prevalence of Chlamydia pneumoniae in atherectomy specimens from patients with coronary heart disease. Clin Infect Dis 1999; 28:988–992.

42. Thomas M, Wong Y, Thomas D, Ajaz M, Tsang V, Gallagher PJ, Ward ME. Relation between direct detection of Chlamydia pneumoniae DNA in human coronary arteries at postmortem examination and histological severity (Stary grading) of associated atherosclerotic plaque. Circulation 1999; 99:2733–2736.

43. Malnick SD, Goland S, Kaftoury A, Schwarz H, Pasik S, Mashiach A, Sthoeger Z. Evaluation of carotid arterial plaques after endarterectomy for Helicobacter pylori infection. Am J Cardiol 1999; 83:1586–1587.

44. Jackson LA, Campbell LA, Kuo CC, Rodriguez DI, Lee A, Grayston JT. Isolation of Chlamydia pneumoniae from a carotid endarterectomy specimen. J Infect Dis 1997; 176:292–295.

45. Ramirez JA. Isolation of Chlamydia pneumoniae from the coronary artery of a patient with coronary atherosclerosis. The Chlamydia pneumoniae/Atherosclerosis Study Group. Ann Intern Med 1996; 125:979–982.

46. Maass M, Bartels C, Engel PM, Mamat U, Sievers HH. Endovascular presence of viable Chlamydia pneumoniae is a common phenomenon in coronary artery disease. J Am Coll Cardiol 1998; 31:827–832.

47. Fong IW, Chiu B, Viira E, Fong MW, Jang D, Mahony J. Rabbit model for Chlamydia pneumoniae infection. J Clin Microbiol 1997; 35:48–52.

48. Moazed TC, Kuo C, Grayston JT, Campbell LA. Murine models of Chlamydia pneumoniae infection and atherosclerosis. J Infect Dis 1997; 175:883–890.

49. Laitinen K, Laurila A, Pyhälä L, Leinonen M, Saikku P. Chlamydia pneumoniae infection induces inflammatory changes in the aortas of rabbits. Infect Immun 1997; 65:4832–4835.

50. Muhlestein JB, Anderson JL, Hammond EH, Zhao L, Trehan S, Schwobe EP, Carlquist JF. Infection with Chlamydia pneumoniae accelerates the development of atherosclerosis and treatment with azithromycin prevents it in a rabbit model. Circulation 1998; 97:633–636.

51. Libby P, Egan D, Skarlatos S. Roles of infectious agents in atherosclerosis and restenosis: An assessment of the evidence and need for future research. Circulation 1997; 96:4095–4103.

52. Lopes-Virella MF. Interactions between bacterial lipopolysaccharides and serum lipoproteins and their possible role in coronary heart disease. Eur Heart J 1993; 14(suppl K):118–124.
53. Nieminen MS, Mattila K, Valtonen V. Infection and inflammation as risk factors for myocardial infarction. Eur Heart J 1993; 14(suppl K):12–16.
54. Cook PJ, Lip GY. Infectious agents and atherosclerotic vascular disease. Q J Med 1996; 89:727–735.
55. Wick G, Schett G, Amberger A, Kleindienst R, Xu Q. Is atherosclerosis an immunologically mediated disease? Immunol Today 1995; 16:27–33.
56. Dechend R, Maass M, Gieffers J, Dietz R, Scheidereit C, Leutz A, Gulba DC. Chlamydia pneumoniae infection of vascular smooth muscle and endothelial cells activates NF-κB and induces tissue factor and PAI-1 expression. A potential link to accelerated atherosclerosis. Circulation 1999; 100:1369–1373.
57. Beatty WL, Morrison RP, Byrne GI. Persistent chlamydiae: From cell culture to a paradigm for chlamydial pathogenesis. Microbiol Rev 1994; 58:686–699.
58. Nakano Y, Inai Y, Yamashita Y, Nagaoka S, Kusuzaki-Nagira T, Nishihara T, Okahashi N, Koga T. Molecular and immunological characterization of a 64-kDa protein of Actinobacillus actinomycetemcomitans. Oral Microbiol Immunol 1995; 10:151–159.
59. Kol A, Galina K. Sukhova, Andrew H. Lichtman, Libby P. Chlamydial heat shock protein 60 localizes in human atheroma and regulates macrophage tumor necrosis factor- and matrix metalloproteinase expression. Circulation 1998; 98:300–307.
60. Birnie DH, Holme ER, McKay IC, Hood S, McColl KE, Hillis WS. Association between antibodies to heat shock protein 65 and coronary atherosclerosis. Possible mechanism of action of Helicobacter pylori and other bacterial infections in increasing cardiovascular risk. Eur Heart J 1998; 19:387–394.
61. Xu Q, Kiechl S, Mayr M, Metzler B, Egger G, Oberhollenzer F, Willeit J, Wick G. Association of serum antibodies to heat-shock protein 65 with carotid atherosclerosis. Clinical significance determined in a follow-up study. Circulation 1999; 100:1169–1174.
62. Van Dam-Mieras MC, Bruggeman CA, Muller AD, Debie WH, Zwaal RF. Induction of endothelial cell procoagulant activity by cytomegalovirus infection. Thromb Res 1987; 47:69–75.
63. Kaukoranta-Tolvanen SS, Laitinen K, Saikku P, Leinonen M. Chlamydia pneumoniae multiplies in human endothelial cells in vitro. Microb Pathog 1994; 16:313–319.
64. Gaydos CA, Summersgill JT, Sahney NN, Ramirez JA, Quinn TC. Replication of Chlamydia pneumoniae in vitro in human macrophages, endothelial cells, and aortic artery smooth muscle cells. Infect Immun 1996; 64:1614–1620.
65. Ward ME. The immunobiology and immunopathology of chlamydial infections. APMIS 1995; 103:769–796.
66. Schachter J. Pathogenesis of chlamydial infections. Pathol Immunopathol Res 1989; 8:206–220.
67. Grayston JT, Wang SP, Yeh LJ, Kuo CC. Importance of reinfection in the pathogenesis of trachoma. Rev Infect Dis 1985; 7:717–725.
68. Brade L, Nurminen M, Mäkelä PH, Brade H. Antigenic properties of Chlamydia trachomatis lipopolysaccharide. Infect Immun 1985; 48:569–572.
69. Ingalls RR, Rice PA, Qureshi N, Takayama K, Lin JS, Golenbock DT. The inflammatory cytokine response to Chlamydia trachomatis infection is endotoxin. Infect Immun 1995; 63:3125–3130.
70. Juvonen J, Juvonen T, Laurila A, Kuusisto J, Alarakkola E, Särkioja T et al. Can degenerative aortic valve stenosis be related to persistent Chlamydia pneumoniae infection? Ann Intern Med 1998; 128:741–744.
71. Patel P, Mendall MA, Carrington D, Strachan DP, Leatham E, Molineaux N, Levy J, Blakeston C, Seymour CA, Camm AJ, et al. Association of Helicobacter pylori and Chlamydia pneumoniae infections with coronary heart disease and cardiovascular risk factors. Br Med J 1995; 311:711–714.
72. Toss H, Gnarpe J, Gnarpe H, Siegbahn A, Lindahl B, Wallentin L. Increased fibrinogen levels are associated with persistent Chlamydia pneumoniae infection in unstable coronary artery disease. Eur Heart J 1998; 19:570–577.
73. Laurila A, Bloigu A, Näyhä S, Hassi J, Leinonen M, Saikku P. Chronic Chlamydia pneumoniae infection is associated with a serum lipid profile known to be a risk factor for atherosclerosis. Arterioscler Thromb Vasc Biol 1997; 17:2910–3913.

74. Gupta S, Leatham EW, Carrington D, Mendall MA, Kaski JC, Camm AJ. Elevated Chlamydia pneumoniae antibodies, cardiovascular events, and azithromycin in male survivors of myocardial infarction. Circulation 1997; 96:404–407.

75. Sinisalo J, Mattila K, Nieminen MS, Valtonen V, Syrjälä M, Sundberg S, Saikku P. The effect of prolonged doxycycline therapy on Chlamydia pneumoniae serological markers, coronary heart disease risk factors and forearm basal nitric oxide production. J Antimicrob Chemother 1998; 41:85–92.

76. Anderson JL, Muhlestein JB, Carlquist J, Allen A, Trehan S, Nielson C, Hall S, Brady J, Egger M, Horne B, Lim T. Randomized secondary prevention trial with azithromycin in patients with coronary artery disease and serological evidence for Chlamydia pneumoniae infection. The Azithromycin in Coronary Artery Disease: Elimination of Myocardial Infection with Chlamydia (ACADEMIC) Study. Circulation 1999; 99:1540–1547.

77. Gurfinkel E, Bozovich G, Daroca A, Beck E, Mautner B. Randomised trial of roxithromycin in non-Q-wave coronary syndromes: ROXIS Pilot Study. Lancet 1997; 350(9075):404–407.

78. Gurfinkel E, Bozovich G, Beck E, Testa E, Livellara B, Mautner B. Treatment with the antibiotic roxithromycin in patients with acute non-Q-wave coronary syndromes: The final report of the ROXIS study. Eur Heart J 1999; 20:121–127.

79. Epstein SE, Zhu J. Lack of association of infectious agents with risk of future myocardial infarction and stroke. Definitive evidence disproving the infection/coronary artery disease hypothesis? Circulation 1999; 100:1366–1368.

80. Grayston JT. Antibiotic treatment trials for secondary prevention of coronary artery disease events. Circulation 1999; 99:1538–1539.

81. Folsom AR. Antibiotics for prevention of myocardial infarction? Not yet! JAMA 1999; 281:461–462.

12
Cellular Immune Responses in Atherosclerosis

Göran K. Hansson
Karolinska Institutet and Karolinska Hospital, Stockholm, Sweden

I. INTRODUCTION

Atherosclerosis is the leading cause of death in the Western world and one of the most rapidly increasing lethal diseases in the developing world (1). It is a slowly progressive disease characterized by focal accumulations of cells, extracellular matrix, and lipids in the intima of large and middle-sized arteries (2,3). This results in narrowing of the lumen and causes hampered blood flow to the end organ with resultant ischemic symptoms such as angina pectoris and intermittent claudication. Moreover, thrombi often develop on the surface of the lesion and may completely occlude the lumen, leading to infarction of the end organ. This is the most common cause of myocardial infarction. Thrombotic material from such lesions may form arterial emboli that can occlude smaller arteries downstream from the "active plaque," which results in sudden ischemic symptoms such as transient ischemic attacks, stroke, and acute gangrene.

Atherosclerosis is in itself a silent pathological process that precipitates clinical manifestations only at a late stage of disease. Clinical research on its pathogenesis has therefore been hampered by the lack of early indicators of the presence of disease and its rate of progression. Furthermore, the mere fact that atherosclerosis is one of the most common diseases that affects mankind causes substantial problems for clinical scientists and epidemiologists attempting to identify markers of disease. Large epidemiological studies have, however, provided important information on atherosclerosis and several risk factors have been identified that are statistically correlated to clinical manifestations of disease. The most important among them are smoking, hypercholesterolemia, high blood pressure, and diabetes. However, it has been estimated that only approximately 50% of the incidence of ischemic heart disease can be explained by these major risk factors. Consequently, there is room for substantial, as yet unidentified, contributing factors.

Experimental research into the molecular and cellular mechanisms of atherosclerosis has provided important information concerning the pathogenesis of the disease. In particular, the recently developed targeted gene deletion technology has provided murine models that have already proven to be very useful in mechanistic research on the pathogenesis of atherosclerosis (4).

While the etiology of the disease has been identified only in individuals who suffer from familial hypercholesterolemia, our current understanding of the disease process is that several different etiologic factors or combinations thereof may lead to a common sequence of events that lead from normal artery to atherosclerotic plaque (3). It involves the accumulation and oxidative modification of circulating low-density lipoproteins (LDLs), activation of endothelial cells at sites of hemodynamic and metabolic strain, entry of mononuclear leukocytes into the intima, activation of macrophages and T lymphocytes, formation of lipid-laden foam cells, and induction of a fibroproliferative response of the smooth muscle cells of the artery (5,6). A common denominator for this process is vascular inflammation, which is discussed in detail in this chapter. Key steps are illustrated in Figure 1.

II. INITIATING EVENTS IN ATHEROGENESIS

Although a large number of early phenomena have been identified in experimental studies of atherosclerosis, the accumulation of lipoproteins in the arterial intima appears to be a sine qua non for this disease. The small dense fraction of LDL is considered particularly atherogenic since it readily penetrates the endothelium and has a tendency to associate with proteoglycans of the extracellular matrix in the arterial wall (7). High circulating LDL levels favor this process by increasing the number of LDL particles that can penetrate the endothelium. Since LDL is the major cholesterol-transporting plasma lipoprotein, serum cholesterol is a risk factor for atherosclerosis.

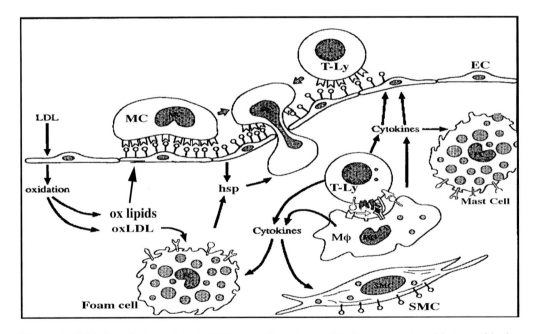

Figure 1 Initiation of atherosclerosis. LDL enters the artery wall in large amounts and is trapped in the subendothelial intima. It undergoes oxidative modification (oxidized LDL, oxLDL), which releases proinflammatory, oxidized lipids that activate endothelial cells to express the vascular cell adhesion molecule-1 (VCAM-1). This serves as a receptor for monocytes and T cells. Oxidized lipids can also induce complement activation and stimulate cells to produce chemokines, both of which will stimulate mononuclear cells to enter the artery. Monocytes differentiate into macrophages, upregulate scavenger receptors, internalize oxLDL, and transform into lipid-laden foam cells. T cells entering the intima may recognize fragments of oxLDL as foreign antigens when presented to them on MHC class II molecules after uptake through scavenger receptors. T cells may also recognize heat shock proteins generated during cell injury, and perhaps also microbial antigens present in the artery wall. T cell activation leads to release of a host of cytokines that in turn activate macrophages and endothelial and smooth muscle cells. Mast cells may also be activated in the intima; this may lead to LDL modification as well as protease secretion.

Once trapped in the artery, LDL may undergo modification by oxidative or proteolytic attack (8). This is accomplished by oxygen radicals and proteases that can be released from activated vascular cells and occasional resident macrophages of the artery. The process is enhanced dramatically in inflammation, when activated macrophages, T cells, and mast cells produce large amounts of radicals and enzymes. Low-density lipoprotein modification tends to increase particle charge, which will force LDLs to detach from the proteoglycans. There is also a tendency toward aggregation of modified LDL particles, leading to large aggregates that can be phagocytized by macrophages. Finally, oxidized LDL is taken up by scavenger receptors on macrophages, leading to intracellular cholesterol accumulation (see below).

When LDL is attacked by oxygen radicals, lipid peroxidation leads to the release of aldehydes that can form covalent bonds with amino groups of polypeptide chains (9). This generates the ligands for scavenger receptors and also serves as B and T cell epitopes (see below). Oxidized lipids, such as PAPC, lyso-PC, 9- and 13-HODE, are proinflammatory and can activate both endothelial cells and macrophages (10,11). Activation of endothelial cells by such lipid species causes expression of leukocyte adhesion molecules (12). Finally, oxysterols derived from cholesterol can activate inflammatory cells (13) and also form aggregates that activate the complement cascade (14). Together, these reactions initiate vascular inflammation, which is a key step in atherogenesis.

III. INFLAMMATION IN ATHEROGENESIS

Endothelial expression of adhesion molecules is the earliest sign of atherosclerosis that can be detected in arterial cells. The vascular cell adhesion molecule-1 (VCAM-1) appears on the luminal endothelium within a few days after induction of hypercholesterolemia in rabbits (15). It is also expressed in early atherosclerosis in genetically hypercholesterolemic mice (16). However, VCAM-1 then disappears from the luminal endothelium after a few weeks and is later expressed by vascular smooth muscle cells in deeper parts of the lesions (17–19).

The VCAM-1 is a receptor for mononuclear leukocytes (monocytes and lymphocytes), which use their VLA-4 ($\alpha 4\beta 1$) integrin to bind to the Ig-like VCAM-1 on the endothelium. Since endothelial VCAM-1 expression is followed by adhesion of mononuclear cells and the appearance of such cells in the intima, this is likely to be important for recruitment of such cells to the forming lesions. In addition, it is possible that VLA-4 expressing leukocytes may bind to fibronectins exposed on the endothelial surface (20). The finding that fatty streak formation is reduced by administering a peptide that blocks VLA-4 supports a role for this integrin in atherogenesis (21).

Table 1 Immune Cells Present in Atherosclerotic Plaques

Cell type	Percent of all cells in lesion	Important functions
Macrophage	30–50	Lipid accumulation; secretion of cytokines, proteases; radical production (oxygen, NO)
T cell	5–20	Antigen recognition; cytokine secretion; macrophage activation; cytotoxicity
Mast cell	>1	LDL modification; protease production

Table 2 Properties of Some Cytokines Found in Atherosclerotic Lesions

Cytokine	Producing cell(s)	Target cell(s)	Effects
IL-1	MΦ, EC, SMC	T cells, MΦ, EC, SMC, mast cells	Adhesion; procoagulant activity; NOS2, COX2 expression, etc.
TNF-α	MΦ, T cells	T cells, MΦ, EC, SMC, mast cells	Adhesion; procoag.; NOS2, COX2; LPL; proteases; metabolism
Interferon-γ	T cells (Th1)	MΦ, EC, SMC, mast cells	Macrophage activ., adhesion; procoag.; NOS2, COX2; proteases; contractile proteins; SR
IL-2	T cells (Th0, Th1)	T cells	Activation, growth
IL-4 (in severe hyperchol.)	T cells (Th2)	T cells, others	Th2 activation; anti-inflamm.; B cell activ.
IL-6	MΦ, EC, SMC	Many	Inflamm., acute phase reaction; B cell stim.
IL-10	T cells, MΦ	T cells, others	Promotes Th2, inhibits Th1
MCP-1	EC, SMC	MC, T cells	Chemotaxis
M-CSF	EC, SMC	MC	MΦ differentiation

For abbreviations, please refer to text.

While VLA-4 is expressed constitutively, VCAM-1 is induced by inflammatory stimuli that act through the transcription factor, NF-κB (22). Such stimuli include endotoxins and proinflammatory cytokines. In addition, oxidized phospholipids such as lysophosphatidylcholine induce monocyte-endothelial adhesion through VCAM-1–dependent mechanisms (12,23). This provides a direct link between LDL oxidation and recruitment of inflammatory cells to the arterial intima.

In addition to VCAM-1, intercellular adhesion molecule-1 (ICAM-1) is also expressed on the surface of atherosclerotic lesions and atherosclerosis-prone areas (16). This adhesion molecule is regulated by inflammatory stimuli acting on NF-κB but the promoter of the ICAM-1 gene also contains a "shear stress–regulated element," i.e., a nucleotide sequence that conveys transcriptional activation upon increases or changes in shear stress on the endothelial surface (24). The ICAM-1 is largely expressed at sites of hemodynamic strain, supporting a role for shear stress–regulated expression of this adhesion molecule (16).

Recruitment of mononuclear cells is thought to require an initial rolling of the leukocyte on the endothelial surface before firm integrin-dependent adhesion can take place. Rolling is mediated by selectins, which are adhesion molecules that bind carbohydrate structures on the cellular counterpart (25). Both P- and E-selectins are inducible in the arterial endothelium; they appear to be important for atherogenesis since compound knockout mice that are hypercholesterolemic but lack both selectins exhibit reduced fatty streak formation (26).

Adhesion is followed by migration of monocytes and T cells into the arterial intima. This process is governed by chemotactic factors. Complement activation may be an important source of such factors, including the C5a peptide. It is generated when the complement cascade is activated, probably on oxysterol aggregates (i.e., aggregates of oxidized cholesterol derivatives) in the arterial intima and forming plaque (14,27). Complement depletion reduces atherosclerosis in experimental animals.

Chemokines are also strong stimuli for leukocyte migration. Particular interest has focused on the monocyte chemotactic protein-1 (MCP-1) and its receptor, CCR2. In spite of its name,

MCP-1 is chemotactic both for T cells and monocytes (28) and it is expressed in atherosclerotic plaques (29). When knockout mice that lack either MCP-1 or CCR2 are crossed with atherosclerosis-prone mice, lesion formation is reduced by up to 80% (30,31). This strongly suggests that chemokine-dependent recruitment is an important early factor in atherosclerosis.

IV. INNATE IMMUNITY—MACROPHAGES, SCAVENGER RECEPTORS, PROTEASES, AND RADICALS

The first stage of the atherosclerotic process—at least in experimental models—is the fatty streak (32,33). This is a cholesterol-rich lesion of the arterial intima. It contains cholesterol both as extracellular lipoproteins and as intracellular droplets in lipid-laden foam cells. The lesion is not particularly elevated from the arterial surface and does not cause any clinical symptoms. It is common in young individuals, as has become evident from autopsy studies of accident victims and war casualties.

In experimental animal models, the subendothelial accumulation of cholesterol and endothelial expression of adhesion molecules is followed by the entry of monocytes and lymphocytes into the subendothelial intima (34). This, in turn, is followed by the differentiation of monocytes into macrophages, upregulation of scavenger receptors, and internalization of modified lipoproteins (5). Macrophage differentiation is dependent on the cytokine, macrophage-colony stimulating factor (M-CSF) (35) but is also enhanced by oxidized lipoproteins (36).

The occurrence of differentiated macrophages in the intima appears to be necessary for atherosclerosis since macrophage-deficient mice do not develop fatty streaks even when severely hypercholesterolemic (37). Such *op/op* mice carry a mutation in the gene for M-CSF and their blood monocytes do not differentiate into tissue macrophages. Among the cells that they lack within the macrophage lineage are osteoclasts. They develop an osteopetrosis-like disease and the defective gene was therefore called *op* before it was identified as the *M-CSF* gene. Even when *op/op* mice are crossed with the severely hypercholesterolemic apoE knockout mouse, hardly any fatty streaks develop. Therefore, the development of macrophages in the artery wall is necessary for atherosclerosis.

The transformation of macrophages into lipid-laden foam cells depends on the activity of scavenger receptors. They are multifunctional receptors that bind ligands with clustered negative charges (38). Such ligands include oxidized lipoproteins but also bacterial endotoxins, several other types of macromolecules, and apoptotic cells and cell fragments. Although scavenger receptors were initially discovered as acetyl-LDL binding receptors (39), they are now considered to be major components in the defense against gram-negative bacteria (38,40).

Scavenger receptors (SRs) constitute a family with several members that have been grouped into the subfamilies A, B, and C. Scavenger receptor-A was the first to be cloned; it is a transmembrane protein with an external C-terminal cysteine-rich domain (SRCR domain, scavenger receptor cysteine-rich domain), which defines motifs common for the entire SR family

Table 3 Candidate Antigens in Atherosclerosis

Antigen	Type
OxLDL	Autoantigen
HSP60	Autoantigen
Chlamydia pneumoniae	Microbial
Cytomegalovirus	Microbial

(38,41). Beneath the SRCR domain is a collagen-like coiled coil that appears to contain the ligand-binding domain (41–43). Scavenger receptor-A ligation results in degradation of the ligand in a lysosomal compartment. However, components of the ligand may associate with MHC class II molecules, appear on the surface of the macrophage, and be recognized as foreign antigens by specific T cells (44,45). Scavenger receptor-A knockout mice succumb to gram-negative infections, supporting a role for this receptor in host defense (46). They show reduced fatty streak formation and their macrophages are less prone to transform into foam cells.

Scavenger receptor-A expression is linked to monocyte-macrophage differentiation but it is also regulated by cytokines. Interferon-γ, tumor necrosis factor-α(TNF-α), and transforming growth factor-β(TGF-β) downregulate SR-A expression (47–49), while M-CSF upregulates it (50). It therefore appears that SR-A activity is a feature of resident macrophages but may disappear during inflammation.

Another scavenger receptor, CD36, exhibits similar structural features and ligand-binding activity as SR-A (40,51). It also acts as a receptor for thrombospondin and individuals with mutations in the *CD36* gene may therefore exhibit defective primary hemostasis and purpural bleedings. Hypercholesterolemic mice that lack CD36 show similar changes in macrophage uptake of oxidized LDL (oxLDL) as those deficient in SR-A, suggesting a role also for this scavenger receptor in atherosclerosis (52). CD36 is regulated partly by the PPARγ transcription factor: oxidized lipids of oxidized LDL can penetrate the cell and ligate PPARγ, which leads to increased CD36 expression (53). This, in turn, enhances uptake of oxidized LDL, resulting in a positive feedback loop for foam cell formation.

A third scavenger receptor, SR-BI, exerts an entirely different functional activity. It acts as a receptor for high-density lipoproteins (HDL), which mobilize cholesterol from cells (54). SR-BI is therefore part of a machinery that eliminates cholesterol from the artery wall, while SR-A and CD36 promote cholesterol deposition in the arterial intima.

A new scavenger receptor, the lectin-like oxLDL receptor-1 (LOX-1) was recently discovered (55). It resembles lectin-like receptors in natural killer (NK) cells, is expressed by endothelial cells but may also appear on smooth muscle and macrophages, is regulated by shear stress and cytokines, and is not related to the SRCR family (56,57).

Macrophages are the main cholesterol-accumulating cells in the atherosclerotic plaque (3,39). In addition, they may promote the development of atherosclerosis in several other ways. They produce a host of cytokines. In particular, the proinflammatory cytokines TNF-α and interleukin-1 (IL-1) have been detected in plaques and appear to be important for disease progression (58,59). These cytokines activate endothelial cells to express leukocyte adhesion molecules and procoagulant factors and initiate a cascade of cytokine secretion that leads to secretion of acute phase reactants such as C-reactive protein (CRP) and IL-6. Furthermore, proinflammatory cytokines stimulate smooth muscle cells to express the cytokine-inducible nitric oxide synthase (iNOS, NOS2) (60) and reduce their content of contractile α-actin protein (61). This reduces vascular contractility; in addition, high levels of nitric oxide (NO) produced through the NOS2 pathway may also cause apoptosis. Similarly, proinflammatory cytokines induce expression of cyclooxygenase-2, which leads to production of a variety of eicosanoids during inflammation and atherogenesis (62). Many of the effects of proinflammatory cytokines are exerted through the transcription factor, NF-κB, the activation of which is increased in the atherosclerotic plaque (63) and enhanced when smooth muscle cells differentiate into the intimal phenotype (64,65).

Growth factors produced by macrophages include the platelet-derived growth factor (PDGF), fibroblast growth factor (FGF), and TGF-β (3), which act on smooth muscle cells to stimulate their cell cycle progression and cell division. After balloon catheter injury to the artery, FGF released from cellular and extracellular stores induce a first wave of smooth muscle cell proliferation (66). In the next phase, PDGF released from platelets on the injured arterial surface chemotactically stimulate smooth muscle cells to migrate from the media into the intima (67). Finally, PDGF secretion by macrophages, smooth muscle cells, and endothelial cells in the intima induces continued smooth muscle proliferation in this compartment (68–70). This mechanism probably drives the formation of the fibrous cap, a structure that encapsulates the foam cell lesion with connective tissue during progression of the fatty streak into a "fibrofatty" atherosclerotic plaque (3,70).

The TGF-β is a growth stimulator for mesenchymal cells, including smooth muscle cells (71). However, its fibrogenic activity is at least as important since TGF-β stimulates collagen formation and hence formation of the fibrous cap (72). Finally, TGF-β is strongly anti-inflammatory (73–75). It is therefore likely that TGF-β counteracts the action of proinflammatory cytokines and that the balance between these two types of signaling molecules may determine the extent of inflammatory and fibrogenic activities in the plaque.

When macrophages are activated by stimuli such as inferferon-γ and endotoxins, they produce factors that can modify lipoproteins (8). These factors include proteases and oxygen free radicals. The latter are generated both through myeloperoxidase activity and nonenzymatic mechanisms (9). Proteolytic attack on LDL can be due to macrophage products but it can also be exerted by chymase, a mast cell enzyme (76). Mast cells have been detected in human and experimental atherosclerotic lesions and may be involved both in lipoprotein modification and in plaque rupture. Their activation is obviously dependent on inflammatory stimuli in the plaque.

V. ADAPTIVE IMMUNITY AND THE ROLE OF SPECIFIC T CELLS

The T cell is an important component of the atherosclerotic lesion. It is present from its start as a fatty streak, is recruited through similar mechanisms as monocytes, and constitutes approximately 10% of all cells in the advanced human plaque (77–81). Most T cells are of the CD4+ type (78) and produce Th1-type cytokines such as interferon-γ (80,82,83).

The concomitant expression of MHC class II molecules by macrophages, endothelial cells, and smooth muscle cells, and of activation markers by adjacent T cells (77) suggests that antigen presentation and immune specific T cell activation is taking place in the plaque. Occasional dendritic cells are also found in plaques (84) and it is possible that they take up plaque antigens, migrate to regional lymph nodes and activate T cells at this location. These T cells may subsequently enter lesions, probably through VLA-4- and chemokine-dependent recruitment, and undergo secondary activation after antigen presentation by macrophages. Antigens that may activate plaque T cells include both endogenous ones such as oxidized LDL and exogenous, microbial antigens. They are discussed below.

T cells affect disease progression both by cell–cell contact mechanisms and by secretion of paracrine factors. The former include cytolytic factors such as granzyme and Fas ligand, which may cause apoptosis of surrounding cells. Among the latter, interferon-γ and IL-2 are detected in almost all advanced human carotid plaques (82). They probably reflect a Th1 effector function, which may be due to local secretion of IL-12 in the lesion (85). Since interferon-γ is a major macrophage-activating cytokine, this is likely to be a major driving force for macrophage activation and inflammation in the plaque. Interestingly, activated T cells are increased at sites of plaque rupture and it is possible that their activation induces acute coronary syndromes by causing macrophage activation, proteolysis, and thrombosis (6,86,87).

T cell cytokines exert important regulatory effects on vascular cells. Interferon-γ inhibits smooth muscle proliferation (61,88) and the expression of α-actin (61) and collagen (89). Such effects are likely to reduce the fibrotic buildup of the plaque cap but also to weaken its tensile strength. It may therefore make the lesion more susceptible to rupture in a situation when macrophage activation leads to secretion of proteases and cytotoxic radicals. Tumor necrosis factor-α, which can be produced by Th1 cells as well as by macrophages, can also inhibit α-actin expression and thus reduce smooth muscle contractility.

Together, interferon-γ and TNF can induce expression of cytokine-inducible NOS2 by macrophages, smooth muscle cells, and other cells. This may serve as a protective mechanism in situations when endothelial dysfunction leads to loss of NO production through the endothelial NO synthase pathway (90,91). However, NOS2 is a high-output enzyme that generates very large amounts of NO. This may induce apoptosis and NO could also react with oxygen radicals to form cytotoxic peroxynitrite (92). Such effects could cause severe damage to cells of the atherosclerotic plaque.

While the proinflammatory Th1 cytokines interferon-γ and TNF therefore may be proatherogenic molecules, Th2 cytokines may have different effects. Interleukin-4 inhibits NOS2 expression (93) but can induce 15-lipoxygenase and therefore promote the formation of oxygen radicals in the lesion (94). Another Th2 cytokine, IL-10, inhibits the Th1 pathway and may therefore reduce plaque inflammation (85). A proatherogenic role for the Th1/interferon-γ pathway is supported by the finding that compound knockout mice that lack interferon-γ receptors and apoE develop less atherosclerosis than interferon-γ receptor–expressing apoE knockout mice (95). Such studies should also be performed to determine the role of the Th2 pathway.

In view of the complexity of T cell subsets, their effector functions and cross-regulatory activities, it is not surprising that studies of compound mutant mice that are hypercholesterolemic and lack specific immunity have been difficult to interpret. RAG-1–/– × apoE–/– mice develop significantly less atherosclerosis than immunocompetent RAG-1+/+ apoE–/– littermates (96). However, the effect is reduced in severe hypercholesterolemia. This may be due to the fact that cellular immune responses switch from a Th1 to a Th2 predominance when the cholesterol load increases (97). One may conclude from studies of gene-modified, immunodeficient, and atherosclerosis-prone mice that while innate immunity is necessary for atherosclerosis, adaptive immunity plays an important modulating role. This conclusion is supported by the recent findings that treatment with polyclonal immunoglobulins at doses that modulate cellular immunity reduces atherosclerosis in apoE knockout mice (98) and that injections of anti-CD40-ligand antibodies reduce atherosclerosis in disease-prone LDL receptor knockout animals (99). Such observations encourage the attempts to use immunomodulation to control progression of atherosclerosis.

VI. CANDIDATE ANTIGENS AND SYSTEMIC IMMUNE RESPONSES

Several antigens have been proposed to be involved in atherosclerosis. The most extensive data are available for oxidized LDL but there is also evidence that heat shock proteins may act as antigens. In addition, microbes may be pathogenic at least partly by inducing immune responses, some of which could involve molecular mimickry with endogenous molecular structures.

A. Oxidized Low-Density Lipoprotein

When LDL accumulates extravascularly, it is prone to undergo oxidative modification (8). This process starts when oxygen radicals attack unsaturated fatty acid residues of triglycerides and phospholipids of the lipoprotein particle. As mentioned above, such oxidized lipids are strongly proinflammatory. Lipid peroxidation leads to release of aldehyde fragments such as malondialdehyde and 4-hydroxynonenal. These short aldehydes may react with the protein moiety of the lipoprotein, particularly by binding to ε-amino groups of lysine. This process generates new epitopes for which tolerance appears not to have developed; structures such as malondialdehyde-lysine are strongly immunogenic and induce high titer antibody production (100). In addition, antibodies develop against oxidized phospholipids. In fact, many cardiolipin antibodies appear to be directed against oxidized structures of the cardiolipin molecule (101).

Both the antigen, oxidized LDL, and anti-oxLDL antibodies are present in the artery wall during atherosclerosis (102,103). It is likely that LDL–anti-oxLDL immune complexes are taken up by Fc receptors and thus contribute to foam cell formation (104). In addition, they may activate the complement cascade and thereby enhance inflammation and the recruitment of mononuclear cells. However, it is also possible that systemic anti-oxLDL antibodies help remove oxLDL from the circulation before it reaches the artery wall (105). The balance between oxidation and elimination of LDL may therefore at least in part depend on systemic elimination vis-à-vis local production in the artery wall.

Both IgM and IgG antibodies to oxLDL are produced during atherosclerosis (97,106). The occurrence of the latter suggests that T cells as well as B cells may recognize oxLDL. This has been verified in cellular immunological studies. T cell clones were obtained from atherosclerotic plaques; when challenged with oxLDL, many of the CD4+ clones recognized it as a classical, HLA-DR–dependent antigen (107). Similarly, apoE knockout mice develop oxLDL-reactive T cells and T cell–dependent B cell responses to oxLDL (97,108,109). The switch from Th1 to Th2 help for anti-oxLDL reactive B cells may be decisive both for the local cellular immune response to oxLDL in the plaque and for the effector properties of the systemic antibody response.

Oxidized LDL antibodies are found in hypercholesterolemic, atherosclerotic experimental animals and they also appear in humans with atherosclerotic disease. Their titers have been found to correlate with the progression of carotid artery atherosclerosis (110) and peripheral atherosclerosis (111) but not with coronary disease in hypercholesterolemic patients (112). The predictive value of such antibodies therefore remains controversial.

If oxLDL is an important autoantigen, one would expect immunization with it to affect disease development. This is actually the case: several experimental studies have shown substantial beneficial effects of oxLDL immunization on atherosclerosis in hypercholesterolemic rabbits and mice (113–115). Although both the antigen preparations and adjuvants administered need to be improved, these findings are encouraging for future research aimed at preventing clinical disease.

B. Heat Shock Proteins

Heat shock proteins are chaperonins that aid protein folding and intracellular transport. They are formed in increased amounts in "cell stress" such as inflammation (116). Therefore, antibodies to heat shock proteins frequently develop in inflammatory and autoimmune diseases (117).

Heat shock protein 60 (HSP60) can be produced by endothelial cells during metabolic strain and vascular inflammation (118). Heat shock protein 60 can elicit antibody production and cellular immune responses, which have been linked to atherosclerosis in the same way as immune responses to oxLDL (119). In addition, human HSP60 exhibits significant structural similarities with microbial heat shock proteins (120). It is therefore possible that microorganisms can affect the atherosclerotic process by molecular mimicry with this protein.

In contrast to the beneficial effects obtained by immunization with oxLDL, immunization with HSP60 has been reported to aggravate atherosclerosis (121). The reason for this difference is unclear but may be due to tissue destruction caused by immune responses against HSP60-expressing vascular cells.

C. Microorganisms

Several microorganisms have been proposed to play a role in atherosclerosis. These suggestions are largely based on seroepidemiological studies; a meta-analysis of these data point to *Chlamydia pneumoniae* and cytomegalovirus as the two most relevant microbes, which should be subjected to further mechanistic and epidemiological studies (122).

Chlamydia pneumoniae was first linked to atherosclerosis in seroepidemiological studies of patients with coronary heart disease and sudden death victims (123). Higher titers of anti–*Chlamydia pneumoniae* antibodies were found in patients than in healthy controls. It was subsequently shown that *Chlamydia pneumoniae* can occur in some macrophages of atherosclerotic lesions (124). Recent animal experiments show that infection with *Chlamydia pneumoniae* may aggravate cholesterol-induced atherosclerosis (125–127) and it has therefore been proposed that this microorganism increases heart disease by acting as an accelerator of the atherosclerotic process. Such an effect could either be due to direct microbial attack of vascular tissue or to immune reactions mounted against the microbe. Support for the latter hypothesis was obtained by the observation that *Chlamydia* heat shock proteins exhibit significant sequence homology to their human counterparts (120).

An entirely different hypothesis for the pathogenic role of *Chlamydia pneumoniae* in heart disease was offered when it was observed that Chlamydia proteins show homologies to α-myosin heavy chain, a cytocontractile protein of the cardiomyocyte (128). According to this proposed scenario, the microbe would induce myocarditis and possibly cardiac arteritis by inducing autoimmune reactions; such an inflammation could aggravate or mimic coronary heart disease and lead to ischemia and sudden death. While the role of *Chlamydia* species in myocarditis is well established, this mechanism remains to be proven for atherosclerotic heart disease.

The seroepidemiological and experimental data that support a role for *Chlamydia pneumoniae* in coronary heart disease have been found sufficiently interesting to justify clinical trials using antibiotics to prevent coronary heart disease. One of these studies (129) found that roxithromycin treatment reduced the incidence of secondary coronary events in patients who had undergone myocardial infarction. In another study, a similar antibiotic, azithromycin, did not provide any clinical effect in patients with coronary artery disease (130). The clinical importance of *Chlamydia pneumoniae* and the benefit of antibiotics in atherosclerotic disease therefore remain unclear and the issue merits further investigations.

Virus species of the herpesvirus family have been linked to atherosclerosis in several studies. A member of the herpes virus family, Marek's disease virus, aggravates cholesterol-induced atherosclerosis in chickens and it was suggested that other members of the family may exert similar effects in man (131). Herpes simplex type I DNA and protein has actually been found in human atherosclerotic plaques (132); however, this virus is ubiquitous and can be identified in many tissues of healthy individuals. In contrast, cytomegalovirus (CMV), which can also be found in human lesions (133), has a more restricted distribution among human individuals and in tissues of healthy individuals. Cytomegalovirus has been linked to transplant arteriosclerosis, i.e., the chronic vascular rejection process that occurs after allogeneic organ transplantation (134–136). However, its role in "garden variety" atherosclerosis remains to be determined.

VII. ACTIVE PLAQUES AND ACUTE ISCHEMIC SYNDROMES

Most atherosclerotic plaques never give rise to clinical symptoms. However, certain plaques located at critical sites, particularly in the coronary and cerebral vasculature, can cause dramatic ischemic syndromes including myocardial infarction and stroke. Autopsy studies in many laboratories have shown that these culprit lesions are sites of mural thrombi (137). Therefore, it is not simply the gradual narrowing of the lumen due to growth of the lesion that causes end-organ is-chemia. Instead, the plaque may undergo an "activation" that involves development of thrombo-genicity.

Recent research has shown that such active plaques are sites of intense inflammation with abundant, activated T cells, macrophages, and mast cells (138–141). They show increased pro-duction of matrix metalloproteinases, which are collagenolytic and elastolytic enzymes, and of reactive radical species (87,142). Since proinflammatory cytokines released by activated T cells and macrophages can induce metalloproteinase expression and radical production in macro-phages, mast cells, smooth muscle cells, and endothelial cells, it appears likely that an immune/inflammatory activation in the plaque leads to tissue proteolysis and cytotoxicity (6).

Such an activity would be expected to reduce the tensile strength of the tissue. Interestingly, plaque fissures and ruptures are found in the majority of culprit lesions in coronary arteries (143). Thus, immune/inflammatory activation results in proteolysis, which in turn causes plaque rup-ture.

Plaque rupture does not usually lead to complete rupture of the artery. Instead, it exposes a small nidus of subendothelial tissue to the circulating blood. Since the extracellular matrix is highly thrombogenic, this will result in the formation of a thrombus. The process is enhanced if tissue factor, the initiator of the external pathway of coagulation, is expressed by cells in the vicin-ity. Interestingly, proinflammatory cytokines induce tissue factor in both endothelial cells, smooth muscle cells, and macrophages (144–146).

Similar to plaque fissures and ruptures, endothelial desquamation can cause thrombosis. This process could be elicited, e.g., by local proteolysis that dissociates endothelial cells from their substratum or by vasospastic events that mechanically damage the endothelium in such a way that the cells detach. Such endothelial desquamation is also observed in many cases of coro-nary thrombosis (87).

Plaque inflammation leads to release of proinflammatory cytokines into the circulation. This, in turn, induces acute phase reactants in a similar manner as for other types of inflamma-tion. Therefore, the acute coronary syndrome is characterized by high levels of acute phase reac-tants such as CRP and fibrinogen, which are useful in the clinical diagnosis of unstable angina pectoris and developing myocardial infarction (147–149). Recent studies of patients with unsta-ble angina point to T-cell activation as an initiating or modulatory event in the inflammatory process (150,151).

VIII. CONCLUSIONS

A large number of experimental and clinical studies have established that the immune system plays an important pathogenetic role in atherosclerosis. Current data imply innate immunity as necessary for lesion formation and this has led investigators to conclude that atherosclerosis is an inflammatory disease. The role of adaptive immunity is more complex—it is present throughout disease development and general immune defects reduce the extent of disease in experimental models. However, specific defects may have entirely different effects and it is likely that certain effector mechanisms of adaptive immunity are proatherogenic while others may be atheroprotec-tive.

Attempts to treat or prevent atherosclerosis by modulating immune activity have been suc-cessful in experimental models. Current interest focuses on specific antigens such as oxLDL, HSP60, and macromolecular components of *Chlamydia pneumoniae* and CMV. In addition, it is possible that modulation of immunologically nonspecific inflammatory reactions may be useful for treating atherosclerosis. Finally, inflammatory markers have already proven to be useful for the diagnosis of active plaques and acute coronary syndromes. All these data imply that the immune system plays an active role in atherosclerosis, which can therefore be viewed as an inflammatory vascular response to a metabolic disturbance.

ACKNOWLEDGMENTS

The author acknowledges the stimulating collaboration of Giuseppina Caligiuri, Antonino Nicoletti, Gabrielle Paulsson, Allan Sirsjö, Sten Stemme, Zhong-qun Yan, and Xinghua Zhou. Our work is supported by the Swedish Medical Research Council (Project 6816), Heart-Lung Foundation, Petrus and Augusta Hedlund Fund, and Johnson Foundation.

REFERENCES

1. Murray CJ, Lopez AD. Global mortality, disability, and the contribution of risk factors: Global Burden of Disease Study. Lancet 1997; 349(9063):1436–1442.
2. Fuster V, Ross R, Topol EJ. Atherosclerosis and Coronary Artery Disease. Philadelphia: Lippincott-Raven, 1996.
3. Ross R. Atherosclerosis: An inflammatory disease. N Engl J Med 1999; 340:115–126.
4. Breslow JL. Mouse models of atherosclerosis. Science 1996; 272:685–688.
5. Hansson GK. Cell-mediated immunity in atherosclerosis. Curr Opin Lipidol 1997; 8:301–311.
6. Libby P, Hansson GK, Pober JS. Atherogenesis and inflammation. In: Chien KR, ed. Molecular Basis of Cardiovascular Disease. Philadelphia: Saunders, 1999:349–366.
7. Camejo G, Hurt-Camejo E, Olsson U, Bondjers G. Proteoglycans and lipoproteins in atherosclerosis. Curr Opin Lipidol 1993; 4:385–391.
8. Steinberg D. Low density lipoprotein oxidation and its pathobiological significance. J Biol Chem 1997; 272:20963–20966.
9. Heinecke JW. Mass spectrometric quantification of amino acid oxidation products in proteins: Insights into pathways that promote LDL oxidation in the human artery wall. FASEB J 1999; 13: 1113–1120.
10. Watson AD, Leitinger N, Navab M, Faull KF, Hörkkö S, Witztum JL, Palinski W, Schwenke D, Salomon RG, Sha W, Subbanagounder G, Fogelman AM, Berliner JA. Structural identification by mass spectrometry of oxidized phospholipids in minimally oxidized low density lipoprotein that induce monocyte/endothelial interactions and evidence for their presence in vivo. J Biol Chem 1997; 272: 13597–13607.
11. Navab M, Berliner JA, Watson AD, et al. The Yin and Yang of oxidation in the development of the fatty streak. A review based on the 1994 George Lyman Duff Memorial Lecture. Arterioscler Thromb Vasc Biol 1996; 16(7):831–842.
12. Kume N, Cybulsky MI, Gimbrone MA. Lysophosphatidylcholine, a component of atherogenic lipoproteins, induces mononuclear leukocyte adhesion molecules in cultured human and rabbit arterial endothelial cells. J Clin Invest 1992; 90:1138–1144.
13. Mattsson-Hultén L, Lindmark H, Diczfalusy U, Björkhem I, Ottosson M, Liu Y, Bondjers G, Wiklund O. Oxysterols present in atherosclerotic tissue decrease the expression of lipoprotein lipase messenger RNA in human monocyte-derived macrophages. J Clin Invest 1996; 97:461–468.
14. Seifert PS, Hugo F, Tranum JJ, ZÑhringer U, Muhly M, Bhakdi S. Isolation and characterization of a complement-activating lipid extracted from human atherosclerotic lesions. J Exp Med 1990; 172(547):547–557.
15. Cybulsky MI, Gimbrone MA. Endothelial expression of a mononuclear leukocyte adhesion molecule during atherosclerosis. Science 1991; 251:788–791.
16. Nakashima Y, Raines EW, Plump AS, Breslow JL, Ross R. Upregulation of VCAM-1 and ICAM-1 at atherosclerosis-prone sites on the endothelium in the apoE-deficient mouse. Arterioscl Thromb Vasc Biol 1998; 18:842–851.

17. Li H, Cybulsky MI, Gimbrone MA, Libby P. Inducible expression of vascular cell adhesion molecule-1 by vascular smooth muscle cells in vitro and within rabbit atheroma. Am J Pathol 1993; 143(1551): 1551–1559.

18. Li H, Cybulsky MI, Gimbrone MA, Libby P. An atherogenic diet rapidly induces VCAM-1, a cytokine-regulatable mononuclear leukocyte adhesion molecule, in rabbit aortic endothelium. Arterioscl Thromb 1993; 13:197–204.

19. Zhou X, Hansson GK. Detection of B cells and proinflammatory cytokines in atherosclerotic plaques of hypercholesterolemic apoE knockout mice. Scand J Immunol. In press.

20. Shih PT, Elices MJ, Fang ZT, Ugarova TP, Strahl D, Territo MC, Frank JS, Kovach NL, Cabanas C, Berliner JA, Vora DK. Minimally modified low-density lipoprotein induces monocyte adhesion to endothelial connecting segment-1 by activating β1 integrin. J Clin Invest 1999; 103:613–625.

21. Shih PT, Brennan ML, Vora DK, Territo MC, Strahl D, Elices MJ, Lusis AJ, Berliner JA. Blocking very late antigen-4 integrin decreases leukocyte entry and fatty streak formation in mice fed an atherogenic diet. Circ Res 1999; 84:345–351.

22. Collins T, Read MA, Neish AS, Whitley MZ, Thanos D, Maniatis T. Transcriptional regulation of endothelial cell adhesion molecules: NF-kappa B and cytokine-inducible enhancers. [Review]. FASEB J 1995; 9(10):899–909.

23. Honda HM LN, Frankel M, Goldhaber JI, Natarajan R, Nadler JL, Weiss JN, Berliner JA. Induction of monocyte binding to endothelial cells by MM-LDL: Role of lipoxygenase metabolites. Arterioscl Thromb Vasc Biol 1999; 19(3):680–686.

24. Gimbrone MA, Nagel T, Topper JN. Biomechanical activation: An emerging paradigm in endothelial adhesion biology. J Clin Invest 1997; 100(suppl):S61–S65.

25. Bevilacqua MP, Nelson RM. Selectins. J Clin Invest 1993; 91(379):379–387.

26. Dong ZM, Chapman SM, Brown AA, Frenette PS, Hynes RO, Wagner DD. The combined role of P- and E-selectins in atherosclerosis. J Clin Invest 1998; 102:145–152.

27. Seifert PS, Hugo F, Hansson GK, Bhakdi S. Prelesional complement activation in experimental atherosclerosis. Terminal C5b-9 complement deposition coincides with cholesterol accumulation in the aortic intima of hypercholesterolemic rabbits. Lab Invest 1989; 60(747):747–754.

28. Taub DD, Proost P, Murphy WJ, Anver M, Longo DL, Van Damme J, Oppenheim JJ. Monocyte chemotactic protein-1 (MCP-1), -2, and -3 are chemotactic for human T lymphocytes. J Clin Invest 1995; 95:1370–1376.

29. Ylä-Herttuala S, Lipton BA, Rosenfeld ME, et al. Expression of monocyte chemoattractant protein 1 in macrophage-rich areas of human and rabbit atherosclerotic lesions. Proc Natl Acad Sci USA 1991; 88(12):5252–5256.

30. Boring L, Gosling J, Cleary M, Charo IF. Decreased lesion formation in CCR2–/– mice reveals a role for chemokines in the initiation of atherosclerosis. Nature 1998; 394:894–897.

31. Gu L, Okada Y, Clinton SK, Gerard C, Sukhova GK, Libby P, Rollins BJ. Absence of monocyte chemoattractant protein-1 reduces atherosclerosis in low density lipoprotein receptor-deficient mice. Molec Cell 1998; 2:275–281.

32. Stary HC, Blankenhorn DH, Chandler AB, et al. A definition of the intima of human arteries and of its atherosclerosis-prone regions. A report from the Committee on Vascular Lesions of the Council on Arteriosclerosis, American Heart Association. Circulation 1992; 85(391):391–405.

33. Stary HC, Chandler AB, Dinsmore RE, et al. A definition of advanced types of atherosclerotic lesions and a histological classification of atherosclerosis. A report from the Committee on Vascular Lesions of the Council on Arteriosclerosis, American Heart Association. Circulation 1995; 92:1355–1374.

34. Hansson GK, Seifert PS, Olsson G, Bondjers G. Immunohistochemical detection of macrophages and T lymphocytes in atherosclerotic lesions of cholesterol-fed rabbits. Arterioscl Thromb 1991; 11(745): 745–750.

35. Brugger W, Kreutz M, Andreesen R. Macrophage colony-stimulating factor is required for human monocyte survival and acts as a cofactor for their terminal differentiation to macrophages in vitro. J Leukocyte Biol 1991; 49:483–488.

36. Frostegård J, Nilsson J, Haegerstrand A, Hamsten A, Wigzell H, Gidlund M. Oxidized low density lipoprotein induces differentiation and adhesion of human monocytes and the monocytic cell line U937. Proc Natl Acad Sci USA 1990; 87(904):904–908.

37. Smith JD, Trogan E, Ginsberg M, Grigaux C, Tian J, Miyata M. Decreased atherosclerosis in mice deficient in both macrophage colony-stimulating factor (op) and apolipoprotein E. Proc Natl Acad Sci USA 1995; 92:8264–8268.
38. Krieger M, Acton S, Ashkenas J, Pearson A, Penman M, Resnick D. Molecular flypaper, host defense, and atherosclerosis. J Biol Chem 1993; 268:4569–4572.
39. Brown MS, Goldstein JL. Lipoprotein metabolism in the macrophage: Implications for cholesterol deposition in atherosclerosis. Annu Rev Biochem 1983; 52(223):223–261.
40. Pearson AM. Scavenger receptors in innate immunity. Curr Opin Immunol 1996; 8(1):20–28.
41. Kodama T, Freeman M, Rohrer L, Zabrecky J, Matsudaira P, Krieger M. Type I macrophage scavenger receptor contains alpha-helical and collagen-like coiled coils. Nature 1990; 343(531):531–535.
42. Rohrer L, Freeman M, Kodama T, Penman M, Krieger M. Coiled-coil fibrous domains mediate ligand binding by macrophage scavenger receptor type II. Nature 1990; 343(570):570–572.
43. Doi T, Higashino Ki, Kurihara Y, et al. Charged collagen structure mediates the recognition of negatively charged macromolecules by macrophage scavenger receptors. J Biol Chem 1993; 268:2126–2133.
44. Abraham R, Singh N, Mukhopadhyay A, Basu SK, Bal V, Rath S. Modulation of immunogenicity of proteins by maleylation to target scavenger receptors on macrophages. J Immunol 1995; 154:1–8.
45. Nicoletti A, Caligiuri G, Törnberg I, Kodama T, Stemme S, Hansson GK. The macrophage scavenger receptor type A directs modified proteins to antigen presentation. Eur J Immunol 1999; 29:512–521.
46. Suzuki H, Kurihara Y, Takeya M, Kamada N, Kataoka M, Jishage K, Ueda O, Sakaguchi H, Higashi T, Suzuki T, Takashima Y, Kawabe Y, Cynshi O, Wada Y, Honda M, Kurihara H, Aburatani H, Doi T, Matsumoto A, Azuma S, Noda T, Toyoda. A role for macrophage scavenger receptors in atherosclerosis and susceptibility to infection. Nature 1997; 386:292–296.
47. Geng YJ, Hansson GK. Interferon-γ inhibits scavenger receptor expression and foam cell formation in human monocyte-derived macrophages. J Clin Invest 1992; 89:1322–1330.
48. Van Lenten BJ, Fogelman AM. Lipopolysaccharide-induced inhibition of scavenger receptor expression in human monocyte-macrophages is mediated through tumor necrosis factor-alpha. J Immunol 1992; 148(112):112–116.
49. Bottalico LA, Wager RE, Agellon LB, Assoian RK, Tabas I. Transforming growth factor-β1 inhibits scavenger receptor activity in THP-1 human macrophages. J Biol Chem 1991; 266(22866):22866–22871.
50. Horvai A, Palinski W, Wu H, Moulton KS, Kalla K, Glass CK. Scavenger receptor A gene regulatory elements target gene expression to macrophages and to foam cells of atherosclerotic lesions. Proc Natl Acad Sci USA 1995; 92(12):5391–5395.
51. Endemann G, Stanton LW, Madden KS, Bryant CM, White RT, Protter AA. CD36 is a receptor for oxidized low density lipoprotein. J Biol Chem 1993; 268(16):11811–11816.
52. Febbraio M, Abumrad NA, Hajjar DP, Sharma K, Cheng W, Pearce SF, Silverstein RL. A null mutation in murine CD36 reveals an important role in fatty acid and lipoprotein metabolism. J Biol Chem 1999; 274:19055–19062.
53. Nagy L, Tontonoz P, Alvarez JGA, Chen H, Evans RM. Oxidized LDL regulates macrophage gene expression through ligand activation of PPARγ. Cell 1998; 93:229–240.
54. Acton S, Rigotti A, Landschulz KT, Xu S, Hobbs HH, Krieger M. Identification of scavenger receptor SR-BI as a high density lipoprotein receptor. Science 1996; 271:518–520.
55. Sawamura T, Kume N, Aoyama T, Moriwaki H, Hoshikawa H, Aiba Y, Tanaka T, Miwa S, Katsura Y, Kita T, Masaki T. An endothelial receptor for oxidized low-density lipoprotein. Nature 1997; 386:73–77.
56. Yamanaka S, Zhang XY, Miura K, Kim S, Iwao H. The human gene encoding the lectin-type oxidized LDL receptor (OLR1) is a novel member of the natural killer gene complex with a unique expression profile. Genomics 1998; 54:191–199.
57. Murase T, Kume N, Korenaga R, Ando J, Sawamura T, Masaki T, Kita T. Fluid shear stress transcriptionally induces lectin-like oxidized LDL receptor-1 in vascular endothelial cells. Circ Res 1998; 83:328–333.
58. Barath P, Fishbein MC, Cao J, Berenson J, Helfant RH, Forrester JS. Detection and localization of tumor necrosis factor in human atheroma. Am J Cardiol 1990; 65(297):297–302.

59. Libby P, Ross R. Cytokines and growth regulatory molecules. In: Fuster V, Ross R, Topol EJ, eds. Atherosclerosis and Coronary Artery Disease. Vol 1. Philadelphia: Lippincott-Raven, 1995:585–594.

60. Geng YJ, Hansson GK, Holme E. Interferon-γ and tumor necrosis factor synergize to induce nitric oxide production and inhibit mitochondrial respiration in vascular smooth muscle cells. Circ Res 1992; 71:1268–1276.

61. Hansson GK, Hellstrand M, Rymo L, Rubbia L, Gabbiani G. Interferon-γ inhibits both proliferation and expression of differentiation-specific α-smooth muscle actin in arterial smooth muscle cells. J Exp Med 1989; 170:1595–1608.

62. Baker CS, Hall RJ, Evans TJ, Pomerance A, Maclouf J, Creminon C, Yacoub MH, Polak JM. Cyclooxygenase-2 is widely expressed in atherosclerotic lesions affecting native and transplanted human coronary arteries and colocalizes with inducible nitric oxide synthase and nitrotyrosine particularly in macrophages. Arterioscler Thromb Vasc Biol 1999; 19:646–655.

63. Brand K, Page S, Rogler G, Bartsch A, Brandl R, Knuechel R, Page M, Kaltschmidt C, Baeuerle PA, Neumeier D. Activated transcription factor nuclear factor-kappa B is present in the atherosclerotic lesion. J Clin Invest 1996; 97:1715–1722.

64. Yan Z-q, Hansson GK. Overepression of inducible nitric oxide synthase by neointimal smooth muscle cells. Circ Res 1998; 82:21–29.

65. Yan Z-q, Sirsjö A, Bochaton-Piallat M-L, Gabbiani G, Hansson GK. Augmented expression of inducible nitric oxide synthase in vascular smooth muscle cells during aging depends on enhanced NF-κB activation. Arterioscler Thromb Vasc Biol. In press.

66. Lindner V, Lappi DA, Baird A, Majack RA, Reidy MA. Role of basic fibroblast growth factor in vascular lesion formation. Circ Res 1991; 68:106–113.

67. Majesky MW, Reidy MA, Bowen PD, Hart CE, Wilcox JN, Schwartz SM. PDGF ligand and receptor gene expression during repair of arterial injury. J Cell Biol 1990; 111:2149–2158.

68. Walker LN, Bowen PD, Ross R, Reidy MA. Production of platelet-derived growth factor-like molecules by cultured arterial smooth muscle cells accompanies proliferation after arterial injury. Proc Natl Acad Sci USA 1986; 83(7311):7311–7315.

69. Ferns G, Raines EW, Sprugel KH, Motani AS, Reidy MA, Ross R. Inhibition of neointimal smooth muscle accumulation after angioplasty by an antibody to PDGF. Science (Wash.) 1991; 253(1129):1129–1132.

70. Schwartz SM, deBlois D, O'Brien ERM. The intima: Soil for atherosclerosis and restenosis. Circ Res 1995; 77:445–465.

71. Battegay EJ, Raines EW, Seifert RA, Bowen PD, Ross R. TGF-beta induces bimodal proliferation of connective tissue cells via complex control of an autocrine PDGF loop. Cell 1990; 63(515):515–524.

72. Nabel EG, Shum L, Pompili VJ, et al. Direct transfer of transforming growth factor β1 gene into arteries stimulates fibrocellular hyperplasia. Proc Natl Acad Sci USA 1993; 90(10759):10759–10763.

73. Wahl SM, Hunt DA, Wong HL, et al. Transforming growth factor-beta is a potent immunosuppressive agent that inhibits IL-1 dependent lymphocyte proliferation. J Immunol 1988; 140(3026):3026–3032.

74. Kähäri VM, Chen YQ, Su MW, Ramirez F, Uitto J. Tumor necrosis factor-α and interferon-γ suppress the activation of human type I collagen gene expression by transforming growth factor-β1. J Clin Invest 1990; 86(1489):1489–1495.

75. Kulkarni AB, Huh CG, Becker D, et al. Transforming growth factor β1 null mutation in mice causes excessive inflammatory response and early death. Proc Natl Acad Sci USA 1993; 90(770):770–774.

76. Kovanen PT. Role of mast cells in atherosclerosis. In: Marone G, ed. Human Basophils and Mast Cells: Clinical Aspects. Basel: Karger, 1995:132–170.

77. Jonasson L, Holm J, Skalli O, Gabbiani G, Hansson GK. Expression of class II transplantation antigen on vascular smooth muscle cells in human atherosclerosis. J Clin Invest 1985; 76(125):125–131.

78. Jonasson L, Holm J, Skalli O, Bondjers G, Hansson GK. Regional accumulations of T cells, macrophages, and smooth muscle cells in the human atherosclerotic plaque. Arteriosclerosis 1986; 6(131):131–138.

79. Hansson GK, Jonasson L, Lojsthed B, Stemme S, Kocher O, Gabbiani G. Localization of T lymphocytes and macrophages in fibrous and complicated human atherosclerotic plaques. Atherosclerosis 1988; 72(135):135–141.

80. Hansson GK, Holm J, Jonasson L. Detection of activated T lymphocytes in the human atherosclerotic plaque. Am J Pathol 1989; 135(169):169–175.

81. Hansson GK. Immune responses in atherosclerosis. In: Hansson GK, Libby P, eds. Immune Functions of the Vessel Wall. Amsterdam: Harwood, 1996:143–159.

82. Geng YJ, Holm J, Nygren S, Bruzelius M, Stemme S, Hansson GK. Expression of macrophage scavenger receptor in atherosclerosis. Relationship between scavenger receptor isoforms and the T cell cytokine, interferon-γ. Arterioscler Thromb Vasc Biol 1995; 15:1995–1202.

83. Frostegård J, Ulfgren A-K, Nyberg P, Hedin U, Swedenborg J, Andersson U, Hansson GK. Cytokine expression in advanced human atherosclerotic plaques: Dominance of proinflammatory (Th1) and macrophage-stimulating cytokines. Atherosclerosis 1999; 145:33–43.

84. Bobryshev YV, Lord RSA. Ultrastructural recognition of cells with dendritic cell morphology in human aortic intima. Contacting interactions of vascular dendritic cells in athero-resistant and athero-prone areas of the normal aorta. Arch Histol Cytol 1995; 58:307–322.

85. Uyemura K, Demer L, Castle SC, et al. Cross-regulatory roles of interleukin (IL)-12 and IL-10 in atherosclerosis. J Clin Invest 1996; 97:2130–2138.

86. van der Wal AC, Becker AE, van der Loos CM, Das PK. Site of intimal rupture or erosion of thrombosed coronary atherosclerotic plaques is characterized by an inflammatory process irrespective of the dominant plaque morphology. Circulation 1994; 89:36–44.

87. Libby P. Molecular bases of the acute coronary syndromes. Circulation 1995; 91:2844–2850.

88. Hansson GK, Holm J, Holm S, Fotev Z, Hedrich HJ, Fingerle J. T lymphocytes inhibit the vascular response to injury. Proc Natl Acad Sci USA 1991; 88(23):10530–10534.

89. Amento EP, Ehsani N, Palmer H, Libby P. Cytokines and growth factors positively and negatively regulate interstitial collagen gene expression in human vascular smooth muscle cells. Arterioscler Thromb 1991; 11:1223–1230.

90. Hansson GK, Geng YJ, Holm J, Hårdhammar P, Wennmalm Å, Jennische E. Arterial smooth muscle cells express nitric oxide synthase in response to endothelial injury. J Exp Med 1994; 180:733–738.

91. Yan Z-q, Yokota T, Hansson GK. Expression of inducible nitric oxide synthase inhibits platelet adhesion to the injured artery. Circ Res 1996; 79:38–44.

92. Stamler JS. A radical vascular connection. Nature 1996; 380:108–110.

93. Bogdan C, Vodovotz Y, Paik J, Xie Q-w, Nathan C. Mechanism of suppression of nitric oxide synthase expression by interleukin-4 in primary mouse macrophages. J Leukocyte Biol 1994; 55:227–233.

94. Conrad DJ, Kuhn H, Mulkins M, Highland E, Sigal E. Specific inflammatory cytokines regulate the expression of human monocyte 15-lipoxygenase. Proc Natl Acad Sci USA 1992; 89(1):217–221.

95. Gupta S, Pablo AM, Jiang X-c, Wang N, Tall AR, Schindler C. IFN-γ potentiates atherosclerosis in apoE knock-out mice. J Clin Invest 1997; 99:2752–2561.

96. Dansky HM, Charlton SA, Harper MM, Smith JD. T and B lymphocytes play a minor role in atherosclerotic plaque formation in the apolipoprotein E-deficient mouse. Proc Natl Acad Sci USA 1997; 94:4642–4646.

97. Zhou X, Paulsson G, Stemme S, Hansson GK. Hypercholesterolemia is associated with a Th1/Th2 switch of the autoimmune response in atherosclerotic apo E-knockout mice. J Clin Invest 1998; 101:1717–1725.

98. Nicoletti A, Kaveri S, Caligiuri G, Bariéty J, Hansson GK. Immunoglobulin treatment reduces atherosclerosis in apo E knockout mice. J Clin Invest 1998; 102:910–918.

99. Mach F, Schönbeck U, Sukhova GK, Atkinson E, Libby P. Reduction of atherosclerosis in mice by inhibition of CD40 signalling. Nature 1998; 394:200–203.

100. Palinski W, Ylä-Herttuala S, Rosenfeld ME, et al. Antisera and monoclonal antibodies specific for epitopes generated during oxidative modification of low density lipoprotein. Arterioscler Thromb 1990; 10(325):325–335.

101. Hörkkö S, Miller E, Dudl E, Reaven P, Curtiss LK, Zvaifler NJ, Terkeltaub R, Pierangeli SS, Branch DW, Palinski W, Witztum JL. Antiphospholipid antibodies are directed against epitopes of oxidized phospholipids. Recognition of cardiolipin by monoclonal antibodies to epitopes of oxidized low density lipoprotein. J Clin Invest 1996; 98:815–825.

102. Ylä-Herttuala S, Palinski W, Rosenfeld ME, et al. Evidence for the presence of oxidatively modified low density lipoprotein in atherosclerotic lesions of rabbit and man. J Clin Invest 1989; 84(1086): 1086–1095.

103. Witztum JL, Steinberg, D. Role of oxidized low density lipoprotein in atherogenesis. J Clin Invest 1991; 88:1785–1792.

104. Griffith RL, Virella GT, Stevenson HC, Lopes VM. Low density lipoprotein metabolism by human macrophages activated with low density lipoprotein immune complexes. A possible mechanism of foam cell formation. J Exp Med 1988; 168(1041):1041–1059.

105. Holvoet P, Perez G, Zhao Z, Brouwers E, Bernar H, Collen D. Malondialdehyde-modified low density lipoprotein in patients with atherosclerotic disease. J Clin Invest 1995; 95:2611–2619.

106. Palinski W, Horkko S, Miller E, et al. Cloning of monoclonal autoantibodies to epitopes of oxidized lipoproteins from apolipoprotein E-deficient mice. Demonstration of epitopes of oxidized low density lipoprotein in human plasma. J Clin Invest 1996; 98(3):800–814.

107. Stemme S, Holm J, Hansson GK. T lymphocytes in human atherosclerotic plaques are memory cells expressing CD45RO and the integrin VLA-1. Arterioscler Thromb 1992; 12(206):206–211.

108. Paulsson G, Zhou X, Törnquist E, Hansson GK. Oligoclonal T cell expansions in atherosclerotic lesions of apoE-deficient mice. Arterioscler Thromb Vasc Biol. In press.

109. Freigang S, Hörkkö S, Miller E, Witztum JL, Palinski W. Immunization of LDL receptor-deficient mice with homologous malondialdehyde-modified and native LDL reduces progression of atherosclerosis by mechanisms other than induction of high titers of antibodies to oxidative neoepitopes. Arterioscler Thromb Vasc Biol 1998; 18:1972–1982.

110. Salonen JT, Ylä-Herttuala S, Yamamoto R, et al. Autoantibody against oxidised LDL and progression of carotid atherosclerosis. Lancet 1992; 339:883–887.

111. Bergmark C, Wu R, de Faire U, Lefvert AK, Swedenborg J. Patients with early-onset peripheral vascular disease have increased levels of autoantibodies against oxidized LDL. Arterioscler Thromb Vasc Biol 1995; 15:441–445.

112. Hulthe J, Wikstrand J, Lidell A, Wendelhag I, Hansson GK, Wiklund O. Antibody titers against oxidized LDL are not elevated in patients with familial hypercholesterolemia. Arterioscler Thromb Vasc Biol 1998; 18:1203–1211.

113. Palinski W, Miller E, Witztum JL. Immunization of low density lipoprotein (LDL) receptor-deficient rabbits with homologous malondialdehyde-modified LDL reduces atherogenesis. Proc Natl Acad Sci USA 1995; 92:821–825.

114. Ameli S, Hultgårdh-Nilsson A, Regnström J, et al. Effect of immunization with homologous LDL and oxidized LDL on early atherosclerosis in hypercholesterolemic rabbits. Arterioscler Thromb Vasc Biol 1996; 16:1074–1079.

115. George J, Afek A, Gilburd B, Levkovitz H, Shaish A, Goldberg I, Kopolovic Y, Wick G, Shoenfeld Y, Harats D. Hyperimmunization of apo-E-deficient mice with homologous malondialdehyde low-density lipoprotein suppresses early atherogenesis. Atherosclerosis 1998; 138:147–152.

116. Xu Q, Wick G. The role of heat shock proteins in protection and pathophysiology of the arterial wall. Mol Med Today 1996; Sept:372–379.

117. Kiessling R, Grînberg A, Ivanyi J, et al. Role of hsp60 during autoimmune and bacterial inflammation. Immunol Rev 1991; 121(91):91–111.

118. Seitz CS, Kleindienst R, Xu QB, Wick G. Coexpression of heat-shock protein 60 and intercellular-adhesion molecule-1 is related to increased adhesion of monocytes and T cells to aortic endothelium of rats in response to endotoxin. Lab Invest 1996; 74(1):241–252.

119. Wick G, Schett G, Amberger A, Kleindienst R, Xu Q. Is atherosclerosis an immunologically mediated disease? Immunol Today 1995; 16(27):27–33.

120. Mayr M, Metzler B, Kiechl S, Willeit J, Schett G, Xu Q, Wick G. Endothelial cytotoxicity mediated by serum antibodies to heat shock proteins of Escherichia coli and Chlamydia pneumoniae: Immune reactions to heat shock proteins as a possible link between infection and atherosclerosis. Circulation 1999; 99:1560–6.

121. Xu Q, Dietrich H, Steiner HJ, et al. Induction of arteriosclerosis in normocholesterolemic rabbits by immunization with heat shock protein 65. Arterioscler Thromb 1992; 12:789–799.

122. Danesh J, Collins R, Peto R. Chronic infections and coronary heart disease: Is there a link? Lancet 1997; 350:430–436.

123. Saikku P, Leinonen M, Mattila K, Ekman MR, Nieminen MS, Mäkelä PH, Huttunen JK, Valtonen V. Serological evidence of an association of a novel Chlamydia, TWAR, with chronic coronary heart disease and acute myocardial infarction. Lancet 1988; 2:983–986.

124. Kuo CC, Gown AM, Benditt EP, Grayston JT. Detection of chlamydia pneumoniae in aortic lesions of atherosclerosis by immunocytochemical stain. Arterioscler Thromb 1993; 13(1501):1501–1504.

125. Muhlestein JB, Anderson JL, Hammond EH, Zhao L, Trehan S, Schwobe EP, Carlquist JF. Infection with Chlamydia pneumoniae accelerates the development of atherosclerosis and treatment with azithromycin prevents it in a rabbit model. Circulation 1998; 24:633–636.

126. Hu H, Pierce GN, Zhong G. The atherogenic effects of chlamydia are dependent on serum cholesterol and are specific to Chlamydia pneumoniae. J Clin Invest 1999; 103:747–753.

127. Moazed TC, Campbell LA, Rosenfeld ME, Grayston JT, Kuo CC. Chlamydia pneumoniae infection accelerates the progression of atherosclerosis in apolipoprotein E-deficient mice. J Infect Dis 1999; 180:238–241.

128. Bachmaier K, Neu N, Maza LM de la, Pal S, Hessel A, Penninger JM. Chlamydia infections and heart disease linked through antigenic mimicry. Science 1999; 283:1335–1339.

129. Gurfinkel E, Bozovich G, Beck E, Testa E, Livellara B, Mautner B. Treatment with the antibiotic roxithromycin in patients with acute non-Q-wave coronary syndromes. The final report of the ROXIS Study. Eur Heart J 1999; 20:121–127.

130. Anderson JLM, JB, Carlquist J, Allen A, Trehan S, Nielson C, Hall S, Brady J, Egger M, Horne B, Lim T. Randomized secondary prevention trial of azithromycin in patients with coronary artery disease and serological evidence for Chlamydia pneumoniae infection: The Azithromycin in Coronary Artery Disease: Elimination of Myocardial Infection with Chlamydia (ACADEMIC) study. Circulation 1999; 99:1540–1547.

131. Nicholson AC, Hajjar DP. Herpesviruses in atherosclerosis and thrombosis. Etiologic agents or ubiquitous bystanders? Arterioscler Thromb Vasc Biol 1998; 18:339–348.

132. Benditt EP, Barrett T, McDougall JK. Viruses in the etiology of atherosclerosis. Proc Natl Acad Sci USA 1983; 80(6386):6386–6389.

133. Hendrix MGR, Salimans MMM, Boven CPA van, Bruggeman CA. High prevalence of latently present cytomegalovirus in arterial walls of patients suffering from grade III atherosclerosis. Am J Pathol 1990; 136:23–28.

134. McDonald K, Rector TS, Braunlin EA, Kubo SH, Olivari MT. Association of coronary artery disease in cardiac transplant recipients with cytomegalovirus infection. Am J Cardiol 1989; 64(359):359–362.

135. Wu T-C, Hruban RH, Ambinder RF, Pizzorno M, Cameron DE, Baumgartner WA, Reitz BA, Hayward GS, Hutchins GM. Demonstration of cytomegalovirus nucleic acids in the coronary arteries of transplanted hearts. Am J Pathol 1992; 140:739–747.

136. Zhou YF, Guetta E, Yu ZX, Finkel T, Epstein SE. Human cytomegalovirus increases modified low density lipoprotein uptake and scavenger receptor mRNA expression in vascular smooth muscle cells. J Clin Invest 1996; 98:2129–2138.

137. Davies MJ, Thomas A. Thrombosis and acute coronary-artery lesions in sudden cardiac ischemic death. N Engl J Med 1984; 310(1137):1137–1140.

138. van der Wal AC, Becker AE, van der Loos CM, Das PK. Site of intimal rupture or erosion of thrombosed coronary atherosclerotic plaques is characterized by an inflammatory process irrespective of the dominant plaque morphology. Circulation 1994; 89(1):36–44.

139. Davies MJ, Woolf N, Rowles P, Richardson PD. Lipid and cellular constituents of unstable human aortic plaques. Basic Res Cardiol 1994; 1(33):33–40.

140. Moreno PR, Falk E, Palacios IF, Newell JB, Fuster V, Fallon JT. Macrophage infiltration in acute coronary syndromes: Implications for plaque rupture. Circulation 1994; 90(2):775–8.

141. Kaartinen M, Penttilä A, Kovanen PT. Accumulation of activated mast cells in the shoulder region of human coronary atheroma, the predilection site of atheromatous rupture. Circulation 1994; 90(1669):1669–1678.

142. Falk E, Shah P, Fuster V. Coronary plaque disruption. Circulation 1995; 92:657–671.
143. Davies MJ, Thomas A. Plaque fissuring: The cause of acute myocardial infarction, sudden ischaemic death and crescendo angina. Br Heart J 1985; 53(363):363–373.
144. Scheibenbogen C, Moser H, Krause S, Andreesen R. interferon-γ-induced expression of tissue factor activity during human monocyte to macrophage maturation. Haemostasis 1992; 22:173–178.
145. Marmur JD, Rossikhina M, Guha A, et al. Tissue factor is rapidly induced in arterial smooth muscle after balloon injury. J Clin Invest 1993; 91(2253):2253–2259.
146. Conway EM, Bach R, Rosenberg RD, Konigsberg WH. Tumor necrosis factor enhances expression of tissue factor mRNA in endothelial cells. Thromb Res 1989; 53(3):231–241.
147. Liuzzo G, Biasucci LM, Gallimore JR, et al. Prognostic value of C-reactive protein and plasma amyloid A protein in severe unstable angina. N Engl J Med 1994; 331:417–424.
148. Liuzzo G, Biasucci LM, Rebuzzi AG, Gallimore R, Caligiuri G, Lanza GA, Quaranta G, Monaco C, Pepys MB, Maseri A. Plasma protein acute-phase response in unstable angina is not induced by ischemic injury. Circulation 1996; 94:2373–2380.
149. Maseri A. Inflammation, atherosclerosis, and ischemic events: Exploring the hidden side of the moon. N Engl J Med 1997; 336:1014–1016.
150. Neri Serneri GG, Abbate R, Gori AM, et al. Transient intermittent lymphocyte activation is responsible for the instability of angina. Circulation 1992; 86:790–797.
151. Caligiuri G, Summaria F, Liuzzo G, Maseri A. Time course of T-lymphocyte activation and of C-reactive protein in unstable angina: Relation to prognosis. Circulation 1996; 94(suppl I):I–571.

13

Cooperative Molecular Interactions in the Regulation of Angiogenesis

Loubna Hassanieh and Peter C. Brooks
University of Southern California School of Medicine, Los Angeles, California

I. INTRODUCTION

The field of vascular biology has grown extensively over the past decade, due in part to the realization of the importance that neovascularization plays in both normal as well as pathological processes. Elegant studies in the field of vascular biology have revealed two general biological mechanisms by which new blood vessels form. The first is called vasculogenesis and is the process by which functional blood vessels develop from precursor cells called angioblasts (1,2). The second mechanism is called angiogenesis and is the process by which new blood vessels sprout from preexisting vessels (3,4). We will not discuss vasculogenesis, but instead, focus on angiogenesis. In particular, we will discuss the expanding body of work that demonstrates unique molecular cooperation between distinct families of molecules that regulate neovascularization.

The critical importance of blood vessel formation for normal physiological processes such as trophoblast implantation, embryonic development, and wound healing has been appreciated for some time (3–5). However, it wasn't until the early 1970s that pioneering work by Dr. Judah Folkman suggested that angiogenesis may also play an important role in the regulation of tumor growth (6,7). These early studies stimulated interest within the scientific community that aberrant neovascularization may contribute to a number of pathological processes such as diabetic retinopathy, rheumatoid arthritis, psoriasis, and tumor growth and metastasis (3–7).

To this end, efforts have been focused on the identification of molecules that regulate angiogenesis. Some of the more widely studied of these angiogenesis regulatory factors can be grouped into four distinct categories (Table 1), including growth factors and their receptors, cell adhesion molecules, proteolytic enzymes, and extracellular matrix (ECM) components (8,9). While we are primarily focused on these particular groups, our discussion is not intended to suggest that these are the only factors involved in angiogenesis, nor that they are necessarily the most important, but rather we use these families as examples to illustrate the important concept of molecular cooperation in the regulation of neovascularization.

As mentioned above, angiogenesis is a complex series of interconnected molecular, cellular, and biochemical events that ultimately result in the formation of new blood vessels. In general, angiogenesis can be organized into three steps or stages (Fig. 1), including an initiation phase where angiogenic cytokines and growth factors are released from a variety of sources (3,5, 7,10). Growth factors are thought to initiate complex signal transduction pathways that ultimately

175

Table 1 General Categories of Angiogenesis Regulatory Molecules[a]

1. Growth Factors and Growth Factor Receptors
2. Cell Adhesion Molecules
3. Proteolytic Enzymes, Protease Inhibitors and Protease Receptors
4. Extracellular Matrix Proteins

[a]General categories or families of molecules that have been shown to regulate the development of new blood vessels.

activate endothelial cells (11,12). Vascular cell activation results in the acquisition of an invasive phenotype that promotes cell–cell disassociation, production of matrix remodeling proteases, and alterations in the expression of cell surface adhesion receptors (3–12). These activated vascular cells remodel ECM components, interact with altered matrix molecules and invade the local interstitium. Once in the interstitial compartment, the vascular cells again remodel their immediate microenvironment, and interact with these modified interstitial ECM components. Vascular cell interactions with these remodeled interstitial components likely lead to morphogenesis and cellular reorganization into tube-like structures. In the final maturation phase of angiogenesis, vascular cells express new matrix components, undergo cell–cell interactions with accessory cells such as pericytes, and differentiate into functional blood vessels (3–12). These newly formed vessels can then provide nutrients, exchange gases, and remove metabolic waste products for proper maintenance of tissues and organs.

Angiogenesis is not a process in which individual molecules function in isolation, but is rather a complex series of molecular, biochemical, and cellular events that function cooperatively to form new vessels. In this regard, the primary focus of this chapter is to examine angiogenesis in terms of molecular cooperation, and to discuss important new insights into the regulation of angiogenesis and neovascular diseases.

II. GROWTH FACTORS AND THEIR RECEPTORS IN ANGIOGENESIS

Studies have implicated growth factor and cytokine stimulation as a critical initiating event in neovascularization (11,12). Some of the more widely studied of these include basic and acidic fibroblast growth factor (FGF), vascular endothelial growth factor (VEGF), platelet-derived growth factor (PDGF), tumor necrosis factor-α (TNF-α), transforming growth factor-β (TGF-β), and insulin and insulin-like growth factors (11,12). It is important to note that this is only a partial list of the large number of factors known to stimulate angiogenesis. Growth factors are expressed by a number of cell types including vascular endothelial cells, smooth muscle cells, stromal cells, inflammatory cells, as well as tumor cells (11,12). The ability of these factors to contribute to angiogenesis depends in part on the concept of molecular cooperation. In its most basic form, these soluble factors bind to their cognate cell surface receptors thereby facilitating signal transduction. For example, VEGF can bind to at least two specific VEGF receptors termed VEGFR-1 (flt1) and VEGFR-2 (KDR/flk-1), while distinct forms of FGF have been shown to interact with at least 4 specific tyrosine kinase receptors (13–15). Direct interactions between these growth factors and their transmembrane tyrosine kinase receptors can regulate a number of processes including cell proliferation, adhesion, migration, protease production, and secretion of ECM components (16–23).

Under normal physiological conditions, angiogenesis is highly regulated. The expression, bioavalability, and activity of these factors must be tightly controlled to avoid aberrant neovascu-

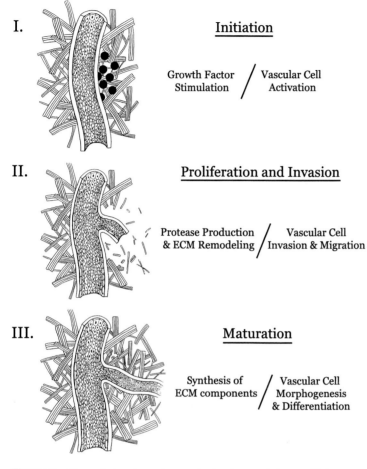

Figure 1 General steps in angiogenesis. Angiogenesis is a multistep process that involves a continuum of interconnected events. In general, the stages can be grouped into three categories including initiation, proliferation/invasion, and maturation. These sequential steps may start by growth factor stimulation of quiescent endothelial cells. Activated endothelial cells in turn remodel their immediate microenvironment, facilitating cellular invasion and migration. In the final stage of maturation, endothelial cells participate in distinct cell–cell and cell–ECM interactions, secrete new ECM molecules, and differentiate into functional vessels.

larization. Given these facts, it is unlikely that a single growth factor or cytokine acts independently to initiate angiogenesis. In fact, it is likely that the expression, biodistribution, and functional activity of these growth factors are regulated by cooperative interactions with other regulatory molecules, including cell adhesion receptors and extracellular matrix components.

III. GROWTH FACTORS AND THEIR RECEPTORS: INTERACTIONS AND MODULATION BY CELL ADHESION MOLECULES

It is well known that angiogenesis can be regulated by signal transduction mechanisms mediated by ligation of endothelial cell tyrosine kinase receptors. As mentioned above, TGF-β has been shown to regulate angiogenesis (11,12,17,21,23). Interestingly TGF-β was shown to block angiogenesis in vitro by inhibiting endothelial cell proliferation (24). In contrast, TGF-β promoted angiogenesis in vivo (25–27). The effects of TGF-β on angiogenesis in vivo are likely due to indirect mechanisms, such as regulating endothelial cell differentiation, as well as expression of ECM proteins and proteases. Recent studies by Munger et al. (28) have shown that integrins αvβ1 and αvβ6 can directly interact with latent TGF-β. This interaction was dependent on an RGD tripeptide motif known to be recognized by many integrin receptors (28). Interestingly, αvβ6-mediated cellular interactions with TGF-β resulted in its activation (28). This novel mechanism by which TGF-β is activated could contribute to angiogenesis by facilitating TGF-β/receptor-mediated signal transduction, since latent TGF-β fails to interact with its receptor.

Platelet-derived growth factor has also been shown to contribute to angiogenesis (29,30). In fact, PDGF regulates both smooth muscle and endothelial cell migration, as well as cell proliferation (16,19,20,31). Another intriguing example of molecular cooperation is illustrated in recent studies by Woodard et al. (31). In these studies, the PDGF receptor was shown to bind to αvβ3 (31). Importantly, this unique interaction between a growth factor receptor and an integrin was shown to promote cell migration (31). Moreover, both αvβ3 and PDGF receptors have been implicated in the regulation of neovascularization (29,31). These studies suggest that molecular associations between members of distinct families of molecules may work in cooperation to potentiate cellular processes that regulate neovascularization. An expanding body of evidence regarding the cooperation between growth factors and integrin signaling is accumulating. There not only appears to exist a convergence of downstream signaling mechanisms, but examples of direct molecular interactions are also emerging (32,34).

To this end, evidence suggests that αvβ3 directly interacts with the insulin receptor substrate-I, an intracellular protein thought to facilitate signal transduction (34,35). Since both insulin as well as insulin-like growth factor-1 have been shown to promote angiogenesis, it is possible that the novel interaction may contribute to cellular proliferation, adhesion, and migration during neovascularization.

Integrins are not the only examples of cell adhesion molecules that regulate growth factor function. Studies have suggested that Ig adhesion molecules may directly interact with growth factor receptors (36,37). In fact, L1/NCAM interacts with FGF receptors (FGFRs) (38). These unique growth factor receptor/cell adhesion molecule interactions may act to regulate angiogenesis by modulating signal transduction pathways. To this end, ligation of FGFRs has been shown to activate signaling molecules, including PLCγ and MAP kinase (31,38,39). Interestingly, MAP kinase activity has recently been demonstrated to contribute to new blood vessel development (40).

IV. INTERACTIONS BETWEEN ANGIOGENIC GROWTH FACTORS AND EXTRACELLULAR MATRIX COMPONENTS

Expression of angiogenic growth factors occurs throughout normal tissues (11,12). Therefore, it is likely that mechanisms exist to control the activity of these angiogenic stimulators. As we have discussed above, direct molecular interactions between tyrosine kinase receptors as well as interactions with distinct cell adhesion molecules may function cooperatively to regulate growth factor activity. A third mechanism that may contribute to the regulation of growth factor activity is direct protein interactions with specific ECM components. The ECM is a complex network of fibrous proteins, proteoglycans, and glycoproteins that interconnect to provide structural as well as biochemical regulatory functions for cells and tissues (41). Recent evidence suggests that direct protein–protein interactions between growth factors and ECM components may provide an important mechanism to regulate growth factor activity (43–50). For example, studies have indicated that TNFα can directly bind to fibronectin and to a lesser extent laminin (45). Furthermore, matrix localization could regulate the capacity of TNF-α to bind to its receptor. Alternatively, the ECM may provide a highly concentrated storage area for TNF-α. These mechanisms may result in regulating both the bioavailability and biological activity of TNF-α.

In addition to TNF-α, bFGF also interacts with the ECM (43,44,47,49). In fact, FGF was shown to bind to heparan sulfate proteoglycans (HSPG), which are known components of the ECM (44,47). Moreover, studies have also suggested that FGF binding to HSPGs may enhance the association of FGF with its receptor and thereby potentiate its mitogenic activity (44,47). Thus, ECM localization of bFGF may act to sequester high levels of growth factors into defined tissue microenvironments. Interestingly, studies have shown that specific proteases including heparanase and plasmin may release ECM-bound FGF (49). Protease-released FGF can bind to its receptor and potentiate mitogenic activity (49). Thus, ECM localization and subsequent release may be essential in the regulation of growth factor bioavailability and activity.

Vascular endothelial growth factor is expressed in a number of forms resulting from alternative splicing of RNA (46,48,50). Specific isoforms that have been described include $VEGF_{125}$, $VEGF_{145}$, $VEGF_{165}$, $VEGF_{185}$, and $VEGF_{206}$. $VEGF_{125}$ exists predominantly in a soluble form whereas $VEGF_{185}$, $VEGF_{145}$, and $VEGF_{206}$ are either cell associated or matrix bound (46,48,50). Interestingly, $VEGF_{165}$ may be present in both soluble and bound forms (46,48,50). Activity of VEGF is thought to be limited due in large part to the expression of its cell surface receptors being primarily confined to endothelial cells (46,48,50). However, like TNF-α and bFGF, VEGF is also capable of binding to ECM components (46,48,50). Interactions of VEGF with the ECM may be mediated by its ability to bind heparan sulfate proteoglycans. However, recent studies by Poltorak et al. (48) have suggested that the $VEGF_{145}$ isoform may bind to the ECM by a mechanism independent from sulfated glycosaminoglycans. In fact, $VEGF_{145}$ was shown to bind to endothelium-secreted ECM that was devoid of sulfated glycosaminoglycans (48). These findings suggest that while HSPGs may facilitate the binding of a number of growth factors, alternative components present in the ECM may also contribute to growth factor–ECM localization.

V. CELL ADHESION MOLECULES AND ANGIOGENESIS

An important characteristic of activated endothelial cells is enhanced expression of cell adhesion molecules (51–55). Cell adhesion molecules can be grouped into at least four distinct families, including cadherins, selectins, immunoglobulin (Ig) super gene family members, and integrins (52,54). Cadherins, selectins, and Ig family members predominantly mediate cell–cell interactions, while members of the integrin family promote cell–matrix interactions (52,54). Integrin receptors, however, can also promote cell–cell interactions (52,54). Traditionally, cell adhesion molecules were thought to contribute to angiogenesis by facilitating cell–cell or cell–ECM interactions. However, exciting new studies have provided intriguing evidence that the view of cell adhesion molecules as molecular glue may be only a small part of their diverse functions. For example, integrins not only facilitate physical associations between other cells and the ECM, but also have the capacity to transmit biochemical information from outside the cell to the interior and from the inside of the cell to the outside, thereby mediating bidirectional signaling (56). Thus, integrins allow cells to sense their immediate extracellular surroundings and, in turn, respond to changes in their dynamic microenvironment. These integrin-mediated signaling pathways have been shown to involve changes in intracellular pH, fluxes in calcium concentrations, and protein phosphorylation (57,58). These biochemical changes may activate signaling molecules including MAP kinases, adapter proteins, and cytoskeletal elements, which in turn regulate processes such as cell adhesion, migration, invasion, gene expression, and differentiation (56–56).

Cadherins, selectins, and members of the Ig superfamily are also thought to contribute to signal transduction pathways (59,60). For example, cadherins interact with intracellular accessory proteins called catenins that help potentiate signal transduction (59,60). Interestingly, studies show that cell adhesion molecules such as integrins and cadherins may function cooperatively to regulate complex cellular behavior such as migration (59,60).

The development of new blood vessels is thought to require adhesive cellular processes, such as endothelial cell adhesion, invasion, and migration. In fact, function-blocking antibodies directed to specific adhesion molecules block endothelial tube formation in vitro and angiogenesis in vivo (52,53,55). While the well-established function of cell adhesion molecules in promoting physical associations likely plays an active role in neovascularization, cooperative molecular interactions with other angiogenesis regulatory molecules may also contribute to the angiogenic cascade.

VI. INTEGRIN–PROTEASE INTERACTIONS IN REGULATION OF ANGIOGENESIS

Recent studies suggest that integrins can interact with an array of molecules other than ECM proteins (Fig. 2). In fact, integrins have been shown to associate with growth factors and growth factor receptors, other cell adhesion molecules, intracellular signaling molecules, cytoskeletal elements, as well as a number of tetraspan transmembrane molecules (61). Interestingly, recent studies have now added a new family of molecules shown to associate with integrins, including proteolytic enzymes and their receptors (62–67).

Two major categories of proteolytic enzymes that contribute to new blood vessel development include serine proteases and members of the matrix metalloproteinase (MMP) family. Recent evidence suggests that serine proteases, such as thrombin, as well as protease receptors, including the urokinase plasminogen activator receptor (uPAR), can directly interact with members of the integrin family (65,67). Thrombin is a multifunctional serine protease which can cleave a

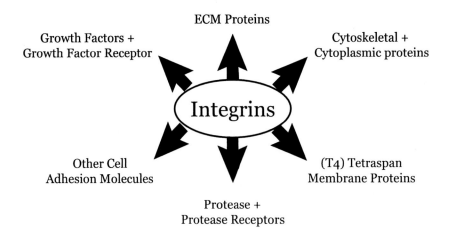

Figure 2   Integrin-mediated molecular interactions. Schematic representation of the diverse set of molecular interactions in which integrin receptors are thought to participate. These molecular interactions may contribute to the mechanisms by which integrins regulate angiogenesis.

number of ECM proteins and convert fibrinogen to fibrin (68,69). Moreover, thrombin can stimulate cellular proliferation, migration, and activation of other proteases including MMPs and the transglutaminase factor XIIIa (70,71). Thus, thrombin may contribute to angiogenesis by regulating a number of mechanisms, including cell proliferation, migration, and ECM remodeling. Interestingly, thrombin contains the integrin tripeptide recognition motif RGD (70). Studies have suggested that the integrin $\alpha v \beta 3$ can specifically interact with thrombin (67,70). In fact, in recent studies by Byzova and Plow, it was shown that prothrombin can specifically bind to $\alpha v \beta 3$ integrin when $\alpha v \beta 3$ is activated (70). Moreover, the related vitronectin receptor αIIb $\beta 3$ can also bind thrombin (70).

In addition to thrombin, another example of a protease (transglutaminase) interaction with integrins is the association of Factor XIIIa with $\alpha v \beta 1$, αIIb $\beta 3$, and $\alpha v \beta 3$ (62,73,74). Factor XIIIa contributes to the stabilization of blood clots by facilitating crosslinking of fibrin monomers (71, 73,74). Factor XIIIa can also contribute to ECM alterations by interacting with fibronectin, collagen, and thrombospondin (71,73,74). Besides protein cross-linking, recent studies by Ueki et al. (62) suggest that Factor XIIIa may contribute to cell adhesion by promoting cellular interactions through integrin receptors such as $\alpha v \beta 3$ and $\beta 1$. Again, molecular cooperation between enzymes and cell adhesion molecules may represent unique mechanisms to regulate neovascularization by regulating endothelial cell adhesion, migration, and proteolytic activity.

The functional activity of proteases can be regulated by cell surface protease receptors (75). For example, the glycosylphosphatidyl inositol (GPI)–linked cell surface receptor uPAR localizes proteolytic activity to close cell–ECM microdomains (75,76). In fact, antagonists of either uPA or uPAR have been shown to block endothelial tube formation in vitro and angiogenesis in vivo (75–77). Interestingly, recent studies have shown that uPAR can associate with the $\alpha v \beta 3$ and $\beta 1$ integrin receptors (65). These novel integrin–uPAR interactions have been suggested to regulate integrin functions such as cellular migration (75–78). Again, unique molecular cooperation between distinct families of angiogenesis regulatory molecules may play important functions during the formation of new blood vessels by coordinating both proteolytic and adhesive cellular mechanisms.

The MMPs are a group of metal dependent, matrix degrading enzymes that collectively remodel most of the components of the ECM (79). Moreover, MMPs have been shown to play an important role in angiogenesis (80,81). In fact, antagonists of MMP activity block endothelial tube formation in vitro and angiogenesis in vivo (82,83). Similar to the serine proteases, MMP activity can be localized to the surface of invasive cells (63,64,79). While a number of serine protease receptors have been identified, little is known concerning similar cell surface receptors for MMPs. Interestingly, recent studies have identified a subfamily of transmembrane MMPs (79). In addition, a novel family of membrane proteins has been identified called ADAMs (84). This family has the unique characteristic of having a disintegrin/integrin-like domain as well as a metalloproteinase domain (84). These membrane proteins combine both cell adhesive functions and proteolytic activity in one molecule. The existence of such a family of molecules suggests the functional importance of molecular cooperation between integrins and MMPs.

To this end, we as well as others have recently identified a unique example of molecular interactions between integrins and MMPs. Studies have indicated that the integrin $\alpha v \beta 3$ can directly bind to MMP-2 (63,64). This unique interaction between MMP-2 and $\alpha v \beta 3$ contributes to the localization of proteolytic activity to the surface of invasive cells (63,64). This protein–protein interaction depends in part on the C-terminal hemopexin-like domain of MMP-2 (64). Moreover, systemic administration of soluble hemopexin domain was shown to disrupt MMP-2/$\alpha v \beta 3$ interactions, thereby inhibiting cell surface collagenolytic activity, angiogenesis, and tumor growth in vivo (64). Interestingly, recent studies by Partridge et al. (85) have provided evidence that MMP-9, a second member of the MMP family, is closely associated with β1 integrins in focal contacts. While not demonstrating a direct protein–protein interaction, these studies suggest that MMP-9 may associate with β1 intergrins (85). The possibility of a MMP-9/β1 interaction is further supported by studies conducted by Pulli et al. (86) that suggest that a short peptide sequence present within the β1 subunit can bind to MMP-9.

In addition to integrins, other cell surface adhesion molecules may contribute to the regulation and localization of proteolytic enzymes. CD44 is a cell surface glycoprotein known to mediate both homophilic cell–cell interactions as well as cell–ECM interactions (87,89). CD44 has been suggested to cooperate with β1 integrins in the regulation of cell adhesion and migration (89). Moreover, studies have also suggested that CD44 may contribute to angiogenesis by regulating endothelial cell adhesion, proliferation, and migration (87–89). Importantly, in studies by Bourguignon and others, evidence was provided that CD44 may contribute to the localization of MMP-9 to the surface of invasive cells (85). Taken together, these findings suggest that unique molecular interactions between cell adhesion molecules and proteolytic enzymes may function to coordinate adhesive and proteolytic activity on the cell surface, which may have a direct impact on angiogenesis in vivo.

VII. MOLECULAR INTERACTIONS BETWEEN INTEGRINS AND TETRASPAN MOLECULES

Tetraspan molecule (TM4) proteins are cell membrane proteins that are thought to span the plasma membrane four times (90). Studies have shown that specific TM4 proteins, including CD9, CD63, CD81, and CD151, can interact with integrins. CD9, CD63, and CD81 have been suggested to regulate cell adhesion and migration (90). Interestingly, CD9, CD63, and CD81 have been shown to interact with integrin α3β1, as well as α6β1 (90). CD151 was also shown to interact with integrin α5β1 (91). In recent studies by Yanez-Mo et al. (92), it was shown that CD81/TAPA-1 and CD151/PETA-3 were specifically associated with endothelial cell–cell junctions (92). Moreover, function-blocking antibodies directed to these membrane proteins blocked endothelial cell migration and invasion into collagen gels (92). These findings suggest that CD151, and CD81–integrin complexes may regulate endothelial cell–cell associations as well as cellular motility, processes known to contribute to vessel formation.

VIII. MOLECULAR INTERACTIONS BETWEEN INTEGRINS AND CYTOSKELETAL/CYTOPLASMIC PROTEINS

Integrin ligation and subsequent receptor clustering have been suggested to promote integrin-dependent signal transduction (93,94). Numerous studies have provided evidence that the cytoplasmic tails of integrins interact with cytoskeletal and cytoplasmic proteins (93,94). Some of these proteins include α-actinin, talin, and filamin (93,94). These proteins have been shown to interact predominantly with the cytoplasmic tails of the β chains of integrins, thereby linking integrins to the actin cytoskeleton (93,94). In addition, integrins interact with cytoplasmic tyrosine kinases including pp125[FAK], and pp59[ILK] (93,94). Moreover, the cytoplasmic adapter proteins paxilin, shc, and caveolin-1 also interact with integrins (93–96). Integrin interactions with these cytoplasmic adapter proteins may depend on integrin ligation of specific ECM components (95,96). This complex set of molecular interactions leads to the activation of MAP kinase and Ras signaling pathways, which have been suggested to regulate cellular processes involved in angiogenesis (93–96).

Studies by Lindberg et al. (97) have identified a novel molecular interaction with β3 integrins. Integrin β3 and αIIb β3 were shown to interact with a protein termed integrin-associated protein (IAP). Integrin-associated protein was later determined to be similar to CD47, a putative 5-pass membrane ion channel that facilitates integrin-dependent calcium entry into endothelial cells (98,99). Importantly, fluxes in intracellular calcium have been suggested to regulate angiogenesis (100). In fact, antagonists of calcium fluxes have been shown to inhibit neovascularization (100). While this is only a partial list of proteins that interact with integrins, it does demonstrate the diversity and complexity of molecular–integrin interactions that may contribute to angiogenesis.

IX.   MOLECULAR INTERACTIONS BETWEEN DISTINCT CELL ADHESION MOLECULES

Homophilic and heterophilic molecular interactions between distinct cell adhesion molecules may contribute to vessel formation. During the initiation of angiogenesis, cell–cell interactions may be disrupted to allow endothelial cell invasion and migration from the preexisting vessels. In contrast, during the maturation phase of angiogenesis, the reestablishment of cell–cell interactions is likely necessary for the formation of a functional vessel (101). In this regard, cell adhesion molecules known to facilitate cell–cell interactions, such as cadherins, selectins, and Ig super gene family members, are likely critical players in the angiogenic cascade.

PECAM-1/CD31 is a member of the Ig super gene family of cell adhesion molecules. Studies by Delisser et al. (102) demonstrated that function-blocking antibodies directed to PECAM-1 block endothelial tube formation in vitro and bFGF-induced angiogenesis in vivo. Interestingly, PECAM-1/CD31 has been shown to directly interact with the vascular integrin αvβ3 (36). This unique interaction between PECAM-1/CD31 and αvβ3 is thought to depend on a protein sequence within domain 2 of PECAM-1/CD31 (36). The unique interaction between PECAM-1/CD31 and αvβ3 may contribute to angiogenesis by regulating endothelial cell adhesion and migration, or perhaps by modulating signal transduction pathways. Other examples of heterotypic interactions between Ig cell adhesion molecules and integrins include LI-CAM and αvβ3, and VCAM-1 and α4β1 (37,103).

Interestingly, studies by Koch et al. (104) have implicated E-selectin as well as VCAM-1 in angiogenesis. In these studies, soluble E-selectin was shown to induce angiogenesis which was dependent on interactions with endothelial cell surface sialy Lewis X (104). In contrast, the ability of soluble VCAM-1 to induce angiogenesis was dependent on interactions with integrin α4β1 (104). Taken together, these findings provide further evidence that unique heterophilic and homophilic molecular interactions between cell adhesion molecules may contribute to the regulation of neovascularization.

X.   MOLECULAR INTERACTIONS BETWEEN CELL ADHESION MOLECULES AND ECM PROTEINS

The vast biochemical information contained within the ECM is transmitted to the cells, in large part, by molecular interactions with integrin receptors. Integrin receptors show both highly selective as well as overlapping binding specificity for distinct ECM components (56).

Direct molecular interactions between integrin receptors and specific ECM proteins have been shown to regulate angiogenesis by a number of biochemical mechanisms. For example, α5β1, which has been suggested to play a role in angiogenesis, binds to the 120-kD cell-binding domain of fibronectin and upregulates the expression of a number of MMPs, including MMP-1, MMP-9 and stromelysin (105). In contrast, ligation of the CS-1 region of fibronectin by integrin $\alpha 4\beta 1$ suppressed MMP expression (105). In other studies, ligation of vitronectin by $\alpha v\beta 3$ integrin resulted in enhanced MMP-2 mRNA and protein levels (106). Importantly, all of these MMPs have been shown to contribute to angiogenesis (80–83). In addition to regulating protease production, studies indicate that integrin ligation of collagen, laminin, fibronectin, and vitronectin can regulate endothelial cell proliferation, adhesion, migration, differentiation, and cell survival (56). Taken together, these unique molecular interactions provide vascular cells with a complex set of mechanisms to tightly control neovascularization.

XI. PROTEOLYTIC ENZYMES AND REGULATION OF ANGIOGENESIS

As mentioned above, two families of proteolytic enzymes that are thought to play critical roles in ECM remodeling include serine proteases and MMPs (80–83). An important example of this concept is the plasminogen activator (PA)–plasmin system (75–78). Critical components of this system include the serine proteases urokinase plasminogen activator (uPA) and tissue plasminogen activator (tPA) (75–78). Both uPA and tPA can convert the zymogen plasminogen to the broad spectrum serine protease plasmin (75–78). In turn, plasmin can degrade a variety of ECM components, including fibronectin, laminin, proteoglycans, and gelatin (75–78). Interestingly, plasmin has been shown to activate zymogen forms of certain MMPs as well as latent elastase (79–81). Thus, molecular cooperation between the PA–plasmin system and MMPs may help regulate proteolytic degradation of the ECM.

Matrix metalloproteinases are a large family of metal-dependent enzymes that, in general, share a common domain structure including a pro-domain, a metal-dependent catalytic domain and a C-terminal hemopexin-like domain (79–83). Matrix metalloproteinases can cleave a variety of ECM components, including distinct forms of collagen, fibronectin, and laminin, as well as some proteoglycans (79–83). While the PA–plasmin system can cleave many of the same substrates as members of the MMP family, distinct differences are also evident. For example, basement membrane collagen type IV is highly resistant to serine proteolytic attack in its native triple helical form (79–83). Since a major component of the subendothelial basement membrane of blood vessels is collagen IV, and since angiogenesis likely involves vascular cells crossing this restrictive barrier, proteolytic remodeling of collagen IV is likely a critical event in facilitating angiogenesis. To this end, both MMP-2 and MMP-9 have the unique ability to specifically cleave native triple helical collagen IV (79–83).

XII. MOLECULAR INTERACTIONS IN REGULATION
OF PROTEOLYTIC ACTIVITY

Proteolytic enzymes play an important role in neovascularization, however, this proteolytic activity must be regulated to prevent excessive proteolytic destruction. Excessive proteolytic degradation may lead to destruction of matrix components, which could in turn hinder cell adhesive processes, such as migration and invasion. Thus, it is likely that a critical balance exists between proteolytic activity and its inhibition to allow optimal ECM remodeling. To this end, at least four naturally occurring inhibitors of MMPs have been identified and are collectively called tissue inhibitors of metalloproteinases (TIMPs) (107). A similar set of naturally occurring protease inhibitors, PAIs (plasminogen activator inhibitors), have been identified for the PA–plasmin system (75,78). These naturally occurring protease inhibitors have been shown to regulate angiogenesis in vivo (108,109). These protease inhibitors can bind specifically to the active sites of their respective enzymes and thereby block catalytic activity (107,81). However, recent evidence suggests that this mode of action may not be the only way these inhibitors function. For example, TIMP-2 can bind to the noncatalytic C-terminal hemopexin-like domain of MMP-2 (107). It has been suggested that this unique molecular interaction stabilizes the proenzyme as well as helps to facilitate localization to the cell surface (107). In other studies, it has been suggested that specific TIMPs may directly regulate cellular growth; however, the mechanisms by which TIMPs facilitate this function is not understood (110). These unique functions and molecular associations add to the potential mechanisms by which proteolytic activity may be controlled.

As mentioned above, the PA–plasmin system also has its own set of protease inhibitors termed PAIs. As with the TIMPs, PAIs can bind to the active site of uPA and block its enzymatic activity (75,81). A number of studies have provided evidence that PAI can bind to ECM proteins such as vitronectin (75,81). In fact, Staffanson et al. (111) demonstrated that PAI can disrupt vascular cell migration by blocking $\alpha v\beta 3$ intergrin access to vitronectin. In studies by Planus et al. (112), it was shown that immobilized PAI-1 can potentiate cell adhesion and migration as a result of interactions with uPA (112). In further studies, it has been suggested that the GPI-linked uPA receptor uPAR can specifically interact with vitronectin (113). Taken together, it is becoming increasingly obvious that while protease–protease inhibitor interactions play an important role in regulating angiogenesis, a number of unique molecular interactions between proteases and cell adhesion molecules may also contribute to the regulation of neovascularization.

XIII. EXTRACELLULAR MATRIX COMPONENTS AND REGULATION OF ANGIOGENESIS

The ECM is a complex mixture of fibrous and adhesive glycoprotein and proteoglycans that are interconnected to form a network-like structure. A partial list of the major components of the ECM includes collagen, laminin, enactin, fibronectin, thrombospondin, fibrinogen, and vitronectin (41,42). Historically, the ECM was thought to primarily function as an inert scaffold to provide structural and mechanical support for cells and tissues. However, a number of biochemical and molecular studies have shown that the ECM can actively regulate a variety of cellular and biochemical processes.

Cellular interactions with the ECM and subsequent activation of signal transduction pathways play critical roles is angiogenesis. For example, disrupting the interactions of integrins $\alpha v\beta 3$, $\alpha v\beta 5$, $\alpha 1\beta 1$, $\alpha 2\beta 1$, $\alpha 5\beta 1$, and $\alpha 6\beta 1$ with ECM proteins has been shown to inhibit angiogenesis (114–117). While integrin–ECM interactions are clearly important in controlling angiogenesis, other molecular interactions with ECM proteins may be of equal importance. As discussed above, ECM proteins bind to a variety of molecules known to regulate angiogenesis, including growth factors. Localization of these angiogenic growth factors to the ECM could modulate their bioavailability, capacity to interact with their receptors, and thus their ability to facilitate angiogenesis.

In addition to localizing growth factors, ECM components bind proteolytic enzymes as well as protease inhibitors. For example, the serine protease thrombin can be localized to the ECM through a short anchorage binding site (amino acids 367–380 of the b chain) (118). This interaction is thought to depend on thrombin's ability to bind to dermatin sulfate within the ECM (118). Importantly, this ECM-bound thrombin was not inhibited by antithrombin III, a physiological inhibitor of thrombin (118). These findings suggest that the ECM-bound thrombin may be protected from interacting with specific inhibitors and thus may remain active and possibly retain its capacity to participate in cellular interactions. These unique interactions may facilitate localized ECM remodeling and/or potentiate cellular mitogenicity mediated by thrombin.

Finally, the ECM may regulate protease activity by sequestering specific protease inhibitors. For example, the serine protease inhibitor PAI-1 has been shown to be bound to the ECM by direct interactions with vitronectin (75,81). Moreover, studies have indicated that TIMP-3, a MMP inhibitor was also associated with the ECM (107). Thus, unique molecular interactions between ECM proteins and integrins, proteases, protease inhibitors, and growth factors may all contribute to the complex mechanisms by which molecular cooperativity may regulate neovascularization.

XIV. CONCLUSIONS

An explosion of biochemical and molecular information over the past decade has clearly demonstrated that angiogenesis is an important and highly complex physiological process. In fact, angiogenesis has been shown to regulate a variety of normal and pathological processes (3–5). Thus, understanding the complex control mechanisms that regulate new blood vessel growth could have profound implications in the development of effective approaches for the treatment of a diverse set of human diseases.

It is becoming increasingly clear that the wide array of molecules that are known to regulate angiogenesis do not necessarily function in isolation, but are rather interconnected in a continuum of biochemical and cellular events (Fig. 3). Understanding these unique molecular interactions involved in angiogenesis may provide novel approaches for the design of effective new drugs to regulate neovascular diseases. For example, an alternative approach for directly targeting proteolytic activity might be to prevent the localization of these enzymes to the cell surface by blocking unique protease–integrin interactions.

In this regard, we have discussed the molecular cooperation among four major families of molecules that are known to regulate angiogenesis, including growth factors and their receptors, cell adhesion molecules, proteolytic enzymes, and extracellular matrix proteins (see Fig. 3). Moreover, instead of focusing on the individual functions of these molecules, we have provided examples of how these diverse sets of proteins may function in a cooperative manner to regulate

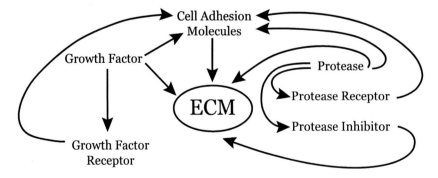

Figure 3 Molecular cooperation between angiogenesis regulatory molecules. Angiogenesis depends on the functions of a number of distinct families of molecules, including cell adhesion molecules, proteases, growth factors, and ECM proteins. Importantly, the functions of these molecules may be tightly regulated by a complex network of molecular interactions. Molecular interactions among these families of molecules may play a critical role in regulating new blood vessel development.

angiogenesis and neovascular diseases. Thus, understanding the development of new blood vessels in terms of molecular cooperation may shed new light on this fascinating and complex physiological process.

REFERENCES

1. Flamme I, Frolich T, Risau W. Molecular mechanisms of vasculogenesis and embryonic angiogenesis. J Cell Physiol 1997; 173:206–210.
2. Tyagi SC. Vasculogenesis and angiogenesis: Extracellular matrix remodeling in coronary collateral arteries and the ischemic heart. J Cell Biochem 1997; 65:388–394.
3. Blood CH, Zetter BR. Tumor interactions with the vasculature: Angiogenesis and tumor metastasis. Biochem Biophys Acta 1990; 1032:89–118.
4. Cockerill GW, Gamble JR, Vadas MA. Angiogenesis: Models and modulators. Int Rev Cytol 1995; 159:113–159.
5. D'Amore PA, Thompson RW. Mechanisms of angiogenesis. Annu Rev Physiol 1987; 49:453–464.
6. Folkman J. The role of angiogenesis in tumor growth. Cancer Biol Semin 1992; 3:65–71.
7. Paku S, Paweletz N. First steps of tumor-related angiogenesis. Lab Invest 1991; 65:334–346.
8. Fox SB, Gatter KC, Harris AL. Tumor angiogenesis. J Pathol 1996; 179:232–237.
9. Auerbach W, Auerbach R. Angiogenesis inhibition: A review. Pharmacol Ther 1994; 63:265–311.
10. Sholley MM, Ferguson GP, Seibel HR, Montour JL, Wilson JD. Mechanisms of neovascularization: Vascular sprouting can occur without proliferation of endothelial cells. Lab Invest 1984; 51:624–634.
11. Leek RD, Harris AL, Lewis CE. Cytokine networks in solid human tumors: Regulation of angiogenesis. J Leukocyte Biol 1994; 56:423–435.
12. Sunderkotter C, Steinbrink K, Goebeler M, Bhardwaj R, Sorg C. Macrophages and angiogenesis. J Leukocyte Biol 1994; 55:410–422.
13. Dvorak HF, Brown LF, Detmar M, Dvorak AM. Vascular permeability factor/vascular endothelial growth factor, microvascular hyperpermeability, and angiogenesis. Am J Pathol 1995; 146:1029–1039.
14. Waltenberger J, Claesson-Welsh L, Siegbahn A, Shibuya M, Heldin CH. Different signal transduction properties of KDR and Flt1, two receptors for vascular endothelial growth factor. J Biol Chem 1994; 269:26988–26995.
15. Soulet L, Lemaitre EC, Blanquaert F, Meddahi A, Barritault D. FGFs and their receptors, in vitro and in vivo studies: New FGF receptor in the brain, FGF-1 in muscle, and the use of functional analogues of low-affinity heparin binding growth factor receptors in tissue repair. Mol Repro Dev 1994; 39: 49–55.
16. Battegay EJ, Rupp J, Iruela-Arispe L, Sage EH, Pech M. PDGF-BB modulates endothelial proliferation and angiogenesis in vitro via PDGF beta-receptors. J Cell Biol 1994; 125:917–928.
17. Yang EY, Moses HL. Transforming growth factor beta 1-induced changes in cell migration, proliferation, and angiogenesis in the chicken chorioallantoic membrane. J Cell Biol 1990; 111:731–741.
18. Rusnati M, Dell'Era P, Urbinati C, Tanghetti E, Massardi ML, Nagamine Y, Monti E, Presta M. A distinct basic fibroblast growth factor (FGF-2)/FGF receptor interaction distinguishes urokinase-type plasminogen activator induction from mitogenicity in endothelial cells. Mol Biol Cell 1996; 7:369–381.
19. Matsumoto K, Ziober BL, Yao CC, Kramer RH. Growth factor regulation of integrin-mediated cell motility. Cancer Metastasis Rev 1995; 14:205–217.
20. Thommen R, Humar R, Misevic G, Pepper MS, Hahn AWA, John M, Battegay EJ. PDGF-BB increases endothelial migration and cord movements during angiogenesis in vitro. J Cell Biochem 1997; 64:403–413.
21. Pepper MS, Belin D, Montesano R, Orci L, Vassalli J-D. Transforming growth factor-beta 1 modulates basic fibroblast growth factor-induced proteolytic and angiogenic properties of endothelial cells in vitro. J Cell Biol 1990; 111:743–755.

22. Patterson C, Perrella MA, Endege WO, Yoshizumi M, Lee M-E, Haber E. Down regulation of vascular endothelial growth factor receptors by tumor necrosis factor-alpha in cultured human vascular endothelial cells. J Clin Invest 1996; 98:490–496.

23. Madri JA, Pratt BM, Tucker AM. Phenotypic modulation of endothelial cells by transforming growth factor-beta depends upon the composition and organization of the extracellular matrix. J Cell Biol 1998; 106:1375–1384.

24. Muller G, Behrens J, Nussbaumer UI, Bohlen P, Birchmeier W. Inhibitory action of transforming growth factor beta on endothelial cells. Proc Natl Acad Sci USA 1987; 84:5600–5609.

25. Roberts AB, Sporn MB, Assoian RH, Smith JM, Roche NS, Wakefield LM, Heine UI, Liotta LA, Falange U, Hehrl JH, Fauci AS. Transforming growth factor type beta: Rapid induction of fibrosis and angiogenesis in vivo, and stimulation of collagen formation in vitro. Proc Natl Acad Sci USA 1986; 83:4167–4171.

26. Yang EY, Moses HL. Transforming growth factor beta 1-induced changes in cell migration, proliferation and angiogenesis in the chicken chorioallantoic membrane. J Cell Biol 1990; 111:731–741.

27. Taipale J, Saharinen J, Hedman K, Keski-Oja J. Latent transforming growth factor beta-1 and its binding protein are components of the extracellular matrix microfibrils. J Histochem Cytochem 1996; 44: 875–889.

28. Munger JS, Huang X, Kawakatsu H, Griffiths MJD, Dalton SL, Wu J, Pittet JF, Kaminski N, Garat C, Matthay MA, Rifkin DB, Sheppard D. The integrin $\alpha v \beta 6$ binds and activates latent TGF beta 1: A mechanism for regulating pulmonary inflammation and fibrosis. Cell 1999; 96:319–328.

29. Nicosia RF, Nicosia SV, Smith M. Vascular endothelial growth factor, platelet-derived growth factor, and insulin-like growth factor-1 promote rat aortic angiogenesis in vitro. Am J Pathol 1994; 145: 1023–1029.

30. Marx M, Perlmutter RA, Madri JA. Modulation of platelet-derived growth factor receptor expression in microvascular endothelial cells during in vitro angiogenesis. J Clin Invest 1994; 93:131–139.

31. Woodard AS, Garcia-Cardena G, Leong M, Madri JA, Sessa WC, Languino LR. The synergistic activity of $\alpha v \beta 3$ integrin and PDGF receptor increases cell migration. J Cell Sci 1998; 111:469–478.

32. Garfinkel S, Hu X, Prudovsky IA, McMahon GA, Kapnik EM, McDowell SD, Maciag T. FGF-1-dependent proliferative and migratory responses are impaired in senescent human umbilical vein endothelial cells and correlate with the inability to signal tyrosine phosphorylation of fibroblast growth factor receptor-1 substrates. J Cell Biol 1996; 134:783–791.

33. Plopper GE, McNamee HP, Dike LE, Bojanowski K, Ingber DE. Convergence of integrin and growth factor receptor signaling pathways within the focal adhesion complex. Mol Biol Cell 1995; 6:1349–1365.

34. Schneller M, Vuori K, Ruoslahti E. $\alpha v \beta 3$ Integrin associates with activated insulin and PDGF beta receptors and potentiates the biological activity of PDGF. EMBO J 1997; 16:5600–5607.

35. Vuori K, Ruoslahti E. Association of insulin receptor substrate-1 with integrins. Science 1994; 266: 1576–1578.

36. Buckley CD, Doyonnas R, Newton JP, Blystone SD, Brown EJ, Watt SM, Simmons DL. Identification of $\alpha v \beta 3$ as heterotypic ligand for CD31/PECAM-1. J Cell Sci 1996; 109:437–445.

37. Montgomety AM, Becker JC, Siu CH, Lemmon VP, Cheresh DA, Pancook JD, Zhao X, Reisfeld RA. Human neural cell adhesion molecule L1 and rat homologue NILE are ligands for integrin $\alpha v \beta 3$. J Cell Biol 1996; 132:475–85.

38. Green PJ, Walsh FS, Doherty P. Promiscuity of fibroblast growth factor receptors. BioEssays 1996; 18:639–646.

39. Miyamoto S, Teramoto H, Gutkind JS, Yamada KM. Integrins can collaborate with growth factors for phosphorylation of receptor tyrosine kinases and MAP kinase activation: Roles of integrin aggregation and occupancy of receptors. J Cell Biol 1996; 135:1633–1642.

40. Eliceiri BP, Klemke R, Stromblad S, Cheresh DA. Integrin $\alpha v \beta 3$ requirement for sustained mitogen-activated protein kinase activity during angiogenesis. J Cell Biol 1998; 140:1255–1263.

41. Nicosia RF, Madri JA. The microvascular extracellular matrix: Developmental changes during angiogenesis in the aortic ring-plasma clot model. Am J Pathol 1987; 128:78–90.

42. Nicosia RF, Bonanno E, Smith M, Yurchenco P. Modulation of angiogenesis in vitro by laminin-entactin complex. Dev Biol 1994; 164:197–206.

43. Hageman GS, Kirchoff-Rempe MA, Lewis GP, Fisher SK, Anderson DH. Sequestration of basic fibroblast growth factor in the primate retinal interphotoreceptor matrix. Proc Natl Acad Sci USA 1991; 88:6706–6710.
44. Aviezer D, Hecht D, Safran M, Eisinger M, David G, Yayon A. Perlecan, basal lamina proteoglycan, promotes basic fibroblast growth factor-receptor binding, mitogenesis, and angiogenesis. Cell 1994; 79:1005–1013.
45. Cahalon L, Hershkoviz R, Gilat D, Miller A, Akiyama SK, Yamada KM, Lider O. Functional interactions of fibronectin and TNF alpha: A paradigm of physiological linkage between cytokines and extracellular matrix moieties. Cell Adhes Comm 1994; 2:269–273.
46. Ferrara N, Houck KA, Jakeman LB, Winer J, Leung DW. The vascular endothelial growth factor family of polypeptides. J Cell Biochem 1991; 47:211–218.
47. Bashkin P, Doctrow S, Klagsbrun M, Svahn CM, Folkman J, Vlodavsky I. Basic fibroblast growth factor binds to subendothelial extracellular matrix and is released by heparitinase and heparin-like molecules. Biochem 1989; 28:1737–1743.
48. Poltorak Z, Cohen T, Sivan R, Kandelis Y, Spira G, Vlodavsky I, Keshet E, Neufeld G. VEGF 145, a secreted vascular endothelial growth factor isoform that binds to extracellular matrix. J Biol Chem 1997; 272:7151–7158.
49. Saksela O, Rifkin DB. Release of basic fibroblast growth factor-heparan sulfate complexes from endothelial cells by plasminogen activator-mediated proteolytic activity. J Cell Biol 1990; 110:767–775.
50. Houck KA, Leung DW, Rowland AM, Winer J, Ferrara N. Dual regulation of vascular endothelial growth factor bioavailability by genetic and proteolytic mechanisms. J Biol Chem 1992; 267:26031–26037.
51. Frater-Schroder M, Risau W, Hallmann R, Gautschi P, Bohlen P. Tumor necrosis factor type alpha, a potent inhibitor of endothelial cell growth in vitro, is angiogenic in vivo. Proc Natl Acad Sci USA 1987; 84:5277–5281.
52. Brooks PC. Cell adhesion molecules in angiogenesis. Cancer Metastasis Rev 1996; 15:187–194.
53. Brooks PC. Role of integrins in angiogenesis. Eur J Cancer 1996; 32A:2423–2429.
54. Stad RK, Buurman WA. Current views on structure and function of endothelial adhesion molecules. Cell Adhes Comm 1994; 2:261–268.
55. Bischoff J. Approaches to studying cell adhesion molecules in angiogenesis. Trends Cell Biol 1995; 5:69–74.
56. Hynes RO. Integrins: Versatility, modulation, and signaling in cell adhesion. Cell 1992; 69:11–25.
57. Yamada KM, Miyamoto S. Integrin transmembrane signaling and cytoskeletal control. Curr Opin Cell Biol 1995; 7:681–689.
58. Sastry SK, Horwitz AF. Integrin cytoplasmic domains: Mediators of cytoskeletal linkages and extra- and intracellular initiated transmembrane signaling. Curr Opin Cell Biol 1993; 5:819–831.
59. Yamada KM, Geiger B. Molecular interactions in cell adhesion complexes. Curr Opin Cell Biol 1997; 9:76–85.
60. Lampugnani MG, Dejana E. Interendothelial junctions: Structure, signaling and functional roles. Curr Opin Cell Biol 1997; 9:674–682.
61. Porter JC, Hogg N. Integrins take partners: Cross-talk between integrins and other membrane receptors. Trends Cell Biol 1998; 8:390–396.
62. Ueki S, Takagi J, Saito Y. Dual functions of transglutaminase in novel cell adhesion. J Cell Sci 1996; 109:2727–2735.
63. Brooks PC, Stromblad S, Sanders LC, von Schalscha TL, Aimes RT, Stetler-Stevenson WG, Quigley JP, Cheresh DA. Localization of matrix metalloproteinase MMP-2 to the surface of invasive cells by interaction with integrin $\alpha v \beta 3$. Cell 1996; 85:683–693.
64. Brooks PC, Silletti S, von Schalscha TL, Friedlander M, Cheresh DA. Disruption of angiogenesis by PEX, a noncatalytic metalloproteinase fragment with integrin binding activity. Cell 1998; 92:391–400.
65. Xue W, Mizukami I, Todd III RF, Petty HR. Urokinase-type plasminogen activator receptors associate with $\beta 1$ and $\beta 3$ integrins of fibrosarcoma cells: dependence on extracellular matrix components. Cancer Res 1997; 57:1682–1689.

66. Deryugina BI, Bourdon MA, Luo G-X, Reisfeld RA, Strongin A. Matrix metalloproteinase-2 activation modulates glioma cell migration. J Cell Sci 1997; 110:2473–2482.

67. Byzova TV, Plow EF. Activation of αvβ3 on vascular cells controls recognition of prothrombin. J Cell Biol 1998; 143:2081–2092.

68. Malik AB, Fenton II JW. Thrombin-mediated increase in vascular endothelial permeability. Semin Thromb Hemost 1992; 18:193–199.

69. Yu JCM, Gotlieb AI. Thrombin promotes aortic endothelial cell spreading and microfilament formation in nonconfluent monolayer cultures. Exp Mol Pathol 1993; 58:139–152.

70. Bar-Shavit R, Sabbah V, Lampugnani MG, Marchisio PC, Fenton II JW, Vlodavsky I, Dejana E. An arg-gly-asp sequence within thrombin promotes endothelial cell adhesion. J Cell Biol 1991; 112:335–344.

71. Tahagi T, Doolittle RF. Amino acid sequence studies on Factor XIIIa and peptides released during its activation by thrombin. Biochem 1974; 13:750–755.

72. Bar-Shavit R, Wilnes GP. Mediation of cellular events by thrombin. Int Rev Exp Pathol 1986; 29:213–241.

73. Greenberg CS, Shuman MA. Specific binding of blood coagulation factor XIIIa to thrombin-stimulated platelets. J Biol Chem 1984; 259:14721–14727.

74. Cox AD, Devine DV. Factor XIIIa binding to activated platelets is mediated through activation of glycoprotein IIb-IIIa. Blood 1994; 83:1006–1016.

75. Blasi F. Urokinase and urokinase receptor: A paracrine/autocrine system regulating cell migration and invasiveness. BioEssays 1993; 15:105–111.

76. Wells JM, Strickland S. Regulated localization confers multiple functions on the protease urokinase plasminogen activator. J Cell Physiol 1997; 171:217–225.

77. Evans CP, Elfman F, Parangi S, Conn M, Cunha G, Shuman MA. Inhibition of prostate cancer neovascularization and growth by urokinase-plasminogen activator receptor blockade. Cancer Res 1997; 57:3594–3599.

78. Wei Y, Lukashev M, Simon DI, Bodary SC, Rosenberg S, Doyle MV, Chapman HA. Regulation of integrin function by the urokinase receptor. Science 1996; 273:1551–1555.

79. Kleiner Jr DE, Stetler-Stevenson WG. Structural biochemistry and activation of matrix metalloproteases. Curr Opin Cell Biol 1993; 5:891–897.

80. Liotta LA, Steeg PS, Stetler-Stevenson WG. Cancer metastasis and angiogenesis: An imbalance of positive and negative regulation. Cell 1991; 64:327–336.

81. Mignatti P, Rifkin DB. Plasminogen activators and matrix metalloproteinases in angiogenesis. Enz Prot 1996; 49:117–137.

82. Moses MA, Langer R. A metalloproteinase inhibitor as an inhibitor of neovascularization. J Cell Biochem 1991; 47:230–235.

83. Moses MA. The regulation of neovascularization by matrix metalloproteinases and their inhibitors. Stem Cells 1997; 15:180–189.

84. Wolfsberg TG, Primakoff P, Myles DG, White JM. ADAM, a novel family of membrane proteins containing a disintegrin and metalloprotease domain: Multipotential functions in cell-cell and cell-matrix interactions. J Cell Biol 1995; 131:275–278.

85. Partridge CA, Phillips PG, Niedbala MJ, Jeffrey JJ. Localization and activation of type IV collagenase/gelatinase at endothelial focal contacts. Am J Physiol 1997; 272:813–822.

86. Pulli T, Koivunenl E, Hyypia T. Cell-surface interactions of echovirus 22. J Biol Chem 1997; 272:21176–21180.

87. Henke CA, Roongta U, Mickelson DJ, Knutson JR, McCarthy JB. CD44-related chondroitin sulfate proteoglycan, a cell surface receptor implicated with tumor cell invasion, mediates endothelial cell migration on fibrinogen and invasion into a fibrin matrix. J Clin Invest 1996; 97:2541–2552.

88. Trochon V, Mabilat C, Bertrand P, Legrand Y, Smadja-Joffe F, Soria C, Delpech B, Lu H. Evidence of involvement of CD44 in endothelial cell proliferation, migration and angiogenesis in vitro. Int J Cancer 1996; 66:664–668.

89. Katagiri YU, Sleeman J, Fujii H, Herrlich P, Hotta H, Tanaka K, Chikuma S, Yagita H, Okumura K, Murakami M, Saiki I, Chambers AF, Uede T. CD44 variants but not CD44s cooperate with β1-con-

taining integrins to permit cells to bind to osteopontin independently of arginine-glycine-aspartic acid, thereby stimulating cell motility and chemotaxis. Cancer Res 1999; 59:219–226.

90. Berditchevski F, Zutter MM, Hemler ME. Characterization of novel complexes on the cell surface between integrins and proteins with 4 transmembrane domains (TM4 proteins). Mol Biol Cell 1996; 7: 193–207.

91. Sincock PM, Mayrhofer G, Ashman LK. Localization of the transmembrane 4 superfamily (TM4SF) member PETA-3 (CD151) in normal human tissues: Comparison with CD9, CD63, and $\alpha 5\beta 1$ integrin. J Histochem Cytochem 1997; 45:515–525.

92. Yanez-Mo M, Alfranca A, Cabanas C, Marazuela M, Tejedor R, Ursa MA, Ashman LK, de Landazuri MO, Sanchez-Madrid F. Regulation of endothelial cell motility by complexes of tetraspan molecules CD81/TAPA-1 and CD151/PETA-3 with $\alpha 3\beta 1$ integrin localized at endothelial lateral junctions. J Cell Biol 1998; 141:791–804.

93. Schlaepfer DD, Hunter T. Integrin signaling and tyrosine phosphorylation: Just the FAKs? Trends Cell Biol 1998; 8:151–157.

94. Hughes PE, Pfaff M. Integrin affinity modulation. Trends Cell Biol 1998; 8:359–364.

95. Wary KK, Mariotti A, Zurzolo C, Giancotti FG. A requirement for caveolin-1 and associated kinase Fyn in integrin signaling and anchorage-dependent cell growth. Cell 1998; 94:625–634.

96. Wary KK, Mainiero F, Isakoff SJ, Marcantonio EE, Giancotti FG. The adaptor protein Shc couples a class of integrins to the control of cell cycle progression. Cell 1996; 87:733–743.

97. Lindberg FP, Gresham HP, Schwarz E, Brown EJ. Molecular cloning of integrin-associated protein: An immunoglobulin family member with multiple membrane spanning domains implicated in $\alpha v\beta 3$-dependent lingand binding. J Cell Biol 1993; 122:485–496.

98. Schwartz MA, Brown EJ, Fazeli B. A 50-kDa integrin-associated protein is required for integrin-regulated calcium entry in endothelial cells. J Biol Chem 1993; 268:19931–19934.

99. Lindberg FP, Lublin DM, Telen MJ, Veile RA, Miller YE, Donis-Keller H, Brown EJ. Rh-related antigen CD47 is the signal-transducer integrin-associated protein. J Biol Chem 1994; 269:1567–1570.

100. Kohn EC, Alessandro R, Spoonster J, Wersto RP, Liotta LA. Angiogenesis: Role of calcium-mediated signal transduction. Proc Natl Acad Sci USA 1995; 92:1307–1311.

101. Hirschi KK, Rohovsky SA, D'Amore PA. Cell-cell interactions in vessel assembly: A model for the fundamentals of vascular remodeling. Transplant Immunol 1997; 5:177–178.

102. DeLisser HM, Christofidou-Solomidou M, Strieter RM, Burdick MD, Robinson CS, Wexler RS, Kerr JS, Garlanda C, Merwin JR, Madri JA, Albelda SM. Involvement of endothelial PECAM-1/CD31 in angiogenesis. Am J Pathol 1997; 151:671–677.

103. Lobb RR, Antognetti G, Pepinsky RB, Burkly LC, Leone DR, Whitty A. A direct binding assay for the vascular cell adhesion molecule-1 (VCAM1) interaction with $\alpha 4$ integrin. Cell Adhes Comm 1995; 3:385–397.

104. Koch AE, Halloran MM, Haskell CJ, Shah MR, Polverini PJ. Angiogenesis mediated by soluble forms of E-selectin and vascular cell adhesion molecule-1. Nature 1995; 376:517–519.

105. Huhtala P, Humphries MJ, McCarthy JB, Tremble PM, Werb Z, Damsky CH. Cooperative signaling by $\alpha 5\beta 1$ and $\alpha 4\beta 1$ integrins regulates metalloproteinase gene expression in fibroblasts adhering to fibronectin. J Cell Biol 1995; 129:867–879.

106. Seftor REB, Seftor EA, Stetler-Stevenson WG, Hendrix MJC. The 72 kDa type IV collagenase is modulated via differential expression of $\alpha v\beta 3$ and $\alpha 5\beta 1$ integrins during human melanoma cell invasion. Cancer Res 1993; 53:3411–3415.

107. Murphy G, Willenbrock F. Tissue inhibitors of matrix metalloendopeptidases. Meth Enzymol 1995; 248:496–509.

108. Soff GA, Sanderowitz J, Gately S, Verrusio E, Weiss I, Brem S, Kwaan HC. Expression of plasminogen activator inhibitor type 1 by human prostate carcinoma cells inhibits primary tumor growth, tumor-associated angiogenesis, and metastasis to lung and liver in an athymic mouse model. J Clin Invest 1995; 96:2593–2600.

109. Anand-Apte B, Pepper MS, Voest E, Montesano R, Olsen B, Murphy G, Apte SS, Zetter B. Inhibition of angiogenesis by tissue inhibitor of metalloproteinase-3. Invest Ophthalmol Vis Sci 1997; 38: 817–823.

110. Nemeth JA, Rafe A, Steiner M, Goolsby CL. TIMP-2 growth-stimulatory activity: A concentration-and cell type-specific response in the presence of insulin. Exp Cell Res 1996; 224:110–115.

111. Stefansson S, Lawrence DA. The serpin PAT-1 inhibits cell migration by blocking integrin $\alpha v \beta 3$ binding to vitronectin. Nature 1996; 383:441–443.

112. Planus E, Barlovatz-Meimon G, Rogers RA, Bonavaud S, Ingber DE, Wang N. Binding of urokinase to plasminogen activator inhibitor type-1 mediates cell adhesion and spreading. J Cell Sci 1997; 110: 1091–1098.

113. Chavakis T, Kanse SM, Yutzy B, Lijnen HR, Preissner KT. Vitronectin concentrates proteolytic activity on the cell surface and extracellular matrix by trapping soluble urokinase receptor-urokinase complexes. Blood 1998; 9:2305–2312.

114. Brooks PC, Montgomery AMP, Rosenfeld M, Reisfeld RA, Hu T, Klier G, Cheresh DA. Integrin $\alpha v \beta 3$ antagonists promote tumor regression by inducing apoptosis of angiogenic blood vessels. Cell 1994; 79:1–20.

115. Senger DR, Claffey KP, Benes JE, Perruzzi CA, Sergiou AP, Detmar M. Angiogenesis promoted by vascular endothelial growth factor: Regulation through $\alpha 1 \beta 1$ and $\alpha 2 \beta 1$ integrins. Proc Natl Acad Sci USA 1997; 94:13612–13617.

116. Bauer J, Margolis M, Schreiner C, Edgell CJ, Azizkhan J, Lazarowski E, Juliano RL. In vitro model of angiogenesis using a human endothelium-derived permanent cell line: Contributions of induced gene expression, G-proteins, and integrins. J Cell Physiol 1992; 153:437–449.

117. Friedlander M, Brooks PC, Shaffer RW, Kincaid CM, Varner JA, Cheresh DA. Definition of two angiogenic pathways by distinct alpha v integrins. Science 1995; 270:1500–1502.

118. Bar-Shavit R, Eldor A, Vlodavsky I. Binding of thrombin to subendothelial extracellular matrix. J Clin Invest 1989; 84:1096–1104.

14

Animal Models of Vasculitis

Ulrich Specks

Mayo Clinic and Mayo Foundation, Rochester, Minnesota

I. INTRODUCTION

The etiology of the systemic vasculitides is largely unknown and their pathogenesis remains incompletely understood. Therefore, current classification schemes for the vasculitides reflect clinical phenomenology and characteristic histopathologic features such as the size of affected vessels, presence of granulomas, or eosinophilic tissue infiltration (1–4).

Animal models have been sought to study cellular and molecular pathomechanisms of vasculitis in vivo and to explore novel mechanisms-based therapeutic modalities. While the validity of extrapolating animal data to human disease can always be challenged, it is obvious that valid animal models allow studies under tightly controlled conditions that can address specific questions about pathogenic mechanisms or the effect of novel therapies that could not be performed in humans. Ideally, the phenotype of an animal model should resemble that of the human disease. In recent years, animal models have provided valuable information about the role of genetic susceptibility, environmental cofactors, proinflammatory mediators, cellular mechanisms, and new mechanism-based treatment modalities for a wide variety of diseases, including autoimmune disorders and vasculitis. Rodent models are particularly appealing because the genetic background of the animals is controlled and the period of gestation and the life span of the animals are relatively short, allowing investigators to assess the disease and effect of interventions readily.

The choice of the species for animal experimentation is influenced by many—mostly practical—considerations. Mice have the advantage that their immune system is very well characterized, and an abundance of secondary reagents facilitating work in the murine system is available. In addition, the techniques for genetic manipulations to generate transgenic or knockout animals to study the biological functions and pathogenic roles of particular molecules is most advanced. The relative disadvantage of mice is their small size, which renders surgical manipulations more difficult and limits the amount of biological material available from an individual animal for laboratory investigations. In this respect, larger animals such as rats, rabbits, or guinea pigs are preferable.

There are essentially two categories of animal models: inbred strains of animals that develop vasculitis spontaneously, and animals in which vasculitis can be induced by certain experimental manipulations. In addition, mice with specific immune defects, such as the severe combined immunodeficiency (SCID) mouse, have been used for the in vivo study of pathogenic mechanisms of human vasculitis. This chapter focuses primarily on rodent disease phenotypes that have been proposed as models for specific types of human vasculitis. The models reviewed are listed in Table 1.

II. INBRED STRAINS OF ANIMALS THAT DEVELOP VASCULITIS SPONTANEOUSLY

A. The MRL/Mp-*lpr/lpr* Mouse

The MRL-*lpr* mouse has been proposed as model of systemic lupus erythematosus (SLE) because of its similarities with the human disease, including autoantibody development, immune complex–mediated glomerulonephritis, and vasculitis. MRL-*lpr* mice are homozygous for the gene *lpr,* which is a defective *fas* gene. The normal *fas*-gene product, Fas, is a tumor necrosis factor (TNF)-type cytokine receptor that transduces a signal causing apoptosis of the Fas-bearing cell when it interacts with its ligand. As Fas-induced apoptosis is involved in clonal deletion of autoreactive lymphocytes, the MRL-*lpr* mice are thought to develop their phenotype as a consequence of inappropriate persistence of autoreactive lymphocytes (5,6). The animals spontaneously develop hypergammaglobulinemia and high levels of IgG autoantibodies, including anti-DNA antibodies, in association with immune-complex mediated glomerulonephritis, vasculitis affecting small and medium-sized arteries and venules, and progressive lymph node and spleen enlargement. The disease has a very reproducible time course. Mild disease is detectable at about 8 weeks, and by about 24 weeks, 50% of the animals die of progressive glomerulonephritis or vasculitis-related hemorrhage.

Even though the MRL-*lpr* mouse represents a very appealing model for SLE and vasculitis, the data derived from this model need to be interpreted with the understanding that it does not exactly mirror the human disease. While increased levels of soluble Fas protein, which might interfere with Fas-induced apoptosis, have been found in some patients with SLE, neither the Fas antigen mutation nor the significant lymphoproliferation of the MRL-*lpr* mice are part of the human disease (7,8).

Nevertheless, the model represents a useful tool to study novel mechanism-based therapies. For instance, it has been used to evaluate gene therapy modalities. Since the mitogen responsiveness of T cells of MRL-*lpr* mice is defective as a result of insufficient interleukin-2 (IL-2) production, Huggins et al. (9) treated MRL-*lpr* mice by oral application of attenuated *Salmonella typhimurium* carrying murine genes encoding IL-2. The slow synthesis and release of IL-2 by these bacteria restored the defective T-cell response to mitogen and suppressed production of anti-dsDNA as well as the development of glomerulonephritis and vasculitis compared with control animals (9). When transforming growth factor-β1 (TGF-β1) was supplemented in the same fashion, the incidence of vasculitis was increased but the autoantibody response and glomerulonephritis were not affected (9). This study demonstrates the feasibility of a novel convenient gene therapy approach to modify autoimmune disease in vivo. At the same time, it underscores the critical importance of vector and route of administration for the outcome of cytokine gene therapy, as the results are quite different from those reported by others who used intramuscular injection of naked DNA (10) or *Vaccinia* virus as vector for the delivery of the cytokines (11).

Most recently Harper et al. (12) have proposed the MRL-*lpr* mouse as a model to study the pathogenicity of antineutrophil cytoplasmic antibodies (ANCAs) directed against myeloperoxidase (MPO). They demonstrated that the development of vasculitis in MRL-*lpr* mice was related to the presence of MPO-ANCAs. While all female MRL-*lpr* mice studied developed anti-(ds)DNA antibodies by 12 weeks, only 22% developed IgG MPO-autoantibodies after 20 weeks. The observed anti-MPO autoantibodies caused a typical perinuclear ANCA staining pattern on ethanol-fixed human neutrophils (P-ANCAs). Unfortunately, it was not shown whether these

Table 1 Rodent Models of Vasculitis

Model designation	Proposed model for	Major insights gained
MRL/Mp-*lpr/lpr* mouse	Systemic lupus erythematosus; MPO-ANCA–associated vasculitis	Defect in T-cell apoptosis leads to autoimmune disease. Different autoantibodies may be associated with different disease phenotype. Infections modulate disease phenotype. Useful tool for therapeutic studies.
McH5-*lpr/lpr* mouse	Granulomatous arteritis	Disease phenotype is restricted by combination of background genes.
SCG/Kj mouse	MPO-ANCA–associated glomerulonephritis	Disease phenotype is restricted by combination of background genes. Genetic defect causing autoimmunity is confined to hematopoietic stem cell compartment.
HgCl$_2$-treated rodents	Autoimmune systemic necrotizing vasculitis	Mast cells involved in early vasculitis phase. Th2 cells instrumental for late phase vasculitis, while Th1 cells are protective. Infections modulate disease phenotype.
MPO-immunized BN rats	MPO-ANCA–associated glomerulonephritis and vasculitis	Anti-MPO alone do not cause disease. Anti-MPO modulate disease severity. Interaction of anti-MPO with target antigen may be required for effect. Location of disease manifestation is determined by location of anti-MPO/MPO interaction.
Autoantibody-immunized Balb/c mice	Variety of autoimmune disorders	Modulation of idiotypic network may contribute to disease development.
Lactobacillus casei–injected C57BL/6 mice	Kawasaki disease	Macrophages and intact complement system are required for this disease. Endothelial cells may play an active role in pathogenesis. Useful tool for therapeutic studies.
Herpesvirus infection of mice (CMV and γHV68)	Large-vessel vasculitis	Infections can induce vasculitic lesions. Inflammatory reaction is modulated by the presence of viral antigen. IFN-γ appears to protect the host from vasculitis. Suggests a link between infection, vascular inflammation and atherogenesis.
Human artery SCID mouse chimera	Human giant cell arteritis	Giant cell arteritis is an antigen-driven T cell–dependent disease. Ideal tool to study mechanism-based therapeutic strategies.

polyreactive autoantibodies also react with the murine homologue of MPO or murine neutrophils. Sixty percent of the anti-MPO–positive mice developed vasculitis, compared with only 18% of the anti-MPO–negative mice. The late phase vasculitis observed in association with anti-MPO autoantibodies was clearly distinct from the early phase immune complex–mediated disease of anti-MPO–negative animals. Anti-MPO–positive mice had a clear survival advantage in comparison with anti-MPO–negative littermates, of which most succumbed to a clinical syndrome consisting of severe lupus nephritis, pulmonary edema, and thrombosis.

The fact that only 60% of anti-MPO–positive mice developed vasculitis suggests that other additional cofactors are required for the development of disease. Indeed, vasculitic lesions were less severe in animals treated with ivermectin and teramycin, implying a disease-modifying role of infections.

Seven hybridomas secreting anti-MPO-IgG were isolated from two MRL-*lpr* mice. For one of these, reactivity with murine neutrophils and activated human neutrophils as well as conformational epitopes of human myeloperoxidase were demonstrated. The authors also refer to yet unpublished data indicating that vasculitis can be induced in cytokine-primed recipients of this monoclonal anti-MPO antibody. Such a transfer experiment would directly support the pathogenicity of MPO-ANCAs in vivo.

B. The McH5-*lpr/lpr* Mouse

Nose et al. (13) have demonstrated that the vasculitis of MRL-*lpr* mice can be genetically segregated from glomerulonephritis, arthritis, and sialadenitis, as well as from autoantibody production. A vasculitis-prone strain, designated McH5-*lpr/lpr* was established by rearranging the genetic background of MRL-*lpr* mice through hybridization with an autoimmune resistant strain of mice, C3H/HeJ-*lpr/lpr* (C3H-*lpr*) (13). They found that 94.4% of McH5-*lpr* mice developed a granulomatous arteritis predominantly involving the kidneys, but only 8.3% of these animals developed glomerulonephritis. This is in contrast to 86 and 98.2% of MRL-*lpr* mice developing vasculitis and glomerulonephritis, respectively. Lymphadenopathy and splenomegaly were equally severe in McH5-*lpr* mice as in MRL-*lpr* mice. Necrotizing small-vessel vasculitis with fibroid degeneration of vessel wall frequently seen in the salivary glands of MRL-*lpr* mice was not detected in McH5-*lpr* mice. Serum levels of anti-DNA and anti-MPO, but not of IgG rheumatoid factors, were significantly lower in McH5-*lpr* mice than in MRL-*lpr* mice. Therefore, autoantibodies, even though associated with the development of glomerulonephritis, may not be required for the development of the granulomatous vasculitis in this particular model (13). Furthermore, the appearance of systemic vasculitis in autoimmune disease as well as the predilection for specific organs appears restricted to a particular combination of background genes (13). Others have corroborated this interpretation using quantitative trait locus mapping studies. Using different strains of backcross mice with distinct clinical phenotypes, various Lpr modifier genes responsible for preferential development of vasculitis, autoantibody production, glomerulonephritis, and lymphoproliferation have been identified (14–17).

C. The SCG/Kj Mouse

Another derivative of the MRL-*lpr* mouse is the recombinant inbred SCG/Kj strain. It was established by Kinjoh and colleagues et al. (18) by selectively mating siblings of (BXSB × MRL/Mp *lpr/lpr*) F1 mice that had developed crescentic glomerulonephritis, and subsequent inbreeding of the progeny for 40 generations. These mice spontaneously develop crescentic glomerulonephritis, necrotizing vasculitis affecting predominantly small arteries and arterioles of spleen, stomach, heart, uterus and ovaries, as well as massive lymphoproliferation at age 4 to 6 weeks. This autoimmune disease leads to premature death in 50% of the mice by the median age of 16 weeks. The renal lesions include scant immune deposits, hypertrophy of the glomerular epithelium, fibrin depositions, and extraglomerular hemorrhage and cellular proliferation within the Bowman's space forming characteristic crescents. Hypergammaglobulinemia and autoantibodies including anti-MPO are also a prominent feature of the autoimmune response. The severity of the glomerular lesions and of the systemic vasculitis is associated with the titers of circulating anti-MPO (18). Because of this association and because the severity of the inflammatory renal lesion is thought to be out of proportion to the observed immune deposits, the SCG/Kj mice have been proposed as a model for MPO-ANCA–associated glomerulonephritis and vasculitis. However, it remains difficult to attribute the lesions solely to anti-MPO as the lesions could not be induced in nude mice by transfer of monoclonal anti-MPO producing hybridomas developed from SCG/Kj mice (19).

When SCG/Kj mice were engrafted with T-cell depleted bone marrow from allogeneic, MHC-compatible, autoimmune-resistent C3H/He donors, the median survival of the recipients was extended by 89% compared with controls and the development of renal lesions was prevented in 50% of the recipients (20). The authors concluded that the molecular genetic lesions responsible for the autoimmune pathology of SCG/Kj mice are confined to the hematopoietic stem cell compartment (20). The authors also documented that the development of the renal lesions could be delayed in SCG/Kj mice subjected to dietary calorie restriction (21).

III. INDUCTION OF VASCULITIS IN RODENTS BY EXPERIMENTAL MANIPULATION

A. Mercuric Chloride–Treated Rodents

Agents such as mercuric chloride ($HgCl_2$), D-penicillamine, or the gold salts can cause an autoimmune disease in certain strains of rats and mice by inducing T cell–dependent polyclonal B-cell activation. In Brown Norway rats, the syndrome resulting from $HgCl_2$ treatment is characterized by lymphoproliferation and hypergammaglobulinemia, with particularly elevated IgE levels, which is taken as an indirect measure of Th2-like cell activity. This autoimmune phenotype is associated with the presence of a variety of IgG autoantibodies, including antibodies against thyroid antigens, single- and double-stranded DNA, glomerular basement membrane (GBM) (78), myeloperoxidase (MPO) (22), and phospholipids (23). Mathieson et al. (24) described a characteristic and reproducible disease phenotype consisting of inflammation and ulceration of the skin at the mucocutaneous junctions, periportal inflammation of the liver, necrotizing leukocytoclastic vasculitis of the gut, and foci of alveolar hemorrhage in the lung, possibly caused by capillaritis.

A genetic predisposition of Brown Norway rats for this autoimmune response to $HgCl_2$ is supported by the observation that Lewis rats failed to develop a similar autoimmune response or comparable tissue lesions in parallel control experiments (24). A similar genetic predisposition for the development of a specific autoimmune response to polyclonal B-cell stimulation by $HgCl_2$ has also been documented in mice (25). B10.S mice are susceptible to develop a systemic autoimmune disorder, and preferentially activate their Th2 cells in response to $HgCl_2$ treatment, whereas B10.D2 mice are resistant to $HgCl_2$-induced systemic autoimmunity and react by preferentially activating their Th1 cells.

In analogy to Harper's observations in MRL-*lpr* mice, modulation of the disease phenotype by infection could be observed in $HgCl_2$-treated Brown Norway rats (12,24). The development of the tissue lesions, but not the autoantibody response, was ameliorated by pretreatment of the experimental animals with antimicrobial agents. This observation clearly indicates that environmental factors, such as infections, may represent essential cofactors for the development of vasculitic lesions in the presence of autoantibodies, which is consistent with clinical observations that link infections to the onset or reactivation of systemic vasculitis. Furthermore, it may explain why different laboratories find variations in disease phenotype as the spectrum of microbial infestation may vary from animal facility to animal facility.

This model has been used extensively to study cellular mechanisms involved in the development of vasculitic tissue lesions. CD8+ T cells are required for the resistance of experimental animals to rechallenge with $HgCl_2$ but not for the initial induction or subsequent spontaneous resolution of the immune response (26). Subsets of CD4+ T cells preferentially expressing the Th1-type cytokines IL-2 and interferon-γ (IFN-γ) (CD4+ CD45RC^{high}) have a protective effect on the development of the tissue lesions that is not associated with a reduction in autoantibody response (27). A dissociation of autoantibody response and tissue lesions was also seen in response to treatment with cyclosporin A (28). While early treatment with cyclosporin A ameliorated the tissue lesions and reduced the autoantibody response, the reduction in autoantibodies seen during late treatment with this drug was associated with an aggravation of tissue lesions. This suggests that anti-GBM and anti-MPO are not required for the development of the tissue lesions in this model. Whereas the late phase of the vasculitis appears Th2 cell–mediated, the speed of onset of tissue injury suggests that cells other than T cells may be involved in the primary induction of vasculitis (29). Indeed, mast cells appear to play a crucial role in the early phase of vasculitis, which is T-cell independent (30). Mast cells are a source for IL-4, which appears to be required for the differentiation of Th2 cells. Interleukin-4 gene expression was detected during the early phase of the disease in the tissue lesion (31), and $HgCl_2$ and other agents were found to directly induce IL-4 expression in mast cells from Brown Norway rats, but not from autoimmune resistant Lewis rats (32). Decomplementation studies using cobra venom factor have indicated that the complement system does not contribute significantly to the induction of autoantibodies or the effector phase of tissue injury (33).

This model has also been used to assess the pathogenic role of MPO-ANCAs. Esnault et al. (22) documented that $HgCl_2$-treated Brown Norway rats develop anti-MPO antibodies synchronously with anti-GBM antibodies. The autoantibody response is detectable after about 10 days of treatment, peaks at 12–15 days, and then resolves spontaneously. The anti-MPO autoimmune response appears independent of the anti-GBM autoimmune response. The rat anti-MPO antibodies recognized human MPO and apparently bind to similar determinants on the MPO heavy chain as human MPO-ANCAs but their cross-reactivity with rat MPO was not reported. No clear relation of the presence of anti-MPO antibodies to the disease phenotype was described even though the authors claim a higher mortality in animals with high titers of anti-MPO. A direct pathogenic role for MPO-ANCAs has not been demonstrated in this model as the disease could not be induced by transfer of serum from experimental animals with circulating antibodies to untreated animals (34). However, the authors were unable to detect anti-MPO antibodies in the recipient rats, rendering it uncertain whether the actual antibody transfer was successful.

The model of $HgCl_2$-induced vasculitis has several features resembling human systemic vasculitis, and it has provided important insights into the cellular mechanisms involved in the development of the tissue lesions. Nevertheless, the role of autoantibodies, particularly of anti-MPO, for the development of vasculitis in this model remains unclear. The polyclonal nature of the antibody response and the coexistence of many different types of antibodies make it difficult to establish any causality between specific antibodies and tissue lesions.

B. Immunization of Brown Norway Rats with Human MPO

Significant clarification of the pathogenic role of MPO-ANCAs has been obtained from a series of elegant studies performed in Brown Norway rats immunized with human MPO (35–41).

The model was originally developed by Brouwer et al. (35) to study pathomechanisms of ANCA-associated necrotizing crescentic glomerulonephritis. It is based on the immunization of Brown Norway rats with 10 µg of human MPO in complete Freund's adjuvant supplemented with 5 mg/ml H37Ra. Two weeks after immunization, the rats developed antibodies that reacted with human MPO and cross-reacted with rat MPO. The rats subsequently underwent unilateral perfusion of the left kidney with lysosomal extract containing MPO, but also PR3 and elastase, and with the substrate for MPO, hydrogen peroxide (H_2O_2). In contrast to control animals, which had been sham-immunized with adjuvant without MPO, the immunized animals developed a proliferative necrotizing crescentic glomerulonephritis closely resembling human disease in the perfused kidney, but not in the contralateral nonperfused kidney (35). Transient immune deposits containing IgG, complement, and MPO detectable 24 hours after perfusion were no longer detectable 4–10 days after perfusion.

This model for the first time provided evidence supporting a pathogenic role of MPO-ANCAs. Lesions did not develop in the absence of MPO-ANCAs. At the same time, these studies indicate that the presence of MPO-ANCAs alone is not sufficient to cause disease, as perfusion with neutrophil lysosomal extract solution and MPO substrate, H_2O_2, was required to develop the lesion. Whether the presence of lysosomal enzymes other than MPO in the perfusate is responsible for the degradation of the immune complexes observed after 24 hours and possibly also for the phenotype of the lesion, remains unclear.

In an attempt to reproduce Brouwer's experiments, Yang et al. (37) immunized Brown Norway rats and spontaneously hypertensive rats with 25 μg of MPO emulsified with TiterMax. They detected similar lesions in perfused kidneys and the lesions were more severe in the hypertensive rats suggesting that hypertension aggravates the lesion (37). However, immune complexes were detected in both strains of rats throughout day 10 after perfusion of the kidneys with MPO and H_2O_2 in the presence or absence of neutral proteases including proteinase 3 (PR3), elastase, and cathepsin G (37). The severity of the observed lesions was proportional to the degree of immune complex deposition, and the authors concluded that this model represents a model of immune complex–mediated rather than ANCA-associated pauci-immune glomerulonephritis (37). These conflicting findings may be the result of differences in immunization protocol or differences in lysosomal extract composition.

When neutrophil lysosomal enzyme extract was infused systemically into Brown Norway rats 2 weeks following immunization with human MPO, all rats developed perivascular mononuclear cell infiltrates, granulomatous inflammation with giant cells, and fibrous tissue deposits in the lungs, as well as a segmental small-vessel vasculitis of the gut (39). Interestingly, other organs, including the kidneys, were not affected by this approach. When single lungs were perfused selectively, the described lesions were limited to the perfused lung (41). These findings suggest that the site of the lesion is determined by the localization of the interaction of MPO-ANCA with its target antigen and possibly the effect of other neutrophil lysosomal enzymes.

The pathogenic role of MPO-ANCAs is further supported by their ability to aggravate subclinical antiglomerular basement membrane (anti-GBM) disease (38) and nephrotoxic serum nephritis in rats (42). These observations are of particular interest because about 30% of patients with anti-GBM autoantibodies also have detectable ANCAs (43). At least those patients with PR3-ANCAs and those with high titers of MPO-ANCAs have all had clinical features of systemic vasculitis in addition to anti-GBM–mediated glomerulonephritis (44–46).

When Brown Norway rats immunized with human MPO were given subnephritogenic doses of rabbit anti-rat GBM, the animals developed severe glomerulonephritis characterized by early onset of severe hematuria, marked proteinuria, and massive glomerular fibrin deposition. Crescent formation and fibrinoid necrosis of capillary loops, significant interstitial mononuclear cell infiltration, tubular necrosis, and atrophy were also detected on day 10 after application (38). In contrast, control-immunized rats given the same dose of anti-rat GBM developed only slight proteinuria and moderate intraglomerular accumulation of macrophages. While these experiments clearly indicate that MPO-ANCAs enhance renal injury, the mechanisms underlying this effect remain speculative. It is possible that anti-GBM/GBM immune complexes as well as MPO-ANCAs may cause neutrophil degranulation with MPO release and binding to negatively charged structures, such as GBM and endothelial cells. Released neutrophil enzymes and reactive oxygen metabolites resulting from the reaction of active MPO with H_2O_2 and halides could cause acute glomerular injury. The focal deposition of MPO/anti-MPO immune complexes is also thought to enhance the recruitment of inflammatory cells with subsequent further production of oxygen radicals and release of proteases. Finally, as suggested by in vitro experiments (47–49), it is possible that circulating anti-MPO increase cytokine synthesis by monocytes and neutrophils, and, thereby, contribute to further recruitment of inflammatory cells to the site of injury.

Using a different system, Kobayashi et al. (42) made observations that seem to corroborate Heeringa's findings. Wistar rats were given rabbit anti-rat MPO or normal rabbit serum in addition to doses of rabbit anti-rat GBM that only induce mild glomerulonephritis by themselves. Rats given rabbit anti-rat MPO and rabbit anti-rat GBM developed a significantly more pronounced glomerular neutrophil influx, fibrin deposition, and proteinuria. Rat MPO could be detected in the glomeruli and anti-rat MPO was eluted from the kidneys, suggesting that the localized interaction of MPO and anti-MPO in the glomeruli may play a significant pathogenic role for the observed enhancement of the glomerular lesion. While these findings seem to support a pathogenic role for anti-MPO and appear to corroborate the notion that local MPO/anti-MPO interactions are instrumental for the observed effects, the significance of the latter model for human ANCA-associated vasculitis remains questionable because of the use of heterologous antisera.

Heeringa et al. (40) have subsequently applied their model to evaluate the role of nitric oxide (NO) radicals as potential mediators of anti-MPO–associated glomerulonephritis. Elevated nitrite and nitrate levels were detected in the urine of experimental animals, indicating enhanced generation of NO. As early as 24 hours after kidney perfusion with neutrophil lysosomal extract and H_2O_2, endothelial NO synthase (eNOS) was markedly reduced as a result of endothelial cell necrosis. Prominent platelet aggregation was also apparent, which is consistent with the beneficial effects eNOS is thought to exert during inflammation by inhibiting platelet aggregation and neutrophil adhesion to the endothelium. Infiltrating neutrophils and monocytes in the glomeruli of perfused kidneys displayed strong expression of inducible NO synthase (iNOS) transiently with a peak at 4 days after kidney perfusion. These findings suggest that during anti-MPO–associated glomerulonephritis, loss of protective NO production by eNOS and increased NO radical production by iNOS contribute to tissue injury. Excessive NO production has also been implicated in the effector phase of tissue injury in the $HgCl_2$-treated Brown Norway rats (50). Specific inhibition of NO synthesis reduced the severity of tissue lesions substantially, but it did not affect the observed neutrophil infiltration or the original autoimmune response (50).

C. Immunization of Mice with Human Autoantibodies

Shoenfeld and coworkers have proposed murine models to investigate the role of autoantibodies in the pathogenesis of vasculitis that are based on idiotypic manipulation of naive animals. This concept has been applied to the study of antiphospholipid antibodies (51), anti-DNA antibodies (52), ANCAs (53,54), and antiendothelial cell antibodies (AECAs) (55). Mice are immunized with affinity-purified human IgG autoantibody (Ab1, idiotype (Id)). These animals develop an anti-Id (Ab2), and after 2–6 months a proportion of animals develops an anti-anti-Id (Ab3) with identical binding characteristics to that of Ab1. Animals with these antibodies develop histopathological abnormalities that resemble autoimmune disease in humans.

The idiotypic manipulation of mice with human PR3-ANCAs and AECAs are of particular interest with respect to the pathogenesis of small-vessel vasculitis (53–55). Mice immunized with an ANCA-enriched affinity-purified IgG fraction of sera from patients with active Wegener's granulomatosis containing PR3-specific antibodies developed mouse anti-human ANCAs (Ab2) with peak titers occurring about 1 month after booster injection. Murine antibodies displaying reactivity with human PR3 (Ab 3) reached peak levels at 4 months. The reported histopathological changes observed in mice immunized with c-ANCA IgG is quite intriguing. In a first experiment, all mice died between 8–15 months from sterile pulmonary abscesses. However, in the second experiment with c-ANCAs from a different patient, mice became ill at 8 months and displayed dense perivascular lymphocytic infiltrates suggestive of vasculitis. The mice also developed proteinuria and diffuse granular immune deposits in the glomeruli in the absence of light microscopic evidence of histopathological changes in the kidneys (53).

While the mice immunized with c-ANCA did not develop antibodies to dsDNA, cardiolipin, histones, or pyruvate dehydrogenase, they did develop antibodies reacting with human MPO (54), as well as high titers of AECAs (53). The contributory role of these antibodies for the development of the described tissue lesions remains unclear.

The authors proposed this model of idiotypic manipulation with PR3-ANCAs as a model for Wegener's granulomatosis (53) and concluded that it indicates a likely pathogenic role of ANCAs in vasculitis (54). However, these conclusions are rather controversial. The reproducibility of the tissue lesions remains unclear (53,56). The lack of granuloma formation and giant cells (54) as well as the presence of significant immune deposits in the kidneys of mice immunized with PR3-ANCAs (53) are not in line with the characteristic Wegener's granulomatosis lesions (57). Furthermore, a possible human PR3 contamination of the human c-ANCA preparation used as the original immunogen cannot be excluded with certainty (56). Finally, the most significant question about the validity of the model is raised by the fact that human PR3-ANCAs do not cross-react with the murine PR3 homologue (58), which may explain why murine PR3 has eluded detection for a long time (56,59,60).

A subsequent study from the same investigators demonstrated that AECAs may be the principal antibody species responsible for the histopathological changes observed in response to immunization of naive mice with IgG fractions of sera from patients with active Wegener's granulomatosis (55). AECA-enriched IgG fractions were prepared from anti-PR3–positive total plasma IgG of patients with active Wegener's granulomatosis by depletion of anti-PR3 reactivity by absorption using purified human PR3. The resulting preparation was PR3-ANCA– and MPO-ANCA–negative. Four months after immunization of BALB/c mice with this preparation, 3 of 10 animals developed significant titers of murine AECAs (Ab 3). Sera of these mice lacked reactivity with human cardiolipin, DNA, PR3, and MPO. Only the animals with a murine AECA response developed perivascular lymphocytic infiltration in lungs and kidneys, similar to the perivascular infiltrate observed in the lungs of mice immunized with human c-ANCAs (53,55). Furthermore, IgG deposits in the vascular walls of the kidneys were detected. The authors conclude that these data provide the first direct evidence for the pathogenicity of AECAs (55). The factors rendering the majority of the animals resistant to antibody production and tissue injury remain unexplained.

These reports indicate that activation of the idiotypic network may induce pathogenic autoantibodies that may influence the phenotype of histopathological lesions. However, to what degree these pathways contribute to the onset or phenotypic modulation of disease remains unknown until the putative primary target antigens for specific autoantibodies (pathogenic idiotypes expressed on environmental antigens, i.e., infectious agents) are identified.

D. *Lactobacillus casei* Injection into C57BL/6 Mice

A murine model of Kawasaki disease has been described resulting from a single intraperitoneal injection of an aqueous suspension of *Lactobacillus casei* cell wall fragments into C57BL/6 mice (61). The animals display a coronary vasculitis with prominent endothelial cell proliferation, stenosis/thrombosis, and aneurysm formation bearing striking similarity with the human disease.

It was shown that macrophage function and an intact complement system are required for the development of the lesions, whereas the role of T cells remains unclear. The prominent endothelial and mural proliferation encountered in both the animal model and the human disease suggests that endothelial cells may play an active role in the pathogenesis. With this rationale, the model was used most recently to assess the efficacy of a novel angiogenesis inhibitor, AGM-1470 (62). The incidence of coronaritis was reduced from 100% of untreated control animals to 30% of animals treated with AGM-1470. Histological severity scores were also much higher in control animals than in the 30% of treated animals that developed vasculitis. These findings provide further support for a significant pathogenic role of vascular cells in Kawasaki disease. This study is exemplary for the use of animal models to study novel agents, both to assess their therapeutic potential and to gain additional insights into cellular mechanisms contributing to the development of end-organ damage.

E. Infection of Mice with Herpesviruses

Several of the animal models described above indirectly imply a disease-modifying role of infections. More direct evidence for the ability of infectious agents to induce vasculitic lesions comes from murine models of herpesvirus infection–mediated vasculitis.

In an effort to further evaluate the pathogenesis of atherosclerotic lesions, Dangler et al. (63) infected BALB/c and C57BL/6 mice with murine cytomegalovirus (CMV). When suckling mice were inoculated at 9 days of age, almost all animals of both strains developed inflammatory lesions of the ascending aorta and pulmonary artery at 8 weeks postinoculation (63). Inflammatory infiltrates of the adventitia and tunica media contained predominantly CD3+, CD4+, and CD8+ lymphocytes. Infiltrates of the intima contained more macrophages (63). The development of inflammatory lesions was independent of an atherogenic diet, but the diet-related arterial lipid accumulation was clearly more severe in infected animals compared with noninfected controls (63).

Berencsi et al. (64) infected irradiated adult BALB/c mice with murine CMV, and were able to induce similar vascular lesions. In contrast, RAG-1–/–mice lacking all functional T and B lymphocytes did not develop any vascular lesions in response to murine CMV infection, indicating that the inflammatory vascular lesions are T and B cell-dependent (64). Presti et al. (65) demonstrated that IFN-γ regulates chronic infection with murine CMV. Within 28–56 days after infection, aortic lesions affecting all layers developed in 5 of 6 interferon-γ receptor–deficient (IFN-γR–/–) mice and in 4 of 10 congenic wild-type control mice. However, within 84 days after inoculation, the aortic lesions had cleared in the wild-type mice, whereas they persisted as long as 154 days in IFN-γR–/– mice. Cytomegalic inclusion bodies and murine CMV antigens were detected in the media of the affected aortas. These data indicate that the lack of IFN-γ responsiveness results in chronic inflammatory lesions of the large elastic arteries, possibly by permitting viral reactivation from latency (65). Arteritic lesions were not detected in IFN-γR–/– mice infected with herpes simplex virus or reovirus serotype 3 8B, suggesting a host response specific to murine CMV infection (65).

Murine models of CMV infection allowing the detailed study of immune mechanisms are of particular relevance because CMV has been implicated in a variety of vascular lesions, including atherosclerosis, abdominal aortic aneurysms, rapidly progressive coronary artery disease, endothelialitis in cardiac transplant patients, and restenosis after coronary angioplasty, and because reactivation of human CMV causes significant morbidity and mortality in immunocompromised hosts.

Mice infected with γ-herpesvirus 68 (γHV68) also develop inflammatory lesions in large vessels (66). Normal 129 or C57BL/6 mice only developed arteritis lesions with detectable γHV68 antigen if infected as weanlings, but not if infected as adults (66). B cell–deficient mice and MHC class II–deficient mice infected as adults developed a mild, predominantly adventitial inflammatory response (66). The most prominent large-vessel vasculitis was induced in IFN-γR–/– and in IFN-γ–/– (66). Mice dying within 1.5–14 weeks after infection displayed severe large-vessel arteritis with narrowing of the aortic lumen by inflammation and thrombus. Surviving infected IFN-γ nonresponsive mice lacked arteritic lesions. Lesions were restricted to the large elastic arteries. All layers of the vessel wall were involved. Inflammatory infiltrates of the adventitia and intima were predominantly mononuclear, whereas neutrophils were present in the media. Viral antigen was detectable in arteritic lesions and correlated well with regions of inflammation within observed skip lesions. Viral antigen was largely restricted to the media and colocalized with smooth muscle cells, suggesting specific tissue tropism. Interestingly, lipid accumulation was detected within arteritic lesions, particularly in the region surrounding the damaged media, irrespective of dietary fat content (66).

Both the murine CMV and γHV68 infection models indicate that IFN-γ has a substantial protective effect against virus-induced chronic vascular damage. Both models are also of interest because they establish and allow further studies of the link between inflammatory lesions of vessels (i.e., vasculitis) and atherogenesis. A link between infections, inflammatory vascular lesions, and atherogenesis has also been suggested by observations derived from rabbit models of *Chlamydia pneumoniae* infection (67,68), from pigs infected with the porcine reproductive and respiratory syndrome virus, a porcine RNA virus (69–71), and from chicken with Marek's disease, an α-herpesvirus–associated vasculitic process with features of atherosclerosis (72).

IV. THE SEVERE COMBINED IMMUNODEFICIENCY MOUSE AS TOOL FOR IN VIVO STUDY OF HUMAN GIANT CELL ARTERITIS

Severe combined immunodeficiency (SCID) mice have defects in humoral and cell-mediated immunity that allow for xenogeneic transplantation without risk of rejection by the recipient animal (73,74). This property was used by Brack et al. (75–77) to develop a very elegant model system for the in vivo study of pathomechanisms and therapeutic strategies in human giant cell arteritis (GCA). Diseased human artery segments obtained from patients with active GCA are implanted subcutaneously into SCID mice (75). The inflammation persists in these xenotransplants for at least 6 weeks, indicating that the implants represent independent functional units, which do not require the influx of cells, mediators, or antigens from the circulation of the host. This model provided convincing evidence that GCA is an antigen-driven T cell–dependent disease in which the activation of tissue-infiltrating T cells and macrophages depends on an infrequent subpopulation of lesional T cells recognizing a locally expressed antigen (75). Interleukin-2 and IFN-γ producing T cells were enriched in the implants, and a narrowing of the T cell receptor repertoire was noted 4 weeks after implantation. Identical T cell receptors were identified in different animals engrafted with artery segments from the same patients. Taken together, these findings suggest that the lesional T cells recognize an antigen that resides within the tissue lesion. When T cell–depleting antiserum was applied to the animals, a reduction of IFN-γ mRNA expression followed by a reduction of IL-1β mRNA expression was observed in the lesions. Adoptive transfer of autologous tissue-derived, but not of peripheral blood T cells amplified IL-2 and IFN-γ mRNA expression in the engrafted temporal artery tissue. These findings underscore the disease relevance of the tissue infiltrating T cells.

This model was subsequently used to study the mechanisms of action of glucocorticoids in vivo (76). One week after administration of dexamethasone to GCA-SCID chimeras a reduction of mRNA expression of IL-2, IL-1β, and IL-6, as well as of inducible NO synthase expression in the tissue lesions was detected. Interferon-γ mRNA expression was only slightly decreased and TGF-β1 mRNA expression was not affected by glucocorticoid treatment. The pattern of "steroid responsive" and "steroid resistant" cytokines suggested an involvement of the NFκB pathway. Subsequent experiments showed that corticosteroid injection caused an induction of the IκBα gene and blocked the nuclear translocation of NFκB in the arterial lesions. When glucocorticoids were applied chronically for 4 weeks, T-cell function was paralyzed as indicated by abolishment of IFN-γ mRNA expression. However, TGF-β1 mRNA expression by tissue macrophages remained unaffected. The latter may provide an explanation for the chronicity of the human disease. This series of experiments would also suggest that in the early phase of the disease patients might benefit from higher doses of glucocorticoids than those currently used (76). Most recently, Rittner et al. (77) have used the model to study free oxygen radical release by macrophages and resulting lipid peroxidation as an important component of tissue damage in GCA. The described experiments clearly identify aldose reductase as an oxidative defense system protecting the tissue from cytopathic effects of lipid peroxidation and, thereby, as a potential novel target for therapeutic intervention (77).

V. SUMMARY

The spontaneous models of vasculitis have clarified that genetic determinants predispose to autoimmunity and vasculitis, and that the development of a specific phenotype with characteristic organ involvement or histopathological features is restricted to a particular combination of background genes. It has also become apparent that cofactors, such as infections, play a significant disease-modifying role. Spontaneous as well as induced vasculitis models have provided evidence for a pathogenic role of MPO-ANCAs. Particularly those models in which anti-MPO are the only important variable have clarified that anti-MPO may directly contribute to the development of vasculitis and glomerulonephritis, that the interaction of anti-MPO with neutrophil lysosomal enzymes including MPO, and possibly its substrate, H_2O_2, is required for the development of lesions, and, finally, that the localization of the lesion is determined by the site of this interaction. Models of infection-mediated vasculitis combined with specific gene "knockout" mice appear to be reproducible tools for the study of pathogenic interactions of infectious organisms with selected components of the host immune system causing inflammatory lesions of vessels. In addition, the SCID mouse represents a very useful tool for the in vivo study of pathogenic mechanisms operative in human vasculitic lesions. Several of these proposed models of vasculitis appear very promising for the evaluation of novel therapeutic modalities, including mechanism-based immune modulation, the use of angiostatins, or gene therapy.

REFERENCES

1. Hunder GG, Arend WP, Bloch DA, et al. The American College of Rheumatology 1990 criteria for the classification of vasculitis: Introduction. Arthritis Rheum 1990; 33:1101–1107.
2. Leavitt RY, Fauci AS, Bloch DA, et al. The American College of Rheumatology 1990 criteria for the classification of Wegener's granulomatosis. Arthritis Rheum 1990; 33:1101–1107.
3. Masi AT, Hunder GG, Lie JT, et al. The American College of Rheumatology 1990 criteria for the classification of Churg-Strauss syndrome (allergic granulomatosis and angiitis). Arthritis Rheum 1990; 33:1094–1100.
4. Jennette JC, Falk RJ, Andrassy K, et al. Nomenclature of systemic vasculitides: The proposal of an international consensus conference. Arthritis Rheum 1994; 37:187–192.
5. Watanabe-Fukunaga R, Brannann CI, Copeland NG, Jenkins NA, Nagata S. Lymphoproliferation disorder in mice explained by defects in Fas antigen that mediates apoptosis. Nature 1992; 356:314–317.

6. Mountz JD, Zhou T, Buethmann H, Wu J, Edwards CK, III. Apoptosis defects analyzed in TcR transgenic and fas transgenic lpr mice. Intern Rev Immunol 1994; 11:321–342.

7. Rose LM, Latchman DS, Isenberg DA. Elevated soluble fas production in SLE correlates with HLA status not with disease activity. Lupus 1997; 6:717–722.

8. Mysler E, Bini P, Drappa J, et al. The apoptosis-1/Fas protein in human systemic lupus erythematosus. J Clin Invest 1994; 93:1029–1034.

9. Huggins ML, Huang F-P, Xu D, Lindop G, Stott DI. Modulation of autoimmune disease in the MRL-lpr/lpr mouse by IL-2 and TGF-b1 gene therapy using attenuated Salmonella typhimurium as gene carrier. Lupus 1999; 8:29–38.

10. Raz E, Dudler J, Lotz M, et al. Modulation of disease activity in murine systemic erythematosus by cytokine gene delivery. Lupus 1995; 4:286–292.

11. Gutierrez-Ramos JC, Andreu JL, Revilla Y, Vinuela E, Martinez C. Recovery from autoimmunity of MRL/lpr mice after infection with an interleukin-2/vaccinia recombinant virus. Nature 1990; 346: 271–274.

12. Harper JM, Thiru S, Lockwood CM, Cooke A. Myeloperoxidase autoantibodies distinguish vasculitis mediated by anti-neutrophil cytoplasm antibodies from immune complex disease in MRL/Mp-lpr/lpr mice: a spontaneous model for human microscopic angiitis. Eur J Immunol 1998; 28:2217–2226.

13. Nose M, Nishimura M, Ito MR, Itoh J, Shibata T, Sugisaki T. Arteritis in a novel congenic strain of mice derived from MRL/lpr lupus mice. Am J Path 1996; 149:1763–1769.

14. Watson ML, Rao JK, Gilkeson GS, et al. Genetic analysis of MRL-lpr mice: Relationship of the Fas apoptosis gene to disease manifestations and renal disease-modifying loci. J Exp Med 1992; 176: 1645–1656.

15. Wang Y, Nose M, Kamoto T, Nishimura M, Hiai H. Host modifier genes affect mouse autoimmunity induced by the lpr gene. Am J Pathol 1997; 151:1791–1798.

16. Vidal S, Kono DH, Theofilopoulos AN. Loci predisposing to autoimmunity in MRL-Fas lpr mice. J Clin Invest 1998; 101:696–702.

17. Gu L, Weinreb A, Wang XP, et al. Genetic determinants of autoimmune disease and coronary vasculitis in the MRL-1pr/1pr mouse model of systemic lupus erythematosus. J Immunol 1998; 161:6999–7006.

18. Kinjoh K, Kyogoku M, Good RA. Genetic selection for crescent formation yields mouse strain with rapidly progressive glomerulonephritis and small vessel vasculitis. Proc Natl Acad Sci USA 1993; 90: 3413–3417.

19. Kinjoh K, Good RA, Taylor J, Nachman P, Falk RJ, Jennette JC. Hybridomas from SCG/Kj mice produce P-ANCA with specificity for myeloperoxidase (MPO) and induce proteinuria in nude mice (abstract). Clin Exp Immunol 1995; 101(suppl 1):37.

20. Cherry NN, Engelman RW, Wang BY, Kinjoh K, El-Badri NS, Good RA. Prevention of crescentic glomerulonephritis in SCG/Kj mice by bone marrow transplantation. Proc Soc Exp Biol Med 1998; 218:223–228.

21. Cherry NN, Engelman RW, Wang BY, Kinjoh K, El-Badri NS, Good RA. Calorie restriction delays the crescentic glomerulonephritis of SCG/Kj mice. Proc Soc Exp Biol Med 1998; 218:218–222.

22. Esnault VLM, Mathieson PW, Thiru S, Oliveira DBG, Martin-Lockwood C. Autoantibodies to myeloperoxidase in brown Norway rats treated with mercuric chloride. Lab Invest 1992; 67:114–120.

23. Marriott JB, Qasim F, Oliveira DBG. Anti-phospholipid antibodies in the mercuric chloride treated Brown Norway rat. J Autoimmun 1994; 7:457–467.

24. Mathieson PW, Thiru S, G. ODB. Mercuric chloride-treated brown Norway rats develop widespread tissue injury including necrotizing vasculitis. Lab Invest 1992; 67:121–129.

25. Doth M, Fricke M, Nicoletti F, Garotta G, Van Velthuysen M-L, Bruijn JA. Genetic differences in immune reactivity to mercuric chloride ($HgCl_2$): Immunosuppression of $H-2^d$ mice is mediated by interferon-gamma ($IFN-\gamma$). 1997.

26. Mathieson PW, Stapleton KJ, Oliveira DBG, Lockwood CM. Immunoregulation of mercuric chloride-induced autoimmunity in Brown Norway rats: A role for $CD8^+$ T cells revealed by in vivo depletion studies. Eur J Immunol 1991; 21:2105–2109.

27. Mathieson PW, Thiru S, Oliveria DBG. Regulatory role of $OX22^{high}$ T cells in mercury-induced autoimmunity in the Brown Norway rat. J Exp Med 1993; 177:1309–1316.

28. Qasim FJ, Mathieson PW, Thiru S, Oliveira DB. Cyclosporin A exacerbates mercuric chloride-induced vasculitis in the Brown Norway rat. Lab Invest 1995; 72:183–190.

29. Qasim FJ, Thiru S, Mathieson PW, Oliveira DBG. The time course and characterization of mercuric chloride-induced immunopathology in the Brown Norway rat. J Autoimmun 1995; 8:193–208.

30. Kiely PDW, Pecht I, Oliveira DBG. Mercuric chloride-induced vasculitis in the Brown Norway rat: αβ T cell-dependent and -independent phases. J Immunol 1997; 159:5100–5106.

31. Gillespie KM, Qasim FJ, Tibbatts LM, Thiru S, Oliveira DBG. Interleukin-4 gene expression in mercury-induced autoimmunity. Scand J Immunol 1995; 41:268–272.

32. Oliveira DBG, Gillespie K, Wolfreys K, Mathieson PW, Qasim F, Coleman JW. Compounds that induce autoimmunity in the Brown Norway rat sensitize mat cells for mediator release and interleukin-4 expression. Eur J Immunol 1995; 25:2259–2264.

33. Mathieson PW, Qasim FJ, Thiru S, Oldroyd RG, Oliveira DBG. Effects of decomplementation with cobra venom factor on experimental vasculitis. Clin Exp Immunol 1994; 97:474–477.

34. Qasim FJ, Mathieson PW, Thiru S, Oliveira DB, Lockwood CM. Further characterization of an animal model of systemic vasculitis. Adv Exp Med Biol 1993; 336:133–137.

35. Brouwer E, Huitema MG, Klok PA, et al. Anti-myeloperoxidase associated proliferative glomerulonephritis: An animal model. J Exp Med 1993; 177:905–914.

36. Brouwer E, Klok PA, Huitema MG, Weening JJ, Kallenberg CGM. Renal ischemia/reperfusion injury contributes to renal damage in experimental anti-myeloperoxidase-associated proliferative glomerulonephritis. Kidney Int 1995; 47:1121–1129.

37. Yang JJ, Jennette JC, Falk RJ. Immune complex glomerulonephritis is induced in rats immunized with heterologous myeloperoxidase. Clin Exp Immunol 1994; 97:466–473.

38. Heeringa P, Brouwer E, Klok PA, et al. Autoantibodies to myeloperoxidase aggravate mild anti-glomerular-basement-membrane mediated glomerular injury. Am J Pathol 1996; 149:1695–1706.

39. Heeringa P, Foucher P, Klok PA, et al. Systemic injection of products of activated neutrophils and H_2O_2 in myeloperoxidase-immunized rats leads to necrotizing vasculitis in the lungs and gut. Am J Pathol 1997; 151:131–139.

40. Heeringa P, van Goor H, Moshage H, et al. Expression of iNOS, eNos, and peroxynitrite-modified proteins in experimental anti-meyloperoxidase associated crescentic glomerulonephritis. Kidney Int 1998; 53.

41. Foucher P, Heeringa P, Petersen AH, et al. Antimyeloperoxidase-associated lung disease. An experimental model. Am J Respir Crit Care Med 1999; 160:987–994.

42. Kobayashi K, Shibata T, Sugisaki S. Aggravation of rat nephrotoxic serum nephritis by anti-myeloperoxidase antibodies. Kidney Int 1995; 47:454–463.

43. Short AK, Esnault VLM, Lockwood CM. Anti-neutrophil cytoplasm antibodies and anti-glomerular basement membrane antibodies: Two coexisting distinct autoreactivities detectable in patients with rapidly progressive glomerulonephritis. Am J Kidney Dis 1995; 26:439–445.

44. Jayne DRW, Marshall PD, Jones SJ, Lockwood CM. Autoantibodies to GBM and neutrophil cytoplasm in rapidly progressive glomerulonephritis. Kindey Intern 1990; 37:956–970.

45. Bosch X, Mirapeix E, Font J, et al. Prognostic implication of anti-neutrophil cytoplasmic autoantibodies with myeloperoxidase specificity in anti-glomerular basement membrane disease. Clin Neph 1991; 36:107–113.

46. Bygren P, Rasmussen N, Isaksson B, Wieslander J. Anti-neutrophil cytoplasm antibodies, anti-GBM antibodies and anti-dsDNA antibodies in glomerulonephritis. Eur J Clin Invest 1992; 22:783–792.

47. Brooks CJ, King WJ, Radford DJ, Adu D, McGrath M, Savage COS. IL-1b production by human polymorphonuclear leucocytes stimulated by anti-neutrophil cytoplasmic autoantibodies: relevance to systemic vasculitis. Clin Exp Immunol 1996; 106:273–279.

48. Casselman BL, Kilgore KS, Miller BF, Warren JS. Antibodies to neutrophil cytoplasmic antigens induce monocyte chemoattractant protein-1 secretion from human monocytes. J Lab Clin Med 1995; 126:495–502.

49. Ralston DR, Marsh CB, Lowe MP, Wewers MD. Antineutrophil cytoplasmic antibodies induce monocyte IL-8 release. Role of surface proteinase-3, α1-antitrypsin, and Fcγ receptors. J Clin Invest 1997; 100:1416–1424.

50. Woolfson RG, Qasim FJ, Thiru S, Oliveira DBG, Neild GH, Mathieson PW. Nitric oxide contributes to tissue injury in mercuric chloride-induced autoimmunity. Biochem Biophys Res Comm 1995; 217:515–521.

51. Bakimer R, Fishman P, Blank M, Sredni B, Djaldetti M, Shoenfeld Y. Induction of primary antiphospholipid syndrome in mice by immunization with human monoclonal anti-cardiolipin antibody (H-3). J Clin Invest 1992; 89:1558–1563.

52. Mendlovic S, Brocke S, Ben-Basat M, et al. Induction of an SLE-like disease in mice by a common anti-DNA idiotype. Proc Natl Acad Sci USA 1988; 85:2260–2264.

53. Blank M, Tomer Y, Stein M, et al. Immunization with anti-neutrophil cytoplasmic antibody (ANCA) induces the production of mouse ANCA and perivascular lymphocyte infiltration. Clin Exp Immunol 1995; 102:120–130.

54. Tomer Y, Gilburd B, Blank M, et al. Characterization of biologically active antineutrophil cytoplasmic antibodies induced in mice. Pathogenetic role in experimental vasculitis. Arthritis Rheum 1995; 38: 1375–1381.

55. Damianovich M, Gilburd B, George J, et al. Pathogenic role of anti-endothelial cell antibodies in vasculitis. J Immunol 1996; 156:4946–4951.

56. Béliveau A, Dagenais P, Ménard HA. Finding a valid model for antineutrophil cytoplasmic antibody-related vasculitis: Comment on the article by Tomer et al. and the letter by Langford and Sneller. Arthritis Rheum 1997; 40:986–990.

57. Langford CA, Sneller MC. Finding a valid model for human Wegener's granulomatosis: Comment on the article by Tomer et al. Arthritis Rheum 1996; 39:1262–1266.

58. Jenne DE, Fröhlich L, Hummel AM, Specks U. Cloning and functional expression of the murine homologue of proteinase 3: Implications for the design of murine models of vasculitis. FEBS Lett 1997; 408:187–190.

59. Goldschmeding R, Cohen-Tervaert JW, Gans ROB, et al. Different immunological specificities and disease associations of c-ANCA and p-ANCA. Neth J Med 1990; 36:114–116.

60. Lucena-Fernandez F, Dalpé G, Dagenais P, et al. Detection of anti-neutrophil cytoplasmic antibodies by immunoprecipitation. Clin Invest Med 1995; 18:153–162.

61. Lehman TJA, Walker SM, Mahnovski V, McCurdy D. Coronary arteritis in mice following the systemic injection of group B Lactobacillus casei cell walls in aqueous suspension. Arthritis Rheum 1985; 28:652–659.

62. Brahn E, Lehman TJA, Peacock DJ, Tang C, Banquerigo ML. Suppression of coronary vasculitis in a murine model of Kawasaki disease using an angiogenesis inhibitor. J Appl Biomater 1999; 90:147–151.

63. Dangler CA, Baker SE, Kariuki Njenga M, Chia SH. Murine cytomegalovirus-associated arteritis. Vet Pathol 1995; 32:127–33.

64. Berencsi K, Endresz V, Klurfeld D, Kari L, Kritchevsky D, Gonczol E. Early atherosclerotic plaques in the aorta following cytomegalovirus infection of mice. Cell Adhes Commun 1998; 5:39–47.

65. Presti RM, Pollock JL, Dal Canto AJ, O'Guin AK, Virgin HW. Interferon gamma regulates acute and latent murine cytomegalovirus infection and chronic disease of the great vessels. J Exp Med 1998; 188:577–88.

66. Weck KE, Dal Canto AJ, Gould JD, et al. Murine gamma-herpesvirus 68 causes severe large-vessel arteritis in mice lacking interferon-gamma responsiveness: a new model for virus-induced vascular disease [see comments]. Nat Med 1997; 3:1346–53.

67. Fong IW, Chiu B, Viira E, Fong MW, Jang D, Mahony J. Rabbit model for Chlamydia pneumoniae infection. J Clin Microbiol 1997; 35:48–52.

68. Laitinen K, Laurila A, Pyhala L, Leinonen M, Saikku P. Chlamydia pneumoniae infection induces inflammatory changes in the aortas of rabbits. Infect Immun 1997; 65:4832–5.

69. Thibault S, Drolet R, Germain MC, D'Allaire S, Larochelle R, Magar R. Cutaneous and systemic necrotizing vasculitis in swine. Vet Pathol 1998; 35:108–16.

70. Rossow KD, Collins JE, Goyal SM, Nelson EA, Christopher-Hennings J, Benfield DA. Pathogenesis of porcine reproductive and respiratory syndrome virus infection in gnotobiotic pigs. Vet Pathol 1995; 32:361–73.

71. Cooper VL, Hesse RA, Doster AR. Renal lesions associated with experimental porcine reproductive and respiratory syndrome virus (PRRSV) infection. J Vet Diagn Invest 1997; 9:198–201.

72. Fabricant CG. Atherosclerosis: The consequence of infection with a herpesvirus. Adv Vet Sci Comp Med 1985; 30:39–66.

73. McCune JM, Namikawa R, Kaneshima H, Shultz LD, Lieberman M, Weissman IL. The SCID-hu mouse: Murine model for the analysis of human hematolymphoid differentiation and function. Science 1988; 241:1632–9.

74. Reddy S, Piccione D, Takita H, Bankert RB. Human lung tumor growth established in the lung and subcutaneous tissue of mice with severe combined immunodeficiency. Cancer Res 1987; 47:2456–60.

75. Brack A, Geisler A, Martinez-Taboada VM, Younge BR, Goronzy JJ, Weyand CM. Giant cell vasculitis is a T cell-dependent disease. Mol Med 1997; 3:530–43.

76. Brack A, Rittner HL, Younge BR, Kaltschmidt C, Weyand CM, Goronzy JJ. Glucocorticoid-mediated repression of cytokine gene transcription in human arteritis-SCID chimeras. J Clin Invest 1997; 99: 2842–50.

77. Rittner HL, Hafner V, Klimiuk PA, Szweda LI, Goronzy JJ, Weyand CM. Aldose reductase functions as a detoxification system for lipid peroxidation products in vasculitis. J Clin Invest 1999; 103: 1007–13.

78. Pusey CD, Bowman C, Morgan A, Weetman AP, Hartley B, Lockwood CM. Kinetics and pathogenicity of autoantibodies induced by mercuric chloride in the brown Norway rat. Clin Exp Immunol 1990; 81:76–82.

15
Historical Perspectives

Eric L. Matteson
Mayo Clinic and Mayo Foundation, Rochester, Minnesota

I. INTRODUCTION

Vasculitis was recognized as a distinct clinical entity about 150 years ago. While the causes of the vasculitides were unknown to the early describers and, indeed, the causes of many remain uncertain, the pathogenesis of several types has become more clearly elucidated.

Many of the forms of idiopathic vasculitis are associated with the authors who wrote an early or classic account of the named disease. Often, descriptions of these diseases can be found that antedate the contributions of these authors, and frequently the author(s) did not realize the uniqueness of the case or appreciate the singular pathophysiology of the disease process they described. Still, it is the contribution of the named authors, e.g., Kussmaul and Maier in polyarteritis nodosa, Takayasu, Horton in giant cell arteritis, Schönlein and Henoch, Wegener, Behçet, Churg and Strauss, and Kawasaki, that stimulated the clear delineation of the disease features and improved understanding of the disease processes with which these authors are associated.

Polyarteritis nodosa was the first noninfectious vasculitis to be described and studied in detail, and has served as the cornerstone for understanding the pathophysiology of other forms of idiopathic vasculitis. In large measure, most forms of vasculitis described subsequently have been characterized and classified on the basis of features either similar to or distinct from polyarteritis.

Diseases of the blood vessels have been recognized since antiquity (Table 1). If physicians of that time observed cases of vasculitis, it appears that they did not recognize their inflammatory nature. The Greco-Roman scholar and physician Claudius Galenus (129–199 AD) described peripheral aneurysms, recognizing especially those occurring as a complication of blood-letting when an artery was accidentally punctured instead of a vein (1). In 1554, the Montpellier professor Antoine Saporta described syphilitic aneurysms (2). Joseph Hodgson more clearly related syphilis to aortitis in his *Treatise on Diseases of Arteries and Veins* published in London in 1815 (3). This report likely represents the first clearly defined example of arteritis. In the same treatise, Hodgson discusses nonsyphilitic inflammation of the "internal coat" of the arteries arising from many causes, including excessive intravascular pressure, puncture, ligature, and systemic inflammation. Hodgson also differentiated the lesions of syphilitic aortitis from those of atherosclerosis (3). Jean-Frédéric (Johann Friedrich) Lobstein in Strassburg named the condition arteriosclerosis (4).

At the end of the 18th century, John Hunter recognized inflammation of the veins (phlebitis) and was also the first to demonstrate the muscularity of arteries (5). He postulated that arterial aneurysms were due not simply to weakness of the arterial wall, but to actual disease of the artery (6).

Table 1 Chronology of Historical Accounts of Primary Vasculitic Diseases and Related
Arterial Pathology

Year	Author	Condition
ca. 170	Claudius Galenus	Peripheral (posttraumatic) aneurysms
1554	Antoine Saporta	Syphilitic aortitis and aortic aneurysm
1761	Giovanni B. Morgagni	Pulseless disease (Takayasu?)
1794	John Hunter	Demonstration of muscularity of arteries; phlebitis
1801	William Heberden	Henoch–Schönlein purpura
1815	Joseph Hodgson	Clear description of arterial inflammation
1833	Jean-Frédéric Lobstein	Arteriosclerosis
1839	James Davy	Pulseless disease (Takayasu)
1852	Karl von Rokitansky	Polyarteritis nodosa
1856	William S. Savoy	Pulseless disease (Takayasu)
1866	A. Kussmaul and R. Maier	Polyarteritis nodosa
1890	Jonathan Hutchinson	Temporal arteritis
1908	Makito Takayasu	Takayasu arteritis
1923	Friedrich Wohlwill	Microscopic polyangiitis
1923	William Ophüls	Granulomatosis, eosinophilia, vasculitis (Churg-Strauss)
1931	Heinz Klinger	Necrotizing granulomatous vasculitis (Wegener)
1932	B. T. Horton, T. B. Magath, and G. E. Brown	Giant cell (temporal) arteritis
1936	Friedrich Wegener	Wegener's granulomatosis
1937	Hulusi Behçet	Behçet syndrome
1949	J. Churg and L. Strauss	Churg–Strauss disease
1961	Tomisaku Kawasaki	Kawasaki disease

Following Hunter's work, others began to attribute certain examples of persistent fevers to inflammation of the arteries. Johann Peter Frank working in Pavia and Vienna recognized macroscopically red and inflamed inner walls of the large arteries, heart, and veins in patients with unremitting fevers (7). In France, François Broussais and Jean-Baptiste Brouillaud came to the conclusion that "angiocarditis" was the correlate of all fevers (8,9). Indeed, the term "rheumatic arteritis" was coined by Bouillaud in 1840 (9), although there is little histological evidence provided in this or subsequent reports to support the conclusion that rheumatic disease was the cause of these lesions.

Into the 20th century, the nature of the inflammatory processes affecting blood vessels remained poorly understood. Much of the debate centered on the question of the anatomical origin of arterial inflammation, i.e., in which layers of the artery inflammation begins. It is difficult to follow this debate without some understanding of the histological notions of the early and mid-19th century. Karl von Rokitansky was of the opinion that arteritis was a process of the adventitia or "outer coat" (or as he terms it, the "Ringfaserschicht," the adventitia with media) (10). Rudolf Virchow, on the other hand, thought that inflammation could begin in the media and intima. In his review of arterial inflammation, Virchow was to lament, "There are few points in clinical pathology, which have gradually become so confused, as the diseases of the vascular system." (11).

II. POLYARTERITIS NODOSA

Kussmaul and Maier gave the first complete description of this form of systemic necrotizing vasculitis in 1866 and assigned the name periarteritis nodosa to it (12). Several earlier authors have been credited with describing aneurysmal lesions of the arteries that may have been inflammatory in nature, but in most cases the clinical and pathological–anatomical picture is not sufficient to conclude that the condition represents polyarteritis nodosa (13–15).

Karl (later Freiherr von) Rokitansky, the great Viennese pathologist, is credited with the initial case report of polyarteritis nodosa in 1852. He described the presence of aneurysmal lesions with nodes in multiple arteries observed at autopsy in a 23-year-old shoemaker's journeyman, Wenzel Plohner (16). Plohner was admitted November 6, 1848 with a 5-day history of bloody diarrhea and fever with abdominal pain, and died January 12, 1849. Rokitansky provides a compelling gross pathological description of the aneurysms seen in specimens obtained at autopsy, which, however, he did not histologically examine (Fig. 1):

> With exception of the aorta and most of its more prominent root branches, further with exception of the brain arteries, all arteries were aneurysmic, that is they were either covered with

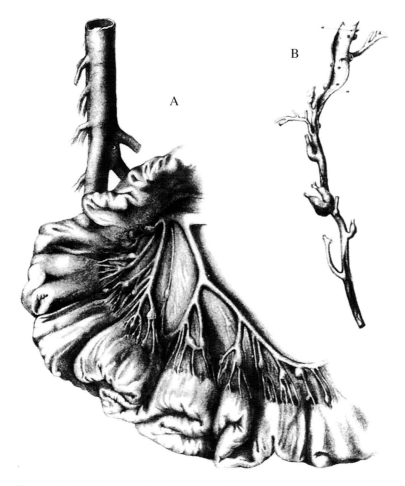

Figure 1   (A) Mesentery from Rokitansky's first case report of polyarteritis nodosa, demonstrating multiple macroscopically apparent arterial nodules. (B) Artery specimen showing larger aneurysms at the branching point of smaller arteries. Rokitansky viewed the aneurysms as located excentrically on the sides of the involved artery, and connected to the lumen of the artery by a small opening, or ostium. In describing the aneurysms, he states, "Larger or smaller, often barely perceptible, needle point sized openings in the vessel lumen led into these, which had the appearance of a delicate vessel ostium (B.a.)." (From Ref. 16.)

more or less numerous oval, round, laterally attached aneurysms the size of millet seeds, hemp seeds, peas or even hazelnuts, which were filled with fibrin thrombi with an appearance from fresh dark red coagulum to rusty brown fibrous tissue. In particular, the aneurysms next to the branching points of the arteries were generally larger (16).

Rokitansky viewed this case as a type of dissecting aneurysm caused by spontaneous tears in the intima and media of smaller arteries. In discussing this case, he recalls two similar cases "from long ago," one with involvement of the hepatic, splenic, and superior mesenteric arteries, and the other with involvement of the gastroepiploica (16).

In 1887, Hans Eppinger, professor of pathological anatomy in Graz, Austria, macroscopically and microscopically analyzed the anatomical specimen of the small bowel and mesentery and coronary arteries described by Rokitansky (17). He found marked thickening of the intima with "cellular deposits" and disruption of all wall layers including the media, elastica, and adventitia, with multiple foci of "disordered cells and twisted fibers" at the sites of the aneurysms (Fig. 2) (17). The appearance of the vessel wall between the aneurysms was described as uninvolved. The description offered by Eppinger is consistent with a necrotizing lesion, although there is no description of inflammatory cells in the specimens nor discussion of inflammation as the primary cause of the affliction. Eppinger viewed the aneurysms as caused by a "congenital debility" of the elastica.

The classic description of polyarteritis nodosa by the internist Adolf Kussmaul and pathologist Rudolf Maier in Freiburg is based on their report of a 27-year-old journeyman tailor (12). The patient, Carl Seufarth, developed acute symptoms of fever, global myalgias, mononeuritis multiplex, abdominal pain and proteinuria. Seufarth succumbed to the illness after a hospitalization of approximately 1 month. About 3 days prior to death, pea-sized nodules were discovered in the subcutaneous skin of the abdomen and chest.

At autopsy, nodules visible to the naked eye along medium-sized arteries were present. The autopsy report introduces the unique nature of the findings:

> *Peculiar mostly nodular thickening (periarteritis nodosa) of countless arteries of and below the caliber of the liver artery and the major branches of the coronary arteries of the heart, principally in the bowel, stomach, kidneys, spleen, heart and voluntary muscles, and to a lesser extent also in the liver, subcutaneous cell tissue and in the bronchial and phrenic arteries* (italics original; translation in Ref. 18).

Microscopic examination demonstrated the intima of the nodularly thickened vessels to be completely intact, while dramatic inflammatory changes were noted in the media and adventitia. The kidneys revealed changes of "acute Bright's disease." "The change affects the interlobular arteries, which have glomeruli at their bifurcations, and it extends into these branches and even into the glomeruli" (18). The drawing of Seufarth's heart demonstrating the macroscopically evident nodular changes in the coronary arteries is reproduced in Fig. 3. Kussmaul and Maier attributed the changes noted in the arteries to "the inflammation of the arteries affecting principally the perivascular sheaths, in which the media also had a part at least in its outer layers," and hypothesized that these inflammatory changes extended to tissues directly surrounding the affected arteries: "and which often attacked neighboring tissues in the opposite direction, for example renal parenchyma, connective and muscle tissue" (18).

Kussmaul and Maier were uncertain of the cause of these changes. Initially, they had speculated that the "countless small nodules" were due to a human form of nematode infestation similar to strongylus, and indeed the first report of their famous case was published under the title "Aneurysma verminosum hominis" (19). They recanted this explanation of the case in the now famous classic report (12).

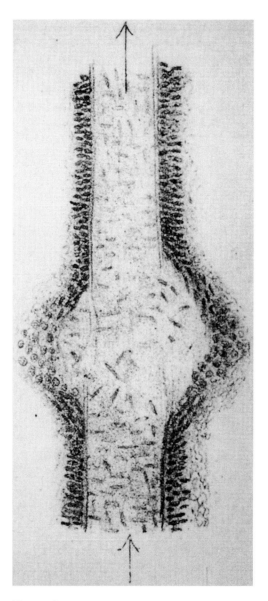

Figure 2 Low-power image of an aneurysmically dilated artery from Rokitansky's case. Eppinger describes marked thickening of the intima and disruption of all wall layers, with multiple foci of "disordered cells and twisted fibers." (From Ref. 17.)

In this same report, Kussmaul and Maier also describe a second patient, Landolin Faist, a 28-year-old day laborer, who spent 13 months in the hospital under the care of Dr. Kussmaul, and even shared a room with the unfortunate Seufarth (12). The exact nature of Faist's illness remains unclear; it is possible that he had polymyositis.

A. Microscopic Polyarteritis

Despite mention in reviews of early literature of a few cases in which the diagnosis was not made on the basis of macroscopic findings (20,21), there are perhaps 1 or 2 of these cases which could be considered microscopic polyangiitis (22,23).

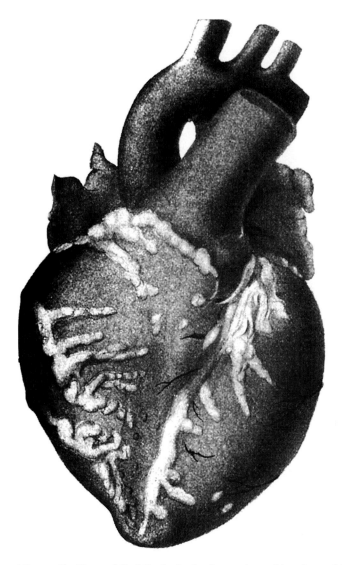

Figure 3 Heart of Carl Seufarth, the first patient with polyarteritis nodosa reported by Kussmaul and Maier. (From Ref. 12.)

Friedrich Wohlwill in Hamburg may be credited with introduction of the term "microscopic polyarteritis nodosa" in his description of two patients with transmural periarteritis and glomeru-lonephritis in his report from 1923 (24). Both patients succumbed to an illness characterized by myalgias, paresis, and glomerulonephritis. In neither case were macroscopic vascular changes ev-ident, nor were the aneurysms and nodules of classic polyarteritis nodosa present. Still, Wohlwill was convinced that the disease he described was a form of polyarteritis nodosa, and concluded that "the overall picture is one of a *well-characterized* and *uniform disease,* which practically de-mands the assumption of an *unified etiology*" (original italics; translation in Ref. 18). Wohlwill also found evidence of venulitis in his specimens, but thought that the venous involvement was "at least in part—distinctly independent of the arteritis, but on the other hand, was a completely uncharacteristic infiltration of the wall with single nuclear elements that bore no similarities to the arterial disease" (18).

B. Nosology of Polyarteritis Nodosa

The term polyarteritis acuta nodosa was introduced by Enrico Ferrari in Trieste in 1903 who observed that the disease had an acute course, and emphasized that the vascular lesions were transmural rather than affecting only the adventitia and media, as thought by Kussmaul and Maier (12, 25). W. E. Carnegie Dickson in Edinburgh introduced the term polyarteritis nodosa to the English language literature in 1908 (26).

The overlap between microscopic polyangiitis and cutaneous polyarteritis nodosa is certainly well recognized (27). Zeek distinguished hypersensitivity vasculitis from classic polyarteritis nodosa. Godman and Churg have stated that "periarteritis nodosa . . . should probably be reserved for the disease picture . . . in which medium-sized arteries are involved with macroscopic nodules" (28). Davson postulated that the presence or absence of glomerulonephritis could distinguish distinctive groups of patients with necrotizing arteritis (29). This view was formalized in the Chapel Hill nomenclature system (30).

C. Etiology of Polyarteritis Nodosa

In the early history of polyarteritis, five principal theories were advanced as to its causation. The most widely debated in the first 50 years was that of syphilis. Although already rejected by Kussmaul and Maier, some other authors suspected syphilis (31,32), but none were able to demonstrate the organism in any of the cases. A second theory was that mechanical factors including hypertension (33–35) or congenital weakness of the internal elastica (17) were causal or of major importance. Ferrari was a proponent of a third theory, that toxic substances, such as alcohol, caused weakness of the arterial walls and so led to the diseases (25).

Most early authors, beginning perhaps with Kussmaul and Maier, favored a fourth theory that some acute infection, likely a bacterium such as *Streptococcus* or *Staphylococcus aureus,* but perhaps also a virus, caused the arterial disease, either by direct effect or by the release of toxins (12,20,24,36–42 and many others). Oskar Klotz in Pittsburgh viewed periarteritis nodosa as a histopathological manifestation common to many infections, stating that it is not a "disease entity, but is only a complication of lesions present in an infection which has many other manifestations" (20). In 1926, William VonGlahn and Alwin Pappenheimer in New York described the differences in the vascular pathology of periarteritis nodosa and the inflammatory blood vessel changes noted in rheumatic fever (43).

Since the turn of the 20th century, authors have speculated about a fifth theory, that periarteritis nodosa may be an allergic reaction to several toxins or infectious agents (40).

Rich called the vasculitic lesions of serum sickness and sulfonamide hypersensitivity periarteritis nodosa (44). The vascular lesions of sulfonamide allergy were reported in 1946 by Lichtenstein and Fox (45) and French (46). To some observers, these allergic reactions to sulfonamides appeared to be similar to periarteritis nodosa (47). However, in 1948, Zeek could provide convincing evidence that primary hypersensitivity vasculitis was a distinct entity from polyarteritis nodosa (48,49). Later, hypersensitivity was viewed as of particular pathoetiological significance in some forms of vasculitis initially viewed as variants of polyarteritis nodosa but which have since been given separate identity. Churg and Strauss are deservedly given recognition for their coherent understanding and description of asthma and allergic angiitis with granuloma formation (50) which bears their names.

III. SCHÖNLEIN–HENOCH PURPURA

William Heberden of London first described what became known as Schönlein–Henoch purpura in his "Commentarii de Marlbaun" of 1801 (51). In Chapter 78 of his *Commentaries on the History and Cure of Diseases* from 1802, entitled "Purpureae Maculae," two cases are presented (52). The first is a 4-year-old boy with red-purple and then yellow swellings on the lower extremities, buttock, and scrotum for about 10 days. The patient was otherwise well. The second was a 5-year-old boy with similar swelling and discoloration especially of the leg, who

> was seized with pains and swellings in various parts, and the penis in particular was so distended, though not discoloured, that he could hardly make water. He had sometimes pains in his belly with vomiting, and at the same time some streaks of blood were perceived in his stools, and the urine was tinged with blood. When the pain attacked his leg, he was unable to walk; and presently the skin of his leg was all over full of bloody points (52).

In both cases the disease was self-limited, although of longer duration in the second child (52).

Although also reported later by others (53,54), the condition does not appear to have been recognized as a distinct entity until Johann Lukas Schönlein in Würzburg called the combination of arthralgias and arthritis associated with a macular rash "peliosis rheumatic" (pelios = livid) in 1837 (55). He distinguished this from purpura hemorrhagica based on the absence of ecchymosis and oral bleeding, and recognized that the exanthem could affect internal organs and could become chronic. In 1874, Eduard Heinrich Henoch in Berlin reported four children with bloody diarrhea, abdominal pain, and rash with painful joints (56). Schönlein and Henoch described the rash as macular but not always purpuric. Henoch also realized that the disease was not always self-limited and could be associated with renal disease and death (57).

The cause of the affliction was uncertain, although already Schönlein had reported on the onset of the purpuric lesions after a preceding cold. William Osler remarked on the similarity between it and serum sickness (58). In 1915, E. Frank in Breslau called the syndrome anaphylactoid purpura (59). Glanzmann (1920) further developed the idea that both infection and sensitization were causal in this and other forms of "post-infective anaphylactoid purpura following otitis and scarlet fever" (60).

IV. WEGENER'S GRANULOMATOSIS

Heinz Klinger in Berlin, a college roommate of Friedrich Wegener, reported the first two cases of the disease Wegener's granulomatosis in 1931 (61). Klinger regarded the illnesses he describes as a form of periarteritis nodosa, and not as a distinct clinical entity. The first case was a 70-year-old physician who presented with nephritis, arthritis, and a history of chronic sinusitis with nasal discharge. At autopsy, invasion of a necrotizing lesion into the base of the skull about the eyes was evident, as was tracheal ulceration. Histological examination revealed vasculitis and granuloma formation, including destruction of the nasal septum. The second case was a 51-year-old carpenter who also presented with bloody sputum, polyarthralgias, and glomerulonephritis (61).

In interpreting his cases, Klinger left no doubt that the oldest vessel or the most advanced vascular changes were also the site at which the disease had its beginnings. These are "sites which are directly exposed to exogenous effects of a noxious agent" (namely, the sites of the respiratory tract) (61).

Two years later, Robert Rössle, then director of the Institute for Pathology at the University of Berlin, where Klinger also made his observations, published two further cases of a form of vasculitis with necrosis of the mucosa of the nose and upper airway occurring among five cases with vasculitic changes that he attributed to rheumatic disease processes (62).

It was Friedrich Wegener in Breslau who, in two publications from 1936 and 1939, established the disease now named for him as a distinct clinical pathological entity (63,64). In the initial, preliminary paper entitled "On generalized, septic vascular diseases," Wegener described three patients (a man, age 38, and two women, ages 33 and 36) who presented with 4–7 month history of fevers, high sedimentation rate, anemia, and rhinitis at the outset, followed by stomatitis, laryngitis, pharyngitis, and trachitis (63). The nasal lesions stood out in the clinical presentation, and granulomatous changes with vasculitis of multiple vessels and organs, as well as glomerulonephritis with periglomerular granuloma in two of the cases dominated the histological findings (63,64).

Wegener interpreted the vascular changes as a form of periarteritis nodosa as described by Kussmaul and Maier (64). Although accompanied by a generalized arteritis like that seen in periarteritis nodosa, both in the preliminary paper of 1936 and the comprehensive treatment of his cases in his paper of 1939, Wegener clearly viewed his cases as unique on the basis of the clinical course and the distinct anatomical changes. He was familiar with the recently reported cases of periarteritis nodosa of Klinger and Rössle, who had interpreted them as rheumatic changes and attributed the disease to an allergic-hypersensitivity process. Wegener was of the opinion that his cases could not be explained on this basis but rather were due to an infectious agent (61,62,64). Wegener understood the granulomatous vasculitis he described as a form of "rheumatoid or rheumatic diseases, respectively" (64). This granulomatous disease typically had a course of 4–7 months, which began with cold symptoms and progressed to necrotic nasal and pharyngeal disease with septic features and progressive renal insufficiency ending in death (63).

V. CHURG–STRAUSS DISEASE

Jacob Churg and Lotte Strauss in New York reported on "allergic granulomatosis, allergic angiitis, and periarteritis nodosa" in 1949 (65), and in more complete form in 1951 (50). A similar constellation of clinical and histopathological findings had been previously reported by numerous authors. In 1923, William Ophüls in San Francisco described the case of a 38-year-old Persian janitor who died after a 6-month history of abdominal pains and night sweats (39). At autopsy, there were multiple granulomatous nodules, especially of the pericardium and peritoneum, eosinophilic infiltration of the bronchi and pulmonary tissue, arteritis and venulitis, and nephritis. Others reported on periarteritis nodosa associated with asthma, a condition that was perceived by these authors as a form of hypersensitivity reaction (66–68).

The credit for defining the clinical syndrome that carries their names goes to Churg and Strauss, who carefully described a series of 13 patients with an illness they identified as a granulomatous vasculitis associated with asthma, fever, and hypereosinophilia, and which is distinct from classic polyarteritis nodosa (50). All patients had asthma beginning between 7–58 years of age that preceded the often fatal illness by an average of 3 years. One patient had rheumatoid arthritis. Recurrent pneumonia was present in virtually every case. Most patients had some type of cutaneous manifestation, generally an erythematous macular papular pustular rash. Cutaneous or subcutaneous nodules were seen in seven cases, and on biopsy in five of these, "allergic granuloma" were found (50). In 9 of 10 autopsied cases there were changes of inflammation like those of periarteritis nodosa, with nodular swellings and associated occlusion of the small arteries of many organs with occasional thrombi. The epicardium of the heart was the site of the most granulomatous lesions. The connective tissues had prominent infiltration with eosinophils and fibrinoid changes with granulomatous (epithelioid and giant cell) reaction in the connective tissue and the blood vessel walls in seven of nine cases with active or healing lesions (50). At the time of publication, Churg and Strauss saw angiitis as the "most malignant expression" of allergic granulomatosis, while other allergic conditions such as Loeffler's syndrome were more benign forms of allergic granulomatosis (50).

VI. GIANT CELL ARTERITIS

The giant cell arteritides consist of two principal clinical syndromes, temporal arteritis and Takayasu's arteritis. These syndromes are usually, but not always, clinically distinct, and both are characterized by a granulomatous vasculitis of medium- and large-sized arteries.

Jonathan Hutchinson in London reported the first clinical description of temporal arteritis in 1890, a case of a "peculiar form of Thrombotic Arteritis of the aged which is sometimes productive of Gangrene" (69). Hutchinson distinguished the disease from atherosclerosis and indeed writes, "I do not . . . feel in the least sure that the advanced calcareous degeneration of old age is a frequent predisponent." The case was of an "old man named Rumbold . . . a tall, fine-looking man rather thin and quite bald. He had been a gentleman servant, having lived in the family of the Earl of Dundonald, and he had, I believe, suffered from gout. . . . He was upwards of eighty and almost in his dotage. I was asked to see him because, as I was told, he had 'red streaks on his head' which were painful and prevented him wearing his hat." Hutchinson identified the red streaks as the temporal arteries. The patient did not develop scalp necrosis and lived for several years "after this without any other manifestation of arterial disease" (69).

In 1932 Horton, Magath, and Brown at Mayo Clinic in Rochester, Minnesota, recognized the presence of a granulomatous arteritis in this disease and subsequently further defined the clinical syndrome (70,71). Already with the publication of the initial two cases, a 55-year-old woman from a southern Minnesota farm, and a 68-year-old man from a farm in Nebraska, these authors were convinced of their uniqueness. They do not cite Hutchinson's account and appear not to have known of it (70). Both patients presented in 1931 with fever, weakness, anorexia, anemia, mild leukocytosis, "and painful areas over the scalp and along the temporal vessels" for about 4–6 weeks. The disease course was characterized by exacerbations and remission. Although Horton et al. did not describe the first case of giant cell arteritis, they may be credited with obtaining the first biopsies of the affected temporal arteries in living patients, and with the histopathological description of the lesions. They found evidence of chronic periarteritis and arteritis with "peculiar circumscribed areas of what appeared to be granulation tissue . . . in the adventitia of the blood vessels which suggested granulomas, and this represented the most characteristic lesion present" (70). In their subsequent report of seven cases, disease features included headache, weakness, fever, night sweats, prominent and nodular temporal arteries, and, in one case, diplopia. "Difficulty in chewing food was invariably present" (71). Horton et al. felt the disease was benign, as "complete recovery occurred in each case," but they go on to note that two of the patients died within 2 years of "unrelated conditions" (71).

Giant cell arteritis was definitively linked to polymyalgia rheumatica by J. Paulley and J. Hughes of Ipswich in 1960, who suggested that the syndrome of "'anarthritic rheumatism' . . . is nothing more than arteritis, in which the classic stigmata of the disease have yet to develop, or have already occurred" (72).

VII. TAKAYASU'S ARTERITIS

Forms of pulseless disease have been described since antiquity. Few of these accounts are complete, but some accounts from the past 200 years or so may support the notion that some acquired diseases leading to arterial occlusion may have a basis in disease processes other than arteriosclerosis or trauma.

In 1761, Giovanni Battista Morgagni, professor of anatomy at the University of Padua, described the case of a woman of about 40 years of age who had no radial pulses for at least 6 years prior to death (73). At autopsy, the radial arteries appeared normal. The proximal aorta was ectatic, while the lower aorta was stenotic. The internal layers of the aorta were yellow and revealed evidence of calcifications (73).

James Davy, a British Army physician and assistant inspector of Army hospitals, is sometimes given credit for the first convincing account of Takayasu's arteritis in 1839 (74). He described two patients with what can be regarded as pulseless disease. The first was an approximately 55-year-old officer who developed pain in the left shoulder at about age 49, and presented about 4 years later to Dr. Davy with faint arm pulses and emaciation. Within 6 months he had developed occasional vertigo, and presumed obstruction of the aortic arch, for

> No pulse could be felt any where in the course of these vessels, neither in the neck, temples, axilla or wrists, and there was a throbbing pulse at the upper part of the sternum, and a slight prominence of the bone there to some little extent (74).

An aneurysm of the aortic arch was diagnosed. The patient did well for 1 1/2 years, and then expired suddenly. At autopsy, a rupture was found in a large aneurysm of the aortic arch, and "all the great vessels rising from the arch were completely closed up at their origin" (74).

In the same account, Davy reports on a second patient, a 36-year-old drummer with the 42d regiment who, "notwithstanding intemperate habits," had enjoyed good health until developing shortness of breath. At hospitalization, no pulses could be detected in the wrists or brachial arteries, while femoral pulses were strong. At autopsy, findings included enlargement of the aortic arch, with irregular thickening and opaqueness of the "inner coat," and thinning of the "middle coat." The left carotid and subclavian arteries were occluded, "firmly plugged up with dense white matter, which it may be inferred was lymph" (74).

An histological examination was not performed in either case. It is unclear whether either of these cases represented Takayasu's disease, as the first may have been degenerative in nature, while the second could have been due to a congenital anomaly.

A convincing account of a disease resembling Takayasu's arteritis is provided by William S. Savory, who reported on a 22-year-old woman admitted to St. Bartholomew's Hospital London in 1854 (75). The patient had been ill for about 5 years with vague symptoms, then developed seizures and was found to be pulseless in all vessels of the head, neck, and upper extremities. During the 13-month hospitalization, she developed blindness of the left eye and a large ulcer appeared on the scalp. The postmortem examination revealed the aorta and vessels of the aortic arch to be thickened and narrowed, "reduced to solid cords." The disease was obviously advanced; aneurysms were not reported. The condition was attributed by Savory to mural inflammation (78).

Makito Takayasu of Kanazawa presented the case of a young woman with retinal arterial changes at the 12th Annual Meeting of the Japanese Society of Ophthalmology in 1908 (76). Judge et al. have published a complete translation of the short paper and subsequent audience discussion, from which it is apparent that Takayasu did not report pulselessness of the peripheral arteries (77). There is an extensive description of the retinal blood vessels:

> there was a wreath-like anastomosis surrounding the optic disc at a distance of 2 or 3 mm and surrounding this was another circular anastomosis. These were anastomotic shunts of arterioles and venules. It was noted that the blood vessels surrounding the optic discs were slightly elevated. Both the surrounding vessels and their branches had 'lumps' here and there which were seen to move from day to day. They were more in the arterioles. There were some slight hemorrhages in areas. However, there was no inflammation (76,77).

It was first Onishi and then Kagoshima who, in the discussion that ensued after Dr. Takayasu's presentation, associated the retinal vascular changes with absent radial pulses in their own patients (77). The first comprehensive description of the histopathological changes of Takayasu's arteritis was by Rudolf Beneke in Halle an der Saale in 1925 (78).

By 1941, the syndrome of pulseless disease occurring especially in young adults was being given a wide variety of names, resulting in considerable confusion. To bring order into the nosology of the disease, and for convenience, Yasuzo Niimi of Nagoya suggested Takayasu be honored by naming the disease for him (79). Shimizu and Sano more completely described the full clinical syndrome and called it "pulseless disease" (80). Caccamise and Okuda introduced the term Takayasu's disease to the English language literature in 1954 (81).

VIII. BEHÇET'S SYNDROME

Behçet's syndrome is likely a disease of antiquity, described by many authors, but awaiting more recent recognition as a distinct pathophysiological entity. Hippocrates described patients with oral and genital mucosal ulcers and eye disease with photophobia and loss of vision (perhaps iritis) (82,83). However, the accounts refer to "fungus excrescences" of the eyelids, a disease feature not consistent with Behçet's syndrome (82,84). Other reports predating Behçet's paper of 1937 may be consistent with cases of Behçet's (85–87).

Hulusi Behçet, professor of dermatology at the University of Istanbul, described two patients with recurrent oral and genital aphthae-like ulcerations and uveitis with hypopyon in 1937 (88). One was a 40-year-old man, the other a 34-year-old woman. Behçet followed the patients for 20 years. One of the patients went to Vienna for a second opinion, where the disease was thought to be due to either tuberculosis or an unidentified parasite. Treatment there with gold and trivalent arsenic was unsuccessful. The patient also underwent iridectomies in Vienna without success (88). Biopsies of ulcers revealed many leukocytes and epithelial cells with saphrophytic rods and cocci, as well as intracellular and extracellular particles that were "suspicious for a virus" on Giemsa and Herzberg staining. The attempt to transmit the organism from this patient to a scarified rabbit cornea caused neither local nor generalized infection. Behçet speculated that the syndrome was caused by an as yet unidentified virus (88), and did not discuss the possibility that the illness was vasculitic in nature.

IX. KAWASAKI DISEASE

In January, 1961, Tomisaku Kawasaki in Tokyo saw the first case of the disease that carries his name. During the following 6 years, he carefully collected clinical and epidemiological information on a total of 50 cases occurring principally in the region around Tokyo Bay, reporting his findings as an acute, febrile mucocutaneous lymph node syndrome of children in 1967 (89).

The main features of the acute syndrome as described by Kawasaki included fever, lymphadenopathy, and mucocutaneous involvement. Detailed case histories are provided for seven patients. The disease course was about 3 weeks, and the disease resolved without complications or recurrence in all the initial patients. Kawasaki could not identify the cause, but suspected that it was either allergic, autoimmune, or infectious. A viral droplet infection seemed likely, but a bacterium was also strongly considered based on the clinical presentation and the frequently present leukocytosis with left shift. Extensive cultures, including cultures of involved excised lymph glands, were not diagnostic, but most (47 of 50) patients were treated with antibiotics. Corticosteroids were given to 22 patients (89).

X. CLASSIFICATION OF VASCULITIS

Early attempts to classify vasculitides further at that time were greatly hampered by lack of understanding of the pathoetiology of these illnesses. Authors, including Kussmaul and Maier, Wegener, Churg and Strauss, and Horton, described vasculitis on the basis of the gross anatomical and histological appearance of the affected blood vessels and the involvement of specific organs. At the same time it must be recognized that even early authors attempted to order the arterial diseases based on pathoetiology (10,11,17).

In 1952, the pathologist Pearl Zeek in Cincinnati defined three periods of evolution in the description and understanding of necrotizing vasculitis (21). The first period from 1866 to 1900 was characterized by numerous publications of case reports, which detailed gross and microscopic pathology and provided speculation about the pathoetiology of the disease. In the second period, from 1900 to 1925, investigators attempted to identify the specific cause of periarteritis, whether infectious in nature or due to an as yet unidentified toxin (21).

The third period defined by Zeek was from 1925 until 1952 (21). By then, the term "periarteritis" was being applied more widely and included the microscopic forms of necrotizing vasculitis, placing them in the same diagnostic category of those of classic periarteritis nodosa. Zeek recognized that considerable confusion had arisen since the time of Kussmaul and Maier regarding the term periarteritis nodosa. In her opinion, this confusion occurred chiefly because the vascular manifestations of allergy were becoming increasingly recognized, and the leukocytoclastic vasculitic changes seen in allergies resembled those described in classic polyarteritis nodosa (21).

In 1953, Zeek presented a classification of necrotizing angiitis based on her own clinical and pathological observations as well as a review of the literature (21). She expanded her earlier observations, incorporating the caliber of blood vessel involved, in her article of 1953 and commented on the similarity between the microscopic form of polyarteritis and hypersensitivity (49). Not all accounts or major forms of vasculitis were considered in this article. For example, Wegener's granulomatosis and Takayasu's arteritis were not even discussed. Zeek classified necrotizing angiitis as (1) hypersensitivity angiitis, (2) allergic granulomatous angiitis, (3) rheumatic arteritis, (4) periarteritis nodosa, and (5) temporal arteritis (21,49).

Later attempts to classify these diseases have built on this historical framework. These classifications systems have been refined by subsequent discoveries and insights about the histopathological features and etiologies of these conditions. A number of schemes have been put forward based on these principles, including those of Lie (90), Churg (91), the Chapel Hill nomenclature (30), and the classification system of the American College of Rheumatology (92).

The observations of early clinicians and investigators are the basis for our current understanding of the pathoetiology and nosology of vasculitis. The challenge they faced as they saw their concepts of vasculitis altered by new information is the challenge we yet face today.

REFERENCES

1. Galenus C. Dissectionis venarum arteriarumque commentarium. Ejusdem de nervis compendium. Antonio Fortolo Ioseriensi interprete. Basel, in aedibus Thomae Wolffii, 1529. See also Galen's Opera Omnia, vol. 7, translated by Carolus Gottlieb Kühn, Leipzig, 1826.
2. Saporta A. Tractus de lue venerea. Ex instructissima biblioteca Ranchiniana eruti, & publici juris facti, cura, & studio Henrici Gras. Lyon: Sumptibus Petri Ravaud, 1624.
3. Hodgson J. Treatise on Diseases of Arteries and Veins. London, 1815.
4. Lobstein JF. Traité d'Anatomie Pathologique. Vol. 2. Paris: Levrault, 1833.
5. Hunter J. A treatise on the blood, inflammation, and gunshot wounds. To which is prefixed a short account of the author's life by Everard Home. London: G Nicoll, 1794.
6. Qvist G. John Hunter 1728–1793. London: William Heinemann, 1981.

7. Frank JP. Grundsätze über die Behandlung der Krankheiten des Menschen. Erster Theil. Von den Fiebern. Mannheim: Schwan & Götz, 1794.

8. Broussais F-J-V. Histoire des phlegmasies ou inflammations chroniques, fondée sur nouvelles observations de clinique et d'anatomie pathologique. 2d ed. Paris: Gobon and Crochard, 1816.

9. Bouillaud J-B. Traité clinique du rhumatisme articulaire, et de la loi de coïncidence des inflammations du coe ur avec cette maladie. Paris: J-B Baillière, 1840.

10. Rokitansky K. Handbuch der pathologischen Anatomie. Vienna: Braumüller and Seidel, 1842.

11. Virchow R. Ueber die akute Entzündung der Arterien. Arch Path Anat Physiol Klin Med 1847; 1:272.

12. Kussmaul A, Maier R. Ueber eine bisher nicht beschriebene eigenthümliche Arterienerkrankung (Periarteritis nodosa), die mit Morbus Brightii und rapid fortschreitender allgemeiner Muskellähmung einhergeht. Dtsch Arch Klin Med 1866; 1:484–518.

13. Michaelis JG. Aneurysmatum cordis disq anat-med. vi. Halle: JC Hendel, 1785.

14. Matani A. De aneurysmaticis praecordiorem morbis anima diversiones juxta exemplar liburnium recusae. xl. Frankfurt and Leipzig, 1776.

15. Pelletan P-J. Clinique chirurgicale, ou mémoires et observations de chirurgie clinique, et sur d'autres objets relatifs à l'art de guérir. Vol. 3. Paris: J-G Dentu, 1810.

16. Rokitansky K. Über einige der wichtigsten Erkrankungen der Arterien. Denkschriften der kaiserlichen Akademie der Wissenschaften (mathematisch-naturwissenschaftliche Classe). Vienna: kaiserlich-königlich Hof- und Staatsdruckerei, 1852; 4:1.

17. Eppinger H. Pathogenesis (Histogenesis und Aetiologie) der Aneurysmen einschliesslich des Aneurysma equi verminosum. Pathologisch-anatomische Studien, Arch Klin Chir 1887; 35:1–563.

18. Matteson EL. Polyarteritis Nodosa and Microscopic Polyangiitis. Translation of the original articles on classic polyarteritis nodosa by Adolf Kussmaul and Rudolf Maier and microscopic polyarteritis nodosa by Friedrich Wohlwill. Rochester, MN: Mayo Clinic Pr, 1998.

19. Kussmaul A, Maier R. Aneurysma verminosum hominis: vorläufige Nachricht. Dtsch Arch Klin Med 1866; 1:125.

20. Klotz OJ. Periarteritis nodosa. J Med Res 1917; 37:1.

21. Zeek PM. Periarteritis nodosa: A critical review. Am J Clin Pathol 1952; 22:777.

22. Fletcher HM. Ueber die sogenannte Periarteriitis nodosa. Beitr Path Anat Allg Path (Ziegler's) 1892; 11:323.

23. Cooke JV. A case of periarteritis nodosa. Proc Path Soc Philadelphia 1911; 15:96.

24. Wohlwill F. Über die nur mikroskopisch erkennbare Form der Periarteriitis nodosa. Arch Path Anat Physiol Klin Med 1923; 246:377.

25. Ferrari E. Ueber Polyarteritis acuta nodosa (sogenannte Periarteritis nodosa), und ihre Beziehungen zur Polymyositis und Polyneuritis acuta. Beitr Pathol Anat 1903; 34:350.

26. Dickson WEC. Polyarteritis acuta nodosa and periarteritis nodosa. J Pathol Bacteriol 1908; 12:31.

27. Diaz-Perez JL, Winkelman RK. Cutaneous periarteritis nodosa. Arch Dermatol 1974; 110:407.

28. Godman G, Churg J. Wegener's granulomatosis. Pathology and review of the literature. Arch Pathol Lab Med 1954; 58:533–553.

29. Davson J, Ball J, Platt R. The kidney in periarteritis nodosa. Q J Med 1948; 17:175–202.

30. Jennette JC, Falk RJ, Andrassy K, Bacon PA, Churg J, Gross WL, Hagen EC, Hoffman GS, Hunder GG, Kallenberg CGM, McCluskey RT, Sinico RA, Rees AJ, van Es LA, Waldherr R, Wiik A. Nomenclature of systemic vasculitides: The proposal of an international consensus conference. Arthritis Rheum 1994; 37:187–192.

31. Schmorl G. Discussant following Marchand F. Ueber das Verhältnis der Syphilis und Arteriosklerose zur Entstehung der Aortenaneurysmen. Verhandl Dtsch Path Gesellsch 1904; 6:203.

32. Versé M. Periarteriitis nodosa und Arteriitis syphilitica cerebralis. Beitr Path Anat Allg Path (Ziegler's), 1906; 40:409.

33. Meyer P. Ueber Periarteriitis nodosa oder multiple Aneurysmen der mittleren und kleineren Arterien. Arch Path Anat Physiol Klin Med 1878; 74:277.

34. Klemperer P, Otani S. Malignant nephrosclerosis. Arch Path 1931; 11:60.

35. Grant RT. Observations on periarteritis nodosa. Clin Sci 1940; 4:245.

36. Lamb AR. Periarteritis nodosa: Clinical and pathological review of disease with report of two cases. Arch Intern Med 1914; 14:481.

37. Lüpke F. Über Periarteriitis nodosa bei Axishirschen. Verhandl Dtsch Gesellsch Inn Med 1906; 10:149.
38. Jaeger A. Die Periarteriitis nodosa: eine vergleichend-pathologische Studie. Arch Path Anat Physiol Klin Med 1909; 197:71.
39. Ophüls W. Periartertiis acuta nodosa. Arch Intern Med 1923; 32:870.
40. Gruber GB. Zur Frage der Periarteriitis nodosa, mit besonderer Berucksichtigung der Gallenblasen- und Nieren-Beteiligung. Arch Path Anat Physiol Klin Med 1925; 258:441.
41. Otani S. Zur Frage nach dem Wesen der sogenannten Periarteriitis nodosa. Frankfurt Ztschr Path 1924; 30:208.
42. von Haun F. Pathohistologische und experimentelle Untersuchungen über Periarteriitis nodosa. Arch Path Anat Physiol Klin Med 1920; 227:90.
43. VonGlahn WC, Pappenheimer AM. Specific lesions of peripheral blood vessels in rheumatism. Am J Pathol 1926; 2:235.
44. Rich AR. The role of hypersensitivity in periarteritis nodosa. Bull Johns Hopkins Hosp 1942; 71:123.
45. Lichtenstein L, Fox LJ. Necrotizing arterial lesions resembling those of periarteritis nodosa and focal visceral necrosis following administration of sulfathiazole. Am J Pathol 1946; 22:665.
46. French AJ. Hypersensitivity in the pathogenesis of the histopathologic changes associated with sulfonamide chemotherapy. Am J Pathol 1946; 22:679.
47. Black-Schaffer B. Pathology of anaphylaxis due to sulfonamide drugs. Arch Pathol 1945; 39:301.
48. Zeek PM, Smith CC, Weeter JC. Studies on periarteritis nodosa. III. The differentiation between the vascular lesions of periarteritis nodosa and of hypersensitivity. Am J Pathol 1948; 24:889.
49. Zeek PM. Periarteritis nodosa and other forms of necrotizing angiitis. N Engl J Med 1953; 248:764.
50. Churg J, Strauss L. Allergic granulomatosis, allergic angiitis, and periarteritis nodosa. Am J Pathol 1951; 27:277.
51. Heberden W. Commentarii de Marlbaun. Historia et curatione. London: Payne, 1801.
52. Heberden W. Purpureae maculae. Commentaries on the History and Cure of Diseases. London, 1802: 395–397.
53. Willian R. On Cutaneous Diseases. London: J Johnson, 1808.
54. Ollivier C. Développement spontané d'ecchymoses cutanées avec œdème aigu cous-cutané, et gastro-entérite; observation recueillie par le docteur Ollivier (d'Angers). Arch Gén Med 1827; 15:206.
55. Schönlein JL. Allgemeine und specielle Pathologie und Therapie. Vol. 2. 3d ed. Würzburg: Herisau, 1837:48.
56. Henoch EHH. Über eine eigenthümliche Form von Purpura. Berl Klin Wochenschr 1874; 11:641.
57. Henoch EHH. Vorlesungen über Kinderkrankheiten. 10th ed. Berlin: Hirschwald, 1899:839.
58. Osler W. Visceral lesions of purpura and allied conditions. Br Med J 1914; 1:517.
59. Frank E. Die essentielle Thrombopenie. Berl Wochenschr 1915; 52:454.
60. Glanzmann E. Die Konzeption der anaphylaktoiden Purpura. Jahrb Kinderh 1920; 91:391.
61. Klinger H. Grenzformen der Periarteritis nodosa. Frankfurt Ztschr Pathol 1931; 42:455.
62. Rössle R. Zum Formenkreis der rheumatischen Gewebsveränderungen mit besonderer Berücksichtigung der rheumatischen Gefässentzündungen. Arch Pathol Anat Physiol Klin Med 1933; 288:780.
63. Wegener F. Über generalisierte, septische Gefässerkrankungen. Verh Dtsch Ges Pathol 1936; 29:202.
64. Wegener F. Über eine eigenartige rhinogene Granulomatose mit besonderer Beteiligung des Arteriensystems und der Nieren. Beitr Pathol 1939; 102:36.
65. Churg J, Strauss L. Allergic granulomatosis (abstr). Am J Pathol 1949; 25:817.
66. Rackemann FM, Greene CC. Periarteritis nodosa and asthma. Trans Assoc Am Physicians 1939; 54:112.
67. Harkavy J. Vascular allergy, III. J Allergy 1942–1943; 14:507.
68. Wilson KS, Alexander HL. The relation of periarteritis nodosa to bronchial asthma and other forms of human hypersensitiveness. J Lab Clin Med 1945; 30:195.
69. Hutchinson J. Diseases of the arteries. On a peculiar form of thrombotic arteries of the aged which is sometimes productive of gangrene. Arch Surg (London) 1890; 1:323.
70. Horton BT, Magath TB, Brown GE. An undescribed form of arteritis of the temporal vessels. Mayo Clin Proc 1932; 7:700.
71. Horton BT, Magath TB. Arteritis of the temporal vessels: Report of seven cases. Mayo Clin Proc 1937; 12:548.

72. Paulley JW, Hughes JP. Giant-cell arteritis, or arteritis of the aged. Br Med J 1960; 2:1562.

73. Morgagni GB. De sedibus et causis morborum per anatomen indagatis. Lib. II, De Morbis Thoracis, Epist Anat Medica XVIII, Absolvitur Sermo de respiratione Laesa a Cordis aut Magnae Arteriae intra Thoracem Aneurysmatibus 34:173; 1761.

74. Davy J. Notice of a case in which the arteria innominata and the left subclavian and carotid arteries were closed without loss of life. In: Researches, Physiological and Anatomical. London: Smith Elder, 1839, and Philadelphia: Waldie, 1840.

75. Savory WS. Case of a young woman in whom the main arteries of both upper extremities and of the left side of the neck were throughout completely obliterated. Med Chir Tr (London) 1856; 39:205.

76. Takayasu M. Case with unusual changes of the central vessels in the retina. [in Japanese]. Acta Soc Ophthalmol Jpn 1908; 12:554.

77. Judge RD, Currier RD, Gracie WA, Figley MM. Takayasu's arteritis and the aortic arch syndrome. Am J Med 1962; 32:379.

78. Beneke R. Ein eigentümlicher Fall schwieliger Aortitis. Arch Path Anat Physiol Klin Med 1925; 254:722.

79. Niimi Y. A case of Dr. Takayasu's disease. [in Japanese]. J Gen Ophthalmol 1941; 35:1404.

80. Shimizu K, Sano K. Pulseless disease. J Neuropathol Clin Neurol 1951; 1:37.

81. Caccamise WC, Okuda K. Takayasu's or pulseless disease. An unusual syndrome with ocular manifestations. Am J Ophthalmol 1954; 37:784.

82. Feigenbaum A. Description of Behçet's syndrome in the Hippocratic third book of endemic diseases. Br J Ophthalmol 1956; 40:355.

83. Jones WHS. Hippocrates, with an English translation by WHS Jones. London: Heinemann, Loeb Classical Library. Vol. 1. 1923:246–247.

84. Adams F. The Genuine Works of Hippocrates translated from the Greek. Vol. 1. London: Sydenham Society, 1849:403–404.

85. Shigeta T. Recurrent iritis with hypopyon and its pathological findings. Acta Soc Ophthalmol Jpn 1924; 28:516.

86. Adamantiadis B. Sur un cas d'iritis à hypopyon recidivante. Ann Oculist 1931; 168:271.

87. Whitwell GPB. Recurrent buccal and vulval ulcers with associated embolic phenomena in skin and eye. Br J Dermatol 1934; 46:414.

88. Behçet H. Über rezidivierende, aphthöse, durch ein Virus verursachte Geschwüre am Mund, am Auge und an den Genitalien. Dermatol Wochenschr 1937; 105:1152.

89. Kawasaki T. Acute febrile mucocutaneous lymph node syndrome in children associated with unusual hand and foot desquamation: Clinical observation of 50 cases. [in Japanese]. Jap J Allerg 1967; 16:178.

90. Lie JT. Illustrated histopathologic classification criteria for selected vasculitis syndromes. Arthritis Rheum 1990; 33:1074.

91. Churg J. Nomenclature of vasculitic syndromes: A historical perspective. Am J Kidney Dis 1991; 18:148.

92. Hunder GG, Arend WP, Bloch DA, Calabrese LH, Fauci AS, Fries JF, Leavitt RY, Lie JT, Lightfoot RW Jr, Masi AT, McShane DJ, Michel BA, Mills JA, Stevens MB, Wallace ST, Zvaifler NJ. The American College of Rheumatology 1990 Criteria for the classification of vasculitis. Arthritis Rheum 1990; 33:1065.

16
Epidemiology of Vasculitis

Jaya K. Rao
Duke University, Durham, North Carolina

Mary Frances Cotch*
National Eye Institute, National Institutes of Health, Bethesda, Maryland

I. INTRODUCTION

Elucidating the epidemiology of the vasculitides is a challenge made complicated by the relative rarity of the respective conditions, difficulty in disease classification, variable time lag between onset of symptoms and diagnosis, and unknown etiologies. Recent progress has been made, however, in describing clinical characteristics, improving treatment options, and estimating incidence and prevalence rates for these syndromes. In this chapter, we describe the key features central to all epidemiological research, present a summary of different types of epidemiological investigations, and provide an overview of the epidemiology of specific vasculitic conditions by citing recently published papers.

II. DEFINING VASCULITIS AND THE EXTENT OF DISEASE

An accurate diagnosis is important to patients, clinicians, and researchers alike. Unfortunately, the diagnosis, reporting, and treatment of vasculitis is hampered by the lack of universal gold standards for these conditions (1,2). To make matters worse, any given type of vasculitis might present atypically or with features of another type. Furthermore, it may be difficult to obtain tissue confirmation because of problems biopsying often-focal vasculitic lesions. Thus, the diagnosis of vasculitis is usually made on the basis of compatible clinical features along with consistent, but not necessarily pathognomic, biopsy or angiography results in patients for whom other diagnoses are excluded (i.e., infections, malignancies). Although several classification schemes based on pathological and/or serological criteria have been proposed (3), universally accepted criteria useful for diagnostic as well as research purposes have yet to be developed for the vasculitides (2,4,5).

Several general principles apply when evaluating investigations of new diagnostic algorithms or tests (6). One looks for an independent and unbiased comparison between findings as

---

* This chapter is the result of independent research and does not represent the views of NIH, DHHS, or the Government.

determined by the diagnostic algorithm (or test) under consideration and those obtained using the commonly accepted gold standard. Both should be applied to the same study population, namely one that includes individuals with a broad clinical spectrum of the disease of interest (i.e., treated, untreated, active, mild, severe, etc.) as well as persons presenting with other commonly confused syndromes that have similar symptoms or clinical features. The process for selecting the patient population and a description of the clinical environment in which the research was performed are critical factors in interpreting the reported sensitivity, specificity, and predictive value of a diagnostic algorithm or tests. For diagnostic tests, in particular, knowledge about the test itself, such as the definition of a normal result, techniques for performing the test, and measurements of test precision, are also important.

III. CHARACTERIZING DISEASE POPULATIONS BY PERSON, PLACE, AND TIME

Epidemiology provides the "who, what, when, and where" associated with a given disease. In addition to estimating incidence and prevalence rates, epidemiologists examine characteristics shared by diseased persons (such as demographic, environmental, or genetic factors) to describe patterns of disease. From this knowledge base, associations between a given factor and the disease as well as interrelationships among multiple factors can be investigated to identify persons at increased risk and generate hypotheses for future study. In this way, epidemiological investigations may complement insights gained from clinical medicine and basic science in directing efforts to improve our understanding about pathogenesis. Different study designs are employed to address specific research questions in the epidemiological study of vasculitis.

IV. CASE REPORTS AND CASE SERIES

Because the vasculitides are relatively rare conditions and their etiologies are unknown, it is often difficult to conduct analytically meaningful population-based studies. Case reports and case series can be quite useful for describing interesting or unusual disease manifestations in a given patient or group of patients, for reporting alleged disease clusters in the context of routine clinical practice, and, if documenting a longitudinal experience, for characterizing the natural history of disease.

Although numerous examples abound in the medical literature, the following two reports may serve as illustrative examples of a case report and case series, respectively. Finkel et al. (7) describe the clinical course of three pediatric patients with systemic vasculitis and evidence of parvovirus B19 infection; all three had resolution of their infection and vasculitis after receiving intravenous immunoglobulin. Jundt et al. (8) describe a series of 46 patients with biopsy-proven temporal arteritis who were seen at a single clinic. Eight patients had occipital neuralgia as an initial presenting feature, and 6 of these 8 patients had normal erythrocyte sedimentation rates. The authors encourage the consideration of giant cell arteritis in the differential diagnosis of elderly persons presenting with occipital pain.

Taken together, a number of case reports may be extremely informative, particularly when the condition is rare. For example, Ramsey-Goldman (9) surveyed the literature and amassed information on the natural history of disease and pregnancy experience in 20 women with Wegener's granulomatosis, 13 women with polyarteritis nodosa and 4 women with Churg–Strauss syndrome. Overall, well-controlled disease resulted in a favorable outcome for both mother and child.

Information from individual reports or a compilation of reports may also stimulate hypotheses for subsequent testing in future analytical epidemiological research. Terai et al. (10) measured the vascular endothelial growth factor (VEGF) in a series of 30 patients with acute Kawasaki disease and found production of VEGF to be increased, therefore suggesting a potential role for VEGF in the pathophysiology of the disease.

V. CASE–CONTROL STUDIES

Case–control designs, particularly useful when studying rare conditions such as vasculitis, are used to investigate the association between disease and a risk factor (or exposure) in a cross-sectional or retrospective manner. Cases are identified because they have disease; controls are chosen to be disease-free and comparable to the cases in every way except for the risk factor of interest. The sample of cases needs to be sufficiently large to rule out the possibility that chance would influence the results (11). The selection of an appropriate control group is critical in minimizing the potential for selection bias. Strategies exist for minimizing this and other biases (11), including the option of selecting all cases and randomly sampling controls from the same population. Another technique is to select retrospectively an unbiased sample of cases and controls from a preestablished cohort (i.e., a nested case–control study). Other strategies to ensure comparability of the control population include matching each case with multiple controls.

Russo et al. (12) used a matched case–control design to examine retrospectively a possible association between infection and the onset of giant cell arteritis. Biopsy-proven cases of giant cell arteritis were sex-matched with a control group of patients who were admitted to the hospital for corrective surgery for hip fracture. The same criteria were used to classify the presence of infection among the cases and the controls. Giant cell arteritis patients were 3.5 times more likely to have evidence of infection compared with sex-matched non–giant cell arteritis controls (OR, 3.5; 95% CI, 1.8–7.0) (12).

Maeno et al. (13) evaluated the role of VEGF in Kawasaki disease by cross-sectionally and longitudinally measuring serum levels of VEGF in 22 patients with Kawasaki disease, 22 febrile children with infection, and 19 healthy children. Although serum VEGF levels were not found to correlate with clinical symptoms or inflammatory markers, children *with* coronary artery lesions had elevated VEGF levels in the subacute stage of their Kawasaki disease, while children *without* coronary artery lesions experienced elevated VEGF levels in the acute stage of Kawasaki disease (13).

VI. COHORT STUDIES

In a cohort study, a group of individuals is selected because of their exposure status and resultant increased likelihood of developing disease. The cohort is then followed to determine the actual incidence of a given outcome (14). In prospective cohort studies, exposure data are accrued longitudinally and outcomes are assessed at a future date. In retrospective cohort studies, information on risk factors or other predictor variables is collected after the outcomes have occurred. In other words, the investigator assembles the cohort, assesses outcome (disease) in all members, and, thereafter, documents past exposures.

In a study of 45 patients with systemic necrotizing vasculitis, retrospective data were supplemented by personal interviews to assess the patients' current status. Study investigators performed survival analysis to identify factors that were predictive of the 24 deaths that occurred over the 5-year follow-up period (15). In multivariate analyses, cardiac or renal involvement was associated with an increased risk of dying (RR, 2.9; 95% CI, 1.3–6.8); comorbid conditions and disease severity were not found to be predictive of prognosis (15).

VII. FAMILY STUDIES

Family studies are often undertaken to determine whether there is an increased risk of disease within a family. However, if familial clustering is found, this does not, by itself, implicate an inherited predisposition to disease since family members often share the same environment. Twin studies comparing the concordance of disease in monozygotic and dizygotic twins are useful to evaluate estimates of heritability (16). Ultimately, molecular genetic studies with use of elaborate statistical models are required to evaluate the independent effects of genes, environmental factors, and possible gene–environment interactions influencing the expression of a disease.

Cuadrado et al. (17) studied a consecutive series of 60 systemic vasculitis patients and their families in London to discover if systemic vasculitis had an allergic component. Compared with a control group of 60 randomly selected patients with other rheumatic disorders and 60 healthy individuals, the prevalence of allergies was significantly higher in the patients with systemic vasculitis and their families. Whether this association between allergy and vasculitis among family members of a vasculitis case is due to a common predisposing genetic factor, a shared environmental factor triggering allergies (which may or may not be related to vasculitis), or a combination of the two is unclear.

Multiple cases of Kawasaki disease have been noted to occur in a family (18–20). Matsubara et al. (20) describe five episodes of Kawasaki disease occurring over a 6-year period in three siblings. Disease in two of the siblings recurred and resulted in coronary artery lesions. In a survey of households having a child with Kawasaki disease, Fujita et al. (19) reported a second-case rate of 2.1% occurring within 1 year after the initial onset of the first case compared with a rate of 0.2% in the general population of children ages 4 and under. Fifty-four percent of these second cases occurred within 10 days of the index case. Sasazuki et al. (18) noted the occurrence of coincident disease to be more likely among twin pairs compared with nontwin siblings, although significant differences between monozygotic twins (14.1%) and dizygotic twins (13.3%) were not observed. These studies suggest that having a genetic predisposition is not sufficient to cause expression of Kawasaki disease.

VIII. POPULATION-BASED STUDIES

Because case series or case–control studies may suffer from referral or selection biases, population-based studies are preferable to estimate the incidence and prevalence rates of disease based on typical (or "generalizable") patients representative of persons in the community. However, even population-based studies may contain biases if, for example, accurate denominator data are not used in estimating the rates or if disease severity is not considered. Estimates of incidence and prevalence are also influenced by the ability of clinicians to accurately and reliably diagnose disease. With the advent of biological markers and recommended diagnostic criteria, increased clinical awareness of vasculitis may result in improvements in diagnosis and a subsequent increase in rates (21).

Pettersson et al. (22) assembled retrospectively a cohort of 719 adults who had diagnostic renal biopsies between 1986 and 1992 in Sweden. From an estimated population of 1.2 million adults, the annual incidence of pauci-immune necrotizing and crescentic glomerulonephritis was estimated at 0.8 per 100,000 persons (71 cases), doubling from 0.6 per 100,000 in 1986 to 1.2 per 100,000 in 1992 (22).

The Norwich Health Authority in the United Kingdom includes a centralized referral hospital, regional hospitals, and 77 general practices covering the entire surrounding population of 414,500 individuals (23). A prospective registry of vasculitis patients has been maintained since 1988. Using this database, Carruthers et al. (24) estimate the annual incidence of Wegener's granulomatosis to be 8.5 per million (95% CI, 5.2–12.9), while the annual incidence of cutaneous vasculitis is estimated to be 38.6 per million (95% CI, 30.6–48.1) (23).

In the United States, Olmstead County, Minnesota, contains one of the best sources of population-based data, largely due to an elaborate and long-standing record-linkage system at the Mayo Clinic and its clinical affiliates. Based on these data, Salvarani et al. (25) reported 245 incident cases of polymyalgia rheumatica in Olmstead County between 1970 and 1991. The average annual age- and sex-adjusted incidence rate of polymyalgia rheumatica was estimated to be 52.5 per 100,000 persons ages 50 and older (95% CI, 45.9–59.2) (25).

IX. HEALTH SERVICES RESEARCH

Health services research is a diverse and growing field of investigation broadly based on the measurement of disease outcomes. Parameters of interest could include functional status, quality of life, costs of care, delivery of care, and patient satisfaction. Although various methodological approaches are employed depending on the research question, it is often difficult or expensive to collect the primary data upon which to base these types of analyses. Instead, secondary data sources, such as hospital databases, pathology records, autopsy results, billing records, and death certificates are used. Because these data are collected routinely for nonresearch purposes, they are often subject to methodological concerns regarding their validity and reliability. Cases may be identified on the basis of assigned diagnostic codes in clinical, administrative, and billing databases, and when possible, should be validated by reviewing a random sample of patient records or physician notes.

Cotch et al. (26) used the National Hospital Discharge Survey, United States Vital Statistics data on deaths, and hospitalizations in the State of New York to estimate the prevalence, annual mortality, and geographical distribution of Wegener's granulomatosis. The prevalence of Wegener's granulomatosis was estimated to be approximately 3.0 per 100,000 persons in the United States (26). Between 1979 and 1988, 1784 death certificates listed Wegener's granulomatosis as a cause of death, resulting in a national average mortality rate of 0.8 death per million persons (26).

The extent to which the disease affects an individual is particularly important when comparing baseline patient characteristics or disease outcomes either cross-sectionally or longitudinally within a given patient and across different study populations. For the vasculitides, as for other chronic systemic diseases requiring toxic therapy, it is often difficult to capture this information (27). A weighted clinical activity index, the Birmingham Vasculitis Activity Score (BVAS), was developed and applied to 213 individuals with systemic vasculitis in the United Kingdom to monitor disease activity and progression over time (28). The same researchers also developed the Vasculitis Damage Index (VDI), applied the VDI to 100 patients with systemic vasculitis, and found it to be a valid and sensitive tool for quantifying disease-related damage (29,30). In a subsequent study, the investigators documented the utility of the VDI in quantifying the severity of systemic vasculitis as measured by damage (31). Although the authors caution against using these scores to compare severity across the different vasculitides, serial use of these indices for a given patient is encouraged. Validation of the BVAS and the VDI in other vasculitis populations is warranted.

X. INTERVENTION STUDIES

In their ideal form, randomized, controlled trials are carefully designed double-blind studies with a rigorous protocol, complete follow-up of all patients, well-defined outcome measures, and adequate statistical power. It is usually difficult to amass enough patients with vasculitis to conduct a randomized controlled trial at a single institution. Thus, patients from multiple academic institutions must have their data combined or be referred to specialized centers, such as the National Institutes of Health, to mount an adequately powered study. Although random treatment allocation within each institution should theoretically eliminate any systematic patient differences among the treatment arms, it is often difficult to prevent subtle differences in implementation within and across enrolling clinicians and at multiple institutions even with a standardized protocol. Therefore, the study protocol should include quality control measures to monitor for differences as the study progresses, and the statistical analysis plan should include methods to examine potential differences by enrolling clinician and clinical center.

When deciding if the results of a randomized trial are applicable to one's own patients, it is important to recognize that the inclusion and exclusion criteria of the trial participants in terms of disease severity, disease activity, and extent of damage, for example, can impact on treatment outcomes. Evaluating treatment strategies in the context of randomized clinical trials for specific vasculitic conditions is a topic covered in other chapters in this text.

XI. SELECTED VASCULITIC SYNDROMES

A. Polymyalgia Rheumatica

In Denmark, all hospitals are legally required to report all new cases of polymyalgia rheumatica to the national patient registry of the Danish Health authorities (32). Elling et al. (32) analyzed these data from 13 of the 16 counties of Demark (approximately 4.3 million people or 80% of the total population) for the years 1982 to 1993, and estimated an incidence rate of 41.3 per 100,000 persons (95% CI, 30–67) aged 50 and older (32). Investigators from South Norway estimated an incidence rate of 112.6 per 100,000 persons (33).

Bahlas et al. (34) studied consecutive patients with polymyalgia rheumatica and/or giant cell arteritis who attended the Edmonton Rheumatic Disease Clinic between 1989 and 1996. Chart audits were performed to obtain demographic and clinical information; these data were supplemented by patient interviews to determine outcomes. Nearly 100% of patients were treated with corticosteroids, and the mean duration of treatment was 28 months; complete remission was achieved in 54% of patients. Seventeen patients developed rheumatoid arthritis subsequent to their diagnosis of polymyalgia rheumatica.

B. Giant Cell Arteritis

In Olmstead County, Minnesota, there were 125 incident cases of giant cell arteritis diagnosed between 1950 and 1991, with an age- and sex-adjusted incidence rate of 17.8 per 100,000 persons ages 50 and older (95% CI, 14.7–21.0) (35). Incident cases were clustered in five peak periods occurring every 7 years. This cyclical finding provides indirect support for the hypothesis of an infectious etiology of giant cell arteritis. Patients with giant cell arteritis were 17.3 times (95% CI, 7.9–33.0) more likely to develop a thoracic aortic aneurysm and 2.4 times (95% CI, 0.8–5.5) more likely to develop an isolated abdominal aortic aneurysm compared with Olmstead County residents of the same age (36).

The age- and sex-adjusted incidence of giant cell arteritis in Jerusalem was estimated to be 10.2 per 100,000 individuals aged 50 and older (95% CI, 8.0–12.3) (37). Baldursson et al. (38), working in Iceland, estimated the incidence to be 27 per 100,000 persons aged 50 years and older (95% CI, 22.7–32.1). In a prospective Danish study, the overall annual incidence of giant cell arteritis was estimated to be 21.5 per 100,000 persons while the incidence among persons aged 50 years and older was 76.6 per 100,000 persons (39).

Using prebiopsy clinical and laboratory data from a cohort of patients who underwent temporal artery biopsies at the Mayo Clinic, Gabriel et al. (40) developed a mathematical model to predict temporal artery biopsy results. Although the model had limited value in predicting positive biopsy results, it identified 60 (11%) of 525 people with ≥95% probability of a negative biopsy (40). This model may be useful to identify patients who *would not* benefit from temporal artery biopsy.

Follow-up was obtained for 95.8% of the 214 patients with giant cell arteritis enrolled in the multicenter 1990 American College of Rheumatology Classification Cohort (41). The survivorship of giant cell arteritis patients in this cohort was virtually identical to that observed in an age-, sex-, and race-matched sample of the general population. The standard mortality ratio (the ratio of observed deaths to the number of expected deaths in the same age group in the population) for patients with giant cell arteritis in Lugo, Spain, was calculated to be 0.80 (95% CI, 0.47–1.13) (42).

C. Takayasu's Arteritis

The clinical features, angiographic findings, and treatment response in a series of 60 patients with Takayasu's arteritis were reviewed by Kerr et al. (43). The majority of patients (97%) were female; the median age at onset of symptoms was 25 years. The median delay between symptom onset and diagnosis was 10 months. Two-thirds of patients had aortic lesions, 32% of whom had involvement of the aortic arch and its branches. Nearly half of the patients who achieved a remission relapsed within 5 years.

In a consecutive series of 120 Japanese patients with Takayasu's arteritis who were followed for a median of 13 years, the overall survival at 15 years after diagnosis was 82.9% (44). The important prognostic predictors of poor long-term outcome in this group were the presence of complications, progressive clinical course, and high erythrocyte sedimentation rate.

Moriwaki et al. (45) performed a retrospective study of 102 Indian and 80 Japanese patients with Takayasu's arteritis. While most patients were affected in their teens or twenties, the female to male ratio was larger in the Japanese series. Other ethnic differences were noted. For example, aortic regurgitation and vertigo were more common in Japanese patients, while hypertension and headache were more common in Indian patients. These clinical differences may relate to differences in aortic involvement: lesions in the aortic arch and its branches were more commonly seen in the Japanese patients, whereas involvement of the abdominal aorta and its branches was more common in the Indian patients.

D. Kawasaki Disease

Kawasaki disease, a common cause of acquired heart disease in children, has defied repeated research efforts to elucidate its etiology (46). Numerous countries have mounted national campaigns to increase physician awareness of the clinical manifestations associated with the condition and to collect data on incident cases.

In Sweden, a 2-year national prospective study was undertaken to estimate the incidence and describe the clinical pattern of disease in patients with Kawasaki disease (47). The incidence of disease was estimated to be 2.9 per 100,000 children under 16 years of age and 6.2 per 100,000 children under 5 years of age. The median age of those affected was 2.2 years. Males were almost 2.5 times as likely as females to manifest disease. In one family, a 10-month-old girl was diagnosed with Kawasaki disease three days before her 2-year-old brother (47).

In Australia, an active national surveillance system was created to collect information on the epidemiology, management, and rate of cardiological sequelae of Kawasaki disease and other rare conditions (48). Over 900 clinicians, mostly pediatricians, were asked monthly to report all new cases of Kawasaki disease, and provide clinical details for each case. Between May 1993 and June 1995, there were 139 confirmed cases, with an estimated annual incidence in 1994 of 3.7 per 100,000 children younger than 5 years old.

In the United States, 58% of hospitals nationwide reported 8014 hospitalizations for Kawasaki disease and 6238 hospitalizations for acute rheumatic fever between 1984 and 1990 (49). Given that these data are not patient-specific and each patient could have multiple hospitalizations, the actual number of patients hospitalized for Kawasaki disease could not be estimated. Despite these limitations, this type of study is useful in providing a broad estimate of disease prevalence over a large geographical area. Using a state-wide computerized hospital reporting system in Washington State, Davis et al. (50) calculated race-specific incidence rates for Kawasaki syndrome and assessed if there was an association of this disease with residential proximity to water (50). The annual incidence rate for Kawasaki syndrome was 15.2 per 100,000 children younger than 5 years. The incidence rate was highest among Asian Americans (33.3 per 100,000 children), followed by African Americans and Caucasians. No association was found with permanent bodies of water.

In Japan, epidemiological surveys of pediatric departments in all hospitals with at least 100 beds are routine. In the 2-year period beginning in January 1993, 65.5% of hospitals reported 11,458 patients with Kawasaki disease for an annual incidence rate of 95.1 per 100,000 children under 5 years old (51). More hospitalizations occurred in winter and summer than in spring and fall. Age-specific incidence rate peaked at 1 year of age (51). One percent of affected children had a sibling with Kawasaki disease, and 3% of children had recurrent disease (52). The mortality rate at 2 years postdiagnosis in this group was 0.08% (52). Because these data have been collected regularly at 2-year intervals since 1970, secular changes can be monitored. Three peak disease patterns occurred in Japan in 1979, 1982, and 1985–1986, which is suggestive of an infectious etiology for this syndrome (53).

E. Polyarteritis Nodosa

Classical polyarteritis nodosa, a disease that is characterized by inflammation and necrosis of medium-sized arteries, is now considered to be an entity distinct from microscopic polyarteritis, a small-vessel vasculitis. The 1990 American College of Rheumatology (ACR) classification criteria for polyarteritis nodosa did not distinguish between these two syndromes. Watts et al. (54) applied the 1990 ACR criteria for polyarteritis nodosa and the Chapel Hill Consensus Conference (CHCC) definition for microscopic polyarteritis to the Norwich vasculitis registry (54). Based on the ACR criteria, the annual incidence of polyarteritis nodosa was estimated to be 2.4 per million (95% CI, 0.9–5.3). The annual incidence of microscopic polyarteritis according to the CHCC definition was estimated to be 3.6 per million (95% CI, 1.7–6.9).

A cohort, assembled by combining patients at three institutions, had data retrospectively collected to evaluate factors predictive of long-term prognosis of patients with systemic necrotizing vasculitis (15). Of 45 patients, 78% had classical polyarteritis, while 18% had Churg–Strauss disease. There was no association between comorbidity, as measured by the Charlson score, and mortality, but cardiac or renal involvement were associated with poorer survival.

The outcomes of 13 patients diagnosed with polyarteritis nodosa and 12 patients with Churg–Strauss syndrome were compared in a retrospective study (55). The study outcome measures included mortality, a vasculitis damage index, and the pain and disability portions of the Health Assessment Questionnaire. Compared with patients with Churg–Strauss syndrome, patients with polyarteritis nodosa had a higher damage index score, more frequent relapses, higher disability and pain scores, and a higher mortality rate.

F. Wegener's Granulomatosis

In 1992, Hoffman et al. (56) reviewed the clinical features and outcomes of 158 patients with Wegener's granulomatosis who were followed at the National Institutes of Health. The mean duration of follow-up was 8 years, and 84% received "standard" treatment with daily oral cyclophosphamide and steroids. Standard treatment resulted in complete remission in 75% of patients, but one or more relapses occurred in 50% of patients after complete remission.

Follow-up information was obtained for 77 (90.6%) of the 85 patients with Wegener's granulomatosis who were part of the American College of Rheumatology vasculitis classification study (57). Overall, the mortality of patients with Wegener's granulomatosis exceeded that of the general population. At 5 years of follow-up, survival of these patients was only 75% of that for the general population. Patients with multisystem disease had a higher mortality compared with those with limited disease, although the difference was not statistically significant.

A survey of 60 patients with well-characterized Wegener's granulomatosis highlighted the impact of this disease on functional status, health-related quality of life, and social functioning (58). Eighty percent reported subnormal energy level with varying degrees of compromised ability to perform activities of daily living. More than half of the patients who were employed prior to the onset of their illness had to modify their work arrangement.

G. Behçet's Syndrome

Genetic and environmental factors may both play a role in the development of Behçet's syndrome, a disease that commonly occurs in the Far and Middle East where there is a high prevalence of HLA-B5 (59). Zierhut et al. (60) conducted a retrospective study of 28 Mediterranean and 11 German patients who were seen for Behçet's syndrome at the University of Tubingen between 1971 and 1993. While genital ulceration was more common in the German patients, ocular manifestations were more common in the Mediterranean patients. Both groups showed a similar association of disease with HLA-B5 antigen, which was present in 66.7% and 54.4% of the German and Mediterranean patients, respectively, compared with a normal HLA-B5 antigen frequency of 5.9% and 16.6%, respectively, in these two ethnic groups.

In Greece, Koumantaki et al. (61) found 80% of 62 patients having Greek ancestry and satisfying the International Study Group criteria for Behçet's disease to carry HLA allele B*5101 compared with 26% of 87 healthy controls matched for age and ethnicity. Although the HLA B*5101 allele may serve as a marker for disease and not be involved directly in its development, the presence of this allele was shown to be associated with a younger age of disease onset and the development of erythema nodosum. Whether this single allele is the only predisposing allele for the HLA-B51 antigen is unknown.

Yazici et al. (62) analyzed data from 152 patients who were newly enrolled in a Behçet's syndrome clinic in Istanbul between 1982 and 1983 to determine the 10-year mortality among these patients. Follow-up information at 10 years was obtained for 79% of the patients, of whom 6 had died during this interval. Two of the six who died were between 15 and 24 years of age, resulting in a higher than expected mortality rate for patients in this age group compared with the general population.

XII. ADVANCING EPIDEMIOLOGICAL AND HEALTH SERVICES RESEARCH

Further progress in understanding the epidemiology of vasculitis would be helpful on several fronts. Efforts to identify specific risk factors for initial onset of disease may aid a more timely diagnosis, and, in turn, treatment of early disease may minimize its extent and severity, decrease the time required to achieve remission, and, possibly, reduce the probability of recurrence. Improving our knowledge of the characteristics predisposing to disease may also inform novel therapeutic strategies whose promise can be evaluated subsequently in randomized clinical trials. Understanding the long-term outcomes of vasculitis, including functional status and patient-reported quality of life, may improve options for tailoring a treatment protocol for a given patient. The latter will become increasingly important given the now chronic (as opposed to fatal) nature of the various vasculitides and the growing emphasis on the role of patient preferences in medical management. Finally, estimates of the direct and indirect costs of vasculitis will demonstrate the impact of these diseases on an individual and societal level.

Advancement of these research goals will be facilitated by the universal acceptance of strict diagnostic criteria, the creation of multicenter disease registries that use standardized data collection procedures, and the development of reliable and valid disease severity indices and quality of life measures. Further epidemiological investigation will complement clinical and basic science research in advancing our understanding of these complex syndromes.

REFERENCES

1. Fries JF, Hochberg MC, Medsger TA, Hunder GG, Bombardier C. Criteria for rheumatic disease. Different types and different functions. The American College of Rheumatology Diagnostic and Therapeutic Committee. Arthritis Rheum 1994; 37(4):454–462.
2. Hoffman GS. Classification of the systemic vasculitides: Antineutrophil cytoplasmic antibodies, consensus and controversy. Clin Exp Rheumatol 1998; 16:111–115.
3. Lie JT. Nomeclature and Classification of Vasculitis: Plus Ca Change, Plus C'est La Meme Chose. Arthritis Rheum 1994; 37(2):181–186.
4. Rao JK, Allen NB, Pincus T. Limitations of the 1990 American College of Rheumatology Classification Criteria in the diagnosis of vasculitis. Ann Intern Med 1998; 129:345–352.
5. Watts RA, Scott DGI. Classification and epidemiology of the vasculitides. Balliere's Clin Rheumatol 1997; 11(2):191–217.
6. Sackett DL, Haynes RB, Guyatt GH, Tugwell P. Clinical Epidemiology: A Basic Science for Clinical Medicine. Boston: Little, Brown, 1991.
7. Finkel TH, Torok TJ, Ferguson PJ, Durigon EL, Zaki SR, Leung DYM, et al. Chronic parvovirus B19 infection and systemic necrotizing vasculitis: Opportunistic infection or aetiologic agent? Lancet 1994; 343:1255–1258.
8. Jundt JW, Mock D. Temporal arteritis with normal erythrocyte sedimentation rates presenting as occipital neuralgia. Arthritis Rheum 1991; 34(2):217–219.
9. Ramsey-Goldman R. The effect of pregnancy on the vasculitides. Scand J Rheumatol 1998; 27(suppl 107):116–117.

10. Terai M, Yasukawa K, Narumoto S, Tateno S, Oana S, Kohno Y. Vascular endothelial growth factor in acute Kawasaki disease. Am J Cardiol 1999; 83:337–339.
11. Fletcher RH, Fletcher SW, Wagner EH. Clinical Epidemiology: The Essentials. 2d ed. Baltimore: Williams & Wilkins, 1988.
12. Russo MG, Waxman J, Abdoh AA, Serebro LH. Correlation between infection and the onset of giant cell (temporal) arteritis syndrome. Arthritis Rheum 1995; 38(3):374–380.
13. Maeno N, Takei S, Masuda K, Akaike H, Matsuo k, Kitajima I. Increased serum levels of vascular endothelial growth factor in Kawasaki disease. Pediatr Res 1998; 44:596–599.
14. Cummings SR, Ernster V, Hulley SB. Designing Clinical Research. In: Hulley SB, Cummings SR, eds. Baltimore: Williams & Wilkins, 1988:63–74.
15. Fortin PR, Larson MG, Watters AK, Yeadon CA, Choquette D, Esdaile JM. Prognostic factors in systemic necrotizing vasculitis of the Polyarteritis Nodosa Group—A review of 45 cases. J Rheumatol 1995; 22:78–84.
16. Khoury MJ, Beaty TH, Cohen BH. Fundamentals of Genetic Epidemiology. New York: Oxford University Press, 1993.
17. Cuadrado MJ, D'Cruz D, Lloyd M, Mujic F, Khamashta MA, Hughes GRV. Allergic disorders in systemic vasculitis: A case-control study. Br J Rheumatol 1994; 33:749–753.
18. Sasazuki T, Harada F, Kawasaki T. Genetic analysis of Kawasaki disease. Prog Clin Biol Res 1987; 250:251–255.
19. Fujita Y, Nakamura Y, Sakata K, Hara N, Kobayashi M, Nagau M. Kawasaki disease in families. Pediatrics 1989; 84:666–669.
20. Matsubara T, Furukawa S, Ino T, Tsuji A, Park I, Yabuta K. A sibship with recurrent Kawasaki disease and coronary artery lesion. Acta Paediatr 1994; 83(9):1002–1004.
21. Watts RA, Carruthers DM, Scott DGI. Epidemiology of systemic vasculitis: Changing incidence or definition? Semin Arthritis Rheum 1995; 25(1):28–34.
22. Pettersson EE, Sundelin B, Heigl Z. Incidence and outcome of pauci-immune necrotizing and crescentic glomerulonephritis in adults. Clin Nephrol 1995; 43(3):141–149.
23. Watts RA, Jolliffe VA, Grattan CEH, Elliott J, Lockwood M, Scott DGI. Cutaneous vasculitis in a defined population: Clinical and epidemiological associations. J Rheumatol 1998; 25:920–924.
24. Carruthers DM, Watts RA, Symmons DA, Scott DGI. Wegener's granulomatosis: Increased incidence or increased recognition? Br J Rheumatol 1996; 35:142–145.
25. Salvarani C, Gabriel SE, O'Fallon WM, Hunder GG. Epidemiology of polymyalgia rheumatica in Olmstead County, Minnesota, 1970–1991. Arthritis Rheum 1995; 38:369–373.
26. Cotch MF, Hoffman GS, Yerg DE, Kaufman GI, Targonski P, Kaslow RA. The epidemiology of Wegener's granulomatosis: Estimates of the five-year period prevalence, annual mortality, and geographic disease distribution from population-based data sources. Arthritis Rheum 1996; 39(1):87–92.
27. Luqmani RA, Exlet AR, Kitas GD, Bacon PA. Disease assessment and management of the vasculitides. Balliere's Clin Rheumatol 1997; 11:423–446.
28. Luqmani RA, Bacon PA, Moots RJ, Janssen BA, Pall A, Emery P, et al. Birmingham Vasculitis Activity Score (BVAS) in systemic vasculitis. Q J Med 1994; 87:671–678.
29. Exley AR, Carruthers DM, Luqmani RA, Kitas GD, Gordon C, Janssen BA, et al. Damage occurs early in systemic vasculitis and is an index of outcome. Q J Med 1997; 90:391–399.
30. Exley AR, Bacon PA, Luqmani RA, Kitas GD, Gordon C, Savage COS, et al. Development and initial validation of the vasculitis damage index for the standardized clinical assessment of damage in the systemic vasculitides. Arthritis Rheum 1997; 40(2):371–380.
31. Exley AR, Bacon PA, Luqmani RA, Kitas GD, Carruthers DM, Moots R. Examination of disease severity in systemic vasculitis from the novel perspective of damage using the vasculitis damage index (VDI). Br J Rheumatol 1998; 37:57–63.
32. Elling P, Olsson AT, Elling H. Synchronous variations of the incidence of temporal arteritis and polymyalgia rheumatica in different regions of Denmark: Association with epidemics of *Mycoplasma pneumonia* infection. J Rheumatol 1996; 23:112–119.
33. Gran JT, Myklebust G. The incidence of polymyalgia rheumatica and temporal arteritis in the County of Aust Agder, South Norway: A prospective study 1987–1994. J Rheumatol 1997; 24:1739–1743.

34. Bahlas S, Ramos-Remus C, Davis P. Clinical outcome of 149 patients with polymyalgia rheumatica and giant cell arteritis. J Rheumatol 1998; 25:99–104.

35. Salvarani C, Gabriel SE, O'Fallon WM, Hunder GG. The incidence of giant cell arteritis in Olmstead County, Minnesota: Apparent fluctuations in a cyclic pattern. Ann Intern Med 1995; 123:192–194.

36. Evans JM, O'Fallon WM, Hunder GG. Increased incidence of aortic aneurysm and dissection in giant cell (temporal) arteritis. Ann Intern Med 1995; 122:502–507.

37. Sonnenblick M, Nesher G, Friedlander Y, Rubinow A. Giant cell arteritis in Jerusalem: A 12-year epidemiologic study. Br J Rheumatol 1994; 33:938–941.

38. Baldursson O, Steinsson K, Bjornsson J, Lie JT. Giant cell arteritis in Iceland. Arthritis Rheum 1994; 37:1007–1012.

39. Boesen P, Sorenson SF. Giant cell arteritis, temporal arteritis, and polymyalgia rheumatica in a Danish county: A prospective investigation, 1982–1985. Arthritis Rheum 1987; 30(3):294–299.

40. Gabriel SE, O'Fallon WM, Achkar AA, Lie JT, Hunder GG. The use of clinical characteristics to predict the results of temporal artery biopsy among patients with suspected giant cell arteritis. J Rheumatol 1995; 22:93–96.

41. Matteson EL, Gold KN, Bloch DA, Hunder GG. Long-term survival of patients with giant cell arteritis classification cohort. Am J Med 1996; 100:193–196.

42. Gonzalez-Gay MA, Blanco R, Abraira V, Garcia-Porrua C, Ibanez D, Riguerio MT, et al. Giant cell arteritis in Lugo, Spain, is associated with low long-term mortality. J Rheumatol 1997; 24:2171–2176.

43. Kerr GS, Hallahan CW, Giordano J, Leavitt RY, Fauci AS, Rottem M, et al. Takayasu arteritis. Ann Intern Med 1994; 120:919–929.

44. Ishikawa K, Maetani S. Long-term outcome for 120 patients with Takayasu's disease: Clinical and statistical analyses of related prognostic factors. Circulation 1994; 90:1855–1860.

45. Moriwaki R, Noda M, Yajima M, Sharma BK, Numano F. Clinical manifestations of Takayasu arteritis in India and Japan: New classification of angiographic findings. Angiology 1997; 48:369–379.

46. Mason WH, Takahashi M. Kawasaki syndrome. Clin Infect Dis 1999; 28:169–187.

47. Schiller B, Fasth A, Bjorkhem G, Elinder G. Kawasaki disease in Sweden: Incidence and clinical features. Acta Pediatr 1995; 84:769–774.

48. Royle JA, Williams K, Elliott E, Sholler G, Nolan T, Allen R, et al. Kawasaki disease in Australia, 1993–1995. Arch Dis Child 1998; 78:33–39.

49. Taubert KA, Rowley AH, Shulman ST. Seven-year national survey of Kawasaki disease and acute rheumatic fever. Pediatr Infect Dis J 1994; 13:704–708.

50. Davis RL, Waller PL, Mueller BA, Dykewicz CA, Schonberger LB. Kawasaki syndrome in Washington State: Race-specific incidence rates and residential proximity to water. Arch Pediatr Adolesc Med 1995; 149:66–69.

51. Yanagawa H, Nakamura Y, Yashiro M, Ojima T, Koyanagi H, Kawasaki T. Update of the epidemiology of Kawasaki disease in Japan from the results of 1993–1994 nationwide survey. J Epidemiol 1996; 6(3):148–157.

52. Yanagawa H, Yashiro M, Nakamura Y, Kawasaki T, Kato H. Epidemiologic pictures of Kawasaki disease in Japan: From the nationwide incidence survey in 1991 and 1992. Pediatrics 1995; 95(4):475–479.

53. Yanagawa H, Yashiro M, Nakamura Y, Hirose K, Kawasaki T. Nationwide surveillance of Kawasaki disease in Japan, 1984 to 1993. Pediatr Infect Dis J 1995; 14(1):69–71.

54. Watts RA, Jolliffe VA, Carruthers DM, Lockwood M, Scott DGI. Effect of classification criteria on the incidence of polyarteritis nodosa and microscopic polyangiitis. Arthritis Rheum 1996; 39(7):1208–1212.

55. Abu-Shakra M, Smythe H, Lewtas J, Badley E, Weber D, Keystone E. Outcome of polyarteritis nodosa and Churg-Strauss syndrome. An analysis of twenty-five patients. Arthritis Rheum 1994; 37(12):1798–1803.

56. Hoffman GS, Kerr GS, Leavitt RY, Hallahan CW, Lebovics RS, Travis WD, et al. Wegener's granulomatosis: An analysis of 158 patients. Ann Intern Med 1992; 116(6):488–498.

57. Matteson EL, Gold KN, Bloch DA, Hunder GG. Long-term survival of patients with Wegener's granulomatosis from the American College of Rheumatology Wegener's granulomatosis classification criteria cohort. Am J Med 1996; 101:129–134.

58. Hoffman GS, Drucker Y, Cotch MF, Locker GA, Easley K, Kwoh K. Wegener's granulomatosis: Patient-reported effects of disease on health, function and outcome. Arthritis Rheum 1998; 41(12):2257–2261.

59. Rigby AS, Chamberlain MA, Bhakta B. Behçet's disease. Ballieres Clin Rheumatol 1995; 9:375–395.

60. Zierhut M, Saal J, Pleyer U, Kotter I, Durk H, Fierlbeck G. Behçet's disease: Epidemiology and eye manifestations in German and Mediterranian patients. German J Ophthalmol 1995; 4:246–251.

61. Koumantaki Y, Stavropoulos C, Spyropoulou M, Messini H, Papademetropoulos M, Giaiaki E. HLA-B*5101 in Greek patients with Behçet's disease. Hum Immunol 1998; 59:250–255.

62. Yazici H, Basaran G, Hamuryudan V, Hizli N, Yurdakul S, Mat C, et al. The ten-year mortality in Behçet's syndrome. Br J Rheumatol 1996; 35:139–141.

17
General Approach to the Diagnosis of Vasculitis

Brian F. Mandell

Cleveland Clinic Foundation, Cleveland, Ohio

I. INTRODUCTION

The differential diagnosis of the vasculitic syndromes includes many diverse disorders that result in organ ischemia, localized inflammation, and/or constitutional symptoms. While acute or sub-acute multisystem dysfunction should heighten concern for the presence of a vasculitic syndrome, nonvasculitic diseases can also present with involvement of multiple organ systems. Conversely, systemic vasculitis can manifest with involvement of a single anatomical region or organ. The pattern of expression of a specific vasculitic disorder may evolve or change over periods of time, independently of therapeutic interventions. For all of these reasons, and the continued controversy over diagnostic criteria, it is difficult at present to devise an evidence-based algorithmic approach to diagnosis, or even accurately describe the operating characteristics of many of the diagnostic tests we utilize. As a general principle, pathological documentation of vasculitis should be pursued whenever feasible. The possibility of a primary infectious or malignant disorder producing the vasculitis should also be considered. Serological or angiographic studies may support the clinical diagnosis of a primary vasculitic syndrome, but should *not* supplant efforts to exclude alternative diagnoses or document the presence and histological pattern of vasculitis. The clinician's ability to confidently diagnose a specific primary vasculitic syndrome is plagued by (1) frequent overlap of clinical patterns of disease among the different syndromes, especially early in the course of the illness; (2) difficulty in obtaining histopathology that is "diagnostic" of a single *specific* vasculitic syndrome; (3) lack of unequivocally diagnostic serological tests; (4) limited understanding of the role that viral and other infectious agents play in the development of some forms of vasculitis; and (5) limitations in our ability to delineate an ideal classification system. Nonetheless, the physician caring for patients with severe multisystem illnesses must quickly define the nature of the disease process. Either delayed or inappropriately aggressive therapeutic intervention may put the patient at risk for an adverse outcome.

II. VASCULITIS OR NOT?

The constitutional and ischemic symptoms and findings induced by the primary vasculitic syndromes, when viewed in isolation, may be identical to those produced by infection, occlusive vascular diseases, or malignancy. Particularly early in the course of an illness, when nonlocalizing constitutional symptoms or involvement of a single organ system may predominate, clinical distinction among these disease processes can be difficult. It is prudent to exclude certain diseases while concurrently attempting to prove the presence of a primary vasculitic disorder. The expected prevalence of an illness in the population, and the physician's prior experience exert critical influences on the derivation, initial hierarchy, and evolution of the differential diagnosis. For example, a previously healthy 48-year-old male who presents with fever, dyspnea, and infiltrates on a chest radiograph most likely has an infectious pneumonia. Although Wegener's granulomatosis, antiglomerular basement membrane disease, and microscopic polyangiitis may present in a similar manner, these uncommon entities are not likely to be the initial focus of concern. If that same patient also has (asymptomatic) glomerulonephritis, as suggested by an active urine sediment, the rank ordered differential diagnosis list will be immediately altered to emphasize pulmonary infections capable of causing glomerulonephritis (e.g., legionella, pneumococcus, and right-sided endocarditis) and certain autoimmune systemic disorders, including some forms of primary systemic vasculitis. Alternatively, the young patient who is found to have multifocal "pneumonia" and coexistent recalcitrant sinus disease, intermittent otitis media, and scleritis is reasonably considered to have a higher likelihood of Wegener's granulomatosis, because no single common illness can easily account for all of these abnormalities. Although uncommon, this diagnosis should therefore be actively pursued from the outset of the evaluation, while other more mundane possibilities are simultaneously excluded. The middle-aged woman who develops palpable purpura, fever, and a foot drop may well have a chronic hepatitis C infection, contracted from forgotten blood transfusions related to her previous hysterectomy. In this scenario, her trivially elevated serum transaminase levels and past medical history may not initially suggest chronic hepatitis, but the pattern of illness is compatible with several disorders, including systemic vasculitis related to viral hepatitis.

The first task of the clinician when approaching the patient with multisystem disease is to accurately catalog areas of disease involvement—by careful history and physical examination. Review of a few basic and directed laboratory studies may be helpful to focus attention toward a nonvasculitic disorder (Table 1). Not all of these tests are required in the evaluation of all patients. Test selection should be based on the patient's clinical presentation and the resultant differential diagnosis. The operating characteristics of each laboratory test, as well as more invasive biopsy studies, strongly depend upon the pretest likelihood of the specific disease that is being sought. "False positive" tests are particularly likely to be obtained when the pretest probability of a specific diagnosis is low. There are no specific blood tests to diagnose vasculitis. Thus, laboratory testing should initially be used to document the type and degree of organ involvement, exclude nonvasculitic disorders, and support the suspected clinical diagnosis. Examination of a freshly obtained urine sample is a mandatory part of the evaluation. This test may provide the only clue to the presence of glomerulonephritis, a serious but usually asymptomatic process.

Many nonvasculitic disorders cause signs, symptoms, and laboratory findings that also occur in patients with systemic vasculitis. A partial categorical list is outlined in Table 2. These diagnoses should be *selectively* considered as warranted by the patient's clinical and laboratory presentation. For example, endovascular infections, including infectious endocarditis (IE), can elicit constitutional symptoms, glomerulonephritis, and vascular occlusion with resultant ischemia and infarction. The type and virulence of the organism, the valvular site of infection, prior antibiotic use, and the underlying status of the patient influence the clinical expression of endocarditis. Infectious endocarditis can mimic several forms of systemic vasculitis. Musculoskeletal, neurological, constitutional, pulmonary, or renal symptoms and findings may dominate the clinical presentation. Laboratory immunological abnormalities may include rheumatoid factor and hypocomplementemia. Immune complexes related to bacterial or viral infections may be present in some patients, em-

Table 1 Selected Laboratory Tests in the Initial Evaluation of Patients with Multisystemic Disease and Possible Vasculitis

Test	Comments
Platelet count	*Thrombocytosis* may parallel the acute phase response.
	Thrombocytopenia not expected in primary vasculitic syndromes. Consider SLE, marrow infiltration, hairy cell leukemia, TTP, DIC, hypersplenism, APLS, HIV, scleroderma renal crisis, heparin-induced thrombocytopenia.
WBC count	*Leukopenia* not expected in primary vasculitis. Consider SLE, leukemia, hypersplenism, sepsis, myelodysplasia, and HIV.
	Eosinophilia common in Churg-Strauss. May occur in Wegener's granulomatosis, rheumatoid arthritis, normotensive scleroderma renal crisis.
ESR	Relatively *low ESR* seen in DIC, liver failure, and hyperviscosity. Frequently low in HSP. May be low in Takayasu's arteritis.
Transaminases	Elevated ALT or AST in liver disease, myositis, rhabdomyolysis, hemolysis, myocardial necrosis.
Anti-GBM	Evaluation of alveolar hemorrhage, with or without GN. Evaluation of normocomplementemic GN.
ANA	Order when there is clinical suspicion of SLE, not a general screening test.
ANCA	Order when there is clinical suspicion of WG, MPA, unexplained normocomplementemic GN without extensive tissue immune deposits.
Drug screen	Unexplained CNS symptoms, myocardial ischemia, vascular spasm, panic attacks with systemic features, tachycardia. Urine screen should be done.
Blood cultures	Febrile, multisystem or wasting illness, pulmonary infiltrates, focal ischemia/infarction. Have low threshold to obtain cultures.
APLA/PTT/RVVT	Unexplained venous or arterial thrombosis, thrombocytopenia.
PPD ($\pm$anergy)	Anyone who may require steroid therapy, has unexplained sterile pyuria or hematuria, granulomatous inflammation, chronic meningitis, or possible exposure to TB.
Angiotensin converting enzyme	Neither sensitive nor specific for sarcoidosis—not a good screening test.
Examination of *fresh* urinary sediment	Perform in everyone with an unexplained febrile or multisystem illness.
Hepatitis serologies	Abnormal transaminases or elevated hepatic alkaline phosphatase, portal hypertension. PAN or MPA syndrome. Unexplained cryoglobulinemia, polyarthritis, cutaneous vasculitis.
Complement C3, C4	Not screening tests for vasculitis. Useful in the differential diagnosis of GN. Low in cryoglobulinemia, may be low in endocarditis. Usually normal in PAN, MPA, HSP, WG. May be low in viral hepatitis–related GN or vasculitis.
Aldolase	Has no specificity–similar organ distribution as LDH.

GN, glomerulonephritis; ANA, antinuclear antibody; ANCA, antineutrophil cytoplasmic antibody; APLA, antiphospholipid antibody; RVVT, Russell viper venom test; TTP, thrombotic thombocytopenic purpura; DIC, disseminated intravascular coagulation; GN, glomerulonephritis; LDH, lactic dehydrogenase.

Table 2 Mimics of Primary Systemic Vasculitis

Infection
  Endocarditis
  Neisseria
  Mycotic aneurysms
  Histoplasmosis
  Syphilis
  Viral hepatitis
  Whipple's disease
Drug toxicity/poisoning
  Cocaine, sympathomimetics
  Allopurinol
  Diphenylhydantoin
  Arsenic
Coagulopathies
  Antiphospholipid antibody syndrome
  Disseminated intravascular coagulation
  Thrombotic thrombocytopenic purpura
Malignancy
  Lymphoma
  Carcinomatosis
  POEMS syndrome
Cardiac myxomas
Generalized atherosclerosis
Cholesterol embolization syndrome
Calciphylaxis
Buerger's disease
Idiopathic hypereosinophilic syndrome
Sarcoidosis

phasizing the necessity of excluding infections, even when vasculitis is demonstrated. The diagnosis of IE is not always straightforward and should be considered in virtually all patients with unexplained multisystem disease. Several diagnostic criteria have been proposed and evaluated (1). At least three sets of blood cultures should be obtained, but cultures have been negative in up to 20% of patients in some series. Identifiable reasons for negative cultures have included inappropriate culture technique, fastidious organisms, prior antibiotic use, and perhaps right-sided valvular disease. Improvements in echocardiographic imaging techniques have led to the present practice of initial screening for endocarditis with transthoracic echocardiography (TTE), followed by transesophageal echocardiography (TEE) if the TTE is negative. Transesophageal echocardiography has detected vegetations in up to 41% of patients with definite endocarditis in whom conventional TTE was negative (2). Incorporation of echocardiography into the diagnostic criteria has improved the sensitivity of clinical diagnosis to between 80–100% in different studies (2), but the specificity is not 100%.

Other, less common intracardiac conditions can also mimic a primary systemic vasculitis. Atrial myxomas represent the most common primary cardiac tumor, but are rare. Similar to patients with IE, those with atrial or ventricular myxomas present with one or more of the clinical triad including constitutional, embolic, and valvular obstructive features (3). Transthoracic echocardiography is the initial study of choice, and has an estimated sensitivity of >90%; TEE may add additional sensitivity and provide more information useful to the cardiac surgeon. Etiologies of noninfective valvular and endocardial vegetations, which can cause similar embolic manifestations, include nonbacterial thrombotic endocarditis, hypereosinophilic syndrome, Libman–Sacks endocarditis, and intracavitary thrombosis. The last two disorders may be associated with the antiphospholipid antibody syndrome. Echocardiography (4) remains the initial study of choice for each of these entities that may cause embolic manifestations.

Some disorders mimic vasculitic syndromes due to the occurrence of regional or diffuse thromboocclusion. Thrombotic thrombocytopenic purpura (TTP) causes diffuse small-vessel occlusions, usually in conjunction with mild–moderate renal dysfunction, fever, and neurological features. The presence of significant thrombocytopenia and a microangiopathic hemolytic anemia should prompt the consideration of this diagnosis in lieu of a primary vasculitis. Thrombosis due to antiphospholipid antibody syndrome (APLS), however, may not be so readily distinguished from a primary vasculitis. The APLS can be associated with thrombotic occlusion of veins and arteries of virtually any caliber, and in any organ distribution (5). Regional ischemia in the absence of constitutional symptoms or markers of systemic inflammation warrants consideration of diseases causing bland thrombosis, or atherosclerosis. However, the systemic reaction to regional ischemic necrosis, or the common concurrence of systemic lupus erythematosus (SLE) with APLS may cause diagnostic confusion. Biopsy of ischemic tissue may reveal relatively noninflammatory thrombosis, or angiography may indicate vascular occlusion without evidence for arteritis; but neither study is entirely satisfactory at distinguishing between thrombosis and vasculopathy. Thrombocytopenia and Coombs'-positive hemolytic anemia may be present in patients with primary or SLE-related APLS, and should suggest a diagnosis other than primary vasculitis.

Antiphospholipid antibodies (APLAs) are detectable in 80–90% of patients with APLS, but can be found in association with other conditions, even when thrombosis is not present (6). The APLAs are generally persistent and of moderate to high titers in patients with APLS, but they may be low or even undetectable. Lupus anticoagulant (LAC) activity should be sought in conjunction with tests for APLA. The LAC may be a more specific test for APLS with thrombosis, and is present in up to 20% of APLA-negative patients who have the syndrome (7). Unfortunately, it is less sensitive than the enzyme-linked immunosorbent assay (ELISA)-based APLA assays. Patients should be screened for the presence of LAC using a phospholipid-sensitive partial thromboplastin time and, if this test is negative, a second test such as the dilute Russell viper venom or kaolin clotting time should be performed. If abnormal, further tests should be utilized to confirm the presence of a LAC and exclude the presence of a factor deficiency or specific factor inhibitor as the cause for the abnormal coagulation test(s). In the future, tests to detect antibodies with specificity to beta2-glycoprotein 1 may become the assays of choice to diagnose APLS. Thrombosis may first be suspected at the time of biopsy or angiogram when searching for vasculitis. Unexplained thrombosis should prompt a work-up for the appropriate hypercoagulable states most consistent with the arterial or venous location of thrombosis. The presence of APLA or LAC, in the absence of venous or arterial thrombosis (or frequent miscarriages), is of unclear significance.

Cholesterol embolization syndrome (40), which may follow an angiographic procedure, lytic therapy of an arterial clot, or large-vessel surgery, can produce symptoms and findings of local ischemia plus laboratory and clinical abnormalities suggestive of a vasculitis. Patients may have fever, livedo reticularis, and rising creatinine—usually a slowly stuttering course. Blood and urine eosinophilia can occur. Acute phase reactants can be elevated, and complement components may be depressed. The setting should suggest the possibility of this diagnosis, which can be histologically proven by finding telltale cholesterol clefts occluding small arteries and arterioles.

Patients should be specifically asked about prescribed, over-the-counter, and illicit drug use. Drug allergies may manifest as fever and constitutional symptoms, or include purpura, pulmonary infiltrates, or interstitial nephritis. Sympathomimetic drugs, including intranasal or oral neosynephrine and ephedrine, may induce spasm and cause Raynaud's disease and/or central neurological dysfunction. Common related sympathomimetic street drugs of abuse include "MOMA," "ecstasy," "CAT," "speed," and "crack cocaine." If the possibility of vascular spasm is considered, as suggested by history or angiography, a urine drug screen for the presence of cocaine, amphetamine, and their metabolites should be promptly performed. Some other drugs reported to cause a systemic vasculitis include allopurinol, minocycline, thiazides, propylthiouracil, and acutane. Discussion with the clinical pathologist prior to test selection may prove to be of value since tests differ among laboratories. The metabolites are rapidly cleared from the circulation, and even a negative urine screen utilizing sensitive chromatographic techniques does not exclude intermittent use of these drugs.

The possibility of malignancy causing systemic symptoms should not be forgotten. Different tumor types have been described in association with a myriad of paraneoplastic syndromes. The most commonly reported association is between leukemias/myelodysplasia and cutaneous small-vessel vasculitis. Paraneoplastic involvement of peripheral nerve is uncommon, but can mimic ischemic neuropathy and a systemic vasculitic syndrome (8). Renal cell carcinoma is frequently cited as a cause of systemic paraneoplastic syndromes, but this is a complication of only 5% of these tumors (9), and many other carcinomas can produce similar diagnostic dilemmas. The presence of significant inflammatory synovitis seems uncommon in paraneoplastic syndromes, although some malignancies, including hairy cell and other leukemias, have been strongly associated with arthritis (10), and case reports have included carcinoma-associated paraneoplastic synovitis (21). The presence of thrombocytopenia or leukopenia should increase concern over a possible malignancy. The frequency of cytopenias besides anemia in patients with primary vasculitic syndromes is difficult to ascertain from the literature, but seems to be quite low. Acute digital spasm and dramatic necrosis have been described in patients with carcinoma (10), as well as with lymphoproliferative related cryoglobulinemia. Regional imaging should be utilized to evaluate a possible mass causing unexplained organ dysfunction or laboratory abnormalities (e.g., stroke syndromes, dyspnea, elevations in alkaline phosphatase, or hematuria without dysmorphic erythrocytes or casts), and any identified infiltration or mass lesion should generally be biopsied, if accessible.

Defined systemic autoimmune disorders such as SLE should be sought using serological tests only if the clinical pretest likelihood of the disease is high. The presence of thrombocytopenia or leukopenia in the setting of a systemic disorder warrants at least consideration of this diagnosis. The antinuclear antibody test is best used to exclude the diagnosis of SLE, when the test is negative. The value of initially screening *all* patients with unexplained multisystem disease for the presence of "abnormal" serological tests, such as anti-RNP, rheumatoid factor, anti-SCL-70, anti-JO-1, ANA, ANCA, etc., is arguable.

In conjunction with excluding the most likely nonvasculitic diseases, it is necessary to attempt documentation of the presence of vasculitis as part of the diagnostic process. A tissue diagnosis of vasculitis is preferred, but not always possible to obtain. Depending upon the suspected diagnosis, certain involved tissues may have a higher or lower likelihood of providing disease specific histopathology. Demonstrating the presence of vasculitis or glomerulonephritis by biopsy may not be sufficient to confirm the final diagnosis. For example, finding mesenteric vasculitis at laparotomy may not distinguish between Wegener's granulomatosis and polyarteritis nodosa. Documenting cutaneous small-vessel vasculitis will not permit distinction between microscopic polyangiitis (MPA), Wegener's granulomatosis (WG), and infection related small-vessel vasculitis. The severity and rate of progression of the patient's illness should dictate the tempo, scope, and degree of invasiveness of the evaluation. This often requires concurrent efforts to confirm or exclude several of the most likely diagnostic possibilities in an acutely ill patient. Infectious and paraneoplastic associations with (secondary) vasculitis are increasingly being recognized, and these are discussed further in the next section.

Histopathology remains the gold standard for the documentation of vasculitis. The pathology results should be coupled with the clinical pattern of disease to make the diagnosis of a specific primary vasculitic syndrome. Although this represents the ideal approach, it is fraught with several pragmatic limitations. Biopsy of accessible tissue, which is not clearly involved by the disease process, should be eschewed since the diagnostic yield is low. It has been estimated that the yields from random biopsy of nonclinically involved muscle or nerve for the diagnosis of polyarteritis nodosa are 29% and 19%, respectively (11). Initial biopsy efforts should be directed toward tissue that is abnormal by clinical, laboratory, or other objective testing. Sural nerve biopsy has become a popular option when attempting to diagnose an arteritis that is affecting medium-sized muscular vessels. The sural nerve is an accessible pure sensory nerve, and its vasa nervorum contains small as well as medium-sized muscular arteries. Nerve conduction studies can identify a diseased ischemic nerve prior to the appearance of clinical symptoms (12). Multiple case reports, however, have emphasized the low diagnostic yield from the biopsy of asymptomatic and electrically normal nerves. Even nerves with abnormal conduction studies have been reported to reveal no diagnostic pathology in 46% of cases (13). In this study, there was notable morbidity associated with the procedure; 13 of 60 patients experienced wound infections or delayed healing, and 3 suffered from new pain in the distribution of the biopsied sural nerve. In a different series of 35 nondiabetic patients with electromyography-confirmed mononeuritis multiplex, only four patients had systemic necrotizing vasculitis. Of these four patients, three had demonstrable vasculitis and one had a nondiagnostic "vasculopathy" on nerve biopsy (14).

Sometimes biopsy of a clinically affected tissue is not feasible. Alternatively, an organ may have suffered ischemic injury with associated necrosis, seem to be the ideal candidate site for biopsy, and not have demonstrable vasculitis on pathology. The absence of arteritis in a surgical sample does not exclude the presence of vasculitis. Sampling error or the presence of occlusive arteritis in vessels proximal to the site of biopsy may explain a "false negative" result. This presents a vexing problem when periluminal ischemia and localized necrosis are demonstrated by endoscopic biopsy of the intestine, but no further pathological diagnosis can be made. In the absence of an acute abdomen, it is difficult to justify an exploratory laparotomy. Thus, biopsy documentation of mesenteric arteritis, the suspected cause of the ischemic bowel disease, may be impractical to obtain. Similarly, only rarely can large-vessel branches of the aorta be sampled. Even when pathological organ specimens can be obtained, it may be difficult to distinguish between true vasculitis and massive transmigration of inflammatory cells into a local area of parenchymal infection, or between vasculitis and angiotrophic malignancies. Special elastin stains may help resolve the former dilemma, while immunophenotyping is often useful in the latter.

The ideal prospective, protocol-directed evaluation of operating characteristics of diagnostic tests, including biopsy, in the different vasculitic syndromes has not been performed. The best diagnostic generalization that can be offered is to biopsy tissue that is clinically involved. When multiple organs are involved, the choice of biopsy site should be dictated by the potential morbidity of the procedure, and the likelihood of obtaining a disease-specific histopathological result. This latter point is discussed below for some of the primary vasculitic syndromes. Even when biopsy is feasible, the sample size must be generous. The vasculitic process may not equally affect all portions of an organ or vessel. The phenomenon of "skip areas" of vasculitic involvement is a well-recognized problem in the diagnosis of giant cell arteritis (temporal arteritis), and generous biopsy of the superficial temporal artery has been recommended (15). The same issue of sample size likely holds true when obtaining a lung, nasal, or sinus biopsy in an effort to document all of the typical pathological features of Wegener's granulomatosis, or a biopsy of symptomatic muscle or nerve in the case of possible vasculitis affecting small and/or medium-sized vessels. Needle, endoscopic, and bronchoscopic biopsies often help to exclude infection, but are generally inferior in yield to excisional biopsies for the diagnosis of vasculitis. Sample size as well as the accessibility of appropriate tissue may play a role in the limitations of the less invasive biopsy techniques.

Antineutrophil cytoplasmic antibodies (ANCAs) with specificity for proteinase 3 (PR3) and myeloperoxidase occur in a high proportion of patients with generalized Wegener's granulomatosis and microscopic polyangiitis, respectively. It is tempting to use these tests in lieu of invasive biopsies, but the sensitivity and specificity of these tests are not perfect. The ANCAs are found in patients with other diseases, including infections, drug-associated vasculitic reactions, and nonvasculitic inflammatory disorders (16). Demonstrating the presence of a circulating ANCA is *not* equivalent to diagnosing vasculitis. Since significant morbidity and mortality may complicate the immunosuppressive therapy of the vasculitic disorders, making the correct diagnosis is of crucial importance. When the pretest likelihood of the diagnosis is extremely high, it may suffice to accept a positive test for anti–PR3 ANCA as strongly supportive of WG. This should only be done in the setting of "classical" WG, after excluding the possibility of coexistent or primary infection. If the diagnosis is made in this manner, any delayed or atypical response to therapy should be pursued with prompt biopsy of an involved organ.

Angiography is a necessary tool in the evaluation of patients who have arteritis or other aneurysmal or occlusive diseases of the aorta and its major branches (e.g., Takayasu's arteritis, sarcoid aortitis, atherosclerosis). It may also aid in diagnosing or following patients with isolated angiitis of the central nervous system, and coronary arteritis due to Kawasaki disease. Complemented by magnetic resonance imaging (MRI), it is possible to obtain images of the large-vessel lumen, and assess arterial wall thickness and associated wall edema, a presumed surrogate of inflammation (24). Magnetic resonance imaging may evolve to become a very useful tool to quantify the severity of arteritis and follow the longitudinal course of the illness. Abdominal angiography is frequently utilized in the evaluation of patients who may have medium-sized vessel arteritis when biopsy has been unrewarding or is not an option. Arteries affected by polyarteritis nodosa (PAN) and other disorders affecting medium-sized muscular arteries may develop microaneurysms or stenoses that can be visualized by angiography. When angiography is used to diagnose systemic necrotizing vasculitis in the absence of pathological evidence of the disease, several caveats must be noted. Angiography has limited spatial resolution; smaller vessels are not well seen. Thus, patients with primarily smaller-vessel disease will not likely have a "diagnostic" angiogram. Only 4 of 30 patients with microscopic polyangiitis, a disease that affects small and medium-sized arteries, had diagnostic renal or celiac angiograms (25). The sensitivity of this test for diagnosing classic PAN is not known, but is most certainly not 100%. Depending upon the definition of microaneurysm, different investigators have reported their presence in 60–90% of patients with PAN (26–28). Aneurysms take time to develop, and may not be present early in the course of the illness. In addition to aneurysms, arteritis may also be associated with stenoses, which may be longer and smoother than typical atherosclerotic lesions, or occlusion (27–29). To maximize the yield from the procedure, angiography should include the celiac, renal, and mesenteric vessels. Lack of clinical involvement of an organ (i.e., no intestinal ischemia) does not exclude the possibility of finding abnormal vessels on angiogram. It has been suggested that the visualization of aneurysms in PAN denotes more severe disease (30); it is unclear whether this may also relate to the actual duration of the illness. Aneurysms may resolve with successful treatment of MPA, PAN, or hepatitis B– or C–related vasculitis (28,31). The presence of visceral microaneurysms is not, however, diagnostic of PAN. They have also been anecdotally described in patients with other forms of vasculitis affecting medium-sized arteries (WG, Churg–Strauss syndrome, Behçet's syndrome). So just as when interpreting a biopsy result of "vasculitis," imaging studies must be considered in the light of the entire clinical profile. Microaneurysms occur in nonvasculitic disorders. Isolated case reports have described aneurysms in patients with atrial myxoma, bacterial endocarditis, peritoneal carcinomatosis, severe arterial hypertension, and following methamphetamine abuse. In a retrospective 10-year survey of 748 patients who underwent abdominal angiography (27), 38 patients had microaneurysms. Seventeen had PAN (in 156 patients the indication for arteriography was possible "arteritis") and seven had severe arterial hypertension. Inadequate data are available to assess the sensitivity, specificity, or predictive value of abdominal angiography in the diagnosis of necrotizing arteritis.

Initiation of empirical glucocorticosteroid therapy is sometimes necessary prior to completion of the diagnostic evaluation. A beneficial response to this intervention should *not* be construed as definitive proof of a primary vasculitic disorder (20), and should not lead to abandonment of an appropriately complete evaluation.

III. SECONDARY VASCULITIS

Many of the disease processes listed in Table 2 are associated with a vasculopathy, or a true vasculitis. Thus, even when vasculitis has been documented, vasculitis may not be the final diagnosis. This is particularly true in the setting of purpura or other manifestations of cutaneous small-vessel vasculitis. Vasculitic involvement of these small vessels has been well described in patients with carcinoma, myelodysplasia, leukemia, endocarditis, viral hepatitis, neisserial and rickettsial infections, and systemic autoimmune processes (e.g., lupus, Sjögren's syndrome, sarcoidosis, inflammatory bowel disease, rheumatoid arthritis). These diagnoses should be considered, in the appropriate clinical setting, even when "vasculitis" has been demonstrated (22). Secondary causes of vasculitis must be excluded before diagnosing a specific primary vasculitic syndrome. The breadth of testing is dependent upon the clinical picture and the pretest probability of a specific primary vasculitic disorder or potential cause of secondary vasculitis. The vasculitides associated with systemic autoimmune disease are discussed in detail in later chapters.

The literature on patients with IE provides multiple caveats relating to the diagnosis of vasculitis without first excluding an underlying chronic infection (17,18). Purpura, mesenteric arterial microaneurysms, glomerulonephritis, retinal vasculitis, cryoglobulinemia, stroke, and arthritis have all been well described in patients with IE. Patients may have a positive rheumatoid factor, cryoglobulinemia, or even high titer ANCA with specificity to PR3 (19). Initial improvement with corticosteroid therapy has been described (20).

Carcinomas have been associated with purpura, fever, and mononeuritis multiplex (21). Secondary vasculitis seems to most commonly involve the small vessels of the skin. In a recent review of 172 adults with cutaneous vasculitis (22), 17 had a systemic necrotizing vasculitis, 4 had malignancy, and 5 had a systemic bacterial infection producing the vasculitis. An additional 20 patients had a defined systemic autoimmune process (e.g., rheumatoid arthritis, SLE, Sjögren syndrome, sarcoidosis), and 11 had "essential" mixed cryoglobulinemia (only 2 were tested for the presence of hepatitis C antibody, 1 was positive). More recent studies have suggested that up to 80% of cases of mixed cryoglobulinemia are due to hepatitis C infection (23). Alternatively, primary vasculitic syndromes including isolated angiitis of the central nervous system (CNS) and Wegener's granulomatosis can occasionally present with localized mass lesions. These examples emphasize the value of a rigorous approach to history-taking, examination, and biopsy when evaluating patients for the presence of these uncommon disorders.

Systemic autoimmune disorders can be associated with a pattern of vasculitis not commonly attributed to the underlying disease. For example, patients with inflammatory bowel disease (IBD) have been described with leukocytoclastic vasculitis, a large-vessel occlusive arteritis (Takayasu's arteritis), and Wegener's granulomatosis (37). Patients with IBD and rheumatoid arthritis may have circulating ANCAs, even in the absence of vasculitis. Patients with systemic lupus erythematosus, rheumatoid arthritis, and sarcoidosis may develop inflammation of the aorta or its major branches.

IV. PRIMARY VASCULITIC DISORDERS

Once vasculitis has been demonstrated, and the more obvious secondary causes eliminated, the clinician's task is to identify the most appropriate diagnostic category that the patient's condition best fits. Diagnostic categorization facilitates predictions of the most likely organs that may be affected by the disease. Accurate diagnosis may also permit a better estimate of the prognosis. In some cases, precise diagnosis may help guide initial therapeutic decisions.

The derivation of a classification scheme of the primary vasculitic syndromes remains an effort in progress. Limited by incomplete knowledge of precipitating triggers and pathogenesis, descriptive classification schemes have primarily focused on the size of the involved blood vessels, the presence or absence (pauci-immune) of significant tissue deposits of immune complexes, the pattern of organ involvement (e.g., upper airway, glomerulus, lung), and the presence or absence of granulomatous inflammation. Patients with infections such as hepatitis C or B, which can produce systemic vasculitic syndromes clinically indistinguishable from PAN or MPA, should be uniquely classified within subsets of secondary vasculitis. Older studies, predating the recognition of hepatitis C, did not make this distinction. An adaptation of one classification scheme (32) is shown in Figure 1. This and other schemes tend to emphasize the characteristics of fulminant or classical disease expression, placing emphasis on the specificity of diagnosis. This frequently leaves the patient with an early, or form fruste, presentation without an appropriate diagnosis if any of the published classification schemes is strictly adhered to. As the patient's disease evolves, an alternative diagnostic category may become more appropriate. For instance, the patient initially diagnosed with MPA on the basis of glomerulonephritis, vasculitic polyneuropathy, alveolar hemorrhage and the presence of P-ANCA, might later be rediagnosed with WG when he develops sinusitis and cavitating pulmonary nodules. The use of "overlap" diagnostic categories in clinical practice highlights the limitations of our current classification systems. Nonetheless, classification schemes remain useful aids to identify patients with fairly homoge-

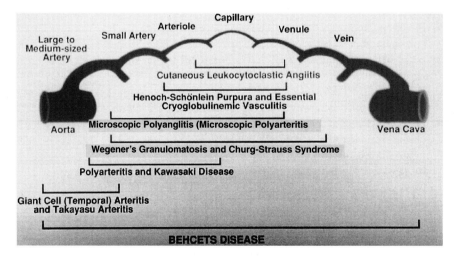

Figure 1 Classification of the systemic vasculitides. (Adapted from Ref. 32.)

neous patterns of disease for participation in clinical trials, and for dictating specific therapies for certain disease groups (i.e., initial combination therapy for patients diagnosed with generalized WG).

After, or simultaneously with, the exclusion of nonvasculitic disorders and the most likely causes of secondary vasculitis, the tentative diagnosis of a primary vasculitic syndrome is made. Detailed descriptions of the individual vasculitic disorders, along with their differential diagnoses, are offered elsewhere in this book. The following comments relate to the diagnostic strategies once a tentative diagnosis of a specific primary vasculitic syndrome is made.

The diagnosis of limited cutaneous vasculitis is absolutely dependent upon the exclusion of the other causes of small-vessel vasculitis. This is the most common type of vasculitis. Small-vessel vasculitis may also be a common component of secondary forms of vasculitis, and may occur in patients with primary vasculitic syndromes affecting predominantly larger vessels. Prior to making the diagnosis of isolated or limited cutaneous vasculitis, other forms of vasculitis must have been ruled out. Purpura generally indicates cutaneous vasculitis, although biopsy may occasionally identify the presence of infiltrative, thrombotic or embolic disorders. Biopsy can also be useful to document the presence or absence of prominent IgA deposition (suggestive of Henoch–Schönlein purpura, HSP), and the deposition of immune complexes at the dermal–epidermal junction (lupus band test). Patients with limited cutaneous vasculitis may not need aggressive treatment. They should receive a detailed physical examination and focused laboratory evaluation, including examination of a freshly obtained urine sediment, stool hemoccult cards, complete blood count, liver enzymes, and hepatitis B and C screening, even in the absence of abnormal transaminase levels. The decision to pursue additional studies should be made on an individual basis. In a recent review of 303 patients with cutaneous vasculitis, almost 100% of patients under the age of 20 had primary vasculitis limited to the skin, or HSP. On the other hand, approximately 40% of adults over 20 years of age had an associated or underlying systemic disorder, and an additional 23% had HSP (22).

The systemic vasculitic disorders that involve the medium-sized muscular arteries (see Figure 1) encompass a wide range of clinical syndromes, various size mixtures of involved vessels, and have several distinct types of histopathology. Some of these syndromes, including classical WG, have predictable enough clinical courses to warrant specific aggressive treatment. This necessitates an aggressive evaluation to confirm the diagnosis of WG, or document the presence of an alternative disorder, in lieu of accepting a more generic diagnosis of necrotizing arteritis.

Classic PAN, the prototypical arteritis affecting medium-sized muscular arteries, is now classified as a non–immune-complex-associated disease affecting only vessels of this size. There are no useful diagnostic serological tests for PAN. Infection with hepatitis B or C or human immunodeficiency virus (HIV), which can cause a PAN-like syndrome, must be excluded. The possible etiological role of other viruses remains to be defined. Purpura, glomerulonephritis, pulmonary capillaritis, and upper airway involvement are not characteristic findings of PAN when a classification scheme based on vessel caliber is strictly adhered to. Their presence in conjunction with documented or suspected medium-sized vessel arteritis should suggest alternative diagnoses, including virus-associated vasculitis and MPA (25). Neurological involvement is common in PAN, and if abnormal sural nerve conduction is documented on electromyography (usually axonal neuropathy), biopsy may demonstrate necrotizing arteritis within the nerve sheath vascular bundle, or only ischemic neuropathy (12). The latter is a suggestive, but not diagnostic, pathological finding. In the absence of readily available, affected organs for biopsy, angiography has been utilized in an effort to demonstrate the presence of microaneurysms in medium-sized arteries. This is a useful but imperfect technique, with still-to-be-defined test characteristics for the diagnosis of PAN. Yet, under the appropriate clinical circumstances, arteriography may provide the only evidence for the presence of a vasculopathy affecting the medium-sized muscular arteries.

Thrombocytopenia and leukopenia are not characteristic of PAN, and their presence in the setting of a polyarteritis-like syndrome suggests an alternative diagnosis such as SLE or hairy cell leukemia. Exclusion of atherosclerotic and thrombotic disease may be difficult, but is necessary. Biopsy of a muscle group with pain suggestive of ischemia (claudication) in the absence of obstructive large-vessel disease may be fruitful. Biopsy of clinically uninvolved muscle is a safe, but fairly low-yield, procedure (11,33). It should be undertaken only if there is no acceptable diseased tissue to biopsy, and arteriography is either unrevealing or unsafe. Insufficient data exist to directly compare the value of open as opposed to a needle muscle biopsy.

Generalized WG is characterized by necrotic, granulomatous inflammation of the lung and upper airway, and glomerulonephritis without extensive immune deposits. Vasculitis affects predominantly the small and medium-sized arteries. Careful attention during the physical examination should be paid to the upper airway, paranasal sinuses, nose, and middle ear; these are areas not affected by classical PAN or MPA. The external eye should also be carefully examined. Glomerulonephritis must be searched for by reviewing freshly obtained urine sediments. Computed tomography (CT) scanning may identify pulmonary and sinus involvement, even when not observed on routine radiographs. ANCA testing has value in the prototypical case (16), but early tissue confirmation of the diagnosis is generally preferable in all but the most classic of circumstances. Vasculitis may at times be difficult to find in the biopsied samples of necrotic lung or upper airway tissue. Small sample size complicates this further; and lesion-directed open lung biopsy has the highest chance of revealing diagnostic pathology. The wide variety of pathological findings seen in the lungs of patients with WG have been described in detail (34). They include the triad of vasculitis, necrotizing inflammation, and granulomas with giant cells. However, all features may not be seen in all specimens. Tissue eosinophilia at times may be significant. It is necessary to exclude the infectious causes of granulomatous inflammation. Biopsy of nerve or kidney is unlikely to provide specific pathological evidence for the diagnosis of WG. Renal biopsy is likely to demonstrate a necrotizing glomerulonephritis with the absence of extensive immune deposits, but no specific findings of WG. Characteristic pathology can at times be found in biopsies of inflammatory lesions in atypical locations, including the lower genitourinary tract (35), skin, or breast.

Microscopic polyangiitis involves medium muscular and smaller arterial beds. Giant cells, which are frequently seen in the inflamed parenchyma of patients with WG, are by definition absent. Upper airway disease is less prominent or absent, but otherwise, patients with MPA may resemble those with WG. Older case series describing patients with "PAN" also included patients with features of MPA, thus accounting for the variable proportion of patients reported as having PAN with glomerulonephritis or alveolar hemorrhage, findings typical of MPA, but not of classic PAN. Patients with MPA may have circulating ANCAs with specificity toward myeloperoxidase and, less often, proteinase 3. However, a positive ANCA, even with myeloperoxidase specificity, is not sufficient to warrant the diagnosis of MPA (16). Renal biopsy generally demonstrates a necrotizing, often proliferative glomerulonephritis without extensive immune complex deposition. Presence of significant immune staining should suggest that the MPA syndrome is secondary to SLE or infection, particularly hepatitis C. Since infection with either hepatitis B or C or HIV can cause a PAN- or MPA-like disease, it is reasonable to exclude these infections in all patients who present with either of these syndromes. Abdominal angiography, if performed, infrequently demonstrates microaneurysms (25).

Churg–Strauss syndrome is a rare vasculitic disorder that clinically and histologically may resemble WG. Patients often have prominent extravascular granulomas, neuropathies, chronic upper airway symptoms and noncavitating pulmonary infiltrates. Patients with Churg–Strauss syndrome (36) invariably have a history of atopy or asthma, often of relatively recent onset. The asthma may abate when the vasculitic phase of the disease begins. Eosinophilia and tissue infiltration with eosinophils is common. Glomerulonephritis is less common and generally less severe than in WG, although renal biopsies may be similar. Cardiac involvement is common, unexplained resting tachycardia should not be ignored. ANCAs, some with antimyeloperoxidase activity, may be present (16), but have no specific diagnostic utility. The diagnosis should be suspected on clinical grounds, and supported by eosinophilia and tissue histopathology of vasculitis, often with prominent eosinophil infiltration. Extravascular granulomatous nodules may occur in the skin.

Giant cell arteritis (GCA) of the elderly is a disorder that affects the extracranial branches of the aorta, as well as the aorta itself. Biopsy of the superficial temporal artery may provide evidence of the characteristic vasculitis with elastic membrane destruction, adventitial cellular infiltration, and giant cells. Giant cells are not uniformly present in all biopsy samples. Skip areas of involvement are typical, and acquisition of a large biopsy specimen is recommended (15). Bilateral temporal artery biopsy seems to increase the diagnostic yield. A particular constellation of symptoms/findings in an elderly patient has a statistically high association with positive superficial temporal artery biopsy: new headache, jaw claudication, and elevated erythrocyte sedimentation rate (ESR). The clinical diagnosis may even be more assured in the coincident presence of polymyalgia rheumatica. When these features rapidly resolve with corticosteroid therapy, the diagnosis of GCA is almost certain. Other types of vasculitis including WG and PAN (38), as well as amyloidosis, have been reported to involve the superficial temporal arteries and cause similar symptoms. A case of atherosclerotic obliterative disease causing amaurosis, unilateral headache, and jaw claudication has been reported (39), carotid artery dissection can cause similar symptoms. There are no specific serologic markers of this disease, and the acute phase response is an imperfect guide to diagnosis (<20% of patients may have a low ESR) or therapy. Giant cell arteritis may cause striking constitutional symptoms, including fevers, wasting, and polymyalgia rheumatica. Peripheral synovitis may occur, but other forms of inflammatory arthritis of the elderly should be excluded (i.e., pseudogout). I generally obtain at least a unilateral biopsy of the superficial temporal artery when the diagnosis of GCA is suspected. Although, a strong argument can be made that the patient should be treated with a trial of corticosteroids, in the setting of the above listed constellation of symptoms, even if the biopsy is negative.

Takayasu's arteritis (TA) and GCA have a similar pattern of vessel involvement. Takayasu's arteritis is diagnosed in younger patients and characteristically affects the more proximal aortic vessels with arch and upper extremity predominance. Tissue-confirmed diagnosis of Takayasu's arteritis is a rarity due to the inaccessibility of suitable biopsy material, except at the time of major vascular surgery. The pathology in Takayasu's arteritis is similar, if not identical, to GCA. The role that vascular magnetic resonance imaging (24) can play in the diagnosis and management of the large-vessel inflammatory disorders remains to be defined. At present, the diagnosis of Takayasu's arteritis is generally made angiographically, but occasionally it is suggested by tissue obtained at the time of aortic or coronary surgery. The possibility that a viral or chlamydial vector is responsible for initiation or perpetuation of these large-vessel diseases remains to be established. The major differential diagnoses include atherosclerosis, fibromuscular dysplasias, sarcoidosis, biochemical disorders of connective tissue, and arterial hypercoagulable states.

V. SUMMARY

The diagnosis of a systemic vasculitic syndrome should be predicated upon clinical evidence obtained from the history and physical examination. The pattern of organ involvement should be delineated as thoroughly as possible by examination, laboratory, and appropriate imaging techniques. The mimics of systemic vasculitis should be excluded, and a tissue diagnosis should be obtained if possible. The site of the biopsy should be determined by the specific suspected diagnosis, coupled with evidence that the site to be biopsied is clinically involved with the disease process. If vasculitis is identified, the secondary causes of vasculitis should be excluded. Testing for specific ANCAs, with identification of the antigen PR3 or myeloperoxidase, should not supplant efforts to obtain a tissue diagnosis, *except* in the most "textbook" cases of Wegener's granulomatosis or microscopic polyangiitis. Giant cell arteritis of the elderly should ideally be diagnosed by biopsy of a superficial temporal artery. Takayasu's arteritis usually must be diagnosed by angiographic demonstration of characteristic stenotic and/or aneurysmal lesions of the major branches of the aortic arch and aorta. The possibility of infection, malignancy, or an unusual drug reaction must always be considered.

REFERENCES

1. Habib G, Derumeaux G, Avierinos JF, Casalta JP, Jamal F, Folot F, Garcia M, Lefevre J, Biou F, Maximovitch-Roadminoff A, Fournier PE, Ambrosi P, Velut JG, Cribier A, Harle JR, Weiller PJ, Raoult D, Luccioni R. Value and limitations of the Duke criteria for the diagnosis of infective endocarditis. JACC 1999; 33(7):2023–2029.
2. Essop R. Transesophageal echocardiography in infective endocarditis: The standard for the 1990s? (editorial) Am Heart J 1995; 130(2):402–404.
3. Markel ML, Waller BF, Armstrong WF. Cardiac myxoma. A review. Medicine 1987; 66(2):114–125.
4. Joffe II, Jacobs LE, Owen AN, Ioli A, Kotler MN. Curriculum in cardiology. Noninfective valvular masses: Review of the literature with emphasis on imaging techniques and management. Am Heart J 1996; 131:1175–1183.
5. Triplett DA. Protean clinical presentation of antiphospholipid-protein antibodies. Thromb Haemost 1995; 74:329–337.
6. Harris EN, Pierangeli SS, Gharavi AE. Review. Diagnosis of the antiphospholipid syndrome: A proposal for use of laboratory tests. Lupus 1998; 7(suppl 2):S144–S148.
7. Triplett DA. Antiphospholipid-protein antibodies: Laboratory detection and clinical relevance. Thromb Res 1995; 78:1–31.
8. Oh SJ. Paraneoplastic vasculitis of the peripheral nervous system. Neurol Clin 1997; 15(4):849–863.
9. Ritchie AWS, Chishol GD. The natural history of renal carcinoma. Semin Oncol 1983; 10:390–400.
10. Nashitz JE, Rosner I, Rozenbaum M, Elias N and Yeshurun D. Cancer associated rheumatic disorders: Clues to occult neoplasia. Semin Arthritis Rheum 1995; 24:231–241.
11. Albert DA, Rimon D, Silverstein MD. The diagnosis of polyarteritis nodosa. I. A literature-based decision analysis approach. Arthritis Rheum 1988; 31(9):1117–1127.
12. Wees SJ, Sunwoo IN, Oh SJ. Sural nerve biopsy in systemic necrotizing vasculitis. Am J Med 1981; 71:525–532.
13. Rappaport WD, Valente J, Hunter GC, Rance NE, Lick S, Lewis T, Neal D. Clinical utilization and complications of sural nerve biopsy. Am J Surg 1993; 166(3):252–256.
14. Hellmann DB, Laing TJ, Petri M, Whiting-O'Keefe Qm, Parry GJ. Mononeuritis multiplex: The yield of evaluations for occult rheumatic diseases. Medicine 1988; 67(3):145–153.
15. Ponge T, Barrier JH, Grolleau JY, Ponge A, Vlasak AM, Cottin S. The efficacy of selective unilateral temporal artery biopsy versus bilateral biopsies for diagnosis of giant cell arteritis. J Rheumatol 1988; 15:997–1000.
16. Hoffman GS, Specks U. Antineutrophil cytoplasmic antibodies: Diagnostic value in systemic vasculitis. Arthritis Rheum 1998; 41:1521–1537.
17. Davis JA, Weisman MH, Dail DH. Vascular disease in infective endocarditis. Report of immune-mediated events in skin and brain. Arch Intern Med 1978; 138:480–483.
18. Trevisani MR, Ricci MA, Michaels RM, Meyer KK. Multiple mesenteric aneurysms complicating subacute bacterial endocarditis. Arch Surg 1987; 122:823–824.
19. Soto A, Jorgensen C, Oksman F, Noel LH, Sany J. Endocarditis associated with ANCA. Clin Exp Rheumatol 1994; 12:203–204.

20. Lawrence EC, Mills J. Bacterial endocarditis mimicking vasculitis with steroid-induced remission. Western J Med 1976; 124:333–334.
21. Poggio ED, Mazzone PJ, Horvath J, Mandell B. Systemic vasculitis and polyarthritis as the presenting feature of renal cell carcinoma. J Clin Rheumatol 1998; 4:266–269.
22. Blanco R, Martinez-Taboada VM, Rodrigues-Valverde V, Garcia-Fuentes M. Cutaneous vasculitis in children and adults: Associated disease and etiologic factors in 303 patients. Medicine 1998; 77:403–418.
23. Agnello V, Chung RT and Kaplan LM. A role for hepatitis C virus infection in type II cryoglobuline-mia. N Engl J Med 1992; 327:1490–1495.
24. Flamm SD, White RD, Hoffman GS. The clinical application of "edema-weighted" magnetic resonance imaging in the assessment of Takayasu's arteritis. Int J Cardiol 1998; 66(suppl 1):S151–S159.
25. Guillevin L, Durand-Gasselin B, Cevallos R, Gayraud M, Lhote F, Callard P, Amourox J, Casassus P and Jarrousse B. Microscopic polyangiitis: Clinical and laboratory findings in 85 patients. Arthritis Rheum 1999; 42:421–430.
26. Travers RL, Allison DJ, Brettle RP, Hughes GR. Polyarteritis nodosa: A clinical and angiographic analysis of 17 cases. Semin Arthritis Rheum 1979; 8:184–199.
27. Hekail P, Kajander H, Pajari R, Stenman S, Somer T. Diagnostic significance of angiographically observed visceral aneurysms with regard to polyarteritis nodosa. Acta Radiol 1991; 32:143–148.
28. Vazquez JJ, San Martin P, Barbado FJ, Gil A, Guerra J, Arnalich F, Garcia Puig J, Sanchez Mejias F. Angiographic findings in systemic necrotizing vasculitis. Angiology 1981; 32(11):773–779.
29. Chatel A, Garnier T, Bigot JM, Toueg C, Lehenon C. Arteriography in polyarteritis nodosa: Diagnostic findings and value of repeated examinations. J Radiol 1979; 60(2):113–120.
30. Ewald EA, Griffin D, McCune WJ. Correlation of angiographic abnormalities with disease manifestations and disease severity in polyarteritis nodosa. J Rheumatol 1987; 14(5):952–956.
31. Darras-Joly C, Lortholary O, Cohen P, Brauner M, Guillevin L. Regressing microaneurysms in 5 cases of hepatitis B virus related polyarteritis nodosa. J Rheumatol 1995; 22(5):876–880.
32. Jennette C, Flak RJ, Andrassy K, Bacon PA, Churg J, Gross WL, Hagen EC, Hoffman GS, Hunder GG, Kallenberg GM, McCluskey RT, Sinico RA, Rees AJ, vanEs LA, Walherr R, Wiik A. Nomenclature of systemic vasculitides: Proposal of an international consensus conference. Arthritis Rheum 1994; 37:187–192.
33. Dahlberg PJ, Lockhart JM, Overholt EL. Diagnostic studies for systemic necrotizing vasculitis. Sensitivity, specificity, and predictive value in patients with multisystem disease. Arch Intern Med 1989; 149:161–165.
34. Travis WD, Hoffman GS, Leavitt RY, Pass HI, Fauci AS. Surgical pathology of the lung in Wegener's granulomatosis. Am J Surg 1991; 15(4):315–333.
35. Goldman HB, Mandell BF, Volk E, Rackley RR and Appell, RA. Urethral diverticulum: An unusual presentation of Wegener's granulomatosis. J Urol 1999; 161:917–918.
36. Guillevin L, Cohen P, Gayraud M, Lhote F, Jarrousse B, Casassus P. Churg-Strauss syndrome: Clinical study and long-term follow-up of 96 patients. Medicine 1999; 78:26–37.
37. Weir A, Taylor-Robinson SD, Poole S, Pignatelli M, Walters JFR, Calam J. Cytoplasmic antineutrophil cytoplasmic antibody-positive vasculitis associated with ulcerative colitis. Am J Gastroenterol 1997; 92(3):506–508.
38. Lie JT. Editorial. When is arteritis of the temporal arteries not temporal arteritis? J Rheumatol 1994; 21(2):186–189.
39. Venna N, Goldman R, Tilak S, Sabin TD. Temporal arteritis-like presentation of carotid atherosclerosis. Stroke 1986; 17(2):325–327.
40. Om A, Ellahham S, and DiScascio, G. Cholesterol embolism: An underdiagnosed clinical entity. Am Heart J 1992; 124:1321–26.

18
Histopathology of Primary Vasculitic Disorders

Johannes Björnsson
Mayo Medical School, Mayo Clinic, and Mayo Foundation, Rochester, Minnesota

I. INTRODUCTION

Numerous unrelated etiologies and pathogenetic pathways may manifest as inflammation of vessels. For the systemic vasculitides, the range of morphological findings is narrower than the clinical spectrum. Morphology is thus only partially reflective of underlying mechanisms and clinical manifestations (1). A certain inflammatory pattern may denote several diseases. Conversely, a given clinical disease or syndrome may manifest itself by more than one inflammatory pattern. Leukocytoclastic vasculitis (LCV) as a *pathological* finding exemplifies this lack of specificity. Leukocytoclastic vasculitis may be identified in such unrelated diseases as drug-induced hypersensitivity vasculitis, Henoch–Schönlein purpura, and Wegener's granulomatosis (2). By the same token, the *disease* giant cell (temporal) arteritis may manifest itself in the biopsy specimen as a transmural granulomatous infiltrate with giant cells or as a nondescript lymphocytic infiltrate in the outer arterial media and adventitia. In diagnostic pathology, therefore, familiarity with the anatomical distribution, vessel size and type, clinical features, and microscopic findings is a prerequisite for meaningful diagnostic interpretation of vasculitic diseases. All parameters must be evaluated and correlated with the morphology before formulating a histopathological diagnosis. A tissue diagnosis that flies in the face of clinical impression is usually wrong. The pathologist's role in the diagnosis of vasculitides is twofold:

1. To confirm the presence or absence of inflammatory injury
2. To characterize and classify the pattern of injury

It is a tenet in the histopathological diagnosis of nonneoplastic diseases that specimens should be initially examined and the pattern of injury determined without prior knowledge of clinical data. The absence of specific and pathognomonic features in most biopsy specimens may lead an already biased pathologist to merely reinforce a clinical impression and possibly perpetuate diagnostic errors. Nevertheless, a definitive diagnosis should never be formulated without correlation with clinical and laboratory findings and consultation with attending physicians. The following review deals with the pathology of the major primary vasculitic syndromes as defined by the American College of Rheumatology in 1990 (3). Each of these clinical entities is discussed under the heading of the predominant histopathological pattern of injury associated with a disease or syndrome.

II. PREDOMINANTLY GRANULOMATOUS VASCULITIS

A. Giant Cell (Temporal) Arteritis

Giant cell arteritis (GCA) is the prototype of a granulomatous vasculitis. The classic appearance is that of transmural inflammation with a predilection for the superficial temporal artery and its branches. Lymphocytes predominate in the infiltrate, accompanied by varying numbers of polymorphonuclear leukocytes, chiefly neutrophils but also eosinophils in approximately 10% of cases. Cellular mucoid intimal thickening causes near-total occlusion of the vascular lumen (Fig. 1a; see color plate). The extent of intimal proliferation correlates with the production of platelet-derived growth factor by macrophages and multinucleated giant cells at the intima–media border (4,5). Epithelioid histiocytes and multinucleated giant cells occupy the junction of intima and media, invariably accompanied by a piecemeal "flea-bitten" destruction of the internal elastic lamina (see Fig. 1b,c; see color plate). Small arterial branches adjacent to the main vessel may be similarly affected (Fig. 2). Lymphocytes may be prominent in the adventitia, often accompanied by fibrotic transformation of the outermost vascular layer (Fig. 3a). In some patients, especially in the early stages of disease, inflammation may be limited to the adventitia. This observation is supported by experimental evidence suggesting that interferon-γ–producing T cells may initially encounter a disease-relevant antigen in the arterial adventitia (6). Multinucleated giant cells are identified in approximately two-thirds of specimens from patients with GCA (7). Their absence

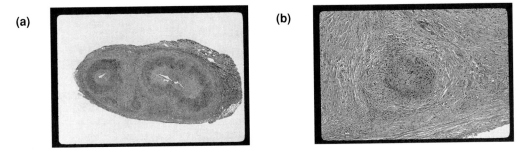

Figure 2   Giant cell (temporal) arteritis. (a) Low-power overview of inflamed main vessel and branches. (b) Detail of small branch of temporal artery with transmural inflammation and luminal occlusion.

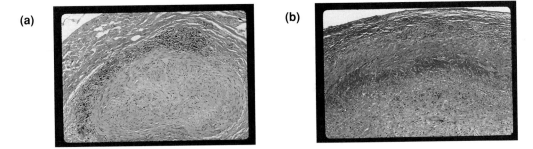

Figure 3   Giant cell (temporal) arteritis. (a) Inflammation limited to the adventitia. (b) Circumferential band-like fibrin deposit in inner media.

does not negate the diagnosis of GCA. The one constant finding is damage to the internal elastic lamina. An intact internal elastic lamina should raise diagnostic possibilities other than GCA. In a minority of patients, a band of fibrinoid deposits is observed in the media (see Fig. 3b). This should not be confused with the transmural fibrinoid necrosis characteristic of polyarteritis nodosa. The relationship between clinical findings and histopathological appearances is variable. A severely ill patient may have mild inflammation on biopsy. Conversely, the histopathological findings may be florid in asymptomatic patients following several weeks of successful treatment with corticosteroids (8,9). Occasionally, attending physicians will postpone corticosteroid treatment until biopsy has been obtained, fearing that a "false-negative" biopsy may result. Such concerns are unnecessary. The structural damage, including inflammatory cells, will persist long after the disappearance of symptoms.

B. Takayasu's Arteritis

Takayasu's arteritis (TA) shares significant histopathological overlap with GCA despite the marked demographic and clinical differences between these entities (10). Affecting chiefly the aorta, including the aortic valve, and its major branches, the inflammation in its early stage is predominantly nonnecrotizing and granulomatous, involving the elastic media of these large vessels. In the usual clinical scenario, the florid stage is characteristically seen on biopsy specimens (Fig. 4a). By the time patients undergo reconstructive vascular surgery, the disease has entered a fibro-obliterative stage (see Fig. 4b) usually with scant inflammation, including the absence of giant cells.

C. Disseminated Giant Cell Arteritis

A small but significant minority of patients with GCA, possibibly as many as 15%, may have evidence of vasculitis involving vessels other than branches of the common carotid arteries (11). The demographics of disseminated GCA are different from the exclusively cranial variant, sometimes affecting children (12). Giant cell aortitis will cause loss of elastic fibers and smooth muscle cells within the media (13), eventuating in aortic dissection (14,15). The histopathology is similar to GCA elsewhere with the added feature of medial elastic destruction (Fig. 5).

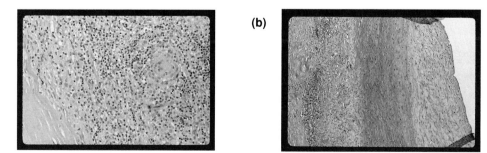

Figure 4   Takayasu's arteritis. (a) Florid granulomatous inflammation of aortic media. (b) Chronic inflammation and intimal fibrosis in axillary artery at reconstructive surgery.

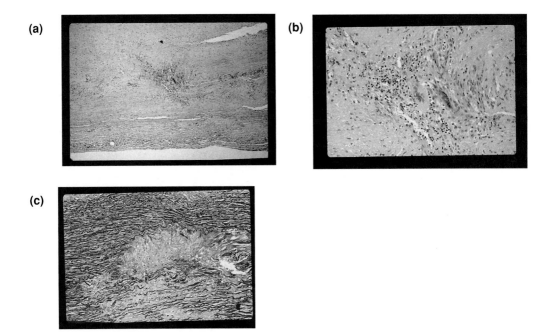

Figure 5 Disseminated giant cell arteritis. (a) Focal inflammatory destruction of aortic media. (b) High-power detail of inflammatory focus with multinucleated giant cells. (c) Absence of elastic fibers (Lawson's elastic–van Gieson stain) demonstrates localized character of inflammatory destruction in aortic media.

D. Central Nervous System Vasculitis

Intracranial, including intracerebral, vessels may be affected by most or all known primary and secondary systemic inflammatory vascular disorders. Primary vasculitis limited to the brain and spinal cord, also known as primary angiitis of the central nervous system (PACNS) is rare. It derives its significance chiefly from its severity and poor outcome. It is preeminently a skip phenomenon, so that a negative brain biopsy does not negate its presence (16). Although a granulomatous histopathology is common (17,18), probably close to half of patients present with nongranulomatous features, with or without necrosis (19,20).

Typically, however, several patterns may coexist with granulomatous inflammation in the same specimen, i.e., lymphocytic and/or necrotizing vasculitis (Fig. 6).

III. PREDOMINANTLY NECROTIZING VASCULITIS

A. Polyarteritis Nodosa

Polyarteritis nodosa (PAN) is the prototype of a necrotizing vasculitis. Limited almost exclusively to the arterial side of the circulation, PAN may affect vessels of all sizes, including capillaries, except large elastic arteries. Considerable confusion and controversy exist regarding the nosology and classification of PAN. From the standpoint of histopathology, the subdivision proposed by the Chapel Hill Conference represents a practical approach (21). In this scheme, the term "polyarteritis nodosa" is reserved for involvement of vessels larger than arterioles. Vasculitis affecting

(a) (b)

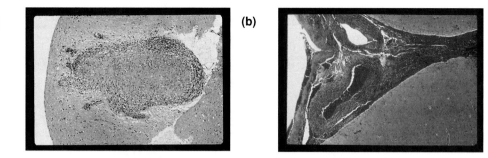

Figure 6   Central nervous system vasculitis. (a) Granulomatous vasculitis within gray matter. (b) Necrotizing vasculitis in leptomeningeal vessels.

arterioles, capillaries (and possibly venules) is termed "microscopic polyangiitis" (MPA). Small, "microscopic" vascular involvement is the defining criterion, so that all patients with microscopic disease, with or without involvement of larger vessels, are placed in the category of MPA. Thus defined, there remains a small group of patients whose disease is limited to medium-sized arteries, or "classic" PAN. From the pathologist's perspective, such division is helpful, since the anatomical differences between medium-sized arteries and capillaries, i.e., lack of discernible three-layered structures in the latter, of necessity impart a different appearance to the vasculitic process. This nosological approach has not, however, met with universal acclaim (22). Microscopic polyangiitis is discussed separately later in this chapter.

In medium-sized arteries, "classic" PAN characteristically causes transmural necrosis, the vascular wall assuming a homogeneous eosinophilic appearance, with obliteration of its distinctive layering. Inflammatory infiltrates, polymorphonuclear leukocytes and, more prominently, lymphocytes, may be heavy or absent, with scattered infiltrates limited to the adventitia (Fig. 7). The necrosis and inflammation may be sectoral, i.e., affecting only part of the circumference of a given arterial segment. Sampling segments only a few microns apart in a given vessel may reveal active necrosis alternating with segments of healing and scarring. Whether sectoral or circumferential, the necrosis gives rise to the characteristic aneurysm formations observed on angiography. Classic systemic PAN as a clinical entity is rare. Not infrequently, however, isolated

(a) (b)

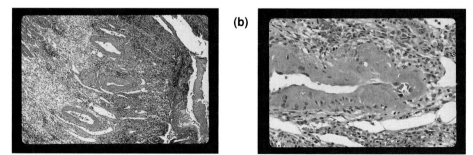

Figure 7   Polyarteritis nodosa. (a) Low-power view of necrotizing vasculitis in ileal mesentery. (b) Transmural fibrinoid necrosis involving portion of vascular circumference and causing thinning of vessel wall.

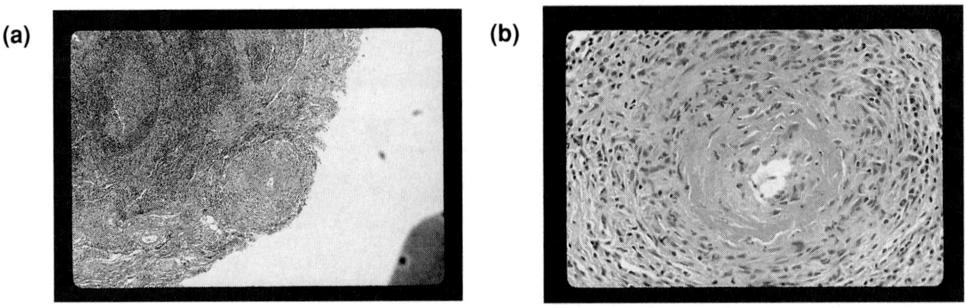

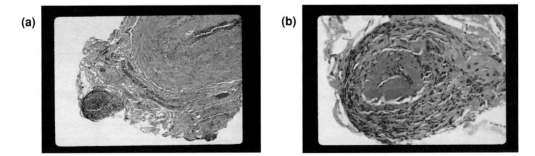

Figure 8 Polyarteritis nodosa. (a) Fibrinoid necrotizing vasculitis incidentally discovered in appendiceal serosa at appendectomy. (b) High-power detail demonstrating fibrinoid necrosis and perivascular inflammation.

lesions of PAN may be discovered in surgical specimens removed for reasons apparently unrelated to a vasculitic process (Fig. 8). These findings may be of significance, e.g., in bowel infarction due to a localized PAN affecting mesenteric arteries (23). In the majority of these cases, however, this finding does not connote a systemic vasculitic syndrome and surgical removal of the affected segment is curative. More frequent is isolated necrotizing vasculitis in branches of the cystic or appendiceal arteries in cholecystectomy or appendectomy specimens (24,25). Possibly, these represent localized immune complex deposition, "Arthus phenomenon." Even if they are a significant finding to be brought to the attention of attending physicians, these localized vasculitic phenomena do not, by themselves, justify a diagnosis of a systemic vasculitic syndrome. Finally, PAN may represent a an unexpected, and sometimes confusing, finding in biopsy obtained to confirm a different vasculitic process (Fig. 9).

Differential diagnosis: Fibrinoid necrotizing vasculitis of medium-sized arteries is a sensitive marker for PAN. Its specificity is less, since identical vascular lesions are seen in the vasculitides accompanying rheumatoid arthritis and systemic lupus erythematosus (SLE).

B. Churg–Strauss Syndrome

Churg–Strauss syndrome (CS), especially early in its course, is characterized by fibrinoid vascular necrosis identical to PAN. With time, however, in contrast to PAN, granulomatous inflamma-

Figure 9 Polyarteritis nodosa. (a) Temporal artery biopsy. The main vessel is intact. (b) High-power detail of small branch of temporal artery demonstrating polyarteritis nodosa.

tion becomes the histological hallmark of CS. Polyarteritis nodosa and Churg-Strauss syndrome share some pathogenetic pathways, in particular myeloperoxidase-specific P-ANCA positivity in the majority of CS patients expressing antineutrophil cytoplasmic antibodies (ANCAs) (26,27). Nevertheless, clinical differences are significant, especially the strong association of CS with asthma and peripheral blood eosinophilia and the lower frequency of necrotizing glomerulonephritis. The histopathology of CS reflects these differences. By the time a patient with CS is biopsied, eosinophil-rich nonnecrotizing granulomatous inflammation is most frequently encountered (Fig. 18.10; see color plate).

C. Wegener's Granulomatosis

Necrotizing granulomas are the histological hallmark of Wegener's granulomatosis (WG). For histopathological confirmation of WG in the upper airways and lungs, identifying vascular inflammation is not required. The diagnostic yield is greatest with open lung biopsies, followed by endoscopic biopsies of the upper airways, including, in particular, the paranasal sinuses. The necrosis is noncaseating, typically assuming irregular ("geographical") outlines (Fig. 18.11; see color plate). The viable tissues bordering the necrotic areas consist of epithelioid histiocytes ("palisading granuloma"), with or without multinucleated giant cells. In the classic syndrome, the upper airways are most frequently affected (87%), followed by the lungs (69%) and kidneys (48%) (28). In addition to palisading granulomas, the tissue manifestations of WG include vasculitis affecting both arteries and capillaries (29,30). The arteritis may be granulomatous, fibrinoid necrotizing, or both (Fig. 18.11c; see color plate). If C-ANCA positivity defines WG and myeloperoxidase-specific P-ANCA positivity defines MPA, pulmonary capillaritis occurs with similar frequency in both. Destructive and infiltrative lesions are, however, more common in WG than in MPA. Such noncapillaritic lesions include bronchiolitis obliterans–organizing pneumonia, peribronchial lymphocytic inflammation, and necrotizing granulomata (31,32). Due to the extensive organ damage and the dismal prognosis of untreated WG (33), prompt and accurate tissue diagnosis is essential. With rare exceptions (34), the renal manifestations of WG are identical to those seen in MPA (see below).

D. Microscopic Polyangiitis

Microscopic polyangiitis (MPA) by definition affects vessels visible only microscopically, i.e., capillaries, arterioles, and venules. In general, these are vascular channels whose outer diameters are less than 500 microns. Vessels of this size lack the well-defined triple layering of their larger counterparts, i.e., a discernible intimal endothelial layer, a continuous internal elastic lamina, a muscular media, and a defined adventitia. Pulmonary capillaries are thus composed of an endothelial layer internal to a discontinuous basal lamina but lack both an elastic lamina and a discernible media. A concentration of inflammatory cells, polymorphonuclear leukocytes and lymphocytes, in and around alveolar septal capillary, therefore, suffices as pulmonary capillaritis (Fig. 18.12a; see color plate). In the lung, this may represent the only histological abnormality in MPA (see above). Patients with Wegener's granulomatosis in addition to capillaritis, often display large geographical necrotizing granulomas.

The renal glomerulus is where the histopathological manifestations of the ANCA-positive small vessel vasculitides, i.e., Wegener's granulomatosis, Churg–Strauss syndrome, and microscopic polyangiitis converge. Although their seminal study from 1954 deals primarily with Wegener's granulomatosis, Godman and Churg (35) recognized that WG, CS and the condition currently termed MPA share a common expression in small vessels, and are thus related. In the kidney, necrotizing glomerulonephritis (GN) is the most frequent and characteristic renal manifestation of MPA. Some authorities even define a specific entity, renal-limited MPA (31). Irrespective of competing classification schemes, necrotizing GN is the defining glomerular lesion in these small-vessel vasculitides. Histologically, the necrosis is segmental, i.e., affects some glomerular capillary tufts and consists of disruptions of the glomerular capillary wall, along with fibrinous and inflammatory exudates, chiefly polymorphonuclear leukocytes (Fig. 18.12b; see color plate). Crescents, composed of parietal epithelium (derived from Bowman's capsule), and mono- and polymorphonuclear leukocytes usually about the external aspect of the affected glomerular segment. The severity of disease dictates the proportion of glomeruli affected and the extent of destruction within a given glomerulus. Depending on the duration of the process, crescents may be predominantly cellular in early lesions, i.e., parietal epithelium and inflammatory cells, or fibrous. Vasculitis of extraglomerular vessels is an inconstant finding in MPA. Extraglomerular vasculitis and/or interstitial renal granulomatous inflammation, with or without necrosis, are more common in both CS and WG (Fig. 13a). Sometimes, however, segmental glomerular necrosis extends proximally into an afferent arteriole (see Fig. 13b).

The necrotizing glomerular lesions of MPA, WG, and CS do not, by definition, display immunoglobulin deposition, i.e., they are "pauci-immune." Not infrequently, however, direct immunufluorescence will reveal weak positivity for IgM and the third component of complement. This finding probably represents passive trapping of large protein molecules in structurally damaged glomeruli. Fibrinogen is characteristically trapped in active cellular crescents.

Differential diagnosis: Glomerular histopathology identical to the small-vessel vasculitides is characteristically seen in several unrelated disease categories. In fact, most glomerulonephritides, whether primary or associated with systemic diseases, may manifest morphologically with segmental necrosis and crescents. The systemic immune complex–mediated connective tissue diseases, primarily systemic lupus erythematosus frequently manifest as necrotizing GN. Anti-glomerular basement membrane antibody–mediated disease (e.g., Goodpasture's syndrome) also presents with necrotizing and crescentic GN. The presence of granular (SLE) and linear (anti-GBM disease) immune deposits in these diseases removes them from the pauci-immune category. The ANCAs are also a useful discriminator between the pauci-immune glomerulonephritides and others.

In interstitial renal vessels, rheumatoid arthritis typically causes a fibrinoid necrotizing vasculitis in its acute stages. The extraglomerular renal appearances of accelerated "malignant" hypertension may be indistinguishable from extraglomerular necrotizing vasculitis.

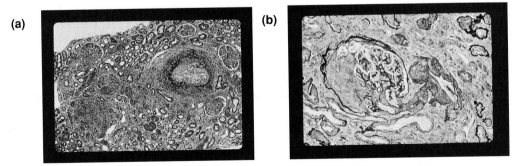

Figure 13 Microscopic polyangiitis. (a) Interstitial renal vessel undergoing fibrinoid necrosis (Masson trichrome stain). (b) Renal glomerulus demonstrating segmental necrosis in continuity with fibrinoid necrosis involving the afferent arteriole entering the glomerulus (Jones methenamine silver stain).

IV. PREDOMINANTLY LEUKOCYTOCLASTIC VASCULITIS

Although not inherent in the designation, the term "leukocytoclastic vasculitis" (LCV) is primarily reserved for inflammation of small arteries and veins. The "leukocytoclasis" refers to breakdown of inflammatory cells leaving small nuclear fragments, "nuclear dust" (karyorrhexis) in and around the vessels (Fig. 18.14a; see color plate). The inflammation is typically transmural, rarely necrotizing, and never granulomatous. Early in its course, LCV may be composed chiefly of polymorphonuclear leukocytes to be replaced later by lymphocytes. Leukocytoclastic vasculitis typically affects the skin.

Hypersensitivity vasculitis (HSV) is the prototype of leukocytoclastic vasculitis. Characterized clinically by a maculopapular or a purpuric rash, HSV shows varying amounts of karyorrhexis and polymorphonuclear leukocytes in and around the walls of the cutaneous vessels. Early in some drug reactions, eosinophils may predominate.

The *differential diagnosis* includes virtually all systemic vasculitides. Thus, patients with Wegener's granulomatosis and skin involvement most commonly manifest as LCV. In a study of 46 patients from the National Institutes of Health who had WG with skin involvement, Barksdale et al. (2) identified LCV in 31%, followed by granulatomous skin inflammation in 19%, and nonspecific ulceration in 4%. In children, LCV is most commonly a manifestation of Henoch–Schönlein purpura (HSP), followed at some distance by hypersensitivity vasculitis. In adults, this relationship is reversed (36). Henoch–Schönlein purpura, a primary systemic vasculitis affecting mainly children, manifests in the skin, gastrointestinal tract, and kidney. The extrarenal histopathology is that of LCV, possible with an accentuation of fibrinoid necrosis. The renal manifestations are largely identical to those of IgA nephropathy (Berger's disease). The characteristic changes are those of proliferative glomerulonephritis, which may affect some (focal) or all (diffuse) glomeruli. Within a single glomerulus, the proliferation may affect some capillary segments (segmental) or the entire glomerulus (generalized) (Fig. 18.14b; see color plate). Necrosis and crescents are seen in a minority of patients. Common to all patients with HSP is the deposition of immunoglobulin-A in the affected organs (Fig. 18.14c; see color plate).

REFERENCES

1. Lie JT. Histopathologic specificity of systemic vasculitis. Rheum Dis Clin North Am 1995; 21:883–909.
2. Barksdale SK, Hallahan CW, Kerr GS, Fauci AS, Stern JB, Travis WD. Cutaneous pathology in Wegener's granulomatosis. A clinicopathologic study of 75 biopsies in 46 patients. Am J Surg Pathol 1995; 19:161–172.
3. Hunder GG, Arend WP, Bloch DA, et al. The American College of Rheumatology 1990 Criteria for the Classification of Vasculitis. Arthritis Rheum 1990; 33(8):1068–1073.
4. Kaiser M, Weyand CM, Bjornsson J, Goronzy JJ. Platelet-derived growth factor, intimal hyperplasia, and ischemic complications in giant cell arteritis. Arthritis Rheum 1998; 41(4):623–633.
5. Weyand CM, Tetzlaff N, Bjornsson J, Brack A, Younge B, Goronzy JJ. Disease patterns and tissue cytokine profiles in giant cell arteritis. Arthritis Rheum 1997; 40(1):19–26.
6. Wagner AD, Bjornsson J, Bartley G, Goronzy JJ, Weyand CM. Interferon-γ-producing T cells in giant cell vasculitis represent a minority of tissue-infiltrating cells and are located distant from the site of pathology. Am J Pathol 1996; 148:1925–1933.
7. Baldursson O, Steinsson K, Björnsson J, Lie JT. Temporal arteritis in Iceland: An epidemiological and histopathological analysis. Arthritis Rehum 1994; 37:1007–1012.

8. Evans JM, Batts KP, Hunder GG. Persistent giant cell arteritis despite corticosteroid treatment. Mayo Clin Proc 1994; 69:1060–1061.

9. Achkar AA, Lie JT, Hunder GG, O'Fallon M, Gabriel SE. How does previous corticosteroid treatment affect the biopsy findings in giant cell (temporal) arteritis? Ann Intern Med 1994; 120:987–992.

10. Lie JT. Occidental (temporal) and oriental (Takayasu) giant cell arteritis. Cardiovasc Pathol 1994; 3(3): 277–240.

11. Lie JT. Aortic and extracranial large vessel giant cell arteritis: A review of 72 cases with histopathologic documentation. Semin Arthritis Rheum 1995; 24:422–431.

12. Kagata Y, Matsubara O, Ogata S, Lie JT, Mark EJ. Infantile disseminated visceral giant cell arteritis presenting as sudden infant death. Pathol Int 1999; 49:226–230.

13. Petursdottir V, Nordborg E, Nordborg C. Atrophy of the aortic media in giant cell arteritis. APMIS 1996; 104:191–198.

14. Evans JM, Bowles CA, Bjornsson J, Mullany CJ, Hunder GG. Thoracic aortic aneurysm and rupture in giant cell arteritis. A descriptive study of 41 cases. Arthritis Rheum 1994; 37(10):1539–1547.

15. Liu G, Shupak R, Chiu BK. Aortic dissection in giant-cell arteritis. Semin Arthritis Rheum 1995; 25: 160–171.

16. Lie JT. Classification and histopathologic spectrum of central nervous system of central nervous system vasculitis. Neurol Clin 1997; 15:805–819.

17. Chu CT, Gray L, Goldstein LB, Hulette CM. Diagnosis of intracranial vasculitis: A multidisciplinary approach. J Neuropathol Exp Neurol 1998; 57(1):30–38.

18. Rhodes RH, Madelaire NC, Petrelli M, Cole M, Karaman B. Primary angiitis and angiopathy of the central nervous system and their relationship to systemic giant cell arteritis. Arch Pathol Lab Med 1995; 119(4):334–349.

19. Younger DS, Calabrese LH, Hays AP. Granulomatous angiitis of the nervous system. Neurol Clin 1997; 15:821–834.

20. Parisi JE, Moore PM. The role of biopsy in vasculitis of the central nervous system. Sem Neurol 1994; 14:341.

21. Jennette JC, Falk RJ, Andrassy K, et al. Nomenclature of systemic vasculitides. Proposal of an international consensus conference. Arthritis Rheum 1994; 37(2):187–192.

22. Lie JT. Nomenclature and classification of vasculitis: plus ça change, plus c'est la même chose. Arthritis Rheum 1994; 37:181–186.

23. Burke AP, Sobin LH, Vimani R. Localized vasculitis of the gastrointestinal trace. Am J Surg Pathol 1995; 19:338–349.

24. Fish DE, Evans DJ, Pusey CD. Gallbladder vasculitis: A report of two cases. Histopathology 1993; 23: 584–585.

25. Nohr M, Laustsen J, Falk E. Isolated necrotizing panarteritis of the gallbladder. Acta Chir Scand 1989; 155:485–487.

26. Travis WD, Fleming MV. Vasculitis of the lung. Pathology (Philadelphia) 1996; 4:23–41.

27. Hoffman GS, Specks U. Antineutrophil cytoplasmic antibodies. Arthritis Rheum 1998; 41(9):1521–1537.

28. Lie JT. Wegener's granulomatosis: Histological documentation of common and uncommon manifestations in 216 patients. Vasa 1997; 26:261–270.

29. Sullivan EJ, Hoffman GS. Pulmonary vasculitis. Clin Chest Med 1998; 19:759–776.

30. Specks U. Wegener's granulomatosis and pulmonary vasculitis. Clin Pulm Med 1995; 2:267–275.

31. Gaudin PB, Askin FB, Falk RJ, Jennette JC. The pathologic spectrum of pulmonary lesions in patients with anti-neutrophil cytoplasmic autoantibodies specific for antiproteinase 3 and anti-meyloperoxidase. Am J Clin Pathol 1995; 104:7–16.

32. Uner AH, Rozum-Slota B, Katzenstein AL. Bronchiolitis obliterans-organizing pneumonia (BOOP)-like variant of Wegener's granulomatosis. A clinicopathologic study of 16 cases. Am J Surg Pathol 1996; 20:794–801.

33. Sullivan EJ, Hoffman GS. Wegener's granulomatosis. Semin Respir Crit Care Med 1998; 19:13–25.

34. Villa-Forte A, Hoffman GS. Wegener's granulomatosis presenting with a renal mass. J Rheumatol 1999; 26:457–458.

35. Godman G, Churg J. Wegener's granulomatosis: Pathology and review of the literature. Arch Pathol 1954; 58:533–553.
36. Blanco R, Martinez-Taboada VM, Rodriguez-Valverde V, Garcia-Fuentes M. Cutaneous vasculitis in children and adults. Assoc diseases and etiologic factors in 303 patients. Med (Baltimore) 1998; 77(6): 403–418.

19

Noninvasive Radiographic Approach to Differential Diagnosis of the Vasculitides

Scott D. Flamm
The Texas Medical Center, Houston, Texas

Richard D. White
Cleveland Clinic Foundation, Cleveland, Ohio

I. INTRODUCTION

Diagnosis of and differentiation among the vasculitides remains squarely based on a detailed clinical history, thorough physical examination, and appropriate laboratory testing. Of these, the physical examination and clinical history will usually form the basis of diagnosis (1). Laboratory testing (i.e., serological acute phase reactants and hematological parameters) may be of benefit when results are abnormal; however, the results are often misleading and do not correlate with disease activity in 50% of patient encounters (2–4). This chapter focuses on the contribution noninvasive imaging provides in differentiating the vasculitides and defining the extent of disease, and discusses new techniques that may provide unique information in defining disease activity and guiding therapy.

The radiographic approach to diagnosis of the vasculitides traditionally has been based on catheter-based techniques. For some of the vasculitides, such as Takayasu's arteritis (TA) and Buerger's disease, conventional angiography has been considered the gold standard for diagnosis. The catheter-driven angiograms provide exquisitely detailed images of the vascular tree lumen, including the small arteries; however, the acquisition of the images requires an invasive procedure and exposes the patient to a significant amount of ionizing radiation. Additionally, the required iodinated contrast material is potentially nephrotoxic. These limitations have opened the door for the newer, noninvasive imaging techniques of ultrasound (US), computed tomography (CT), and magnetic resonance imaging (MRI) as adjuncts to and possible replacements for catheter-based techniques in the diagnostic evaluation of patients with vasculitis.

Ultrasound, CT, and MRI all have finite resolution that limits their imaging of small arteries. They are most adept at imaging the large and medium-sized arterial vessels; small-vessel vasculitides necessarily must be addressed using conventional catheter angiography. This chapter is limited to discussing those vasculitides involving the medium-sized and large vessels, including TA, giant cell arteritis (GCA), and infectious vasculitides such as syphilitic arteritis.

II. IMAGING TECHNIQUES

A. Ultrasound

Ultrasound is a noninvasive technique that has found widespread practical application in imaging of the human body. Ultrasound imaging requires no ionizing radiation or intravenous contrast agents. In addition, the ultrasonic sound waves employed have no known deleterious effects in humans and imaging can be performed real-time and, if necessary, portably.

For imaging of the vasculitides, US has its greatest utility in evaluation of the medium-sized, more peripheral arteries, with lesser utility for the large arteries (5). The abdominal aorta is accessible when a limited amount of overlying bowel gas is present. However, evaluation of the abdominal aorta is often limited to a simple analysis of size. The low-frequency transducer needed to penetrate the typical distances encountered limits evaluation of wall thickness and wall characterization. As a result, US of the abdominal aorta is usually limited to follow-up evaluation of abdominal aortic aneurysms looking for changes in size (Fig. 1). The pelvic arteries, too, are relatively deep in the soft tissues of the pelvis and, similar to the abdominal aorta, also may be difficult to evaluate with ultrasound.

Interposition of air between the chest wall and aorta impedes full evaluation of the thoracic aorta, particularly the arch and descending portion. Transthoracic echocardiography can visualize the proximal ascending aorta when an adequate acoustic window is present, but is limited in certain groups of patients. Specifically, patients with retrosternal fibrosis and scarring from prior median sternotomy or thoracotomy, obese patients with abundant chest-wall adipose tissue, and patients with hyperinflated lungs from chronic obstructive pulmonary disease frequently have poor acoustic windows that significantly limit evaluation with US techniques. Transesophageal echocardiography produces detailed images of the thoracic aorta (with the frequent exception of the aortic arch), but is unable to evaluate the abdominal aorta; it will not be discussed further as it is not a "noninvasive" technique.

The previously mentioned limitations of US restrict its use for evaluating the large arteries; however, it is ideally suited to study the medium-sized branch vessels of the aorta. Specific vascular regions that have been investigated with US include the common carotid, proximal internal and external carotid, temporal, and femoral arteries. The use of high-frequency transducers provides detailed information regarding wall thickness and intimal surface characteristics. Under ideal conditions, US can even discriminate between adventitial and medial involvement, and identify areas of perivascular edema (6).

B. Computed Tomography

Computed tomography has been a mainstay of noninvasive imaging for over 20 years. Its advantages include the ability to image large areas of the human body, relatively rapid data acquisition, and relatively high spatial resolution. The recent development of spiral acquisition techniques has enabled even faster scanning along with improved volumetric three-dimensional (3-D) reconstruction capabilities. The limitations to CT include exposure to ionizing radiation and potentially nephrotoxic contrast agent, the practical limitation of acquiring data in the axial plane, and the lack of functional information, such as blood flow dynamics or heart valve function. Despite these limitations, CT may provide important details regarding the degree and nature (e.g., calcification) of wall thickening and extent of disease (7,8). The addition of 3-D reconstruction techniques contributes angiogram-like images highlighting areas of stenosis, occlusion, or aneurysmal dilation (9).

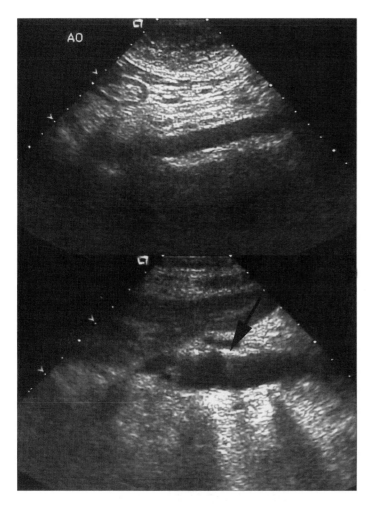

Figure 1 Ultrasound images of the abdominal aorta. The upper panel is a longitudinal view of the aorta in a young adult. The aortic wall has a smooth luminal surface, but the resolution is insufficient to measure the wall thickness or differentiate the three layers. The lower panel is a longitudinal view from an elderly adult with atherosclerosis; the luminal surface is irregular and focal echogenic areas that cause shadowing identify areas of calcification (black arrow).

C. Magnetic Resonance Imaging

Magnetic resonance imaging is the most comprehensive of the available noninvasive imaging techniques. Similar to CT, MRI can image large areas of the human body in the transaxial plane, but is also capable of directly acquiring images in sagittal and coronal planes, and complex oblique orientations.

Spin-echo (or "black-blood") imaging can provide excellent anatomical information about vessel anatomy, wall thickness, and characteristics of the tissue comprising the thickened arterial walls. Recent studies have suggested MRI's ability to identify inflammatory changes within the vessel walls after the administration of the MRI contrast agent, gadolinium, or with the use of newer sequences that are "edema-weighted." Gradient-echo sequences that are gated to the electrocardiogram produce cinematic, movie-like images that provide functional information, such as cardiac valve function and vessel blood flow dynamics. Finally, fast magnetic resonance angiography (MRA) techniques generate angiogram-like images during a patient's single breathhold of 10–15 duration. These images can be acquired in any orientation to focus on the vessels of interest and provide detailed evaluation of the vessel lumen and stenoses with quality approaching that of a conventional, catheter-based angiogram (Fig. 2). Notably, this information may be obtained without exposing patients to ionizing radiation or nephrotoxic contrast agents.

Despite the multiple advantages MRI has over other less comprehensive noninvasive imaging techniques, it has not gained widespread acceptance for a variety of reasons. Currently, MRI may be more expensive than CT or ultrasound to perform, is less widely available, and the imaging results may be equally or more operator-dependent than CT or US. Further, high-resolution imaging with definition comparable to US may be unduly time consuming.

III. IMAGING FINDINGS OF THE VASCULITIDES

A. Takayasu's Arteritis

Takayasu's arteritis is characterized principally by circumferential wall thickening that has a smooth intimal surface. The wall thickening typically affects the thoracic and/or abdominal aorta

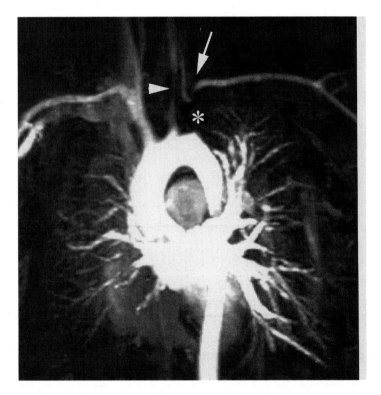

Figure 2 Magnetic resonance angiography of the thoracic aorta and arch branch vessels. This young female with TA has a long, severe stenosis of the left common carotid artery (arrowhead) and complete occlusion of the proximal left subclavian artery (asterisk) with subclavian "steal" phenomenon, i.e., the left vertebral artery has retrograde flow providing blood supply to the mid- and distal left subclavian artery (arrow). The detail obtained is less than that of a conventional angiogram, but the MRA can be instrumental in planning further therapy, whether it be medical, catheter-based, or surgical.

and primary branch vessels, resulting in luminal narrowing and stenoses. Vessels may become occluded when disease involvement is severe. The most common patterns of involvement have been well classified by Numano et al. (10), with the most typical pattern consisting of wall thickening of the ascending aorta, aortic arch, and extending into the arch branch vessels.

The normal aortic wall has a thickness of 1–2 mm, which may increase up to 7 or 8 mm or greater in acute TA. Chronic scarring will often decrease the wall thickening compared to the early or acute stages, though the thickness of the wall typically does not return to normal. The wall thickening in TA is often characterized by a well-demarcated, abrupt transition between the normal and abnormal segments of aortic wall. This is in contrast to other conditions, such as atherosclerosis, where wall thickening is patchy and the transition zones gradual.

While few longitudinal studies have been performed and some disagreements exist regarding the phases of disease activity, in general, the luminal caliber of the aorta and branch vessels should be normal or near-normal in the early phases of the disease with scarring and stenoses occurring with disease progression. Many patients will develop some degree of ectasia, but only a minority will have true aneurysmal dilation of the aorta and/or arch branch vessels. Thus, aneurysms may be considered the exception and not the rule (11,12).

Aortic wall thickening can involve the aortic root and valve, and aortic insufficiency has been consistently described in approximately 25% of patients with TA. Pulmonary artery involvement has also been described, though the incidence in reported series varies widely up to 86%, likely reflecting the chronicity of disease in the studied population (13–15). Both pulmonary artery aneurysms and stenoses have been described, with or without wall thickening (16). The wide variation in manifestations of pulmonary artery involvement makes pulmonary artery abnormalities a less specific and reliable feature in diagnosing TA (Fig. 3).

Ultrasound has only a limited role in the evaluation of TA, as it is unable to visualize the majority of affected vessels (thoracoabdominal aorta and proximal branch vessels) in a consistent

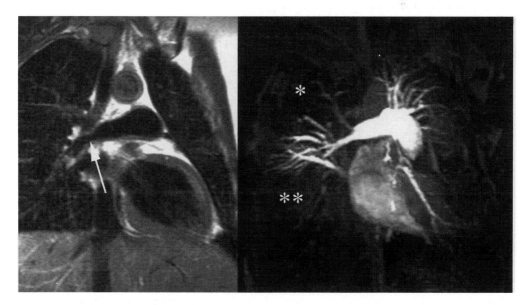

Figure 3 Magnetic resonance imaging and MRA of pulmonary artery involvement in a young female with TA. On the left is a spin-echo MRI demonstrating wall thickening with stenosis of the right pulmonary artery (arrow). On the right is an MRA of the pulmonary arteries showing the severe stenosis of the distal right pulmonary artery and paucity of blood flow to the upper (asterisk) and lower (double asterisk) lobes of the right lung.

and reliable fashion. As such, it cannot be used reliably to make a definite initial assessment or to follow the course of disease activity or response to therapy. It has found a niche role in assessing disease involvement in the carotid and femoral arteries (though the latter are less frequently involved). High-resolution images of the common and proximal internal and external carotid arteries can be obtained using high-frequency transducers to demonstrate the long segmental uniform wall thickening typically seen in TA. These findings can easily be distinguished from the irregular-surfaced, focal plaques of atherosclerosis.

Computed tomography is valuable for defining the extent of disease involvement in TA (7). Imaging is performed relatively rapidly and provides data describing the extent of involvement of the entire thoracoabdominal aorta and proximal branch vessels. Computed tomography can easily define areas of wall thickening for those vessels that are imaged perpendicular to their long axes (e.g., the ascending and descending aorta and common carotid arteries) (Fig. 4). It performs less well in areas where the vessels run parallel to the imaging plane, such as the aortic arch, subclavian arteries, renal arteries, etc. The angiogram-like images produced from 3-D reconstruction techniques can help surmount these difficulties by providing information about luminal narrowing and length of stenosis (17).

Unfortunately, CT provides no functional information regarding the aortic and pulmonary valves, critical structures that may be involved in TA. An additional limitation in evaluating TA is that while CT can define the degree of wall thickening present, it does not provide any direct evidence of disease activity. Computed tomography defines only the extent and degree of wall thickening, but not the presence or absence of inflammatory activity; however, disease activity has been determined retrospectively based on follow-up studies (18). On the other hand, CT is optimal for the delineation of arterial wall calcification, which may be helpful in staging TA and differentiating it from other causes of wall thickening, such as atherosclerosis.

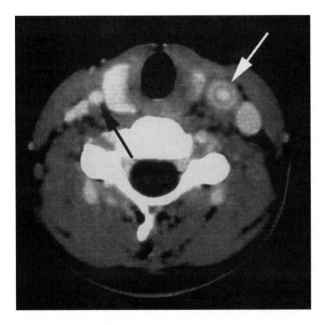

Figure 4   Axial CT scan image from the lower neck of a young woman with TA. The thickened wall of the left carotid artery (white arrow) is easily contrasted with the normal wall of the right carotid artery (black arrow). Note that despite significant thickening of the wall of the left carotid artery, the lumen of the vessel is not narrowed.

Similar to angiographic evaluation of TA, MRI can assess luminal caliber of large and medium-sized arteries, but without the burden of ionizing radiation or iodinated contrast agent. The primary disadvantage of MRI compared with angiography is its inability to accurately define small branch vessels. Moreover, MRI can classify stenoses only qualitatively. The primary advantage for MRI is its ability to perform an examination of the entire extent of the thoracoabdominal aorta and medium-sized branch vessels in an examination of <1 hour. Further, MRI has the added capability of evaluating wall thickness, an assessment that angiography cannot perform reliably (Fig. 5). The degree of wall thickening correlates loosely with disease activity as moderately to markedly thickened walls are more likely to represent acute or subacute disease activity, while thinner walls likely reflect less severe disease activity, more indolent activity, or scarring (19–22).

While arterial wall visualization is an advantage compared with angiography, it does not address the issue of disease activity, insofar as wall thickening alone may reflect either active inflammation or scar tissue. Recently, two different approaches have been used to assess disease activity in TA. The first approach uses gadolinium enhancement on T1-weighted images in areas of wall thickening. Gadolinium is an extracellular contrast agent that accumulates in areas of increased vascularity such as tumors and vascular malformations, and in areas of increased vascular permeability as is seen in infection or inflammation. Preliminary results in patients with TA suggest that gadolinium enhancement in areas of wall thickening may be a marker of acute disease activity, while lack of enhancement suggests inactive disease. One group of investigators studied 14 patients with gadolinium-enhanced MRI and found correlation of MRI features with disease activity in all patients. Three of the fourteen patients had persistent clinical disease activity after treatment; despite a normal erythrocyte sedimentation rate, MRI findings concurred with

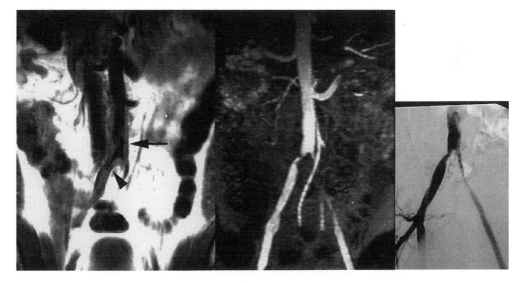

Figure 5   Aorto-iliac involvement in a young male with TA. On the left is a spin-echo MRI demonstrating the characteristic wall thickening (arrow) of the distal abdominal aorta and common iliac arteries resulting in a severe stenosis of the proximal right common iliac artery (arrowhead). The left common iliac artery is out of the plane of imaging on this image. In the middle is the corresponding MRA highlighting the focal stenosis of the right common iliac artery, as well as the long severe stenosis of the left common iliac artery. On the right is the conventional catheter-based contrast angiogram that reveals finer detail than the MRA, but does not provide information about wall abnormalities.

ongoing disease activity, suggesting that MRI may be a more useful adjunctive test than acute phase reactants (23).

The second approach to characterizing disease activity uses similar logic, but a different surrogate imaging marker of inflammation. T2- and STIR-weighted sequences ("edema-weighted" MRI techniques) are sensitive to extracellular fluid, which manifests as increased signal intensity compared with surrounding normal tissue. These sequences have been used to identify tissue edema in entities such as cerebral stroke, neoplasia, and acute myocardial infarction. Inflammatory tissue also is characterized by edema, and the edematous changes are likely a surrogate marker of inflammation. In preliminary work in patients with TA, edema-weighted imaging identified inflammation in areas of wall thickening. The degree of inflammation identified correlated with disease activity and with response to therapy (24) (Fig. 6). Both of these approaches, gadolinium-enhanced and edema-weighted MRI, if successfully applied in larger studies, suggest that noninvasive imaging may provide a more reliable way to assess disease activity than current approaches.

B. Giant Cell Arteritis

Pathology specimens from patients with GCA are frequently indistinguishable from TA, as both reveal characteristic giant cell formations and extensive inflammatory changes. Giant cell arteritis is distinguished from TA primarily by an arbitrary dividing line based on age of onset, with TA <40 years and GCA >40 years (25,26). In addition, GCA has a somewhat different distribution of vessel involvement; GCA frequently affects the temporal artery, whereas temporal artery involvement is rare in TA. The distribution of involvement of the aorta and branch vessels has been

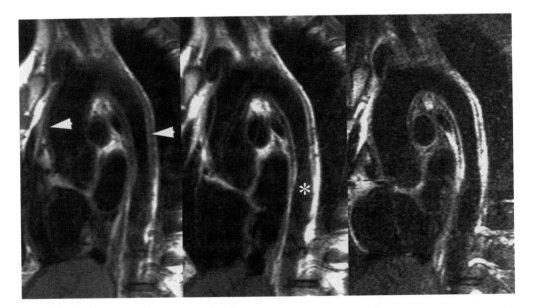

Figure 6   Magnetic resonance imaging of the thoracic aorta in a young female with TA. From left to right the images are T1-, T2-, and STIR-weighted, respectively. The T1-weighted image demonstrates the marked wall thickening in the ascending and descending thoracic aorta (arrowheads) in this patient with active TA. Both the T2- and STIR-weighted images demonstrate increased signal intensity (bright) consistent with edema and active inflammation. The asterisk on the middle image denotes the zone of abrupt transition between abnormal and normal aortic wall.

less well studied and characterized in GCA compared with TA, although GCA seems to affect the majority of the thoracic aorta more frequently and is considerably more likely to result in true aneurysm formation. Patients with GCA are also significantly more prone to aortic dissection and rupture, which, unfortunately, may be the initial and fatal presentation of disease (27).

In addition to developing thoracic aortic aneurysms, GCA appears to have a predilection for involvement of the mid- to distal subclavian arteries, usually with severe, long segmental stenosis (Fig. 7). The degree of wall thickening in GCA is less prominent than in TA and symptom manifestation (e.g., claudication) may be more insidious than TA, likely as a result of the reduced physical activity in older patients.

To date, US has been the imaging modality of choice, as GCA typically affects the temporal artery. Ultrasound is ideal to study GCA, as the temporal artery is superficial and lends itself to detailed examination with high-frequency transducers placed directly over the indurated, erythematous, inflamed vessel (28). Ultrasound can easily identify the smooth-surfaced, circumferential wall thickening surrounded by soft-tissue erythema and edema that characterizes GCA, though the diagnostic benefit of US over the combination of history and clinical examination alone is debated (29). Magnetic resonance angiography can be useful in demonstrating the vascular stenoses and/or occlusions that occur with GCA, though neither CT nor MRI has demonstrated any added value in evaluating the inflammatory wall changes in the temporal arteries (30). High-resolution MRI using surface coils has the potential to provide new diagnostic information,

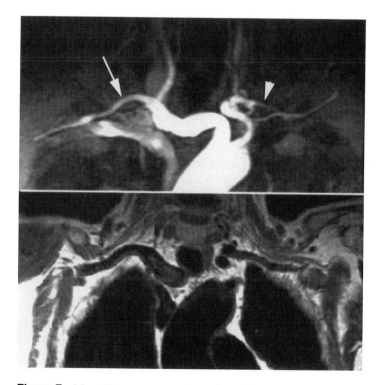

Figure 7 Magnetic resonance angiography and MRI of the subclavian arteries in an elderly female with GCA. The upper panel MRA shows stenoses of the mid- to distal subclavian arteries; the left subclavian artery is occluded just after the origin of the vertebral artery (arrowhead), while the right subclavian artery is diffusely narrowed (arrow). In the lower panel, the corresponding spin-echo MRI demonstrates the wall thickening of the respective subclavian arteries.

similar to the use of edema-weighted MRI in TA, however, detailed studies have yet to be performed.

Similar to its use in TA, US has little role in the evaluation of the central arteries in GCA. Alternatively, both CT and MRI have depicted the characteristic wall thickening and aneurysm formation seen in the thoracic aorta. As mentioned previously, the wall thickening is less prominent than in TA, and the marked thickening seen in acute TA has not been described to the same extent in GCA. The aortic wall is frequently more lobulated and irregular in GCA than in TA, and many patients with GCA have disease that is virtually indistinguishable from atherosclerosis on either CT or MRI using current techniques. It is unclear whether atherosclerosis is part of the spectrum of GCA or if many patients have overlapping disease states.

C. Infectious/Syphilitic Arteritis

Involvement of the aorta and branch vessels is usually a late manifestation of syphilis. Presently aortic "lues" is encountered only rarely, as effective early treatment has been available for decades. Textbook accounts of aortic syphilis typically describe aneurysms of the ascending aorta and "pencil fine" calcifications of the wall in the distal ascending aorta as seen on plain chest x-rays (31). Only case report descriptions exist in the modern literature using CT and MRI. The characteristics are similar to what is described in GCA: mild, irregular-surfaced wall thickening of the ascending aorta and aortic arch in combination with ectasia to aneurysmal dilation of the affected regions (32,33).

Both CT and MRI may be helpful in differentiating syphilitic involvement from atherosclerosis, but are unlikely to be specific. The diagnosis will depend on confirmation with the appropriate history and positive laboratory tests.

IV. DIFFERENTIAL CONSIDERATIONS

In general, the imaging findings for the arteritides discussed in this chapter comprise aneurysms, stenoses, and areas of wall thickening or scarring. Differentiating TA from GCA will most often be made on clinical factors alone with reported accuracy of 95% (1). However, some patients in the diagnostic "gray" zone or those in whom an arteritis is unsuspected may be differentiated by some imaging features alone. Imaging features differentiating TA and GCA are presented in Table 1.

V. CONCLUSIONS

Computed tomography, MRI, and US are important diagnostic techniques in the initial evaluation and follow-up of patients with arteritis of the large and medium-sized arteries. Computed tomography and US will likely persist as the primary noninvasive imaging modalities because of their ubiquity within the healthcare system and their ease of application and reproducibility. Magnetic resonance imaging will likely gain a larger role as the technology becomes more widely distributed and familiarity with the newer techniques increases. The advantages of combined morphological and functional analysis, along with the potential ability to identify and monitor disease activity (with inflammation-sensitive techniques) all in one study suggests a promising future for MRI as a noninvasive imaging technique in the evaluation of vasculitides.

Table 1 Imaging Features Differentiating TA and GCA

	Takayasu's arteritis	Giant cell arteritis
Thoracic aorta	Wall thickening is more prominent in the acute stages Stenoses are common Aneurysms, dissection, and rupture are rare	Wall thickening is less prominent Aneurysms, dissection, and rupture are more common
Aortic valve	Aortic insufficiency common	Aortic insufficiency common
Aortic arch branch vessels	Typically involves the proximal arteries with stenosis and/or occlusions resulting in vertebral "steal" syndrome	Mid to distal subclavian artery stenoses more typically involved
Temporal artery	Rarely involved	Characteristically involved
Pulmonary arteries	Highly variable reported prevalence and manifestations—probably not reliable for differential consideration	Rarely involved
Abdominal aorta	Stenoses of the renal, mesenteric, and common iliac arteries are common, particularly in the Southeast Asian populations (e.g., India, Thailand)	Less commonly involved

REFERENCES

1. Michel BA, Arend WP, Hunder GG. Clinical differentiation between giant cell (temporal) arteritis and Takayasu's arteritis. J Rheumatol 1996; 23:106–111.
2. Kerr GS, Hallahan CW, Giordano J, Leavitt RY, Fauci AS, Rottem M, et al. Takayasu arteritis. Ann Intern Med 1994; 120:919–929.
3. Hoffman GS. Treatment of resistant Takayasu's arteritis. Rheum Dis Clin North Am 1995; 21:73–80.
4. Lagneau P, Michel JB, Vuong PN. Surgical treatment of Takayasu's disease. Ann Surg 1987; 205:157–166.
5. Buckley A, Southwood T, Culham G, Nadel H, Malleson P, Petty R. The role of ultrasound in evaluation of Takayasu's arteritis. Rheumatol 1991; 18:1073–1080.
6. Pariser KM. Takayasu's arteritis. Curr Opin Cardiol 1994; 9:575–580.
7. Park JH, Chung JW, Im JG, Kim SK, Park YB, Han MC. Takayasu arteritis: Evaluation of mural changes in the aorta and pulmonary artery with CT angiography. Radiology 1995; 196:89–93.
8. Sharma S, Taneja K, Gupta AK, Rajani M. Morphologic mural changes in the aorta revealed by CT in patients with nonspecific aortoarteritis (Takayasu's arteritis). Am J Roentgenol 1996; 167:1321–1325.
9. Park JH, Chung JW, Lee KW, Park YB, Han MC. CT angiography of Takayasu arteritis: Comparison with conventional angiography. J Vasc Intervent Radiol 1997; 8:393–400.
10. Hata A, Noda M, Moriwaki R, Numano F. Angiographic findings of Takayasu arteritis: New classification. Int J Cardiol 1996; 54(suppl):S155–S163.
11. Hall S, Barr W, Lie JT, Stanson AW, Kazmier FJ, Hunder GG. Takayasu arteritis. A study of 32 North American patients. Medicine (Baltimore) 1985; 64:89–99.
12. Cho YD, Lee KT. Angiographic characteristics of Takayasu arteritis. Heart Vessels 1992; 7(suppl): 97–101.
13. Yamato M, Lecky JW, Hiramatsu K, Kohda E. Takayasu arteritis: Radiographic and angiographic findings in 59 patients. Radiology 1986; 161:329–334.

14. Moriwaki R, Numano F. Takayasu arteritis: Follow-up studies for 20 years. Heart Vessels Suppl 1992; 7(suppl):138–145.

15. Yamada I, Numano F, Suzuki S. Takayasu arteritis: Evaluation with MR imaging. Radiology 1993; 188:189–94.

16. Paul JF, Hernigou A, Lefebvre C, Bletry O, Piette JC, Gaux JC, et al. Electron beam CT features of the pulmonary artery in Takayasu's arteritis. Am J Roentgenol 1999; 173:189–93.

17. Yamada I, Nakagawa T, Himeno Y, Numano F, Shibuya H. Takayasu arteritis: Evaluation of the thoracic aorta with CT angiography. Radiology 1998; 209:103–109.

18. Hayashi K, Fukushima T, Matsunaga N, Hombo Z. Takayasu's arteritis: Decrease in aortic wall thickening following steroid therapy, documented by CT. Br J Radiol 1986; 59:281–283.

19. Yamada I, Numano F, Suzuki S. Takayasu arteritis: Evaluation with MR imaging. Radiology 1993; 188:89–94.

20. Choe YH, Lee WR. Magnetic resonance imaging diagnosis of Takayasu arteritis. Int J Cardiol 1998; 66(suppl)1:S175–S179.

21. Matsunaga N, Hayashi K, Sakamoto I, Matsuoka Y, Ogawa Y, Honjo K, et al. Takayasu arteritis: MR manifestations and diagnosis of acute and chronic phase. J Magnet Resonance Imag 1998; 8(2):406–414.

22. Matsunaga N, Hayashi K, Sakamoto I, Ogawa Y, Matsumoto T. Takayasu arteritis: Protean radiologic manifestations and diagnosis. Radiographics 1997; 17:579–594.

23. Kim J, Choe YH, Han BK, oh EM, Kim DK, Do YS, et al. Takayasu arteritis: Assessment of disease activity with contrast-enhanced MR imaging (abstr). Arthritis Rheum 1998; 41(suppl):S34.

24. Flamm SD, White RD, Hoffman GS. The clinical application of "edema-weighted" magnetic resonance imaging in the assessment of Takayasu's arteritis. Int J Cardiol 1998; 66(suppl 1):S151–S159.

25. Hunder GG, Bloch DA, Michel BA, Stevens MB, Arend WP, Calabrese LH, et al. The American College of Rheumatology 1990 criteria for the classification of giant cell arteritis. Arthritis Rheum. 1990; 33:1122–1128.

26. Arend WP, Michel BA, Bloch DA, Hunder GG, Calabrese LH, Edworthy SM, et al. The American College of Rheumatology 1990 criteria for the classification of Takayasu arteritis. Arthritis Rheum 1990; 33:1129–1134.

27. Evans JM, Bowles CA, Bjornsson J, Mullany CJ, Hunder GG. Thoracic aortic aneurysm and rupture in giant cell arteritis. A descriptive study of 41 cases. Arthritis Rheum 1994; 37:1539–1547.

28. Schmidt WA, Kraft HE, Vorpahl K, Volker L, Gromnica-Ihle EJ. Color duplex ultrasonography in the diagnosis of temporal arteritis. N Engl J Med 1997; 337:1336–1342.

29. Hunder GG, Weyand CM. Sonography in giant-cell arteritis (editorial; comment). N Engl J Med 1997; 337:1385–1386.

30. Mitomo T, Funyu T, Takahashi Y, Murakami K, Koyama K, Kamio K. Giant cell arteritis and magnetic resonance angiography. Arthritis Rheum 1998; 41:1702.

31. Lande A, Berkmen YM. Aortitis: Pathologic, clinical and arteriographic review. Radiol Clin North Am 1976; 14:219–240.

32. Lindsay JJ. Diagnosis and treatment of diseases of the aorta. Curr Prob Cardiol 1997; 22:485–542.

33. Beachley MC, Ranniger K. Radiographic findings in aneurysms of the aorta. Crit Rev Clin Radiol Nucl Med 1976; 7:291–338.

20

Angiography of Vasculitis

Anthony W. Stanson

Mayo Clinic and Mayo Foundation, Rochester, Minnesota

I. BACKGROUND AND TECHNIQUE

The traditional diagnostic modality of angiography should be appreciated for its pivotal contributions to our understanding of the diagnosis of vascular diseases in this emerging era of alternative imaging procedures: ultrasound (US), computed tomographic (CT) scanning, and magnetic resonance imaging (MRI). These current imaging modalities have not yet fully been implemented in their capability to display the pathological features of arterial disease.

An angiogram outlines the lumen of the vessel being injected with contrast material. Irregularities of contour and caliber provide diagnostic information about vascular anatomy and disease. The distribution of lesions and the specific vascular segments involved give additional diagnostic clues. And finally, a solid medical history and physical examination compensate for the frequent unavailability of histopathology when making diagnostic interpretations from the imaging study.

The wall of the vessel is not adequately depicted by angiography. However, the vessel wall can be seen if it is sufficiently calcified (end stage of arteriosclerosis) or if the vessel is at least partially surrounded by air (e.g., the lungs) such as with most of the left border of the thoracic aorta and the proximal brachiocephalic arteries. The other imaging modalities do provide information about the walls of vessels and important diagnostic information may be observed. Therefore, at times, it may be important to have more than one imaging study performed. This will depend on the disease entity being evaluated.

Angiography is an invasive procedure, and therefore carries an inherent, although small, risk to the patient. Puncture site complications are the most frequent, occurring in about 1 in 500 patients. The risk is increased if selective injections of the brachiocephalic arteries are performed in patients beyond the seventh decade of life; it approaches 0.7%. However, angiographic complications occur less frequently today than they did a decade ago because of improvements in catheter technology and digital filming. Also, in the current era, dedicated specialists perform most angiographic procedures.

The advantages of angiography are its unsurpassed spatial and contrast resolution that allows detection of small degrees of abnormalities in vessel lumen morphology. When small arterial beds must be critically studied, no other imaging modality is satisfactory. The angiogram also provides a global view of the entire territory beyond the catheter and within the field size of the filming area. If repeat injections are necessary, either for a different angle or to extend the field of view, they may be performed rapidly and safely. Currently, most angiography is performed under a digital format that does not quite have the high level of spatial resolution as former film technology. Improvements in computer technology are likely to improve image resolution in the future.

An advantage of invasive angiographic techniques is in providing opportunities for therapeutic intervention: balloon catheter dilatation of stenotic and occluded arterial lesions. This technique is not often applied to lesions of vasculitis, but in patients with GCA and Takayasu's disease it is an option. It is not advocated in the active disease state because of the possibility of inciting further occlusive changes. Once disease becomes quiescent, even arterial occlusions may be successfully treated. Long-term patency has been disappointing, but one would wonder if the success might be higher if reliable clinical markers for disease activity were available. Occasionally, a ruptured aneurysm of polyarteritis or Behçet's disease may be therapeutically controlled by catheter embolization.

Disadvantages of angiography, beyond the occasional complications listed above, are profound allergy to the contrast material, which is rare, and renal toxicity to contrast material in patients with elevated serum creatinine.

II. MAJOR TYPES OF VASCULITIS

The vast majority of patients with vasculitis encountered in our practice have one of four diseases: extracranial temporal arteritis (giant cell arteritis, GCA), Takayasu's disease, polyarteritis (nodosa) (PAN), and Buerger's disease. These diseases present with arterial abnormalities in arterial beds that are large enough to be studied by angiography.

A. Giant Cell Arteritis

There is a group of patients with temporal arteritis, 10–15%, who manifest extracranial arterial disease involving the peripheral arteries (1,2). The most commonly affected arteries are the proximal arteries of the upper extremities. These include the subclavian arterial segments, usually limited to the segments distal to the vertebral artery origins, the entire axillary segments, and the proximal brachial arteries. More distal involvement rarely occurs. Also, rarely, the femoral arteries and their branches, including extension into the tibial arteries, may be involved. The arterial lesions are often present bilaterally, but are nearly always asymmetric in appearance (Fig. 1). At times the angiographic appearance on one side is nearly normal while advanced disease is pres-

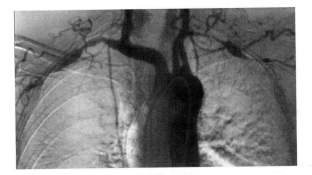

Figure 1   Giant cell arteritis in a 67-year-old female. Aortic arch injection shows bilateral subclavian and axillary artery lesions of stenoses and early aneurysm formation. In the subclavian artery segments, the disease is present distal to the vertebral artery origins.

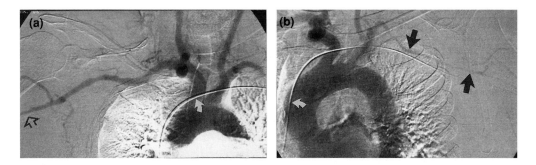

Figure 2   Giant cell arteritis in a 73-year-old female. This study is an intravenous digital subtraction arteriogram with injection of contrast material from a catheter (curved arrow) in the right atrium. There is marked asymmetry in the degree of involvement in the subclavian and axillary arteries segments with a moderate degree of disease on the right side (a) and severe, diffuse stenotic disease (arrows) on the left side (b). In A, note that the stenotic disease process (open arrow) continues up to the brachial artery junction.

ent on the opposite side (Fig. 2). But the findings are almost never found to be unilaterally present. The importance of high-quality, arterially injected angiograms becomes evident in patients with minimal abnormalities. In such cases, an intravenous digital subtraction angiogram (as well as imaging studies of ultrasound, CT scanning and MR scanning) will not allow a correct diagnosis to be made in a timely manner. Multiple additional angiographic technical factors (beyond the scope of this chapter) must be employed to assure diagnostic accuracy.

The classic angiographic appearance of peripheral arteries in GCA is that of stenotic lesions, although sometimes occlusions and rarely aneurysmal changes are also found. Most often, the lumina of the arteries affected show smooth, elongated, tapered caliber reduction ranging from near occlusion to slight narrowing (Fig. 3). The tapered nature of the stenoses occurs at both the proximal and distal ends. Sometimes the diseased segment is many centimeters in length with a marked reduction in lumen diameter that at times may have the false appearance of occlusion. The pattern of the lesions is one of alternating zones of caliber alterations, sometimes mixed with intervening normal, or near-normal caliber. These specific angiographic appearances are not found in any other disease state except Takayasu's disease, which usually has lesions in the aorta and in the proximal branches, which almost always distinguishes it from GCA.

Occlusions also occur, but are less frequently found than stenoses. The most common site for an occlusion to be found is at the distal axillary segment into the zone of the proximal brachial artery (Fig. 4). Collateral refilling may be difficult to appreciate unless an adequate volume of contrast material is injected and delayed filming is obtained. Because of the relatively short time interval between the occlusive process and the angiogram, the collateral arteries are often not large and numerous.

In those rare cases when aneurysmal lesions are present, the segments affected are relatively short and fusiform in shape (Fig. 5). They are not large in diameter. However, rarely in the aorta, a focal aneurysm of a destructive nature is found. It usually has the eccentric, irregular appearance of a false aneurysm. Also, in rare instances, aortic dissection may accompany the early presentation of the disease. In some patients, after several years, a diffuse aneurysm of the thoracic aorta develops, sometimes complicated by dissection (3,4). Although an angiogram could be employed to detect this late consequence of GCA, other imaging methods are more cost effective.

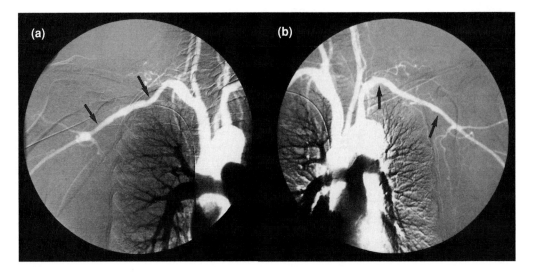

Figure 3 Giant cell arteritis in a 65-year-old female. This is an intravenous digital arteriogram with the venous catheter placed in the right atrium. There is mild irregularity in the subclavian and axillary segments bilaterally (arrows). Two injections were made in the oblique position: (a) is the right side, (b) is the left. Note the high-quality contrast opacification as a manifestation of normal cardiac function in this patient.

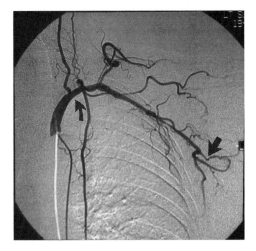

Figure 4 Giant cell arteritis in a 68-year-old female. Selective left subclavian arteriogram shows slight narrowing of the subclavian artery beginning at the origin of the vertebral artery (curved arrow). The luminal irregularity continues into the axillary artery segment where there is occlusion (arrow) at the brachial artery junction.

Extension of the disease process into the distal branches of the upper extremities and involvement of any of the arteries of the lower extremities is not commonly encountered in patients with GCA. However, angiographic abnormalities will be found in about 15% of patients with GCA (unpublished data). The arterial lesions are predominantly those of stenoses and occlusions. Long, smoothly outlined stenotic segments and an alternating pattern of tapered caliber changes are typically identified. In the lower extremities, the involved segments usually start at the femoral bifurcation and may extend to the feet (Figs. 6 and 7).

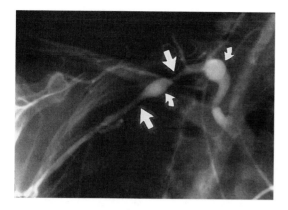

Figure 5 Giant cell arteritis in a 59-year-old female. Innominate artery injection shows stenoses (arrows) and early aneurysm formation (curved arrows) in the right subclavian and axillary artery segments. In this case, disease is present (aneurysm) in the subclavian artery proximal to the origin of the vertebral artery.

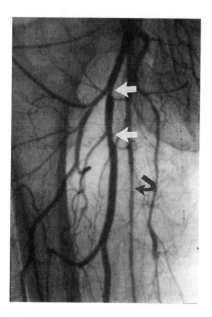

Figure 6 Giant cell arteritis in a 64-year-old female. Right femoral arteriogram shows segmental stenosis of the superficial femoral artery (curved arrow) and stenoses involving a deep femoral branch (arrows).

The differential diagnosis mainly includes Takayasu's disease. At times, GCA and Takayasu's disease are indistinguishable by arteriography, especially if a global study is not performed. However, marked differences in the age of onset, almost always make the distinction easy.

Arteriosclerosis is another disease that can simulate some of the findings of GCA. Certainly in this elderly population, the prevalence of arteriosclerosis mandates that its presence must be considered in the differential diagnosis (Fig. 8). Likewise, artifacts of patient positioning, such as when the shoulder is elevated and the pectoralis minor muscle causes an abrupt angular, eccentric focal stenosis, may result in an incorrect diagnosis (see Fig. 12). When arteriosclerosis causes

(a)

(b)

(c)

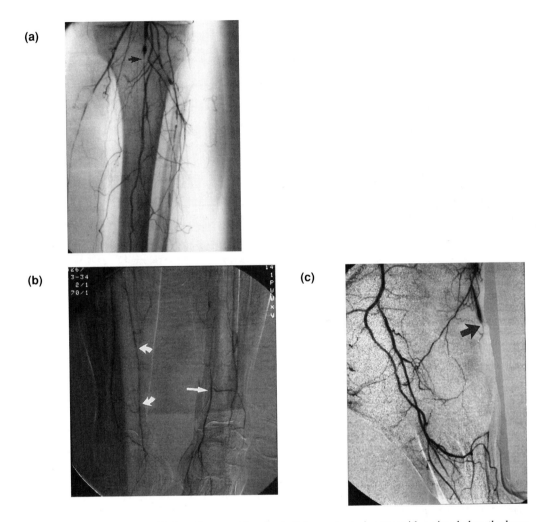

Figure 7   Giant cell arteritis in a 63-year-old male. Left femoral arteriogram with a view below the knee (a) shows marked stenosis of the posterior tibial trunk (arrow) and occlusions of the anterior and posterior tibial arteries. Both lower legs are included in (b). The occluded left posterior tibial artery refills above the ankle (arrow). The right posterior tibial artery has multiple areas of stenoses (curved arrows). Lateral view of the foot (c) shows occlusion of the dorsalis pedis artery (arrow).

stenosis in the brachiocephalic arteries, it most often affects the proximal portion, while the axillary segments and the axillary–brachial junctions are rarely the dominant area of involvement. Also, the lesions of arteriosclerosis are more irregular in their margins, shorter in length, and eccentric in position compared with the adjacent walls. The stenotic lesions of GCA spare the proximal branches of the aorta, such as the common carotids, the innominate, and the subclavian (proximal to the vertebral artery origins), as well as the visceral and common iliac arteries. That is not to say that these segments are spared of the disease process, indeed, they are not. Disease involvement may be identified at pathology, by ultrasound, CT, or MR scanning because the wall of the artery can be evaluated by all of these methods. But rather, evidence of the typical arterial lesions beyond the first order branches is not found angiographically.

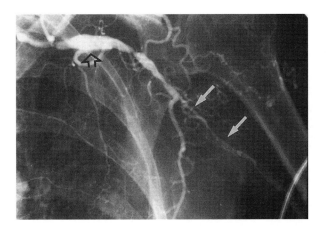

Figure 8 Giant cell arteritis in a 65-year-old female. Left subclavian arteriogram shows severe disease in the axillary artery segment extending to the proximal brachial artery with marked narrowing (arrows) of this arterial segment. There is also slight ectasia at the subclavian–axillary junction (open arrow). This is an example of a mixed pattern of disease with arteriosclerosis and GCA.

B. Takayasu's Disease

The angiographic findings in Takayasu's disease can be quite similar to GCA in some patients. However, a more complete angiographic survey, including the entire aorta and the primary branches, will almost always allow the distinction between these two diseases to be made from the global arteriographic pattern (Figs. 9 and 10). It is the constellation of findings that separates almost all cases of Takayasu's disease from other diseases.

Aortic involvement can be detected in nearly every case. There are two different patterns of findings: stenotic lesions and aneurysmal changes. The lesions may be very difficult to appreciate unless careful attention is paid to the lumen caliber along the course of the aorta (Figs. 9–11). An alteration in diameter of even 1 mm may be an indicator of disease involvement in a young patient in whom the aortic caliber should be uniform except at the region near the isthmus and distal to major branches (Fig. 12). About 25–40% of patients with Takayasu's disease have aneurysmal lesions in the aorta and branches. Even in this setting, stenotic lesions usually coexist. A rare complication of Takayasu's disease is aortic dissection.

Patterns of lesion distribution have shown differences among ethnic groups in Asia; thoracic arterial lesions predominate in Japan, while abdominal arterial disease is more prevalent in Korea and China. In North America, arteriographic abnormalities are found in both distributions (5–8).

The brachiocephalic arteries manifest stenotic or aneurysmal lesions by arteriography. They are almost always evident at the primary branch level in addition to more distal locations. This is an important distinction from GCA. However, in some patients, the lesions may be difficult to detect proximally and if they are only detected distally, a mistaken diagnosis of GCA could be made (Figs. 13–15). Again, the importance of high-quality angiographic techniques, including global imaging, is stressed.

An adequate angiographic study of the visceral arteries must show the proximal segments of all the arteries and therefore a lateral view of the abdominal aorta must be included to detect disease of the celiac, superior mesenteric, and inferior mesenteric arteries (see Figs. 10b and 11c). The renal arteries will be well seen on the anterior projection of the aortogram (Fig. 16). The lesions are predominantly stenotic in nature and rarely are found to extend far from the origins. About one-third of the patients will show occlusion of one or more of the visceral arteries. Addi-

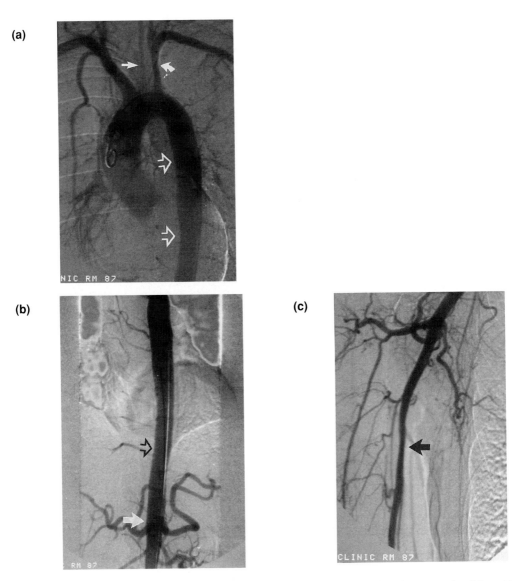

Figure 9   Takayasu's disease in a 30-year-old female. (a) Aortic arch injection shows ectasia of the mid-ascending aortic segment. There is diffuse narrowing of the left common carotid artery (arrow) and slight narrowing of the left subclavian artery proximal to the vertebral (curved arrow). There is also luminal irregularity of the descending segment of the aorta with slight expansion of the proximal portion (upper open arrow) and slight narrowing of the lower segment (lower open arrow). (b) Aortogram of the low thoracic zone extending into the upper abdominal segment shows slight narrowing of the lower thoracic aortic segment (open arrow) and slight expansion of the upper abdominal segment (arrow). (c) Right upper extremity arteriogram shows slight narrowing at the proximal brachial artery (arrow).

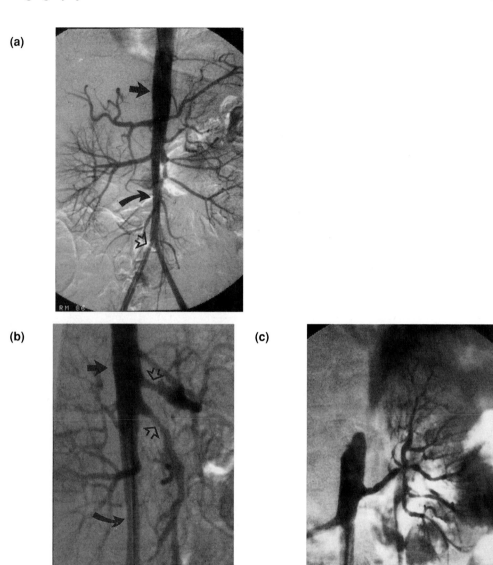

Figure 10 Takayasu's disease in a 11-year-old female. (a) There is slight ectasia of the thoracolumbar junction of the aorta (arrow) and there is slight narrowing of the infrarenal segment (curved arrow). There is also narrowing of the right common iliac artery (open arrow) compared with the left one. (b) Lateral view of the abdominal aortogram again shows slight ectasia of the upper aortic segment (arrow) and slight narrowing of the infrarenal segment (curved arrow). There is also narrowing of the celiac artery (upper open arrow) and of the superior mesenteric artery (lower open arrow). (c) Selective left renal artery injection shows extensive stenotic lesions throughout the branches.

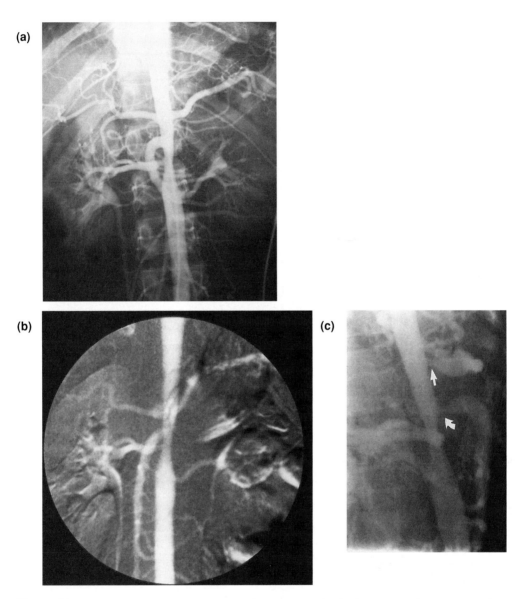

Figure 11 Takayasu's disease in a 17-year-old female. (a) Abdominal aortogram shows segmental narrowing of the paravisceral aortic segment. (b) Intravenous digital subtraction arteriogram of the midabdominal aortic segment is a high-quality examination in this patient with normal cardiac function. Compare to figure 1a. (c) Lateral view of the abdominal aorta shows high-grade stenosis at the origin of the celiac (arrow) and of the superior mesenteric (curved arrow) arteries. Also note the stenosis of the abdominal aorta.

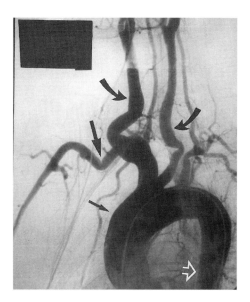

Figure 12 Takayasu's disease in a 21-year-old female. There is ectasia of the ascending segment of the aorta (arrow) and of the innominate artery and of both common carotid arteries (curved arrows). There is also luminal irregularity of the right subclavian and axillary segments. Note the decrease in caliber of the proximal descending thoracic aortic segment (open arrow). The focal, eccentric narrowing (large arrow) of the right axillary artery is extrinsic compression from the pectoralis minor muscle. This artifact is produced by shoulder elevation.

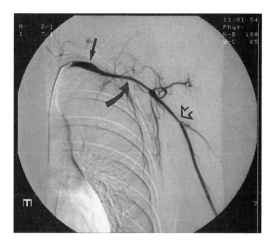

Figure 13 Takayasu's disease in a 31-year-old female. Selective injection of left subclavian artery shows slight expansion of the subclavian near the axillary junction (arrow) and diffuse narrowing with smooth walls of the axillary artery segment (curved arrow) extending to the brachial artery junction (open arrow).

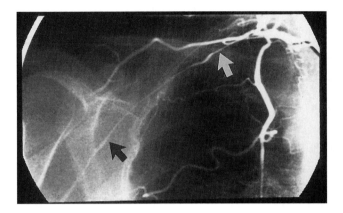

Figure 14 Takayasu's disease in a 40-year-old female. Right subclavian artery injection shows diffuse stenosis of the distal subclavian and axillary artery segments (arrows) extending to the brachial artery level.

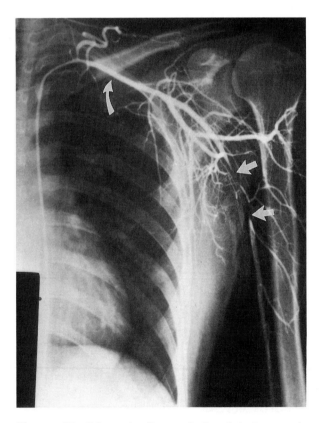

Figure 15 Takayasu's disease. Left subclavian arteriogram shows high-grade stenosis at the axillary–brachial junction with near-occlusion (arrows). There is also narrowing of a lesser degree involving a short zone at the subclavian–axillary junction (curved arrow).

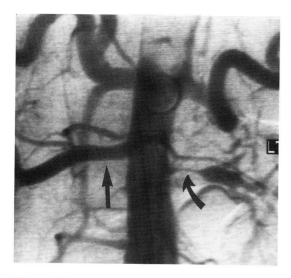

Figure 16 Takayasu's disease. High-grade short segmental stenosis of the left main renal artery (curved arrow). There is slight narrowing of the proximal right main renal artery (arrow).

tional angiographic changes that may be found include secondary changes to the occlusive arterial disease. This includes extensive collateral arteries refilling distally to occluded arterial beds. If the kidneys are involved with renal artery lesions, atrophy may be present (see Fig. 10c).

Takayasu's disease may extend to the iliac arteries (see Fig. 10a) and even into the femoral artery distributions, although it is rarely seen to do so. The lesions are those of stenoses.

The differential diagnosis of Takayasu's disease includes a variety of other diseases depending upon the appearance and location of the arterial abnormality. Caliber alteration in the aorta at the proximal descending thoracic segment may be a normal finding at the region of the ligamentum arteriosum. Stenosis near this location may be evidence of a congenital coarctation. At the thoracoabdominal region, stenosis may represent yet another site of congenital coarctation or of aortic dysplasia secondary to neurofibromatosis. Slight ectasia of the abdominal aorta may also be found in patients with neurofibromatosis as well as in some patients with Takayasu's disease. Associated visceral artery stenosis may be present in all three of these disease conditions. Indeed, such vascular abnormalities in the abdominal area may present a diagnostic challenge. Thus, the importance of extending the angiographic study to include the thoracic aortic branches is evident.

In patients with minimal aortic caliber alteration and stenoses in the distal brachiocephalic branches, distinguishing GCA from Takayasu's disease may be difficult. Careful attention to the pattern of arterial abnormalities throughout the branches, especially looking for slight caliber changes in the common carotid arteries usually secures the correct diagnosis. Focal stenosis of the distal subclavian or proximal axillary artery segments from thoracic outlet compression may cause misinterpretation (see Fig. 12). Therefore, neutral arm and shoulder position during angiography is important to prevent such artifacts from being recorded. At times, confusion arises in distinguishing between Takayasu's disease and early atherosclerosis when at least two of the brachiocephalic arteries have a tapered stenosis or occlusion proximally. Atheromatous lesions may be present in patients who smoke as early as during the fourth decade. These atheromatous lesions may be smooth and tapered in appearance in a young patient (Fig. 17). If an occlusion is present also, then it may be difficult to make the correct diagnosis. However, if the lesions are

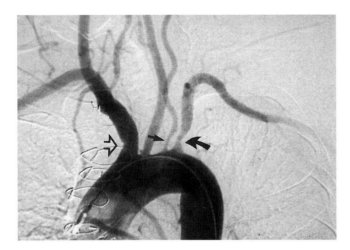

Figure 17 Atheromatous disease in a 46-year-old male. There are stenotic lesions near the origins of the anomalous left vertebral artery (arrow) and the left subclavian artery (curved arrow). There are also small atheromatous plaques at the origins of the innominate artery (open arrow) and at the origin of the left carotid artery. This patient is a heavy smoker and atheromatous lesions in patients of this age and younger who smoke may be misinterpreted as arteritis.

only stenotic, then the appearance of the artery immediately beyond the stenotic focus holds the clue: an abrupt change in caliber indicates an atheromatous lesion.

The coronary and pulmonary arteries may also be affected in Takayasu's disease (Fig. 18). The lesions are predominantly those of stenoses and occlusion. The incidence reported is variable from 5–30% depending upon the country of origin of the report. Of course, the true incidence cannot be known unless all possible arterial beds are included in the angiographic study.

C. Polyarteritis Nodosa

The most common type of necrotizing vasculitis encountered at angiography is PAN (9,10). The angiographic findings are those of stenoses, occlusions, and aneurysms of various sizes, number, and distribution. Approximately 70% of patients with a clinical diagnosis of PAN have positive angiographic findings.

The angiographic findings of so-called microaneurysms are the most widely recognized lesion typical of classic PAN (Figs. 19–22) but in some cases the aneurysms may be large and rupture is not uncommon. However, stenotic and occlusive lesions are more commonly found than are aneurysms in patients with PAN (Figs. 23–26). Indeed, in the absence of aneurysms, the diagnosis could be missed by an inexperienced observer. The viscera are most commonly affected, but PAN is a widespread arterial disease and lesions may also be found in the intercostal and lumbar arteries and other branches in the retroperitoneal area (Fig. 27), such as capsular branches of the renal arteries. When performing an angiogram for the diagnosis of PAN, it may be found necessary to inject all the visceral arteries: renal, superior mesenteric, inferior mesenteric, hepatic, and splenic arteries. The involvement may be limited to only one of these arterial beds. Rarely, the involvement is predominantly in the hands or feet (Fig. 28). In these locations, the lesions are occlusive in nature but sometimes aneurysms are found.

In a recent review of our patients with PAN, 56 patients had angiograms available for study (11). Aneurysms were found in 27 of the patients and arterial ectasia of slight to moderate degree was identified in another 7 patients. The remaining 22 patients had only evidence of arterial le-

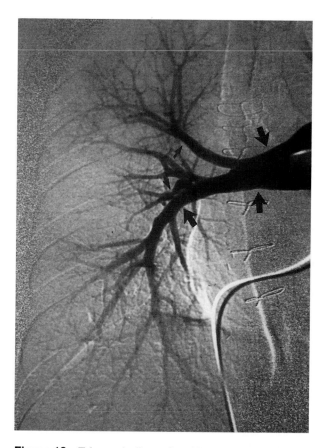

Figure 18 Takayasu's disease in a 21-year-old female. Right pulmonary arteriogram shows diffuse narrowing of the right main pulmonary artery and the proximal branches (arrows).

sions of stenosis and occlusion. In total, 55 of the 56 patients had evidence of stenotic and occlusive lesions. Arterial lesions were usually found in multiple vascular beds, but in the group with visceral artery disease, 60% of the patients had at least one organ free of lesions. Arterial lesions were present in the viscera in most of the patients, but in nine patients, there was also involvement in muscular branches of the thorax, abdomen, or pelvis. An additional nine patients had involvement of the extremities.

There were 5 of the 56 patients who presented with rupture of a large aneurysm arising from a visceral artery. These were successfully treated by transcatheter embolization (12). The diagnosis of rupture and identification of hemorrhage was made by CT scanning. The diagnosis could also have been made by MRI, but CT is much faster and less expensive to produce.

D. Kawasaki Disease

Kawasaki disease, or syndrome, is a necrotizing vasculitis that appears somewhat like PAN, but it occurs in young children. The arterial pattern of Kawasaki disease is that of aneurysms, usually segmental in appearance, and at times huge in size relative to the native artery. The involved arterial zones may be widespread as in PAN (Fig. 29), but the predominant site of involvement is the coronary arteries (13,14). In this vascular bed, angiography has traditionally been the diagnostic imaging modality of choice, but ultrasound, MR, and electron beam CT scanning are also able to detect coronary artery aneurysms, although areas of a minimal degree of involvement

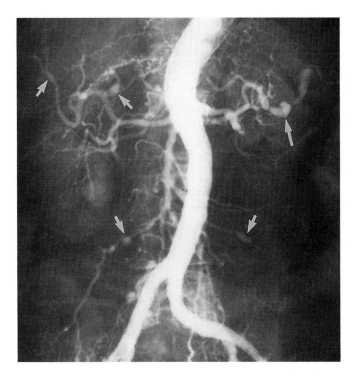

Figure 19 Polyarteritis nodosa in a 69-year-old female. Abdominal aortogram shows multiple aneurysms in the distribution of the hepatic, splenic, and superior mesenteric arteries (arrows).

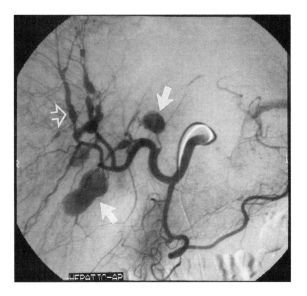

Figure 20 Polyarteritis nodosa in a 97-year-old female. Hepatic arteriogram shows multiple aneurysms in the hepatic artery distribution. Some of these are huge relative to the involved artery segment (arrows). Others are fusiform in shape (open arrow).

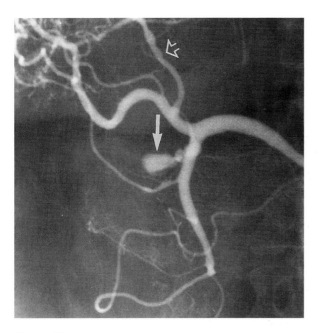

Figure 21 Polyarteritis nodosa in a 68-year-old male. Common hepatic arteriogram showing a localized view of the gastroduodenal artery, which has a large aneurysm of a proximal small branch (arrow). Slight ectasia noted in the left hepatic artery (open arrow).

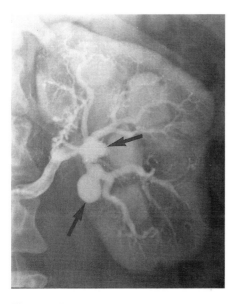

Figure 22 Polyarteritis nodosa in a 32-year-old female. Left renal arteriogram shows large eccentric aneurysms (arrows) involving the primary branches.

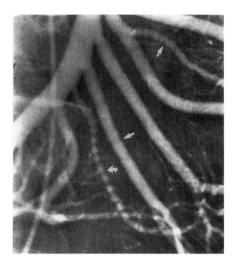

Figure 23 Polyarteritis nodosa in a 34-year-old male. Superior mesenteric arteriogram shows three branches with luminal irregularities. There is severe involvement in one branch (curved arrow) with multiple stenotic foci. Two other branches show minimal luminal irregularity (arrows).

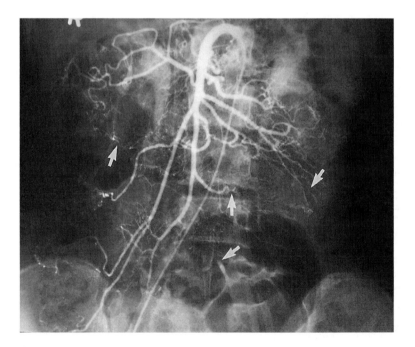

Figure 24 Polyarteritis nodosa in a 19-year-old female. Superior mesenteric arteriogram shows diffuse stenotic and occlusive lesions (arrows) but without aneurysms.

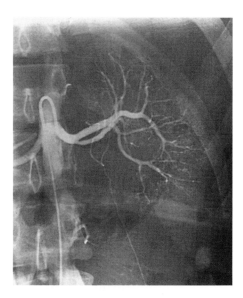

Figure 25 Polyarteritis nodosa in a 19-year-old female. Left renal arteriogram shows multiple stenoses and occlusions of renal artery branches.

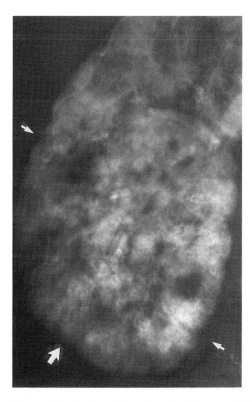

Figure 26 Polyarteritis nodosa in a 25-year-old female. Right renal arteriogram in the parenchymal phase shows multiple scattered small infarcts (arrows).

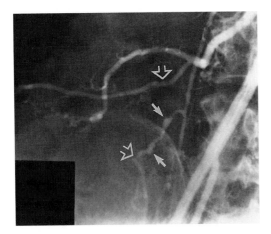

Figure 27 Polyarteritis nodosa in a 32-year-old female. Retroperitoneal arterial branches in the right lower quadrant show areas of ectasia (arrows) and stenoses (open arrows).

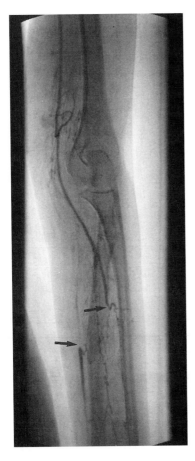

Figure 28 Polyarteritis nodosa in a 19-year-old female. Left upper extremity arteriogram shows occlusion of the arteries in the forearm (arrows).

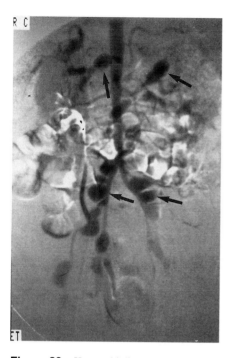

Figure 29   Kawasaki disease in a 2-month-old infant. Abdominal aortogram shows extensive aneurysmal disease present in the hepatic artery branches, left renal artery, and branches of both iliac arteries (arrows).

would be best detected by angiography. The role of angiography is important to consider when trying to detect early arterial involvement.

E.   Behçet's Disease

Behçet's disease is rarely encountered in North America because it is not one of the endemic areas. About one-quarter of the cases are associated with venous thrombosis for which ultrasound is the diagnostic modality of choice while venography is rarely employed. The diagnostic findings of venous occlusion are nonspecific in patients with Behçet's disease. Arterial lesions are rare and are usually found to be aneurysms, which may become complicated by occlusion or rupture. The most common location is the aorta, followed by the pulmonary arteries and the larger arteries of the extremities (15). The arteriographic appearance of these aneurysms is not specific for Behçet's disease, but rather they have the appearance of a false aneurysm because of the irregular contour of the wall. When found to be multiple in the pulmonary bed, the diagnosis of Behçet's disease should be suspected as almost no other condition causes this outside of infectious processes (16).

Diagnostic modalities of CT, MRA, and ultrasound are well suited to detect and evaluate aneurysms of Behçet's disease. Angiography may be necessary to identify small aneurysms and it offers a treatment option. Therapeutic catheter intervention may be applied in an attempt to control hemorrhage in cases of rupture or to prevent rupture in patients with large or symptomatic aneurysms.

F. Buerger's Disease

The arterial occlusive lesions of Buerger's disease may be difficult to diagnose angiographically because the early pattern of distal limb involvement may simulate other diseases. However, in a young patient who smokes cigarettes, distal limb arterial occlusions should raise the possibility of Buerger's disease in every case. There are very specific angiographic findings in this disease, which unfortunately occur in only the minority of patients. Other diagnostic imaging modalities are not adequate to establish an accurate diagnosis of Buerger's disease.

The first angiographic pattern of the disease is that of distal limb arterial stenoses and occlusions (Fig. 30). Occlusive disease in the feet and hands must be present before any consideration can be given to a more proximal lesion in establishing the diagnosis. There is always a skip pattern of occlusive disease in the early stages and some normal arterial segments are found within the affected anatomical level. The findings are bilateral though not often particularly symmetrical (Fig. 31). As the process progresses centrally, the same type of arterial lesions that are found initially in the lower legs and forearms appear more proximally (Fig. 32). Rarely, iliac and visceral artery involvement is found. It is not uncommon for an entire arterial segment, such as the posterior tibial, to be occluded flush to its origin while the companion artery, such as the peroneal, is normal. This feature is often found among the arteries of the lower legs and forearms. Stenotic arterial lesions are common, the appearance being of two types. The first is that of smooth narrowing (of short segments) similar to that seen in other types of vasculitis. The second is a unique appearance found almost only in patients with Buerger's disease: a narrowed, tortuous, irregular pathway through the lumen of the artery (Fig. 33). At times, this has the appearance of a corkscrew, but it is rarely so uniformly symmetrical.

An associated finding in patients with Buerger's disease is preservation of the vasa vasorum of the occluded artery, which becomes a prominent collateral to the distal circulation. Often in these cases, the vasa vasorum is found to have somewhat of a corkscrew appearance because

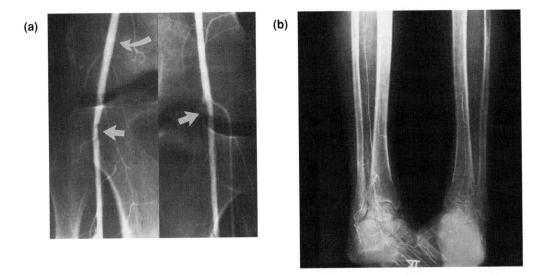

Figure 30 Buerger's disease in a 22-year-old female. (a) Bilateral femoral arteriogram shows irregularity of the lumen of the popliteal artery segments (arrows) and ectasia of the right popliteal artery (curved arrow). (b) Extensive arterial occlusive disease involving the lower legs and feet. All major arteries have occlusive disease.

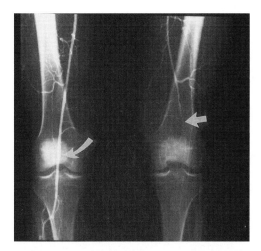

Figure 31 Buerger's disease in a 49-year-old male. Bilateral femoral arteriography shows occlusion of the left popliteal artery (arrow) and slight expansion of the right popliteal artery (curved arrow).

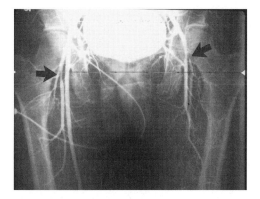

Figure 32 Buerger's disease in a 34-year-old male. Bilateral femoral arteriography shows stenotic lesions proximally in the deep femoral arteries (arrows).

of tortuosity associated with high flow and thus this corkscrew appearance is not specific for Buerger's disease (see Fig. 33b).

Another associated finding, which is not common and not widely appreciated, is ectatic segments of arteries within the diseased bed. If this finding is present, it is usually found in the popliteal and digital distributions (see Figs. 30a and 31).

As a constellation of findings, the arteriographic findings of Buerger's disease usually are quite specific, and the diagnosis is confidently made by an experienced physician (17–19). Occasionally, the disease presents for the first time relatively late in life and the diagnosis may become difficult to establish in the presence of peripheral arteriosclerosis.

The differential diagnosis includes sequelae of thromboembolic disease, early arteriosclerosis of diabetes, obliterative arterial disease of scleroderma, ergotamine toxicity, PAN, and exposure to cocaine.

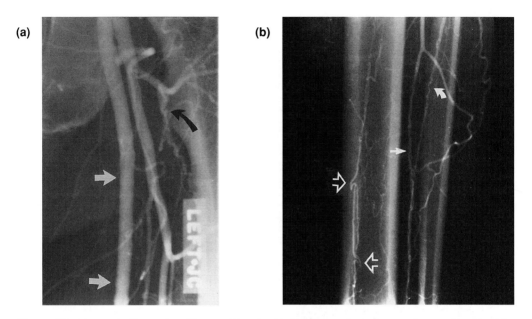

Figure 33 Buerger's disease in a 58-year-old male. (a) Left femoral arteriogram shows a branch of the deep femoral artery (curved arrow) with marked corkscrew irregularity indicating direct angiographic evidence of Buerger's disease. There is also a mild degree of luminal irregularity of the superficial femoral artery (arrows). (b) Left femoral arteriogram shows marked irregularity of the lumen of the peroneal artery (arrow) and of the anterior tibial artery (curved arrow) in a corkscrew-like pattern. There is also reduction in caliber. This represents direct angiographic evidence of Buerger's disease. Also, note the vasa vasorum (open arrows) of the occluded posterior tibial artery.

III. MISCELLANEOUS DISEASES

Occasionally, patients with other types of vasculitis, such as Wegener's granulomatosis, Churg-Strauss syndrome, and others, may come to angiography. Vascular lesions are not often found. But when they are, the appearance of lesions is similar to those of the more common forms of vasculitis.

IV. CONCLUSIONS

Angiography has been the main imaging modality for many years for the diagnosis of arteritis and, indeed, for many other vascular diseases. It maintains its essential role in those diseases with predominant small-vessel involvement, such as PAN and Buerger's disease. In those diseases with predominantly large-vessel involvement, such as Behçet's disease, Takayasu's disease, and GCA, angiographic findings are the template upon which new and noninvasive imaging modalities are measured. Additional advantages of these new modalities are that they have the ability to display additional findings, such as wall thickening, inflammation, thrombosis, as well as physiological information of flow, velocity, and age of thrombosis.

REFERENCES

1. Stanson A, Klein R, Hunder G. Extracranial angiographic findings in giant cell (temporal) arteritis. Am J Roentgenol 1976; 127:957–963.
2. Brack A, Martinez-Taboada V, Stanson A, Goronzy J, Weyand C. Disease Pattern in Cranial and Large-Vessel Giant Cell Arteritis. Arthritis Rheum 1999; 42:311–317.
3. Evans J, Bowles C, Bjornsson J, Mullany C, Hunder G. Thoracic aortic aneurysm and rupture in giant cell arteritis: A descriptive study of 41 cases. Arthritis Rheum 1994; 37:1539–1547.
4. Evans JM, O'Fallon WM, Hunder GG. Increased incidence of aortic aneurysm and dissection in giant cell (temporal) arteritis: A population-based study. Ann Intern Med 1995; 122:502–507.
5. Lupi-Herrera E, Sanchez-Torres G, Marcushamer J, et al. Takayasu's arteritis. Clinical study of 107 cases. Am Heart J 1977; 93:103.
6. Hall S, Barr W, Lie J, Stanson A, Kazmier F, Hunder G. Takayasu arteritis: A study of 32 North American patients. Medicine (Baltimore) 1985; 64:89–99.
7. Yamato M, Lecky JW, Hiramatsu K, et al. Takayasu arteritis: Radiographic and angiographic findings in 59 patients. Radiology 1986; 161:329–334.
8. Ishikawa K. Diagnostic approach and proposed criteria for the clinical diagnosis of Takayasu's arteriopathy. J Am Coll Cardiol 1988; 12:964–972.
9. Hunder GG, Lie JT. Vasculitic syndromes. Intern Med 1994; 307:2430–2441.
10. Valente RM, Hall S, O'Duffy JD, Conn DL. Vasculitis and related disorders. In Kelley WN, ed. Textbook of Rheumatology. Philadelphia: Saunders, 1997:1079–1122.
11. Stanson AW, Friese JL, Johnson CM, McKusick MA, Breen JF, Sabater EA, Andrews JC. Polyarteritis nodosa: spectrum of angiographic findings. RadioGraphics 2001; 21:151–159.
12. Achkar AA, Stanson AW, Johnson CM, Srivatsa SS, Dale LC, Weyand CM. Rheumatoid vasculitis manifesting as intra-abdominal hemorrhage. Mayo Clin Proc 1995; 70:565–569.
13. Fukushige J, Nihill MR, McNamara DG: Spectrum of cardiovascular lesion in mucocutaneous lymph node syndrome: Analysis of eight cases. Am J Cardiol 1980; 45:98.
14. Suzuki A et al. Coronary artery lesions of Kawasaki's disease. Cardiac catheterization findings of 100 cases. Pediatr Cardiol 1986; 7:3.
15. Park JH, Han MC, Bettmann MA. Arterial manifestations of Behçet disease. Am J Rheumatol 1984; 143:821–825.
16. Numan F, Islak C, Berkmen T, Tuzun H, Cokyuksel O. Behçet disease: Pulmonary arterial involvement in 15 cases. Radiology 1994; 192:465–468.
17. Wolf Ea, Sumner DS, Standness DE Jr. Disease of the mesenteric circulation in patients with thromboangiitis obliterans. Vasc Surg 6:218, 1973.
18. Suzuki S, et al. Buerger's disease (thromboangiitis obliterans): An analysis of the arteriograms of 119 cases. Clin Radiol 33:235, 1982.
19. Hagen B, Lohse S. Clinical and radiologic aspects of Buerger's disease. Cardiovasc Intervent Radiol 7:283, 1984.

21
Kawasaki Disease

Karyl S. Barron
National Institute of Allergy and Infectious Diseases, National Institutes of Health, Bethesda, Maryland

I. INTRODUCTION

Kawasaki disease (KD) is an acute febrile illness of childhood and is the primary cause of acquired heart disease in children in the United States and Japan. Initially described by Dr. Tomasaku Kawasaki in 1967 (1), the syndrome was thought to be a benign, self-limited febrile illness. It is now recognized to be a systemic vasculitis occurring predominantly in small and medium-sized muscular arteries, especially the coronary arteries. Specific epidemiological evidence suggests an infectious etiology, but a causative organism or toxin has not been identified. A current theory describes KD as an immunologically mediated generalized vasculitis that is triggered in a susceptible host by a variety of common infectious agents prevalent in the community (2). Morbidity and mortality of the disease are most often due to cardiac sequelae, and treatment is based on prevention of coronary artery aneurysm formation.

II. CLINICAL FEATURES

The principal diagnostic criteria for KD are shown in Table 1 along with other associated manifestations. Five of the six criteria, with fever being an absolute, must be present for diagnosis. In addition, the illness should not be explained by other known disease processes. "Atypical" cases may be diagnosed with fewer criteria when coronary artery aneurysms are noted by echocardiography or angiography.

    The fever associated with KD is generally high and spiking (usually to 104 °F, 40 °C, or higher), and persists in the untreated patient for 1 to 2 weeks or longer. Kawasaki disease should be considered in the differential diagnosis of a young child with unexplained fever. Bilateral conjunctival injection usually begins shortly after the onset of the fever. It typically involves the bulbar conjunctivae more than the palpebral conjunctivae and is not associated with an exudate (Fig. 1). Typical changes of the lips and oral cavity include erythema and fissuring of the lips, erythema of the oropharyngeal mucosa, and strawberry tongue, with prominent papillae and erythema. Oral ulcerations are not a feature of this disease. Early in the disease there may be brawny induration of the hands and feet and erythema confined to the palms and soles. In the convalescent stage of the disease, characteristic periungual desquamation of the fingers and toes occurs and may involve the entire hand or foot (Fig. 21.2; see color plate). Interestingly, the rash, peripheral edema,

Table 1 Characteristics of Kawasaki Disease

Principal diagnostic criteria*
  Fever lasting more than 5 days
  Conjunctival injection
  Oropharyngeal changes
    Erythema, swelling, and fissuring of the lips
    Diffuse erythema of the oropharynx
    Strawberry tongue
  Peripheral extremity changes
    Erythema of the palms and soles
    Induration of the hands and feet
    Desquamation of the skin of the hands and feet
  Polymorphous rash
  Cervical lymphadenopathy, usually a single node >1.5 cm
Associated manifestations
  Irritability
  Sterile pyuria, meatitus
  Perineal erythema and desquamation
  Arthralgias, arthritis
  Abdominal pain, diarrhea
  Aseptic meningitis
  Hepatitis
  Obstructive jaundice
  Hydrops of the gallbladder
  Uveitis
  Sensorineural hearing loss
  Cardiovascular changes

*Five of the six principal criteria, with fever being an absolute, must
 be present for a diagnosis.

and desquamation are reminiscent of the skin changes observed in some patients undergoing immunotherapy with interleukin-2 (3). Beau's lines (transverse grooves) of the nails occurs several months later as a testament to the acute illness. Skin involvement is frequently seen early in the disease and is polymorphous and nonspecific. The typical rash is macular or morbilliform and involves the trunk and extremities (Fig. 21.3; see color plate). Rarely, the rash may be pustular, but it is neither vesicular nor bullous in nature. A large portion of children will initially develop erythema of the perineum, which evolves into desquamation within 48 h (Fig. 21.4; see color plate). Cervical lymphadenopathy is considered a principal finding when at least one lymph node is more than 1.5 cm in diameter. The lymphadenopathy is usually unilateral and is the least common among the five principal clinical findings.

A number of other features are characteristic of KD, although not included in the diagnostic criteria. Extreme irritability is common, especially in young infants. Central nervous system involvement may also include aseptic meningitis, facial palsy, subdural effusion, and symptomatic and asymptomatic cerebral infarction (4). Pulmonary infiltrates and pleural effusions may be present. Gastrointestinal manifestations include hepatomegaly, which may be associated with jaundice (5), hydrops of the gallbladder (6), diarrhea, and pancreatitis (7). Renal manifestations range from sterile pyuria (most likely secondary to urethral inflammation), with or without proteinuria, to acute renal insufficiency with interstitial nephritis proven by biopsy (8). Arthritis and arthralgia may also be seen in the first week of illness and are usually polyarticular, involving the

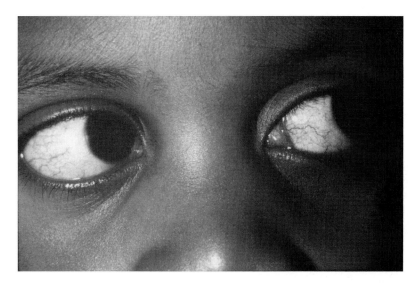

Figure 1   Bilateral, nonpurulent conjunctival injection is one of the clinical criteria in the diagnosis of Kawasaki disease.

hands, knees, and ankles. A pauciarticular arthritis involving the knees, ankles, or hips frequently occurs in the second or third week of illness. Ocular findings range from inflammatory, nonpurulent conjunctival injection to anterior uveitis (9). Sensorineural hearing loss has been reported, albeit in conjunction with aspirin therapy (10). An interesting feature in some patients is erythema and induration at the site of a recent vaccination with bacille Calmette–Guérin (BCG) (Fig. 5). While BCG immunization is rarely administered in the United States, it is commonly administered to children in Japan. Takayama et al. (11) reported erythema at the site of BCG inoculation in 36% of 295 KD patients. The cause of this reaction is unknown.

The clinical features of KD mimic many childhood illnesses, and the differential diagnosis includes infections, toxicosis, drug reactions, connective tissue diseases, and malignancy, as summarized in Table 2.

III. CARDIAC DISEASE

Cardiovascular manifestations can be prominent in the acute phase of the disease and are the leading cause of long-term morbidity. In this phase, pericardial effusion is detected by echocardiography in approximately 30% of patients and usually resolves spontaneously without specific therapy. Myocarditis is also common in the acute phase and may be manifested by tachycardia out of proportion to the degree of fever and gallop rhythm. Myocarditis can be detected clinically using imaging techniques, and it has been found to be very common in the acute phase of KD, as diagnosed by left ventricular dilatation and reduced contractility on echocardiogram, by presence of elevated antimyosin antibody titers, and by uptake of gallium or labeled white blood cells with radionuclide cardiac imaging (12). The severity of carditis is not necessarily linked with the presence of coronary artery dilatation. Congestive heart failure and atrial and ventricular arrhythmias can occur in the setting of KD. Electrocardiogram findings include decreased R-wave voltage, ST-segment depression, and T-wave flattening or inversion. Myocardial inflammation may also cause slowed conduction, resulting in prolongation of P–R and/or Q–T intervals (13). When

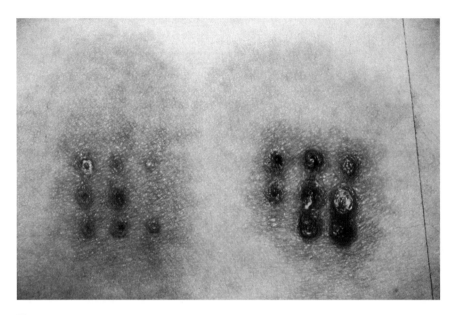

Figure 5 Erythema and induration at the site of a recent bacille Calmette–Guérin (BCG) vaccination in a patient with Kawasaki disease.

valvular involvement occurs it is usually mitral, although aortic valve involvement has been described (14). Recent evidence suggests that mitral regurgitation may be present in 30% of patients, although it is usually mild (15).

Coronary artery lesions are responsible for most of the morbidity and mortality of the disease. They developed in approximately 20% of patients prior to the widespread use of intravenous γ-globulin (IVGG), but now occur in less than 10%. Aneurysms usually appear from 1–4 weeks after the onset of illness, and it is rare to detect new lesions after 6 weeks (Fig. 6). Factors associated with an increased risk of developing coronary artery aneurysms include male gender; age less than 1 year; other signs or symptoms of pericardial, myocardial, or endocardial involvement, including arrhythmias; prolonged fever; recurrence of fever; elevated white blood cell count; increased level of cytokines, including interleukin-6, interleukin-8, and tumor necrosis factor; and elevated β-thromboglobulin, an indicator of increased platelet activation (13,16–19).

Coronary artery aneurysms are described as small (4 mm), medium (4–8 mm), or giant (>8 mm), and are more commonly proximal than distal. Aneurysms may be fusiform or saccular (near-equal axial and lateral diameters). Ectasia of the vessels (vessel size larger than age-matched controls) is also a common finding. Aneurysms are most easily detected by transthoracic two-dimensional echocardiography, but other imaging techniques are being evaluated (20–25).

The natural history, or fate, of the coronary aneurysms is the critical issue of KD. Most ectatic coronary lesions and small aneurysms regress, whereas moderate aneurysms remain unchanged, regress, or progress to stenosis or obstruction (26–28). Giant aneurysms rarely regress in size. Kato (29) investigated the various factors that could affect the prognosis of coronary aneurysms and found that the most important factor to predict the prognosis was the size of the coronary aneurysms. By discrimination analysis, the risk factors for coronary aneurysms to develop into ischemic heart disease included the size of aneurysms greater than 8 mm and the shape of large diffuse or saccular aneurysms. Coronary aneurysms developing in patients older than 2 years of age were also less likely to regress. Pathology of the coronary artery in KD several years after onset demonstrates marked intimal proliferation, and in some patients, calcification deposits

Table 2 Differential Diagnosis of Kawasaki Disease

Infection
  Bacterial
    Streptococcus spp.
    Staphylococcus spp.
    Proprionibacterium acnes
  Spirochetal
    Leptospira spp.
  Rickettsial
    Rocky Mountain spotted fever
  Viral
    Measles
    Adenovirus
    Parainfluenza
    Epstein–Barr virus
    Cytomegalovirus
    Retroviruses
  Fungal
    Candida spp.
Toxicosis
  Mercury
Drug reactions
  Antibiotics
  Antifungals
  Anticonvulsants
Connective tissue disease
  Systemic onset juvenile rheumatoid arthritis
  Other vasculitides
Malignancy
  Leukemia
  Lymphoma

of protein-like material and hyalinized degeneration in the thickened intima, which are quite similar to arteriosclerotic lesions (29).

While some aneurysms appear to regress to a normal size by echocardiography, these vessels most likely remain abnormal, as response to pharmacological dilation may remain impaired (30). Pathologically regressed aneurysms may reveal abnormal intimal proliferation (31) and, in fact, may also be associated with narrowed lumens and calcified arterial walls, despite the fact that these changes may not be apparent on arteriography (25). Therapy with IVGG has decreased the incidence of giant aneurysms (26), which rarely regress and frequently develop complicating thromboses, stenosis, or total occlusion. Myocardial infarction may result; when it occurs, it is most likely to be in the first year, with 40% occurring in the first 3 months of illness (32). Symptoms of myocardial infarction in the young child include inconsolable crying, vomiting, dyspnea, cardiovascular collapse, and shock. Chest pain has been described by children who can communicate the symptom (13). There are case reports of young adults suffering from myocardial infarction over a decade after their initial disease (33–35), and others with coronary artery aneurysms who were not known to have had KD as children (36,37).

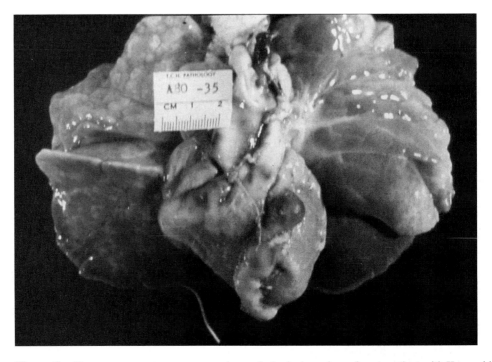

Figure 6   Giant coronary artery aneurysms in a pathological specimen from a patient with Kawasaki disease.

Blood vessels other than the coronary arteries may also be involved, including the abdominal aorta (38), the superior mesenteric (39), axillary, subclavian, brachial, iliac, and renal arteries, with resultant distal ischemia and necrosis (Fig. 7). Peripheral extremity ischemia occurs infrequently, but may result in gangrene of the affected area. Vasculitis with resultant vessel spasm is thought to be responsible (40).

IV. EPIDEMIOLOGY

Eighty percent of cases of KD occur in children less than 5 years of age. Worldwide, the peak incidence is in children 2 years of age and younger, with boys affected 1.5 times as often as girls. Recurrences occur in 1–3% of cases (12), and familial incidence is approximately 2% (41). Although all racial groups are represented, children of Asian ancestry continue to predominate, with the incidence in the Japanese being highest at approximately 50–200 per 100,000 children less than 5 years of age (nonepidemic vs. epidemic years) (12,42). The incidence in the United States ranges from 6–15 per 100,000 children younger than 5 years of age (43), with Asian Americans being proportionately overrepresented and white Americans underrepresented. In North America, cases occur throughout the year, with larger numbers occurring in late winter to early spring (44). Mortality rates have been shown to be higher in boys, with most deaths occurring in the first 2 months of illness. Nakamura et al. (45) has shown that if deaths in the first few months of illness

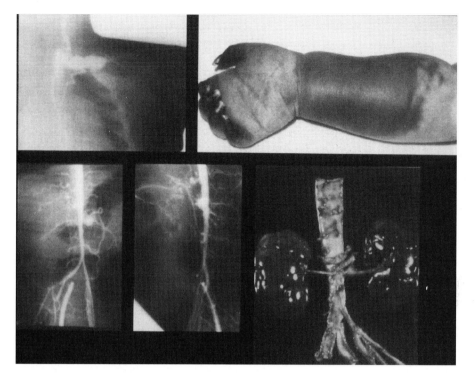

Figure 7 Aneurysms can occur in arteries other than the coronary arteries in Kawasaki disease. (Top left) Radiograph of an aneurysm of the subclavian artery. (Top right) Vasculitis with probable vasospasm of peripheral arteries in Kawasaki disease may lead to compromised perfusion distal to the lesion with consequent ischemic changes as seen in this infant's arm. (Bottom right) Aneurysm of the take-off of the renal artery and areas of infarction in the upper pole of the kidney. (Bottom left) Arteriogram revealing aneurysm of renal artery.

are excluded, the death rate for both boys and girls was not statistically different from that for the control population. With the institution of therapy with IVGG, case fatality has improved from 2–0.3% or less (46).

V. LABORATORY FINDINGS

Laboratory evaluation early in the course of disease reveals a leukocytosis with a left shift, normochromic, normocytic anemia, increased sedimentation rate, increased α_1-antitrypsin (as an acute phase reactant), and depressed albumin. Thrombocytosis occurs in the subacute stage of the disease, with platelet counts frequently reaching $1,000,000/\mu L$ or greater. Lipid metabolism has been found to be abnormal in the acute stage, with a decrease in high-density lipoprotein cholesterol and total cholesterol. Months later, total cholesterol levels return to normal, but high-density lipoprotein levels may remain depressed for several years (47,48). A mild hepatitis may be evident by elevated transaminases, and direct bilirubin and urobilinogen may be elevated secondary to hydrops of the gallbladder with functional biliary tract obstruction. Urinalysis may reveal mild proteinuria, probably secondary to fever, and sterile pyuria, probably a reflection of urethral involvement. Cerebrospinal fluid shows a mononuclear pleocytosis with normal protein and glucose. Joint fluid shows predominantly polymorphonuclear neutrophilic leukocytes with 50,000–300,000 cells/mm^3 (46).

Although we have yet to determine the initiating factor, immune activation may play a major role in KD pathogenesis. Acute phase leukocytosis is accompanied by increased numbers of circulating helper T cells, increased monocytes and macrophages, and polyclonal activation of B cells (2,49–51). Other findings associated with aberrant immune regulation include increased levels of serum interleukin-1 (52), interleukin-2 (53), soluble interleukin-2 receptors (54), interleukin-4 (55), interleukin-6 (56), interleukin-10 (55,57), tumor necrosis factor-α (TNF-α) (49, 58), interferon-γ (59), and soluble CD30 serum antigen (60). Furukawa et al. (61) reported that serum levels of p60-soluble TNF receptor levels may also be useful for determining the severity of vascular damage during acute KD and that patients with KD and high TNF receptor levels seem to be susceptible to coronary artery lesions even if they receive therapy with IVGG. CD14+ T cells are increased, as are the percentages of monocytes and macrophages (compared with the total number of monocytes) and B cells (2,49–51). Antineutrophil cytoplasmic antibodies may be present, however it seems likely that these antibodies are nonspecific epiphenomena associated with generalized immune activation and polyclonal B-cell activation, rather than pathogenically important agents (62). Finally, recent studies show that elevation of plasma endothelin-1 (63) or urine neopterin (64) may be markers of activation of the cellular immune response and thus may serve as predictors of coronary artery aneurysm development.

VI. DISEASE MECHANISMS

Although the etiological agent of the disease remains a mystery, epidemiological data indicate that there may be an infectious cause. Many organisms and toxins have been reported as possible agents in the disease: *Staphylococcus* spp., *Streptococcus* spp., *Candida* spp., *Rickettsia* spp., retroviruses, Epstein–Barr virus, and others (65) (see Table 2). Enterotoxins and exotoxins of staphylococci and streptococci have recently been identified from cultures, predominantly of the rectum and oral pharynx, in a small cohort of children with KD. Although Leung et al. (66) speculated that these toxins may be acting as superantigens in the disease process, others have failed to confirm this association (67,68). Virus-like particles with reverse transcriptase activity (69), extracellular products of oral Streptococcus viridans strains (70), antibodies to heat-shock protein 65 (71), and Epstein–Barr virus genome isolated from renal cells and aorta (72,73) have all been described in children with KD. Unfortunately, none of these hypotheses has been proven as yet. Conventional methods for detection of an infectious agent have failed to yield the cause of KD. With the advent of new molecular biology techniques, it is now possible to look for infectious agents by molecular cloning. By creating a cDNA library from a patient with KD, Rowley et al. (74) have preliminary evidence of novel cDNAs that may provide further support for an infectious etiology.

Kawasaki disease has a high incidence in the Japanese as well as disproportionately high attack rate among Japanese Americans. For this reason, a number of investigators have searched for evidence of genetic susceptibility. Whereas some reports suggest a major histocompatibility antigen association with susceptibility to KD (75,76), others have failed to find a significant association (77,78).

The pathological consequences of immune system activation in KD are well described, consisting primarily of findings one would expect from a vasculitis that affects small and medium-sized blood vessels. Skin biopsy specimens from children in the acute stage of KD are characterized by extensive edema of the capillaries. The predominant cellular infiltrate is mononuclear (79). HLA-DR has been found to be expressed on the epidermal keratinocyte surface, on walls of small blood vessels, as well as coronary artery endothelium in KD patients (80,81).

VII. MANAGEMENT AND FOLLOW-UP

Treatment in the acute phase of the disease is aimed at limiting inflammation, especially the coronary arterial wall and myocardium. Later, therapy is aimed at preventing coronary thrombosis by inhibiting platelet aggregation. Specific therapy awaits the discovery of the causative agent.

Treatment with IVGG in various regimens has been shown to significantly reduce the incidence of coronary artery aneurysm formation, as well as abate the fever and reduce myocardial inflammation (82–84). In the United States, the standard of care is 2 g/kg IVGG as a single infusion (85). Aspirin is given concurrently at a dose of 80–100 mg/kg/day orally until the fever has subsided. In children with KD, absorption of aspirin may be impaired and monitoring serum concentrations can be helpful in apparent nonresponders or in certain other circumstances (13). After the child becomes afebrile the dosage is then reduced to 3 to 5 mg/kg/day, which is sufficient for the antiplatelet effect. This low dose of aspirin is then continued for approximately 6–8 weeks and then discontinued when the platelet count has returned to normal and if there is no evidence of coronary artery abnormalities. If coronary artery abnormalities are detected, low-dose aspirin therapy should be continued indefinitely and the patient referred to a pediatric cardiologist for long-term follow-up. The risks of aspirin in children with KD are similar to those reported in other settings: transaminase elevation, gastritis, transient hearing loss, and, rarely, Reye's syndrome. These risks may be increased in KD; aspirin binding studies suggest that the hypoalbuminemia of KD predisposes to toxic free salicylate levels despite measured values within the therapeutic range (86). To reduce the risk of developing Reye's syndrome, aspirin therapy should be temporarily discontinued if the child develops varicella or influenza.

If the fever persists despite treatment with IVGG, a second dose of IVGG at 1 g/kg may result in defervescence, although it is unknown whether retreatment prevents the development of coronary artery lesions (87).

Intravenous γ-globulin therapy in KD is not free of toxicity. Gamma-globulin is a biological agent derived from pooled donor plasma, and potentially important product-manufacturing differences exist. Its safety profile is generally favorable, but minor side effects such as fever, headache, and rash occur in 1–15% of cases, depending upon the brand (12). In addition, there have been reports of aseptic meningitis, hemolysis, and disseminated intravascular coagulation, possibly related to antibodies present in IVGG (88). The greatest potential concern is transmission of blood-borne pathogens. Elaborate sterilization procedures, including lyophilization, pasteurization, and addition of solvent detergents, are generally effective in rendering the product free of at least lipid-soluble viruses. Nonetheless, an apparent manufacturing breach led to more than 100 cases of hepatitis C in recipients of a single brand of IVGG in 1994, although none occurred in children with KD (89). Finally, IVGG is expensive; the wholesale cost is $25–75 U.S. per gram, with the average child receiving about 30 gr (12).

A subgroup of patients with KD is resistant to IVGG therapy; these patients are at greatest risk of development of coronary artery aneurysms and long-term sequelae of the disease. No effective treatment for these patients with refractory disease has been established. Wright et al. (90) described preliminary results showing that some patients with IVGG-resistant KD can be treated safely with intravenous pulse steroid therapy. Further prospective studies are needed to confirm these findings and other anecdotal reports of steroid efficacy and safety in KD.

Unfortunately, at this time, there is no sensitive scoring system to enable early prediction of which children will develop coronary abnormalities. Therefore, the current recommendation is that all children diagnosed with KD within 10 days of onset of fever should receive IVGG and aspirin as early as possible.

Children with Kawasaki disease should not receive live virus vaccines (e.g., measles–mumps–rubella) for at least 5 months after treatment with intravenous γ-globulin, because the preparation may contain neutralizing antibodies, thus preventing the proper immune response.

The mechanism of action of IVGG in KD is unknown. Therapy with IVGG may act in several ways to abate the inflammatory response, including Fc receptor blockade, neutralization of an infectious agent or toxin, provision of negative feedback to B cells secreting immune globulin, prevention of platelet adhesion to vascular wall endothelium, and induction of an anticytokine effect (91,92). The clinical benefit of IVGG in KD is generally so prompt that it is very tempting to conclude that cytokine downregulation, which could occur over a very short time course, is the best explanation. In support of this theory is a report by Takata et al. (93) that demonstrated an inhibitory effect of pooled human immunoglobulin on interleukin-12 and interferon-γ production.

Additional therapeutic options have been suggested for KD; however, no formal consensus as to efficacy has been achieved. In response to reports of elevated TNF-α and soluble TNF receptor levels in acute KD (49,58,61), pentoxifylline (thought to block TNF-α production) has been tried in combination with IVGG (94). This preliminary study, which reported efficacy in reducing the incidence of coronary artery lesions when administered early in the course of KD, awaits confirmation by other investigators.

The duration, frequency, and best imaging methods for long-term follow-up are still a matter of debate. Of greatest concern are those children with initial coronary artery aneurysms, because thrombosis or segmental stenosis may occur in the chronic phase of the disease. The American Heart Association has recommended guidelines for long-term follow-up (95). Children with multiple aneurysms, giant aneurysms, or known coronary artery obstruction require close follow-up and possible long-term anticoagulation therapy. Stress testing in the adolescent years is important, especially in those patients with a history of coronary artery involvement, because abnormalities may require limitations in physical activity and may indicate the need for angiography to assess the degree of coronary artery stenosis or obstruction. Long-term follow-up of these patients has yet to determine an increased risk of development of atherosclerosis; however, careful follow-up seems prudent. Despite normal arteriographic findings in some coronary aneurysms, the sites of regressed aneurysms may show a reduced vasodilative reactivity, indicating a great concern of the possibility of development of localized stenosis and arteriographic changes regardless of the arteriographic improvement on follow-up studies (96).

Severe coronary artery complications of KD have been treated by a variety of coronary artery bypass procedures (97–99). Coronary artery bypass grafting (CABG) is technically feasible in patients as young as 8 months (12). Revascularization has long-term benefits in selected patients; however, there is a small population of patients in whom revascularization procedures are not successful or not possible because of the extent of their disease. This has led to consideration of cardiac transplantation in these patients (100,101). The most common indications for transplantation include very severe left ventricular dysfunction secondary to infarctions, severe arrhythmias, and extensive distal multivessel coronary disease.

VIII.   SUMMARY

Kawasaki disease is an immunologically mediated diffuse vasculitis of childhood with generally self-limited clinical features. Morbidity and mortality are primarily due to cardiovascular complications, specifically, the development of coronary artery aneurysms. Current therapy with aspirin and IVGG has significantly improved the long-term morbidity of affected children. Although immune system activation occurs in the acute stage of the disease, the initiating factor is yet to be identified.

REFERENCES

1. Kawasaki T. Acute febrile mucocutaneous lymph node syndrome with lymphoid involvement with specific desquamation of the fingers and toes in children [in Japanese]. Jpn J Allergy 1967; 16:178–222.
2. Barron K, DeCunto C, Montalvo J, Orson F, Lewis D. Abnormalities of immunoregulation in Kawasaki syndrome. J Rheumatol 1988; 15:1243–1249.
3. Gaspari AA, Lotze MT, Rosenberg SA, Stern JB, Katz SI. Dermatologic changes associated with interleukin-2 administration. JAMA 1987; 258:1624–1629.
4. Fujiwara S, Yamano T, Hattori M, Fujiseki Y, Shimada M. Asymptomatic cerebral infarction in Kawasaki disease. Pediatr Neurol 1992; 8:235–236.
5. Bader-Meunier B, Hadchouel M, Fabre M, Arnoud MD, Dommergues JP. Intra-hepatic bile duct damage in children with Kawasaki disease. J Pediatr 1992; 120:750–752.
6. Falcini F, Trapani S, Pampaloni A, Ienuso R, Pollini I, Bartolozzi G. Hydrops of the gallbladder requiring cholecystectomy in Kawasaki syndrome. Clin Exp Rheumatol 1993; 11:99–100.
7. Lanting W, Mulnos W, Kamani N. Pancreatitis heralding Kawasaki disease. J Pediatr 1992; 121:743–744.
8. Veiga P, Pieroni D, Maier W, Field L. Association of Kawasaki disease and interstitial nephritis. Pediatr Nephrol 1992; 6:421–423.
9. Germaine B, Moroney J, Guggino G, Cimino L, Rodriquez C, Bocanegra T. Anterior uveitis in Kawasaki disease. J Pediatr 1980; 97:780–781.
10. Sundel R, Cleveland S, Beiser A, Newburger J, McGill T, Baker A, Koren G, Novak R, Harris J, Burns J. Audiologic profiles of children with Kawasaki disease. Am J Otol 1992; 13:512–515.
11. Takayama J, Yanase Y, Kawasaki T. A study on erythematous change at the site of the BCG inoculation (in Japanese). Acta Pediatr Jpn 1982; 86:567–572.
12. Barron KS, Shulman ST, Rowley A, Taubert K, Myones BL, Meissner HC, Peters J, Duffy CE, Silverman E, Sundel R: Report of the National Institutes of Health Workshop on Kawasaki disease. J Rheumatol 1999; 26:170–190.
13. Dajani A, Taubert K, Gerber M, Shulman S, Ferrieri P, Freed M, Takahashi M, Bierman F, Karchmer A, Wilson W, et al. Diagnosis and therapy of Kawasaki disease in children. Circulation 1993; 87:1776–1780.
14. Nakano H, Nojima S, Saito A, Ueda K. High incidence of aortic regurgitation following Kawasaki disease. J Pediatr 1985; 107:59–63.
15. Usami H, Ryo S, Harada K, Okuni M. Mitral regurgitation in the acute phase of Kawasaki disease. In: Takahashi M, Taubert K, eds. Proceedings of the Fourth International Symposium on Kawasaki Disease, Dallas, TX. American Heart Association, 1993:370–373.
16. Asai T. Evaluation method for the degree of seriousness of Kawasaki disease. Acta Paediatr Jpn 1983; 25:170–175.
17. Burns JC, Glode MP, Clarke SH, Wiggins J, Hathaway WE. Coagulopathy and platelet activation in Kawasaki syndrome: Identification of patients at high risk for development of coronary artery aneurysms. J Pediatr 1984; 105:206–211.
18. Nakano H, Ueda K, Saito A, Tsuchitani Y, Kawamori J, Miyake T, Yoshida T. Scoring method for identifying patients with Kawasaki disease at high risk of coronary artery aneurysms. Am J Cardiol 1986; 58:739–742.
19. Lin CY, Lin CC, Hwang B, Chiang BN. Cytokines predict coronary aneurysm formation in Kawasaki disease patients. Eur J Pediatr 1993; 152:309–312.

20. Schwartz S, Gillam L, Weintraub A, Sanzobrino B, Hirst J, Hsu T, Fisher J, Marx G, Fulton D, McKay R, Pandian W. Intracardiac echocardiography in humans using a small-sized (6F), low frequency (12.5Mhz) ultrasound catheter. J Am Coll Cardiol 1993; 21:189–198.

21. Suzuki A, Arakaki Y, Sugiyama H, Ono Y, Yamagishi M, Kimura K, Kamiya T. Observation of coronary arterial lesion due to Kawasaki disease by intravascular ultrasound. In: Kato H, ed. Kawasaki Disease. New York: Elsevier, 1995:451–459.

22. Sugimura T, Kato H, Yokoi H, Inoue O, Sato N, Akagi T, Hashino K, Kawano T, Nobuyoshi M. Intravascular ultrasound study in Kawasaki disease: Assessment of coronary and systemic arterial pathology, and application for coronary intervention. In: Kato H, ed. Kawasaki Disease. New York: Elsevier, 1995:460–465.

23. Ishikawa S, Takamoto S, Nozaki Y, Iwasaki A, Kim YW, Okuyama K, Kawauchi A. Evaluation of coronary artery aneurysm in children with Kawasaki disease: transesophageal doppler color flow mapping. In: Takahashi M, Taubert K, eds. Proceedings of the Fourth International Symposium on Kawasaki Disease, Dallas, TX. American Heart Association, 1993:402–403.

24. Fujiwara M, Yoshibayashi M, Ono Y, Kurosaki K, Suzuki A, Kamiya T, Takamiya M, Naito H. Usefulness of UFCT to detect myocardial damage due to stenotic lesion. In: Kato H, ed. Kawasaki Disease. New York: Elsevier, 1995:494–497.

25. Uemura S, Hirayama K, Suzuki H, Yoshida S, Handa S, Takeuchi T, Kasamatsu M, Koike M. Coronary angiography and segmental cine MRI in a single breath-hold to detect the coronary arterial aneurysm following Kawasaki disease. In: Kato H, ed. Kawasaki Disease. New York: Elsevier, 1995: 531–538.

26. Akagi T, Rose V, Benson L, Newman A, Freedom R. Outcome of coronary artery aneurysm after Kawasaki disease. J Pediatr 1992; 121:689–694.

27. Tzen K-T, Wu M-H, Wang J-K, Lue N-C, Lee C-Y, Chien S-C. Prognosis of coronary arterial lesions in Kawasaki disease treated without intravenous immunoglobulin. Acta Paediatr Sin 1997; 38:32–37.

28. Fukushige J, Takahashi N, Ueda K, Hijii T, Igarashi H, Ohshima A. Long-term outcome of coronary abnormalities in patients after Kawasaki disease. Pediatr Cardiol 1996; 17:71–76.

29. Kato H. Long-term consequences of Kawasaki disease: Pediatrics to adults. In: Kato H, ed. Kawasaki Disease. New York: Elsevier, 1995:557–566.

30. Sugimura T, Kato H, Inoue O, Takagi J, Fukuda T, Sato N. Vasodilatory response of the coronary arteries after Kawasaki disease: Evaluation by intracoronary injection of isosorbide dinitrate. J Pediatr 1992; 121:684–688.

31. Sasaguri Y, Kato H. Regression of aneurysms in Kawasaki disease: A pathologic study. J Pediatr 1992; 100:225–231.

32. Kato H, Ichinose E, Kawasaki T. Myocardial infarction in Kawasaki disease: Clinical analyses in 195 cases. J Pediatr 1986; 108:923–927.

33. Kodama K, Okayma H, Tamura A, Suetsugu M, Honda T, Doiuchi J, Hamada N, Nomoto R, Akamatsu A, Jo T. Kawasaki disease complicated by acute myocardial infarction due to thrombotic occlusion of coronary aneurysms 19 years after onset. Intern Med 1992; 31:774–777.

34. Kato H, Inoue O, Kawasaki T, Fujiwara H, Watanabe T, Toshima H. Adult coronary artery disease probably due to childhood Kawasaki disease. Lancet 1992; 340:1127–1129.

35. Kagawa K, Misao J, Fujiwara H, Fujiwara T. Silent myocardial ischemia in adults as sequelae of Kawasaki disease. In: Kato H, ed. Kawasaki Disease. New York: Elsevier, 1995:624–628.

36. Shaukat N, Syed A, Mebewu A, Freemont A, Keenan D. Myocardial infarction in a young adult due to Kawasaki disease: A case report and review of the late cardiological sequelae of Kawasaki disease. Int J Cardiol 1993; 39:222–226.

37. Smith B, Grider D. Sudden death in a young adults: Sequelae of childhood Kawasaki disease. Am J Emerg Med 1993; 11:381–383.

38. Fukuda M, Matsushima H, Yoshii H, Uchida M, Furukawa S. Abdominal aneurysm in Kawasaki disease: A case report. In: Kato H, ed. Kawasaki Disease. New York: Elsevier, 1995:416–421.

39. Nemoto S, Toyoda S, Katayama A, Sakuma S, Hamada R. Ultrasonographic evaluation of abdominal vessels in Kawasaki disease. Acta Paediatr Jpn 1993; 35:68–71.

40. Tomita S, Chung K, Mas M, Gidding S, Shulman S. Peripheral gangrene associated with Kawasaki disease. Clin Infect Dis 1992; 14:121–126.

41. Fujita Y, Nakamura Y, Sakata J, Hara N, Kobayashi M, Nagai M, Yanagawa H, Kawasaki T. Kawasaki disease in families. Pediatrics 1989; 84:666–669.

42. Yashiro M, Nakamura Y, Hirose K, Yanagawa H: Surveillance of Kawasaki disease in Japan, 1984–1994. In: Kato H, ed. Kawasaki Disease. New York: Elsevier, 1995:115–21.

43. Taubert K. Epidemiology of Kawasaki disease in the United States and worldwide. Prog Pediatr Cardiol 1997; 6:181–185.

44. Khan AS, Holman RC, Clarke MJ, Vernon LL, Gyurik TP, Schonberger LB. Kawasaki syndrome surveillance United States, 1991–1993. In: Kato H, ed. Kawasaki Disease. New York: Elsevier, 1995: 80–84.

45. Nakamura Y, Yanagawa H, Kawasaki T. Mortality among children with Kawasaki disease in Japan. N Engl J Med 1992; 326:1246–1249.

46. Sundel R, Newburger J. Kawasaki disease and its cardiac sequelae. Hosp Pract 1993; 28:51–66.

47. Newburger J, Burns J, Beriser A, Loscalzo J. Altered lipid profile after Kawasaki syndrome. Circulation 1991; 84:625–631.

48. Chiang AN, Hwang B, Shaw GC, Lee BC, Lu JH, Meng CCL, Chou P. Changes in plasma levels of lipids and lipoprotein composition in patients with Kawasaki disease. Clin Chim Acta 1997; 260: 15–26.

49. Furukawa S, Matsubara T, Jujoh K, Yone K, Sagomara T, Sasai K, Kato H, Yabuta K. Peripheral blood monocyte/macrophage and serum necrosis factor in Kawasaki disease. Clin Immunol Immunopathol 1988; 48:247–251.

50. Leung D, Siegel R, Grady S, Krensky A, Meade R, Reinherz E, Geha R. Immunoregulatory abnormalities in mucocutaneous lymph node syndrome. Clin Immunol Immunopathol 1982; 23:100–112.

51. Leung D, Chu E, Wood N, Grady S, Krensky A, Meade R, Geha R. Immunoregulatory T cell abnormalities in mucocutaneous lymph node syndrome. J Immunol 1983; 130:2002–2004.

52. Maury C, Salo E, Pelkonen P. Circulating interleukin-1 beta in patients with Kawasaki disease [letter]. N Engl J Med 1988; 319:1670–1671.

53. Lin CY, Lin CC, Hwang B, Chiang BN. The changes of interleukin-2, tumour necrotic factor and gamma-interferon production among patients with Kawasaki disease. Eur J Pediatr 1991; 150:179–182.

54. Barron K, Montalvo J, Joseph A, Hilario M, Saadeh C, Giannini E, Orson F. Soluble interleukin-2 receptors in children with Kawasaki disease. Arthritis Rheum 1990; 33:1371–1377.

55. Hirao J, Hibi S, Andoh T, Ichimura T. High levels of circulating interleukin-4 and interleukin-10 in Kawasaki disease. Int Arch Allergy Immunol 1997; 112:152–156.

56. Ueno Y, Takano N, Kanehane H, Yokoi T, Yachie A, Miyawaki T, Taniguchi W. The acute phase nature of interleuykin-6: Studies in Kawasaki disease and other febrile illnesses. Clin Exp Immunol 1989; 76:337–342.

57. Kim DS, Lee HK, Noh GW, Lee SI, Lee KY. Increased serum interleukin-10 level in Kawasaki disease. Yonsei Med J 1996; 37:125–130.

58. Sakaguchi M, Kato H, Nishiyori A, Sagawa K, Itoh K. Production of tumor necrosis factor-alpha by Vβ2⁻ or Vβ8⁻ CD4⁺ T cells in Kawasaki disease. In: Kato H, ed. Kawasaki Disease. New York: Elsevier, 1995:206–212.

59. Rowley A, Shulman S, Preble O, Poiesz B, Ehrlich G, Sullivan J. Serum interferon concentration and retroviral serology in Kawasaki syndrome. Pediatr Infect Dis J 1988; 7:663–665.

60. Vagliasindi C, Spinozzi F, Sensi L, Radicioni M, De Rosa O, Solinas L, Vaccaro R, Bertotto A. Soluble CD30 serum antigen in Kawasaki disease. Acta Paediatr 1997; 86:317–318.

61. Furukawa S, Matsubara T, Umezawa Y, Okumura R, Yabuta K. Serum levels of p60 soluble tumor necrosis factor receptor during acute Kawasaki disease. J Pediatr 1994; 124:721–725.

62. Nash MC, Shah V, Dillon MJ. ANCA are not increased in Kawasaki disease. In: Kato H, ed. Kawasaki Disease. New York: Elsevier, 1995:248–251.

63. Ayusawa M, Karasawa K, Yamashita T, Noto N, Yamaguchi H, Sumitomo N, Izumi H, Okada T, Harada K. Plasma endothelin-1 level in acute phase of Kawasaki disease. In: Kato H, ed. Kawasaki Disease. New York: Elsevier, 1995:391–395.

64. Iizuki T, Minatogawa Y, Suzuki H, Itoh M, Nakamine S, Hatanake Y, Uemura S, Koike M. Urinary

neopterin as a predictive marker of coronary artery abnormalities in Kawasaki syndrome. Clin Chem 1993; 39:600–604.

65. Barron K. Kawasaki disease: Epidemiology, late prognosis, and therapy. Rheum Dis Clin North Am 1991; 17:907–919.

66. Leung D, Meissner H, Fulton D, Kotzin B, Schlievert P. Toxic shock syndrome toxin-secreting *Staphylococcus aureus* in Kawasaki syndrome. Lancet 1993; 342:1385–1388.

67. Marchette NJ, Cao X, Kihara S, Martin J, Melish ME. Staphylococcal toxic shock syndrome toxin-1, one possible cause of Kawasaki syndrome? In: Kato H, ed. Kawasaki Disease. New York: Elsevier, 1995:149–155.

68. Terai M, Miwa K, Williams T, Kabat W, Fukuyama M, Okajima Y, Igarashi H, Shulman S. Failure to confirm involvement of staphylococcal toxin in the pathogenesis of Kawasaki disease. In: Kato H, ed. Kawasaki Disease. New York: Elsevier, 1995:144–148.

69. Lin CY, Chen IC, Cheng TI, Liu WT, Hwang B, Chiang B. Virus-like particles with reverse transcriptase activity associated with Kawasaki disease. J Med Virol 1992; 38:175–182.

70. Takada H, Kawabeta Y, Tamura M, Matsushita K, Igarashi H, Ohkuni H, Todome Y, Uchiyama T, Kotani S. Cytokine induction by extracellular products of oral viridans group Streptococci. Infect Immun 1993; 61:5252–5260.

71. Yokota S, Tsubaki K, Kuriyama T, Shimizu H, Ibe M, Mitsuda Y, Aihara Y, Kosug K, Nomaguchi H. Presence in Kawasaki disease of antibodies of mycobacterial heat-shock protein HSP65 and autoantibodies to epitopes of human HSP65 cognate antigen. Clin Immunol Immunopathol 1993; 67:163–170.

72. Muso E, Fujiwara H, Yoshida R, Hosokawa R, Yashiro M, Hongo Y, Matumiya T, Yamabe H, Kikuta H, Hironaki T, et al. Epstein-Barr virus genome positive tubulointerstitial nephritis associated with Kawasaki disease-like coronary artery aneurysms. Clin Nephrol 1993; 40:7–15.

73. Kikuta H, Sakiyama Y, Matsumoto S, Hamada I, Yazaki M, Iwaki T, Nakano M. Detection of Epstein-Barr virus DNA in cardiac and aortic tissues from chronic, active Epstein-Barr virus infections associated with Kawasaki disease-like coronary artery aneurysms. J Pediatr 1993; 123:90–92.

74. Rowley AH, Rowe CL, Eckerley CA, Baker SC. Isolation of novel cDNAs from the serum of patients with acute Kawasaki syndrome. In: Kato H, ed. Kawasaki Disease. New York: Elsevier, 1995:187–192.

75. Barron K, Silverman E, Gonzales J, St. Clair M, Anderson K, Reveille J. Major histocompatibility complex class II alleles in Kawasaki syndrome: Lack of consistent correlation with disease or cardiac involvement. J Rheumatol 1992; 19:1790–1793.

76. Kato S, Kumira M, Tsuji K, Kusakawa S, Asai T, Juji T, Kawasaki T. HLA antigens in Kawasaki disease. Pediatrics 1978; 61:252–255.

77. Fildes N, Burns J, Newburger J, Klitz W, Begovich B. The HLA class II region and susceptibility to Kawasaki disease. Tissue Antigens 1992; 39:99–101.

78. Iwasa M, Sahashi N, Kamura H, Ando T. Association of Kawasaki disease with human lymphocyte antigen. In: Takahashi M, Taubert K, eds. Proceedings of the Fourth International Symposium on Kawasaki Disease, Dallas, TX. American Heart Association; 1993:217–218.

79. Hirose S, Hamashima Y. Morphologic observations on the vasculitis in the mucocutaneous lymph node syndrome: A skin biopsy study of 27 patients. Eur J Pediatr 1978; 129:17–27.

80. Sato N, Sagawa K, Sasaguri Y, Inoue O, Kato H. Immunopathology and cytokine detection in the skin lesions of patients with Kawasaki disease. J Pediatr 1993; 122:198–203.

81. Leung D. Immunologic aspects of Kawasaki syndrome. J Rheumatol 1990; 17(suppl 24):15–18.

82. Newburger JW, Takahashi M, Burns JC, Beiser AS, Chung KJ, Duffy CE, Glode MP, Mason WH, Reddy V, Sanders SP, et al. Treatment of Kawasaki syndrome with intravenous gamma globulin. N Engl J Med 1986; 315:341–347.

83. Barron KS, Murphy DJ, Silverman ED, Ruttenberg HD, Wright GB, Franklin W, Goldberg SJ, Higashino S, Cox DG, Lee M. Treatment of Kawasaki syndrome: A comparison of two dosage regimes of intravenous immune globulin. J Pediatr 1990; 117:638–644.

84. Kao C, Hsieh K, Wang Y, Chen C, Liao S, Wan S, Yeh S. Tc-99m HMPAO imaging to detect carditis

and to evaluate the results of high dose gamma globulin treatment in Kawasaki disease. Clin Nucl Med 1992; 17:623–626.

85. Newburger JW, Takahashi M, Beiser AS, Burns JC, Bastian J, Chung KJ, Colan SD, Duffy CE, Fulton DR, Glode MP, et al. A single infusion of gamma globulin as compared with four infusions in the treatment of Kawasaki syndrome. N Engl J Med 1991; 324:1633–1639.

86. Koren G, Silverman E, Sundel R, Edney P, Newburger JW, Klein J, Robieux I, Laxer R, Giesbrecht E, Burns JC. Decreased protein binding of salicylates in Kawasaki disease. J Pediatr 1991; 118:456–459.

87. Sundel R, Burns J, Baler A, Beiser A, Newburger J. Gamma globulin retreatment in Kawasaki disease. J Pediatr 1993; 123:1633–1639.

88. Duhem C, Dicato MA, Ries F. Side-effects of intravenous immune globulin. Clin Exp Immunol 1994; 97(suppl 1):79–83.

89. Outbreak of hepatitis C associated with intravenous immunoglobulin administration—United States, October 1993–June 1994. MMWR Morb Mortal Wkly Rep 1994; 43:505–509.

90. Wright DW, Newburger JW, Baker A, Sundel RP. Treatment of immune globulin-resistant Kawasaki disease with pulsed doses of corticosteroids. J Pediatr 1996; 128:146–149.

91. Barron K, Sher M, Silverman E. Intravenous immunoglobulin therapy: Magic or black magic? J Rheumatol 1992; 19(suppl 33):94–97.

92. Shulman ST. IVGG therapy in Kawasaki disease: mechanism(s) of action. Clin Immunol Immunopathol 1989; 53:S141–146.

93. Takata Y, Seki S, Dobashi H, Takeshita S, Nakatani K, Kamezawa Y, Hiraide H, Sekine I, Yoshioka S. Inhibition of Il-12 synthesis of peripheral blood mononuclear cells (PBMC) stimulated with a bacterial superantigen by pooled human immunoglobulin: Implications for its effect on Kawasaki disease (KD). Clin Exp Immunol 1998; 114:311–319.

94. Furukawa S, Matsubara T, Umegawa Y, Motohashi T, Ino T, Yabuta K. Pentoxifylline and intravenous gamma globulin combination therapy for acute Kawasaki disease. Eur J Pediatr 1994; 153:663–667.

95. Dajani A, Taubert K, Takahashi M, Bierman F, Freed M, Ferrieri P, Gerber M, Shulman S, Karchmer A, Wilson W, et al. Guidelines for long-term management of patients with Kawasaki disease. Circulation 1994; 89:916–922.

96. Suzuki A, Arakaki Y, Sugiyama H, Ono Y, Yamagishi M, Kimura K, Kamiya T. Observation of coronary arterial lesion due to Kawasaki disease by intravascular ultrasound. In: Kato H, ed. Kawasaki Disease. New York: Elsevier, 1995:451–459.

97. Kitamura S, Kameda T, Seki T, Kawachi K, Endo M, Takeuchi Y, Kawasaki T, Kawashima Y. Long-term outcome of myocardial revascularization in patients with Kawasaki coronary artery disease: A multicenter cooperative study. J Thoracic Cardiovasc Surg 1994; 107:663–673.

98. Maeno Y, Sato N, Kato H. Long-term therapeutic strategies in patients with Kawasaki disease who suffered from old myocardial infarction. In: Kato H, ed. Kawasaki Disease. New York: Elsevier, 1995:517–521.

99. Sugimura T, Kato H, Inoue O, Sato N, Akagi T, Kazue T, Hashino K, Kiyomatsu Y. Long-term consequences of Kawasaki disease: Serial coronary angiography and 10–20 years follow-up study. In: Kato H, ed. Kawasaki Disease. New York: Elsevier, 1995:574–579.

100. Checchi P, Pahl E, Rosenfeld E, Radley-Smith E, Shulman ST. The worldwide experience with cardiac transplantation for Kawasaki disease. In: Kato H, ed. Kawasaki Disease. New York: Elsevier, 1995:522–526.

101. Koutlas TC, Wernovsky G, Bridges ND, Suh EJ, Godinez RI, Nicolson SC, Spray TL, Gaynor JW. Orthotopic heart transplantation for Kawasaki disease after rupture of a giant coronary artery aneurysm. J Thorac Cardiovasc Surg 1997; 113:217–218.

22
Henoch–Schönlein Purpura

Paul J. DeMarco*
Balboa Naval Medical Center, San Diego, California

Ilona S. Szer
Children's Hospital of San Diego and University of California School of Medicine, San Diego, La Jolla, California

I. EPIDEMIOLOGY

Although well described in all age groups, Henoch–Schönlein purpura (HSP) is much less frequent in adults than in children. In school-aged children, the incidence of HSP is as high as 13.5 per 100,000. Girls and boys are affected equally and the median age of onset is 4 years (1). Controversy exists regarding seasonal increase in its occurrence with reports of peaks in the spring, fall, and winter months. In 50% of the children, HSP is preceded by an upper respiratory tract infection. Multiple organisms have been implicated in triggering HSP, including streptococci, *Mycoplasma pneumoniae*, *Yersinia*, *Legionella*, *Helicobacter pylori*, Epstein–Barr virus, hepatitis B, varicella, adenovirus, cytomegalovirus, and parvovirus B19. Several case reports link vaccinations against typhoid, paratyphoid A and B, measles, cholera, and yellow fever with the subsequent development of HSP. This suggests that more than one infectious agent may trigger the expression of the disease. In addition, allergens such as drugs (penicillin, ampicillin, erythromycin, lisinopril, enalapril, acetylsalicylic acid, quinine, and quinidine) as well as foods, exposure to cold, and insect bites have been implicated as potential triggers (2).

II. CLINICAL FEATURES

The diagnosis of HSP in children requires the presence of palpable purpura (Fig. 22.1; see color plate), with a normal platelet count. Although most children have the classic triad of purpura, colicky abdominal pain, and arthritis, up to 50% of children may present with symptoms other than purpura (Table 1), including abdominal pain, arthritis, and importantly, testicular swelling (which must be differentiated from testicular torsion). Multiple manifestations of HSP have been described, including pulmonary hemorrhage, which although exceedingly rare, may be fatal. In a

---

*The views expressed in this article are those of the authors and do not reflect the official policy or position of the Department of the Navy, Department of Defense, or the United States Government.

Table 1 Clinical Manifestations of HSP

	% at onset	% during course
Purpura (nl platelet count)	50	100
Subcutaneous edema	10–20	20–46
Arthritis (large jts)	25	60–84
Gastrointestinal disorder	30	85
Renal disorder	?	10–50
Genitourinary (ddx torsion) disorder	?	2–35
Pulmonary (TLCO) disorder	?	95
Pulmonary hemorrhage	?	rare, may be fatal
CNS (headache, organic brain, seizures)	?	rare, may be fatal

recent study, 95% of children with active disease had decreased carbon monoxide diffusion capacity that resolved when purpura resolved (3).

It is interesting to note that the clinical spectrum differs in younger children and older children (Table 2); renal disease occurs less often in children who are less than 2 years of age while subcutaneous edema is more common in this age group than in children older than 2 years (4).

Similar to other rheumatic conditions of childhood, the course of HSP may be quite variable. It may be thought of as monophasic in the majority (>80%) of children, polyphasic in 10–20%, or may become chronic and continuous in less than 5%.

A. Cutaneous Manifestations

Palpable, nonthrombocytopenic purpura is a prerequisite to the diagnosis and occurs in 100% of patients, but may be a presenting sign in only 50%. Dependent areas of the body, such the buttocks and the lower extremities, are the most common sites of the rash. Edema of the hands (Fig. 2), feet, scalp, and ears is a common (20–46%) early finding.

B. Joint Involvement

Arthralgia or arthritis is the second most common symptom of HSP. Acute arthritis most frequently affects the knees and the ankles and occurs in 60–84% of the patients. Arthritis and arthralgia may precede the rash in 25% of children. The arthritis is transient and self-limited but may be painful and may produce occasional inability to ambulate. There are no permanent sequelae in regard to joint space narrowing and erosions.

Table 2 Influence of Age on Clinical Manifestations in Children

	<2 years old, % involved	>2 years old, % involved
Renal	23	43
GI	29	75
Arthritis	56	73
Scalp edema	59	19
Other edema	71	51

Source: Ref. 4.

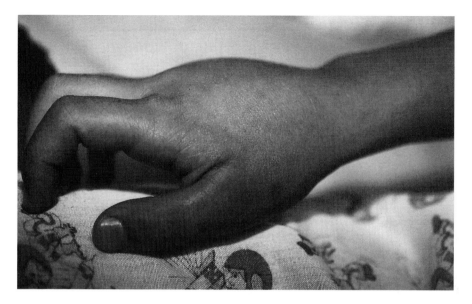

Figure 2 Painful, unilateral edema over the dorsum of the hand in a 12-year-old boy with purpura, abdominal pain, and microscopic hematuria.

C. Gastrointestinal Involvement

Gastrointestinal (GI) signs and symptoms have been reported in up to 85% of patients and include colicky pain, nausea, vomiting, and gastrointestinal bleeding. Up to a third of the patients with HSP and GI manifestations experience hematemesis and 50% have occult bleeding, but major hemorrhage occurs in only 5%, and intussusception in 2%. Most cases of abdominal pain are due to submucosal and intramural extravasation of fluid and blood into the intestinal wall, which may lead to localized ulceration of the mucosa and may be associated with diffuse arterial inflammation and fibrinoid necrosis. Endoscopic studies commonly reveal hemorrhagic, erosive duodenitis. Less frequently, gastric, jejunal, colonic, and rectal erosions have been demonstrated. In a recent study (5), upper GI endoscopy revealed abnormalities in 6 of 7 children with HSP, while sigmoidoscopy revealed abnormalities in 1 of 4 of the patients. The mucosal changes were more marked in the second part of the duodenum rather than in the bulb or in the stomach. Endoscopic findings included redness, swelling, petechiae or hemorrhage, as well as erosions and ulceration of the mucosa. Histology of the mucosal biopsy specimens revealed nonspecific inflammation with positive staining for IgA in the capillaries but no evidence of vasculitis.

Radiographic findings are nonspecific and may include thickening of bowel wall, blurring of bowel folds due to edema of the wall, scalloping due to local hemorrhage of bowel wall, filling defects in bowel wall due to vascular occlusion in the submucosa, bleeding into the mesentery, and intussusception. Sudden increase in intensity of abdominal pain may be secondary to intussusception, bowel infarct, perforation, pancreatitis, or hydrops of the gallbladder. Intussusception is reported in 2% of children with HSP while other GI complications are extraordinarily rare. The cause of intussusception may be bowel wall edema or a submucosal hematoma. The HSP-related intussusception is ileoileal in 65% of cases compared with idiopathic intussusception which is usually ileocolic. As a result, ultrasonography (US) is more helpful in the diagnosis of intussusception in children with HSP rather than barium enema which may miss the ileoileal location. In a recent study (6) of 14 children with HSP and abdominal pain, high-resolution US provided information at three levels:

1. Acute abdominal pain was associated with US evidence of edema and hemorrhagic changes of the intestinal wall in all cases. The enteric wall appeared thickened (3–11 mm). Lesions were diffuse in 6 children and focal in others (duodenal in 5, jejunal in 2, and ileal in 1).
2. US was a convenient means to follow the evolution of the disease. There was extension of lesions in 5 patients and resolution in the remaining 9 children in whom US showed progressive decrease of parietal thickening, reexpansion of small bowel lumen, and reappearance of peristalsis.
3. In each case, US detected surgery-requiring complications: ileoileal intussusception in 3 patients and perforation in 1.

D. Renal Involvement

The incidence of renal involvement in HSP ranges between 10 and 50% (4). Children over 9 years of age develop glomerulonephritis more often than their younger peers. Reportedly, children with bloody stools have a 7.5-fold increased risk for renal disease compared with children whose stools are hemoccult negative. The overall prognosis for renal disease is favorable, with a 1.1–4.5% incidence of persistent involvement and an approximate < 1% progression to end-stage renal failure. Generally, renal involvement occurs within 3 months of onset of the rash. Persistence of rash for 2 to 3 months is associated with a slightly increased risk of nephropathy.

Clinical expression of nephritis ranges from transient isolated microscopic hematuria to rapidly progressive glomerulonephritis. Hematuria is detected in virtually all children with HSP-associated nephritis. Proteinuria, nephrotic syndrome, hypertension, and renal insufficiency are uncommon. Up to 15% of children with the combination of hematuria and proteinuria may develop progressive renal insufficiency. Up to 50% of children who present with nephrotic syndrome and evidence of renal insufficiency develop renal failure within 10 years (7).

Similar to clinical expression, renal histopathology ranges from minimal change to severe crescentic glomerulonephritis (GN). Electron microscopy may reveal mesangial, subendothelial, and subepithelial deposits. Immunofluorescent studies reveal diffuse glomerular deposition of immunoglobulin A (IgA), C3, fibrin, IgG, properdin, and IgM.

Henoch–Schönlein purpura and IgA nephropathy, the latter described almost exclusively in young adults, appear to be related disorders on the same spectrum (7). It is important to note that 30% of adult patients with IgA nephropathy have rash and joint symptoms similar to HSP. An increased serum IgA level is seen in both disorders and renal biopsy findings are identical. However, HSP is a systemic syndrome while IgA nephropathy is primarily localized to the kidney. The age of onset is the major difference between these two histologically similar illnesses, and prognosis remains favorable for HSP and guarded for IgA nephropathy. Yet unknown is whether adults with IgA nephropathy had HSP as children (8).

E. Genitourinary Involvement

Extrarenal genitourinary involvement has been described in HSP and may precede the rash. Acute scrotal swelling, secondary to inflammation and hemorrhage of the scrotal vessels, has been reported in 2–35% of children. The frequency of 18% was recently reported by Chamberlain and Greenberg (9) who reviewed the medical records of 61 children with HSP and found that 10 had scrotal involvement on physical examination and one patient reported purpuric lesions and scrotal edema 2 days prior to the onset of generalized rash. The differentiation of scrotal edema from acute torsion of the spermatic cord is a challenge in children who have scrotal involvement as the first sign of HSP (10). In testicular involvement from HSP, normal or increased Doppler and radionuclide flow are expected, while in idiopathic testicular torsion, both the Doppler flow on the affected side and the uptake of radionuclide are decreased. Evaluation of boys with testicular swelling should include one or both of these techniques, which may reveal features of vasculitis and may avoid the need for surgical exploration (10). True testicular torsion is rare in HSP but when it occurs, it represents a surgical emergency since vascular insufficiency may lead to infarction and death of the Leydig cells within 10 h unless blood supply is restored.

F. Central Nervous System Involvement

Central nervous system involvement is exceedingly rare but has been described. The most common manifestation is headache, followed by subtle encephalopathy with minimal changes in mental status, labile mood, apathy, and hyperactivity. Seizures, subdural hematomas, cortical hemorrhage, intraparenchymal bleeding, and infarction have been documented. Peripheral neuropathy may also occur, but is rare (11).

G. Pulmonary Involvement

Chaussain et al. (3) documented impairment of lung diffusion capacity in the majority of children with HSP during the active phase of the illness. In a study of 29 children, 28 had significant decrease of lung transfer for carbon monoxide (56.8% of predicted TLCO). During the subsequent longitudinal follow-up, TLCO normalized in all children who recovered completely but remained abnormal in patients who had evidence of persistent disease activity. The authors concluded that decreased TLCO measurement may reflect an alteration of the alveolar-capillary membrane secondary to circulating immune complexes and thus serves as a parameter of disease activity. None of the patients in this study had clinically apparent pulmonary distress. However, massive pulmonary hemorrhage has been reported in HSP. Olson et al. (12) described four children with severe pulmonary bleeding of whom one died of massive pulmonary hemorrhage. Although an autopsy was not performed, previous reports of postmortem pulmonary specimens in HSP have revealed periarterial infiltrates and fibrinoid necrosis of the lungs.

H. HSP in Adults

It has been suggested that HSP differs in the adult and pediatric populations. However, numerous studies published over the last 30 years have not provided convincing data delineating clear distinctions. Different results appear to be due to variations in population characteristics, outcome measures, and inclusion criteria. Table 3 is a summary of the available data that highlight clinical characteristics in presumed adult HSP. It is difficult to make comparisons among studies, given the lack of uniform adherence to defining criteria such as those proposed by the American College of Rheumatology (ACR) (24) or use of standard nomenclature, such as proposed by the Chapel Hill Consensus Conference (19).

Early studies are most difficult to evaluate regarding significant differences between adults and children. Bernhardt (13) first studied and defined HSP in adults, citing the second case report of this vasculitis occurring in a 36-year-old woman in 1808 originally described by Willan. In the 18 patients studied by Bernhardt, many had renal involvement with more severe associated morbidity. The first large population study to define HSP in adults included 77 patients (14). Forty-nine percent of the cases presented with renal disease with either abnormalities of urinary

Table 3 HSP in Adults: Clinical Characteristics of Study Populations

Author (ref.)	Bernhardt (13)	Cream (14)	Bar-On (15)	Roth (16)	Tancrede-Bohin (21)	Blanco (22)	Uthman (20)
Study period (yrs)	1956–1966	1956–1968	1959–1969	1968–1983	1985–1993	1975–1994	1986–1996
No. patients	18	77	21	9	57	46	10
Mean age (yrs)	45	43.7	34	48	52	53	37
% male	72	50	57	ND[a]	49	80	82
% purpura	100	100	100	100	100	94	100
% arthritis	88	56	76	67	33	37	100
% GI sx	94	53	66	67	19	57	100
% renal sx	83	50	57	100	49	85	90
% renal biopsy	28	0	38	100	23	13	ND[a]
% CRF[b]	30	10	22	22	7	13	20

[a]ND = not delineated within the study population.
[b]CRF = chronic renal failure, as denoted by need for dialysis or impaired creatinine clearance.

sediment (16 of 77), acute nephritis (19 of 77) or progressive renal disease (3 of 77); biopsy was obtained only in patients with progressive renal disease. The mortality from renal disease was 4%. Although Cream et al. (14) concluded that the prevalence and mortality of HSP in adults was comparable to that in children, many textbooks reference this article to substantiate the claim that renal disease is more severe in adults. These authors did conclude adults were more likely to develop skin necrosis and "there is little to be gained in dividing what is probably a spectrum of disease" (14). Further attempts to assess HSP in adults and severity of renal disease include a study by Bar-On and Rosenmann (15) in which 10 of 21 patients developed renal disease; 8 of 10 had renal biopsies and 2 patients progressed to renal failure. These two patients had diffuse glomerulonephritis. The authors concluded that renal biopsy characteristics at presentation are predictive of outcome and that renal disease runs its course independent of treatment and response of other organ systems. Roth et al. (16) further studied the spectrum of adult HSP and reached similar conclusions. Although only nine patients are reported, all had renal biopsies and seven had mesangial deposition of IgA. Renal outcomes were favorable short term, but the study did not provide long-term follow-up.

Balland et al. (17) reported retrospective clinical observations of 14 adults with HSP and renal disease. Histologic characteristics were noted from seven renal biopsies. A triad of nonthrombocytopenic purpura, joint pain, and renal abnormalities were the inclusion criteria. Of these patients, ages 29–89 years, 4 of 14 died. Although these four patients shared common elements of glomerular involvement and interstitial infiltration, the lesions varied from mesangial hypercellularity to crescent formation (two of four biopsies). Long-term follow-up was not available on surviving patients. The authors concluded that glomerular crescent formation correlated with fatal outcome.

Using more stringent inclusion criteria that included a minimum of a 12-month follow-up period, Fogazzi et al. (18) studied long-term outcome in adult HSP. All 16 patients fulfilled well-defined classification criteria including age >15 years, purpura, renal disease, and glomerular IgA deposition on immunofluorescence studies of renal biopsies. After a mean follow-up of 90.5 months, 3 of 16 patients required chronic dialysis while 50% had renal dysfunction. Although no clinical features predicted renal disease, high IgA levels correlated with a favorable clinical course. The investigators concluded that adult HSP nephritis carries a high long-term risk of renal dysfunction.

In an effort to underscore and define the differences between hypersensitivity vasculitis (HV) and HSP, Michel et al. (19) generated a subanalysis of the ACR Vasculitis Subcommittee data on HV and HSP and observed differences in cohorts of patients either younger than or older than 20 years. The age cutoff was based on its ability to distinguish between HV and HSP as delineated by the subcommittee's findings; the population was defined by 60 "children" and 25 adults. Although the data were not collected to evaluate the difference between children and adults, this study analysis notes adults were statistically more likely to have melena, hematuria, impairment in renal function, cutaneous ulceration, and prior medication use. In HV, renal dysfunction (blood urea nitrogen >40 or creatinine >1.5 mg/dL) occurred in 28% of all patients, compared with 11% of all patients with HSP, suggesting a possible bias due to age and related comorbidities, such as hypertension. The study criteria, however, have been criticized for the age-dependent criterion, which makes it difficult to define an adult with HSP and, therefore, a child with HV. The study may have selected more severely affected adults for a diagnosis of HSP, and less severely affected children for HV (20).

In a retrospective analysis of 57 French patients diagnosed with HSP whose ages were greater than 15 years, the prognosis did not seem worse for adults. Tancrede-Bohin et al. (21) defined the population by the presence of purpura and skin biopsies that revealed IgA deposition in dermal vessel walls. They noted no difference in the age distribution of the 51% of the patients without hematuria or proteinuria; 23% (13 of 57) had IgA-associated glomerulonephritis on biopsy and 26% had minor abnormalities or no abnormalities in renal function or on biopsy. Furthermore, of the 25 patients with a mean follow-up of 19 months, a minority had recurrent symptoms and only 2 of the 13 patients with GN went on to develop progressive renal failure. Within the adult group, purpura above the waist, pyrexia, elevated acute phase reactants, and antecedent upper respiratory infection were statistically significantly associated with IgA glomerulonephritis.

The only investigation to compare adults and children was retrospective and included 46 Spanish adults and 116 children. Blanco et al. (22) defined "children" as less than 20 years old. This study specifically sought to determine if age at onset altered clinical presentation and course and used the criteria as defined by Michel et al. Adults showed a higher frequency of melena, renal disease, and joint symptoms, and lower frequency of fever. Eighty-five percent of the adults developed nephropathy vs. 25% of children; renal insufficiency developed in 13% of the adults but none of the children. Relapse rates were essentially the same for adults and children (36% and 42.6%, respectively) with both groups having a relatively good outcome. Follow-up was an average of 1.5–2 years.

The currently available data regarding the differences between adults and children with HSP are not compelling. Although there is some suggestion of more morbidity with regard to renal disease, HSP appears to remain largely a self-limiting, reversible disease entity. Severity of extrarenal disease also does not seem to correlate with either age or presence of renal disease. Further multicenter studies are needed to best define any meaningful differences between adults and children with HSP.

III. LABORATORY FEATURES AND INVESTIGATIONS

The diagnosis of HSP is based on clinical signs and symptoms. Skin biopsy, if obtained, shows leukocytoclastic vasculitis with neutrophils and neutrophil debris within and around vessel walls, necrosis of vessel walls, and deposits of pink amorphous fibrin within and around the small-ves-

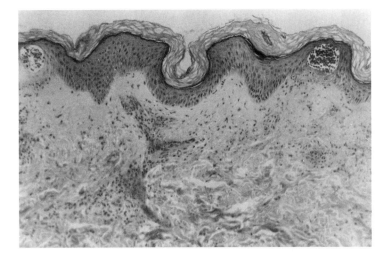

Figure 3 Skin section obtained from a 5-year-old girl with purpura reveals a neutrophillic vasculitis involving small dermal vessels. The infiltrate is primarily localized to the upper dermis. (H & E stain, 40×.) (Courtesy of Dr. Glenn Billman.)

sel walls (Figs. 3 and 4). Immunofluorescence studies may show IgA and C3 along the small vessels of the skin and in the renal glomeruli. Routine laboratory studies are usually normal and abnormalities reflect particular organ involvement or bleeding. There are no diagnostic studies, although an elevated serum level of IgA, in the appropriate clinical setting, is suggestive of HSP. Laboratory evaluation is aimed at excluding other disorders and assessing the extent of organ involvement.

IV. DIAGNOSIS

An entity known as acute hemorrhagic edema (AHE) of childhood has been described almost exclusively in the European literature. It is said to affect children under 24 months of age and may or may not represent HSP in infants (23). The manifestations of AHE are edema and ecchymotic, target-like purpura on the limbs and face. Most patients have a history of either a recent illness, drug exposure, or immunizations. Systemic symptoms, such as bloody stools or renal involvement, seem to occur less frequently in AHE than HSP, although these symptoms are also uncommon in infants and toddlers thought to have HSP. Spontaneous and complete resolution occurs within 1–3 weeks, but 1–3 recurrences are frequent. Leukocytoclastic vasculitis is seen when a skin biopsy is obtained. It is not known whether AHE is an IgA-related vasculitis.

Recently, a subcommittee of the American College of Rheumatology defined criteria for the classification of several forms of vasculitis in adults, including hypersensitivity vasculitis (Table 4) and HSP (Table 5) (24). Because the two entities share many clinicopathological features and HSP is often considered a type of HV, Michel et al. (19) compared the characteristics of HV and HSP as separate and definable clinical syndromes, using the ACR study database. Both disorders share the common feature of leukocytoclastic vasculitis of small vessels with prominent skin involvement. Major differences with respect to frequency and type of organ involvement were found, suggesting that indeed these are distinct entities that carry different prognoses. Although hematuria and proteinuria were more often seen in HSP, elevated blood urea nitrogen and creati-

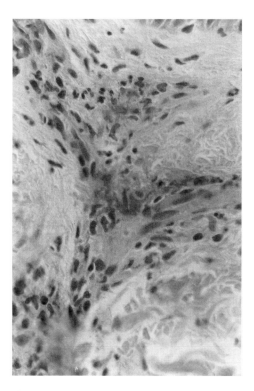

Figure 4 Same sample of dermal biopsy as in Figure 3 demonstrates a perivascular neutrophilic infiltrate with nuclear fragmentation, endothelial cell swelling, and deposition of fibrin within and around the vessel wall representing an eosinophilic fibrinoid change. (H & E stain, 250×.) (Courtesy of Dr. Glenn Billman.)

Table 4 1990 Criteria for Classification of Hypersensitivity Vasculitis[a]

Criterion	Definition
Age at disease onset >16 years	Development of symptoms after age 16
Medication at disease onset	Medication was taken at the onset of symptoms that may have been a precipitating factor
Palpable purpura	Slightly elevated purpuric rash over one or more areas of the skin; does not blanch with pressure and is not related to thrombocytopenia
Maculopapular rash	Flat and raised lesions of various sizes over one or more areas of the skin
Biopsy including arteriole and venule	Histological changes showing granulocytes in a perivascular or extra vascular location

[a]For purposes of classification, a patient shall be said to have hypersensitivity vasculitis if at least three of the five criteria are present. The presence of any three or more criteria yields a sensitivity of 71% and a specificity of 83.9%.
Source: Ref. 24.

Table 5   Criteria for Differentiating HSP from Hypersensitivity Vasculitis

Criterion	Definition
Palpable purpura	Slightly elevated purpuric rash over one or more areas of the skin not related to thrombocytopenia
Bowel angina	Diffuse abdominal pain worse after meals or bowel ischemia usually including bloody diarrhea
GI bleeding	GI bleeding, including melena, hematochezia, or positive test for occult blood in the stool
Hematuria	Gross hematuria or microhematuria (>1/hpf)
Age at onset <20	Development of first symptoms at age 20 or less
No medications	Absence of any medication at onset of disease that may have been a precipitating factor

The presence of any three or more of the six criteria yields a correct classification of HSP cases of 87.1%. The presence of two or fewer criteria yields a correct classification of HV cases in 74.2%.
Source: Ref. 24.

nine as factors reflecting functional renal impairment (and likely to reflect worse prognosis) were significantly more frequent in HV. Generally, important organ involvement was found more often in HV (pleuritis, pericarditis, congestive heart failure, and more extensive involvement of skin, mucosa, and muscle). Similarly, tests that classically reveal active inflammatory processes, i.e., erythrocyte sedimentation rate (ESR) and C4 levels, were more frequently abnormal in patients with HV than those with HSP. Frank arthritis was significantly more common in HSP whereas arthralgia was reported more frequently in HV. In adults, HSP tended to affect organs more extensively and the prognosis appeared to be worse with regard to renal disease when compared with children and adolescents with HSP. In summary, this study corroborates the concept that HV and HSP are distinct clinical disorders within the broader group of small-vessel vasculitis with prominent skin involvement.

V.   MANAGEMENT

Treatment of HSP is largely supportive and includes adequate hydration and monitoring of vital signs. Nonsteroidal antiinflammatory drugs (NSAIDs) help with joint pain and do not worsen the purpura. However, it is prudent to avoid NSAIDs in the setting of renal insufficiency. Steroids are helpful in the management of painful edema but there is no absolute requirement for such treatment.

A.   Treatment of Abdominal Pain

In a retrospective analysis, Rosenblum and Winter (25) evaluated the effect of corticosteroids on the duration of abdominal pain in 43 children with HSP and abdominal pain. Twenty-five patients received oral prednisone at a dose of 2 mg/kg/day and 18 children served as controls. Results showed that during the first 24 h, abdominal pain resolved in 44% of children who received steroids compared with spontaneous resolution in only 14% of children who were not treated. Over the next 24 h, 65 vs. 45%, respectively, no longer had abdominal pain. After 72 h, 75% of patients in both groups were well. It is this experience that has influenced many physicians to treat abdominal pain with corticosteroids. In addition, similar observations by Allen et al. (4) included the finding that painful edema and arthritis resolved either with or without steroids within 24–48 h after onset and that steroids had no effect on either purpura or renal disease. Of note, none of the patients with abdominal pain who received steroids developed intussusception.

To further address this issue, Glasier et al. (26) designed another retrospective study of 22 children admitted to the hospital with abdominal pain. Their findings agreed with Rosenblum and Winter (25) and Allen et al. (4); 20 of 22 (91%) children recovered with or without steroids (26). Multiple case reports suggest improvement of abdominal pain, melena, and massive hemorrhage with the use of steroids. This is supported by many physicians who have "successfully" treated children with steroids who were hospitalized for abdominal pain. However, to date, no placebo-controlled study has been done and we are left with experience and reason, but not definitive proof, to support recommendations to treat with steroids.

B. Prevention of Delayed Nephritis

Buchanec et al. (27) reported the results of a retrospective study of 32 children with HSP and no evidence of renal involvement. Twenty-three patients received corticosteroids (prednisone 2 mg/kg/day) and 10 did not. Of the treated children, only 1 (5%) developed nephritis, while in the untreated group, 5 patients (50%) developed renal manifestations. These authors concluded that immediate treatment with steroids prevented renal disease. Mollica et al. (28), employed a modified prospective, open, nonrandomized design to study 84 children who received corticosteroids and 84 children did not. The results over 2 years of follow-up showed no renal involvement in any of the treated children, while in the nonintervention group, 10 children developed hematuria ($p < 0.001$) and of those, four still had hematuria 12 months later and two developed renal insufficiency 18 months after onset. This study was immediately followed by retrospective observations of Saulsbury (29) who had treated 20 children without renal disease with steroids and did not treat 30 children without renal disease. In both groups, there was a 20% frequency of subsequent renal involvement within 3 months of initial presentation, suggesting that pretreatment with steroids did not prevent the onset of delayed nephritis in children with HSP.

The seemingly confusing results regarding prevention of delayed onset of renal disease are difficult to interpret. One explanation may be an inherent flaw in the design of each study; none of the studies were placebo-controlled or randomized, and two of three were retrospective observations. There were also inconsistencies regarding the timing of corticosteroid administration among the studies, further contributing to difficulty in interpreting the results.

C. Poor Prognostic Signs

The controversy regarding management of HSP nephritis is centered primarily on children whose disease is associated with a high risk for renal insufficiency and/or failure. For the majority of children with HSP, renal involvement is transient, but for the 1–5% who develop chronic renal disease and up to 1% who may go on to renal failure, management that would predictably prevent this sequela is uncertain.

To examine which patients are at highest risk, the study of Allen et al. (4) provides multiple insights. Forty children had no renal findings, 24 presented with hematuria only, and 10 had hematuria and proteinuria. One year later, 80% of the children who had no renal involvement at onset and 71% of mildly affected children remained well. In contrast, only 40% of those who presented with severe involvement were free of renal findings. In a similar study by Niaudet et al. (7), none of the children with mild initial renal findings (hematuria only or proteinuria < 1 g/day) developed renal disease more than 1 year later. However, of the patients who presented with either nephrotic syndrome, renal insufficiency, and/or renal failure, a significant number went on to chronic renal failure (Table 6). The same authors then correlated biopsy findings with clinical

Table 6 Correlations Between Initial Clinical Manifestations and Renal Outcome in HSP After One Year of Follow-Up[a]

Manifestation	N	Clinical remission	Minimal urinary abnormalities	Persistent nephropathy	Renal failure
Hematuria	2	2	0	0	0
Proteinuria (<1 g/d)	16	7	6	3	0
Proteinuria (>1 g/d)	42	17	10	9	6
Nephrotic syndrome	64	32	14	10	8
Nephrotic syndrome and renal failure	27	8	2	2	15
Total	151	66	32	24	29

[a]Only children whose initial renal biopsy results were available were included.
Source: Ref. 7.

Table 7 Correlations Between Initial Renal Biopsy Results and Renal Outcome in HSP After One Year of Follow-Up[a]

Biopsy finding	N	Clinical remission	Minimal urinary abnormalities	Persistent nephropathy	Renal failure
Mesangiopathic GN	2	2	0	0	0
Focal segmental GN	47	26	15	4	2
Proliferative endocapillary GN	13	8	3	1	1
Endocapillary and extracapillary GN					
crescents <50%	21	11	3	6	1
crescents >50%	68	19	11	13	25
Total	151	66	32	24	29

[a]Only children whose initial renal biopsy results were available are included.
Source: Ref. 7.

renal manifestations and reported significant association of proliferative glomerulonephritis with >50% crescents with the development of future renal failure (Table 7).

In summary, the presence of hematuria with nephrotic-range proteinuria confers a 15% risk of renal failure, while nephrosis with renal insufficiency and documentation of >50% crescentic glomerulonephritis may lead to renal failure in up to 50% of patients with renal HSP after a 10-year course. Aggressive treatment should therefore be attempted to prevent late sequelae. Children with nephrotic-range proteinuria, nephrotic syndrome, and signs of renal insufficiency should undergo renal biopsy to determine the extent of renal involvement.

D. Treatment of Severe Nephritis

Multiple studies have recommended various treatment modalities for patients with severe renal involvement, including pulse or oral corticosteroids alone or in combination with cytotoxic or other immunosuppressive agents, such as azathioprine, cyclophosphamide, or cyclosporine; plasmapheresis, high-dose IV IgG, danazol, and fish oil (Table 8) (28–34). The studies suffer from small numbers of subjects, retrospective analysis of data, and lack of placebo-controlled groups. In addition, renal biopsy findings are inconsistently available, and interventions are given at different times in the course of the illness. It is therefore difficult to draw meaningful conclusions from these reports. Nonetheless, a recent uncontrolled study suggests that the natural history of

Table 8 Renal Outcome in HSP: Conclusions from Literature Review

Author (Ref.)	Source	Conclusion (study design)
Levy et al. (30)	Adv Nephrol 6:183, 1976	Improved with steroids (pilot).
Counahan et al. (31)	BMJ 2:11, 1977	No improvement with steroids (retrospective analysis).
Mollica et al. (28)	Eur J Pediatr 151:140, 1992	Steroids prevent delayed renal disease (open, nonrandomized, controlled, prospective trial).
Saulsbury (29)	Pediatr Nephrol 7:69, 1993	Steroids do not prevent delayed renal disease (retrospective analysis).
Rostoker et al. (32)	Ann Intern Med 120:476, 1994	High-dose IgG stabilizes poor renal function in HSP/IgA nephropathy (open prospective cohort study).
Oner et al. (33)	Pediatr Nephrol 9:6, 1995	Triple therapy may be effective in severe HSP nephritis (see text, pilot).
Rostoker et al. (34)	Nephron 69:327, 1995	Low-dose IgG slows progression of renal disease (open, uncontrolled, prospective trial).

severe HSP nephritis may be changed favorably. Oner et al. (33) treated 12 children with HSP and biopsy-proven rapidly progressive crescentic glomerulonephritis with a combination of methyl-prednisolone at 30 mg/kg/day for three consecutive days, followed by oral corticosteroids at 2 mg/kg/day, cyclophosphamide at 2 mg/kg/day for 2 months and dipyridamole at 5 mg/kg/day for 6 months (33). At the 3-month evaluation, glomerular filtration rate (GFR) normalized in 11 of 12, nephrosis resolved in 8 of 12, and hematuria was no longer detectable in 9 of 12 children. Furthermore, at 30 months after treatment, only one patient had persistent nephrotic syndrome and one child developed renal failure.

VI. PATHOGENESIS

Henoch–Schönlein purpura is thought to be an immune complex–mediated small-vessel vasculitis. Serological studies document elevated levels of IgA in 50% and activation of the alternate pathway of the complement system. IgA levels become elevated either because of increased production or decreased clearance. It is hypothesized that an unknown antigen(s) stimulates IgA production, activating pathways leading to vasculitis. Levels of C3 and C4 complement components are normal. Histopathology of the skin and other affected organs reveals polymorphonuclear cells in the vessel wall, with IgA, C3, and immune complexes seen in venules, arterioles, and capillaries (4).

In HSP, complement-fixing immune complexes (ICs) are present in the circulation and deposited on the interior of blood vessels of the skin. Immune complexes are capable of activating complement, leading to the formation of chemotactic factors such as C5a, which in turn recruit polymorphonuclear neutrophil (PMN) leukocytes at the site of deposition. Release of lysosomal enzymes follows ingestion of immune complexes by PMNs resulting in vessel damage. The C5b-9 complex, also known as membrane attack complex (MAC) was recently colocalized with IgA and C3 on vessel walls of the skin and on capillary walls and mesangium of glomeruli of patients with HSP-related nephritis. Kawana and Nishiyama (35) assessed the degree of in vivo terminal pathway activation through the measurement of serum concentrations of the terminal complement complex (TCC). The results show that vascular endothelial cells in each MAC-positive case were injured even in papillary dermal vessels in which no PMNs could be detected but C5b-9 deposition was seen. This suggests that not only leukocytes but also MAC are necessary for endothelial cells to incur damage. Using the C5b-9 enzyme immunoassay, the serum concentration of C5b-9 was shown to be significantly increased in most HSP patients. Complement activation leading to terminal complement sequence is thus shown to occur in the circulation as well as the skin of patients with HSP. Immune complexes may contribute to terminal complement activation. Terminal complement complex increased significantly at the time of disease flare-up but dropped to the normal range during remission and showed close correlation with disease activity. The authors conclude that the assay for TCC should prove useful in monitoring the activity of HSP. Routine assessment of complement activation, i.e., C3, C4, and CH50, showed no abnormality. However, the measurement of plasma anaphylatoxins C3a and C4a in 46 patients with HSP and IgA nephropathy showed significant correlation with plasma creatinine and urea levels (36). In addition, a positive correlation between C3a and creatinine was reported. These observations suggest a role for anaphylatoxin determination as a sensitive indicator of complement activation and a useful tool in monitoring the activity of disease in affected patients. Similar to this study, a group of investigators from Heidelberg, Germany (37), investigated the possibility that the local inflammatory and thrombotic process may be regulated by increased biosynthesis of vasoactive prostanoids, including thromboxane A2 (TxA2), a potent vasoconstrictor and platelet agonist, prostacyclin, a vasodilator and platelet antagonist, and prostaglandin E2, a mediator of inflammation. The results of their study of 14 children with HSP revealed that both thromboxane A2 and prostacyclin were significantly increased during the acute phase of the disease and again during subsequent recurrences of HSP. Of note, both patients with nephrotic syndrome had the highest concentrations of renal thromboxane A2. The enhanced TxA2 formation is consistent with phasic platelet activation in HSP. The increased prostacyclin biosynthesis likely reflects endothelial cell damage and may be a response of the vascular endothelium to modulate platelet–vessel wall and leukocyte–vessel wall interactions.

There have been several reports suggesting that the deficiency of C4 complement and/or deletion of C4 genes represent genetic risk factors in both IgA nephropathy and HSP-associated nephritis. In particular, the C4B isotype deficiency has been reported in these patients. To further clarify the genetic structure of deleted C4 genes, Jin et al. (38) investigated the DQB and DRB genes, which are located near the C4 loci, to identify a possible linkage and to find the associated allele. The results show that locus II deletion of C4 was the risk factor for these diseases in this group of Japanese patients and that the deleted gene can be either C4A or C4B. The authors found neither specific isotype nor specific allotype deficiency suggesting that it is the C4 deletion per se that renders the patient susceptible to nephritis.

The role of cytokine regulation in the pathogenesis of various types of glomerulonephritis has been widely reported. The role of interleukin-6 (IL-6) in immune complex–induced mesangial proliferative GN in both IgA nephropathy and systemic lupus erythematosus (SLE) has been documented, and urinary excretion of IL-6 as an index of the disease activity has been emphasized, especially in IgA nephropathy. The study of Wu et al. (39) demonstrates a similar finding, namely increased excretion of IL-6 in children with HSP. However, these authors also found IL-6 in other types of nephropathies and in normal individuals and suggested that IL-6 excretion is related to inflammation and is not a marker for specific glomerulonephropathies. This study also identified tumor necrosis factor-α (TNF-α) and IL-1β in urine of patients with IgA nephropathy. Since these cytokines were not simultaneously detected in the serum, the authors postulated that they were locally produced by the inflamed glomeruli and excreted in the urine, and that concentrations of urinary TNF-α and IL-1β may be used as markers of active nephritis.

That serum levels of IgA are elevated in children with HSP is well known. To investigate the mechanism(s) leading to this finding, Kondo et al. (40) studied 12 children with HSP. Serum IgA levels were significantly elevated within 2 weeks (5–14 days) after onset while serum levels

COLOR
PLATES

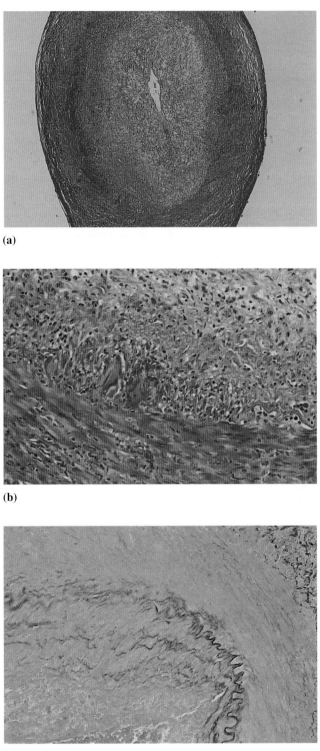

Figure 18.1 *Giant cell (temporal) arteritis*. (a) Symmetric mucoid intimal proliferation with near-total occlusion of lumen. (b) Epithelioid histiocytes and multinucleated giant cells at intima–media junction. (c) Lawson's elastic–van Gieson stain highlights partial inflammatory destruction of internal elastic lamina.

(a)

(b)

(c)

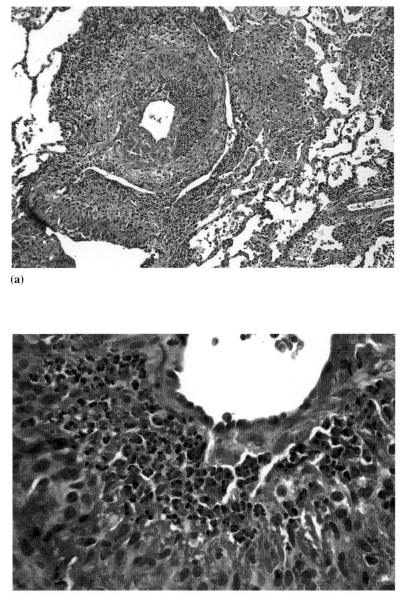

Figure 18.10 *Churg-Strauss syndrome*. (a) Open-lung biopsy showing vasculitis and interstitial inflammation. (b) High-power detail demonstrating eosinophil-rich granulomatous vasculitis.

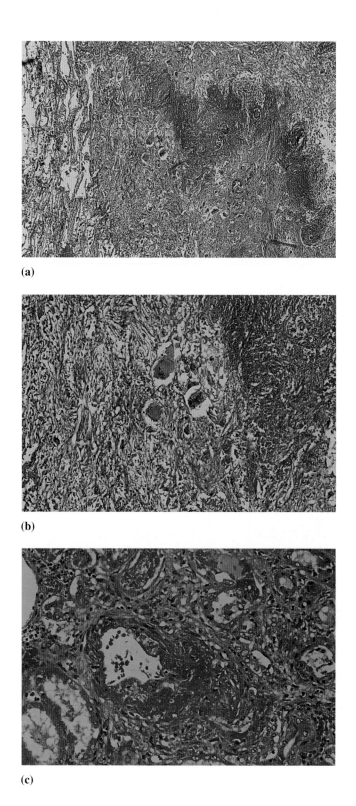

Figure 18.11 *Wegener's granulomatosis*. (a) Open-lung biopsy showing extensive coagulative necrosis. (b) High-power detail demonstrating basophilic necrosis bordered by multinucleated giant cells. (c) Fibrinoid necrosis in interstitial renal vessel (arcuate artery).

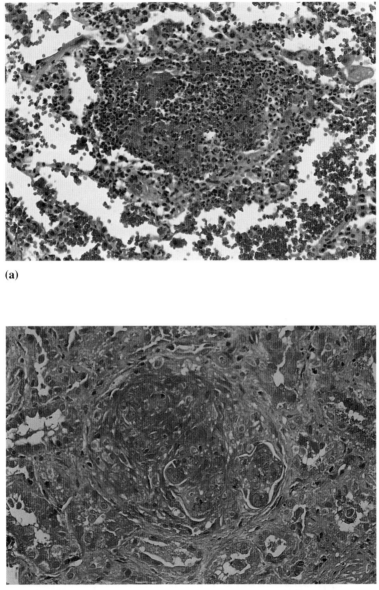

(a)

(b)

Figure 18.12 *Microscopic polyangiitis.* (a) Open-lung biopsy demonstrating distended and engorged alveolar capillaries with predominantly polymorphonuclear mural infiltrates. (b) Renal glomerulus demonstrating capillary compression, necrosis, and cellular crescent (Masson trichrome stain).

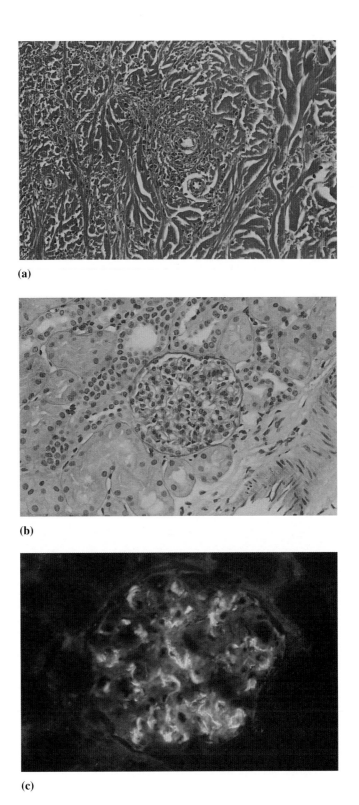

Figure 18.14 *Henoch-Schönlein purpura.* (a) Leukocytoclastic vasculitis in and around dermal vessel. (b) Diffuse proliferative glomerulonephritis without necrosis (periodic acid–Schiff reaction). (c) Immunoglobulin-A deposits in glomerular mesangium (direct immunofluorescence).

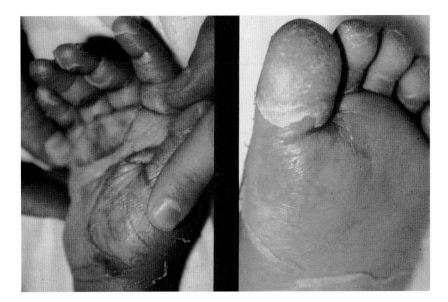

Figure 21.2 Periungual desquamation is a feature of the convalescent stage of disease and may involve the palms and soles.

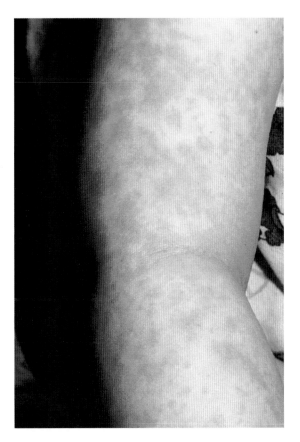

Figure 21.3 A polymorphous rash occurs early in patients with Kawasaki disease and often appears as nonpruritic, erythematous plaques.

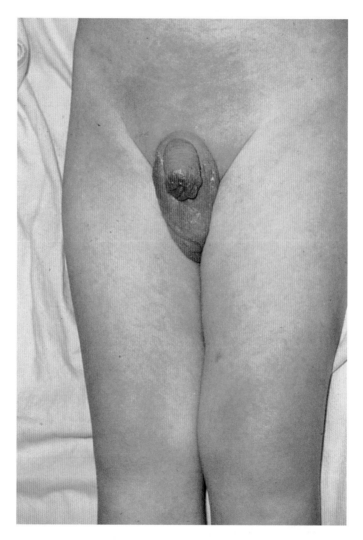

Figure 21.4 Perineal erythema and desquamation is a common finding in Kawasaki disease.

of both IgG and IgM were normal. Although the percentage of surface IgA-bearing B cells is not increased, the numbers of IgA-secreting cells significantly increased within 2 weeks of onset. These data provide strong evidence for a selective triggering of IgA-secreting cells that appears to correlate with disease activity. Ault et al. (41) reported a significant association of C4B deficiency in patients with HSP-related glomerulonephritis (19% of children with glomerulonephritis had C4B deficiency vs. 3% of controls). Because the complement system plays a crucial role in the solubilization and clearance of immune complexes, deficiency of C4B complement component may predispose to renal disease. Using radial immunodiffusion and enzyme-linked immunoabsorbent assay (ELISA), Saulsbury (42) investigated the heavy and light chain composition of serum IgA and IgA-rheumatoid factors in 34 children with HSP. As expected, serum IgA concentrations were elevated. The predominant subclass was IgA1, while levels of IgA2 remained normal. The majority of the patients (19 of 34) had circulating rheumatoid factors composed primarily of IgA1. There were no IgG or IgM rheumatoid factors. Determination of the light chain composition of serum IgA1 was similar in both patients and controls. However, the IgA1 rheumatoid factors were enriched in κ light chains. The predominance of IgA1 is not surprising since 80–90% of serum IgA is the IgA1 subclass. Similar findings were reported in patients with IgA nephropathy, underscoring the similarity between the disorders.

During the last several years, there has been a profusion of articles characterizing the spectrum of antineutrophil cytoplasmic antibodies (ANCAs) associated with systemic vasculitis syndromes and a variety of inflammatory disorders. It is now apparent that ANCAs are a family of related but distinct autoantibodies. The putative role for ANCAs in the pathogenesis of both HSP and IgA nephropathy was suggested by one group of investigators who detected IgA ANCAs in 55% of patients with HSP and 15% of patients with Berger's nephropathy (43). However, in a study by O'Donoghue et al. (44), this finding was not confirmed. Indeed, of the 30 children with early HSP, none had ANCAs. Similarly, of the 100 adult patients with IgA nephropathy, only two were found to have ANCAs. Both of these patients had IgG antimyeloperoxidase antibodies (pANCA) and even though both had persistent microscopic hematuria with slowly progressive renal failure, neither had glomerular crescents nor focal necrosis, which are classically associated with pANCA. It appears, therefore, that IgA ANCAs are not involved in the pathogenesis of HSP or in the pathogenesis of glomerular injury in IgA nephropathy, even in patients who develop rapidly progressive renal insufficiency. The detection of IgG antimyeloperoxidase antibodies in a small minority of patients raised the possibility that a small subset of IgA-related renal disorders shares the immunopathogenic mechanisms with other systemic vasculitides classically associated with ANCAs. O'Donaghue et al. further studied the relationship of specific IgG autoantibodies directed against glomerular antigens in the serum of patients with active HSP. Sixty-one percent of children with HSP complicated by nephritis had IgG antiglomerular antibodies compared with one-sixth of children without overt renal involvement (45). The finding that IgG antibodies were not detected during remission or in patients without renal manifestations further supports the hypothesis that IgG antibodies may play a direct role in renal injury.

VII. SUMMARY

Henoch–Schönlein purpura is the most common vasculitis syndrome of childhood. It is generally a benign disorder that follows an intercurrent illness, usually of the upper respiratory tract. Most children have a self-limited course and serious systemic disease and sequelae are infrequent. It is characterized by a spectrum of clinical findings, including purpuric rash, particularly over dependent areas of buttocks and lower extremities, arthritis affecting primarily the large joints, abdominal cramping with bloody stools, and microscopic and/or gross hematuria. The spectrum of the clinical expression of HSP may vary from only minimal petechial rash to severe gastrointestinal, renal, neurological, pulmonary, and joint disease.

The currently available data regarding the important differences in disease outcome between adults and children with HSP is not compelling. Although there is some suggestion of greater renal morbidity in adults, HSP appears to remain largely a self-limiting, reversible disease entity for patients of all ages. Severity of extrarenal disease also does not seem to correlate with either age or renal disease. Further large multicenter studies are needed to better define significant differences between HSP in adults and children.

REFERENCES

1. Robson WLM, Leung AKC. Henoch-Schönlein purpura. Adv Pediatr 1994; 41:163–194.
2. Szer IS. Henoch-Schönlein purpura. Current Science. Curr Opin Rheumatol 1994; 6:25–31.
3. Chaussain M, De Boissieu D, Kalifa G, Epelbaum S, Niaudet P, Badoual J, Gendrel D. Impairment of lung diffusion capacity in HSP. J Pediatr 1992; 121:12–16.
4. Allen DM, Diamond LK, Howell DA. Anaphylactoid purpura in children (Henoch-Schönlein syndrome). Am J Dis Child 1960; 99:147–168.
5. Kato S, Shibuya H, Neganuma H, Nekagawa H. Gastrointestinal endoscopy in Henoch-Schönlein purpura. Eur J Pediatr 1992; 151:482–484.
6. Couture A, Veyrac C, Baud C, Galifer RB, Armelin I. Evaluation of abdominal pain in Henoch-Schönlein syndrome by high frequency ultrasound. Pediatr Radiol 1992; 22:12–17.
7. Niaudet P, Murcia I, Beaufils H, Broyer M, Habib R. Primary IgA nephropathies in children: Prognosis and treatment. Adv Nephrol 1993; 2:121–140.
8. Nakamoto Y, et al. Primary IgA glomerulonephritis and Schönlein-Henoch purpura nephritis: Clinicopathological and immuno-histochemical characteristics. Q J Med 1978; 47:495–516.
9. Chamberlain RS, Greenberg LW. Scrotal involvement in Henoch-Schönlein purpura: A case report and review of the literature. Pediatr Emerg Care 1992; 8:213–215.
10. Singer JI, Kissoon N, Gloor J. Acute testicular pain: Henoch-Schönlein purpura versus testicular torsion. Pediatr Emerg Care 1992; 8:51–53.
11. Belman AL, Eicher CR, Moshe SL, Mezey AP. Neurologic manifestations of Schönlein-Henoch purpura: Report of three cases and review of the literature. Pediatrics 1985; 75:687–692.
12. Olson JC, Kelly KJ, Pan CG, Wortmann DW. Pulmonary disease with hemorrhage in Henoch-Schönlein purpura. Pediatrics 1992; 89:1177–1181.
13. Bernhardt JP. La nephropathie du syndrome de Schönlein-Henoch chez l'adulte. Praxis 1968; 3:70–87.
14. Cream JJ, Gumpel JM, Peachey RDG et al. Schönlein-Henoch purpura in the adult. Q J Med 1970; 39:461–472.
15. Bar-On H, Rosenmann E. Schönlein-Henoch syndrome in adults. Israel J Med 1972; 10(8):1702–1715.
16. Roth DA, Wilz DR, Theil GB. Schönlein-Henoch syndrome in adults. Q J Med 1985; 55:145–152.
17. Ballard HS, Eisinger RP, Gallo G. Renal manifestations of the Henoch-Schönlein syndrome in adults. Am J Medicine 1970; 49:328–335.
18. Fogazzi GB, Pasquali S, Moriggi M, et al. Long-term outcome of Schönlein-Henoch nephritis in the adult. Clin Nephrol 1989; 31(2):60–66.
19. Michel BA, Hunder GG, Bloch DA and Calabrese LH. Hypersensitivity vasculitis and Henoch-Schönlein purpura: A comparison between the two disorders. J Rheumatol 1992; 19:721–728.
20. Rodriguez-Valverde V, Blanco R, Martinez-Taboada VM. Henoch-Schönlein purpura in adulthood and childhood [letter]. Arthritis Rheum 1997:1518–1519.
21. Tancrede-Bohin E, Ochinisky S, Vignon-Pennamen MD, et al. Schonlein-Henoch purpura in adult patients. Predictive factors for IgA glomerulonephritis in a retrospective study of 57 Cases. Arch Dermatol 1997; 133:438–442.
22. Blanco R, Martinez-Taboada VM, Rodriguez-Valverde V et al. Henoch-Schönlein purpura in adults and childhood. Arthritis Rheum 1997; 40:859–864.

23. Ince E, Mumcu Y, Suskan E, Yalcinkaya F, Tumer N, Cin SC. Infantile acute hemorrhagic edema: A variant of leucocytoclastic vasculitis. Pediatr Dermatol 1995; 12(3):224–227.

24. Calabrese LH, Michel BA, Bloch DA, Arend WP, Edworthy SM, Fauci AS, Fries JF, Hunder GG, Leavitt RY, Lie JT, et al. The ACR 1990 criteria for the classification of hypersensitivity vasculitis. Arthritis Rheum 1990; 33:1108–1113.

25. Rosenblum ND, Winter HS. Steroid effects on the course of abdominal pain in children with HSP. Pediatr 1987; 79:1018–1021.

26. Glasier CM, Siegel MJ, McAlister WH, et al. Henoch-Schönlein syndrome in children: Gastrointestinal manifestations. Am J Rheumatol 1981; 136:1081–1085.

27. Buchanec J, Galanda V, Belakova S, Minarik M, Zibolen M. Incidence of renal complications in Schönlein-Henoch purpura syndrome in dependence of early administration of steroids. Int J Nephrol 1988; 20:409–412.

28. Mollica F, Li Volti S, Garozzo R, Russo G. Effectiveness of early prednisone treatment in preventing the development of nephropathy in anaphylactoid purpura. Eur J Pediatr 1982; 151:140–144.

29. Saulsbury FT. Corticosteroid therapy does not prevent nephritis in Henoch-Schönlein purpura. Pediatr Nephrol 1993; 7:69–71.

30. Levy M, Broyer M, Arsan A, et al. Anaphylactoid purpura nephritis in childhood: Natural history and immunopathology. Adv Nephrol 1976; 6:183–189.

31. Counahan R, Winterborn MH, White RHR, et al. Prognosis of Henoch-Schönlein nephritis in children. Br Med J 1977; 2:11–14.

32. Rostoker G, Desvaux-Belghiti D, Pilatte Y, et al. High-dose immunoglobulin therapy for severe IgA nephropathy and Henoch-Schönlein purpura. Ann Intern Med 1994; 120:476–484.

33. Oner A, Tinaztepe K, Erdogan O. The effect of triple therapy on rapidly progressive type of Henoch-Schönlein nephritis. Pediatr Nephrol 1995; 9:6–10.

34. Rostoker G, Desvaux-Belghiti D, Pilatte Y, et al. Immunomodulation with low-dose immunoglobulins for moderate IgA nephropathy and Henoch-Schönlein purpura. Nephron 1995; 69:327–334.

35. Kawana S, Nishiyama S. Serum SC5b-9 (terminal complement complex) level, a sensitive indicator of disease activicty in patients with Henoch-Schönlein purpura. Dermatology 1992; 184:171–176.

36. Abou-Ragheb HHA, Williams AJ, Brown CB, Milford-Ward A. Plasma levels of the anaphylatoxins C3a and C4a in patients with IgA nephropathy/Henoch-Schönlein nephritis. Nephron 1992; 62:22–26.

37. Tonshoff B, Momper R, Schweer H, Scharer K, Seyberth HW. Increased biosynthesis of vasoactive prostanoids in Schönlein-Henoch purpura. Pediatr Res 1992; 32:137–140.

38. Jin DK, Kohsaka T, Koo JW, Ha IS, Cheong HI, Choi Y. Complement 4 Locus II gene deletion and DQA1'0301 gene: Genetic risk factors for IgA nephropathy and Henoch-Schönlein nephritis. Nephron 1996; 73:390–395.

39. Wu TH, Wu SC, Huang TP, Yu CL, Tsai CY. Increased excretion of tumor necrosis factor alpha and interleukin 1b in urine from patients with IgA nephropathy and Schönlein-Henoch purpura. Nephron 1996; 74:79–88.

40. Kondo N, Kasahara K, Shinoda S, Orii T. Accelerated expression of secreted alpha-chain gene in anaphylactoid purpura. J Clin Immunol 1992; 12:193–196.

41. Ault BH, Stapleton FB, Rivas ML, Waldo FB, Roy III S, McLean RH, Bin J, Wyatt RJ. Association of Henoch-Schönlein purpura glomerulonephritis with C4B deficiency. J Pediatr 1990; 117:753–755.

42. Saulsbury FT. Heavy and light chain composition of serum IgA rheumatoid factor in Henoch-Schönlein purpura. Arthritis Rheum 1992; 35:1377–1380.

43. Shaw G, Ronda N, Bevan JS, Esnault V, Griffiths DFR, Rees A. antineutrophil cytoplasmic antibodies (ANCA) of IgA class correlate with disease activity in adult Henoch-Schönlein purpura. Nephrol Dial Transplant 1992; 7:1238–1241.

44. O'Donoghue DJ, Nusbaum P, Noel LH, Halbwachs-Mecarelli L, Lesavre Ph. Antineutrophil cytoplasmic antibodies in IgA nephropathy and Henoch-Schonlein purpura. Nephrol Dial Transplant 1992; 7: 534–538.

45. O'Donoghue DJ, Jewkes F, Postlethwaite RJ, Ballardie FW. Autoimmunity to glomerular antigens in Henoch-Schönlein nephritis. Clin Sci 1992; 83:281–287.

23

Microscopic Polyangiitis: Pathogenesis

Peter Heeringa, J. Charles Jennette, and Ronald J. Falk
University of North Carolina, Chapel Hill, North Carolina

I. INTRODUCTION

Approximately 50 years ago, in an attempt to differentiate vasculitis into clinical and pathological categories, Zeek et al. (1,2) described a form of small-vessel vasculitis that they called hypersensitivity angiitis. This form of vasculitis differed from periarteritis nodosa in that it involved vessels other than arteries and frequently affected capillaries in the lungs and kidneys. In 1954, Godman and Churg (3) confirmed the distinctive clinical and pathological characteristics of this form of vasculitis, but preferred the term microscopic periarteritis because they did not find evidence for an allergic response in their patients with this category of vasculitis. The 1993 Chapel Hill Consensus Conference on the Nomenclature of Systemic Vasculitis adopted the name microscopic polyangiitis for Zeek's hypersensitivity angiitis and Godman and Churg's microscopic periarteritis (4). This designation was preferred over microscopic polyarteritis because, in some patients, microscopic polyangiitis affects capillaries (e.g., alveolar and glomerular capillaries) and venules (e.g., dermal venules) with no identifiable involvement of arteries. The Chapel Hill Nomenclature System also requires that microscopic polyangiitis have few or no immunoglobulin deposits in vessel walls, which distinguishes microscopic polyangiitis from a number of other small-vessel vasculitides that appear to be mediated by immune complexes localized in vessel walls (e.g., cryoglobulinemic vasculitis and Henoch–Schönlein purpura) or by antibodies directed against constituents of vessel walls (e.g., Goodpasture's syndrome). This paucity of immunoglobulin is the basis for the designation pauci-immune small-vessel vasculitis, which refers to a category of necrotizing small-vessel vasculitis with little or no immunoglobulin localization that includes not only microscopic polyangiitis but also Wegener's granulomatosis and Churg–Strauss syndrome (4,5). The pathological similarity among these three categories of small-vessel vasculitis suggested to Godman and Churg that they share the same pathogenic mechanism (3), and this is supported further by their association with antineutrophil cytoplasmic autoantibodies (4–8).

II. PATHOGENIC IMPLICATIONS OF THE PATHOLOGY

The acute vasculitic lesions of all forms of pauci-immune small-vessel vasculitis are characterized by segmental fibrinoid necrosis (Figs. 1 and 2), influx of predominantly neutrophils, and conspicuous karyorrhexis, especially of neutrophils (leukocytoclasia), caused by apoptosis and

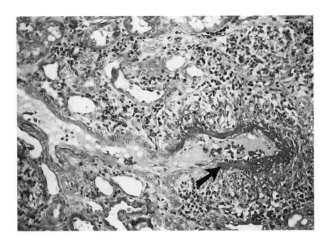

Figure 1   Necrotizing vasculitis affecting an interlobular artery in a patient with microscopic polyangiitis. Note that the fibrinoid necrosis (arrow) and adjacent inflammation are confined to the segment of the artery to the right while the segment to the left is uninvolved. (Trichrome stain.)

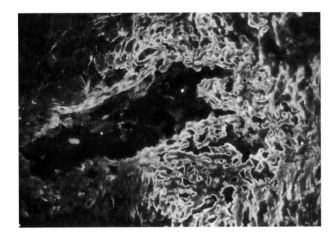

Figure 2   Direct immunofluorescence microscopy demonstrating fibrin in a zone of vasculitic fibrinoid necrosis.

necrosis (5–7). Eosinophils may be conspicuous. As the lesions progress over time, the leukocyte infiltrate is dominated by mononuclear leukocytes (Fig. 3), mainly monocyte/macrophages and T lymphocytes, and they eventually evolve into fibrotic lesions. Wegener's granulomatosis and Churg–Strauss syndrome share indistinguishable histological vasculitic lesions with microscopic polyangiitis, but also have distinctive pathological and clinical characteristics that distinguish these categories of pauci-immune small-vessel vasculitis from microscopic polyangiitis (4,5). Specifically, patients with Wegener's granulomatosis have necrotizing granulomatous inflammation and patients with Churg–Strauss syndrome have blood eosinophilia and asthma. Thus, although the pathogenesis of the small-vessel vasculitis may be the same in these three categories of vasculitis, some modification of the efferent or afferent limb of disease induction must be different in Wegener's granulomatosis and Churg–Strauss syndrome to account for the disease manifestations that these processes have that differ from those in microscopic polyangiitis.

The acute pathological lesion in microscopic polyangiitis indicates that very destructive lytic

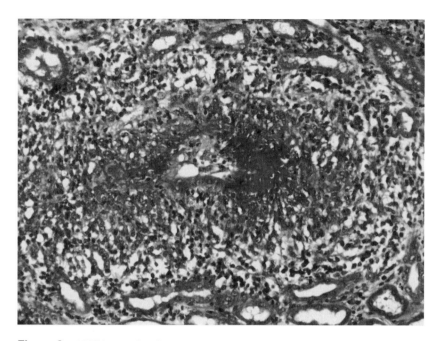

Figure 3 ANCA-associated small-vessel vasculitis with extensive mural and perivascular infiltration by predominantly mononuclear leukocytes. (Mason trichrome stain.)

and necrotizing factors are involved in causing the tissue injury. The fibrinoid necrosis (see Fig. 1 and 2) results from the spillage of plasma into the tissue adjacent to the lumen, where thrombogenic factors, such as collagen and necrotic debris, activate the coagulation cascade leading to the formation of fibrin. The activated coagulation cascade is a marker for activation of other interconnected humoral inflammatory mediator systems, such as the kinin system. Immunohistological examination of the acute lesions demonstrates the fibrinogen and fibrin, but reveals only low-level complement activation and little or no immunoglobulins. In addition to the extensive lytic destruction of cells and extracellular matrix, the conspicuous karyorrhexis documents extensive death of endogenous cells and infiltrating leukocytes. Neutrophils are the only inflammatory cells that are known to cause this pattern of destructive lytic injury, and thus, whatever the pathogenic mechanism is in microscopic polyangiitis, it must have a component of recruitment and activation of neutrophils, at least during the initial phase of injury. Within days, most of the vasculitic lesions contain a predominance of mononuclear leukocytes, including monocytes, macrophages, and T lymphocytes. This, of course, is the natural histological evolution of any acute inflammatory process. The neutrophils quickly die out, and the monocytes that come in with the initial wave of neutrophils persist and transform into macrophages that release cytokines that orchestrate the evolution of the acute inflammatory response into a chronic inflammatory response with a predominance of additional monocytes, macrophages, and T lymphocytes. At sites of severe or persistent injury, the chronic inflammatory response ultimately engenders fibrosis by the recruitment and activation of fibroblasts.

Therefore, sites of vasculitis in microscopic polyangiitis begin as acute necrotizing inflammation and evolve through chronic inflammation to fibrosis. The last two phases are stereotypical responses to any type of acute injury, and may be independent of the etiological pathogenic events. Any explanation of the pathogenesis of microscopic polyangiitis must account for the critical initial acute destructive injury.

III. PATHOGENIC IMPLICATIONS OF THE SEROLOGY

Over the past 15 years, it has become evident that the pauci-immune small-vessel vasculitides are strongly associated with the presence of autoantibodies directed against lysosomal constituents of neutrophils and monocytes (5–8). This category of autoantibodies is now collectively known as antineutrophil cytoplasmic antibodies (ANCAs). The first description of ANCAs dates back to 1982 when Davies et al. (9) reported that sera from a small number of patients with segmental necrotizing glomerulonephritis reacted with the cytoplasm of neutrophils. These observations were largely unnoticed until, in 1985, van der Woude et al. (10) showed that ANCAs are sensitive serological markers for Wegener's granulomatosis. Later, the presence of ANCAs was established in microscopic polyangiitis, Churg–Strauss syndrome, and idiopathic pauci-immune necrotizing crescentic glomerulonephritis (11–13).

The original, and still routinely used, technique to screen sera for the presence of ANCAs is indirect immunofluorescence on ethanol-fixed neutrophils. The ANCAs produce two staining patterns on this substrate, cytoplasmic (C-ANCA) and perinuclear (P-ANCA) (11). The major target antigen recognized by C-ANCA–positive sera has been identified as proteinase 3 (PR3), which is a 29-kDa serine proteinase localized in the azurophilic granules of neutrophils and the lysosomes of monocytes (14–17). The enzyme is slightly cationic (isoelectric point of 9.1) and has proteolytic activity on several physiological substrates, such as extracellular matrix proteins (18).

In patients with vasculitis, P-ANCA sera usually are specific for myeloperoxidase (MPO) which, like PR3, is localized in the azurophilic granules of neutrophils and lysosomes of monocytes (11). Myeloperoxidase is a 140-kDa, highly cationic protein (isoelectric point of >11) involved in the generation of reactive oxygen species (19). The P-ANCA staining pattern produced by sera positive for MPO was found to be an artifact of the ethanol fixation, which causes cationic cytoplasmic proteins to shift toward the negatively charged nuclear membrane. Upon fixation of neutrophils with a cross-linking fixative, such as formalin, these sera produce a cytoplasmic staining pattern (11).

Most patients with Wegener's granulomatosis have PR3-ANCAs, whereas most patients with microscopic polyangiitis or Churg–Strauss syndrome have MPO-ANCAs; however, either type of ANCA can occur in any of the clinicopathological categories of pauci-immune small-vessel vasculitis (4–8).

The etiology and pathogenesis of pauci-immune small-vessel vasculitis, including microscopic polyangiitis, is still unknown. However, the close association with ANCAs, together with the shared histopathological features, has prompted the hypothesis that the underlying pathogenesis is the same in all forms of pauci-immune small-vessel vasculitis, and that this somehow involves ANCAs. Most immune responses have both an antibody-mediated (B cell) and a cell-mediated (T cell) component, and there is evidence that the ANCA immune response is no exception because T cells with reactivity against PR3 or MPO can be identified in patients with ANCA-associated small-vessel vasculitis (20,21). Whether these T cells are only involved in the efferent (immunogenic) phase of ANCA induction or are also involved in the afferent (pathogenic) phase of pauci-immune small-vessel vasculitis has not been determined.

IV. PATHOGENIC IMPLICATIONS OF CLINICAL OBSERVATIONS

As just noted, the fact that ANCAs occur in over 80% of patients with pauci-immune small-vessel vasculitis raises the possibility that they have a pathogenic role. This is further supported by the observation that the titer of ANCAs correlates to a degree with clinical activity and response to treatment (6,8). Although this is consistent with a cause and effect relationship, it would also occur with an epiphenomenon that was secondary to active disease, as is the case with the erythrocyte sedimentation rate. The effectiveness of aggressive immunosuppressive therapy in ANCA disease also suggests immune mediation, although this could be an immune mechanism that does not involve ANCAs. In addition, immunosuppressive agents have nonspecific antiinflammatory effects, such as depression of leukocyte production and function, and thus may cause disease remission by abrogating secondary mediator events rather than primary (etiological) immunological events. The apparent effectiveness of pooled intravenous immune globulin in patients with ANCA vasculitis is somewhat more supportive of an antibody-mediated pathogenic process (22). The most compelling clinical evidence that ANCAs cause vasculitis is the observation that certain drugs, such as aminoguanidines, thiouracils, hydralazine and penicillamine (23–31), and environmental exposures, e.g., to silica (32–38), are capable of inducing ANCA formation that is associated with the development of pauci-immune small-vessel vasculitis or the closely related pauci-immune necrotizing and crescentic glomerulonephritis. These clinical observations suggest a pathogenic relationship between ANCAs and microscopic polyangiitis but do not prove this or identify the mechanism by which ANCA could cause vascular inflammation.

V. PATHOGENIC IMPLICATIONS OF IN VITRO STUDIES

A. ANCA-Mediated Neutrophil Activation

In 1990, Falk et al. (39) demonstrated that ANCA can activate primed neutrophils leading to the production of reactive oxygen metabolites and the release of lysosomal proteolytic enzymes, including the ANCA antigens themselves (Fig. 4). Since then, numerous studies have been reported in which these phenomena are further elaborated (40,41). Stimulation of neutrophils by ANCA requires prior priming of the cells by proinflammatory cytokines, such as tumor necrosis factor (TNF) and interleukin-1β (IL-1β). Priming results in the expression of the target antigens of ANCA, i.e., PR3 and MPO, on the surface of the neutrophil making them accessible for interaction with the anti-PR3 and anti-MPO antibodies. Interestingly, primed neutrophils expressing PR3 and MPO occur in the peripheral blood of patients with active ANCA-associated small-vessel vasculitis. If interaction between ANCA and primed neutrophils occurs in the circulation, massive systemic release of lytic enzymes and oxygen radicals would ensue. However, it has been demonstrated that this process only occurs when neutrophils are adherent to a surface. This adherence particularly involves β-integrins. In support of this, Ewert et al. (42) have shown that endothelial injury induced in vitro by ANCA-induced neutrophil activation requires β-integrin ligation. Thus, ANCA-induced neutrophil activation in vivo probably takes place at sites of local cytokine release where neutrophils are primed and endothelial cells activated, and in small vessels where neutrophils are in close contact with vessel walls. A recent study showed that ANCA-induced reactive oxygen production and degranulation is markedly enhanced in the presence of extracellular arachidonic acid (43). It appeared that ANCAs are potent activators of the 5-lipoxygenase pathway in neutrophils, inducing the production of large amounts of leukotriene B4. Leukotriene B4 is a potent chemoattractant for neutrophils and may trigger an autocrine loop of cell activation, resulting in increased oxygen metabolite production and degranulation.

In addition to oxygen metabolite production and degranulation, ANCA can stimulate neutrophils to secrete cytokines such as IL-8 and IL-1β (44,45). The ANCA-induced IL-8 production by neutrophils may amplify the recruitment of additional neutrophils, whereas IL-1β production may be involved in the transition from acute to chronic inflammation.

The mechanisms responsible for ANCA-mediated neutrophil activation are not completely

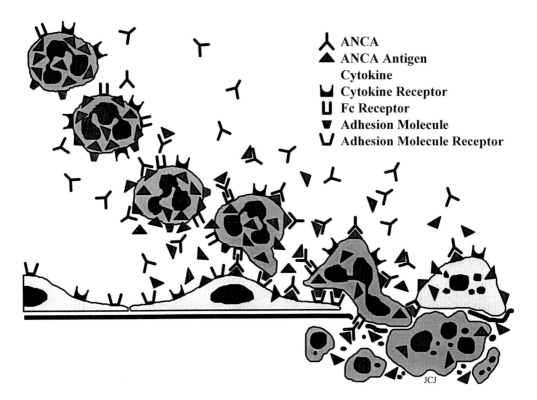

Figure 4 Diagram depicting hypothetical events in the induction of necrotizing vasculitis by the synergistic interaction of ANCA with other inflammatory stimuli that prime neutrophils by inducing the expression of ANCA antigens on the surface of neutrophils. Beginning at the upper left, normal neutrophils with no ANCA antigens on the surface are primed by cytokines, resulting in expression of ANCA antigens at the neutrophil cell surface where they can interact with the Fab'2 of ANCA. Neutrophils then can be activated by direct ANCA Fab'2 binding, as well as by engagement of Fc receptors by ANCA complexed with ANCA antigens in the fluid microenvironment of the neutrophil and on vascular surfaces. At the bottom right, neutrophil activation ultimately results in endothelial cell and neutrophil apoptosis and necrosis, as well as lytic disruption of vessel wall matrix material. Similar events would occur for monocytes, which also contain ANCA-antigens. (From Ref. 6.)

clear. As mentioned before, neutrophils express the ANCA antigens on the cell membrane upon priming with proinflammatory cytokines. In addition, the ANCA antigens are also expressed on the cell surface of apoptotic neutrophils and are recognized by ANCA. Binding of ANCAs to primed or apoptotic neutrophils may lead to further activation of the same or a second neutrophil, which appears to depend on the interaction of the Fc portion of the antibody with Fc receptors on the neutrophils or Fab'2 recognition of antigen (Fig. 4). Blocking the Fc$_\gamma$RIIa receptor with specific monoclonal antibodies inhibits ANCA-mediated neutrophil activation to a large extent (46,47). A study by Kocher et al. demonstrated an important role for the FcRIIIb (48). However, in other studies F(ab)$_2$ fragments of the antibodies also induced neutrophil activation suggesting that Fc$_\gamma$R independent processes are involved as well (49).

Because the ANCA antigens PR3 and MPO are also constituents of granules from monocytes, these cells are likely to be targets for ANCA activation as well (50). However, the effects of ANCAs on monocytes have not been extensively studied. It has been reported that monocytes can be activated to produce reactive oxygen metabolites by ANCAs (50). In addition, it has been shown that ANCAs stimulate monocytes to produce monocyte chemoattractant protein-1 and IL-8 (51,52). In vivo, ANCA-induced MCP-1 and IL-8 secretion may play an important role by amplification of local monocyte and neutrophil recruitment. Even if neutrophils and monocytes are activated equally by ANCA, it is conceivable that the initial leukocyte response at a site of new ANCA-induced injury would be predominated by neutrophils because they outnumber monocytes in the circulation; however, once the destruction is induced and the lesion begins to mature, the neutrophils would die out but the monocytes would persist and transform into macrophages. As mentioned earlier, these activated macrophages would then orchestrate the chronic inflammatory and fibrotic response to the acute injury, resulting in resolution or scarring.

The cytokine dependency of ANCA-mediated neutrophil activation in vitro is of particular interest because it correlates well with some features of the clinical presentation of ANCA-associated small-vessel vasculitis, including microscopic polyangiitis. In clinically quiescent patients, high ANCA titers can be present suggesting that ANCAs alone are not sufficient to induce disease activity (53). Furthermore, in many patients, onset and exacerbations are preceded by signs and symptoms of infections, and there is an increased incidence of ANCA-associated small-vessel vasculitis during winter months (54). These observations support the hypothesis that nonspecific immune activation leading to cytokine production and priming of neutrophils is required for the onset of disease activity in vivo.

B. Interaction of ANCAs with Their Target Antigens

Besides their capacity to activate neutrophils, ANCAs may also affect the enzymatic properties of their target antigens. This has been demonstrated for anti-PR3 antibodies and recently also for anti-MPO antibodies.

Binding of anti-PR3 to PR3 can inhibit the irreversible inactivation of PR3 by α_1-antitrypsin although most anti-PR3–positive sera also inhibit the enzymatic activity of PR3 (55–57). Binding of PR3-ANCAs to PR3 may interfere with the clearance of PR3 released from neutrophils and may lead to the longer persistence of anti-PR3–PR3 complexes in tissues. Subsequently, dissociation of active PR3 from these complexes may contribute to tissue injury. Interestingly, in a longitudinal study of patients with Wegener's granulomatosis, it was found that disease activity correlated with the amount of inhibitory activity of the antibodies on the inactivation of PR3 by α_1-antitrypsin rather than with the anti-PR3 titer itself (56,57).

Ceruloplasmin has been identified as a physiological inhibitor of MPO enzymatic activity, preventing the production of hypochlorous acid (58). Recently, Griffin et al. (59) demonstrated that this inhibition can be disrupted in the presence of anti-MPO antibodies isolated from patients with microscopic polyangiitis and Wegener's granulomatosis. In this study, the majority of the anti-MPO antibodies (76%) did not themselves inhibit MPO activity, suggesting that steric hindrance following binding of the antibodies near the active site is responsible for the inhibitory effect. Interestingly, the capacity of anti-MPO antibodies derived from Wegener's granulomatosis patients to reverse the ceruloplasmin-mediated inhibition of MPO activity was much less marked as compared with anti-MPO antibodies derived from MPA patients. These results suggest different anti-MPO epitope specificities in Wegener's granulomatosis and microscopic polyangiitis, which may influence disease manifestations.

C. Interaction Between ANCAs and Endothelial Cells

Myeloperoxidase and PR3 are cationic proteins with isoelectric points of >11 and 9.1, respectively. Upon release from activated neutrophils, these enzymes may bind to anionic structures such as basal membranes or the luminal surface of endothelial cells. Subsequently, ANCAs may bind, resulting in opsonization and complement activation, enhanced influx of inflammatory cells, and antibody-dependent cellular cytotoxicity. Activation of such effector pathways in vivo may aggravate the inflammatory process and eventually cause vessel wall destruction. In vitro studies have shown that ANCAs bind to endothelial cells previously incubated with MPO or PR3, and can induce complement-dependent endothelial cell lysis (42,60,61). Furthermore, incubation with PR3 and elastase enhances IL-8 production by endothelial cells and triggers endothelial cell apoptosis (62,63). Although the effects of ANCAs were not studied, these observations may be of pathophysiological importance because in renal biopsies of ANCA-associated vasculitides MPO, PR3 and elastase are localized extracellularly on endothelial and tubular cells (64).

Most evidence indicates that the ANCA antigens MPO and PR3 are specific for cells of the monomyeloid lineage. Some studies, however, suggest that PR3 may be expressed by other cell types as well, including endothelial cells (65). In endothelial cells, increased PR3 expression and translocation of the enzyme to the cell membrane has been reported after stimulation with either TNF-α, interferon-γ (IFN-γ) or IL-1β (65). Addition of anti-PR3 antibodies in the presence of primed neutrophils results in cytotoxicity of these primed endothelial cells (66). These observations suggest that PR3 is available for interaction with the autoantibodies on endothelial cells at inflammatory sites. However, other studies have not been able to demonstrate PR3 expression by cytokine-treated endothelial cells (67). Thus, the role of this phenomenon in the pathophysiology of ANCA-associated small-vessel vasculitis is controversial. In addition, within vascular lesions in microscopic polyangiitis and other forms of ANCA-associated vasculitis, deposits of immunoglobulin are absent or scanty. Therefore, direct or indirect binding of ANCA to endothelial cells as a pathophysiological mechanism in the development of ANCA-associated vasculitis has been disputed. However, the absence of detectable immunoglobulin deposits in fully developed vascular lesions does not exclude a role for immune complexes in the initial phase of the disease process or a role for low levels of immune complex deposits.

D. T-Cell Reactivity in ANCA-Associated Small-Vessel Vasculitis

This absence or paucity of immunoglobulin deposits in vascular lesions in microscopic polyangiitis and other forms of ANCA-associated small-vessel vasculitis has raised the possibility that T cell–mediated immunity is involved in the pathogenesis of ANCA-associated small-vessel vasculitis (68). In addition, levels of soluble IL-2 receptor are elevated in Wegener's granulomatosis patients and increase preceding major relapses, providing more indirect prove for a role of activated T cells in ANCA-associated small-vessel vasculitis (69). The target antigens of these autoreactive T cells have not been identified. Proteinase 3 and MPO are likely candidates. Although T-cell reactivity to PR3 and MPO has been found to be more frequent and stronger in Wegener's granulomatosis patients than in healthy controls, not all Wegener's granulomatosis patients respond to PR3 or MPO. As noted earlier, the presence of activated T cells and their products is to be expected in any patient with severe inflammatory injury of more than a few days' duration, and thus does not prove a causal relationship to the initial injury that led to the inflammation. Therefore, the role of T cells with specificity for PR3 and MPO in the pathophysiology of ANCA-associated small-vessel vasculitis is unresolved.

E. Infections and ANCA-Associated Small-Vessel Vasculitis

There is considerable circumstantial evidence suggesting a role for infections in the pathophysiology of ANCA-associated small-vessel vasculitis. As mentioned before, relapses in disease activity are often preceded by infections, for example, chronic nasal carriage of *Staphylococcus au-*

reus has been shown to be an important risk factor for the development of relapses in Wegener's granulomatosis. Furthermore, antimicrobial treatment reduces the incidence of relapses in Wegener's granulomatosis (70).

There are several ways by which infections may play a role in ANCA-associated vasculitis. At the site of an infection, inflammatory mediators such as TNF-α are released causing activation of the endothelium and priming of neutrophils. Thus, infections may be the trigger creating the environment in which ANCA-mediated neutrophil activation can occur. Furthermore, microbial components have been shown to be effective T-cell independent B-cell mitogens that may induce autoreactive B-cells to produce ANCA. In addition, a role for microbial antigens acting as superantigens has been suggested. Superantigens, in a non–antigen specific manner, cause selective expansion of T cells bearing particular T-cell receptor Vβ chain variable regions whereas conventional antigens usually stimulate T cells expressing several V gene products. So far, studies in ANCA-associated small-vessel vasculitis regarding the T-cell receptor repertoire have been inconclusive. In one study, abnormal expansions of T cells, especially CD4+ T cells, using particular Vα and Vβ gene products were found. In another study, increased Vβ 2.1 gene usage was demonstrated in vasculitis patients and was most marked in microscopic polyangiitis. In both studies, there was no correlation with any specific clinical feature or disease activity. Considering this, it should be noted that the results may have been biased by the use of peripheral blood lymphocytes. Studies examining the T-cell Vβ gene usage of lesional T cells would provide interesting information regarding the antigenic stimulus of those T cells but have not been done so far. Thus, the causal relationship between microbial antigens and T-cell reactivity in ANCA-associated diseases remains speculative.

VI. PATHOGENIC IMPLICATIONS OF IN VIVO STUDIES

In order to substantiate a pathophysiological role for ANCA, in vivo animal models are required. In such models, a direct relation between antibodies reacting with autologous PR3 and MPO on the one hand and disease manifestations similar to those in human pauci-immune small-vessel vasculitis on the other should be demonstrable. However, in the case of PR3, development of an animal model is hampered by the fact that human anti-PR3 antibodies only react with neutrophils of baboons, and not with those of lower species. In addition, immunization of rats or mice with human PR3 does not result in antibodies reacting with rat or mouse neutrophils. Recently, the murine equivalent of human PR3 was detected in mice and cloned (71,72). However, again monoclonal and polyclonal antibodies to human PR3 did not recognize cloned mouse PR3.

Antihuman PR3 has been induced in mice by idiotypic manipulation (73,74). In these studies, mice were immunized with affinity-purified PR3-IgG from two separate Wegener's granulomatosis patients. After 2 weeks, the mice developed anti-idiotypic, and after 4 months anti-anti-idiotypic antibodies reacting with human PR3. In addition, sera derived from these mice also reacted with human MPO and endothelial cell surface proteins. Interestingly, a number of these mice developed sterile microabscesses in the lungs after 8 months. It is, however, unclear whether these antibodies also recognize murine PR3. Thus, the real autoimmune nature of this model awaits further study.

In the case of anti-MPO–associated vasculitis/glomerulonephritis, several animal models have been described to date (75).

Exposure to mercuric chloride (HgCl₂) of susceptible rat strains, usually of the TH2-responder type such as the Brown Norway (BN) rat, induces an autoimmune syndrome mediated by a T cell–dependent polyclonal B-cell activation. As part of this polyclonal B-cell activation, antibodies to MPO occur, as do antibodies to nuclear antigens, constituents of the glomerular basement membrane and other antigens (76). Necrotizing leukocytoclastic vasculitis occurs in multiple organs in $HgCl_2$-treated Brown Norway rats, particularly in the submucosal vessels of the duodenum and caecum. Pretreatment with broad-spectrum antibiotics diminished $HgCl_2$-induced vasculitis. This suggested that the microbial load of the animals contributes to, but is not entirely responsible for, $HgCl_2$-induced vasculitis. Thus, the model of $HgCl_2$-induced vasculitis has several characteristics that resemble aspects of human microscopic polyangiitis. First, as in humans, it features necrotizing vasculitis involving small to medium-sized vessels accompanied by fibrinoid necrosis of the vessel wall and inflammatory cell infiltration. Second, there is evidence that bacteria contribute to vascular injury in this model. Third, autoantibodies develop, similar to those present in humans. Despite these analogies to human disease, the model has also some important dissimilarities. In humans, necrotizing crescentic glomerulonephritis is a prominent feature of microscopic polyangiitis and other ANCA-associated small-vessel vasculitides but is not observed in $HgCl_2$-induced vasculitis. Furthermore, a range of autoantibodies is induced in this model, which precludes any conclusion as to the pathophysiological role of anti-MPO antibodies alone in this model.

In SCG/Kj mice, derived from the F1 hybrid of B×SB and MRL/lpr mice, crescentic glomerulonephritis and necrotizing vasculitis develop spontaneously in ±50% of mice (77). In agreement with findings in human microscopic polyangiitis, immune deposits are scanty or absent. Sera derived from SCG/Kj mice produce a P-ANCA staining pattern on human and murine neutrophils and react with a murine neutrophil extract and human MPO by enzyme-linked immunosorbent assay (ELISA). Again, however, the anti-MPO response is part of a polyclonal autoimmune response.

Induction of a selective autoimmune response to MPO is a more direct method of studying the pathophysiological role of anti-MPO antibodies. Immunization of Brown Norway (BN) rats results in an immune response to human MPO that cross-reacts with autologous rat MPO but immunization alone does not induce any lesions (78,79). When, 2 weeks after immunization, the products of activated neutrophils, i.e., proteolytic enzymes (proteinase 3, elastase), MPO, and its substrate hydrogen peroxide (H_2O_2) are perfused into the left kidney, the MPO-immunized rats develop necrotizing crescentic glomerulonephritis and vasculitis (78). At 1 day after perfusion, immune deposits are clearly present along the glomerular basement membrane (GBM), but at 4 and 10 days after perfusion, the lesions lack immune deposits. These studies suggest that ANCA-associated vascular inflammation may develop after transient focal immune complex formation along the GBM. The absence of immune deposits in the later stages of this model may be due to degradation of immune complexes by proteolytic enzymes released from activated neutrophils. However, the pauci-immune character of this model has been disputed by others (79).

Kobayashi et al. (80) reported that anti-GBM nephritis in rats is aggravated by the administration of heterologous rabbit anti-rat MPO antibodies. In these studies, the administration of rabbit anti-rat MPO antibodies together with rabbit anti-rat GBM antibodies resulted in an increased influx of neutrophils and more extensive fibrin depositions compared with rats injected with normal rabbit antibodies and rabbit anti-rat GBM antibodies. However, no evidence for crescent formation and vasculitis was found. To extend these observations, Heeringa et al. (81) injected a subnephritogenic dose of anti-GBM antibodies in rats previously immunized with human MPO. These rats developed severe glomerulonephritis characterized by the early occurrence of hematuria and severe proteinuria at day 10. In this model, MPO-immunized rats developed renal lesions characterized by fibrinoid necrosis of glomerular capillaries, extensive fibrin deposition, interstitial and intraglomerular accumulation of monocytes/macrophages and crescent formation. In control-immunized rats injected with the anti-GBM antibodies only mild glomerulonephritis was found without evidence for crescent formation, suggesting that the autologous anti-rat MPO antibodies are responsible for the exacerbation of the anti-GBM disease in this model.

Therefore, in rats, it appears that anti-MPO autoantibodies can synergize with low levels of immune complexes (78) and subnephritogenic anti-GBM antibodies (81) to cause severe necrotizing vascular inflammation that could not be caused by the priming events alone.

VII. HYPOTHESIS FOR THE PATHOGENESIS OF MICROSCOPIC POLYANGIITIS

Based on the currently available clinical, pathological, and experimental data, we hypothesize that microscopic polyangiitis and the other forms of ANCA-associated pauci-immune small-vessel vasculitis are caused by the synergistic interaction between ANCAs and other proinflammatory stimuli, such as high levels of circulating or microenvironmental cytokines. This initiates an initial phase of acute neutrophil-rich necrotizing vascular inflammatory injury that evolves into a phase that is rich in mononuclear leukocytes (monocytes, macrophages, and T cells) that ultimately may progress to fibrosis or resolution.

REFERENCES

1. Zeek PM, Smith CC, Weeter JC. Studies on periarteritis nodosa. III. The differentiation between the vascular lesions of periarteritis nodosa and of hypersensitivity. Am J Pathol 1948; 24:889–917.
2. Zeek PM. Periarteritis nodosa: a critical review. Am J Clin Pathol 1952; 22:777–790.
3. Godman GC, Churg J. Wegener's granulomatosis. Pathology and review of the literature. Arch Pathol Lab Med 1954; 58:533–553.
4. Jennette JC, Falk RJ, Andrassy K, Bacon PA, Churg J, Gross WL, Hagen EC, Hoffman GS, Hunder GG, Kallenberg CG, et al. Nomenclature of systemic vasculitides. Proposal of an international consensus conference. Arthritis Rheum 1994; 37:187–192.
5. Jennette JC, Falk RJ. Small vessel vasculitis. N Engl J Med 1997; 337:1512–1523.
6. Jennette JC, Falk RJ. Pathogenesis of the vascular and glomerular damage in ANCA-positive vasculitis. Nephrol Dial Transplant 1998; 13(suppl 1):16–20.
7. Jennette JC. Antineutrophil cytoplasmic autoantibody-associated diseases: A pathologist's perspective. Am J Kidney Dis 1991; 18:164–170.
8. Kallenberg CG, Brouwer E, Weening JJ, Tervaert JW. Anti-neutrophil cytoplasmic antibodies: Current diagnostic and pathophysiological potential. 1994; Kidney Int 46:1–15.
9. Davies DJ, Moran JE, Niall JF, Ryan GB. Segmental necrotising glomerulonephritis with antineutrophil antibody: Possible arbovirus aetiology? Br Med J Clin Res Ed 1982; 285:606–606.
10. van der Woude FJ, Rasmussen N, Lobatto S, Wiik A, Permin H, van Es LA, van der Giessen M, van der Hem GK, The TH. Autoantibodies against neutrophils and monocytes: Tool for diagnosis and marker of disease activity in Wegener's granulomatosis. Lancet 1985; 1:425–429.
11. Falk RJ, Jennette JC. Anti-neutrophil cytoplasmic autoantibodies with specificity for myeloperoxidase in patients with systemic vasculitis and idiopathic necrotizing and crescentic glomerulonephritis. N Engl J Med 1988; 318:1651–1657.
12. Cohen Tervaert JW, Goldschmeding R, Elema JD, van der Giessen M, Huitema MG, van der Hem GK, The TH, von dem Borne AE, Kallenberg CG. Autoantibodies against myeloid lysosomal enzymes in crescentic glomerulonephritis. Kidney Int 1990; 37:799–806.
13. Cohen Tervaert JW, Goldschmeding R, Elema JD, Limburg PC, van der Giessen M, Huitema MG, Koolen MI, Hene RJ, The TH, van der Hem GK, et al. Association of autoantibodies to myeloperoxidase with different forms of vasculitis. Arthritis Rheum 1990; 33:1264–1272.
14. Goldschmeding R, van der Schoot CE, ten Bokkel Huinink D, Hack CE, van den Ende ME, Kallenberg CG, von dem Borne AE. Wegener's granulomatosis autoantibodies identify a novel diisopropylfluorophosphate-binding protein in the lysosomes of normal human neutrophils. J Clin Invest 1989; 84:1577–1587.

15. Niles JL, McCluskey RT, Ahmad MF, Arnaout MA. Wegener's granulomatosis autoantigen is a novel neutrophil serine proteinase. Blood 1989; 74:1888–1893.

16. Ludemann J, Utecht B, Gross WL. Anti-neutrophil cytoplasm antibodies in Wegener's granulomatosis recognize an elastinolytic enzyme. J Exp Med 1990; 171:357–362.

17. Jennette JC, Hoidal JH, Falk RJ. Specificity of anti-neutrophil cytoplasmic autoantibodies for proteinase 3. Blood 1990; 75:2263–2264.

18. Rao NV, Wehner NG, Marshall BC, Gray WR, Gray BH, Hoidal JR. Characterization of proteinase 3, a neutrophil serine proteinase. J Clin Invest 1991; 266:9540–9548.

19. Weiss SJ. Tissue destruction by neutrophils. N Engl J Med 1989; 320:365–376.

20. Brouwer E, Stegeman CA, Huitema MG, Limburg PC, Kallenberg CG. T cell reactivity to proteinase 3 and myeloperoxidase in patients with Wegener's granulomatosis (WG). Clin Exp Immunol 1994; 98: 448–453.

21. Griffith ME, Coulthart A, Pusey CD. T cell responses to myeloperoxidase (MPO) and proteinase 3 (PR3) in patients with systemic vasculitis. Clin Exp Immunol 1996; 103:253–258.

22. Jordan SC. Treatment of systemic and renal-limited vasculitic disorders with pooled intravenous immune globulin. J Clin Immunol 1995; 15:76S–85S.

23. Dolman KM, Gans ROB, Vervaat TJ, Zevenbergen G, Maingay D, Nikkels RE, Donker AJM, von dem Borne AEGK, Goldschmeding R. Vasculitis and antineutrophil cytoplasmic autoantibodies associated with propylthiouracil therapy. Lancet 1993; 342:651–652.

24. Vogt BA, Kim Y, Jennette JC, Falk RJ, Burke BA, Sinaiko A. Antineutrophil cytoplasmic autoantibody-positive crescentic glomerulonephritis as a complication of treatment with propylothiouracil in children. J Pediatr 1984; 124:986–988.

25. Tanemoto M, Miyakawa H, Hanai J, Yago M, Kitaoka M, Uchida S. Myeloperoxidase-antineutrophil cytoplasmic antibody-positive crescentic glomerulonephritis complicating the course of Grave's disease: Report of three adult cases. Am J Kidney Dis 1995; 26:774–780.

26. D'Cruz D, Chesser AM, Lightowler C, Comer M, Hurst MJ, Baker LR, Raine AE. Antineutrophil cytoplasmic antibody-positive crescentic glomerulonephritis associated with anti-thyroid drug treatment. Br J Rheumatol 1995; 34:1090–1091.

27. Whittier F, Spinowitz B, Wuerth JP, Cartwright K. Pimagedine Safety Profile in patients with type I diabetes mellitus, J Am Soc Nephrol 1999; 10:184A.

28. Merkel PA. Drugs associated with vasculitis. Curr Opin Rheumatol 1998; 10:45–50.

29. Short AK, Lockwood CM: Antigen specificity in hydralazine associated ANCA positive systemic vasculitis. Q J Med 1995; 88:775–783.

30. Karpinski J, Jothy S, Radoux V, Levy M, Baran D. D-penicillamine-induced crescentic glomerulonephritis and antimyeloperoxidase antibodies in a patient with scleroderma. Case report and review of the literature. Am J Nephrol 1997; 17:528–532.

31. Gaskin G, Thompson EM, Pusey CD. Goodpasture-like syndrome associated with anti-myeloperoxidase antibodies following penicillamine treatment. Nephrol Dial Transplant 1995; 10:1925–8.

32. Slavin RE, Swedo JL, Brandes D, Gonzalez-Vitale JC, Osornio-Vargas A. Extrapulmonary silicosis: A clinical, morphologic, and ultrastructural study. Hum Pathol 1985; 16:393–412.

33. Gregorini G, Ferioli A, Donato F, Tira P, Morassi L, Tardanico R, Lancini L, Maiorca R. Association between silica exposure and necrotizing crescentic glomerulonephritis with P-ANCA and anti-MPO antibodies: A hospital-based case-control study. In WL Gross, ed. ANCA-Associated Vasculitides: Immunological and Clinical Aspects, New York: Plenum Press, 1993:435–440.

34. Nuyts GD, van Vlem E, De Vos A, Daelemans RA, Rorive G, Elseviers MM, Schurgers M, Segaert M, D'Haese PC, De Broae ME. Wegener granulomatosis is associated to exposure to silicon compounds: A case-control study. Nephrol Dial Transplant 1995; 10:1162–1165.

35. Wichman I, Sanchez-Roman J, Morales J, Castillo MJ, Ocana C, Nunez-Roldan A. Antimyeloperoxidase antibodies in individuals with occupational exposure to silica. Ann Rheum Dis 1996; 55:205–207.

36. Gregorini G, Tira P, Frizza J, D'Haese PC, Elseviers MM, Nuyts G, Maiorca R, De Broe ME. ANCA-associated diseases and silica exposure. Clin Rev Allergy Immunol 1997; 15:21–40.

37. Tervaert JW. Stegeman CA. Kallenberg CG: Silicon exposure and vasculitis. Curr Opin Rheumatol 1998; 10:12–17.

38. Hogan SL, Satterly KK, Dooley MA, Nachman PH, Jennette JC, Falk RJ. Silica exposure with ANCA-associated glomerulonephritis and lupus nephritis. J Am Soc Nephrol 2000; 12:134–142.

39. Falk RJ, Terrell RS, Charles LA, Jennette JC. Anti-neutrophil cytoplasmic autoantibodies induce neutrophils to degranulate and produce oxygen radicals in vitro. Proc Natl Acad Sci USA 1990; 87:4115–4119.

40. Charles LA, Caldas MLR, Falk RJ, Terrell RS, Jennette JC. Antibodies against granule proteins activate neutrophils in vitro. J Leuk Biol 1991; 50:539–546.

41. Brouwer E, Huitema MG, Mulder AH, Heeringa P, van Goor H, Tervaert JW, Weening JJ, Kallenberg CG. Neutrophil activation in vitro and in vivo in Wegener's granulomatosis. Kidney Int 1994; 45:1120–1131.

42. Ewert BH, Jennette JC, Falk RJ: Anti-myeloperoxidase antibodies stimulate neutrophils to damage human endothelial cells. Kidney Int 1992; 41:375–383.

43. Grimminger F, Hattar K, Papavassilis C, Temmesfeld B, Csernok E, Gross WL, Seeger W, Sibelius U. Neutrophil activation by anti-proteinase 3 antibodies in Wegener's granulomatosis: Role of exogenous arachidonic acid and leukotriene B4 generation. J Exp Med 1996; 184(4):1567–1572.

44. Cockwell P, Brooks CJ, Adu D, Savage CO. Interleukin-8: A pathogenetic role in antineutrophil cytoplasmic autoantibody-associated glomerulonephritis. Kidney Int 1999; 55(3):852–863.

45. Brooks CJ, King WJ, Radford DJ, Adu D, McGrath M, Savage CO. IL-1 beta production by human polymorphonuclear leucocytes stimulated by anti-neutrophil cytoplasmic autoantibodies: Relevance to systemic vasculitis. Clin Exp Immunol 1996; 106(2):273–279.

46. Mulder AH, Heeringa P, Brouwer E, Limburg PC, Kallenberg CG. Activation of granulocytes by anti-neutrophil cytoplasmic antibodies (ANCA): A Fc gamma RII-dependent process. Clin Exp Immunol 1994; 98:270–278.

47. Porges AJ, Redecha PB, Kimberly WT, Csernok E, Gross WL, Kimberly RP. Anti-neutrophil cytoplasmic antibodies engage and activate human neutrophils via Fc gamma RIIa. J Immunol 1994; 153:1271–1280.

48. Kocher M, Edberg JC, Fleit HB, Kimberly RP. Antineutrophil cytoplasmic antibodies preferentially engage Fc gammaRIIIb on human neutrophils. J Immunol 1998; 161:6909–6914.

49. Kettritz R, Jennette JC, Falk RJ: Crosslinking of ANCA-antigens stimulates superoxide release by human neutrophils. J Am Soc Nephrol 1997; 8:386–394.

50. Charles LA, Falk RJ, Jennette JC: Reactivity of antineutrophil cytoplasmic autoantibodies with mononuclear phagocytes. J Leuk Biol 1992; 51:65–68.

51. Ralston DR, Marsh CB, Lowe MP, Wewers MD. Antineutrophil cytoplasmic antibodies induce monocyte IL-8 release. Role of surface proteinase-3, alpha 1-antitrypsin, and Fcgamma receptors. J Clin Invest 1997; 100(6):1416–1424.

52. Casselman BL, Kilgore KS, Miller BF, Warren JS. Antibodies to neutrophil cytoplasmic antigens induce monocyte chemoattractant protein-1 secretion from human monocytes. J Lab Clin Med 1995; 126(5):495–502.

53. Cohen Tervaert JW, Huitema MG, Hene RJ, Sluiter WJ, The TH, van der Hem GK, Kallenberg CG. Prevention of relapses in Wegener's granulomatosis by treatment based on antineutrophil cytoplasmic antibody titre. Lancet 1990; 336:709–711.

54. Falk RJ, Hogan S, Carey TS, Jennette JC. Clinical course of anti-neutrophil cytoplasmic autoantibody-associated glomerulonephritis and systemic vasculitis. The Glomerular Disease Collaborative Network [see comments]. Ann Intern Med 1990; 113:656–663.

55. van de Wiel BA, Dolman KM, van der Meer-Gerritsen CH, Hack CE, von dem B, Goldschmeding R. Interference of Wegener's granulomatosis autoantibodies with neutrophil Proteinase 3 activity. Clin Exp Immunol 1992; 90:409–414.

56. Dolman KM, Stegeman CA, van de Wiel BA, Hack CE, von dem B, Kallenberg CG, Goldschmeding R. Relevance of classic anti-neutrophil cytoplasmic autoantibody (C-ANCA)-mediated inhibition of proteinase 3-alpha 1-antitrypsin complexation to disease activity in Wegener's granulomatosis. Clin Exp Immunol 1993; 93:405–410.

57. Daouk GH, Palsson R, Arnaout MA. Inhibition of proteinase 3 by ANCA and its correlation with disease activity in Wegener's granulomatosis. Kidney Int 1995; 47(6):1528–1536.

58. Segelmark M, Persson B, Hellmark T, Wieslander J. Binding and inhibition of myeloperoxidase (MPO): A major function of ceruloplasmin? Clin Exp Immunol 1997; 108:167–174.

59. Griffin SV, Chapman PT, Lianos EA, Lockwood CM. The inhibition of myeloperoxidase by ceruloplasmin can be reversed by anti-myeloperoxidase antibodies. Kidney Int 1999; 55:917–925.

60. Vargunam M, Adu D, Taylor CM, Michael J, Richards N, Neuberger J, Thompson RA. Endothelium myeloperoxidase-antimyeloperoxidase interaction in vasculitis. Nephrol Dial Transplant 1995; 7: 1077–1081.

61. Savage CO, Pottinger BE, Gaskin G, Pusey CD, Pearson JD. Autoantibodies developing to myeloperoxidase and proteinase 3 in systemic vasculitis stimulate neutrophil cytotoxicity toward cultured endothelial cells. Am J Pathol 1992; 141:335–342.

62. Berger SP, Seelen MA, Hiemstra PS, Gerritsma JS, Heemskerk E, van der Woude FJ, Daha MR. Proteinase 3, the major autoantigen of Wegener's granulomatosis, enhances IL-8 production by endothelial cells in vitro. J Am Soc Nephrol 1996; 7:694–701.

63. Yang JJ, Kettritz R, Falk RJ, Jennette JC, Gaido ML. Apoptosis of endothelial cells induced by the neutrophil serine proteases proteinase 3 and elastase. Am J Pathol 1996; 149:1617–1626.

64. Mrowka C, Csernok E, Gross WL, Feucht HE, Bechtel U, Thoenes GH. Distribution of the granulocyte serine proteinases proteinase 3 and elastase in human glomerulonephritis. Am J Kidney Dis 1995; 25:253–261.

65. Mayet WJ, Schwarting A, Orth T, Duchmann R, Meyer zBK. Antibodies to proteinase 3 mediate expression of vascular cell adhesion molecule-1 (VCAM-1). Clin Exp Immunol 1996; 103:259–267.

66. Mayet WJ, Schwarting A, Meyer zum Buschenfelde KH. Cytotoxic effects of antibodies to proteinase 3 (C-ANCA) on human endothelial cells. Clin Exp Immunol 1994; 97:458–465.

67. King WJ, Adu D, Daha MR, Brooks CJ, Radford DJ, Pall AA, Savage CO. Endothelial cells and renal epithelial cells do not express the Wegener's autoantigen, proteinase 3. Clin Exp Immunol 1995; 102: 98–105.

68. Cunningham MA, Huang XR, Dowling JP, Tipping PG, Holdsworth SR. Prominence of cell-mediated immunity effectors in "pauci-immune" glomerulonephritis. J Am Soc Nephrol 1999; 10(3):499–506.

69. Stegeman CA, Cohen TJ, Huitema MG, Kallenberg CG. Serum markers of T cell activation in relapses of Wegener's granulomatosis. Clin Exp Immunol 1993; 91:415–420.

70. Stegeman CA, Cohen TJ, de Jong PE, Kallenberg CG. Trimethoprim-sulfamethoxazole (co-trimoxazole) for the prevention of relapses of Wegener's granulomatosis. Dutch Co-Trimoxazole Wegener Study Group. N Engl J Med 1996; 335(1):16–20.

71. Aveskogh M, Lutzelschwab C, Huang MR, Hellman L. Characterization of cDNA clones encoding mouse proteinase 3 (myeloblastine) and cathepsin G. Immunogenetics 1997; 46:181–191.

72. Jenne DE, Frohlich L, Hummel AM, Specks U. Cloning and functional expression of the murine homologue of proteinase 3: Implications for the design of murine models of vasculitis. FEBS Letters 1997; 408:187–190.

73. Blank M, Stein TM, Kopolovic J, Wiik A, Meroni PL, Conforti G, Shoenfeld Y. Immunization with anti-neutrophil cytoplasmic antibody (ANCA) induces the production of mouse ANCA and perivascular lymphocyte infiltration. Clin Exp Immunol 1995; 102:120–130.

74. Tomer Y, Gilburd B, Blank M, Lider O, Hershkoviz R, Fishman P, Zigelman R, Meroni P, Wiik A, Shoenfeld Y. Characterization of biologically active antineutrophil cytoplasmic antibodies induced in mice. Arthritis Rheum 1995; 47:454–463.

75. Heeringa P, Brouwer E, Cohen TJ, Weening JJ, Kallenberg CG: Animal models of anti-neutrophil cytoplasmic antibody associated vasculitis. Kidney Int 1998; 53:253–263.

76. Esnault VL, Mathieson PW, Thiru S, Oliveira DB, Martin-Lockwood C. Autoantibodies to myeloperoxidase in brown Norway rats treated with mercuric chloride. Lab Invest 1992; 67:114–120.

77. Kinjoh K, Kyogoku M, Good RA. Genetic selection for crescent formation yields mouse strain with rapidly progressive glomerulonephritis and small vessel vasculitis. Proc Natl Acad Sci USA 1993; 90: 3413–3417.

78. Brouwer E, Huitema MG, Klok PA, de Weerd H, Tervaert JW, Weening JJ, Kallenberg CG. Anti-myeloperoxidase-associated proliferative glomerulonephritis: An animal model. J Exp Med 1993; 177:905–914.

79. Yang JJ, Jennette JC, Falk RJ. Immune complex glomerulonephritis is induced in rats immunized with heterologous myeloperoxidase. Clin Exp Immunol 1994; 97:466–473.
80. Kobayashi K, Shibata T, Sugisaki T. Aggravation of rat nephrotoxic serum nephritis by anti-myeloperoxidase antibodies. Kidney Int 1995; 47:454–463.
81. Heeringa P, Brouwer E, Klok PA, Huitema MG, van den Born J, Weening JJ, Kallenberg CG. Autoantibodies to myeloperoxidase aggravate mild anti-glomerular-basement-membrane-mediated glomerular injury in the rat. Am J Pathol 1996; 149:1695–1706.

24
Microscopic Polyangiitis: Clinical Aspects

Paul A. Bacon
University of Birmingham Medical School, Birmingham, England

Dwomoa Adu
Queen Elizabeth Hospital, Edgbaston, Birmingham, England

I. HISTORY: ORIGINS OF MICROSCOPIC POLYANGIITIS

Microscopic polyangiitis (MPA) has only recently been accepted as a distinct disease, separate from polyarteritis nodosa (PAN) (1). Polyarteritis nodosa was described a century ago as a rare (probably new) disease. Further case descriptions expanded the concept of vasculitis, lumping virtually all idiopathic vasculitides under the same umbrella. However, the last 50 years has seen a process of peeling off one entity after another, again making classic PAN a rare disease. Wegener's granulomatosis (WG) and Churg–Strauss syndrome (CSS), two other illnesses with similar renal involvement to MPA, were also split off from PAN. Better understanding of clinical, histopathological, and pathogenetic aspects of MPA has justified its unique and separate identity among the vasculitides. Renal involvement was included in the early descriptions of PAN, and subsequent widespread use of the microscope lead to recognition of small-vessel disease. "Polyarteritis nodosa" was studied extensively in the United Kingdom, where patients were frequently recognized to have glomerular inflammation (2). Further work by the Hammersmith group (3) defined the clinical features of "microscopic polyarteritis" as a syndrome that was recognized by nephrologists as a common, distinct form of small-vessel vasculitis and a major cause of rapidly progressive glomerulonephritis (GN). Other specialties were slower to classify MPA separately from PAN. The proceedings of the Chapel Hill Consensus Conference (CHCC) have led to widespread acceptance of the term "microscopic polyangiitis," which emphasizes small-vessel vasculitis in MPA.

II. DEFINITION

Microscopic polyangiitis is defined as a predominantly small-vessel necrotizing vasculitis with dominant involvement of glomerular and also pulmonary capillaries. However, concurrent arteritis of muscular arteries may occur as well (1). By contrast, PAN is a disease of only medium-sized or small muscular arteries that excludes GN and pulmonary capillaritis.

III. NOMENCLATURE AND DIAGNOSTIC CRITERIA

There are no diagnostic criteria for MPA that have been tested for specificity and sensitivity. The Chapel Hill Nomenclature, perhaps combined with a better understanding of the role of antineutrophil cytoplasmic antibodies (ANCAs) in pathogenesis and diagnosis, may lead to improved criteria for classification of vasculitides.

Microscopic polyangiitis is regarded as one of the "ANCA-associated vasculitides" and ANCA is found in approximately 85% of patients with MPA. In contrast, ANCA is infrequent (0–10%) in PAN (4,5). The ANCA patterns are helpful in distinguishing MPA from WG. Most patients with MPA have antibodies that produce perinuclear ("P") immunofluorescence when applied to ethanol-fixed neutrophils. These P-ANCAs are usually specific for myeloperoxidase (MPO). However, 10–15% of sera in MPA may be C-ANCA–positive with PR3 specificity (5), the most common pattern in WG. Thus, ANCA serology can be useful, but is not sufficiently specific to be the principal determinant of diagnosis.

IV. EPIDEMIOLOGY

A detailed study of all the cases of systemic vasculitis presenting from a stable population in Norfolk, in eastern England, revealed a higher total frequency of vasculitis than expected. The total incidence of all systemic vasculitides was 42 cases per million (6). The 8 cases who met the American College of Rheumatology (ACR) criteria (7) for PAN also satisfied the CHCC definition for MPA (but not for PAN), giving a total annual incidence for MPA of 5.2 per million (8). Recognition of MPA is increasing, in part because of the widespread use of ANCA testing in suspect cases. Thus, the apparent incidence of MPA in Leicester, United Kingdom, increased from 0.5 to 3.3 per million after the introduction of ANCA testing (9). There is a clinical impression that the ANCA-related vasculitides are more common in Northern European Caucasian populations. A survey from Sweden showed a higher than predicted incidence of 16 cases per million population—with MPA being 4 times as frequent as WG (10). Cases have been reported from India and Israel (11,12), and we have seen cases from the tropical north of Australia as well as Malaysia. Ethnic differences have been observed in our own studies. Microscopic polyangiitis was most frequent in whites and was infrequent in blacks or in individuals from the Indian subcontinent. Data from the United States are similar, with MPA reported to be much more common in whites as compared with blacks (14). Additional data are required before the geographical distribution and effects of ethnicity on MPA can be established. A role for MPA being precipitated by infection has been suggested based on seasonal variation in incidence in a Swedish series and the reported association with influenza vaccination (13).

V. CLINICAL FEATURES

A. General

Microscopic polyangiitis affects males more than females (M/F 1.8:1) (3,16), and is more common in older patients (mean age ~50 years). It is a multisystem disease. Systemic features may antedate diagnosis for up to 1 or more years (15). Constitutional features, such as malaise, weight loss, myalgias, and arthralgias, are seen in half to three-quarters of patients at presentation (3,16). Hypertension occurs in approximately 20% of cases. Skin involvement is present in at least two-thirds of patients, frequently manifesting as purpura but also as livedo, nodules, or urticaria (5). Over 60% have neurological involvement, particularly mononeuritis multiplex. Central nervous system (CNS) disease may present as a stroke.

B. Renal

The clinical presentation of MPA renal disease is usually asymptomatic microscopic hematuria and proteinuria (80% of patients). Gross hematuria is uncommon (6% of patients).

The characteristic lesion is a necrotizing crescentic glomerulonephritis. This distinguishes the disease from PAN, but is identical to the lesion seen in WG or renal-limited vasculitis. Half of MPA cases have renal insufficiency at presentation. Over 90% of patients eventually have renal disease, and in most series, no fewer than 30% of patients were oliguric by the time the diagnosis was made (5). In the elderly, rapidly progressive renal failure is frequent. In a French series (5), 10% required long-term dialysis and, overall, one-third died. Renal impairment was a major contribution to mortality. The prognosis was worse in those treated with only corticosteroids, compared with corticosteroids plus cyclophosphamide.

C. Pulmonary

Lung involvement is characteristic of MPA and, in the absence of treatment, carries a poor prognosis. Mortality is greatest in the setting of the pulmonary–renal syndrome (17). This presentation must be distinguished from that seen in WG or in Goodpasture's syndrome. In MPA, the pulmonary lesion is a small-vessel vasculitis, with fibrinoid necrosis of capillaries, leading to alveolar septal disruption, blood filling alveoli, and the clinical sequelae of dyspnea, cough, and/or hemoptysis. The absence of hemoptysis does not exclude lung involvement. On occasion, a surprisingly large intraalveolar hemorrhage can occur, with major falls in circulating hemoglobin levels, without hemoptysis. The chest radiograph shows a typical "bat's wing" alveolar filling pattern. Diffuse pulmonary hemorrhage requires urgent aggressive therapy. The relative risk of death in MPA has been calculated to be 8 times higher in those patients with pulmonary hemorrhage (18).

D. Outcome

It is clear that MPA is a serious disease with a significant risk of either death or end-stage renal failure. This provides the rationale for aggressive therapy, even though the evidence base for this is less satisfying than desirable (19). In those patients who initially respond to therapy, there is an important risk of relapse. Relapse was described in 36% of patients in the series by Savage et al. (3) and in 26% of a recent study by Gordon et al. (20). The relapse rate may be less when care is provided in units that specialize in systemic vasculitis. In spite of this impression, relapse rates of 29, 34, and 46% have recently been described from the United States, France, and Sweden, respectively (21,5,22). This has important implications in regard to long-term surveillance, duration of therapy, and choice of medications for treatment.

E. Renal Biopsy

The characteristic renal histopathology is focal thrombosis of glomerular capillaries with fibrinoid necrosis of a segment of the glomerular tuft (23). This is accompanied by rupture of the glomerular basement membrane and adjacent extracapillary proliferation. Between 15 and 20% of biopsies show extensive extracapillary proliferation (crescent formation). Healed glomerular lesions are characterized by sharply defined segmental scars in which disrupted glomerular capillary loops can be seen. Glomerular immune deposits of immunoglobulin and complement are sparse. In about

20% of the patients, there is an acute vasculitis affecting arterioles as well as arteries (24). Most biopsies also show a tubulointerstitial infiltrate with lymphocytes and eosinophils, often around affected glomeruli. The severity of renal impairment correlates more closely with the severity of tubular damage than with the extent of glomerular disease.

Electron microscopy of glomeruli, arteries, and arterioles shows that the earliest changes are endothelial swelling and degeneration with focal detachment of the endothelium and subendothelial deposits of fibrin (23). With more advanced lesions, there is more widespread denudation of endothelium with intraluminal fibrin deposits and occasional thrombi. At this stage, polymorphonuclear leukocytes and monocytes are found both in the vessel lumen and within and around the walls.

Immunohistological studies of renal biopsies in both WG and MPA have shown infiltrating monocytes/macrophages and neutrophils within glomeruli and in crescents. CD3- and IL-2R-positive T cells were also identified in crescents, in the periglomerular area, and in the interstitium (23,26). The glomerular endothelium in biopsies from patients with WG and MPA expresses vascular cell adhesion molecule-1 (VCAM-1) (27) which colocalizes with macrophage infiltrates (28). The VCAM-1 expression by the glomerular endothelium may be important in selectively recruiting monocytes/macrophages and T lymphocytes that express VLA-4 (CD49d/CD29). This adhesion molecule may be involved in the genesis of this type of glomerular inflammation.

VI. ASCERTAINMENT OF DISEASE ACTIVITY AND DAMAGE

Detailed assessment of disease status is important in all forms of systemic vasculitis. It is important to distinguish disease activity due to current active inflammation from fixed damage that has resulted from disease. The latter represents the "scars" of disease that conceptually will not heal and will require different types of therapy. Damage includes all scars that have occurred since the onset of disease, including those due to intercurrent events, such as infection and drug toxicity, since these all contribute to the overall perception of disease by the patient. Finally, to get a comprehensive estimate of disease severity from the patient's point of view, it is necessary to determine the patient's functional status. These three factors together, activity, damage, and function, give a global measure of disease severity (29–37). Ideally, assessment would include an estimate of disease cost, both to health providers and to the individual.

Significant damage is detectable in many patients by 6 months. This may involve several systems and is a major contributor to ultimate disease severity and mortality (33). Although acute mortality from MPA and other forms of vasculitis have markedly diminished, 5-year follow-up data emphasize that these remain severe diseases with significant accelerated mortality (34,35).

VII. LABORATORY FEATURES

Acute phase proteins can be useful serial tests to help in the assessment of disease activity. However, these studies are nonspecific, and the values increase due to many different causes of tissue injury or inflammation.

von Willebrand's factor (vWF) is released from activated or damaged endothelium and platelets. von Willebrand's factor is increased in vasculitis. However, the value of serial testing is diminished by the tendency of vWF to remain elevated after clinical measures of disease activity have improved.

Antineutrophil cytoplasmic antibody serology has been used by many investigators to follow disease activity. Its use as a guide to treatment decision making is controversial. Data from clinics that follow this approach have shown that ANCA titers (by enzyme-linked immunosorbent assay, ELISA) are usually elevated at the time of disease flare or relapse (40). However, in an individual patient, the elevation may occur well before or immediately after other evidence of a flare, limiting its value in ascertaining disease activity (41,42). In addition, a minority of patients are persistently ANCA-negative and others may have a persistently elevated ANCA titer despite control of disease activity. Improvements in ANCA assay methodology with standardization of antigens may alter these perceptions in the future. Comparison of ANCA with specific clinical parameters may also improve our understanding of these antibodies. For example, it has been suggested that ANCA titers reflect renal disease more accurately than disease activity in other systems. Persistently elevated anti-MPO titers have been associated with development of chronic renal failure and thus may be a predictor of poor outcome (43).

VIII. MANAGEMENT

A. General Approach

In an aggressive disease such as MPA, it is important to start therapy for a disease flare as early as possible, to control disease activity, and prevent the early development of organ damage and disability. The initial treatment of active disease is aggressive. However, such powerful therapy is usually not necessary for the duration of illness. Current treatment recommendations have endorsed a phased regimen that utilizes different approaches at different stages of disease. Maximal disease suppression is advocated for the initial active phase of disease, followed by a less aggressive, less toxic regimen once disease activity is controlled. Long-term maintenance therapy should be considered to prevent relapse. If remission is not achieved, a return to a more aggressive regimen is usual. The European Vasculitis Collaboration is currently conducting large-scale controlled trials based on regimens tailored to disease extent and severity (44). Long-term treatment of the individual, rather than the disease label, has become increasingly important now that acute mortality can usually be prevented.

B. Induction Regimens

Cyclophosphamide (CP) remains the standard therapy for disease induction, in both MPA and WG. The risk of death has been estimated to be over 5 times less in CP-treated patients compared with those treated with corticosteroids alone (18). The internationally accepted standard is the daily oral CP regimen described by the National Institutes of Health (NIH) group (45). However, this approach is not used long term, as had been initially proposed. Cyclophosphamide at a dose of at least 2 mg/kg/day is combined with oral prednisolone, starting at 1 mg/kg/day for 1 month before commencing dose reduction. This regimen, with appropriate dose modifications for renal failure, is widely used. Studies over the past 10 years have explored an alternative approach of giving CP as intermittent pulses (46). Our standard pulse regimen, based on its successful use in systemic rheumatoid vasculitis (47), starts with a 2-week pulse interval. This may be important to its use in primary vasculitis (1°SNV) with renal involvement such as MPA and WG, since experiments with a 4-week dose interval have been less successful (48,49). A controlled trial in 1°SNV, including MPA, compared this pulse regimen with the standard oral regimen. There were no significant differences between treatment groups (50). There was a trend to earlier remission, but there were also more late relapses in the pulse group. A similar observation was noted in a recent French study (51).

Various adjuvant therapies are frequently added for severe disease. None of these interventions have been evaluated in controlled studies. Several such studies are in progress. Pulse high-dose methylprednisolone, provided over 3–5 days, carries a high risk of infection in these sick patients. Plasma exchange may be of benefit to those patients who present with dialysis-dependent renal failure (52). Intravenous immunoglobulin (IVIg) has also been frequently used. This may have palliative effects in patients with vasculitis flares complicated by infection (53,54). Some IVIg preparations have a deleterious effect on renal function. This probably relates to their high sucrose content. The utility of IVIg remains controversial.

C. Maintenance Therapy

A principal concern in planning long-term treatment for MPA is knowing when it is safe to switch from CP to less potent and less toxic therapy, to avoid CP long-term toxicity (55). The response to standard oral therapy can require as long as 2 years to achieve complete remission (45). However, marked palliation is achieved much sooner and new disease activity is usually absent well before that time. Most authorities advocate switching to an agent such as azathiaprine (AZA) or methotrexate (MTX) after 3–6 months. Preliminary results from a large European study that employed AZA for maintenance suggest this approach is as safe and effective as 12 months of daily CP therapy.

In MPA, relapse is not uncommon. In addition, AZA, even when employed in low doses (1–2 mg/kg/day), is not devoid of long-term toxicity. A small study has suggested that cyclosporin A can be useful (56), but this drug is nephrotoxic and cannot be generally recommended. Currently there is no ideal nontoxic, effective maintenance therapy for MPA. Studies of agents that block tumor necrosis factor (TNF) are ongoing. Prevention of carriage of microorganisms, useful in WG (57), has not been tried in MPA, nor has methotrexate.

The obvious treatment choice for disease flares is to return to standard induction regimens. The prognosis is often better in relapse and less damage usually accrues (32), perhaps because these patients are often being followed closely and present earlier in a flare. This may make them good candidates for study with alternative newer drugs that are less toxic.

D. New Therapies

Methotrexate and leflunamide, both useful in WG, have not been formally studied in MPA, but may have a role in induction or maintenance regimes (58,59). Mycophenolate is another agent with promise (60). Targeting adhesion molecules to prevent inflammatory cell recruitment or TNF-α blockade to diminish endothelial cell activation are currently under investigation.

IX. SUMMARY

Microscopic polyangiitis has only recently been accepted as a distinct form of systemic vasculitis. Effective empirical therapy has been derived from past experience with other vasculitides, such as WG and PAN. The pathogenesis of MPA is becoming better understood, but the etiology of this disease remains elusive. Disease-specific, effective therapies will emerge as we come to understand the mechanisms of vascular injury in MPA and related disorders.

REFERENCES

1. Jennette JC, Falk RJ, Andrassy K, Bacon PA, Churg J, Gross WL, Hagen EC, Hoffman GS, Hunder GG, Kallenberg CGM, McCluskey RT, Sinico RA, Rees AJ, Vanes LA, Waldherr R, Wiik A. Nomenclature of systemic vasculitides. Proposal of an international consensus conference. Arthritis Rheum 1994; 37:187.

2. Davson J, Ball J, Platt R. The kidney in periarteritis nodosa. Q J Med 1948; 17:175.
3. Savage C, Winearls C, Evans D, Rees A, Lockwood C. Microscopic polyarteritis: presentation, pathology and prognosis. Q J Med 1985; 56:467.
4. Guillevin L, Lhote F, Amouroux J, Gherardi R, Callard P, Casassus P. Antineutrophil cytoplasmic antibodies, abnormal angiograms and pathological findings in polyarteritis nodosa and Churg-Strauss syndrome: Indications for the classification of vasculitides of the polyarteritis nodosa group. Br J Rheum 1996; 35:958.
5. Guillevin L, Durand-Gasselin B, Cevallos R, Gayraud M, Lhote F, Callard P, Amouroux J, Casassus P, Jarousse B. Microscopic polyangiitis. Clinical and laboratory findings in eighty-five patients. Arthritis Rheum 1999; 42:421.
6. Scott DGI, Watts RA. Classification and epidemiology of systemic vasculitis. Br J Rheumatol 1994; 33:897.
7. Lightfoot RW, Michel BA, Bloch DA, Hunder GG, Zvaifler NJ, Mcshane DJ, Arend WP, Calabrese LH, Leavitt RY, Lie JT, Masi AT, Mills JA, Stevens MB, Wallace SL. The American College of Rheumatology 1990 criteria for the classification of polyarteritis nodosa. Arthritis Rheum 1990; 33:1088.
8. Watts RA, Jolliffe VA, Carruthers DM, Lockwood M, Scott DGI. Effect of classification on the incidence of polyarteritis nodosa and microscopic polyangiitis. Arthritis Rheum 1996; 39:1208.
9. Andrews M, Edmunds M, Campbell A, Walls J, Feehally J. Systemic vasculitis in the 1980's: Is there an increasing incidence of Wegeners granulomatosis and microscopic polyarteritis? J R Coll Physicians Lond 1990; 24:284.
10. Tidman M, Olander R, Svalander C, Danielsson D. Patients hospitalized because of small vessel vasculitides with renal involvement in the period 1975–95: Organ involvement, anti-neutrophil cytoplasmic antibodies patterns, seasonal attack rates and fluctuation of annual frequences. J Intern Med 1998; 244:133.
11. Handa R, Aggarwal P, Biswas A, Wig N, Wali JP. Microscopic polyangiitis associated with antiphospholipid syndrome. Rheumatology 1999; 38:478.
12. Gur H, Tchakmakjian L, Eherenfeld M, Sidi Y. Polyarteritis nodosa: A report from Israel. Am J Med Sci 1999; 317:238.
13. Kelsall JT, Chalmers A, Sherlock CH, Tron VA, Kelsall AC. Microscopic polyangiitis after influenza vaccination. J Rheum 1997; 24:1198.
14. Falk RJ, Hogan S, Carey TS, Jennette JC. Clinical course of anti-neutrophil cytoplasmic autoantibody-associated glomerulonephritis and systemic vasculitis Ann Int Med 1990; 113:656.
15. Schleiffer T, Burkhard B, Klooker P, Brass H. Clinical course and symptomatic prediagnostic period of patients with Wegener's granulomatosis and microscopic polyangiitis. Ren Fail 1998; 20:519.
16. Adu D, Howie A, Scott D, Bacon P, McGonigle R, Michael J. Polyarteritis and the kidney. Q J Med 1987; 62:221.
17. Niles JL, Bottinger EP, Saurina GR, Kelly KJ, Pan GL, Collins AB, McCluskey RT. The syndrome of lung hemorrhage and nephritis is usually an ANCA-associated condition. Arch Intern Med 1996; 156:440.
18. Hogan SL, Nachman PH, Wilkman AS, Jennette JC, Falk RJ. Prognostic markers in patients with antineutrophil cytoplasmic autoantibody-associated microscopic polyangiitis and glomerulonephritis. J Am Soc Nephrol 1996; 7:23.
19. Jindal KK. Management of idiopathic crescentic and diffuse proliferative glomerulonephritis: Evidence-based recommendations. Kidney Int 1999; 55:33.
20. Gordon M, Luqmani RA, Adu D, Greaves I, Richards N, Michael J, Emery P, Howie AJ, Bacon PA. Relapses in patients with a systemic vasculitis. Q J Med 1993; 86:779.
21. Nachman PH, Hogan SL, Jennette JC, Falk RJ. Treatment response and relapse in antineutrophil cytoplasmic autoantibody-associated microscopic polyangiitis and glomerulonephritis. J Am Soc Nephrol 1996; 7:33.
22. Westman KWA, Bygren PG, Olsson H, Ranstam J, Wieslander J. Relapse rate, renal survival, and cancer morbidity in patient with Wegener's granulomatosis or microscopic polyangiitis with renal involvement. J Am Soc Nephrol 1998; 9:842.
23. D'Agati V, Chander P, Nash M, Mancilla-Jimnez R. Idiopathic microscopic polyarteritis nodosa: Ultrastructural observations on the renal vascular and glomerular lesions. Am J Kidney Dis 1986; 7:95.

24. Adu D, Howie AJ. Vasculitis in the kidney. Curr Diag Pathol 1995; 2:73.

25. Adu D, Howie AJ, Scott DGI, Bacon PA, McGonigle RJS, Michael J. Polyarteritis and the kidney. Q J Med 1987; 62:221.

26. Noronha IL, Kruger C, Andrassy K, Ritz E, Waldherr R. In situ production of TNF-α, IL-1β and IL-2R in ANCA positive glomerulonephritis. Kidney Int 1993; 43:682.

27. Pall AA, Howie AJ, Adu D, et al. Glomerular vascular cell adhesion molecule-1 expression in renal vasculitis J Clin Pathol 1996; 49:238.

28. Rastaldi MP, Ferrario F, Tunesi S, Yang L, D'Amico G. Intraglomerular and interstitial leukocyte infiltration, adhesion molecules, and interleukin-1a expression in 15 cases of anti neutrophil cytoplasmic autoantibody-associated renal vasculitis Am J Kidney Dis 1996; 27:48.

29. Luqmani R, Bacon P, Moots R, Janssen B, Pall A, Emery P. Birmingham Vasculitis Activity Score (BVAS) in systemic necrotising vasculitis. Q J Med 1994; 87:671.

30. Exley A, Bacon P, Luqmani R, Kitas G, Gordon C, Savage C, Adu D. Development and initial validation of the vasculitis damage index (VDI) for the standardized clinical assessment of damage in the systemic vasculitides. Arthritis Rheum 1997; 40:371.

31. Abu-Shakra M, Smythe H, Lewtas J, Badley E, Weber D, Keystone E. Outcome of polyarteritis nodosa and Churg-Strauss syndrome: An analysis of 25 patients. Arthritis Rheum 1994; 37:1798.

32. Exley A, Carruthers D, Luqmani R, Kitas G, Gordon C, Janssen B, Savage C, Bacon P. Damage occurs early in systemic vasculitis and is an index of outcome. Q J Med 1997; 90:391.

33. Exley AR, Bacon PA, Luqmani RA, Kitas GD, Carruthers DM, Moots R. Examination of disease severity in systemic vasculitis from the novel perspective of damage using the vasculitis damage index (VDI) Br J Rheumatol 1998; 37:57.

34. Matteson EL, Gold KN, Bloch DA, Hunder GG. Long-term survival of patients with Wegener's granulomatosis from the American College of Rheumatology Wegener's Granulomatosis Classification Criteria Cohort. Am J Med 1996; 101:129.

35. Anderson G, Coles ET, Crane M, et al,. Wegener's granuloma. A series of 265 British cases seen between 1975 and 1985. A report by a subcommittee of the British Thoracic Society. Q J Med 1992; 83:427.

36. Ware JE, Sherbourne CD. The MOS 36-item short-form health survey (SF-36). 1. Conceptual-framework and item selection. Med Care 1992; 30:473.

37. Raza K, Wilson A, Carruthers DM, Reay C, Amft N, Bacon PA. Impaired SF36 in patients with primary systemic necrotizing vasculitis (1°SNV): Influence of factors besides disease activity and damage. Arthritis Rheum. In press.

38. Reinhold-Keller E, Kekow J, Schnabel A, Schmitt W, Heller M, Beigel A, Duncker G, Gross W. Influence of disease manifestation and antineutrophil cytoplasmic titer on the response to pulse cyclophosphamide therapy in patients with Wegener's granulomatosis. Arthritis Rheum 1994; 37:919.

39. Guillevin L, Lhote F, Gayraud M, Cohen P, Jarousse B, Lortholary O, Thibult N, Casassus P. Prognostic factors in polyarteritis nodosa and Churg-Strauss syndrome: A prospective study in 342 patients. Medicine (Baltimore) 1996; 75:17.

40. Kyndt X, Reumaux D, Bridoux F, Tribout B, Bataille P, Hachulla E, Hatron PY, Duthilleul P, Vanhille P. Serial measurements of antineutrophil cytoplasmic autoantibodies in patients with systemic vasculitis. Am J Med 1999; 106:527.

41. Kallenberg CGM, Brouwer E, Weening JJ, Tervaert JWC. Anti-neutrophil cytoplasmic antibodies: current diagnostic and pathophysiological potential. Kidney Int 1994; 46:1.

42. Jayne DRW, Gaskin G, Pusey CD, Lockwood CM. ANCA and predicting relpase in systemic vasculitis. Q J Med 1995; 88:127.

43. Franssen CFM, Stegeman CA, Oost Kort WW, Kallenberg CGM, Limburg PC, Tiebosch A, DeJong PE, Tervaert JWC. Determinants of renal outcome in anti-myeloperoxidase-associated necrotizing crescentic glomerulonephritis. J Am Soc Nephrol 1998; 9:1915.

44. N Rasmussen. Consensus therapeutic regimens for ANCA-associated systemic vasculitis. The European Community Systemic Vasculitis Study Group. Lancet 1997; 349:1029.

45. Hoffman GS, Kerr GS, Leavitt RY, Hallahan CW, Lebovics RS, Travis WD, Rottem M, Fauci AS. Wegener granulomatosis: An analysis of 158 patients. Ann Intern Med 1992; 116:488.

46. Kitas G, Bacon PA, Luqmani RA. Therapy of other vasculitis syndromes. In van de Putte L, Furst D, van Irel P, Williams J, eds. Therapy of Systemic Rheumatic Disorders. New York: Marcel Dekker, 1997:585.

47. Scott DGI, Bacon PA. Intravenous cyclophosphamide plus methylprednisolone in treatment of systemic rheumatoid vasculitis. Am J Med 1984; 76:377.

48. Hoffman GS, Leavitt RY, Fleisher TA, Minor JR, Fauci AS. Treatment of Wegener's granulomatosis with intermittent high-dose intravenous cyclophosphamide. Am J Med 1990; 89:403.

49. Reinhold-Keller E, Kekow J, Schnabel A. Effectiveness of cyclophosphamide pulse treatment in Wegener's granulomatosis. Adv Exp Med Biol 1993; 336:483.

50. Adu D, Pall A, Luqmani RA, Richards NT, Howie AJ, Emery P, Michael J, Savage COS, Bacon PA. Controlled trial of pulse versus continuous prednisolone and cyclophosphamide in the treatment of systemic vasculitis. Q J Med 1997; 90:401.

51. Guillevin L, Cordier JF, Lhote F, Cohen P, Jarrousse B, Royer I, Lesavre P, Jacquot C, Bindi P, Bielefeld P, Desson JF, Detree F, Dubois A, Hachulla E, Hoen B, Jacomy D, Seigneuric C, Lauque D, Stern M, Longy-Boursier M. A prospective, multi-center, randomized trial comparing steroids and pulse cyclophosphamide versus steroids and oral cyclophosphamide in the treatment of generalized Wegener's granulomatosis. Arthritis Rheum 1997; 40:2187.

52. Pusey CD, Rees AJ, Evans DJ, Peters DK, Lockwood CM. Plasma exchange in focal necrotizing glomerulonephritis without anti-GBM antibodies. Kidney Int 1991; 40:757.

53. Jayne DRW, Black CM, Davies M, Fox C, Lockwood CM. Treatment of systemic vasculitis with pooled intravenous immunoglobulin. Lancet 1991; 337:1137–1139.

54. Richter C, Schnabel A, Csernok E, de Groot K, Reinhold-Keller E, Gross WL. Treatment of anti-neutrophil cytoplasmic antibody ANCA)-associated systemic vasculitis with high-dose intravenous immunoglobulin. Clin Exp Immunol 1995; 101:2–7.

55. Talar-Williams C, Hijazi YM, Walther MM et al. Cyclophosphamide-induced cystitis and bladder cancer in patients with Wegener granulomatosis. Ann Intern Med 1996; 124:477.

56. Haubitz M, Koch KM, Brunkhorst R. Cyclosporin for the prevention of disease reactivation in relapsing ANCA-associated vasculitis. Nephrol Dial Transplant 1998; 13:2074.

57. Stegman CA, Tervaert JWC, Sluiter WJ, Manson WL, deJong PE, Kallenberg CGM. Association of chronic nasal carriage of *Staphylococcus aureus* and higher relapse rates in Wegener granulomatosis. Ann Intern Med 1994; 120:12.

58. Sneller MC, Hoffman GS, Talar-Williams C, Kerr GS, Hallahan CW, Fauci AS. An analysis of forty-two Wegener's granulomatosis patients treated with methotrexate and prednisolone. Arthritis Rheum 1995; 38:608.

59. Metzler C, Reinhold-Keller E, Schmitt W, Gross WL. Maintenance of remission with leflunomide in 11 patients with Wegener's granulomatosis. Arthritis Rheum 1997; 40:808.

60. Nowack R, Birck R, VanderWoude FJ. Mycophenolate mofetil for systemic vasculitis and IgA nephrology. Lancet 1997; 349:774.

25
Wegener's Granulomatosis: Pathogenesis

Paul Cockwell
Queen Elizabeth Hospital, Birmingham, England

Caroline O.S. Savage
University of Birmingham Medical School, Birmingham, England

I. INTRODUCTION

Wegener's granulomatosis (WG) is one of three similar disorders, with microscopic polyangiitis (MPA) and Churg–Strauss syndrome, among the primary small-vessel vasculitides (1). WG is characterized histologically by granulomatous inflammation and vasculitis of the upper and lower respiratory tract and systemic vasculitis with a predilection for the kidneys and lungs. Wegener's granulomatosis usually begins with limited organ involvement (of the upper respiratory tract) that progresses to systemic disease (generalized WG). Autoantibodies with specificity against the neutrophil cytoplasmic granule enzyme proteinase 3 (PR3-ANCA) are present in virtually all patients with generalized WG and together with presence of circulating T cells which proliferate in vitro, when exposed to PR3, indicate an autoimmune-based pathogenesis. The etiology of WG remains unknown, but in the past 15 years, many processes that may sustain and amplify the disease have been identified.

II. HISTOPATHOLOGY

Histological, immunohistochemical, and molecular analysis of diseased tissue has provided a basis for our understanding of the pathogenesis of WG. Most studies have focused on renal biopsy tissue; analyses of head, neck, and lung biopsy material are limited to histological studies only.

A. Upper Respiratory Tract

The upper respiratory tract is usually the first site of clinical disease in most patients (2). There are no immunohistochemical or molecular data from studies on the upper respiratory tract to permit comparison of cell infiltrates and immune mediators in limited disease with affected sites in generalized WG.

In the largest histological study, the definitive features of WG were only present in the minority of biopsies from the head and neck (3). Vasculitis, necrosis, and granulomatous inflammation were found in 26, 33, and 42%, respectively, of all biopsy specimens. The changes associated with these findings included microabscesses and scattered giant cells. Neutrophils, eosinophils, and mononuclear cells (including lymphocytes) were all present. These results are at variance with a recent study of nasal biopsies from 11 patients with WG, where leukocytoclastic capillaritis and granulomas were identified in 73 and 100% of biopsies, respectively (4), although similar profiles of infiltrating cells were identified.

B. Lung

The typical lung findings are necrotizing vasculitis and focal granulomatous inflammation. The vasculitis can affect both capillaries and medium-sized vessels. Other patterns of lung involvement may include brochiolitis obliterans–organizing pneumonia (BOOP)-type fibrosis (5), alveolar hemorrhage secondary to pulmonary capillaritis (6), and interstitial fibrosis (7). No clinical features distinguish these variants and they are probably secondary manifestations of the primary disease. Ultrastructural studies on pulmonary vasculitis provided conceptual impetus for understanding the pathogenesis of WG. The presence of lysed leukocytes and extruded nuclei within capillaries in the lungs was noted by Donald et al. in 1976 (8) and led to the prescient suggestion that cytophilic circulating antibodies were responsible for this finding.

C. Kidney

Wegener's granulomatosis causes a focal, segmental, thrombotic, and necrotizing glomerulonephritis that progresses to a crescentic glomerulonephritis (GN) with periglomerular and focal interstitial inflammatory infiltrates. This is the classical lesion of vasculitic GN (9). In the early stages, thrombosis may be present within intact glomerular capillary loops at sites where glomerular mesangial and/or endocapillary hypercellularity and extravascular leukocyte accumulation are absent. Indeed, the first identifiable changes affect the vascular endothelium itself, with swelling, necrosis, and loss of adherence (10,11), suggesting that these cells are targets for initial injury. By immunohistochemistry there is absence of immunoglobulin at these sites of active disease (12). Data on the kinetics of cytokine expression and leukocyte infiltration are reviewed below.

Renal WG is usually impossible to differentiate from MPA, although arteritis is more common in MPA and glomerular necrosis and sclerosis more common in WG (13). The presence of "granulomas" within the kidney is controversial and these lesions may be whole inflamed glomeruli, although giant cells are present at extracapillary, glomerular, and periglomerular sites (11). Acute tubular damage is common in vasculitic glomerulonephritis and interstitial infiltrates of inflammatory cells are usually present. These may accumulate secondary to downstream ischemia, proteinuria, glomerular produced proinflammatory cytokines, and/or vasculitis of the peritubular capillary network.

III. HUMORAL AUTOIMMUNITY

A. Antineutrophil Cytoplasmic Autoantibodies

There is an established association between autoantibodies against the neutrophil cytoplasmic enzyme proteinase 3 (PR3-ANCAs) and WG (14,15). There is a positive correlation between ANCA titres and disease activity, while disease relapse is often (albeit not always) preceded by a rise in ANCA titre (16–18). These observations have led to in vitro studies that indicate a role for ANCAs in the pathogenesis of WG.

The ANCAs are a potent tool in diagnosis and in the laboratory, but the absence of circulating ANCAs in half of the cases with early disease suggest they are a consequence rather than a cause of the initial inflammation. Molecular mimicry, denaturation or breakdown of PR3 may render it antigenic; subsequent production of ANCAs may then be involved in triggering systemic disease with its emphasis on vascular inflammation (Fig. 1). If interactions between ANCAs and small numbers of neutrophils are sufficient to initiate microvascular lesions, absence of ANCAs at these sites may not be surprising. This would also explain the clinical and histological parallels with MPA.

B. Neutrophil and Monocyte Activation by Anti-PR3 ANCAs

In vitro PR3-ANCA (and MPO-ANCA) activates tumor necrosis factor-α (TNF-α)–primed neutrophils to degranulate and produce reactive oxygen species (19). Priming of neutrophils is required to translocate the antigens to the cell surface where they are accessible for ANCAs. The ANCA antigen is ligated by the $F(ab')_2$ component of the immunoglobulin G (IgG) molecule, which then triggers neutrophil activation by binding to Fc_γ receptors and activating downstream signaling pathways (20). Some studies have suggested that human $F(ab')_2$ may be sufficient to activate neutrophils; however, in one study, presence of contaminating monocytes may have allowed ANCA-sensitized monocytes to cross-stimulate neutrophils (21), while in another study, mouse monoclonal $F(ab')_2$ fragments were ineffective although the intact monoclonal antibody and human $F(ab')_2$ fragments stimulated a neutrophil respiratory burst, suggesting inconsistencies in the response (22). Increased relative amounts of the IgG3 subclass of ANCAs may be present in active WG and relate to an increased capacity to induce the respiratory burst through a higher affinity for $F\gamma RII$ receptors than other IgG isotypes (23).

However, other studies have found that ANCA is predominantly of the IgG1 and IgG4 subclasses (24). An important route for the effect of ANCAs may be through arachidonic acid dependent 5'-lipoxygenase pathway–induced production of leukotriene B4, a neutrophil chemoattractant, which also causes autocrine production of reactive oxygen intermediates and degranulation (25). Involvement of the protein kinase $\beta2$ isoform has also been identified (26). In addition, ANCAs may ligate antigens as they become expressed on the surface of neutrophils undergoing apoptosis (27). Phagocytosis of such ANCA-opsonized neutrophils by tissue macrophages may elicit release of macrophage-derived proinflammatory molecules, further enhancing tissue damage.

Ligation of neutrophils within the microvasculature by ANCAs may trigger damage of vascular endothelium (Fig. 2). Within the glomerulus in WG, the majority of neutrophils are activated (28) and retained within capillary loops adjacent to endothelium (29). Enhanced F-actin polymerization and reduced neutrophil deformability may promote neutrophil stasis within vessels (30). In vitro ANCA promotes the adhesion of neutrophils to endothelial cells (ECs) (31) and the production of proinflammatory cytokines (32), and activates primed neutrophils to lyse cultured ECs (33).

Proteinase 3-ANCA can stimulate production of interleukin-8 (IL-8) and monocyte chemoattractant protein-1 (MCP-1) from monocytes (34,35). These chemokines attract neutrophils and mononuclear cells, respectively, to inflammatory sites. Anti-PR3-ANCA–induced monocyte IL-8 release can be inhibited by up to 80% by α_1-proteinase inhibitor (α_1-PI), which is a physiological inhibitor of PR3. Recent evidence that ANCAs stimulate neutrophil IL-8 production and that the released IL-8 inhibits local neutrophil-transendothelial migration suggests a role for frustrated neutrophil trafficking in the pathogenesis of WG (29). This and other mechanisms, including F-actin polymerization and increased rigidity, may operate to localize neutrophils within the microvasculature where, in an activated form, they may cause bystander damage to ECs.

Other mechanisms of EC injury in WG may include charge mediated–binding of PR3 to ECs. Ligation by ANCAs may then trigger damage through antibody-dependent cellular cytotoxicity (ADCC) (36). Proteinase 3 may be expressed by ECs with cell surface translocation in response to TNF-α (37) where ANCA ligation and ADCC may then occur (38). Recently PR3-

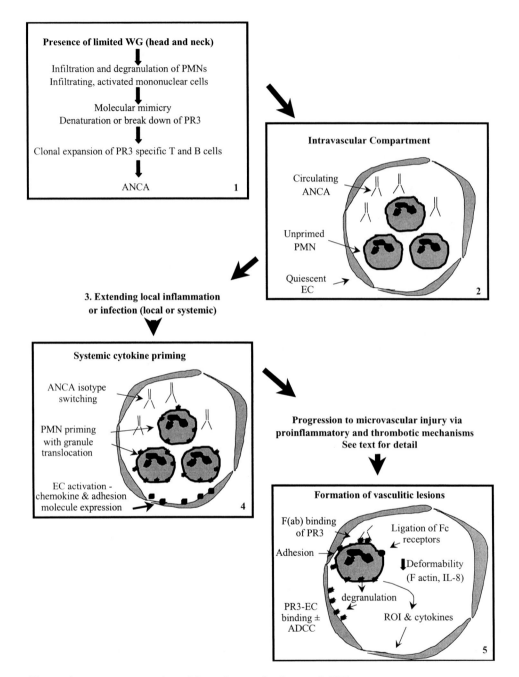

Figure 1   Schematic overview of the pathogenesis of systemic WG.

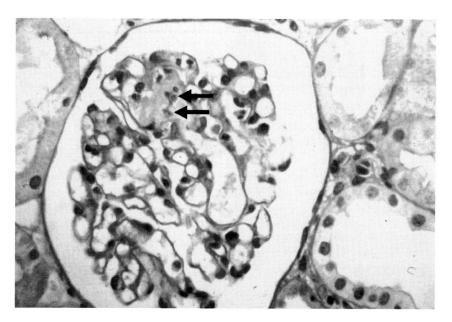

Figure 2   The earliest visible changes by light microscopy of ANCA-associated glomerulonephritis: capillary loop thrombosis with intravascular neutrophils (arrowed). Original magnification ×400.

ANCA has been shown to induce preformed phosphoinositide hydrolysis–related signal transduction pathways in human ECs and lead to dose-dependent increases in transendothelial protein leak (39). Three other laboratories, however, have independently failed to demonstrate PR3 expression by ECs (40,41).

C.   Antigenic Targets of Anti–PR3-ANCA

Proteinase 3-ANCA may bind to a number of antigenic epitopes, some close to the active site of the enzyme. Peptides of several linear PR3 regions identified as contributing to PR3 antigenic epitopes inhibit the binding of IgG PR3-ANCA (42). Previous studies, however, had indicated that ANCA recognized conformational rather than linear epitopes on PR3 (43). Circulating PR3-ANCA may noncompetitively inhibit the esterolytic and proteolytic effects of PR3 (44), although these interactions have not been confirmed (45). This inhibition may occur through binding to α_1-PI sites (46). In addition, other studies show that ANCA from patients with WG specifically interfered with the binding of α_1-PI and enhanced PR3 proteolytic activity. An anti-idiotypic antibody (5/7 Id), found in 50% of sera from patients with WG (47) inhibits PR3-ANCA-antigen–binding activity in vitro, although there is no correlation between prevalence of 5/7 Id expression and disease activity or organ manifestations.

D.   Antiendothelial Cell Antibodies

Endothelial cell damage in WG may be mediated by antibodies to the cells themselves (AECAs) (48). Del Papa et al. (49) identified the presence of AECAs in 28 out of 62 patients with primary small-vessel vasculitis (49). The AECAs may be directed against determinants constitutively expressed on the EC surface and cytotoxic to ECs in the presence of peripheral blood mononuclear cells. IgG AECA from patients with WG can upregulate adhesion molecule, cytokine, and chemokine production (50,51). This is achieved by release of at least two AECA-induced soluble mediators from ECs, one of which is IL-1; this behaves in an autocrine and paracrine fashion to upregulate E-selectin, VCAM-1 and ICAM-1 (51,52).

IV. INFLAMMATORY MEDIATORS

A number of inflammatory mediators have been studied in WG, both circulating and in situ (within the kidney). Expression of these mediators is not specific for WG, and also occurs in MPA and other systemic autoimmune diseases. They do, however, show the role of endothelial activation and leukocyte- and tissue-produced cytokines in sustaining and amplifying tissue injury.

A. Circulating Cytokines and Adhesion Molecules

Increased levels of circulating cytokines, such as TNF-α (53), IL-1β, IL-6, and interferon-γ (IFN-γ) (54,55), elevated levels of soluble adhesion molecules (56), and markers of EC damage and activation of the coagulation cascade (57) indicate systemic immune activation with endothelium involvement. The β1 isoform of transforming growth factor (TGF) is overexpressed in WG and correlates with disease activity (58). Transforming growth factor-β1 is a potent translocation factor for PR3 and, like TNF-α, increases PR3 membrane expression on primed neutrophils by up to 51%. Proteinase 3 activates latent TGF-β, indicating a role for autocrine and paracrine proinflammatory mechanisms.

B. Cytokine, Chemokine, and Adhesion Molecule Expression In Situ

Tumor necrosis factor-α–, IL-1β–, and/or IL-2R–positive cells are present in renal biopsies from patients with WG and MPA (59). By in situ hybridization there is increased TNF-α mRNA and IL-1β mRNA in infiltrating mononuclear cells, epithelial cells of Bowman's capsule and some tubules. Local production of these cytokines may prime ECs in vitro and upregulate local expression of chemokines and adhesion molecules. The presence and pattern of distribution of IL-1β has been confirmed by others (60,61).

Leukocytes circulate to inflammatory sites by a series of molecular interactions coordinated by chemokines and adhesion molecules, expressed by resident cells, including ECs, and by infiltrating cells (62,63). A number of studies have shown the presence of chemokines specific for neutrophils (29) and mononuclear cell subsets (64,65) in renal biopsies from patients with WG. The adhesion molecules necessary for successful trafficking are also present (61,66), and functional assays indicate that T cells adhere to renal biopsy material from patients with WG (67).

V. INFILTRATING LEUKOCYTES AND CELL-MEDIATED IMMUNITY

The accumulation of circulating leukocytes at extravascular sites is a prominent feature of vasculitic glomerulonephritis (Fig. 3). Careful analysis of human biopsy material and information from animal models of GN demonstrate that lesions often evolve from being neutrophil- to

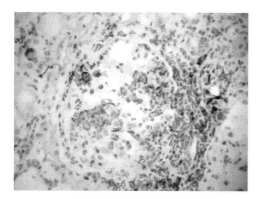

Figure 3 Heavy infiltration of macrophages (by anti-CD68) within the glomerulus in ANCA associated glomerulonephritis. Original magnification ×400.

mononuclear cell–rich, reflecting changing expression over time of endothelial-expressed surface and secreted recruitment molecules.

A. Neutrophils

Neutrophils are the first tissue-infiltrating leukocytes at inflammatory sites. They cause tissue damage (68,69) and recruit further waves of neutrophils and mononuclear cells (70). In patients with severe WG, Brouwer et al. (28) identified 7.4 ± 6.4 neutrophils per glomerular cross section. A high proportion of these cells, as measured by their ability to produce hydrogen peroxide (H_2O_2), were activated. In another study, the majority of neutrophils within the glomerulus were localized within capillary loops (29).

B. Mononuclear Cells

Macrophages and T cells are the major infiltrating cell types in established lesions. Many accumulate within Bowman's space, where together with proliferating parietal epithelial cells, they constitute crescents. Macrophages themselves may also proliferate within the glomerulus or Bowman's space, driven by G-CSF (71). The natural history of a glomerular crescent is variable. It can either progress to fibrosis and scarring or resolve (72). One marker of crescent progression to fibrosis is disruption of Bowman's capsule (73). Many of the T cells present are activated, as shown by expression of IL-2R– (74) and HLA-DR–positivity (75,76). Their presence suggests a role for cell-mediated immunity. Indeed, Cunningham et al. (77) have recently shown the presence of T cells, the majority of which are memory cells, together with macrophages and endothelial derived tissue factor (TF) in patients with ANCA-associated glomerulonephritis. Tissue factor has an important role in augmenting delayed-type hypersensitivity responses and is produced by both macrophages and endothelial cells within the inflamed glomerulus. Unlike other studies that show a greater number of CD4+ than CD8+ cells, there were equal numbers of both. In animal models, crescentic glomerulonephritis can be induced by T cells sensitized to an antigen planted in the glomerulus (78). The in vitro evidence for antigen-specific T-cell proliferation in WG is reviewed below.

Mononuclear cells also accumulate in the tubulointerstitium in large numbers (61). The tubulointerstitium has a central role in disease progression in immune and inflammatory glomerulonephritis (66). In most renal diseases, damage to the tubulointerstitium is regarded as the best marker of likely progression to end-stage renal failure.

C. Platelets

Platelets have a role in the initiation of thrombosis within the glomerulus. Scanning electron microscopy studies have shown the presence of platelets in interlobular vessels in vasculitic lesions of patients with early WG. These lesions were associated with intimal disruption (79). Recently, evidence that platelets can be involved at the initiation of an inflammatory process has been supported by data from Henn et al. (80). They showed that platelets rapidly express CD40 ligand on stimulation, which induces endothelium to secrete the chemokines IL-8 and MCP-1 and the adhesion molecules E-selectin, ICAM-1, and VCAM-1. These studies should encourage further work on the role of platelets in inflammation in WG.

VI.   ANTIGEN-SPECIFIC T-CELL PROLIFERATION

In vitro T-cells from WG patients proliferate to PR3. In 1995, Ballieux et al. (81) demonstrated increased proliferative responses of human T cells to purified PR3 and to azurophil granules of neutrophils, although the statistical analysis of these data has been criticized (82). In 1996, Griffiths et al. (83) showed that T cells from patients with PR3-ANCA and MPO-ANCA proliferated in response to PR3 and MPO, respectively, and recently King et al. (84) showed significant proliferative responses to both heat-inactivated and native PR3 preparations, as well as to -granules, by T cells isolated from patients with WG. Responses to PR3 peptides were detected in one patient.

T cells with highly restricted T-cell receptor (TCR) V gene usage may directly mediate autoimmune diseases. Expanded and diminished populations of T cells using TCR $V\alpha$ or $V\beta$ gene products are present in patients with WG indicating exposure of patients to antigens with the ability to stimulate and eliminate specific subsets of T cells (85). These T-cell expansions occurred more frequently in the CD4+ subset, the predominant population of tissue-infiltrating T cells in most studies on WG. Further support for a T-cell-driven process is provided by isotype switching of IgG antibodies in relapse and remission (86). A recent analysis of IgM autoantibodies to PR3 from clonal lymphoblastoid cell lines derived from B cells from patients with WG showed evidence of somatic mutations indicative of a selective maturation process, providing evidence for generation of antibodies by an antigen-driven process (87).

VII.   Th RESPONSES

Th1 cells and their inflammatory cytokines, IFN-γ and TNF-α, may have a critical role in the development of autoimmune disease. Th2 cytokines, such as IL-4, may have a protective effect (88). Identification of a specific Th response in WG may direct development of novel immunotherapies to skew the Th response.

Evidence is now accumulating for a Th1 response in systemic WG. CD4+ HLADR+ cells from patients with active WG exhibit 10-fold increased secretion of the Th1 cytokine IFN-γ when stimulated by anti-CD2/anti-CD28 compared with stimulated cells from normal controls, but not of the Th2 cytokines IL-4, IL-5, and IL-10 (89). Monocytes from patients with WG also exhibit increased production of IL-12, the major inducer of IFN-γ. The Th2 cytokine IL-10 has a dose-dependent blocking effect on IFN-γ production by peripheral blood mononuclear cells from patients with active WG.

In T-cell clones generated from nasal biopsy specimens and brochoalveolar lavage (BAL) fluid from patients with generalized WG, Th1 cytokine profiles predominate (90). Both polyclonal CD4+ and CD8+ T cells from peripheral blood and BAL fluid produce Th1 cytokines. This pattern of cytokine production may be promoted by activation-induced upregulation of the ligands B7-1 and B7-2 and lack of CD28 expression on T cells from patients with WG (91). CD28 expression promotes the production of Th2 cytokines, and T cells from such patients also show altered CD4+/CD8+ ratios consistent with increased expression of B7 ligands on CD8+ cells.

VIII. THE ENDOTHELIUM

The endothelium has a role in the pathogenesis of WG both as a target for injury and as an active participant in inflammation. Endothelial cell activation can be triggered by proinflammatory cytokines and other products of inflammation, including coagulation proteins and proteolytic enzymes (92). In situ studies have identified evidence for EC activation in WG, particularly through expression of mediators that direct leukocyte trafficking (29,61,64,66), and the evidence for endothelium as a target for disease is reviewed above.

Vascular endothelium from vessels of different sizes and organs shows morphological and functional differentiation (93,94) and this heterogeneity of vascular endothelium may partly explain why the systemic vasculitis of WG affects particular vascular beds. Also, leukocyte extravasation occurs at the level of postcapillary venules in organs such as the skin, but occurs through capillaries in inflamed lung and renal glomeruli where space constraints suggest that leukocyte rolling cannot occur (95) and higher intravascular pressures prevail compared with the postcapillary bed. It may be pertinent that the kidneys, a major site of injury in WG, receive one-fifth of the cardiac output and have two capillary beds arranged in series—the glomerular and peritubular beds.

IX. INFECTIONS

Relapses of disease often follow systemic infections (96), and nasal carriage of *Staphylococcus aureus* is a risk factor for development of relapse (97). Antibiotic treatment reduces the incidence of relapse in WG (98). The mechanism by which infection promotes relapse is unclear although several mechanisms may exist. Infection may promote cytokine production that is responsible for the local and systemic priming of neutrophils and activation of endothelial cells. *S. aureus* may act as a T-cell independent B-cell mitogen to induce autoreactive B-cell ANCA production (99), or microbial superantigens may drive selective T-cell expansion.

X. GENETIC FACTORS

A number of genetic predispositions are possible determinants of disease occurrence and clinical course. The PiZ allele of the (α_1-PI) gene is the predominant genetic variant responsible for subnormal concentrations of α_1-PI (100). The α_1-PI is protective against the effects of proteolytic enzymes released from leukocytes undergoing degranulation. Studies from Sweden and France have shown a high incidence of PiZ heterozygosity in patients with PR3-ANCA–positive vasculitis (101,102). Carriage of the PiZ phenotype may be associated with more generalized vasculitis and the risk of a fatal outcome (103). It is unclear, however, if carriage of the PiZ gene is a risk factor for the occurrence of WG. Allelic differences in FcγRII receptors could account for differences in the magnitude of the oxidative bursts (20), although this has not been substantiated (104).

There are conflicting data on the association of WG with specific HLA antigens. Most studies were performed in a limited number of patients and associations have been described with HLA-B8 (105), -DR2 (106), DR1-DQ1 (107) and -DQ7 antigens (108). In some studies, no association has been demonstrated (109). The largest study of HLA antigens was performed in two centers in the Netherlands (110). This showed a significant decrease in frequency of HLA-DR13 in patients with WG when compared with controls. The authors speculated a protective role for HLA-DR13 against the development of systemic vasculitis, possibly through modulating the response of autoreactive T cells.

XI. ANIMAL MODELS

There are no models of noninfective granulomatous systemic disease with vasculitis that are analogous to WG. There are several other models of ANCA-associated disease, and these have recently been the subject of a detailed review (111). Collectively, they indicate a role for priming by infection (112), ischemia, and reactive oxygen intermediates in triggering disease (113,114). One model proposed as specific for WG is based on the generation, in mice, of antiidiotype and anti-antiidiotype antibodies following injection with affinity-purified human anti-PR3 IgG (115). These animals develop sterile pulmonary microabscesses and die between 8 and 15 months after immunization. Although antibodies from these animals induce adhesion of human neutrophils and trigger a respiratory burst, it has not been demonstrated that they recognize mouse PR3 (116).

XII. CONCLUSIONS

There is no clear evidence for the cause of WG, although many speculate that the disease may be triggered by infection in genetically susceptible individuals. The evolution from limited disease to a systemic process is of particular interest; interactions of ANCA with neutrophils may be central to this process but evidence for a role at disease onset is limited. Recent work increasingly demonstrates cell-mediated immune processes and this area will remain a focus of intense interest.

REFERENCES

1. Jennette JC, Falk RJ, Andrassy K, Bacon PA, Churg J, Gross WL, Hagen EC, Hoffman GS, Hunder GG, Kallenberg CGM, McCluskey RT, Sinico RA, Rees AJ, van Es LA, Waldheer R, Wiik A. Nomenclature of systemic vasculitides. Proposal of an international consensus conference. Arthritis Rheum 1994; 37:187–192.
2. Fauci A, Wolff S. Wegener's granulomatosis. Medicine (Baltimore) 1973; 52:535–561.
3. Devaney K, Travis W, Hoffman G, Leavitt R, Lebovics R, Fauci A. Interpretation of head and neck biopsies in Wegener's granulomatosis. Am J Surg Pathol 1990; 14:555–564.
4. Matsubara O, Yoshimura N, Doi Y, Tamura A, Mark E. Nasal biopsy in the early diagnosis of Wegener's (pathergic) granulomatosis. Virchows Arch 1996; 428:13–19.
5. Uner A, Rozum-Slota B, Katzenstein A-L. Bronchiolitis obliterans-organizing pnuemonia (BOOP)-like variant of Wegener's granulomatosis. Am J Surg Pathol 1996; 20:794–801.

6. Mark E, Ramirez J. Pulmonary capillaritis and hemorrhage in patients with systemic vasculitis. Arch Pathol Lab Med 1985; 109:413–418.

7. Nada A, Torres V, Ryu J, Lie J, Holley K. Pulmonary fibrosis as an unusual clinical manifestation of a pulmonary-renal vasculitis in elderly patients. Mayo Clin Proc 1990; 65:1197–1198.

8. Donald KJ, Edwards RL, McEvoy JDS. An ultrastructural study of the pathogenesis of tissue injury in limited Wegener's granulomatosis. Pathology 1976; 8:161–169.

9. Adu D, Howie AJ. Vasculitis and the kidney. Curr Diag Pathol 1995; 2:73–77.

10. Weiss MA, Crissman JD. Renal biopsy findings in Wegener's granulomatosis: Segmental necrotizing glomerulonephritis with glomerular thrombosis. Hum Pathol 1984; 15:943–956.

11. Antonyvych A, Sabnis SG, Tuur SM, Sesterhenn IA, Balow JE. Morphological differences between polyarteritis and Wegener's granulomatosis using light, electrical and immunohistochemical techniques. Mod Pathol 1989; 2:349–359.

12. Ronco P, Verroust P, Mignon F, Kourilsky O, Vanhille P, Meyrier A, Mery J, Morel-Maroger L. Immunopathological studies of polyarteritis nodosa and Wegeners granulomatosis: A record of 43 patients with 51 biopsies. Quart J Med 1983; 10:141–148.

13. Franssen C, Gans R, Arends B, Hageluken C, ter Wee P, Gerlag P, Hoorntje S. Differences between anti-myeloperoxidase and anti-proteinase 3-associated renal disease. Kidney Int 1995; 47:193–199.

14. van der Woude FJ, Rasmussen N, Lobatto S, Wiik A, Permin H, van Es LA, van der Giessen M, van der Hem GK, The TH. Autoantibodies against neutrophils and monocytes: Tool for diagnosis and marker of disease activity in Wegener's granulomatosis. Lancet 1985; i:425–429.

15. Savage COS, Winearls CG, Jones S, Marshall PD, Lockwood CM. Prospective study of radioimmunoassay for antibodies against neutrophil cytoplasm in diagnosis of systemic vasculitis. Lancet 1987; i:1389–1393.

16. Cohen Tervaert JW, van der Woude FJ, Fauci AS, Ambrus JL, Velosa J, Keane WF, Meijer S, van der Giessen M, The TH, van der Hem GK, Kallenberg CGM. Association between active Wegener's granulomatosis and anticytoplasmic antibodies. Arch Intern Med 1989; 149:2461–2465.

17. Cohen Tervaert JW, Huitema MG, Hene RJ, Sluiter WJ, The TH, van der Hem GK, Kallenberg CGM. Prevention of relapses in Wegener's granulomatosis by treatment based on antineutrophil cytoplasmic antibody titre. Lancet 1990; 336:709–711.

18. Egner W, Chapel HM. Titration of antibodies against neutrophil cytoplasmic antigens is useful in monitoring disease activity in systemic vasculitis. Clin Exp Immunol 1990; 82:244–249.

19. Falk RJ, Terrell RS, Charles LA, Jennette JC. Anti-neutrophil cytoplasmic autoantibodies induce neutrophils to degranulate and produce oxygen radicals in vitro. Proc Natl Acad Sci USA 1990; 87:4115–4119.

20. Porges AJ, Redecha PB, Kimberly WT, Csernok E, Gross WL, Kimberly RP. Anti-neutrophil cytoplasmic antibodies engage and activate human neutrophils via $Fc\gamma RIIa$. J Immunol 1994; 153:1271–1280.

21. Keogan MT, Esnault VLM, Green AJ, Lockwood CM, Brown DL. Activation of normal neutrophils by anti-neutrophil cytoplasm antibodies. Clin Exp Immunol 1992; 90:228–234.

22. Kettritz R, Jennette J, Falk R. Crosslinking of ANCA-antigens stimulates superoxide release by human neutrophils. J Am Soc Nephrol 1996; 8:386–394.

23. Mulder AHL, Heeringa C, Brouwer E, Limburg PC, Kallenberg CGM. Activation of granulocytes by anti-neutrophil cytoplasmic antibodies (ANCA): a $Fc\gamma RII$-dependent process. Clin Exp Immunol 1994; 98:270–278.

24. Segelmark M, Wieslander J. IgG subclasses of antineutrophil cytoplasm antibodies (ANCA). Nephrol Dial Transplant 1993; 8:696–702.

25. Grimminger F, Hattar K, Papavassiliis C, Temmesfield B, Csernok E, Gross W, Seeger W, Sibelius U. Nuetrophil activation by anti-proteinase 3 antibodies in Wegener's granulomatosis: Role of exogenous arachidonic acid and leukotriene B4 generation. J Exp Med 1996; 184:1567–1572.

26. Radford D, Lord J, Savage C. Investigation of the signalling pathways involved in the activation of neutrophils by ANCA. J Am Soc Nephrol 1998; 9:429A.

27. Gilligan H, Bredy B, Brady H, Hebert M-J, Slayter H, Xu Y, Rauch J, Shia M, Akoh J, Levine J. Antineutrophil cytoplasmic autoantibodies interact with primary granule constituents on the surface of apoptotic neutrophils in the absence of neutrophil priming. J Exp Med 1996; 184:2231–2241.

28. Brouwer E, Huitema MG, Mulder AHL, Heeringa P, Van Goor H, Cohen Tervaert JW, Weening JJ, Kallenburg CGM. Neutrophil activation in vitro and in vivo in Wegener's granulomatosis. Kidney Int 1994; 45:1120–31.

29. Cockwell P, Brooks C, Adu D, Savage COS. Interleukin 8: A pathogenetic role in antineutrophil cytoplasmic autoantibody-associated glomerulonephritis. Kidney Int 1999; 55:852–863.

30. Tse W, Nash G, Savage C, Adu D. ANCA decreases neutrophil deformability through actin polymerization. Implications for microvascular injury. J Am Soc Nephrol 1998; 9:488A.

31. Keogan MT, Rifkin I, Lockwood CM, Brown DL. Anti-neutrophil cytoplasm antibodies increase neutrophil adhesion to cultured human endothelium. Adv Exp Med Biol 1993; 336:115–119.

32. Brooks CJ, King WJ, Radford D, Adu D, McGrath M, Savage COS. IL-1β production by human polymorphonuclear leucocytes stimulated by anti-neutrophil cytoplasmic autoantibodies: Relevance to systemic vasculitis. Clin Exp Immunol 1996; 106:273–279.

33. Savage COS, Pottinger BE, Gaskin G, Pusey CD, Pearson JD. Autoantibodies developing to myeloperoxidase and proteinase 3 in systemic vasculitis stimulate neutrophil cytotoxicity towards cultured endothelial cells. Am J Pathol 1992; 141:335–342.

34. Ralston D, Marsh C, Lowe M, Wewers M. Antineutrophil cytoplasmic antibodies induce monocyte IL-8 release. Role of surface proteinase 3, α1-antitrypsin and Fcγ receptors. J Clin Invest 1997; 100:1416–1424.

35. Casselman BL, Kilgore KS, Miller BF, Warren JS. Antibodies to neutrophil cytoplasmic antigens induce monocyte chemoattractant protein-1 secretion from human monocytes. J Lab Clin Med 1995; 126:495–502.

36. Savage COS, Gaskin G, Pusey CD, Pearson JD. Anti-neutrophil cytoplasm antibodies (ANCA) can recognize vascular endothelial cell-bound ANCA-associated autoantigens. J Exp Nephrol 1993; 1:190–195.

37. Mayet WJ, Csernok E, Szymkowiak C, Gross WL, Meyer zum Buschenfelde KH. Human endothelial cells express proteinase-3, the target of anticytoplasmic antibodies in Wegener's granulomatosis. Blood 1993; 82:1221–1229.

38. Mayet WJ, Schwarting A, Meyer zum Buschenfelde KH. Cytotoxic effects of antibodies to proteinase 3 (c-ANCA) on human endothelial cells. Clin Exp Immunol 1994; 97:458–65.

39. Sibelius U, Hatta K, Schenkel A, Noll T, Csernok E, Gross W, Mayet W-J, Piper H-M, Seeger W, Grimminger F. Wegener's granulomatosis: Anti proteinase 3 antibodies are potent inductors of human endothelial signalling and leakage response. J Exp Med 1998; 187:597–503.

40. King WJ, Adu D, Daha MR, Brooks CJ, Radford DJ, Pall AA, Savage COS. Endothelial cells do not express the Wegener's autoantigen proteinase 3. Clin Exp Immunol 1995; 102:98–105.

41. Prendergraft WF, Yang JJ, Reeves HM, Falk RJ, Preston GA. Endothelial cells do not express proteinase 3 (PR3) and myeloperoxidase (MPO). J Am Soc Nephrol 1997; 8:543A.

42. Williams Jr R, Staud R, Malone C, Payabyab J, Byres L, Underwood D. Epitopes on proteinase-3 recognized by antibodies from patients with Wegener's granulomatosis. J Immunol 1994; 152:4722–4737.

43. Bini P, Gabay JE, Teitel A, Melchior M, Zhou J, Elkon KB. Antineutrophil cytoplasmic autoantibodies in Wegener's granulomatosis recognize conformational epitope(s) on proteinase 3. J Immunol 1992; 149:1409–1415.

44. Daouk G, Palsson R, Arnaout M. Inhibition of proteinase 3 by ANCA and its correlation with disease activity in Wegener's granulomatosis. Kidney Int 1995; 47:1528–1536.

45. Baslund B, Szpirt W, Eriksson S, Elzouki A-N, Wiik A, Wieslander J, Petersen J. Complexes between proteinase 3, a$_1$ antitrypsin and proteinase 3 anti-neutrophil cytoplasm autoantibodies: a comparison between a$_1$-antitrypsin PiZ allele carriers and non-carriers with Wegener's granulomatosis. Eur J Clin Invest 1996; 26:786–792.

46. van der Wiel BA, Dolman KM, Hack CE, von dem Borne AEGK, Goldschmeding R. Interference of Wegener's granulomatosis autoantibodies with the regulation of neutrophil proteinase 3. In: Gross WL, ed. ANCA Associated Vasculitis. London: Plenum, 1993.

47. Strunz H, Csernok E, Gross W. Incidence and disease associations of a proteinase 3-antineutrophil

cytoplasmic antibody idiotype (5/7 Id) whose antiidiotype inhibits proteinase 3-antineutrophil cytoplasmic antibody antigen binding activity. Arthritis Rheum 1997; 40:135–142.

48. Savage COS, Pottinger B, Gaskin G, Lockwood CM, Pusey CD, Pearson J. Vascular damage in Wegener's granulomatosis and microscopic polyarteritis: presence of anti-endothelial cell antibodies and their relation to anti-neutrophil cytoplasm antibodies. Clin Exp Immunol 1991; 85:14–19.

49. Del Papa N, Meroni PL, Barcellini W, Sinico A, Radice A, Tincani A, D'Cruz D, Nicoletti F, Borghi MO, Khamashta MA, Hughes GRV, Balestrieri G. Antibodies to endothelial cells im primary vasculitides mediate in vitro endothelial cytotoxicity in the presence of normal peripheral blood mononuclear cells. Clin Immunol Immunopathol 1992; 63:267–274.

50. Del Papa N, Guidali L, Sironi M, Schoenfeld Y, Mantovani A, Tincani A, Balestrieri G, Radice A, Sinico R, Meroni PL. Anti-endothelial cell IgG antibodies from patients with Wegener's granulomatosis bind to human endothelial cells in vitro and induce adhesion molecule and cytokine expression. Arthritis Rheum 1996; 39:758–766.

51. Carvalho D, Savage C, Isenberg D, Pearson J. IgG antiendothelial cell autoantibodies from patients with systemic lupus erythematosus stimulate the release of two endothelial cell-derived mediators which enhance adhesion molecule expression and leukocyte adhesion in an autocrine fashion. Arthritis Rheum 1999; 42:631–640.

52. Carvalho D, Savage C, Black C, Pearson JD. IgG antiendothelial cell autoantibodies from scleroderma patients induce leukocyte adhesion to human vascular endothelial cells in vitro. J Clin Invest 1996; 97:111–119.

53. Deguchi Y, Shibata N, Kishimoto S. Enhanced expression of the tumor necrosis factor/cachectin gene in peripheral blood mononuclear cells from patients with systemic vasculitis. Clin Exp Immunol 1990; 81:311–314.

54. Grau GE, Roux-Lombard P, Gysler C, Lambert C, Lambert PH, Dayer JM, Guillevan L. Serum cytokine changes in systemic vasculitis. Immunology 1989; 68:196–198.

55. Kekow J, Szymkowiak CH, Gross WL. Involvement of cytokines in granuloma formation within primary systemic vasculitis. In: Romagni S, ed. Cytokines: Basic Principles and Clinical Applications. New York: Raven, 1992:342–348.

56. Pall AA, Adu D, Drayson M, Richards NT, Michael J. Circulating soluble adhesion molecules in systemic vasculitis. Nephrol Dial Transplant 1994; 9:770–774.

57. Hergessel O, Andrassy K, Nawroth P, Gabat S. Endothelial dysfunction and activation of haemostasis (anticardiolipin antibodies, thrombin-antithrombin complexes (TAT), prothrombin fragments (F1+2), D-Dimers) as markers of disease activity in patients with systemic necrotizing vasculitis. Thromb Haemost 1993; 69:953.

58. Csernok E, Szymkowiak C, Mistry N, Daha M, Gross W, Kekow J. Transforming growth factor-beta (TGF-β) expression and interaction with proteinase 3 (PR3) in anti-neutrophil cytoplasmic antibody (ANCA)-associated vasculitis. Clin Exp Immunol 1996; 105:104–111.

59. Noronha IL, Kruger C, Andrassy K, Ritz E, Waldherr R. In situ production of TNF-α, IL-1β and IL-2R in ANCA-positive glomerulonephritis. Kidney Int 1993; 43:682–692.

60. Jenkins DAS, Wojtacha DR, Swan P, Fleming S, Cumming AD. Intrarenal localization of interleukin-1β mRNA in crescentic glomerulonephritis. Nephrol Dial Transplant 1994; 9:1228–1233.

61. Rastaldi MP, Ferrario F, Tunesi S, Yang L, D'Amico G. Intraglomerular and interstitial leukocyte infiltration, adhesion molecules, and interleukin-1α expression in 15 cases of anti-neutrophil cytoplasmic autoantibody-associated renal vasculitis. Am J Kidney Dis 1996; 27:48–57.

62. Springer TA. Traffic signals on endothelium for lymphocyte recirculation and leukocyte emigration. Annu Rev Physiol 1995; 57:827–872.

63. Cockwell P, Savage C. Chemokines and their receptors in leukocyte trafficking and renal inflammation. Nephrol Dial Transplant 1997; 12:1307–1310.

64. Cockwell P, Howie AJ, Adu D, Savage COS. in situ analysis of CC chemokine mRNA in human glomerulonephritis. Kidney Int 1998; 54:827–836.

65. Rovin BH, Rumancik M, Tan L, Dickerson J. Glomerular expression of monocyte chemoattractant protein-1 in experimental and human glomerulonephritis. Lab Invest 1994; 71:536–542.

66. Roy-Chaudhury P, Wu B, King G, Campbell M, Macleod AM, Haites NE, Simpson JG, Power DA. Adhesion molecule interactions in human glomerulonephritis: Importance of the tubulointerstitium. Kidney Int 1996; 49:127–134.

67. Chakravorty SJ, Howie AJ, Cockwell P, Adu D, Savage COS. T cell lymphocyte adhesion mechanisms within the inflamed kidney. Am J Pathol 1999; 154:503–514.

68. Johnson RJ, Couser WG, Chi EY, Adler S, Klebanoff SJ. New mechanism for glomerular injury. Myeloperoxidase-hydrogen peroxide-halide system. J Clin Invest 1987; 79:1379–1387.

69. Couser WG. Pathogenesis of glomerulonephritis. Kidney Int 1993; 44:S19–S26.

70. Cassatella MA. The production of cytokines by polymorphonuclear neutrophils. Immunol Today 1995; 16:21–26.

71. Yang N, Isbel N, Nikolic-Paterson D, Li Y, Ye R, Atkins R. Local macrophage proliferation in human glomerulonephritis. Kidney Int 1998; 54:143–151.

72. Downer G, Phan SH, Wiggins RC. Analysis of renal fibrosis in a rabbit model of crescentic nephritis. J Clin Invest 1988; 1988:998–1006.

73. Silva FG, Hoyer JR, Pirani CL. Sequential studies of glomerular crescent formation in rats with antiglomerular basement membrane-induced glomerulonephritis and the role of coagulation factors. Lab Invest 1984; 51:404–415.

74. Li HL, Hancock WW, Dowling JP, Atkins RP. Activated (IL-2R+) intraglomerular mononuclear cells in crescentic glomerulonephritis. Kidney Int 1991; 39:793–798.

75. Bolton WK, Innes DJ, Sturgill BC, Kaiser DL. T-cells and macrophages in rapidly progressive glomerulonephritis: Clinicopathologic correlations. Kidney Int 1987; 32:869–876.

76. Nolasco FEB, Cameron JS, Hartley B, Coelho A, Hildreth G, Reuben R. Intraglomerular T cells and monocytes in nephritis: Study with monoclonal antibodies. Kidney Int 1987; 31:1160–1166.

77. Cunningham M, Huang X, Dowling J, Tipping P, Holdsworth S. Prominence of cell-mediated immunity effectors in "pauci-immune" glomerulonephritis. J Am Soc Nephrol 1999; 10:499–506.

78. Rennke H, Klein P, Sandstrom D, Mendrick D. Cell-mediated immne injury in the kidney: Acute nephritis induced in the rat by azobenzenearsonate. Kidney Int 1994; 45:1044–1056.

79. Novak RF, Christiansen RG, Sorensen ET. The acute vasculitis of Wegener's granulomatosis in renal biopsies. Am J Pathol 1982; 78:367–371.

80. Henn V, Slupsky JR, Grafe M, Anagnostopolous I, Forster R, Muller-Berghaus G, Kroczek RA. CD40 ligand on activated platelets triggers an inflammatory reaction of endothelial cells. Nature 1998; 391:591–594.

81. Ballieux BEPB, Van der Burg SH, Hagen EC, Van der Woude FJ, Melief CJM, Daha MR. Cell-mediated autoimmunity in patients with Wegener's granulomatosis (WG). Clin Exp Immunol 1995; 100:186–193.

82. Mathieson PW, Oliviera DBG. The role of cellular immunity in systemic vasculitis. Clin Exp Immunol 1995; 100:183–185.

83. Griffiths M, Coulthart A, Pusey C. T cell responses to myeloperoxidase and proteinase 3 in patients with systemic vasculitis. Clin Exp Immunol 1996; 102.

84. King WJ, Brooks CJ, Holder R, Hughes P, Adu D, Savage COS. T lymphocyte responses to anti-neutrophil cytoplasmic autoantibody are present in patients with ANCA-associated systemic vasculitis and persist during disease remission. Clin Exp Immunol 1998; 112:539–546.

85. Giscombe R, Grunewald J, Nityanand S, Lefvert A. T cell receptor (TCR) V gene usage in patients with systemic necrotizing vasculitis. Clin Exp Immunol 1995; 101:213–219.

86. Jayne DRW, Weetman AP, Lockwood CM. IgG subclass distribution of autoantibodies to neutrophil cytoplasmic antigens in systemic vasculitis. Clin Exp Immunol 1991; 84:476–481.

87. Sibilia J, Benlagha K, Ronco P, Vanhille P, Brouet J-C, Mariette X. Structural analysis of human antibodies to proteinase 3 from patients with Wegener granulomatosis. J Immunol 1997; 159:712–719.

88. Sacca R, Cuff CA, Ruddle NH. Mediators of inflammation. Curr Opin Cell Biol 1997; 9:851–857.

89. Ludviksonn B, Sneller M, Chua K, Talar-Williams C, Langford C, Ehrhardt R, et al. Active Wegener's granulomatosis is associated with HLA-DR+ CD4+ T-cells exhibiting an unbalanced Th1-type T cell cytokine pattern. J Immunol 1998; 160:3602–3609.

90. Csernok E, Trabandt A, Muller A, Wang G, Moosig F, Paulsen J, Schnabel A, Gross W. Cytokine pro-

files in Wegener's granulomatosis. Predominance of Type 1 (Th1) in the granulomatous inflammation. Arthritis Rheum 1999; 42:742–750.

91. Moosig F, Csernok E, Wang G, Gross W. Costimulatory molecules in Wegener's granulomatosis (WG): Lack of expression of CD28 and preferential up-regulation of its ligands B7-1 (CD80) and B7-2 (CD86) on T cells. Clin Exp Immunol 1998; 114:113–118.

92. Cockwell P, Tse WY, Savage COS. Activation of endothelial cells in thrombosis and vasculitis. Scand J Rheumatol 1997; 26:145–150.

93. Steinhoff G, Behrend M, Schrader B, Duijvestijn AM, Wonigeit K. Expression patterns of leukocyte adhesion ligand molecules on human liver endothelia. Am J Path 1993; 142:481–488.

94. Fleming S, Jones DB. Antigenic heterogeneity of renal endothelium. J Pathol 1989; 158:319–323.

95. Downey GP, Worthen GS, Henson PM, Hyde D. Neutrophil sequestration and migration in localized pulmonary inflammation. Am Rev Respir Dis 1993; 147:168–176.

96. Pinching AJ, Rees AJ, Pussell BA, Lockwood CM, Mitchison RS, Peters DK. Relapses in Wegener's granulomatosis: The role of infection. Br Med J 1980; 281:836–838.

97. Stegeman CA, Cohen Tervaert JW, Sluiter W, Manson W, De Jong P, Kallenberg CGM. Association of chronic nasal carriage of *Staphylococcus aureus* and higher relapse rates in Wegener's granulomatosis. Ann Intern Med 1992; 113:12–17.

98. Stegeman CA, Cohen Tervaert JW, De Jong P, Kallenberg CGM. Trimethoprim (Co-trimoxazole) for the prevention of relapses of Wegener's granulomatosis. N Engl J Med 1996; 335:16–20.

99. Fleischer B, Schrezenmeier H. T cell stimulation by *Staphylococcal* enterotoxins. J Exp Med 1988; 167:1697–1707.

100. Crystal R. α_1-antitrypsin deficiency deficiency, emphysema and liver disease: Genetic basis and startegies for therapy. J Clin Invest 1990; 85:1343–1352.

101. Elzouki A-N, Segelmark M, Wieslander J, Eriksonn S. Strong link between the alpha-1-antitrypsin PiZ allele and Wegener's granulomatosis. J Intern Med 1994; 236:543–548.

102. Esnault VLM, Testa A, Audrain M, Roge C, Barner JH, Sesboue R, Martin JP, Lesavre P. Alpha 1 anti-trypsin genetic polymorphism in ANCA-positive systemic vasculitis. Kidney Int 1993; 43:1329–1332.

103. Segelmak M, Elzouki A, Weislander J, Eriksson S. The PiZ gene of α_1-antitrypsin as a determinant of outcome in Pr3-ANCA-positive vasculitis. Kidney Int 1995; 48:844–850.

104. Tse WY, Abadeh S, McTiernan A, Jefferis R, Savage COS, Adu D. No association between neutrophil FCγRIIa allelic polymorphism and antineutrophil cytoplasmic antibody (ANCA)-positive systemic vasculitis. Clin Exp Immunol 1999; 117:198–205.

105. Katz P, Alling DW, Haynes BF, Fauci AS. Association of Wegener's granulomatosis with HLA-B8. Clin Immunol Immunopathol 1979; 14:268–270.

106. Elkon KB, Sutherland DC, Rees AJ, Hughes GRV, Batchelor JR. HLA frequencies in systemic vasculitis. Increase in HLA-DR2 in Wegener's granulomatosis. Arth Rheum 1983; 26:102–105.

107. Papiha S, Murty G, Ad Hia A, Mains B, Venning M. Association of Wegener's granulomatosis with HLA antigens and other genetic markers. Ann Rheum Dis 1992; 51:246–248.

108. Spencer SJW, Burns A, Gaskin G, Pusey CD, Rees AJ. HLA class II specificities and the development and duration of vasculitis with antibodies to neutrophil cytoplasmic antigens. Kidney Int 1992; 41:1059–1063.

109. Zhang L, Jayne D, Zhao M, Lockwood C, Oliveira D. Distribution of MHC class II alleles in primary systemic vasculitis. Kidney Int 1995; 47:294–298.

110. Hagen E, Stegeman C, D'Amaro J, Schreuder G, Lems S, Cohen Tervaert J, De Jong G, Hene R, Kallenberg C, Daha M, Van der Woude F. Decreased frequency orf HLA-DR13DR6 in Wegener's granulomatosis. Kidney Int 1995; 48:801–805.

111. Heeringa P, Brouwer E, Cohen Tervaert J, Weening J, Kallenberg C. Animal models of anti-neutrophil cytoplasmic autoantibody associated vasculitis. Kidney Int 1998; 53:253–263.

112. Mathieson P, Thiru S, Oliviera D. Mercuric chloride treated Brown Norway rats develop widespread tissue injury including necrotizing vasculitis. Lab Invest 1992; 67:121–129.

113. Brouwer E, Huitema MG, Klok PA, de Weerd H, Cohen Tervaert W, Weening JJ, Kallenberg CGM. Antimyeloperoxidase-associated proliferative glomerulonephritis: An animal model. J Exp Med 1993; 177:905–914.

114. Brouwer E, Klok P, Huitema M, Weening J, Kallenberg C. Renal ischemia/reperfusion injury con-
      tributes to renal damage in experimental anti-myeloperoxidase-associated proliferative glomeru-
      lonephritis. Kidney Int 1995; 47:1121–1129.
115. Blank M, Tomer Y, Stein M, Kopolovic J, Wiik A, Meroni P, Conforti G, Schonfeld Y. Immunization
      with anti-neutrophil cytoplasmic antibody (ANCA) induces the production of mouse ANCA and
      perivascular lymphocyte infiltration. Clin Exp Immunol 1995; 102:120–130.
116. Tomer Y, Gilburd B, Blank M, Lider O, Hershkovic R, Fishman P, Zigelman R, Meroni P, A, Schoen-
      feld Y. Characterisation of biologically active antineutrophil cytoplasmic antibodies induced in mice.
      Arth Rheum 1995; 38:1375–1381.

26
Wegener's Granulomatosis: Clinical Aspects

Gary S. Hoffman
Cleveland Clinic Foundation, Cleveland, Ohio

Wolfgang L. Gross
University of Lubeck, Bad Bramstedt, Germany

I. EPIDEMIOLOGY AND SOCIOECONOMIC IMPACT

Wegener's granulomatosis (WG) affects at least 1 in 30,000 people in the United States (1). A retrospective review of hospitalizations in a Norwegian community suggested that prevalence in that country may be as great as 1 in 20,000 (2). The great majority of patients are adults, although individuals of all age groups can be affected. Most large studies do not reveal significant gender differences (3–5). Although WG is recognized predominantly in Caucasians, it also occurs in persons of all other ethnic and racial backgrounds. African-American patients are relatively underrepresented, comprising less than 8% of patients in the United States, while contributing 11% of the general population.

Limited information is available about the geographical distribution of WG. In one survey that assessed cases per regional address (zip) codes in New York State, it was apparent that the prevalence of disease was clearly higher (up to 7 per 100,000) in certain counties compared with others where no cases were identified. It is uncertain whether apparent clustering of cases represents common exposure to important disease precipitants (1). Rigorous epidemiological investigations to identify environmental agents that may play a role in causing disease have not been conducted. Predominant involvement of the airways and the presence of neutrophilic alveolitis at disease onset has led to speculation that an inhaled agent may trigger disease expression. A recent case-controlled study compared 101 patients with WG with healthy individuals and other patients with chronic diseases. A standardized interviewer-administered questionnaire was used in an attempt to identify unique environmental exposures, particularly "inhalants," that patients may have noted prior to disease onset. Although striking differences were not apparent among people with WG, healthy controls, and diseases other than WG, there were statistically significant differences in regard to WG patients having a greater degree of exposure to fumes, insecticides, and particulate airborne matter (6). Others have suggested that inhalation of silica and grain particles may increase the risk of developing WG (7–9). Speculation about respiratory infections being a trigger for WG has been advanced since 1931 (10–13). A very provocative observation in this regard has been made in patients with established WG, who have nasal carriage of *Staphylococcus aureus*. These individuals had a sixfold increase in disease relapse, compared with patients in whom chronic nasal carriage of *S. aureus* did not occur (14). The authors have made an argument for *S. aureus* playing a role in relapse, but not in causing initial disease expression. Whether infections or noninfectious environmental exposures are significant in initiation or perpetuation of WG is uncertain. At least as important is the possibility of there being unique abnormalities of host responses to exogenous factors.

Reports of mortality in WG have varied considerably, in part because of differences in study methods, particularly inclusion criteria and treatment. In the United States, a national and New York State survey noted that hospitalization for WG was associated with a 10–11% mortality (1). In a similar survey from the United Kingdom, 50% mortality was noted over a 12-year follow-up period (5). In studies where care is provided by specialty units, uniquely devoted to serving patients with vasculitis, mortality from disease or treatment has been reported to be as low as 12–13% over mean or median follow-up periods of 7–8 years (3,15). As might be expected, patients who are elderly (greater than 50–60 years) tend to be less resilient in coping with both disease and treatment. Mortality tends to be higher in this group then among younger individuals. The most common cause of death has become secondary infection (15,16).

Although once considered a disease with almost certain short-term mortality, treatment has converted WG into a chronic illness, for which there is now recognized significant morbidity, both from illness and from treatment. Consequently, assessment of disease impact should not be restricted to only analyses of mortality. A survey of patients who have had disease for a median of 5 years noted that approximately 80% required continued immunosuppressive therapy for maintenance of disease control or remission, 80% had to modify normal activities of daily living, and 50% who were employed at the time of diagnosis needed to modify their job requirements or accept total disability (31%). Within 1 year of diagnosis, patients suffered a 26% reduction in income as a result of these changes. Extrapolation of the costs of hospitalization and the impact of partial or complete disability suggested that the financial impact of WG in the United States considerably exceeded $30 million per year. These figures from the United States do not take into account the cost of outpatient care or the impact of deaths, which occur in approximately 10% of patients who are hospitalized for WG nationwide (17).

II. CLINICAL FEATURES

WG can mimic many other disorders—clinically, radiographically, and pathologically. The diagnosis is highly likely if patients present with typical features of disease affecting the upper respiratory tract, lungs, and kidneys, have a biopsy with distinctive histopathological features, and their sera contain antineutrophil cytoplasmic antibodies (ANCAs). However, many patients do not have classical features at disease onset. Early manifestations may be diagnosed as sinusitis due to allergy or infection, pneumonia, lung cancer or other malignancies, rheumatoid and other forms of arthritis, or idiopathic nephritis. In such cases, the diagnostic challenge may be considerable.

Along with the classical clinical-pathological *triad* of *necrotizing inflammation with granulomas* and/or *vasculitis* of the upper and lower respiratory tract, plus *glomerulonephritis,* WG may also involve joints, skin, peripheral nerves, skeletal muscle, heart, brain and eyes (Fig. 1). A strict diagnosis of WG depends on (1) characteristic clinical signs and symptoms, (2) histological demonstration of characteristic features that cannot be attributed to infection, and/or (3) compatible clinical features and the detection in serum of ANCAs (usually "C," cytoplasmic type, and antibody specific for proteinase 3, PR3). The diagnosis should not rely on any one of these variables alone. The yield of finding classical histopathological features of WG varies with the site and size of biopsy. The ANCA sensitivity varies (50–75%) depending on disease severity and distribution of organ involvement, especially in regard to glomerulonephritis, wherein ANCA is usually positive.

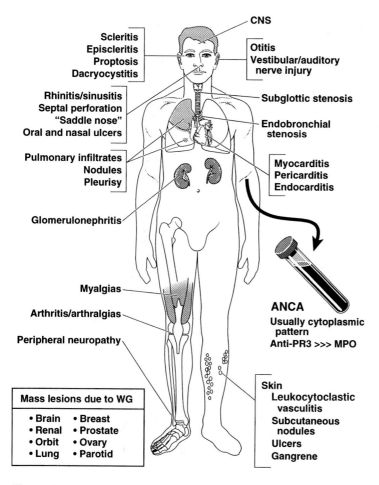

Figure 1   The clinical spectrum of Wegener's granulomatosis.

Upper airway and focal pulmonary features may evolve over several months and even years, only later to be followed by the overt presentation of severe systemic disease, including glomerulonephritis. In cases that evolve slowly or remain localized to the upper airway (approximately 10%), the diagnosis WG may not be made until some time after upper airway presentation, failed therapies with antibiotics, or after a biopsy reveals features that suggest WG.

On the other hand, WG may occasionally present without obvious ear, nose, and throat disease or pulmonary nodular lesions. The first manifestations may be a severe pulmonary–renal syndrome. In this regard, it is important to realize that there are overlapping features shared by WG and microscopic polyangiitis (MPA) (Chapter 24) (e.g. glomerulonephritis, skin vasculitis, pulmonary infiltrates/vasculitis) that may not allow clear distinction of these diseases, unless upper airway disease becomes apparent or a biopsy reveals granuloma.

Nasal and sinus manifestations include obstruction (mucosal swelling), pain, serosanguinous or purulent discharge and epistaxis. Examination may reveal mucosal irregularity ("cobblestone" or "granular" appearance), ulcers, thick crusts, friable mucosa and septal perforation. In many patients, the clinical diagnosis can be confirmed by characteristic findings in a biopsy (18,19). Facial pain due to sinusitis and nasal chondritis with swelling or collapse of the nasal

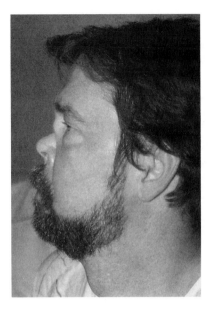

Figure 2 Nasal deformity ("saddlenose") that has resulted from chronic destructive inflammatory changes in Wegener's granulomatosis. This deformity may be mimicked by similar changes that are seen in relapsing polychondritis.

bridge ("saddle nose") may appear early or late in the course of the illness (Fig 2). In the *oral cavity and oropharynx*, gingival involvement can lead to ulcerative stomatitis, hyperplastic gingivitis, or lingual ulcerations.

Laryngeal (subglottic) symptoms such as pain, hoarseness, cough, dyspnea, wheezing, and/or increasing stridor are frequently due to reddish, friable, circumferential narrowing just below the vocal cords. In time, such lesions may become a bland cicatrix.

Otological manifestations include chondritis, serous or suppurative otitis media, mastoiditis, vertigo, and sensorineural deafness (20,21).

Eye disease may be due to nasolacrimal duct inflammation and obstruction, episcleritis, scleritis, retroorbital masses or pseudotumors that cause proptosis, compression of the optic nerve and blindness, or entrapment of extraocular muscles, leading to diploplia (Fig. 3). Less frequently, orbital involvement may result from the spread of purulent bacterial sinusitis. Wegener's granulomatosis may also involve the retinal arteries, leading to profound visual loss or field cuts. (22–24).

Lung involvement includes bronchial stenosis, which may cause atelectasis and/or obstructive pneumonia. Single or multiple pulmonary nodules, with or without cavitation, may be symptomatic or asymptomatic (Fig. 4a) (3,25–27). Pulmonary capillaritis/alveolitis may be associated with diffuse lung hemorrhage and severe respiratory insufficiency. The three most consistent features for recognition of alveolar hemorrhage are hemoptysis, infiltrates on the chest roentgenogram, and anemia. Plain radiographs and computerized axial tomography (CAT) scans typically show an alveolar or mixed alveolar–interstitial pattern (Fig. 4b). A distribution like that in pulmonary edema is most common, but focal and sometimes migratory shadows are also observed.

Nervous system disease can be due to vasculitis, mass-like lesions or extension of lesions from contiguous sites, e.g., ears, nose, and throat (ENT). Lesions that originate in the sinuses and middle ear may spread by direct extension to the retropharyngeal area and base of the skull. This can lead to cranial neuropathy, proptosis, diabetes insipidus, or meningitis (28–30).

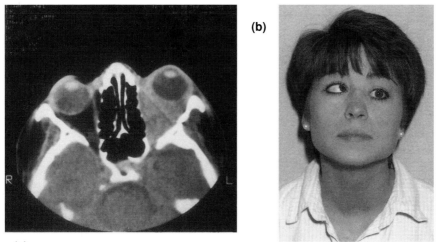

(b)

(a)

Figure 3   (a) CAT scan image of a left retro-orbital pseudotumor that has caused restriction of extra-ocular muscles. When asked to look to the left, the patient (b) is unable to abduct the left eye.

(a)

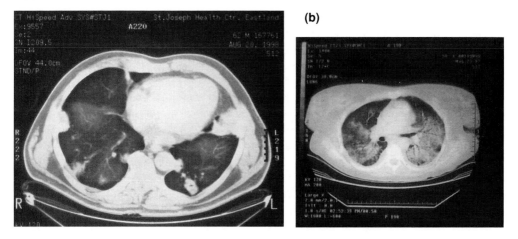

(b)

Figure 4   (a) CAT scan of the lung demonstrates multifocal nodules, including a left posterior lesion with early cavitation. (b) Reveals multifocal areas of diffuse pulmonary infiltrate, which on biopsy revealed pulmonary hemorrhage, capillaritis and necrosis. Among patients who have an established diagnosis of Wegener's and are receiving immunosuppressive therapy, this presentation needs to be distinguished from opportunistic infection or drug-induced pneumonitis, secondary to agents such as methotrexate or cyclophosphamide.

Musculoskeletal features of WG are quite pleomorphic and can be the source of diagnostic consternation. In some series, myalgias and/or arthralgias, frank arthritis and/or myositis represent the second most frequent symptom complex (after ENT-region symptoms) in WG. These rheumatic manifestations may occur in up to two-thirds of patients. In one large series, 28% had nonerosive and nondeforming polyarthritis. Sacroiliitis was found in 3 of 50 and polychondritis in 2 of 50 WG patients. Rheumatoid factor was present in half of the patients tested. In the Lubeck, Germany, cohort of 186 patients, episodes of arthralgia, myalgia, or arthritis occurred as the presenting symptom in two-thirds of cases and over time occurred in three-fourths of all cases. The most common complaint was myalgia (45%), followed by frank arthritis (21%), mainly in the larger joints (monoarthritis, 10%; oligoarthritis, 5%; polyarthritis, 6%). Joint pain can follow a migratory or additive pattern and can be mild or profound and even disabling. When an additive, symmetric pattern occurs, it is frequently misdiagnosed as rheumatoid arthritis. This error is often reinforced by the high frequency of rheumatoid factor in WG. Approximately 90% of patients with rheumatic symptoms have a generalized form of the disease, often associated with overt features of vasculitis (3,31–34).

Skin involvement may occur as palpable purpura due to leukocytoclastic vasculitis. Tender subcutaneous nodules, papules, livedo reticularis, and pyoderma gangrenosum are less common and may rarely be a presenting feature (35,36). All patients who present with any type of cutaneous vasculitis should be evaluated for ENT, pulmonary, renal, and other visceral features of disease.

In many patients who appear to have regional ENT disease, a transition to a more generalized and even fulminant course may be heralded by constitutional symptoms, such as weight loss, fever, and night sweats. Such symptoms may be associated with striking laboratory abnormalities, including markedly elevated erythrocyte sedimentation rate (ESR) and C-reactive protein (CRP), leukocytosis, and thrombocytosis. Life-threatening or critical organ-threatening disease may at first become manifest by widespread palpable purpura, pneumonitis, pulmonary hemorrhage, peripheral neuropathy, or glomerulonephritis. Glomerulonephritis may lead to dialysis dependency within several days to weeks. In fulminant WG, all of these features can occur simultaneously or in rapid sequence. In the absence of rapid diagnosis and immediate immunosuppressive therapy, this disease presentation is immediately life-threatening. Most patients follow a clinical course between the extremes of having a regional disease pattern vs. fulminant generalized disease.

The pulmonary–renal presentation of WG can often be distinguished from other pulmonary–renal syndromes by obtaining information about prior or persistent upper airway involvement. In addition, immunohistochemistry on lung biopsies (e.g., via bronchoscopy) or kidney specimens in WG reveal a few or no immune deposits, thus excluding immune complex–mediated and anti-basement membrane antibody–mediated pulmonary and pulmonary–renal vasculitic syndromes. Most patients with such "pauci-immune" pulmonary–renal vasculitic syndromes have either C-ANCA (Ab usually directed to proteinase 3, i.e., PR3-ANCA) or P-ANCA (Ab usually directed to myeloperoxidase, i.e., MPO-ANCA) (25,27,36–38). It is noteworthy that very similar lesions can be due to another ANCA-associated vasculitis, microscopic polyangiitis (39–42). Microscopic polyangiitis is most often associated with antibodies to MPO. In addition, unlike WG, MPA is *not* characterized by chronic upper airway injury or pulmonary nodules.

III. LABORATORY FINDINGS

Until 1985, no laboratory test existed that was highly specific for WG. Disease activity was evaluated according to the clinical picture and *serological markers of inflammation* (ESR, CRP). In addition, the degree of anemia, leukocytosis, occasional mild to moderate eosinophilia, and thrombocytosis crudely correlated with the disease activity. Wegener's granulomatosis patients with regional ENT abnormalities may have little to no abnormalities of routine laboratory parameters, compared with those with severe systemic illness, who often have profound changes, which might include "leukemoid" reactions.

In contrast to the larger family of systemic autoimmune diseases, patients with WG usually lack (1) antinuclear antibodies (ANAs), (2) evidence for complement consumption, and (3) cryoglobulins. However, rheumatoid factor is present in up to 60% of patients. The most important routine laboratory study in patients with WG is the urinalysis. An abnormal urine may be the first sign of glomerulonephritis, and occurs prior to a rise in serum creatinine.

Antineutrophil cytoplasmic antibodies were first reported in 1982 in patients with glomerulonephritis, who lacked evidence of immune deposits. Subsequent work by a Danish–Dutch collaboration (43) delineated an association between a certain type of ANCA (C-ANCA) with WG. The clinical utility of C-ANCA as a diagnostic marker for WG was recently confirmed in a large prospective European study that utilized sera from vasculitis and control patients (sensitivity 60%, specificity 95%) (44). However, in another prospective single-center study in which ANCA was employed as a routine screening test for WG (defined according to American College of Rheumatology criteria) in patients with unproven, but initially suspected vasculitis, the sensitivity of C-ANCA was only 28% (98% specificity for WG). The sensitivity rose to 83% if the diagnosis of WG was supported by biopsy features that were characteristic of the disease (45). A meta-analysis of 15 studies comprised 13,652 patients, of which 736 had WG. The pooled sensitivity of ANCA for WG was 66% and specificity was 98% (46). Taken together, these data show that the value of ANCA testing is limited by a rather low sensitivity. The greatest utility of ANCA testing may be in patients with suspected WG, in whom the pretest probability of disease is high (47). Proper testing should always include antigen-specific reactivity (e.g., PR3, MP0, or other antigens). Rising titers should alert the clinician to an increased risk of exacerbations. However, flaws in the association of titer change and disease activity have led to recommendations not to utilize ANCA titers alone as an indication to alter therapy (48–50).

IV. HISTOPATHOLOGY AND DIAGNOSIS

For a long time, it was believed that open biopsies of pulmonary lesions were necessary to obtain adequate specimens for histopathological demonstration of WG. However, the majority of WG patients present first with symptoms involving the upper airway. Although all of the characteristic histological features of WG may not be present in the majority of ENT biopsies, important diagnostic information can be found in nasal and sinus specimens, especially when infection and malignancy have been ruled out.

The characteristic pathological features of WG are granuloma formation, with histiocytic epithelioid cells, often including giant cells. Additionally, plasma cells, lymphocytes, neutrophils, and sometimes eosinophils may be present (51). Vessels can be involved in the form of nongranulomatous or granulomatous arteritis, phlebitis, perivasculitis, or giant cell vasculitis (10,52). Fienberg (53) has described pulmonary lesions, in the absence of vasculitis, as an "idiopneumonic pathergic granulomatosis" (54). Micronecrosis, usually with neutrophils (microabscesses), constitutes the early phase in the development of *organized palisading granuloma*. There is then a progression of disease from micronecrosis to macronecrosis (= widespread necrosis), and then to fibrosis (55). Areas of macronecrosis may be surrounded by palisading histiocytes or diffuse granulomatous tissue (Fig 5).

The microscopic findings in the kidneys are also quite varied. Here too, the above-described vascular lesions and disseminated granulomas can be occasionally found. However, much more common is proliferative crescentic focal glomerulitis (56) with necrosis and thrombosis of individual loops or larger segments of the glomerulus. Sometimes almost all glomeruli are destroyed, and this is accompanied by capsular adhesion and proliferation (Fig. 6). In some instances, a diffuse, i.e., extracapillary, mesangioproliferative glomerulonephritis may be observed as well.

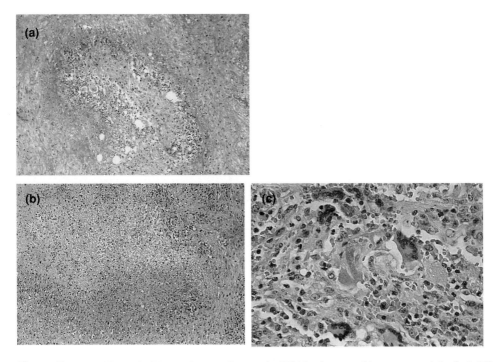

Figure 5   Lung biopsy in Wegener's granulomatosis: Within the same biopsy, one might find different pathological characteristics of disease such as necrotizing vasculitis (a, 100×), geographic necrosis (b, 100×) for which the borders of necrotic tissue appear to have the irregularity of continents or regions on the map and granuloma formation that often includes the presence of giant cells (c, 400× magnification).

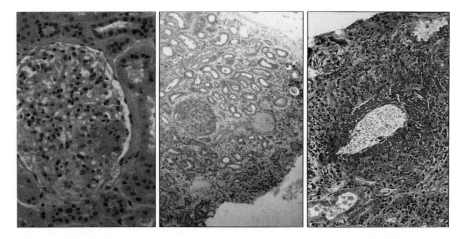

Figure 6   Renal disease in Wegener's granulomatosis: The most common early histopathological lesion is focal segmental glomerulonephritis (a), which when properly treated may not progress to chronic renal impairment. However, when crescentic, necrotic, and sclerotic changes have already occurred (b), restoration of normal renal function even with aggressive treatment is unlikely. Occasionally frank vasculitis (c) of medium-sized intrarenal vessels may be seen as well. (Reproduced with permission of authors and publishers. Hoffman GS. Wegener's granulomatosis. In: Rheumatology, 2nd ed. St. Louis: Mosby.)

V. TREATMENT

Once it has been determined that a patient has WG, treatment can be customized to suit unique clinical circumstances. At one time, it was believed that all patients with WG had immediate life-threatening disease that justified an aggressive approach, generally consisting of high-dose daily corticosteroids plus daily cyclophosphamide. This approach was based upon older literature that had documented 50% mortality at 5-month and 82% mortality at 1-year follow-up in patients who had not received any treatment (57). Median survival time of 12.5 months had been reported among patients treated with only glucocorticoids (58). There is no question that aggressive therapy with prednisone (approximately 1 mg/kg/day) and cyclophosphamide (approximately 2 mg/kg/day) dramatically changed the prognosis, such that in the most encouraging of series, 80–86% survival was observed 7–8 years from the time of diagnosis and treatment (3,15). In addition, in a large National Institutes of Health (NIH) series, 75% of all treated patients achieved complete remission and almost all patients experienced marked improvement (3). However, over the years, we have learned a great deal about the treatment of WG. There are marked variations in presentation, course of illness, and tendency for disease to relapse. There is also profound morbidity that has resulted from having converted WG to a chronic disease that often requires extended treatment with potentially dangerous medications.

The observation that at least 20% of patients may have WG restricted to the upper airway and have a course of illness that is indolent has led to questions about the utility of less aggressive pharmacological treatment. It has been suggested that trimethaprim/sulfamethoxizole might be an effective means of treating mild forms of WG that do not produce serious critical-organ-system involvement, such as pulmonary hemorrhage or glomerulonephritis (59). Anecdotal reports initially appeared to support the notion that such treatment was effective. However, subsequent studies suggested that if such is the case, the frequency with which antibiotic therapy produced remission was low and such treatment should not be considered as the principal means of therapy in patients with serious organ system disease (60,61). Similar conflicting data have been reported in regard to the same antibiotic therapy being effective in reducing the frequency of disease relapses, following induction of remission with more conventional therapy (14,62). At present, the role of antibiotic therapy in treating disease or maintaining remission is uncertain and controversial.

During the late 1980s and early 1990s, increasing numbers of reports were being published supporting the utility of methotrexate (MTX) in mild forms of WG, defined as not including diffuse pulmonary hemorrhage or rapidly progressive glomerulonephritis. Methotrexate had been shown to be immunosuppressive in regard to decreasing B-cell number and function, suppressing neutrophil leukotriene and superoxide production, and impairing chemotaxis and neutrophil adhesion to endothelial cells (63–70). It has subsequently been demonstrated that certain patients who do not have immediately life-threatening disease can be effectively treated with daily corticosteroid and weekly MTX therapy (62,71,72). The best results have been reported when patients received 0.3 mg/kg as an initial dose (not to exceed 15 mg once a week), which was gradually increased to 20 to 25 mg per week, as tolerated. Because MTX is excreted through the kidneys, doses were reduced in the setting of renal impairment and MTX was considered to be contraindicated if serum creatinine exceeded 2.5 mg/dL. The combination of corticosteroids and MTX, provided in this fashion, resulted in 71% of patients achieving remission of disease, and an additional 12% having marked improvement. Unfortunately, approximately 40% of patients experienced relapses at 2-year follow-up, during which time glucocorticoids were tapered and discontinued, and/or MTX was tapered to <15 mg per week. Approximately 5% of patients on this regimen developed MTX-associated pneumonitis. Although there are clear limitations to the utility of MTX, it has emerged as a reasonable alternative to cyclophosphamide in the treatment of patients with milder forms of disease.

Attempts to minimize the toxicity of cyclophosphamide and still retain its striking benefits led to studies of high-dose monthly intravenous cyclophosphamide. The results of such studies have been discordant and controversial. In general, most reports have agreed that high-dose intravenous cyclophosphamide is capable of producing either marked improvement or remission in the great majority of patients in whom it is provided. However, several investigations have demonstrated an unacceptably high relapse rate in the course of tapering corticosteroids and/or decreasing the frequency of cyclophosphamide therapy to less than once monthly (73,74). Others have suggested that both means by which cyclophosphamide may be administered provide comparable results (75,76). Although this area remains one of significant controversy (77), all authors would agree that when WG presents as an immediately life-threatening illness, it is critical to induce remission with the most effective therapy available (cyclophosphamide) and later sustain remission with an effective and safer form of therapy than cyclophosphamide.

This goal has been successfully approached by three different groups who have recently demonstrated that induction of remission with cyclophosphamide (daily therapy) may be effectively followed by converting cyclophosphamide, after several months, to either MTX (62,78) or azathioprine (79). This strategy has led to remission induction and maintenance of remission in over 80% of patients followed for periods of 1 1/2 to 2 years. Additional studies have continued attempts to identify other effective forms of therapy. Mixed results have been reported with adjunctive use of intravenous immunoglobulin (80–83).

Increasing appreciation for the role of mononuclear cells in initiating and perpetuating WG has led to new experimental therapies. Ludviksson et al. (84) have demonstrated that CD4+ T cells and monocytes from patients with active disease express much higher concentrations of T-cell and monocyte activation markers than noted in either patients with WG in remission or normal controls. Different experimental approaches have demonstrated that CD4+ and CD8+ T cells from granulomatous lesions in the nose and from bronchoalveolar lavage express increased quantities of the Th1 cytokine interferon-γ (IFN-γ) (84a). Kobold et al. (85) have also demonstrated close correlation between disease activity and plasma concentrations of interleukin-6 (IL-6) and the unique monocyte activation product, neopterin. It appears that the Th1 lymphocyte pathway is particularly favored during active WG, resulting in increased concentrations of tumor necrosis factor-α (TNF-α) and interferon-γ (Th1 cytokines). The combination of these cytokines and activation of monocytes (producing IL-1, IL-12 and IL-18) are important components to setting the stage for granuloma formation. Th1 cytokines are effective stimuli for neutrophils, leading to their activation, which results in expression of neutrophil cytoplasmic antigens on the cell surface, where they are accessible to ANCA (Fig. 7). These interrelationships suggest that interfering with either monocyte and/or Th1 lymphocyte activation might be palliative in the treatment of WG. Trials of IL-10 (an inhibitor of monocytes) and etanercept (TNF-α receptor-fusion protein) are currently in clinical trials. These are exciting opportunities that may provide more selective, and hopefully less toxic, therapies for patients with WG. A great deal of work will be required before investigators will be able to determine efficacy, as well as the potential consequences of diminishing immune surveillance.

VI. GENERAL PRINCIPLES OF THERAPY

It is obvious that provision of early proven therapy for WG is critically important. However, under the best of circumstances, in the setting of units dedicated to only the treatment of vasculitis, significant permanent morbidity still occurs. In a large series from the National Institutes of Health (3), 86% of patients had clinically important persistent morbidity from the effects of disease and 42% of patients had permanent morbidity that was attributed directly to therapy. Rapidly pro-

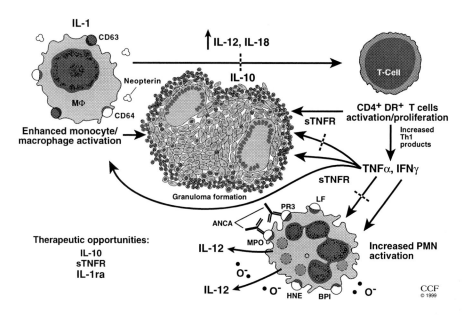

Figure 7   Current concepts about the pathogenesis of Wegener's granulomatosis. Increasing emphasis on the Th1 pathway has led to ongoing treatment trials that focus on Th1 inhibition.

gressive renal failure and dialysis can be avoided when the diagnosis is immediately suspected and appropriate treatment quickly provided. However, in those instances where acute need for dialysis occurs, effective therapy may still result in important recovery of renal function in 22–70% of patients followed for at least 3 years (86–89). Whether plasmapheresis provides additional benefit to the usual therapies provided for WG is uncertain. Two controlled trials have produced opposite results (90–92).

Providing excellent care for patients with WG, who usually have multisystem disease, not only requires internal medicine subspecialists who are familiar with the immunological, rheumatological, renal, and pulmonary complications of the disease, but also surgical colleagues. This is obvious in regard to patients who require lung biopsies, sinus drainage procedures, myringotomy tubes, hearing aids, surgical intervention for subglottic stenosis, ophthalmological care for orbital or retroorbital disease, and renal transplantation.

Also, ENT surgical consultants can be of great benefit in educating patients about the importance of nasal and sinus "hygiene," including irrigation of sinuses with cleansing solutions to minimize crusting and secondary *S. aureus* superinfection. The treatment of subglottic stenosis is particularly difficult in WG. Subglottic stenosis develops in about 23% of patients, of whom approximately one-fourth may require tracheostomy. Until recent years, only modest degrees of palliation were achieved with various means of dilatation. The advent of intralesional injection of long-acting corticosteroids, combined with gentle progressive dilatation has led to marked improvement in outcomes (93).

Engaging the services of a urologist may be extremely important in the care of patients who have been treated with daily cyclophosphamide and have developed hematuria that might not be related to glomerulonephritis. Although daily cyclophosphamide may be life-saving therapy, it is responsible for a 50% frequency of cystitis in patients who have received chronic therapy. In addition, 5% of patients treated in this fashion have been noted to develop transitional cell carcinoma of the bladder at 10-year follow-up and are expected by Kaplan-Meier projections to have a 16% frequency of bladder cancer at 15-year follow-up. Because hematuria appears grossly and microscopically the same whether it be from cystitis or bladder cancer, the distinction between etiologies requires cystoscopic evaluation and biopsy. Dependence on only urine cytology is inadequate. The limited sensitivity for findings of dysplasia (43%) or atypia (29%) in bladder cancer does not allow for a high degree of confidence in ruling out malignancy (94).

Physicians who care for patients with WG should recall the potential enduring mutagenic effects of cytotoxic medications that are currently in use. In addition to causing a marked increase in the risk of bladder cancer (33-fold increase), cyclophosphamide therapy is also known to increase the likelihood of lymphomas (11-fold increase), leukemia, and myelodysplasia (3). The latency period between treatment and manifestations of these abnormalities can be years, even long after cyclophosphamide had been discontinued.

The patient can play an important role in maximizing chances for a good outcome. For those patients who do not have an abnormal urine sediment, it is advised that physicians or nurses teach patients how to dipstick their own urine to detect blood and protein. At the first indication of hematuria, the patient should be instructed to notify their physician. It is then imperative for the physician to examine a fresh urine sediment for evidence of red blood cell casts, which are highly suggestive of new-onset glomerulonephritis. Relapses from renal disease or new-onset renal disease is usually a clinically silent process. Renal relapses may occur in the absence of evidence of disease activity in other organ systems. It is reasonable to ask the patient to routinely dipstick their urine every 2 weeks. Patients and physicians should emphasize the importance of access to the treating physician. It should not be assumed that upper respiratory or pulmonary symptoms are due to the same process that is "going around" the family or the work environment. New onset or worsening of musculoskeletal symptoms should also not be assumed to be "old age arthritis" or poor conditioning.

VII. *PNEUMOCYSTIS CARINII* PNEUMONIA

Unless prophylaxis against *Pneumocystis carinii* pneumonia is provided, 6% of patients treated with aggressive immunosuppressive therapies for vasculitis will develop this life-threatening complication. The high mortality rates of immunocompromised hosts who experience this infection have led to recommendations for *Pneumocystis* prophylaxis in the setting of severe systemic autoimmune disease treated with cytotoxic agents and corticosteroids in doses that are likely to produce sustained lymphopenia (95,96).

VIII. RENAL TRANSPLANTATION

A past history of WG is not a contraindication to renal transplantation. Such therapy should be considered when the potential recipient has experienced sustained remission on little or no immunosuppressive therapy. Although only limited information on renal transplantation in WG is available, the data suggest that prognosis for renal and patient survival is comparable to that in other transplant populations (97–99).

IX. SUMMARY

Medical progress during the past 30 years has dramatically alltered the course of WG. Life-saving, albeit toxic, therapies are better understood and protocols have been modified to reduce the risks of treatment with corticosteroids and alkylating agents. Studies are in progress that explore the utility of biological agents that may have precise immunoregulatory effects, and lack the toxicities of current therapies.

REFERENCES

1. Cotch MF, Hoffman GS, Yerg DE, Kaufman GI, Targonski P, Kaslow RA. The epidemiology of Wegener's granulomatosis. Arthritis Rheum 1996; 39:87–91.
2. Haugeberg G, Bie R, Bendvold A, Larsen AS, Johnsen V. Primary vasculitis in a Norwegian hospital community: A retrospective study. Clin Rheumatol 1998; 17:364–367.
3. Hoffman GS, Kerr GS, Leavitt RY, Hallahan CW, Lebovics RS, Travis WD, Rottem M, Fauci AS. Wegener's granulomatosis: An analysis of 158 patients. Ann Intern Med 1992; 116:488–498.
4. Bajema IM, Hagen EC, van der Woude FJ, Bruijn JA. Wegener's granulomatosis: A meta-analysis of 349 literary case reports. J Lab Clin Med 1997; 129:17–22.
5. Anderson G, Coles ET, Crane M, Douglas AC, Gibbs AR, Geddes DM, Peel ET, Wood JB. Wegener's granulomatosis. A series of 265 British cases seen between 1975 and 1985. A report by a subcommittee of the British Thoracic Society Research Committee. Q J Med 1992; 83:427–438.
6. Duna GF, Cotch MF, Galperin C, Hoffman DB, Hoffman GS. Wegener's granulomatosis: Role of environmental exposures. Clin Exp Rheum 1998; 16:669–674.
7. Gregorini G, Ferioli A, Donato F, Tira P, Morassi L, Tardanico R, Lancini L, Maiorca R. Adv Exp Med Biol 1993; 336:435–440.
8. Nuyts GD, Van Vlem E, De Vos A, Daelcmans RA, Rorive G, Elseviers MM, Schurgers M, Segaert M, D'Haese PC, De Broe ME. Wegener granulomatosis is associated to exposure to silicon compounds: A case-control study. Nephrol Dial Transplant 1995; 10:1162–1165.
9. Cohen Tervaert JW, Stegeman CA, Kallenberg CGM. Silicon exposure and vasculitis. Curr Opin Rheumatol 1998; 10:12–17.
10. Klinger H. Grenzformen der Panarteritis nodosa. Z Path 1931; 42:455.
11. George J, Levy Y, Kallenberg CGM, Shoenfeld Y. Infections and Wegener's granulomatosis: A cause and effect relationship? Q J Med 1997; 90:367–373.
12. Jennette JC, Falk RJ. Antineutrophil cytoplasmic autoantibodies and associated diseases: A review. Am J Kidney Dis 1990; 15:517–529.
13. Raynnauld J-P, Block D, Fries JF. Seasonal variation in onset of Wegener's granulomatosis, polyarteritis nodosa and giant cell arteritis. J Rheumatol 1993; 20:1524–1526.
14. Stegeman CA, Cohen Tervaert JW, De Jong PE, Kallenberg CGM for the Dutch Co-trimoxazole Wegener Study Group. Trimethoprim/sulfamethoxazole (co-trimoxazole) for the prevention of relapses of Wegener's granulomatosis. N Engl J Med 1996; 335:16–20.
15. Reinhold-Keller E, Beuge N, Latza U, de Groot K, Rudert H, Nolle B, Heller M, Gross WG. An interdisciplinary approach to the care of 155 patients with Wegener's granulomatosis. Arthritis Rheum 2000; 43:1021–1032.
16. Krafcik SS, Covin RB, Lynch JP III, Sitrin RG. Wegener's granulomatosis in the elderly. Chest 1996; 109:430–437.
17. Hoffman GS, Drucker Y, Cotch MF, Locker GA, Easley K, Kwoh K. Wegener's granulomatosis: Patient-reported effects of disease on health, function, and income. Arthritis Rheum 1998; 41:2257–2262.
18. Devaney KO, Travis WD, Hoffman GS, Leavitt R, Lebovics R, Fauci AS. Interpretation of head and neck biopsies in Wegener's granulomatosis. Am J Surg Pathol 1990; 14:555–564.
19. Del Buono EA, Flint A. Diagnostic usefulness of nasal biopsy in Wegener's granulomatosis. Hum Pathol 1991; 22:107–110.
20. D'Cruz DP, Baguley E, Asherson RA, Hughes GRV. Ear, nose, and throat symptoms in subacute Wegener's granulomatosis. Br Med J 1989; 299:419–422.
21. Murty GE. Wegener's granulomatosis: Otorhinolaryngological manifestations. Clin Otolaryngol 1990; 15:385–393.

22. Charles SJ, Meyer PAR, Watson PG. Diagnosis and management of systemic Wegener's granulomatosis presenting with anterior ocular inflammatory disease. Brit J Ophthalmol 1991; 75:201–207.

23. Satorre J, Antle M, O'Sullivan R, White VA, Nugent R, Rootman J. Orbital lesions with granulomatous inflammation. Can J Ophthalmol 1991; 26:174–195.

24. Duncker G, Nölle B, Asmus R, Koltze H, Rochels R. Orbital involvement in Wegener's granulomatosis. In: Gross WL, ed. ANCA-Associated Vasculitides. New York: Plenum, 1993:315–318.

25. Specks U, DeRemee RA, Gross WL. Die Wegener'sche granulomatose: Systemerkrankung mit bevorzugtem befall des respirationstraktes. Pneumologie 1989; 43:648–659.

26. Travis WD, Hoffman GS, Leavitt RY, Pass HI, Fauci AS. Surgical pathology of the lung in Wegener's granulomatosis. Am J Surg Pathol 1991; 15:315–333.

27. Aberle DR, Gamsu G, Lynch D. Thoracic manifestations of Wegener's granulomatosis: Diagnosis and course. Radiology 1990; 174:703–709.

28. Rosete A, Cabral A, Kraus R, Alarcon-Segovia D. Diabetes insipidus secondary to Wegener's granulomatosis: Report an review of the literature. J Rheumatol 1991; 18:761–765.

29. Greenan TJ, Grossman RI, Goldberg HI. Cerebral vasculitis: MR imaging and angiographic correlation. Radiology 1992; 182:65–72.

30. Nishino H, Rubino FA, DeRemee A, Swanson JW, Parisi JE. Neurological involvement in Wegener's granulomatosis: An analysis of 324 consecutive patients at the Mayo Clinic. Ann Neurol 1993; 33:4–9.

31. Alcalay M, Azais I, Pallier B, Touchard G, Patte F, Brugier IC, Debiais F, Preud'homme JL, Ingrand P, Babin P. Les manifestations articulaires de la maladie de Wegener. Revue Rheum 1990; 57:845–853.

32. Gross WL, Schmitt WH, Csernok E. Antineutrophil cytoplasmic autoantibody-associated diseases: A rheumatologist's perspective. Am J Kidney Dis 1991; 18:175–179.

33. Handrock K, Gross WL. Relapsing polychondritis as a secondary phenomenon of primary systemic vasculitis. Ann Rheum Dis 1993; 52:895–897.

34. Noritake DT, Weiner SR, Bassett LW, Paulus HE, Weisbart R. Rheumatic manifestations of Wegener's granulomatosis. J Rheumatol 1987; 14:949–951.

35. Frances C, Du LT, Piette JC, Saada V, Boisnic S, Wechsler B, Bletry O, Godeau P. Wegener's granulomatosis. Dermatological manifestations in 75 cases with clinicopathologic correlation. Arch Dermatol 1994; 130:861–867.

36. Dreisin RB. New perspectives in Wegener's granulomatosis. Thorax 1993; 48:97–99.

37. Lombard CM, Duncan SR, Rizk NW, Colby TV. The diagnosis of Wegener's granulomatosis from transbronchial biopsy specimens. Hum Pathol 1990; 21:838–842.

38. Cordier J-F, Valeyre D, Guillevin L, Loire R, Brechot J-M. Pulmonary Wegener's granulomatosis. A clinical imaging study of 77 cases. Chest 1990; 97:906–912.

39. Falk RJ, Jennette JC. A nephrological view of the classification of vasculitis. Adv Exp Med Biol 1993; 336:197–208.

40. Jennette JC, Falk RJ. Pathogenic potential of anti-neutrophil cytoplasmic autoantibodies. Lab Invest 1994; 70:135–137.

41. Weiss MA, Crissman JD. Renal biopsy findings in Wegener's granulomatosis: Segmental necrotizing glomerulonephritis with glomerular thrombosis. Hum Pathol 1984; 15:943–956.

42. Wegener F. Wegener's granulomatosis. Thoughts and observations of a pathologist. Eur Arch Otorhinolaryngol 1990; 247:133–142.

43. van der Woude FJ, Lobatto S, Permin HA, van Es LA, van der Giessen M, van der Hem GK, The TH. Autoantibodies against neutrophils and moncytes: Tool for diagnosis and marker of disease activity in Wegener's granulomatosis. Lancet 1985; 1:425–429.

44. Hagen EC, Andrassy K, Csernok E, Daha MR, Gaskin G, Gross WL, Lesavre P, Lüdemann J, Pusey CD, Rasmussen N, Savage COS, Sinico RA, Wiik A, van der Woude FJ. The value of indirect immunofluorescence and solid phase techniques for ANCA detection: A report on the first phase of an international cooperative study on the standardization of ANCA assays. J Immunol Methods 1993; 159:1–16.

45. Rao JK, Allen NB, Feussner JR, Weinberger M. A prospective study of antineutrophil cytoplasmic antibody (cANCA) and clinical criteria in diagnosing Wegener's granulomatosis. Lancet 1995; 346:926–931.

46. Rao JK, Weinberger M, Oddone EZ, Allen NB, Lansman P, Feussner JR. The role of antineutrophil cy-

toplasmic antibody (cANCA) testing in the diagnosis of Wegener's granulomatosis. Ann Intern Med 1995; 123:925–932.

47. Edgar JDM, McMillan SA, Bruce JN, Caulan SK. An audit of ANCA in routine clinical practise. Postgrad Med J 1995; 71:605–612.

48. Gross WL, Csernok E. Immunodiagnostic and pathophysiologic aspects of antineutrophil cytoplasmic antibodies in vasculitis. Curr Opin Rheumatol 1995; 7:11–19.

49. Kerr GS, Fleisher TA, Hallahan CW, Leavitt RY, Fauci AS, Hoffman GS. Limited prognostic value of changes in antineutrophil cytoplasmic antibody titer in patients with Wegener's granulomatosis. Arthritis Rheum 36:365–71, 1993.

50. Hoffman GS, Specks U. Antineutrophil cytoplasmic antibodies. Arthritis Rheum 1998; 41:1521–37.

51. Wegener F. Die pneumogene allgemeine Granulomatose—sog. Wegener'sche Granulomatose. In: Staemmler M, Kaufmann E, eds. Lehrbuch der Speziellen Pathologischen Anatomie. Berlin: De Gruyter, 1967:225ff.

52. Walton EW. Giant cell granuloma of the respiratory tract (Wegener's granulomatosis). Br Med J 1958:265–270.

53. Fienberg R. Pathergic granulomatosis. Am J Med 1955; 19:829.

54. Gross WL. Wegener's granulomatosis. New aspects of the disease course, immundiagnostic procedures, and stage-adapted treatment. Sarcoidosis 1989; 6:15–29.

55. Mark EJ, Matsubara O, Tan-Liu NS, Fienberg R. The pulmonary biopsy in the early diagnosis of Wegener's (pathergic) granulomatosis: A study based on 35 open lung biopsies. Hum Pathol 1988; 19:1065–1071.

56. Zollinger U. Die Herdglomerulitis beim Wegener-Syndrom in Niere und ableitenden Harnwegen. In: Doerr W, Uhlinger E, eds. Spezielle Pathologische Anatomie. Berlin: Springer, 1966:386.

57. Walton EW. Giant cell granuloma of the respiratory tract (Wegener's granulomatosis). Br J Rheumatol 1958; 2:265–270.

58. Hollander D, Manning RT. The use of alkylating agents in the treatment of Wegener's granulomatosis. Ann Intern Med 1967; 67:393–398.

59. De Remee RA, McDonald TJ, Weiland LH. Wegener's granulomatosis: Observations on treatment with antimicrobial agents. Mayo Clin Proc 1985; 60:27–32.

60. Reinhold-Keller E, DeGroot K, Rudert H, Nolle B, Heller M, Gross WL. Response to trimethoprim/sulfamethoxazole in Wegener's granulomatosis depends on the phase of disease. Q J Med 1996; 89:15–23.

61. Hoffman GS. Immunosuppressive therapy is always required for the treatment of limited Wegener's granulomatosis. Sarcoid Vasc Diff Lung Dis 1996; 13:249–252.

62. De Groot K, Reinhold-Keller E, Tatsis E, Paulsen J, Heller M, Nolle B, Gross WL. Therapy for the maintenance of remission in 65 patients with generalized Wegener's granulomatosis. Methotrexate versus trimethoprim/sulfamethoxazole. Arthritis Rheum 1996; 39:2052–2061.

63. Firestein GS, Bullough D, Gruber H, Mullane K: Selectin-mediated anti-inflammatory effects of adenosine and an adenosine kinase inhibitor. Arthritis Rheum 1993; 36:48.

64. Palmblad J, Lindstrom P, Lerner R. Leukotriene B4 induced hyperadhesiveness of endothelial cells for neutrophils. Biochem Biophys Res Commun 1990; 848–851.

65. Cronstein BN, Eberle MA, Gruber HE, Levin RI: Methotrexate inhibits neutrophil function by stimulating adenosine release from connective tissue cells. Proc Natl Acad Sci USA 1991; 88:2441–2445.

66. Walsdorfer U, Christophers E, Schroder JM. Methotrexate inhibits polymorphonuclear leukocyte chemotaxis in psoriasis. Br J Dermatol 1983; 108:451–456.

67. Sperling RI, Coblyn JS, Larkin JK, Benincaso AI, Austen KF, Weinblatt ME. Inhibition of leukotriene B4 synthesis in neutrophils from patients with rheumatoid arthritis by a single oral dose of methotrexate. Arthritis Rheum 1990; 33:1149–1155.

68. Alarcon GS, Schrohenloher RE, Bartolucci AA, Ward JR, Williams HJ, Koopman WJ. Suppression of rheumatoid factor production by methotrexate in patients with rheumatoid arthritis. Arthritis Rheum 1990; 33:1156–1161.

69. Olsen NJ, Callahan LF, Pincus T. Immunologic studies of rheumatoid arthritis patients treated with methotrexate. Arthritis Rheum 1987; 30:481–488.

70. Wascher TC, Hermann J, Brezinschek HP, Brezinschek R, Wilders-Truschnig M, Rainer F, Krejs GJ.

Cell-type specific response of peripheral blood lymphocytes to methotrexate in the treatment of rheumatoid arthritis. Clin Invest 1994; 72:535–540.

71. Hoffman GS, Leavitt RY, Kerr GS, Fauci AS. The treatment of Wegener's granulomatosis with glucocorticoids and methotrexate. Arthritis Rheum 1992; 35:6112–6118.

72. Sneller MC, Hoffman GS, Talar-Williams C, Kerr GS, Hallahan CW, Fauci AS. An analysis of 42 Wegener's granulomatosis patients treated with methotrexate and prednisone. Arthritis Rheum 1995; 38:608–613.

73. Hoffman GS, Leavitt RY, Fleisher TA, Minor JR, Fauci AS. Treatment of Wegener's granulomatosis with intermittent high dose intravenous cyclophosphamide. Am J Med 1990; 89:403–410.

74. Reinhold-Keller E, Beuge N, de Groot K, Latza U, Rudert H, Nolle B, Heller M, Gross WL. An interdisciplinary approach to the care of patients with Wegener's granulomatosis. Arthritis Rheum 2000; 43:1021–1032.

75. Falk RJ, Hogan S, Carey TS, Jennette JC and The Glomerular Disease Collaborative Network. Clinical course of antineutrophil cytoplasmic autoantibody-associated glomerulonephritis and systemic vasculitis. Ann Intern Med 1990; 113:656–663.

76. Guillevin L, Cordier JF, Lhote F, Cohen P, Jarrousse B, Royer I, Lesavre P, Jacquot C, Bindi P, Bielefeld P, Desson JF, Detree F, Dubois A, Hachulla E, Hoen B, Jacomy D, Seigneuric C, Lauque D, Stern M, Longy-Boursier M. A prospective, multicenter, randomized trial comparing steroids and pulse cyclophosphamide versus steroids and oral cyclophosphamide in the treatment of generalized Wegener's granulomatosis. Arthritis Rheum 1997; 40:2187–2198.

77. Hoffman GS. Treatment of Wegener's granulomatosis: Time to change the standard of care? Arthritis Rheum 1997; 40:2099–2104.

78. Langford CA, Talar-Williams C, Barron KS, Sneller MC. A staged approach to the treatment of Wegener's granulomatosis: Induction with glucocorticoids and daily cyclophosphamide switching to methotrexate for remission maintenance. Arthritis Rheum 1999; 42:2666–2673.

79. Luqmani R, Jayne D, EUVAS. A multicenter randomized trial of cyclophosphamide versus azathioprine during remission in ANCA-associated systemic vasculitis. Arthritis Rheum 1999; 42(S):928.

80. Blum M, Andrassy K, Adler D, Hartmann M, Volcker HE. Early experience with intravenous immunoglobulin treatment in Wegener's granulomatosis with ocular involvement. Graefes Arch Clin Exp Ophthal 1997; 235:599–602.

81. Richter C, Schnabel A, Cernok E, DeGroot K, Reinhold-Keller E, Gross WL. Treatment of antineutrophil cytoplasmic antibody (ANCA)-associated systemic vasculitis with high-dose intravenous immunoglobulin. Clin Exp Immunol 1995; 101:2–7.

82. Jayne DRW, Esnault VLM, Lockwood CM. ANCA anti-idiotype antibodies and the treatment of systemic vasculitis with intravenous immunoglobulin. J Autoimmun 1993; 6:207–219.

83. Rossi F, Jayne DRW, Lockwood CM, Kazatchkine MD: Anti-idiotypes against antineutrophil cytoplasmic antigen autoantibodies in normal human polyspecific IgG for therapeutic use and in remission sera of patients with systemic vasculitis. Clin Exp Immunol 1991; 83:298–303.

84. Ludviksson BR, Sneller MC, Chua KS, Talar-Williams C, Langford CA, Ehrhardt RO, Fauci AS, Strober W. Active Wegener's granulomatosis is associated with HLA-DR+ CD4+ T cells exhibiting an unbalanced Th1-type T cell cytokine pattern: Reversal with IL-10. J Immunol 1998; 160:3602–3609.

84a. Csernok E, Trabandt A, Muller A, Wang G, Moosig F, Schnabel A, Gross WL. Cytokine profiles in Wegener's granulomatosis: predominance of type 1 (Th1) in the granulomatous inflammation. Arthritis Rheum 1999; 42:742–750.

85. Kobold ACM, Kallenberg CGM, Cohen Tervaert JW. Monocyte activation in patients with Wegener's granulomatosis. Ann Rheum Dis 1999; 58:237–245.

86. Andrassy K, Erb A, Koderisch J, Waldherr R, Ritz E. Wegener's granulomatosis with renal involvement: Patient survival and correlations between initial renal function, renal histology, therapy and renal outcome. Clin Nephrol 1991; 35:139–147.

87. Mekhail TM, Hoffman GS. Long-term outcome of Wegener's in patients with renal disease requiring dialysis. J Rheumatol 2000; 27:1237–1240.

88. Nachman PH, Hogan SL, Jennette JC, Falk RJ. Treatment response and relapse in antineutrophil cytoplasmic autoantibody-associated microscopic polyangiitis and glomerulonephritis. J Am Soc Nephrol 1996; 7:33–39.

89. Geffriaud-Ricouard C, Noel LH, Chauveau D, et al. Clinical spectrum associated with antineutrophil cytoplasmic antibodies. Defined antigen specificities in 98 selected patients. Clin Nephrol 1993; 39:125.

90. Pusey CD, Rees AJ, Evans DJ, Peters DK, Lockwood CM. Plasma exchange in focal necrotizing glomerulonephritis without anti-GBM antibodies. Kidney Int 1991; 40:757–763.

91. Cole E, Cattran D, Magil A, Greenwood C, Math M, Churchill D, Sutton D, Clark W, Morrin P, Posen G, Bernstein K, Dyck R and the Canadian Apheresis Study Group. A prospective randomized trial of plasma exchange as additive therapy in idiopathic crescentic glomerulonephritis. Am J Kidney Dis 1992; 20:261–269.

92. Glassock RJ. Intensive plasma exchange in crescentic glomerulonephritis: Help or no help? Am J Kidney Dis 1992; 20:270–275.

93. Langford CA, Sneller MC, Hallahan CW, Hoffman GS, Kammerer WA, Talar-Williams C, Fauci AS, Lebovics RS. Clinical features and therapeutic management of subglottic stenosis in patients with Wegener's granulomatosis. Arthritis Rheum 1996; 39:1754–1760.

94. Talar-Williams C, Hijazi YM, Walther MM, Linehan WM, Hallahan CW, Lubensky I, Kerr GS, Hoffman GS, Fauci AS, Sneller MC. Cyclophosphamide-induced cystitis and bladder cancer in patients with Wegener's granulomatosis. Ann Intern Med 1996; 124:477–484.

95. Ognibene FP, Shelhamer JH, Hoffman GS, Kerr GS, Reda D, Fauci AS, Leavitt RY. Pneumocystis carinii pneumonia: A major complication of immunosuppressive therapy in patients with Wegener's granulomatosis. Am J Respir Crit Care Med 1995; 151:795–799.

96. Godeau B, Mainardi JL, Roudot-Thoraval F, Hachulla E, Guillevin L, Huong Du LT, Jarrousse B, Remy P, Schaeffer A, Piette JC. Factors associated with Pneumocystis carinii pneumonia in Wegener's granulomatosis. Ann Rheum Dis 1995; 54:991–994.

97. Nyberg G, Akesson P, Norden G, Wieslander J. Systemic vasculitis in a kidney transplant population. Transplantation 1997; 63:1273–1277.

98. Wrenger E, Pirsch JD, Cangro CB, D'Alessandro AM, Knechtle SJ, Kalayoglu M, Sollinger HW. Single-center experience with renal transplantation in patients with Wegener's granulomatosis. Transplant Int 1997; 10:152–156.

99. Rostaing L, Modesto A, Oksman F, Cisterne JM, Le Mao G, Durand D: Outcome of patients with antineutrophil cytoplasmic autoantibody-associated vasculitis following cadaveric kidney transplantation. Am J Kidney Dis 1997; 29:96–102.

27

Churg–Strauss Syndrome: Clinical Aspects

Loïc Guillevin, François Lhote, and Pascal Cohen
Hôpital Avicenne, Université Paris–Nord, Bobigny, France

I. INTRODUCTION

Churg–Strauss syndrome (CSS) was first described in 1951 (1) from an autopsy series of patients thought to have been affected by polyarteritis nodosa (PAN). The main characterisitics of the disease were the presence of asthma, eosinophilia, and histopathological manifestations comprising vasculitis of small-sized vessels, arterioles, and venules associated with granuloma. Churg–Strauss syndrome is now considered to be a well-defined vasculitis, clearly distinct from other small- and/or medium-sized-vessel vasculitides. In this chapter, we review the clinical aspects, outcome, and treatment of CSS.

II. CLASSIFICATION

Different systems have been devised and, for CSS, all of them can be applied adequately for classification purposes. The American College of Rheumatology (ACR) described a group of clinical and biological symptoms that are shown in Table 1 (2). In the Chapel Hill Nomenclature (3), CSS is included among the group of small-sized vessel vasculitides. Other criteria, described by Lanham et al. (4), are really useful for diagnosis. These criteria are the association of asthma, peripheral blood eosinophils >1500/mm^3 and symptoms of systemic vasculitis involving at least two extrapulmonary sites. In most, but not all, patients CSS is associated with the presence of antineutrophil cytoplasm antibodies (ANCAs). The ANCAs seem more often to be observed in small-vessel vasculitis but, unlike Wegener's granulomatosis where cytoplasmic (anti-proteinase 3)-ANCA are found (5), the fluorescence pattern is perinuclear (p-) and antimyeloperoxidase (MPO) antibodies are found in the majority of ANCA-positive patients.

III. EPIDEMIOLOGY

Churg–Strauss syndrome is a rare disease and very few descriptions of large series have been published. Recently, we reported on a series of patients observed over 32 years (6) and the Mayo Clinic has reported its experience with CSS from 1974 to 1992 (7).

In Norwich County, United Kingdom, the annual incidence of the disease, measured between 1988 and 1994, was 2.4 per million inhabitants (8). When the incidence of CSS was com-

Table 1 Churg–Strauss Syndrome: 1990 Criteria of the American College of Rheumatology

Asthma
Blood eosinophilia >10%
History of allergy
Mononeuropathy or polyneuropathy
Pulmonary infiltrates, nonfixed
Paranasal sinus abnormality
Extravascular eosinophils on biopsy

Four or more of the 6 items listed here can be used for the classification of Churg–Strauss syndrome.

pared between urban areas and the countryside, the authors noted that 5.1 per million in rural areas were affected with CSS vs. 1.8 per million in urban areas. The authors postulated a role for pollens or pesticides in disease pathogenesis.

If we consider the published series of vasculitides, formerly called the "PAN-group" (9), 10–26% of the patients presented with CSS (10–14). In the prospective series of the French Vasculitis Study Group, CSS was present in 19.1% of patients (12,15,16). According to Lie's pathological analysis (17), only 40 of 1337 autopsied patients with vasculitis had CSS.

The mean age of occurrence of CSS is 48.2 ± 14.6 years at the time of diagnosis (6). Age of occurrence is lower than for PAN or microscopic polyangiitis (MPA). The sex ratio is around 1 with 53% of patients being males in our series (6).

IV. CLINICAL MANIFESTATIONS

Churg–Strauss syndrome occurs after two long prodromic phases (4). During the first period, asthma and other allergic manifestations occur and precede the second period that consists of eosinophilia and lung infiltrates. The third period is the disease itself. The clinical manifestations of CSS may occur several years after the onset of asthma. A systematic inquiry showed that 63.8% of patients had a personal history of allergy (6) and one out of four patients (18) had a familial history of allergy. It can be difficult to define the exact time of CSS onset; the clinical manifestations appear within a few weeks with progressive worsening of asthma, and simultaneously other general symptoms: fever, weight loss, and fatigue. The main clinical manifestations of CSS are summarized in Table 2 (4,6,18–22).

A. Pulmonary Manifestations

1. Asthma

Asthma is one of the major symptoms of CSS. It is widely accepted that asthma is an essential element for diagnosis. However, we have very rarely observed patients who presented with other allergic manifestations (e.g., rhinitis, allergic dermatitis) or who developed asthma simultaneously with systemic manifestations of vasculitis. Asthma occurred 8.86 ± 10 years before the first symptoms of vasculitis (6). Asthma often occurs late in the life of patients, at around 30 years, but, in other patients, asthma begins during infancy. In half of the patients, asthma is severe and requires steroids, at least by spray and more often orally. Asthma becomes more severe during the weeks preceding vasculitis, becomes corticosteroid-dependent, and patients often need to be hospitalized to treat asthma attacks or respiratory failure. Although severe, asthma is rarely the cause

Table 2 Frequency (%) of Main Clinical Manifestations of Churg–Strauss Syndrome (372 Patients)

Parameter	Chumbley et al. (19) 1977	Literature review (4) 1984	Lanham et al. (4) 1984	Guillevin et al. (18) 1987	Gaskin et al. (21) 1991	Haas et al. (20) 1991	Abu-Shakra et al. (22) 1994	Guillevin et al. (6) 1999
n	30	138	16	43	21	16	12	96
Sex, M/F	21/9	72/66	12/4	24/19	14/7	12/4	6/6	45/51
Age, mean	47	38	38	43	46	42	48	48
Range	15–69			7–66	23–69	17–74	28–70	17–74
Asthma	100	100	100	100	100	100	100	100
General symptoms				72		100	100	70
Lung infiltrates	27	74	72	77	43	62	58	38
ENT manifestations: allergic rhinitis, sinusitis	70	69	70	21	70	10	83	47
Mononeuritis multiplex	63	64	66	67	58	75	92	78
GI manifestations	17	62	59	37	15	56	8	33
Cardiac manifestations	16	52	47	49	43	56	42	30
Rheumatic manifestations	20	46	51	28		31	42	41
Myalgias			68			43	33	54
Skin manifestations	66				50	68	67	51
Purpura	27	46	48	28		25		31
Nodules	20	33	30	21		25		19
Kidney manifestations		42	49	16	80	31	8	16
Pleuritis		29	29			25		

of death. When vasculitis occurs, the asthma is usually controlled by steroids and the other manifestations of vasculitis predominate.

2. Lung Hemorrhage

As in other small-vessel vasculitides, lung capillaritis may occur, characterized by lung hemorrhage (23,24). Diagnosis is based on the association of hemoptysis, lung infiltrates, and anemia. Computed tomography (CT) scanning is very useful for establishing the diagnosis of minor forms of lung hemorrhage (Fig. 1).

3. Pleural Effusion

In retrospective studies (4,25), pleural effusions were detected in 25–65% of the cases. In a meta-analysis of prospective studies (25), pleural effusion was observed in only 3% of the patients. The effusion can be unilateral or bilateral and is often asymptomatic. The fluid is an exudate. Lactic acid dehydrogenase levels can be above normal in the pleural fluid and glucose can be low. The main characteristic is the presence of eosinophils which can exceed 85% of all white blood cells. Vasculitis and infiltration of the pleura by eosinophils can be found. Churg–Strauss syndrome can on rare occasions be diagnosed by pleural biopsy (6).

4. Lung Infiltrates

Lung x-ray is abnormal in 38–70% of the cases (4). Opacities are unilateral or bilateral and transitory nonfixed. When they are localized in the periphery of the lungs, they mimic chronic eosinophilic pneumonia. Infiltrates are migratory and regress spontaneously or following corticosteroid therapy. Infiltrates of the parenchyma are composed of eosinophils and may be due, in rare cases, to alveolar hemorrhage.

5. Miscellaneous

Palsy of the phrenic nerve has been described in rare cases (26) and is considered to be due to nerve vasculitis.

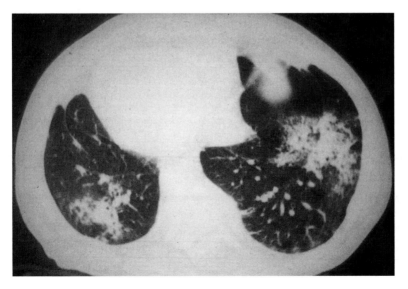

Figure 1   Lung CT scan showing bilateral infiltrates due to alveolar hemorrhage.

B. Central Nervous System Involvement

1. Peripheral Neuropathy

Peripheral neuropathy occurs in the majority of CSS patients (6,18,27). Pain and hypoesthesia may precede the first objective sensory or motor manifestations of neuropathy. Peripheral neuropathy is present in 53–75% of patients (4,7,11,12,18,20). Mononeuritis multiplex more often affects the legs than the arms and predominates in the superficial and deep peroneal nerves. Palsy of these latter nerves was present in 65.6% of our patients and in 82.8% of patients who presented with mononeuritis multiplex (6). Electromyography shows axonal nerve involvement. This technique often detects more extensive involvement than the clinical symptoms would indicate.

Cubital, radial, and median nerves can also be involved. Although cranial nerve palsies are rare, the cranial nerves II, III, VI, and VIII are sometimes affected. Sensory and/or motor involvement can be observed.

At the onset of the disease, palsies are rapidly progressive. Only superficial sensitivity is affected. In rare cases, symmetric palsy mimicking Guillain–Barré syndrome is present (28). Some severe palsies do not improve and are responsible for major morbidity. During the first months of overt disease, several attacks of palsies may occur. After a period of stability, palsies regress but the extent of recovery cannot be predicted, regardless of the initial intensity of the palsy. Recovery from sensory deficits is less frequent than motor recovery and sensory sequelae are common.

2. Central Nervous System

Central nervous system involvement can be present. It occurred in 8.3% of our patients (6), usually early during the course of the disease. Clinical manifestations are not specific—strokes with motor or sensory deficit, meningeal or brain hemorrhage, sometimes due to choroid plexus vasculitis (29), cognitive dysfunction, epilepsy—reflect the presence of brain vascultis. Computed tomography scans show infarcts, magnetic resonance images contain multiple T_2-weighted enhancing lesions, localized to cortical and subcortical white matter areas (Fig. 2). When angiography is performed, caliber irregularities of vessels (Fig. 3) suggest the presence of vasculitis.

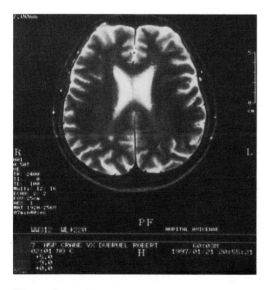

Figure 2 Brain CT scan showing T_2-weighted enhanced lesions suggestive of brain vasculitis.

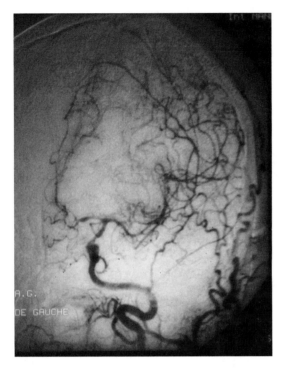

Figure 3 Brain angiogram showing multiple stenoses and irregularities in a patient who presented with stroke occurring in the course of Churg–Strauss syndrome.

C. Skin Manifestations

Skin manifestations are frequent, 40–70% of the cases (4,6,30), and are the consequence of small-vessel involvement. They reflect the presence of vasculitis or extravascular granuloma. They are the first manifestation of vasculitis in <5% of the cases (6). Vascular purpura is the most frequent skin manifestation occurring in 31–50% of the cases (4,6). Other cutaneous manifestations have been reported including livedo reticularis (6.2%) (6), urticarial lesions (9.3%) (6), Raynaud's phenomenon, patchy skin necrosis, infiltrated papules, vesicles or bullae and toe or finger ischemia. Nodules are observed in roughly 30% of the patients (31). They are red or violaceous, predominantly localized on fingers, foreskin, skull, and extensor surface of the elbows and forearm. They are often bilateral and symmetrical. Skin biopsies show extravascular granulomas, which are not specific for CSS and can also be present in patients with other vasculitides or inflammatory bowel disease (31).

D. Gastrointestinal Involvement

Gastrointestinal (GI) manifestations are present in 31.2% of patients. The first GI manifestation is usually abdominal pain (30–60%) (4,6). Nausea, vomiting, and diarrhea are less frequent. Bowel hemorrhage and melena or hematemesis are present in 6.2 and 3.1% of patients, respectively (6). Bowel perforation is the most severe manifestation and is one of the major causes of death (4,6). Vasculitis and granuloma can be present throughout the GI tract, but more frequently in the small intestine and/or colon. Endoscopy and biopsies may show the presence of pseudopolyps (32). The presence of several duodenal and jejunal ulcers may evoke the diagnosis. Biopsies may show vasculitis and/or an eosinophilic infiltration of the GI tract. When inflammatory infiltrates are found predominantly in the mucosa, anemia, hypoalbuminemia, and steator-rhea may be present (32). Angiography may reveal the presence of vessel stenoses and microaneurysms. The sensitivity of angiography in this setting is not defined. The severity of abdominal pain and symptoms suggesting peritonitis or bowel ischemia may necessitate surgery. Only four patients out of a series of 96 patients were so affected: bowel ischemia was found in two, appendicitis in one, and ischemic colitis in one (6). Gastrointestinal manifestations have been demonstrated to be one of the factors of poor prognosis for CSS (16).

E. Cardiac Manifestations

Cardiac involvement is one of the most severe manifestations of CSS and is the most frequent cause of death. In the literature, its frequency varies between 15 and 84.6% (1,4,18,20,33). In our patients (6), 22.9% had pericarditis and 13.4% had myocardial involvement. Pericardial involvement is rarely complicated by tamponade. Endocarditis usually does not occur. Endomyocardial fibrosis has been described very rarely (1); this entity has been observed in hypereosinophilic syndrome but usually not in CSS, despite the presence of eosinophilia. Cardiac involvement is the consequence of several different mechanisms: vasculitis of coronary artery branches, extravascular granuloma, and interstitial eosinophilic infiltrates. In Churg and Strauss's series, eosinophilic infiltration was the most common histological observation (1); epicardial and myocardial granuloma were also present. Necrotizing vasculitis of the pericardium has also been found in pericardial biopsies of two patients (6,34).

Cardiac insufficiency develops rapidly and is often severe. It was the cause of death of 3 of 11 patients reported by Churg and Strauss (1) and 13 of our 96 patients (6). Angina pectoris is rare, despite frequent coronary vasculitis. Myocardial infarction is also rare (35). Electrocardiograms shows abnormalities due to ischemia or cardiomyopathy. Under treatment, these abnormalities may disappear (36). When coronary angiography is performed, stenoses, microaneurysms, and/or thromboses are rarely observed (36) because the vasculitis predominantly affects small vessels. Nevertheless, angiograms are sometimes abnormal (35,37), reflecting the possible extension of the disease to medium-sized arteries. In the case of cardiomyopathy, endomyocardical biopsies usually do not provide the diagnosis. Echocardiography shows diminished contractile parameters that are not specific to vasculitis.

F. Muscle and Joint Involvement

Arthralgias are frequent and often occur during the first days or weeks. Arthritis with local inflammatory findings is rare and joint deformity and radiographic erosions not occur. Although all joints can be affected by arthralgias, they predominate in the larger articulations.

Myalgias are frequent (53.6–68.7%) (4,6) and usually regress quickly under treatment. Sometimes myalgias are so intense that they mimic polymyositis (38).

G. Renal Involvement

Renal involvement is infrequently observed in CSS. In our series of 96 patients (6), the kidney was affected in only 16.5% (6). In other series, the frequency was probably overestimated (4). Proteinuria and hematuria should, nonetheless, be assessed in every patient. When present, glomerulonephritis is usually extracapillary with crescents, segmental and focal (39). For some of these cases, the outcome of rapid progressive glomerulonephritis was renal failure with the need for temporary or prolonged hemodialysis (39). Glomerulonephritis is associated with the presence of p-ANCA (anti-MPO). In CSS, there is usually absence of renal vasculitis involving medium-sized arteries. Consequently, angiograms usually do not show microaneurysms. We have demonstrated that, in ANCA-positive patients, there is no justification to perform angiography before renal biopsy (40). Renal involvement is one of the items included in the five-factors score (FFS) that has been a useful guide to estimating prognosis in CSS. Shortened survival is clearly correlated with renal involvement (16).

Ureteral involvement has been also described in CSS (41). Stenosis is usually observed in the lower part of the ureters and more rarely in the upper part. Anuria and/or renal insufficiency are the consequence of unilateral or bilateral stenoses.

H. ENT and Ophthalmological Symptoms

Maxillary sinusitis is one of the major symptoms of CSS and is one of the ACR classification criteria for CSS. Allergic rhinitis and/or sinus polyposis are frequent (70% of the patients) (4). A history of chronic sinusitis preceded CSS in 62.5% of our patients (6). Ear, nose, and throat (ENT) manifestations of CSS and those of Wegener's granulomatosis can be the similar. However, bone destruction is not observed in CSS and the prognosis of CSS ENT manifestations overall is good (6). Ear, nose, and throat symptoms are not considered in the FFS.

The eye can also be involved, and uveitis, retinal vasculitis, episcleritis and/or conjunctival nodules have been described (42). Ischemic optic neuropathy can complicate CSS. Temporal artery involvement is also observed, with necrotizing vasculitis of temporal artery branches (43).

I. Miscellaneous

Mediastinal or peripheral lymph nodes containing eosinophils have been observed on rare occasions (4).

V. LIMITED FORMS OF CHURG–STRAUSS SYNDROME

Churg–Strauss syndrome is a systemic disease that our cause constitutional symptoms, such as fever, weight loss, malaise, muscular-skeletal pain, and eosinophilia. In addition to the systemic disease, limited forms have been reported (17), localized to one organ and usually associated with constitutional symptoms. A history of allergy is found in the majority of patients, but asthma may be absent at the time of diagnosis. The GI tract and the heart are the organs most frequently involved. The clinical manifestations of GI involvement are eosinophilic cholecystitis, eosinophilic enteritis, and mesenteric artery vasculitis. Cardiac failure has also been observed. Some rare cases of peripheral skin nodules (44) and ureteral stenosis have also been described. The outcome for survival depends on the organ involved.

VI. PRECIPITATING FACTORS

The etiology of CSS remains unknown. Nevertheless, various authors have incriminated certain precipitating factors in the etiology of some cases of CSS (6,18,44,45). These putative "triggering" factors are very diverse and it is not possible to identify a common antigen among the suspected drugs, particles, and hyposensitization treatments. It is suggested that every hyposensitization treatment, allergen, or drug implicated in the occurrence of the initial disease flare or in relapses be discontinued. Suspected precipitating factors were observed in 24 of our patients (6).

There have recently been several case reports of CSS occurring in the course of leukotriene antagonist drug therapy for chronic asthma. Zafirlukast and montelukast are two drugs in this group that have been suspected precipitants of CSS (46–50).

In addition to certain drug or environmental agents possibly playing a role in disease expression, a rapid decrease of the corticosteroid dose or abrupt withdrawal of treatment for asthma may play a role in the occurrence of CSS.

VII. LABORATORY FINDINGS AND COMPLEMENTARY INVESTIGATIONS

The main biological characteristics are eosinophilia, the presence of an inflammatory syndrome, and ANCA positivity. Increases in acute phase reactants, e.g., erythrocyte sedimentation rate (ESR) and C-reactive protein (CRP), are common and were present in 80% of our patients (6). Eosinophilia is usually >1500/mm^3. The mean eosinophil count in our patients was 7193 ± 6706/mm^3 (6); the maximum eosinophil count in the literature was 50,000/mm^3 (51).

Antineutrophil cytoplasmic antibodies were present in 47.6–85% of patients (mean = 59.2%) (6,21,52,53). The immunofluorescence pattern is usually perinuclear and very rarely cytoplasmic. By enzyme-linked immunosorbent assay (ELISA), MPO is usually the "targeted" antigen in p-ANCA–positive patients. Rheumatoid factor can be found in 53.6% of the patients (4,20). When performed, bronchoalveolar lavage fluid contains eosinophils. After corticosteroid therapy, eosinophil levels decrease very quickly, sometimes in less than a week. The ANCA titer is not correlated with outcome, but the persistence of ANCA might be associated with increased risk of relapses.

Pulmonary abnormalities were seen on x-rays in 37.5% of our patients (6), and included bilateral and "migratory" infiltrates and patchy alveolar opacities. Sinusitis may be observed on x-rays but is seen more clearly on CT scans. Angiography is not systematically performed but is done in patients with GI manifestations or for diagnostic purposes. Stenoses and microaneurysms are less frequent than in PAN but can be observed in 33% of the selected patients in whom this complementary investigation was done (6). Although CSS predominantly affects small vessels, microaneurysms and stenoses, when present on angiograms, reflect medium-sized arterial involvement, demonstrating the range of vessel involvement in this illness.

VIII. OUTCOME

The prognosis of CSS has improved dramatically since the introduction of corticosteroids and, in some cases, cytotoxic therapies. With treatment, remission is rapidly obtained in >80% of patients (88.6% of our patients). Relapses occurred in 25.5% of our patients during the first year, in half of cases, and later in the others, after a mean follow-up period of 69.3 months (6). The clinical symptoms of relapse differ from the first manifestations of CSS in half of the patients and they can be severe and sometimes responsible for death. Some patients experience several relapses within several years after the first manifestations. The 10-year survival rate was 79.4% for our patients (6). Some symptoms are correlated with increased mortality and are taken into account in the FFS to assess disease severity and approximate prognosis. (16). Cardiac involvement is the primary cause of death of CSS patients and the main causes of death are cardiac failure, mesenteric infarction, and iatrogenic complications. Asthma usually persists after recovery from vasculitis and often requires maintenance treatment with corticosteroids. Sequelae of CSS can be neurological, such as the consequence of severe peripheral neuropathy or cerebral ischemia. Cardiac insufficiency is also a major concern in the long term and cardiac transplantation may be necessary in some patients. Renal insufficiency may lead to chronic dialysis.

IX. TREATMENT

Corticosteroids, sometimes in conjunction with cytotoxic agents, are the most effective treatment of CSS.

A. Steroids

Churg–Strauss syndrome responds well to corticosteroids, which represent the treatment of choice. The initial management should include high doses (12,54,55). The administration of methylprednisolone pulses (usually 15 mg/kg intravenously over 60 min repeated at 24-h intervals for 1–3 days) has become widely used at the onset of therapy for severe systemic vasculitis (55,56) because of its rapid action and relative safety, especially in the presence of life-threatening organ involvement or severe mononeuritis multiplex. Corticosteroids (prednisone or prednisolone) are given at the dose of 1.0 mg/kg/day. One or more methylprednisolone pulses are sufficient to obtain dramatic attenuation of asthma and general symptoms, and the disappearance of eosinophilia. In an ongoing trial in which good-prognosis patients are treated with corticosteroids alone, a clinical remission was obtained in >90%. We recommend decreasing the daily dose by 5 mg every 10 days until a level equivalent to half the initial dosage is reached. This dose is then maintained for 3 weeks and then further decreased by 2.5 mg every 10 days, to approximately 15 mg/day. A more careful tapering schedule was followed for doses <15 mg/day. The daily dose was decreased by 1 mg every 10 days, until stopping treatment. Nevertheless, it is often impossible to completely stop corticosteroids because of the residual asthma that may require low doses (5–10 mg) of prednisone and/or inhaled corticosteroids.

B. Cytotoxic Therapy

The indication of cytotoxic drugs, especially cyclophosphamide, must be based on well-defined prognostic factors (16). According to FFS (16), the majority of CSS patients would not have factors of poor prognosis. In that case, cyclophosphamide would only be prescribed as second-line treatment, in the case of failure of the initial treatment or relapse.

1. Cyclophosphamide

A low dose has conventionally been defined as 2 mg/kg/day or less for 1 year and, in combination with corticosteroids, represented the traditional treatment of PAN. Although this regimen is an effective treatment for vasculitic disease, it has a low therapeutic/toxic index. Major side effects associated with daily cyclophosphamide administration include drug-induced cystitis (56), bladder fibrosis, bone-marrow suppression, ovarian failure and/or neoplasm (bladder cancer and hematological malignancies) (57). Severe infections represent a major cause of mortality of systemic vasculitis patients, especially while they are receiving high doses of corticosteroids with adjunctive immunosuppressive drugs (58). In an attempt to decrease the morbidity associated with daily cyclophosphamide administration, protocols utilizing intermittent treatment with larger doses have been developed. Pulse cyclophosphamide therapy is now being used increasingly for systemic necrotizing vasculitis (59–61) and is preferred by some investigators to oral cyclophosphamide. The cyclophosphamide content of each pulse, as well as both the total number and the frequency of the pulses, should be adjusted according to the patient's condition, renal function, hematological data, and the disease's response to previous therapies. For CSS, we recommend an initial dose of 0.6 g/m^2, given at intervals of 2 weeks for 1 month, then every month for 6 to 12 months. High-dose pulse cyclophosphamide may be particularly dangerous in patients with renal failure. Lowering the dose according to renal function would be prudent. Intense hydration and the use of sodium 2-mercaptoethanesulfonate (mesna) is recommended during pulse therapy. The indication of cyclophosphamide for CSS should be adapted to the FFS and given only to patients with FFS >0.

Chumbley et al. (19) reported a 90% 1-year survival rate and a 62% 5-year survival rate. In our study of 96 patients, the 78-month survival rate was 72.3% (6). On these two series, the major cause of death was cardiac involvement, primarily congestive heart failure and much less frequently myocardial infarction. In the literature review by Lanham et al. (4), the cause of death could be identified in 50 cases: nearly half of the patients (48%) died of cardiac failure or myocardial infarction. Other causes of death were renal failure in 18%, cerebral hemorrhage in 16%, GI perforation or hemorrhage in 8%, status asthmaticus in 8%, and respiratory failure in 2%.

C. Other Treatments

There are presently no data to support the systematic prescription of plasma exchange in CSS. Intravenous immunoglobulins, 1 g/kg for 2 days, can also be prescribed as has been done for other ANCA-related vasculitides (62,63). This treatment is not recommended as a first-line therapy, but may be useful for patients refractory to more conventional treatment. Cyclosporine has been given in anecdotal cases of CSS (64,65). One patient who received cyclosporine to prevent cardiac graft rejection suffer did not relapse (64). Interferon-α has recently been utilized, with success (66) in 4 patients with severe CSS. Such treatment merits evaluation in a larger series of patients.

REFERENCES

1. Churg J, Strauss L. Allergic granulomatosis, allergic angiitis and periarteritis nodosa. Am J Pathol 1951; 27:277–294.
2. Masi A, Hunder G, Lie J, et al. The American College of Rheumatology 1990 criteria for the classification of Churg-Strauss syndrome (allergic granulomatosis angiitis). Arthritis Rheum 1990; 33:1094–1100.
3. Jennette JC, Falk RJ, Andrassy K, et al. Nomenclature of systemic vasculitides. Proposal of an international consensus conference. Arthritis Rheum 1994; 37:187–192.
4. Lanham J, Elkon K, Pusey C, Hughes G. Systemic vasculitis with asthma and eosinophilia: A clinical approach to the Churg-Strauss syndrome. Medicine (Baltimore) 1984; 63:65–81.
5. Kallenberg CG. Antineutrophil cytoplasmic antibodies (ANCA) and vasculitis. Clin Rheumatol 1990; 9:S132–S35.
6. Guillevin L, Cohen P, Gayraud M, Lhote F, Jarrousse B, Casassus P. Churg-Strauss syndrome. Clinical study and long-term follow-up of 96 patients. Medicine 1999; 78:26–37.
7. Sehgal M, Swanson J, DeRemee R, Colby T. Neurologic manifestations of Churg-Strauss syndrome. Mayo Clin Proc 1995; 70:337–341.
8. Watts RA, Carruthers DM, Scott DG. Epidemiology of systemic vasculitis: Changing incidence or definition? Semin Arthritis Rheum 1995; 25:28–34.
9. Fauci A, Haynes B, Katz P. The spectrum of vasculitis: Clinical, pathologic, immunologic and therapeutic considerations. Ann Intern Med 1978; 89:660–676.
10. Frohnert P, Sheps S. Long term follow-up study of polyarteritis nodosa. Am J Med 1967; 43:8–14.

11. Guillevin L, Lê THD, Godeau P, Jais P, Wechsler B. Clinical findings and prognosis of polyarteritis nodosa and Churg-Strauss angiitis: A study in 165 patients. Br J Rheumatol 1988; 27:258–264.

12. Guillevin L, Lhote F, Jarrousse B, Fain O. Treatment of polyarteritis nodosa and Churg-Strauss syndrome. A meta-analysis of 3 prospective controlled trials including 182 patients over 12 years. Ann Med Interne (Paris) 1992; 143:405–416.

13. Leib E, Restivo C, Paulus H. Immunosuppressive and corticosteroid therapy of polyarteritis nodosa. Am J Med 1979; 67:941–947.

14. Rose G, Spencer H. Polyarteritis nodosa. Q J Med 1957; 26:43–81.

15. Guillevin L, Fain O, Lhote F, et al. Lack of superiority of steroids plus plasma exchange to steroids alone in the treatment of polyarteritis nodosa and Churg-Strauss syndrome. A prospective, randomized trial in 78 patients. Arthritis Rheum 1992; 35:208–215.

16. Guillevin L, Lhote F, Gayraud M, et al. Prognostic factors in polyarteritis nodosa and Churg-Strauss syndrome. A prospective study in 342 patients. Medicine (Baltimore) 1996; 75:17–28.

17. Lie J. Limited forms of Churg-Strauss syndrome. Pathol Annu 1993; 28:199–220.

18. Guillevin L, Guittard T, Blétry O, Godeau P, Rosenthal P. Systemic necrotizing angiitis with asthma: Causes and precipitating factors in 43 cases. Lung 1987; 165:165–172.

19. Chumbley L, Harrison E, DeRemee R. Allergic granulomatosis and angiitis (Churg-Strauss syndrome). Mayo Clin Proc 1977; 52:477–484.

20. Haas C, Géneau C, Odinot J, et al. L'angéite allergique avec granulome: Syndrome de Churg et Strauss. Etude rétrospective de 16 observations. Ann Med Interne (Paris) 1991; 142:135–142.

21. Gaskin G, Ryan J, Rees A, Pusey C. Antimyeloperoxydase antibodies in vasculitis. Relationship to ANCA and clinical diagnosis. APMIS 1990; 98, S19:33.

22. Abu-Shakra M, Smythe H, Lewtas J, Badley E, Weber D, Keystone E. Outcome of polyarteritis nodosa and Churg-Strauss syndrome. Arthritis Rheum 1994; 37:1798–1803.

23. Lai R, Lin S, Lee P. Churg-Strauss syndrome presenting with capillaritis and diffuse alveolar hemorrhage. Scand J Rheumatol 1998; 27:230–232.

24. Leatherman J, Davies S, Hoidal J. Alveolar hemorrhage syndromes: Diffuse microvascular lung hemorrhage in immune and idiopathic disorders. Medicine 1984; 63:65–81.

25. Lhote F, Cohen P, Chemlal K, Jarrousse B, Guillevin L. Les manifestations pleurales au cours de la périartérite noueuse, de la maladie de Wegener et du lupus érythémateux systémique. Ann Med Interne (Paris) 1992; 143:228–232.

26. Herreman G, Ferme I, Puech H, Caubarrère I. Angéite granulomateuse de Churg et Strauss avec paralysie phrénique. Deux observations. Presse Med 1980; 9:3631.

27. Cohen-Tervaert J, Kallenberg C. Neurologic manifestations of systemic vasculitides. Rheum Dis Clin North Am 1993; 19:913–40.

28. Ng K, Yeung H, Loo K, Chan H, Wong C, Li P. Acute fulminant neuropathy in a patient with Churg Strauss syndrome. Postgrad Med J 1997; 73:236–238.

29. Chang Y, Kargas S, Goates J, Horouplan D. Intraventricular and sub-arachnoid hemorrhage resulting from necrotizing vasculitis of the choroid plexus in a patient with Churg Strauss syndrome. Clin Neuropathol 1993; 12:84–87.

30. Davis M, Daoud M, McEvoy M, Su D. Cutaneous manifestations of Churg Strauss syndrome: A clinicopathologic correlation. J Acad Dermatol 1997; 37:199–203.

31. Finan M, Winkelmann R. The cutaneous extravascular necrotizing granuloma (Churg Strauss granuloma) and systemic disease: A review of 27 cases. Medicine (Baltimore) 1983; 62:148–158.

32. Suen K, Burton J. The spectrum of eosinophilic infiltration of the gastrointestinal tract and its relationship to other disorders of angiitis and granulomatosis. Hum Pathol 1979; 10:31–43.

33. Guillevin L, Lhote F, Gallais V, et al. Gastrointestinal tract involvement in polyarteritis nodosa and Churg-Strauss syndrome. Ann Méd Interne 1995; 146:260–267.

34. Sharma A, de Varennes B, Sniderman A. Churg-Strauss syndrome presenting with marked eosinophilia and pericardial effusion. Can J Cardiol 1993; 9:329–330.

35. Kozak M, Gill E, Green L. The Churg Strauss syndrome. A case report with angiographically documented coronary involvement and a review of the literature. Chest 1995; 107:578–580.

36. Isaka N, Araki S, Shibata M, et al. Reversal of coronary artery occlusions in allergic granulomatosis and angiitis (Churg-Strauss syndrome). Am Heart J 1994; 128:609–13.

37. Hasley P, Follansbee N, Couleman J. Cardiac manifestations of Churg Strauss syndrome: Report of a case and review of the literature. Am Heart J 1990; 120:996–999.

38. De Vlam K, De Keyser F, Goemaere S, Praet M, Veys E. Churg-Strauss syndrome presenting as polymyositis. Clin Exp Rheumatol 1995; 13:505–507.

39. Gaskin G, Clutterbuck E, Pusey C. Renal disease in the Churg Strauss syndrome. Diagnosis, management and outcome. Contrib Nephrol 1991; 94:58–65.

40. Guillevin L, Lhote F, Brauner M, Casassus P. Antineutrophil cytoplasmic antibodies (ANCA) and abnormal angiograms in polyarteritis nodosa and Churg Strauss syndrome: Indications for the diagnosis of microscopic polyangiitis. Ann Méd Interne (Paris) 1995; 146:548–550.

41. Azar N, Guillevin L, Huong DL, Herreman G, Meyrier A, Godeau P. Symptomatic urogenital manifestations of polyarteritis nodosa and Churg Strauss angiitis: Analysis of 8 of 165 patients. J Urol 1989; 142:136–138.

42. Nissim F, Von der Valde J, Czernobilsky B. A limited form of Churg-Strauss syndrome. Ocular and cutaneous manifestations. Arch Pathol Lab Med 1982; 106:305–7.

43. Généreau T, et al. Temporal artery biopsy: a diagnostic tool for systemic necrotizing vasculitis. Arthritis Rheum. Arthritis Rheum 1999; 42:2674–2681.

44. Churg A, Brallas M, Cronin S, Churg J. Formes frustes of Churg Strauss syndrome. Chest 1995; 108:320–323.

45. Phanupak P, Kohler P. Onset of polyarteritis nodosa during allergic hyposensitization treatment. Am J Med 1980; 68:1866–1872.

46. Drazen J, Israel E, O'Byrne P. Treatment of asthma with drugs modifying the leukotriene pathway. N Engl J Med 1999; 340:197–206.

47. Honsinger R. Zafirlukast and Churg Strauss syndrome (letter). JAMA 1998; 279:1949.

48. Katz R, Papernik M. Zafirlukast and Churg-Strauss syndrome. JAMA 1998; 279:1949.

49. Knoell D, Lucas J, Allen J. Churg Strauss syndrome associated with zafirlukast. Chest 1998; 114:332–334.

50. Wechsler M, Garpestad E, Flier S, et al. Pulmonary infiltrates, eosinophilia and cardiomyopathy following corticosteroid withdrawal in patients with asthma receiving zafirlukast. JAMA 1998; 279:455–457.

51. Hübner C, Dietz A, Stremmel W, Stiehl A, Andrassy K. Macrolide-induced Churg Strauss syndrome in a patient with atopy (letter). Lancet 1997; 350:563.

52. Guillevin L, Visser H, Noël LH, et al. Antineutrophil cytoplasm antibodies in systemic polyarteritis nodosa with and without hepatitis B virus infection and Churg Strauss syndrome—62 patients. J Rheumatol 1993; 20:1345–1349.

53. Cohen-Tervaert J, Goldschmeding R, Elema JD, von den Borne A, Kallenberg CG. Antimyeloperoxidase antibodies in the Churg Strauss syndrome. Thorax 1991; 46:70–71.

54. Cogan E, Schandené L, Crusiaux A, Cochaux P, Velu T, Goldman M. Clonal proliferation of type 2 helper T cells in a man with the hypereosinophilic syndrome. N Engl J Med 1994; 330:535–538.

55. De Toffol B, Gaymard B, Adam G, Larmande P, Autret A. Pneumonie infiltrante chronique à éosinophiles suivie d'une angéite de type Churg Strauss. Ann Méd Interne (Paris) 1989; 140:334–335.

56. Stillwell T, Benson R. Cyclophosphamide-induced hemorrhagic cystitis: A review of 100 patients. Cancer 1988; 61:451–457.

57. Baker G, Kahl L, Zee B, Stolzer B, Agarwal A, Medsger TJ. Malignancy following treatment of rheumatoid arthritis with cyclophosphamide. Long-term case-control follow-up study. Am J Med 1987; 83:1–9.

58. Jarrousse B, Guillevin L, Bindi E, et al. Increased risk of Pneumocystis carinii pneumonia in patients with Wegener's granulomatosis. Clin Exp Rheumatol 1993; 11:615–621.

59. Guillevin L, Lhote F, Cohen P, et al. Corticosteroids plus pulse cyclophosphamide and plasma exchanges versus corticosteroids plus pulse cyclophosphamide alone in the treatment of polyarteritis nodosa and Churg-Strauss syndrome patients with factors predicting poor prognosis. A prospective, randomized trial in sixty-two patients. Arthritis Rheum 1995; 38:1638–1645.

60. Gayraud M, Guillevin L, Cohen P, et al. Treatment of good-prognosis polyarteritis nodosa and Churg-Strauss syndrome: Comparison of steroids and oral or pulse cyclophosphamide in 25 patients. Br J Rheumatol 1997; 36:1290–1297.

61. Luqmani R, Exley A, Kitas G, Bacon P. Disease assessment and management of the vasculitides. Bailliere's Clin Rheum 1997; 11:423–446.
62. Hamilos D, Christensen J. Treatment of Churg Strauss syndrome with high-dose intravenous immunoglobulins. J Allergy Clin Immunol 1991; 88:823–824.
63. Jayne DR, Lockwood CM. Intravenous immunoglobulin as sole therapy for systemic vasculitis. Br J Rheumatol 1996; 35(11):1150–3.
64. Henderson R, Hasleton P, Hamid B. Recurrence of Churg Strauss vasculitis in a transplanted heart. Br Heart J 1993; 70:553.
65. McDermott E, Powell R. Cyclosporin in the treatment of Churg-Strauss syndrome. Ann Rheum Dis 1998; 57:256–257.
66. Tatsis E, Schnabel A, Gross W. Interferon alpha treatment in four patients with the Churg Strauss syndrome. Ann Intern Med 1998; 129:370–374.

28

Giant Cell Arteritis: Pathogenesis

Cornelia M. Weyand and Jörg J. Goronzy

Mayo Clinic and Mayo Foundation, Rochester, Minnesota

I. INTRODUCTION

Giant cell (temporal) arteritis (GCA) is an inflammatory vasculopathy that manifests in medium-sized and large arteries. The disease displays a stringent tropism for arteries with well-developed elastic membranes and essentially spares capillaries, arterioles, and veins. Not all territories in the arterial tree are equally susceptible to this vasculitis; at highest risk are the upper extremity branches of the aorta and cranial arteries. Histomorphologically, GCA is a panarteritis that is associated with the formation of multinucleated giant cells in about 50% of all cases (1). Typical histological features include the arrangement of highly activated macrophages in granulomas, focal disintegration of the muscularis, and fragmentation of the elastic lamina. There is a trend for tissue-infiltrating immune cells to form complex structures in the vicinity of the internal and external elastic laminae. Although giant cells have led to the common name of this vasculitis, the presence of these macrophage polykaryons is not essential for the diagnosis of GCA. This vasculitic process can present with diffuse mononuclear cell infiltrates without granulomatous reaction, and the blood vessel inflammation can be segmental, producing patchy lesions.

There is evidence that GCA is a heterogeneous syndrome that includes multiple subtypes of disease. In part, the phenotypic heterogeneity reflects the vascular bed targeted by the disease, e.g., large-vessel GCA vs. cranial GCA (2). Also, there is support of the concept that polymyalgia rheumatica (PMR) is a forme fruste of GCA and represents a subtype with dominant systemic illness and minimal vascular involvement (3). Giant cell arteritis in all its variations is not limited to arterial wall inflammation, but consistently has additional systemic manifestations. Highly upregulated acute phase responses are closely correlated with the systemic illness, and the prompt response of GCA to therapy with corticosteroids likely relates to the sensitivity of systemic inflammatory pathways to this immunosuppression. Both features of GCA, the systemic component and the explicit responsiveness to steroid therapy, provide useful clues to the etiopathogenesis of this inflammatory vasculopathy (Table 1).

In the last decade, advances in genetics and molecular biology have provided the unprecedented opportunity to readdress the pathophysiology of GCA. Although a single cause or etiological agent has not yet been identified, substantial progress has been made in understanding disease pathways in this arteritis. Molecular events in the vascular lesions have been carefully dissected and support the notion that vascular pathology is the result of a dialogue between the host's immune system and the arterial wall. It is now appreciated that vascular morbidity is mainly a consequence of a hyperproliferative reaction of arterial wall cells forming lumen-

Table 1 Clues to the Pathogenesis of Giant Cell Arteritis

Very restricted tissue tropism with targeting of the branches of the proximal aorta
Nonrandom geographical distribution of disease incidence
Manifests exclusively in individuals older than 50 years
Granuloma formation without fibrinoid necrosis
Vascular morbidity largely related to luminal occlusion with ischemia of different organ systems
Vascular lesions composed of T cells and macrophages; B cells are absent
HLA association
Persistance of vascular infiltrates despite successful treatment of systemic symptoms
Markedly upregulated acute phase response
Disease with multiple phenotypes, a forme fruste, polymyalgia rheumatica, lacks clinically overt vascular
   inflammation

---

occlusive neointima. The emerging paradigm is that GCA develops as T lymphocytes encounter antigen in the arterial wall and cause immunological injury. This immune response by itself does not jeopardize the integrity of the blood vessel wall. However, the artery responds to the injury with a tissue repair program that promotes more damage than healing (4).

II. DISEASE MODEL FOR GIANT CELL ARTERITIS

The disease model shown in Figure 1 attempts to integrate the pathogenic studies of GCA, the enormous expansion in the knowledge of the immune system, and the progress in vascular biology. Like all disease models, it cannot demand exclusiveness but it provides a framework for accumulated data from different fields of investigation.

   The model proposes that GCA results from an antigen-specific immune response occurring in the wall of medium-sized and large arteries (5). The antigen may be exogenous, endogenous, or altered self-antigen. The manifestation of antigen-specific immune reactivity in the vessel wall is a function of multiple risk factors, including age, immunogenetics of the host, and the nature of the antigen. Antigen recognition in the blood vessel wall is preceded by a phase of immune stimulation in the periphery that generates highly activated monocytes. These monocytes then serve as reservoirs for antigenic material. Upon their interaction with activated vasa vasorum and infiltration into the blood vessel wall, the activated monocytes disseminate this antigenic material to sites where it is encountered by antigen-specific T cells. T cells recognize processed antigen on monocyte surfaces, thereby initiating a series of events that results in the generation of immune effector cells with tissue injurious characteristics. If insufficient antigen is transported to the artery, the disease process will mainly be limited to the periphery with minor immune stimulation in the vessel. The clinical equivalent to this scenario is polymyalgia rheumatica. The nature of the vascular immune response and, consequently, the downstream effects are determined by the microenvironment in which it evolves. Cellular and noncellular components of the arterial wall enter into a crosstalk with the infiltrating immune cells. As a result of this dialogue, immune functions are modulated and signals are given to the arterial wall components. Most importantly, a program of injury response is set into action and, depending on the reaction pattern, different forms of vascular pathology emerge. Immune responses localized in the aorta will primarily favor tissue destructive pathways resulting in aortic aneurysm formation. In arteries with a different wall composition (i.e., temporal arteries), defense reaction to injury will involve the mobilization, migration, and proliferation of myofibroblasts and will result in the creation of lumen-obstructive intima. This disease model predicts that various antigens can function as an instigator for the im-

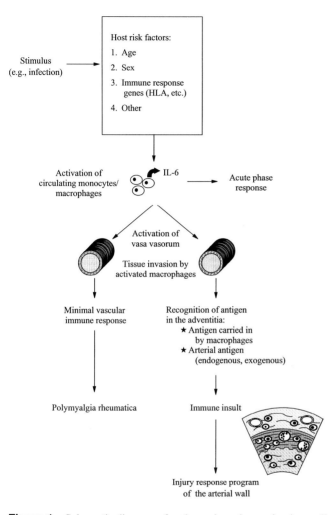

Figure 1 Schematic diagram of pathogenic pathways in giant cell arteritis.

munological injury and that the amount and nature of the antigen eliciting an immune reaction in the vascular wall is only one of the components determining the disease process. It is likely that the complex chain of events underlying the clinical syndrome of GCA can be intersected at multiple levels, defining promising opportunities for therapeutic interventions.

III. RISK FACTORS

The incidence of GCA varies greatly in different geographical regions of the world. The highest incidence rates have been measured in Northern Europe and in Minnesota, a state with a population of mainly Northern European descent, with estimates of about 20 cases annually per 100,000 persons older than 50 years of age (6,7). Incidence rates are about 10-fold lower in Blacks and Hispanics, suggesting striking differences in disease risk among ethnic groups (8,9). In the Northern Italian population, disease risk is intermediate with yearly incidence rates of about 6 cases per 100,000 individuals (10). In Asian countries, GCA and PMR are distinctly infrequent.

Nonrandomness in the geographical and ethnic distribution of GCA is highly suggestive of genetic risk determinants but it could also indicate a contribution of environmental factors. Evidence for disease-risk genes has come from studies exploring the representation of *HLA-DRB* genes in GCA/PMR (11,12). In both conditions, donors expressing *HLA-DR4* alleles are enriched. Sequence comparison of disease-associated and non–disease associated *HLA-DR* polymorphisms has led to the hypothesis that amino acid positions located directly in the antigen binding site of HLA dimers confer the highest risk, supporting the notion that antigen binding and presentation are critical steps in the disease. It can be expected that other genes with a role in the immune system can modulate the susceptibility of the host to develop GCA.

GCA is markedly age-restricted. Essentially no cases have been reported in individuals younger than 50 years of age and the likelihood of being diagnosed with this vasculitis increases continuously with age (13). With aging, the immune system undergoes dramatic changes, generally described as immunosenescence (14). Multiple processes are suspected to contribute to the decline in immunocompetence in the elderly but a major factor has been attributed to deteriorating thymic function and output. Functional consequences of immunosenescence include a progressive loss of antivaccine responses, increased risk for infections, and reduced antitumor immunity. Coincidentally, older individuals have a higher incidence of clonal disorders and more frequently have autoantibodies. How, exactly, age-related perturbations in the immune system affect immunoreactivity in hosts with GCA has not been investigated.

IV. SYSTEMIC MANIFESTATIONS

Besides vascular lesions, GCA patients consistently have signs of systemic inflammation. Monocytes in the circulation have been found to be constitutively activated and synthesize interleukin-6 (IL-6) protein (15). Interleukin-6 is a potent inducer of acute phase reactants, providing an excellent explanation for the highly upregulated acute phase response in GCA. Laboratory abnormalities in untreated disease are typical for an abrupt acute phase reaction. A close relation between muscle pain/stiffness with plasma IL-6 levels has been reported in patients with PMR, and plasma IL-6 concentrations have been shown to be exquisitely sensitive to corticosteroid suppression with rebounding elevated IL-6 levels by 24 after a dose of oral steroids (16).

Production of IL-6 by circulating monocytes/macrophages emphasizes the systemic nature of the disease. This component of the syndrome is equally developed in PMR and GCA, supporting the notion that it is independent from florid vasculitis and likely precedes vascular lesions. Both disease components, the systemic inflammatory illness and the emergence of arteritic infiltrates, differ in their sensitivity to steroid therapy, providing additional evidence for the concept that these two aspects of the disease process are independently regulated.

In PMR patients, the systemic component overshadows the vascular involvement. However, in other patients, the systemic inflammatory illness is dominant but coexists with overt vasculitis. In these patients, the clinical pattern is often not that of cranial ischemia but fever of unknown origin, weight loss, night sweats, anemia, and wasting. Analysis of tissue cytokine patterns in temporal arteries have indicated that patients with cranial ischemia and patients with wasting syndrome can be distinguished based upon the production of interferon-γ (IFN-γ) in the vascular lesions (17). In patients with wasting syndrome, acute phase responses appear to be even more activated than in patients with cranial ischemia (18).

V. NATURE OF THE IMMUNOLOGICAL INJURY

Multiple lines of evidence have led to the conclusion that the center of the immune response in the vascular lesions lies in the adventitia (Fig. 2). The adventitia supports the vasa vasorum, mi-

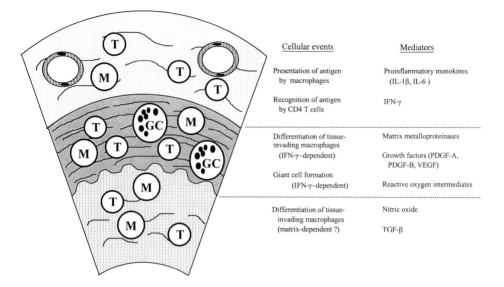

Cellular events	Mediators
Presentation of antigen by macrophages	Proinflammatory monokines (IL-1β, IL-6)
Recognition of antigen by CD4 T cells	IFN-γ
Differentiation of tissue-invading macrophages (IFN-γ–dependent)	Matrix metalloproteinases
	Growth factors (PDGF-A, PDGF-B, VEGF)
Giant cell formation (IFN-γ–dependent)	Reactive oxygen intermediates
Differentiation of tissue-invading macrophages (matrix-dependent ?)	Nitric oxide
	TGF-β

Figure 2 Immune insult in giant cell arteritis. Immune events in the artery are compartmentalized with a close correlation between the topography of the vessel wall and immune pathways. T-cell activation by antigen occurs in the adventitia with subsequent differentiation of macrophages in the media and intima to assume specialized effector functions.

crocapillaries that supply the vessel wall with nutrients and oxygen. CD4+ T cells bearing activation markers accumulate in the areas surrounding the vasa vasorum (19). Most importantly, these T cells are the producers of IFN-γ, a key player in the vascular immune reaction. In arteries from patients with PMR and no apparent cell infiltration or histomorphological vascular wall destruction, in situ production of cytokines can be documented (3). However, the adventitial immune response is aborted and is limited to IL-2 production without IFN-γ. Possible explanations include decreased levels of immunogen and reduced frequencies of antigen-specific precursor T cells. Antigen-presenting cells displaying immunogenic peptides on their surface have not been formally identified, but macrophages producing high amounts of IL-1β and IL-6 are the most likely candidates. Vasa vasorum can be assumed to be their port of entrance (20). Preactivation of tissue-invading monocytes in the periphery would enhance their antigen-presenting capability; however, the origin of the antigen initiating an adventitial immune response has not been demonstrated. Alternatives include that the antigen travels to the adventitia in macrophages that have phagocytosed it outside of the blood vessel wall and begin to display it as a result of their activation. Antigen could be trapped in the adventitial tissue as a result of directed or unintentional deposition from the bloodstream. Finally, arterial wall components could become antigenic. The hypothesis that constituents of the artery acquire immunogenicity, possibly reflecting age-related alterations, is attractive but experimental data are lacking. Extracts prepared from temporal arteries of GCA and PMR patients activate T cell lines generated from vascular infiltrates, strongly supporting the idea that antigens eliciting the vascular lesions are shared among patients and are present in PMR arteries (21).

T cells assumed to contact antigen in the adventitia are classical T-cell receptor α/β T cells that undergo clonal expansion in the arterial wall (22). Their repertoire is limited; identical T-cell clonotypes have been isolated from right- and left-side temporal arteries and from nonadjacent lesions in the vessel wall.

It is important to note that the immune response in the adventitia has not been associated with structural changes in this layer, correlating with the observation that macrophages accompanying adventitial T cells have an inflammatory but not a tissue destructive phenotype, e.g., they produce inflammatory cytokines but no matrix metalloproteinases and no oxygen radicals (20).

An unresolved but fascinating issue is how the immune reaction in the adventitia distally regulates the vascular inflammation occurring in the media and intima. Cytokines released by activated cells are prime candidates for facilitating this communication. The major T-cell products in the artery are IL-2 and IFN-γ, and concentrations of these cytokines produced in the tissue have been associated with differences in clinical manifestations (17). Specifically, cranial ischemia presenting as ocular symptoms or jaw claudication has been correlated with high IFN-γ production, whereas dominant systemic disease is typical for patients with low IFN-γ transcription. The IFN-γ levels are also predictive for the presence of multinucleated giant cells, a cell type usually not encountered in the adventitia (23).

VI. DAMAGE TO THE ARTERIAL WALL

One of the downstream effects of antigen-driven T-cell activation in GCA is vessel wall destruction. Smooth muscle cells disappear and the elastic membranes undergo fragmentation. Nevertheless, aneurysm formation and vessel rupture do not occur in cranial arteries but are limited to patients with aortitis (24). Progress has been made in identifying pathways of tissue injury in the lesions but much work remains to be done. Disintegration of the elastic laminae requires enzymatic action and metalloproteinases are abundantly expressed in the inflamed arterial wall (20,25,26). Loss of smooth muscle cells is less well understood, but potential mechanisms include apoptosis and necrosis.

Only recently a novel pathway of tissue injury in GCA arteries, lipid peroxidation of cellular membranes, has been described. Lipid peroxidation products are generated by reactive oxygen intermediates targeting lipid components of the cell membrane (27,28). While toxic oxygen metabolites are difficult to detect in the tissue due to their extremely short half-life, aldehydes formed by their interaction with lipid groups are easily identified through antibodies binding to 4-hydroxynoneal. In temporal arteries, medial smooth muscle cells and infiltrating inflammatory cells were both affected by oxidation-mediated membrane damage. However, mitochondria are highly active in tissue-infiltrating cells, indicating that these cell populations do not experience oxidative damage. Experimental evidence has been provided that some of the cells can protect themselves from oxidative stress by upregulating aldose reductase (28). Aldose reductase metabolizes toxic aldehydes, thus functioning as a detoxifier for oxidative damage. There is preliminary evidence that the oxidative injury in GCA also includes nitration. Nitric oxide–dependent tyrosine nitration can be demonstrated, particularly in areas of granuloma formation (Weyand et al., unpublished data).

VII. THE ARTERY'S PERSPECTIVE

Consequences of vascular wall inflammation are not limited to tissue destruction. On the contrary, in many cases of GCA, the predominant outcome of vasculitis is luminal obstruction (Fig. 3; see color plate). Specifically, the intima, normally a single-cell layer with barrier function, increases in thickness due to proliferation of myofibroblasts and excessive deposition of extracellular matrix, eventually causing obstruction of the lumen. Intimal hyperplasia results from the artery's response to inflammatory injury and represents a repair mechanism. Recognizing that the artery is not just passive in arteritis has been conceptually important in studying GCA. In this context, it is important to realize that the arterial wall has several options in responding to the immune insult. Upregulation of protective proteins, such as heat-shock proteins, occurs. The artery's response pattern also includes generative processes, including tissue proliferation and healing. The most fascinating aspect is that the artery's response may actually be maladaptive, exacerbating injury and creating novel pathology.

Thickening of the intimal layer has been extensively studied in atherosclerotic disease (29) and is now also understood as an important component of transplant vasculopathy. Marked progress has been made in identifying the cellular components involved and intense research is currently focusing on elucidating the underlying molecular events.

Intimal hyperplasia in GCA has features that distinguish it from atherosclerotic vascular disease. In particular, hyperproliferation in inflamed arteries of GCA patients is a fast process with concentric progression that almost obliterates the lumen. In contrast, in response to the atherosclerotic plaque, intimal proliferation progresses slowly and asymmetrically. It is possible that arteries, ranging from coronary arteries to temporal arteries, have evolved a program by which they communicate, interact, and react to the presence of immune cells and other insults. The consequences of this response-to-injury program is clinically one of the most important aspects of vascular disease.

How the arterial wall senses the injury is not known. Cells resembling smooth muscle cells become mobile, begin to proliferate, and initiate secretory activities. The origin of these cells has not been unequivocally identified and possibilities range from dedifferentiated medial smooth muscle cells to adventitial cells or even rare smooth muscle cells trapped in the intima (30). Growth, migration, and matrix production of these cells is under the control of growth factors. Also, metalloproteinases are required for the mobilization and penetration of these cells through the tissue. Recent studies have demonstrated that all of these components are present in temporal arteries in GCA. Platelet-derived growth factor (PDGF)-A and PDGF-B are both abundantly expressed, and tissue expression levels are closely related to the degree of luminal stenosis (31). Tissue production of PDGF has also been associated with the occurrence of ischemic symptoms, supporting the concept that vascular obstruction is one of the critical outcomes in this arteritis.

In contrast to transplantation vasculopathy and atherosclerosis, resident cells of the wall contribute minimally to PDGF production in GCA arteries; infiltrating mononuclear cells are the major cellular source of PDGF. Most interestingly, multinucleated giant cells also synthesized PDGF. This study provided the first evidence that multinucleated giant cells have secretory capabilities in addition to having roles in tissue digestion and debris removal (31).

Multinucleated giant cells also produce vascular endothelial growth factor (VEGF), an angiogenesis factor with the ability to support the growth of new capillaries (23). The normal arterial wall is a rather avascular tissue with vasa vasorum restricted to the adventitia. With florid panarteritis, new capillaries are formed throughout the wall with a majority forming in the hyperplastic intima. It has been proposed that multinucleated giant cells regulate multiple steps in the arterial response-to-injury program, including the release of tissue-mobilizing metalloproteinases, the provision of proliferation-inducing growth factors, and the production of angiogenesis factors. Tissue production of angiogenesis factors can probably be complemented by mediators in the circulation, such as haptoglobin (32).

VIII. MECHANISMS OF ACTION OF CORTICOSTEROIDS

One of the characteristic features of GCA is the prompt improvement of symptoms upon initiation of corticosteroid therapy. In PMR, the explicit sensitivity of clinical symptoms has been suggested as a diagnostic criterion to distinguish PMR from other inflammatory diseases. There is little, if any, evidence that corticosteroids can be replaced in treating GCA, emphasizing the unique role of steroid-mediated immunosuppression in this vasculitis. Understanding the mechanisms of action of this treatment could thus provide valuable insights into pathogenic pathways.

Studies of in vivo effects of glucocorticoids in the inflamed arterial wall required the establishment of an appropriate experimental system. Such a system was created when temporal arteries harvested from patients were successfully implanted into severe combined immunodeficiency mice. These chimeric mice can then be treated with corticosteroids and molecular events can be compared in explants from control and treated animals.

Steroid therapy is not able to deplete the transmural inflammatory infiltrates, but it alters functional activities of tissue-invading cells (33). Steroid injection is accompanied by the suppression of many inflammatory mediators. However, some of the mediators are steroid resistant and very high doses of steroids have to be administered to inhibit steroid-responsive cytokines. The T-cell product IFN-γ and the macrophage product transforming growth factor-β (TGF-β) are hardly affected by steroids, while IL-1β, IL-6, and IL-2 transcripts are downregulated. Comparison of the promoter regions of steroid-responsive and steroid-resistant genes revealed an association of steroid responsiveness with the presence of NF-κB binding sites. Studies in tissue sections from explanted temporal arteries of steroid-treated mice chimeras have demonstrated a lack of nuclear NF-κB (33). Cytoplasmic trapping of the transcription factor could be attributed to the induction of the physiological inhibitor IκBα (34).

These data provide an explanation for the promptness of the therapeutic effects seen with glucocorticoids, which is often combined with normalization of the acute phase reaction, a process involving a series of NF-κB-dependent genes (Fig. 4). The persistence of inflammatory lesions and the continued production of some of the proinflammatory mediators also explains

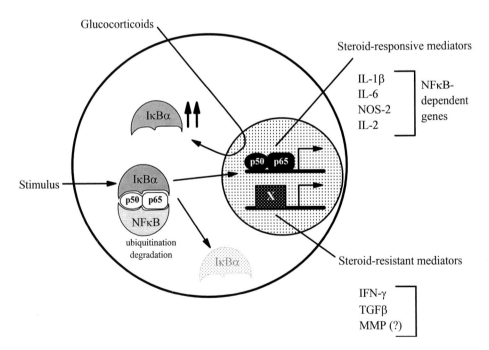

Figure 4 Mechanism of steroid-induced immunosuppression. Glucocorticoids upregulate the production of the NFκB-binding protein IκB and therefore prevent the nuclear translocation of active NKκB upon cell stimulation. Cytoplasmic trapping of NF-κB leads to the repression of NF-κB-dependent cytokines and mediators.

why GCA patients have to been treated chronically and do not tolerate early and abrupt withdrawal of steroids.

If the major mechanism of steroids in GCA and PMR is the inhibition of the NF-κB, then NF-κB-regulated gene activation appears to be variable among patients (35). A recent prognostic treatment trial in PMR has indicated that steroid requirements differ among patients. The need for steroid medication was estimated by measuring the occurrence of disease flares with dose reduction. A subset of patients had a short and uncomplicated disease course with excellent response to therapy and no recurrence of disease activity upon tapering. A second subset of patients responded well initially when steroid doses were high but experienced recurrent pain and stiffness when doses were decreased. Finally, one subset of patients was only partially responsive to initial steroid treatment. Differences in steroid doses required for clinically satisfactory management correlated with pretreatment erythrocyte sedimentation rates and with the degree of steroid-induced inhibition of IL-6 synthesis. It remains to be explored whether differences in inflammatory activity and insensitivity to steroid-mediated suppression of NF-κB reflect genuine heterogeneity of disease pathways or diversity in the responsiveness to a fundamentally identical disease initiator.

Lessons learned from studying therapeutic effects of steroids in GCA and PMR can be integrated into the disease model discussed earlier in this chapter (see Fig. 1). The two disease components, the systemic inflammatory reaction and the vascular lesions, appear to respond differently to corticosteroid therapy. The rapid improvement occurs despite persistent vascular infiltrates and almost certainly is related to inhibiting the release of proinflammatory cytokines in the periphery. Thus, steroids are clearly insufficient to eradicate the disease instigator. Nevertheless, they remain powerful therapeutic instruments to relieve symptoms and patients can eventually be taken off steroids while sustaining clinical remission.

IX. SUMMARY AND FUTURE CHALLENGES

The vascular pathology characteristic of GCA results from an immune insult (see Fig. 2) that initiates a reaction pattern in the arterial wall leading to structural changes, some of which are critically involved in luminal occlusion and subsequent ischemia (see Fig. 3). The precise mechanisms triggering the immune stimulation are not yet known but evidence suggests that arterial wall inflammation is preceded by activation of immune cells in the circulation and an intense acute phase response (see Fig. 1). In the artery, activated T cells localize preferentially in the vicinity of vasa vasorum, indicating a critical role of the adventitia in this vasculitis. Through the production of IFN-γ, these T cells can regulate and control the activity of macrophages, of which several functional subsets are represented in the artery. A close correlation between macrophage effector function and arterial wall layer suggests a direct contribution of the arterial microenvironment in the recruitment and differentiation of these effector cells. Tissue-damaging effector functions of macrophages include the release of metalloproteinases and the production of reactive oxygen metabolites. The arterial wall resident cells react to the immune insult by the induction of pathways that are not protective or regenerative but are maladaptive. Clinically, the most important maladaptive response is the mobilization, migration, and proliferation of smooth muscle cells to form lumen-obstructive neointima (see Fig. 4). This ill-fated injury response is supported by the formation of new microcapillaries. Growth factors regulating intimal hyperplasia and neoangiogenesis derive from tissue-invading macrophages, placing ultimate control of the arterial injury response program to the immune system. Evidence has been provided that clinical patterns of GCA are variable and attempts are being made to correlate the heterogeneity of the immune insult and diverse arterial response patterns to variations in clinical disease. Future challenges include the identification of the antigen driving the immune insult, with the potential outcome that arteritis is a common pathway triggered by multiple different antigens. Efforts should focus on identifying host risk elements, such as genetic susceptibility and environmental factors, that determine the initial immune stimulation, control the influx of cells into the arterial wall, regulate the persistence of immune reactivity, and modulate the artery's response to the immune insult.

REFERENCES

1. Lie JT. Illustrated histopathologic classification criteria for selected vasculitis syndromes. American College of Rheumatology Subcommittee on Classification of Vasculitis. Arthritis Rheum 1990; 33:1074–1087.
2. Brack A, Martinez-Taboada V, Stanson A, Goronzy JJ, Weyand CM. Disease pattern in cranial and large-vessel giant cell arteritis. Arthritis Rheum 1999; 42:311–317.
3. Weyand CM, Hicok KC, Hunder GG, Goronzy JJ. Tissue cytokine patterns in patients with polymyalgia rheumatica and giant cell arteritis. Ann Intern Med 1994; 121:484–491.
4. Weyand CM, Goronzy JJ. Arterial wall injury in giant cell arteritis. Arthritis Rheum 1999; 42:844–853.
5. Brack A, Geisler A, Martinez-Taboada VM, Younge BR, Goronzy JJ, Weyand CM. Giant cell vasculitis is a T cell-dependent disease. Mol Med 1997; 3:530–543.
6. Machado EB, Michet CJ, Ballard DJ, Hunder GG, Beard CM, Chu CP, O'Fallon WM. Trends in incidence and clinical presentation of temporal arteritis in Olmsted County, Minnesota, 1950–1985. Arthritis Rheum 1988; 31:745–749.
7. Nordborg E, Bengtsson BA. Epidemiology of biopsy-proven giant cell arteritis (GCA). J Intern Med 1990; 227:233–236.
8. Smith CA, Fidler WJ, Pinals RS. The epidemiology of giant cell arteritis. Report of a ten-year study in Shelby County, Tennessee. Arthritis Rheum 1983; 26:1214–1219.
9. Gonzalez EB, Varner WT, Lisse JR, Daniels JC, Hokanson JA. Giant-cell arteritis in the southern United States. An 11-year retrospective study from the Texas Gulf Coast. Arch Intern Med 1989; 149: 1561–1565.
10. Salvarani C, Macchioni P, Zizzi F, Mantovani W, Rossi F, Castri C, Capozzoli N, Baricchi R, Boiardi L, Chiaravalloti F. Epidemiologic and immunogenetic aspects of polymyalgia rheumatica and giant cell arteritis in northern Italy. Arthritis Rheum 1991; 34:351–356.
11. Weyand CM, Hicok KC, Hunder GG, Goronzy JJ. The HLA-DRB1 locus as a genetic component in giant cell arteritis. Mapping of a disease-linked sequence motif to the antigen binding site of the HLA-DR molecule. J Clin Invest 1992; 90:2355–2361.
12. Weyand CM, Hunder NN, Hicok KC, Hunder GG, Goronzy JJ. HLA-DRB1 alleles in polymyalgia rheumatica, giant cell arteritis, and rheumatoid arthritis. Arthritis Rheum 1994; 37:514–520.
13. Hunder GG, Bloch DA, Michel BA, Stevens MB, Arend WP, Calabrese LH, Edworthy SM, Fauci AS, Leavitt RY, Lie JT. The American College of Rheumatology 1990 criteria for the classification of giant cell arteritis. Arthritis Rheum 1990; 33:1122–1128.
14. Miller RA. The aging immune system: Primer and prospectus. Science 1996; 273:70–74.
15. Wagner AD, Goronzy JJ, Weyand CM. Functional profile of tissue-infiltrating and circulating CD68+ cells in giant cell arteritis. Evidence for two components of the disease. J Clin Invest 1994; 94:1134–1140.
16. Roche NE, Fulbright JW, Wagner AD, Hunder GG, Goronzy JJ, Weyand CM. Correlation of interleukin-6 production and disease activity in polymyalgia rheumatica and giant cell arteritis. Arthritis Rheum 1993; 36:1286–1294.
17. Weyand CM, Hicok KC, Hunder GG, Goronzy JJ. Tissue cytokine patterns in patients with polymyalgia rheumatica and giant cell arteritis. Ann Intern Med 1994; 121:484–491.
18. Cid MC, Font C, Oristrell J, de la Sierra A, Coll-Vinent B, Lopez-Soto A, Vilaseca J, Urbano-Marquez A, Grau JM. Association between strong inflammatory response and low risk of developing visual loss and other cranial ischemic complications in giant cell (temporal) arteritis. Arthritis Rheum 1998; 41:26–32.

19. Wagner AD, Bjornsson J, Bartley GB, Goronzy JJ, Weyand CM. Interferon-gamma-producing T cells in giant cell vasculitis represent a minority of tissue-infiltrating cells and are located distant from the site of pathology. Am J Pathol 1996; 148:1925–1933.

20. Weyand CM, Wagner AD, Bjornsson J, Goronzy JJ. Correlation of the topographical arrangement and the functional pattern of tissue-infiltrating macrophages in giant cell arteritis. J Clin Invest 1996; 98: 1642–1649.

21. Martinez-Taboada V, Hunder NN, Hunder GG, Weyand CM, Goronzy JJ. Recognition of tissue residing antigen by T cells in vasculitic lesions of giant cell arteritis. J Mol Med 1996; 74:695–703.

22. Weyand CM, Schonberger J, Oppitz U, Hunder NN, Hicok KC, Goronzy JJ. Distinct vascular lesions in giant cell arteritis share identical T cell clonotypes. J Exp Med 1994; 179:951–960.

23. Kaiser M, Younge BR, Bjornsson J, Weyand CM, Goronzy JJ. Formation of new vasa vasorum in vasculitis: Production of angiogenic cytokines by multinucleated giant cells. Am J Pathol 1999; 155:765–774.

24. Evans JM, O'Fallon WM, Hunder GG. Increased incidence of aortic aneurysm and dissection in giant cell (temporal) arteritis. A population-based study. Ann Intern Med 1995; 122:502–507.

25. Nikkari ST, Hoyhtya M, Isola J, Nikkari T. Macrophages contain 92-kd gelatinase (MMP-9) at the site of degenerated internal elastic lamina in temporal arteritis. Am J Pathol 1996; 149:1427–1433.

26. Sorbi D, French DL, Nuovo GJ, Kew RR, Arbeit LA, Gruber BL. Elevated levels of 92-kd type IV collagenase (matrix metalloproteinase 9) in giant cell arteritis. Arthritis Rheum 1996; 39:1747–1753.

27. Rittner HL, Kaiser M, Brack A, Szweda LI, Goronzy JJ, Weyand CM. Tissue destructive macrophages in giant cell arteritis. Circ Res 1999; 84:1050–1058.

28. Rittner HL, Hafner V, Klimiuk PA, Szweda LI, Goronzy JJ, Weyand CM. Aldose reductase functions as a detoxification system for lipid peroxidation products in vasculitis. J Clin Invest 1999; 103:1007–1013.

29. Ross R. Atherosclerosis—an inflammatory disease. N Engl J Med 1999; 340:115–26.

30. Barker SG, Talbert A, Cottam S, Baskerville PA, Martin JF. Arterial intimal hyperplasia after occlusion of the adventitial vasa vasorum in the pig. Arterioscler Thromb 1993; 13:70–77.

31. Kaiser M, Weyand CM, Bjornsson J, Goronzy JJ. Platelet-derived growth factor, intimal hyperplasia, and ischemic complications in giant cell arteritis. Arthritis Rheum 1998; 41:623–633.

32. Cid MC, Grant DS, Hoffman GS, Auerbach R, Fauci AS, Kleinman HK. Identification of haptoglobin as an angiogenic factor in sera from patients with systemic vasculitis. J Clin Invest 1993; 91:977–985.

33. Brack A, Rittner HL, Younge BR, Kaltschmidt C, Weyand CM, Goronzy JJ. Glucocorticoid-mediated repression of cytokine gene transcription in human arteritis-SCID chimeras. J Clin Invest 1997; 99: 2842–2850.

34. Scheinman RI, Cogswell PC, Lofquist AK, Baldwin ASJ. Role of transcriptional activation of I kappa B alpha in mediation of immunosuppression by glucocorticoids. Science 1995; 270:283–286.

35. Weyand CM, Fulbright JW, Evans JM, Hunder GG, Goronzy JJ. Corticosteroid requirements in polymyalgia rheumatica. Arch Intern Med 1999; 159:577–584.

29
Giant Cell Arteritis: Clinical Aspects

Gene G. Hunder
Mayo Clinic and Mayo Foundation, Rochester, Minnesota

Robert M. Valente
Arthritis Center of Nebraska, Lincoln, Nebraska

I. INTRODUCTION

Giant cell arteritis (GCA), a relatively common form of vasculitis in the United States and Europe, is also referred to as temporal arteritis, cranial arteritis, and Horton's disease (1–4). It affects persons over 50 years of age and approximately 90% of patients are over 60 years of age when the disease begins (5). Giant cell arteritis involves the cranial branches of the arteries originating from the arch of the aorta most prominently, but is often more generalized (6,7).

II. EPIDEMIOLOGY

Published incidence rates have varied considerably depending on ethnic background of the population studied. Highest rates have been reported in northern Europe and in the United States in populations of similar derivation (5,8–12). In Iceland, one of the highest rates, 50 cases per year per 100,000 population over age 50, has been noted (8). In Olmsted County, Minnesota, an average annual incidence of 17.8 cases per 100,000 persons over age 50 was found, producing a prevalence rate of 1 per 500 persons aged 50 years and older (5). Several studies suggest that the incidence rate is increasing. In Olmsted County, the rate increased from 6.2 to 19.1 per 100,000 persons per year over a 42-year study period (5). In the same study, a clustering of cases of giant cell arteritis in five peaks about 7 years apart was noted (Fig. 1). The cause of the clusters is uncertain but could represent involvement in the development of this condition by some infectious agent (13). Recent studies in Denmark have also shown considerable variation in the incidence of GCA (14). Age-specific rates show a progressive increase after age 50 (5). Autopsy studies suggest that giant cell arteritis may be even more frequent. Arteritis was found in 1.6% of 889 patients dying over the age of 50 in which sections of the temporal artery and two transverse sections of the aorta were examined (15).

Incidence rates of the closely related syndrome polymyalgia rheumatica (PMR) have been reported less widely but appear to be greater than for GCA. In Olmsted County, Minnesota, an average annual incidence rate of 52.5 per 100,000 persons 50 years of age and older. The prevalence was approximately 1 per 200 persons age 50 and above (16).

425

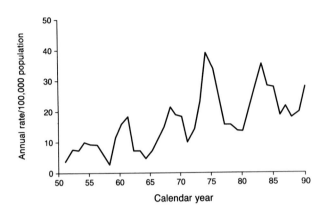

Figure 1   Annual incidence rates of giant cell arteritis in Olmsted County, Minnesota, per 100,000 people 50 years of age or older showing a cyclic pattern. Rates were calculated using a centered 3-year moving average. (Modified from Ref. 16.)

III. CLINICAL FEATURES

The mean age at onset of GCA is about 70 years, with a range of 50 to greater than 90 years (5,17). Women are affected about twice as frequently as men. The onset is usually gradual over several weeks, but may be abrupt. Clinical features of GCA are extremely variable. Constitutional symptoms, including progressive tiredness and loss of appetite and weight, are present in many patients and may be the initial manifestations. Low-grade fever has been noted in up to half of patients, and about 15% have a higher temperature elevation producing clinical findings of a "fever of unknown origin" (FUO) (18). The initial manifestations in 100 consecutive temporal artery–positive biopsy cases are listed in Table 1.

   At some time during the course of the disease, most patients with GCA have symptoms related the involved arteries (17). Clinical features in 100 patients with GCA are listed in Table 2.

Table 1   Initial Manifestation in 100 Patients with Giant Cell Arteritis

Manifestation	No. of Patients
Headache	32
Polymyalgia rheumatica	25
Fever	15
Visual symptoms without loss	7
Weakness, malaise, or fatigue	5
Tenderness over arteries	3
Myalgias	4
Weight loss or anorexia	2
Jaw claudication	2
Permanent loss of vision	1
Tongue claudication	1
Sore throat	1
Vasculitis on angiogram	1
Stiffness of hands and wrists	1
	100

Source: Ref. 17.

Table 2 Giant Cell Arteritis: Clinical Findings in 100 Patients

Finding	Number
Sex (female/male)	69/31
Duration of manifestations before diagnosis (months)[a]	7 (1–48)
Onset (gradual/sudden)	64/36
Weight loss or anorexia	50
Malaise, fatigue, or weakness	40
Fever	42
Polymyalgia rheumatica	39
Other musculoskeletal pains	30
Synovitis	15
Symptoms related to arteries	83
Headache	68
Visual symptoms	
Transient	
Fixed	16
Jaw claudication	14
Swallowing claudication or dysphagia	45
Tongue claudication	8
Limb claudication	6
Signs related to arteries	4
Artery tenderness	66
Decreased temporal artery pulsations	27
Erythematous, nodular, or swollen scalp arteries	46
Large artery bruits	23
Decreased large artery pulses	21
Ophthalmological	7
Visual loss	20
Ophthalmoscopic	14
Extraocular muscle weakness	18
Raynaud's phenomenon	2
Central nervous system abnormalities	3
Sore throat	15
	9

[a]Shown as mean with range in parentheses.
Source: Ref. 17.

Headache is the most frequent symptom and is present in about two-thirds or more of patients. It is usually present early in the course of the disease. The discomfort is often localized to the temporal areas but may be frontal, occipital, or more diffuse. It is often severe, but may be mild. At times, headache may become less marked or change location even before treatment is started. It is a type of headache that the patient has not experienced before (17,19).

Loss of vision is the most important early manifestation of GCA because of its devastating consequences (20,21). It is caused by ischemia of the optic nerve or tracts secondary to arteritis of the branches of the ophthalmic or posterior ciliary arteries and occasionally is caused by occlusion of the retinal arterioles. Arterial lesions in the distal cervical region or base of brain rarely result in infarction of the occipital cortex causing central blindness (21). The initial visual changes may be transitory (amaurosis fugax) but later become fixed (20). Early visual loss is usually unilateral and likely to be partial (20). But if the arteritis is not recognized and treated, the visual loss is often progressive and becomes bilateral within a few weeks or less (21). However, complete bilateral blindness is uncommon (20). The incidence of permanent loss of vision in recent series is about 20% (20,21). Ophthalmoscopic examination in patients without visual loss is generally normal. The early funduscopic appearance seen in those with visual loss is ischemic optic neuritis with slight pallor and edema of the optic disc and scattered cotton-wool patches and small hemorrhages (Fig. 2). Later, optic atrophy occurs. Diplopia and ptosis are also seen (20,21). In a 5-year follow-up study of 245 patients with GCA, Aiello et al. (20) found visual loss in 34 cases (14%). In 32 of these patients, the visual deficit developed before glucocorticoid therapy for GCA was begun. In the two other patients, the visual loss occurred after the diagnosis was made and therapy was started. Visual loss progressed in three patients after initiation of oral glucocorticoids, and in five others, vision improved after beginning prednisone. After a 5-year follow-up it was determined that the probability of developing visual loss after initiating treatment was 1% (Kaplan-Meier technique), and the probability of additional loss was 13% in patients with GCA who had a visual deficit at the time therapy was begun.

Intermittent claudication, or ischemic muscle pain, may occur in the jaw muscles, the extremities, and occasionally, the muscles of the tongue or those involved in swallowing (18). In jaw claudication, the discomfort is noted especially when chewing meat or other firm foods. It is generally bilateral, but may involve only one side. In some instances, spasm of the muscles of mastication may result and make opening of the mouth painful or not possible. A rare case of dysarthria due to GCA was recently reported (22). Claudication of the tongue or swallowing apparatus may occur with or without jaw pain. Sore throat and cough, usually nonproductive, occur in approximately 8% of cases (23). Examination of the upper airway usually shows little to explain the findings. Rarely, more severe vascular involvement may cause gangrene of the scalp or tongue (24).

Neurological findings have been described in up to 30% of patients (19,25). Other than visual loss, peripheral neuropathies and strokes or transient ischemic attacks are most common. Peripheral neurological manifestations include mononeuropathies and polyneuropathies. These are likely secondary to involvement of nutrient arteries, but little pathological documentation has

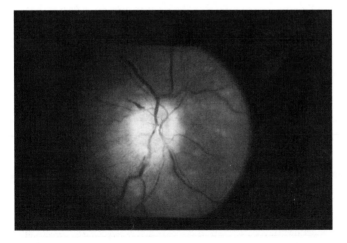

Figure 2   Ophthalmoscopic view of the acute phase of ischemic optic neuropathy as seen in patients with giant cell arteritis and loss of vision. The optic disc is pale and swollen, the retinal veins are dilated, and a flame-shaped hemorrhage is visible.

been reported. Brain stem events and hemiparesis are caused by narrowing or occlusion of the carotid or vertebrobasilar arteries. In our experience, these episodes usually occur in patients who do not have occlusive changes in the subclavian arteries. Caselli (26) described three patients with GCA who had multiinfarct dementia. In these patients, the lesions were found mainly in the posterior part of the brain and cerebellum.

Occlusive lesions develop in large proximal extremity arteries in about 15% of cases (7). Generally, these involve the upper extremity arteries, including the subclavian, axillary, and brachial arteries (27–30). The most common manifestations are arm claudication and reduced or absent arm pulses and blood pressures in one or both arms. Bruits over the subclavian, axillary, and brachial arteries are audible in many instances. The arms may become cool and cyanotic with use, but frank gangrene of the extremities is a rare occurrence. Cervical bruits are also likely to be present in such cases, but brain stem events or hemiparesis are less frequent in such patients. Angina pectoris, congestive heart failure, and myocardial infarction secondary to coronary arteritis occur in rare instances (31).

Polymyalgia rheumatica is a clinical syndrome closely linked to GCA (10,16,32,33). The population affected, sex ratio of involved persons, and age at onset are the same as in GCA. Polymyalgia rheumatica is characterized by the presence of proximal aching and morning stiffness and pain with movement of the proximal joints. The discomfort limits the patient's activities and frequently is severe enough to confine the patient to bed. Constitutional symptoms including fatigue and malaise are usually present. Low-grade fever occurs in a minority. The symptoms of PMR appear to be due to proximal synovitis and tenosynovitis (34). Patients with PMR and also GCA often also have peripheral joint synovitis (35–37). Criteria for the diagnosis of PMR usually include the presence of aching and morning stiffness lasting one-half hour or more, located in two of the three areas commonly affected (shoulder girdle, hip girdle, and neck or torso), accompanied by an elevated erythrocyte sedimentation rate or C-reactive protein (16). Polymyalgia rheumatica as a syndrome occurs 2 to 3 times more commonly than GCA (38). Thus, most patients with PMR have no overt clinical evidence of vasculitis throughout the course of their illness. However, in others, GCA and PMR may develop simultaneously or PMR may develop at some other time during the course of GCA. In some instances, for example, symptoms of PMR may be noted initially late in the course of GCA when the patient has been treated with prednisone and the dose has been subsequently reduced to low levels. Temporal artery biopsies obtained in patients with PMR who have no manifestations of vasculitis are found to be positive in about 10–15% of cases. In a minority of patients with PMR, more prominent distal tenosynovitis may develop, confusing the diagnosis. Some evidence points to the presence of a subclinical vasculitis in PMR (39).

Thoracic aortic aneurysms and dissection of the aorta are important late complications in GCA (40–42) (Fig. 3). A series from our center included 41 patients with this manifestation (Tables 3 and 4) (40). In three patients, the thoracic aortic aneurysms developed before GCA was diagnosed, in five near the time of the diagnosis, and in 33 after the diagnosis of GCA (median of 7 years after diagnosis). Sixteen patients developed acute aortic dissection, which caused death in eight. Nineteen patients also had aortic valve insufficiency due to aortic root dilation. Fifteen of these latter patients developed congestive heart failure. Eighteen patients underwent 21 surgical procedures for the aneurysm and/or aortic valve replacement or repair. Aortitis was documented histologically in 10 cases at surgery or autopsy. In the 33 who developed thoracic aortic findings subsequent to the diagnosis of GCA, 20 had discontinued prednisone therapy when the thoracic symptoms became manifest. However, in about half there was clinical evidence of active vasculitis, and most had elevated erythrocyte sedimentation rates, providing a clue to the presence of an underlying active vasculitis. In a subsequent population-based survey, 11 of 96 patients with GCA were found to have thoracic aortic aneurysms (41). Compared with all persons of the same

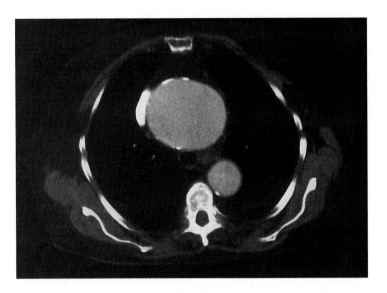

Figure 3   CT examination of the chest of a patient with giant cell arteritis with ascending thoracic aortic aneurysm. Transverse view shows eccentric dilation of ascending thoracic aorta.

Table 3   Cardiothoracic Manifestations in 41 Patients with Giant Cell Arteritis

Manifestation	No. of Patients
Aortic valve insufficiency murmur	19
Dyspnea on exertion	15
Chest pain from acute dissection	8
Sudden cardiac death from acute dissection	8
Paroxysmal nocturnal dyspnea	7
Peripheral edema	7
Angina pectoris	6
Orthopnea	5
Limb claudication	4
Arterial bruit	3
Pulmonary rales	4
Palpitations	2

Source: Ref. 40.

age and sex living in the same community, patients with GCA were 17.3 times more likely to develop thoracic aortic aneurysm and 2.4 times more likely to develop isolated abdominal aortic aneurysm.

IV.   LABORATORY FINDINGS

Laboratory tests reflect the inflammatory processes. A mild to moderate normochromic anemia is usually present. Acute phase reactant serum proteins are generally elevated to high levels (43–47).

Table 4 Initial Manifestation Related to the Thoracic Aorta in 41 Patients with Giant Cell Arteritis

Manifestation	No. of Patients
Asymptomatic aortic aneurysm	14
Dyspnea on exertion	8
Chest pain (acute dissection)	7
Asymptomatic aortic valve insufficiency	4
Sudden death (acute dissection)	4
Paroxysmal nocturnal dyspnea	1
Dysphagia (large aneurysm causing esophageal distortion)	1
Hemiparesis (cerebral embolus)	1
Leg pain (acute aortic dissection causing iliac artery occlusion)	1

Source: Ref. 40.

The erythrocyte sedimentation rate (ESR) is usually markedly elevated. Levels to 100 mm in 1 hour (Westergren method) are common, but occasionally, untreated biopsy-proven cases may have normal results (48,49). Some authors prefer the C-reactive protein (CRP) test as a more reliable diagnostic test and for following patients' therapy because it is not influenced as much by nonspecific changes such as anemia or significantly increased serum gamma globulins. Platelet counts are also often elevated. Recent studies have suggested that plasma interleukin-6 concentrations are more sensitive and specific as an indicator for the presence of vasculitis than other acute phase reactants (50–52). This cytokine is released from monocytes and macrophages and, when elevated, should directly indicate the presence of active vasculitis if other causes of inflammation have been excluded. The leukocyte and differential counts are generally normal. Serum complement and gamma globulins are normal or may be slightly increased (43). Tests for antinuclear antibodies and rheumatoid factor are usually normal.

Liver function tests have been found to be mildly to moderately abnormal in about one-third of patients with GCA (17,53–55). Increased serum aspartate transaminase (AST) and alkaline phosphatase are the most commonly reported tests but others may be abnormal as well. Function returns to normal with therapy.

Renal function tests are normal. Urinalysis is also usually normal, but red cells and red cell casts have been found in some instances (7,56). These do not appear to indicate significant renal vasculitis.

In patients with GCA and PMR, tests for muscle inflammation are normal, including serum creatine kinase and electromyograms. Muscle biopsies are normal or show mild atrophy (57).

Other tests reported to be increased include plasma factor VIII/von Willebrands factor, endothelial adhesion molecules, and anticardiolipin antibodies (58–65). While these tests likely reflect the pathological processes, they have not been shown clearly to be helpful in the diagnosis or management of patients with GCA.

V. DIAGNOSIS

A diagnosis of GCA should be considered in patients above 50 years of age who have a new form of headache along with systemic symptoms, those with abrupt visual loss without other explanation, in patients with polymyalgia rheumatica, unexplained fever or anemia, and high erythrocyte sedimentation rate, and those who have vascular manifestations such as outlined above. The symptoms of GCA vary in severity from one patient to another and may even improve without specific treatment. Thus, the patient should be questioned carefully about recent as well as current symptoms. The arteries of the head, neck, upper torso, and arms should be examined for tenderness, enlargement, or thrombosis and auscultated for bruits. Both the anterior and parietal branches of the superficial temporal arteries should be palpated. The occipital, facial, and posterior auricular arteries also should be palpated. When examining the scalp, a temporal artery that "rolls" under the examiner's finger rather than collapsing is usually abnormal. A tender or erythematous temporal artery has stronger diagnostic significance. However, the examiner needs to make sure that the artery itself is tender rather than the temporalis muscle or other scalp structures.

Artery biopsy is recommended in all patients suspected of having giant cell arteritis. The temporal artery is readily accessible and biopsied most frequently, but a specimen of the occipital or facial artery can also be taken for histological study if clearly abnormal. Giant cell arteritis tends to affect arteries in an irregularly intermittent fashion (66). Thus, a clinically abnormal segment of artery should be chosen for biopsy if possible. If the temporal artery is clearly visibly and palpably abnormal on examination, only a small specimen of that region needs to be removed for histological examination (Figs. 4 and 5). However, when the arteries are normal on examination, it is important to biopsy a longer, 3- to 4-cm segment of temporal artery and examine the specimen at several levels to obtain adequate sampling. In most instances, we recommend biopsy of the second side also if the first is normal on histological review. When possible, temporal artery biopsy should be carried out before starting on glucocorticoid treatment, although the inflammatory infiltrate is slow to resolve and biopsy can readily be carried out up to 2 weeks or perhaps more after initiating therapy if necessary (67,68). Mathematical models using clinical and laboratory data have not been highly sensitive to date in predicting a positive temporal artery biopsy (69). However, in one analysis of 535 patients with temporal artery biopsies, the presence of synovitis, a relatively low erythrocyte sedimentation rate, absence of jaw claudication, and absence of temporal artery tenderness predicted a 95% probability of a temporal artery biopsy showing no vasculitis (69).

Biopsy findings characteristic of this disease include infiltration of the vessel wall, especially the inner media near the internal elastic membrane, with lymphocytes, macrophages, and multinucleated giant cells (70). The internal elastic membrane becomes fragmented as a result of the inflammation. Occasional neutrophils and eosinophils may be present. Intimal thickening, but

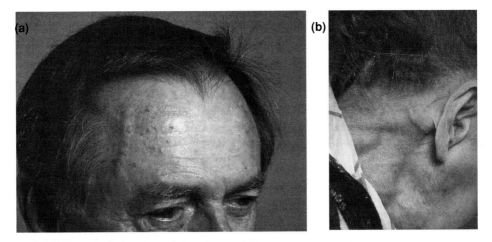

Figure 4   (a) Giant cell arteritis involving the temporal artery. The anterior branch of the right superficial temporal artery is visibly swollen. Tenderness was noted on examination. (b) In a different patient with giant cell arteritis, the posterior auricular artery was noted to be swollen, an uncommon finding.

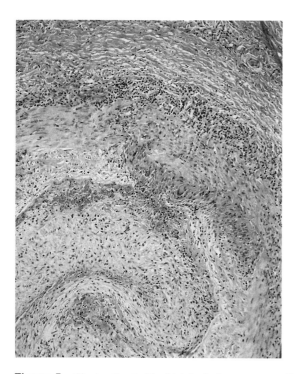

Figure 5 Giant cell arteritis, histological appearance. Transverse section of temporal artery, occluded lumen is at bottom left. Intense lymphocytic infiltration of the media is visible. Giant cells are visible near the inner media. (Hematoxylin and eosin, original magnification ×100.) (Courtesy of Dr. Johannes Bjornsson.)

with little inflammatory cell infiltration, is present in most cases. These classic findings are present in about 50% of positive cases examined by usual means. The other 50% show a similar inflammatory process with predominantly lymphocytes and macrophages but no giant cells. In some instances a panarteritis is seen. Thus, giant cells are not a required finding to make the diagnosis if clinical findings are compatible. Similar histopathological changes are present in other involved arteries (7,28).

Ultrasound examination of the temporal arteries has been of interest for some time (71–73). Recently color duplex ultrasonography of the temporal arteries has been reported to be helpful in the diagnosis of GCA. Schmidt et al. (73) found ultrasonographic abnormalities in most patients with GCA. Using color duplex ultrasonography, they noted a "halo" around the arterial lumen in the majority of patients given the diagnosis of GCA but not others (Fig. 6). If further studies show this finding to be as specific for GCA as these authors suggest, temporal artery biopsy may not be necessary in patients manifesting this change. In other patients, ultrasound alterations may help the clinician choose the best site of the temporal artery to biopsy. This test is noninvasive, available in many centers and may prove to enhance diagnosis of GCA. However, more experience is necessary before we recommend eliminating temporal artery biopsy in any case suspected of GCA (74,75).

An angiogram should be considered if large arteries are involved (7,29). This will help determine the extent of the vasculitis and the help separate GCA from a nonvasculitic cause such as atherosclerosis. As noted, GCA tends to affect the upper extremity arteries more commonly than the iliac vessels whereas the opposite is true in atherosclerosis. An arteriogram provides the best detail of large vessels (Fig. 7), but intravenous digital subtraction angiography may suffice in

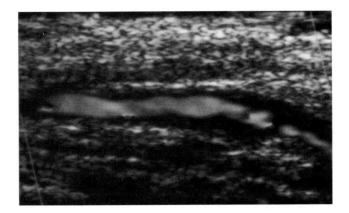

Figure 6 Duplex ultrasonography of the anterior branch of the right superficial temporal artery in a patient with giant cell arteritis. A clear hypoechoic "halo" is present over a portion of the artery (right side in the sonogram) where the temporal artery was visibly and palpably enlarged.

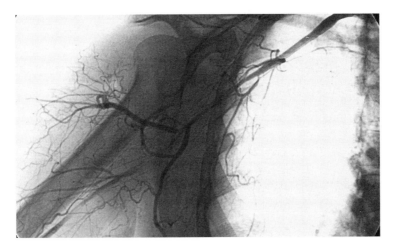

Figure 7 Giant cell arteritis of larger arteries. Arch aortogram. Right subclavian and axillary arteries are affected. Areas of smooth-walled segmental constrictions are visible. Distal axillary artery becomes occluded. Collateral vessels refill the brachial artery distal to the occlusion.

some cases. Magnetic resonance imaging (MRI) and computed tomography scans may help determine large artery involvement, but overall vascular changes are not defined as well by these procedures as arteriography (Fig. 8).

In patients with PMR without clinical evidence of GCA by history or physical examination, a decision regarding temporal artery biopsy is more difficult and should be based on the findings in each patient. If the musculoskeletal symptoms are mild and stable or of recent onset and a temporal artery ultrasound examination is normal, we recommend close follow-up without temporal artery biopsy. If a temporal artery ultrasound examination is abnormal, especially if a halo is present, a temporal artery biopsy should be obtained.

In most patients, there is little difficulty in distinguishing GCA from other forms of vasculitis because of the age, different clinical manifestations, distribution of lesions, and organ involvement. In occasional instances, however, other forms of vasculitis may involve the temporal

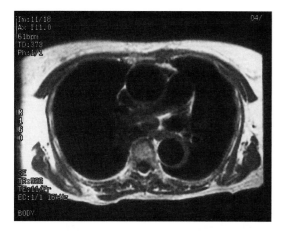

Figure 8 MRI of the chest in a patient with active giant cell arteritis. Thickened wall of descending thoracic aortic wall is visible and indicates aortitis.

artery and mimic GCA to the degree that a temporal artery biopsy is done and is found to show vasculitis (76,77). In most of these cases, however, the histopathology is different than in GCA. For example, in several forms of vasculitis, including polyarteritis nodosa, microscopic polyangiits, Churg–Strauss vasculitis, hypersensitivity vasculitis, and Wegener's granulomatosis, the biopsy findings characteristically show prominent artery wall infiltration by neutrophils or eosinophils in contrast to the typical lymphocytes, macrophages, and multinucleated giant cells in GCA (70,76). Takayasu's arteritis, which involves many of the same arteries as GCA and shares the same vascular histological appearance, occurs most commonly in patients of Asian ethnicity and begins before the age of 40. In Takayasu's arteritis, the temporal artery has not been shown to be affected frequently. Occasionally, amyloidosis causes jaw or arm claudication mimicking vasculitis. In such cases, the temporal artery biopsy shows the presence of amyloid deposits in amyloidosis, but no vasculitis (78).

Criteria for the classification of GCA have been formulated (79). These criteria differentiate this disease from other types of vasculitis and should be used in all studies of GCA to help describe the patient population in the investigation (Table 5).

VI. ASCERTAINMENT OF DISEASE ACTIVITY

Although the clinical presentations of GCA may vary widely from an FUO, unexplained anemia, thrombocytosis, or elevated ESR, to PMR or jaw pain, there is usually little difficulty determining the presence of active disease at the time of diagnosis. However, the ascertainment of active disease is often more difficult later in the course of the disease after a period of prednisone treatment, when this drug is being withdrawn to avoid adverse side effects. If a relapse occurs accompanied by fever, or vascular-related symptoms, the diagnosis of active disease can be straightforward. But a frequent experience in GCA is that during the period of prednisone withdrawal, blood tests show an elevated ESR or CRP but the patient has no symptoms, or only nonspecific complaints such as fatigue, which may be related to the treatment. In such instances, ascertainment of active disease is difficult or impossible with tests available today. Another temporal artery biopsy or arteriogram is impractical in most instances and unlikely to fundamentally help.

Table 5 1990 Criteria for the Classification of Giant Cell (Temporal) Arteritis (Traditional Format)[a]

Criterion	Definition
1. Age at disease onset ≥50 years	Development of symptoms or findings beginning at age 50 or older
2. New headache	New onset of or new type of localized pain in the head
3. Temporal artery abnormality	Temporal artery tenderness to palpation or decreased pulsation, unrelated to arteriosclerosis of cervical arteries
4. Elevated erythrocyte sedimentation rate	Erythrocyte sedimentation rate ≥50 mm/h by the Westergren method
5. Abnormal artery biopsy	Biopsy specimen with artery showing vasculitis characterized by a predominance of mononuclear cell infiltration or granulomatous inflammation, usually with multinucleated giant cells

[a]For purposes of classification, a patient with vasculitis shall be said to have giant cell (temporal) arteritis if at least three of these five criteria are present. The presence of any three or more criteria yields a sensitivity of 93.5% and a specificity of 91.2%.
Source: Ref. 79.

There is no experience with ultrasound regarding in the temporal artery in relapses. Interleukin-6 determinations may provide some guidance in this situation, but more experience is needed (80). Other acute phase reactants and hematological tests have not provided better answers. This is an area needing further study and development.

VII. MANAGEMENT

Once the diagnosis of GCA is established, prednisone or a related glucocorticoid should be started. Patients strongly suspected of the disease, especially those with recent or impending vascular complications such as visual loss, may be started on therapy immediately before a temporal artery biopsy. Glucocorticoids rapidly suppress the symptoms and prevent most subsequent vascular occlusions (20). However, the influence of glucocorticoids on the vascular wall inflammatory processes appears to be much more gradual and biopsies may be obtained later as noted above (67,68). In patients who have lost vision or who appear to be at immediate risk, intravenous pulses of glucocorticoid therapy can be given and later switched to oral treatment, although no data are available to show that parenteral therapy is more effective that oral therapy alone. We recommend starting between 40 and 60 mg of prednisone per day in a single or divided dose (81). If the patient does not clearly respond within 3 to 5 days, the dose can be increased by 10–20 mg/day temporarily. Although experience has shown that some patients are also likely to respond to lower doses, there are currently no reliable clinical or laboratory markers available to identify such patients before therapy is started. After 2 weeks, the dose can be reduced to 50 mg/day and at the end of 4 weeks, to 40 mg/day. The patient's reversible symptoms usually subside rapidly within a few days to a week or two. Thereafter, the prednisone dose can be reduced by approximately 10% of the daily dose each week or two as long as the symptoms and laboratory tests remain normal. Below the daily dose of 20 mg/day, the length between decrements can be increased to 2–4 weeks as appropriate to the patient's course. Below 10 mg/day, we recommend reducing the dose

1 mg/month as tolerated. The ESR or CRP can be obtained at monthly intervals to follow the patient along with a brief clinical assessment of the patients progress. If the ESR or CRP levels become mildly elevated again without a relapse of symptoms, the prednisone dose may be held at its current level for another 2–4 weeks and the laboratory tests repeated again. If normal at that time, the reduction schedule can be resumed. If the patient's symptoms return along with a significant increase in the ESR or CRP, the prednisone dose can be elevated again to a previous level that suppressed the manifestations. If has been our practice, later in the course of the disease, after several months of prednisone therapy, to attempt to gradually reduce the prednisone dose further even if the ESR or CRP are only slightly elevated provided no symptoms of GCA are present. If major adverse effects of prednisone have developed and it appears not possible to reduce prednisone because of active disease, a cytotoxic drug such as methotrexate may be added (82–84). However, available studies have not shown a clear steroid sparing for this or other drugs (85). A better therapeutic armamentarium for this disease is needed.

Most patients are eventually able to discontinue prednisone therapy. In our studies, the average duration of therapy is about 2 years, much of which is at low prednisone doses (86). But because of adverse reactions to glucocorticoids that occur in the majority of patients, the lowest dose possible must be used and a program to prevent osteoporosis should be instituted. Although most patients subsequently appear to do well, occasional relapses occur. Thus, the patients need to be followed periodically. In view of the high frequency of the development of aortic aneurysms after several years a chest x-ray is recommended at yearly intervals. Overall, there appears to be no increased mortality rate in patients with GCA compared with age-matched population.

VIII. SUMMARY

Giant cell arteritis is a vasculitis of unknown etiology that affects middle-aged and older persons. In some populations, it is the most common form of vasculitis. Although its clinical picture is extremely variable, early diagnosis is imperative because vascular occlusions caused by the vasculitis may result in blindness, stroke, and other severe problems. Fortunately, GCA responds quickly to glucocorticoid therapy. These drugs rapidly suppress reversible symptoms and laboratory test alterations associated with the disease and prevent further vascular occlusions. However, they appear to have a more gradual effect on some components of the inflammatory processes in the vessel walls. Temporal artery biopsy is recommended to confirm the diagnosis in all cases, preferably before treatment is started, but afterwards if necessary. Many patients have mild relapses of the disease as the glucocorticoid dose is being reduced, and some have them later. Most can discontinue this therapy within about 2 years. However, the majority of patients develop adverse effects from glucocorticoid therapy (86). Periodic long-term monitoring is indicated because of the high frequency of the development of aneurysm of the thoracic aorta.

REFERENCES

1. Gilmour JR. Giant-cell arteritis. J Pathol Bacteriol 1941; 53:263–277.
2. Horton BT, Magath TB, Brown GE. An undescribed form of arteritis of the temporal vessels. Proc Staff Meet Mayo Clin 1932; 7:700–701.
3. Kilbourne ED, Wolff HH. Cranial arteritis: A critical evaluation of the syndrome of "temporal arteritis" with report of a case. Ann Intern Med 1946; 24:1–10.
4. McMillan GC. Diffuse granulomatous aortitis with giant cells: Associated with partial rupture and dissection of the aorta. Arch Pathol 1950; 49:63–69.

5. Salvarani C, Gabriel SE, O'Fallon WM, et al. The incidence of giant cell arteritis in Olmsted County, Minnesota: Apparent fluctuations in cyclic pattern. Ann Intern Med 1995; 123:192–194.

6. Wilkinson IMS, Russell RWR. Arteries of the head and neck in giant cell arteritis: A pathological study to show the pattern of arterial involvement. Arch Neurol 1972; 27:378–391.

7. Klein RG, Hunder GG, Stanson AW, et al. Large artery involvement in giant cell (temporal) arteritis. Ann Intern Med 1975; 83:806–812.

8. Baldursson O, Steinsson K, Bjornsson J, et al. Giant cell arteritis in Iceland. An epidemiologic and histologic analysis. Arthritis Rheum 1994; 37:1007–1012.

9. Nordborg E, Bengtsson B-A. Epidemiology of biopsy-proven giant cell arteritis (GCA). J Intern Med 1990; 227:233–236.

10. Gran JT, Myklebust G. The incidence of polymyalgia rheumatica and temporal arteritis in the county of Aust Agder, South Norway: A prospective study 1987–94. J Rheumatol 1997; 24(9):1739–1743.

11. Boesen P, Sorensen SF. Giant cell arteritis, temporal arteritis and polymyalgia rheumatica in a Danish county: A prospective investigation, 1982–1985. Arthritis Rheum 1987; 30:294–299.

12. Barrier J, Pion P, Massari R, et al. Epidemiologic approach to Horton's disease in Department of Loire-Atlantique: 110 cases in 10 years (1970–1979). Rev Med Interne 1983; 3:13–20.

13. Espy MJ, Gabriel SE, Bjornsson J, et al. The role of parvovirus B19 in the pathogenesis of giant cell arteritis: A preliminary evaluation. Arthritis Rheum 1999; 42:1255–1258.

14. Elling P, Olsson AT, Elling H. Synchronous variations of the incidence of temporal arteritis and polymyalgia rheumatica in different regions of Denmark: Association with epidemics of Mycoplasma pneumoniae infection. J Rheumatol 1996; 23(1):112–119.

15. Ostberg G. Temporal arteritis in a large necropsy series. Ann Rheum Dis 1971; 30:224–235.

16. Salvarani C, Gabriel SE, O'Fallon WM, et al. Epidemiology of polymyalgia rheumatica in Olmsted County, Minnesota, 1970–1991. Arthritis Rheum 1995; 38:369–373.

17. Calamia KT, Hunder GG. Clinical manifestations of giant cell arteritis. Clin Rheum Dis 1980; 6:389–403.

18. Calamia KT, Hunder GG. Giant cell arteritis (temporal arteritis) presenting as fever of undetermined origin. Arthritis Rheum 1981; 24:1414–1418.

19. Casselli RJ, Hunder GG, Whisnant JP. Neurologic disease in biopsy-proven giant cell (temporal) arteritis. Neurology 1988; 38:352–359.

20. Aiello PD, Trautmann JC, McPhee TJ, et al. Visual prognosis in giant cell arteritis. Ophthalmology 1993; 100:550–555.

21. Hayreh SS, Podhajsky PA, Zimmerman B. Ocular manifestations of giant cell arteritis. Am J Ophthalmol 1998; 125(4):509–520.

22. Lee CC, Su WW, Hunder GG. Dysarthria associated with giant cell arteritis. J Rheumatol 1999; 26(4):931–932.

23. Larson TS, Hall S, Hepper NGG, et al. Respiratory tract symptoms as a clue to giant cell arteritis. Ann Intern Med 1984; 101:594–597.

24. Rudd JC, Fineman MS, Sergott RC. Ischemic scalp necrosis preceding loss of visual acuity in giant cell arteritis. Arch Ophthalmol 1998; 116(12):1690–1691.

25. Caselli RJ, Hunder GG. Giant cell (temporal) arteritis. Neurol Clin 1997; 15(4):893–902.

26. Caselli RJ. Giant cell (temporal) arteritis: A treatable cause of multi-infarct dementia. Neurology 1990; 40:753–755.

27. Hamrin B. Polymyalgia arteritica. Acta Med Scand 1972; (suppl) 533.

28. Lie JT. Aortic and extracranial large vessel giant cell arteritis: A review of 72 cases with histopathologic documentation. Semin Arthritis Rheum 1995; 24:422–431.

29. Stanson AW, Klein RG, Hunder GG. Extracranial angiographic findings in giant cell (temporal) arteritis. Am J Roentgenol 1976; 127:957–963.

30. Brack A, Martinez-Taboada V, Stanson A, Goronzy JJ, Weyand CM. Disease pattern in cranial and large-vessel giant cell arteritis. Arthritis Rheum 1999; 42(2):311–317.

31. Freddo T, Price M, Kase C, Goldstein MP. Myocardial infarction and coronary artery involvement in giant cell arteritis. Optom Vis Sci 1999; 76(1):14–18.

32. Bahlas S, Ramos-Remus C, Davis P. Clinical outcome of 149 patients with polymyalgia rheumatica and giant cell arteritis. J Rheumatol 1998; 25(1):99–104.

33. Weyand CM, Fulbright JW, Evans JM, Hunder GG, Goronzy JJ. Corticosteroid requirements in polymyalgia rheumatica. Arch Intern Med 1999; 159(6):577–584.

34. Salvarani C, Cantini F, Olivieri I, Barozzi L, Macchioni L, Niccoli L, Padula A, De Matteis M, Pavlica P. Proximal bursitis in active polymyalgia rheumatica. Ann Intern Med 1997; 127(1):27–31.

35. Salvarani C, Cantini F, Macchioni P, Olivieri I, Niccoli L, Padula A, Boiardi L. Distal musculoskeletal manifestations in polymyalgia rheumatica: A prospective follow-up study. Arthritis Rheum 1998; 41(7):1221–1226.

36. Salvarani C, Gabriel S, Hunder G. Distal extremity swelling with pitting edema in polymyalgia rheumatica. Arthritis Rheum 1996; 39:73–80.

37. Salvarani C, Hunder GG. Musculoskeletal manifestations in a population-based cohort of patients with giant cell arteritis. Arthritis Rheum 1999; 42:1259–1266.

38. Hunder GG. Giant cell arteritis and polymyalgia rheumatica. Med Clin North Am 1997; 81(1):195–219.

39. Weyand CM, Hicok KC, Hunder GG, et al. Tissue cytokine patterns in patients with polymyalgia rheumatica and giant cell arteritis. Ann Intern Med 1994; 121:484–491.

40. Evans JM, Bowles CA, Bjornsson J, et al. Thoracic aortic aneurysm and rupture in giant cell arteritis. A descriptive study of 41 cases. Arthritis Rheum 1994; 37:1539–1547.

41. Evans JM, O'Fallon WM, Hunder GG. Increased incidence of aortic aneurysm and dissection in giant cell (temporal) arteritis: A population-based study. Ann Intern Med 1995; 122:502–507.

42. Lie JT. Aortic and extracranial large vessel giant cell arteritis: A review of 72 cases with histopathologic documentation. Semin Arthritis Rheum 1995; 24(6):422–431.

43. Malmvall B-E, Bengtsson B-A, Kaijser B, et al. Serum levels of immunoglobulin and complement in giant cell arteritis. JAMA 1976; 236:1876–1878.

44. Kyle V. Laboratory investigations including liver in polymyalgia rheumatica/giant cell arteritis. Baillieres Clin Rheumatol 1991; 5(3):475–484.

45. Pountain GD, Calvin J, Hazleman BL. Alpha 1-antichymotrypsin, C-reactive protein and erythrocyte sedimentation rate in polymyalgia rheumatica and giant cell arteritis. Br J Rheumatol 1994; 33(6):550–554.

46. Salvarani C, Macchioni P, Boiardi L, Rossi F, Casadei Maldini M, Mancini R, Beltrandi E, Spacca C, Lodi L, Portioli I. Soluble interleukin 2 receptors in polymyalgia rheumatica/giant cell arteritis. Clinical and laboratory correlations. J Rheumatol 1992; 19(7):1100–1106.

47. Hachulla E, Salie R, Parra HJ, Hatron PY, Gosset D, Fruchart JC, Devulder B. Serum amyloid A concentrations in giant-cell arteritis and polymyalgia rheumatica: A useful test in the management of the disease. Clin Exp Rheumatol 1991; 9(2):157–163.

48. Zweegman S, Makkink B, Stehouwer CD. Giant-cell arteritis with normal erythrocyte sedimentation rate: Case report and review of the literature. Netherlands J Med 1993; 42(3–4):128–131.

49. Neish PR, Sergent JS. Giant cell arteritis. A case with unusual neurologic manifestations and a normal sedimentation rate. Arch Intern Med 1991; 151(2):378–380.

50. Roche NE, Fulbright JW, Wagner AD, et al. Correlation of interleukin-6 production and disease activity in polymyalgia rheumatica and giant cell arteritis. Arthritis Rheum 1993; 36:1286–1294.

51. Weyand CM, Fulbright JW, Evans JM, et al. Corticosteroid requirements in polymyalgia rheumatism. Arch Intern Med 1999; 159:577–584.

52. Weyand CM, Fulbright JW, Hunder GG, Goronzy JJ. Corticosteroid requirements in giant cell arteritis. Submitted for publication.

53. Ilan Y, Ben-Chetrit E. Liver involvement in giant cell arteritis. Clin Rheumatol 1993; 12(2):219–222.

54. Kyle V, Wraight EP, Hazleman BL. Liver scan abnormalities in polymyalgia rheumatica/giant cell arteritis. Clin Rheumatol 1991; 10(3):294–297.

55. Rousselet MC, Kettani S, Rohmer V, Saint-Andre JP. A case of temporal arteritis with intrahepatic arterial involvement. Pathol Res Pract 1989; 185(3):329–331.

56. Sherard RK, Coleridge ST. Giant-cell arteritis. J Emerg Med 1986; 4(4):293–299.

57. Brooke MH, Kaplan H. Muscle pathology in rheumatoid arthritis, polymyalgia rheumatica, and polymyositis: A histochemical study. Arch Pathol 1972; 94:101–118.

58. Persellin ST, Daniels TM, Rings LJ, et al. Factor VIII-von Willebrand factor in giant cell arteritis and polymyalgia rheumatica. Mayo Clin Proc 1985; 60:457–462.

59. Olsson A, Elling P, Elling H. Serologic and immunohistochemical determination of von Willebrand factor antigen in serum and biopsy specimens from patients with arteritis temporalis and polymyalgia rheumatica. Clin Exp Rheumatol 1990; 8:55–58.

60. Meyer O, Nicaise P, Moreau S, de Bandt M, Palazzo E, Hayem G, Chazerain P, Labarre C, Kahn MF. Antibodies to cardiolipin and beta 2 glycoprotein I in patients with polymyalgia rheumatica and giant cell arteritis. Revue du Rhumatisme, English Edition 1996; 63(4):241–247.

61. Manna R, Latteri M, Cristiano G, Todaro L, Scuderi F, Gasbarrini G. Anticardiolipin antibodies in giant cell arteritis and polymyalgia rheumatica: A study of 40 cases. Br J Rheumatol 1998; 37(2):208–210.

62. Nordborg E, Nordborg C. The inflammatory reaction in giant cell arteritis: An immunohistochemical investigation. Clin Exp Rheumatol 1998; 16(2):165–168.

63. Carson CW, Beall LD, Hunder GG, et al. Serum ELAM-1 is increased in vasculitis, scleroderma, and systemic lupus erythematosus. J Rheumatol 1992; 20:809–814.

64. Macchioni P, Boiardi L, Meliconi R, Salvarani C, Grazia Uguccioni M, Rossi F, Pulsatelli L, Facchini A. Elevated soluble intercellular adhesion molecule 1 in the serum of patients with polymyalgia rheumatica: Influence of steroid treatment. J Rheumatol 1994; 21(10):1860–1864.

65. Coll-Vinent B, Vilardell C, Font C, Oristrell J, Hernandez-Rodriguez J, Yague J, Urbano-Marquez A, Grau JM, Cid MC. Circulating soluble adhesion molecules in patients with giant cell arteritis. Correlation between soluble intercellular adhesion molecule-1 (sICAM-1) concentrations and disease activity. Ann Rheum Dis 1999; 58(3):189–192.

66. Klein RG, Campbell RJ, Hunder GG, Carney JA. Skip lesion in temporal arteritis. Mayo Clin Proc 1976; 51(8):504–510.

67. Achkar AA, Lie JT, Hunder GG, et al. How does previous corticosteroid treatment affect the biopsy findings in giant cell (temporal) arteritis? Ann Intern Med 1994; 120:987–992.

68. Evans JM, Batts KP, Hunder GG: Persistent giant cell arteritis despite corticosteroid treatment. Mayo Clin Proc 1994; 69:1060–1061.

69. Gabriel SE, O'Fallon WM, Achkar AA, et al. The use of clinical characteristics to predict the results of temporal artery biopsy among patients with suspected giant cell arteritis. J Rheumatol 1995; 22: 93–96.

70. Lie JT. Illustrated histopathologic classification criteria for selected vasculitis syndromes. American College of Rheumatology Subcommittee on Classification of Vasculitis. Arthritis Rheum 1990; 33(8): 1074–1087.

71. Puechal X, Chauveau M, Menkes CJ. Temporal doppler-flow studies for suspected giant-cell arteritis. Lancet 1995; 345:1437–1438.

72. Barrier J, Potel G, Renaut-Hovasse H, et al. The use of Doppler flow studies in the diagnosis of giant cell arteries: Selection of temporal artery biopsy site is facilitated. JAMA 1982; 248:2158–2159.

73. Schmidt WA, Kraft HE, Vorpahl K, Völker L, Gromnica-Ihle EJ. Color duplex ultrasonography in the diagnosis of temporal arteritis. N Engl J Med 1997; 337:1336–1342.

74. Hall S, Persellin S, Lie JT, O'Brien PC, et al. The therapeutic impact of temporal artery biopsy. Lancet 1983; 2:1217–1220.

75. Hall S, Hunder GG. Is temporal artery biopsy prudent? Mayo Clin Proc 1984; 59(11):793–796.

76. Lie JT: When is arteritis of the temporal arteries not temporal arteritis? J Rheum 1994; 21:186–189.

77. Lie JT. Temporal artery biopsy diagnosis of giant cell arteritis: Lessons from 1109 biopsies. Anat Pathol 1996; 1:69–97.

78. Gertz MA, Kyle RA, Griffing WL, et al. Jaw claudication in primary systemic amyloidosis. Medicine 1986; 65:173–179.

79. Hunder GG, Bloch DA, Michel BA, et al. The American College of Rheumatology 1990 Criteria for the Classification of Giant Cell Arteritis. Arthritis Rheum 1990; 33:1122–1128.

80. Hunder GG, Weyand CM. Sonography in giant-cell arteritis. N Engl J Med 1997; 337:1385–1386.

81. Hunder GG, Sheps SG, Allen GL, et al. Daily and alternate-day corticosteroid regimens in treatment of giant cell arteritis: Comparison in a prospective study. Ann Intern Med 1975; 82:613–618.

82. van der Veen MJ, Dinant HJ, van Booma-Frankfort C, van Albada-Kuipers GA, Bijlsma JW. Can methotrexate be used as a steroid sparing agent in the treatment of polymyalgia rheumatica and giant cell arteritis? Ann Rheum Dis 1996; 55(4):218–223.

83. Hernandez-Garcia C, Soriano C, Morado C, Ramos P, Fernandez-Gutierrez B, Herrero M, Banares A, Jover JA. Methotrexate treatment in the management of giant cell arteritis. Scand J Rheumatol 1994; 23(6):295–298.

84. Feinberg HL, Sherman JD, Schrepferman CG, Dietzen CJ, Feinberg GD. The use of methotrexate in polymyalgia rheumatica. J Rheumatol 1996; 23(9):1550–1552.

85. De Silva M, Hazleman BL. Azathioprine in giant cell arteritis/polymyalgia rheumatica: A double-blind study. Ann Rheum Dis 1986; 45(2):136–138.

86. Proven A, Gabriel S, Hunder G. Treatment outcome in a cohort of patients with giant cell arteritis. In preparation.

30
Takayasu's Arteritis: Pathogenesis

Yoshinori Seko
University of Tokyo, Tokyo, Japan

I. INTRODUCTION

Takayasu's arteritis (TA) is an acute inflammatory disease of unknown etiology, characterized by stenotic lesions in the aorta and its main branches that usually occurs in young women. However, it seems that older (middle-aged) cases of Takayasu's arteritis with chronic ongoing vasculitis are now being found more often, at least in Japan. Histopathological analysis in the acute phase of TA reveals extensive inflammation characterized by massive cell infiltration, destruction of the media, the adventitia around the vasa vasorum, and intimal hyperplasia, causing stenotic lesions. When destructive changes of the vessel wall predominate, it occasionally causes dilated lesions presenting as aneurysms (1). Vascular inflammation sometimes persists even after acute inflammation apparently subsides. Local vasculitis may latently occur without apparent inflammatory manifestations in the periphery, resulting in vascular damage that may evolve into lesions with pathological features resembling atherosclerotic aortic aneurysm. There is evidence of an association between Takayasu's arteritis and specific human leukocyte antigen (HLA) genes such as *HLA-B52, -B39,* and *MICA* (2–10). A recent report describes a close correlation between serum levels of inflammatory cytokines such as interleukin (IL)-6 and RANTES (regulated on activation, normal T cell expressed and secreted) with disease activity (11), suggesting a role of activated monocytes and T cells in the pathogenesis of TA. Some of the immunological mechanisms relevant in TA may also be involved in the formation of atherosclerotic aortic aneurysms (12–14). However, the precise mechanism of vessel injury as well as the primary cause that triggers the autoimmune process involved in both vascular diseases are still unknown and remain to be clarified.

We have investigated two aspects of the cell-mediated immunological mechanism. First, we have examined the mechanism of vascular cell injury by immune effector cells, especially the role of the pore-forming protein (perforin), one of the most important cytolytic effector molecules with which killer lymphocytes directly injure target cells. Second, we have investigated T-cell activation, more precisely the distribution of T-cell receptors (TCRs) and the expression of HLA antigens, and costimulatory signals for T-cell activation, which are mainly mediated by members of the immunoglobulin and tumor necrosis factor (TNF) receptor/ligand superfamilies.

II. PHENOTYPIC ANALYSIS OF INFILTRATING CELLS IN AORTIC TISSUE WITH TAKAYASU'S ARTERITIS

Investigation of the cell-mediated immunopathology was designed to analyze the characteristics of the infiltrating cells and the immunological responses of the target cells in aortic tissue from patients with Takayasu's arteritis. First, we analyzed the phenotypes of the infiltrating cells and found that most consisted of TCR γδ+ T-lymphocytes (about 31% of the total cells), CD16+ natural killer (NK) cells (20%), CD8+ cytotoxic T lymphocytes (CTLs) (15%), CD4+ T-helper cells (Th cells) (14%), CD14+ monocytes/macrophages (13%), and CD20+ B-cells (15). There was a markedly higher percentage of γδ T-lymphocytes in the artery than in peripheral blood, and the number of infiltrating αβ and γδ T-lymphocytes was almost the same. In sharp contrast, the infiltrating cells in samples from aortic aneurysms consisted of monocytes/macrophages (31%), NK cells (29%), CTLs (12%), and Th cells (6%). There were few γδ T-lymphocytes or B cells (15). The percentage of the infiltrating macrophages and γδ T-lymphocytes were quite different between the two diseases, suggesting that distinct immunological mechanisms had triggered the cell infiltration.

III. EXPRESSION OF CYTOLYTIC FACTOR PERFORIN IN INFILTRATING CELLS IN AORTIC TISSUE WITH TAKAYASU'S ARTERITIS

Killer cells such as NK cells and T cells, especially CTLs and γδ T-lymphocytes, are known to play a major part in cell-mediated cytotoxicity against virus-infected cells, tumor cells, or cells expressing foreign antigens. These lymphocytes are thought to kill target cells directly with the effector molecules contained in their cytoplasmic granules, one of which is named pore-forming protein or perforin (16,17). Perforin is expressed by infiltrating lymphocytes in various inflammatory diseases as well as lymphocytes under physiological conditions, plays a critical role in cytolysis, and can be a good marker for killer cells (18–24). Perforin-mediated lytic pathways as well as Fas-Fas ligand pathways play an essential role in CTL cytotoxicity (25). It is thought that killer cells recognize and adhere to the target cells followed by an exocytotic discharge of perforin in response to surface binding. After perforin monomers are released, they insert into the target bi-layer cell membrane, polymerize, and assemble into transmembrane pores. This, in turn, causes colloid-osmotic injury to the target cells. Perforin pores and the membrane attack complex of complement (which consist of C5b, 6, 7, 8, and C9) have very similar microstructure. In addition, perforin and C9 have high molecular homology (17). It is interesting that the effector molecules of cytolysis involved in cell-mediated and humoral immunological mechanisms are similar.

To analyze in more detail the characteristics of the tissue-infiltrating cells, especially their pathogenic role, we examined the expression of perforin in CTLs, NK cells, and γδ T-lymphocytes by double-immunostaining (15). Figure 1 shows that perforin was clearly expressed in the peripheral cytoplasmic granules of CTLs, NK cells, and γδ T-lymphocytes. Furthermore, to confirm that these killer cells had the potential to damage the aortic vascular cells by releasing perforin, we examined the expression of perforin molecules in the infiltrating cells by immunoelectron microscopy (15). Massive amounts of perforin molecules were released from the surface of an infiltrating cell and directly onto the surface of an aortic vascular cell, which was in contact with the infiltrating cell. This shows direct evidence that perforin molecules were secreted from the infiltrating cells and passed across the narrow extracellular space to reach the surface of the vascular cell and may indicate that perforin-mediated direct target cell damage occurred. Perforin was also clearly expressed in the peripheral cytoplasm and on the surface of another infiltrating cell.

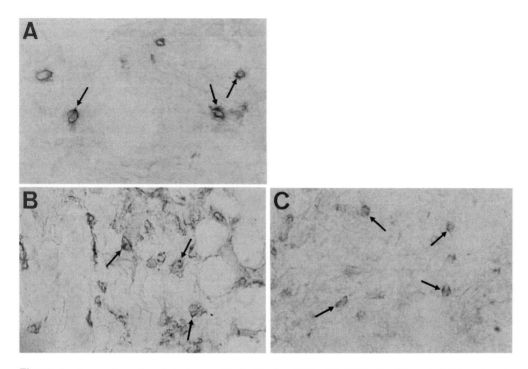

Figure 1   Expression of perforin (arrows) in infiltrating CTLs (A), NK cells (B), and γδ T-lymphocytes (C) in aortic tissue from a patient with Takayasu's arteritis. Double-staining by an enzyme antibody method was performed for perforin and surface markers; CD8 (panel A), CD16 (panel B), and TCR γδ (panel C). (Original magnification, ×200.) (Modified from Ref. 15.)

Next, we examined the expression of perforin in infiltrating cells in the aortic tissue from atherosclerotic aortic aneurysm by double-immunostaining for perforin and the surface markers CD8 and CD16. We found again that there was clear expression of perforin in the peripheral cytoplasmic granules of CTLs and NK cells (26). Because there were only few infiltrating γδ T-lymphocytes in the aortic tissue, we did not study the expression of perforin in γδ T-lymphocytes. Immunoelectron microscopic studies also demonstrated that the infiltrating cells released massive amounts of perforin molecules directly onto the surface of arterial vascular cells (26). These findings provided evidence that at least a part of the infiltrating cells in the aortic tissue consisted of killer cells and strongly suggested that these killer cells played a critical role in the vascular cell injury of atherosclerotic aortic aneurysm as well as Takayasu's arteritis.

IV. EXPRESSION OF HEAT-SHOCK PROTEIN-65 IN AORTIC TISSUE WITH TAKAYASU'S ARTERITIS

Heat-shock proteins (HSPs) are a highly conserved group of proteins found in various cells in most organisms. The synthesis of these proteins is known to be increased in response to environmental stresses, such as temperature changes, irradiation, ischemia/reperfusion, inflammation, and viral infection. Evidence has accumulated that γδ T-lymphocytes can recognize mycobacterial antigens, especially HSP-65 (27–29), and may play a role in various autoimmune diseases (30,31). Because there was marked increase of γδ T-lymphocyte infiltration in aortic tissue with

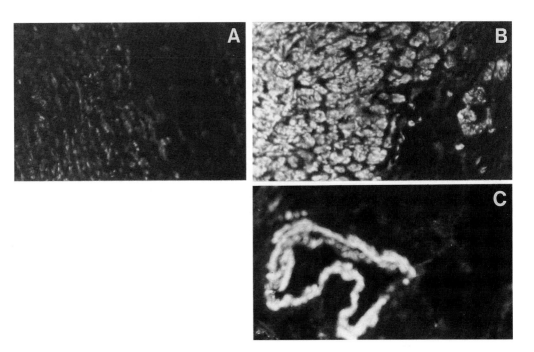

Figure 2 Expression of HSP-65 in aortic tissue from a patient with Takayasu's arteritis stained by immunofluorescence. Aortic tissue from a normal subject (A). Aortic tissue from a patient with Takayasu's arteritis (B and C). Note that the expression of HSP-65 was markedly increased in the media (B) and in some of the vasa vasorum (C) in Takayasu's arteritis. (Original magnification, ×200.) (From Ref. 15.)

Takayasu's arteritis, we examined the expression of HSP-65 in the aortic tissue. There was weak expression of HSP-65 only in the media of aortic tissue from normal subjects (Fig. 2A). In contrast, the expression of HSP-65 in the media was markedly increased in aortic tissue from patients with Takayasu's arteritis (Fig. 2B). Some of the vasa vasorum also strongly expressed HSP-65 (Fig. 2C). We found enhanced expression of HSP-65 in aortic tissue from all patients with Takayasu's arteritis studied (15).

Markedly increased expression of HSP-65 in the media and vasa vasorum supported the participation of γδ T-lymphocytes in Takayasu's arteritis. There was only weak or slightly increased expression of HSP-65 in the media and the vasa vasorum of aortic tissue with atherosclerotic aortic aneurysm. In this context, it is interesting that aneurysmal tissue also contains very low γδ T-lymphocytes. Xu et al. (32) reported that immunization with HSP-65 induced arteriosclerotic lesions in normocholesterolemic rabbits. The authors also reported that serum anti–HSP-65 antibodies were significantly increased in patients with carotid atherosclerosis (33). However, there was no evidence that dominant population of the infiltrating T cells bear TCR γδ and that HSP-65 is strongly induced in the arteriosclerotic lesions. It is uncertain that HSP-65–induced arteriosclerotic lesions can be a model for human atherosclerosis. Hohlfeld et al. (31) reported a case of polymyositis highly responsive to steroid therapy that was mainly mediated by γδ T-lymphocytes. The authors demonstrated that all muscle fibers strongly expressed HSP-65 as well as HLA class I. Aggarwal et al. (34) reported increased levels of serum antibodies against *Mycobacterium tuberculosis* antigens, especially HSP-65, in patients with Takayasu's arteritis. Recently, Moraes et al. (35) reported that peripheral lymphocytes from a patient with Takayasu's arteritis were reactive to HSP-65. These data suggest a possible pathogenic role of HSP-65 in

Takayasu's arteritis. Considering that the number of patients with Takayasu's arteritis has increased since bacille Calmette-Guérin (BCG) vaccination was started in the 1950s, it has been hypothesized that BCG vaccination in the susceptible host might contribute to the pathogenesis of Takayasu's arteritis (36).

V. EXPRESSION OF HLA CLASS I, CLASS II, AND INTERCELLULAR ADHESION MOLECULE-1 IN AORTIC TISSUE WITH TAKAYASU'S ARTERITIS

T cells are thought to recognize antigens presented by syngeneic major histocompatibility complex (MHC) antigens on antigen-presenting cells (APCs). Furthermore, cell adhesion molecules expressed on both immune cells and target cells are thought to play an essential role in cell–cell interactions in the immune responses. Among them, intercellular adhesion molecule-1 (ICAM-1), which belongs to the immunoglobulin superfamily and is a ligand for lymphocyte function–associated antigen-1 (LFA-1), is thought to be induced by cytokines on various target cells at the site of inflammation and to play an important role in the recognition, adhesion, and cytotoxicity of killer lymphocytes (37–41) (Fig. 3). To clarify the immunological mechanism that may cause persistent vascular cell damage, especially the pathophysiology of T-cell–mediated autoimmune process in Takayasu's arteritis, we analyzed the expression of HLA class I, class II, and ICAM-1 in aortic tissue. Figure 4 shows a representative immunohistochemical stainings for HLA class I, class II, and ICAM-1 in the aortic tissue from a normal subject and from a patient with Takayasu's arteritis. The expression of these antigens (especially HLA class I) was moderately to strongly increased in the vasa vasorum of vessel wall collected from patients with Takayasu's arteritis.

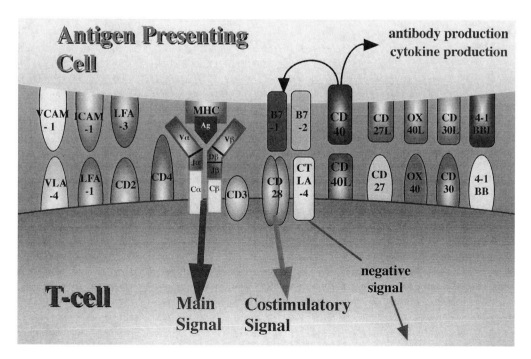

Figure 3   Scheme showing interactions between T cells and antigen-presenting cells.

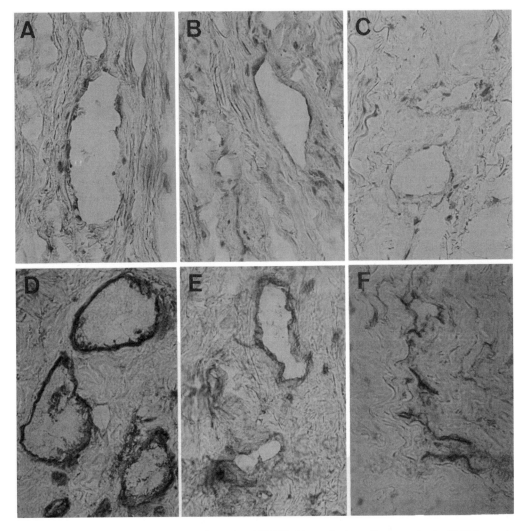

Figure 4 Expression of HLA class I, class II, and ICAM-1 in aortic tissue from a patient with Takayasu's arteritis stained by immunoperoxidase. Aortic tissue from a normal subject (A–C) and that from a patient with Takayasu's arteritis (D–F) were stained for HLA class I, class II, and ICAM-1, respectively. The expression of these antigens was moderately to markedly increased in the vasa vasorum of aortic tissue from a patient with Takayasu's arteritis. (Original magnification, ×200.) (From Ref. 15.)

VI. RESTRICTED USAGE OF TCR AV-BV GENES IN INFILTRATING CELLS IN AORTIC TISSUE WITH TAKAYASU'S ARTERITIS

It is thought that foreign antigens such as viruses are digested and degraded into peptide fragments in the cytoplasm of APCs and then presented on the cell surface by MHC antigens. In general, T-cells specifically recognize processed antigens in association with MHC molecules through their TCRs. The TCR α chain consists of variable (AV), joining (AJ), and constant regions (AC), and the β chain consists of variable (BV), diversity (BD), joining (BJ), and constant regions (BC). The specificity of TCR to the antigen is defined by the variable, diversity, and joining gene elements, which are rearranged and joined during T-cell differentiation (see Fig. 4). Evidence has accumulated that infiltrating T cells involved local immune responses in various autoimmune diseases (42–44), allograft rejection (45), and malignant tumors (46) use a limited range of TCR genes, strongly suggesting that these T cells specifically interact with a given antigen and play a pivotal role in the immunopathology. To further characterize the infiltrating cells, especially the antigen specificity of infiltrating αβ T-cells in Takayasu's arteritis in comparison with atherosclerotic aortic aneurysm, we analyzed the expression of TCR AV and BV genes by reverse transcription-polymerase chain reaction (RT-PCR) (47). Figure 5 shows the results of Southern blot analysis of PCR-amplified products obtained from infiltrating cells in aortic tissue with atherosclerotic aortic aneurysm and Takayasu's arteritis. Almost all TCR AV and BV genes were expressed in infiltrating lymphocytes from three different patients with aortic aneurysm. This indicated that the PCR could successfully amplify AV and BV gene transcripts. In sharp contrast, only a limited number of AV and BV genes were preferentially expressed in the aortic tissue with Takayasu's arteritis. This observation suggests that distinct immunological mechanisms are involved in the pathogenesis of these two aortic diseases. Although the number of patients studied was not enough to determine whether there were specific patterns in the expression of AV and BV genes among patients, AV2, AV16, AV17, BV7, and BV13.1 were rearranged in three of four patients. The restricted usage of both TCR AV and BV genes by infiltrating cells in Takayasu's arteritis could be an indication that a specific antigen in the groove of MHC molecule in the aortic tissue was targeted. Conversely, the polyclonal expression of TCR AV-BV genes in atherosclerotic aortic aneurysm may indicate nonspecific T-cell recruitment by inflammatory cytokines rather than by antigen-specific T-cell infiltration. Swanson et al. (48) have also reported polyclonal expression of TCR BV genes in human atheroma, supporting our results. However, it

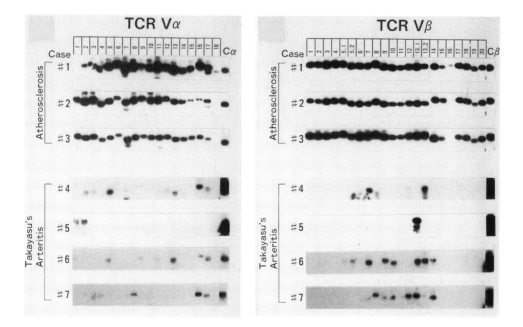

Figure 5 Southern blot analysis of the expression of TCR AV and BV gene segments in aortic tissue from patients with atherosclerotic aortic aneurysm (1–3) and Takayasu's arteritis (4–7). Polymerase chain reaction (PCR) was performed using each of the 18 TCR-AV family-specific as well as an AC-specific 5′-primer and a common AC 3′-primer, or each of the 22 TCR-BV family-specific as well as a BC-specific 5′-primer and a common BC 3′-primer. Amplified DNA was hybridized with a ^{32}P-labeled 5′-AC or 5′-BC primer. (From Ref. 47.)

remains possible that antigen-specific T-cells were present at low frequencies in the atherosclerotic tissue.

To investigate the T-cell clonality in more detail, especially to examine whether there was a difference in T-cell clonality within the same vascular lesion of Takayasu's arteritis, we analyzed the TCR BV clonality in two separate sections of the aortic tissue by RT-PCR and then by a single-stranded conformation polymorphism (SSCP). We found that there were several clear bands of expressed TCR BV clones in each of the examined BV subfamily. Some of the BV subfamilies were not represented. This indicated that the expression of TCR BV clones was restricted because polyclonal expression of TCR genes should produce a smear pattern and no banding. In addition, patterns of the bands of expressed TCR BV clones in separate pieces from the same lesion were almost the same, strongly suggesting that TCR BV clonality of the infiltrating cells in the two parts were shared.

VII. EXPRESSION OF COSTIMULATORY MOLECULES IN AORTIC TISSUE WITH TAKAYASU'S ARTERITIS

It is thought that T cells need to receive two signals from APCs to be activated. The main signal is provided by TCR engagement with the antigen/MHC complex, and the second signal is provided by costimulatory receptor-ligand pairs expressed on T-cells and APCs (see Fig. 3). Among them, the molecules B7-1 and B7-2, which belong to the immunoglobulin superfamily, are the most extensively characterized and appear to be critical (49–53). Other costimulatory molecules belonging to the TNF receptor/ligand superfamily have been identified and have been characterized over the past several years (54,55). These molecules include CD27/CD27 ligand (CD27L, CD70), CD30/CD30L (CD153), CD40/CD40L (CD154), OX40 (CD134)/OX40L, and 4-1BB (CD137)/4-1BBL. Evidence has accumulated that costimulatory molecules belonging to the TNF receptor/ligand superfamily play a pivotal role in T-cell–mediated immune responses, T-cell–dependent help for B cells, and humoral immune responses. To investigate the T-cell–mediated immunological mechanism of vascular injury in Takayasu's arteritis, we analyzed the expression of these costimulatory molecules on infiltrating cells as well as in the aortic tissue. We found that there was moderate to strong expression of B7-1, B7-2, CD40, CD27L, CD30L, and OX40L in the lesions of Takayasu's arteritis. We also found that at least some of the infiltrating immunocytes in the aortic lesion expressed the counterparts CD28, CD40L, CD27, CD30, and OX40. Expression of these costimulatory molecules in aortic tissue and their counterparts on the infiltrating cells in aortic lesions of Takayasu's arteritis provided further evidence for the involvement of T-cell–mediated immunological mechanism in the disease process.

VIII. SUMMARY

1. The infiltrating cells in Takayasu's arteritis mainly consist of γδ and αβ T-cells and NK cells, whereas there are only few infiltrating γδ T-cells in atherosclerotic aortic aneurysms.
2. Perforin is expressed by γδ T-cells, CTLs, and NK cells in Takayasu's arteritis, and by CTLs and NK cells in atherosclerotic aortic aneurysms. Infiltrating cells could injure vascular cells by releasing perforin.
3. As expected, the expression of HSP-65 as well as HLA class I and II is enhanced in the lesion of Takayasu's arteritis.
4. TCR αβ gene usage in infiltrating cells in Takayasu's arteritis is restricted, whereas that in atherosclerotic aortic aneurysm is broad.

5.   TCR BV clonality of infiltrating cells in Takayasu's arteritis was similar within isolated sections of the lesion.
6.   Costimulatory molecules are moderately to strongly expressed in lesions of Takayasu's arteritis.

In conclusion, these findings suggest that a specific antigen may be involved in the vascular injury in Takayasu's arteritis. Identification of such a specific antigen could facilitate a better understanding of the pathological mechanism of Takayasu's arteritis as well as the development of immunotherapy for Takayasu's arteritis.

REFERENCES

1.   Seko Y, Yazaki Y, Uchimura H, Isobe M, Tsuchimochi H, Kurabayashi M, Yoshizumi M, Ouchi Y, Tada Y, Kurihara H, Takaku F. A case of Takayasu's disease with ruptured carotid aneurysm. Jpn Heart J 1986; 27:523–531.
2.   Numano F, Isohisa I, Kishi U, Arita M, Maezawa H. Takayasu's disease in twin sisters. Possible genetic factors. Circulation 1978; 58:173–177.
3.   Numano F, Isohisa I, Maezawa H, Juji T. HL-A antigens in Takayasu's disease. Am Heart J 1979; 98: 153–159.
4.   Takeuchi Y, Matsuki K, Saito Y, Sugimoto T, Juji T. HLA-D region genomic polymorphism associated with Takayasu's arteritis. Angiology 1990; 41:421–426.
5.   Yoshida M, Kimura A, Katsuragi K, Numano F, Sassazuku T. DNA typing of HLA-B gene in Takayasu's arteritis. Tissue Antigens 1993; 42:87–90.
6.   Kimura A, Kobayashi Y, Takahashi M, Ohbuchi N, Kitamura H, Nakamura T, Satoh M, Sasaoka T, Hiroi S, Arimura T, Akai J, Aerbajinai W, Yasukochi Y, Munano F. MICA gene polymorphism in Takayasu's arteritis and Buerger's disease. Int J Cardiol 1998; 66:S107–S113.
7.   Charoenwongse P, Kangwanshiratada O, Boonnam R, Hoomsindhu U. The association between the HLA antigens and Takayasu's arteritis in Thai patients. Int J Cardiol 1998; 66:S117–S120.
8.   Kitamura H, Kobayashi Y, Kimura A, Numano F. Association of clinical manifestations with HLA-B alleles in Takayasu arteritis. Int J Cardiol 1998; 66:S121–S126.
9.   Mehra NK, Jaini R, Balamurugan A, Kanga U, Prabhakaran D, Jain S, Talwar KK, Sharma BK. Immunogenetic analysis of Takayasu artetritis in Indian patients. Int J Cardiol 1998; 66:S127–S132.
10.   Rodriguez-Reyna TS, Zuniga-Ramos J, Salgado N, Hernandez-Martinez B, Vargas-Alarcon G, Reyse-Lopez PA, Granadoz J. Intron 2 and exon 3 sequences may be involved in the susceptibility to develop Takayasu arteritis. Int J Cardiol 1998; 66:S135–S138.
11.   Noris M, Daina E, Gamba S, Bonazzola S, Remuzzi G. Interleukin-6 and RANTES in Takayasu arteritis. A guide for therapeutic decisions? Circulation 1999; 100:55–60.
12.   Jonasson L, Holm J, Skalli O, Bondjers G, Hansson GK. Regional accumulation of T cells, macrophages, and smooth muscle cells in the human atherosclerotic plaque. Arteriosclerosis 1986; 6:131–138.
13.   Emeson EE, Robertson AL Jr. T lymphocytes in aortic and coronary intimas. Their potential role in atherogenesis. Am J Pathol 1988; 130:369–376.
14.   Hansson GK, Jonasson L, Seifert PS, Stemme S. Immune mechanisms in atherosclerosis. Arteriosclerosis 1989; 9:567–578.
15.   Seko Y, Minota S, Kawasaki A, Shinkai Y, Maeda K, Yagita H, Okumura K, Sato O, Takagi A, Tada Y, Yazaki Y. Perforin-secreting killer cell infiltration and expression of a 65-kD heat-shock protein in aortic tissue of patients with Takayasu's arteritis. J Clin Invest 1994; 93:750–758.
16.   Young JDE. Killing of target cells by lymphocytes: A mechanistic view. Physiol Rev 1989; 69:250–314.
17.   Shinkai Y., Takio K, Okumura K. Homology of perforin to the ninth component of complement (C9). Nature 1988; 334:525–527.
18.   Young LHY, Klavinskis LS, Oldstone MBA, Young JDE. In vivo expression of perforin by CD8[+] lymphocytes during an acute viral infection. J Exp Med 1989; 169:2159–2171.

19. Young LHY., Peterson LB, Wicker LS, Persechini PM, Young JDE. In vivo expression of perforin by CD8$^+$ lymphocytes in autoimmune disease: Studies on spontaneous and adoptively transferred diabetes in nonobese diabetic mice. J Immunol 1989; 143:3994–3999.

20. Seko Y, Shinkai Y, Kawasaki A, Yagita H, Okumura K, Takaku F, Yazaki Y. Expression of perforin in infiltrating cells in murine hearts with acute myocarditis caused by coxsackievirus B3. Circulation 1991; 84:788–795.

21. Kawasaki A, Shinkai Y, Yagita H, Okumura K. Expression of perforin in murine natural killer cells and cytotoxic T lymphocytes in vivo. Eur J Immunol 1992; 22:1215–1219.

22. Kawasaki A, Shinkai Y, Kuwana Y, Furuya A, Iigo Y, Hanai N, Itoh S, Yagita H, Okumura K. Perforin, a pore forming protein detectable by monoclonal antibodies, is a functional marker for killer cells. Int Immunol 1990; 2:677–684.

23. Nakata M., Smyth MJ, Norihisa Y, Kawasaki A, Shinkai Y, Okumura K, Yagita H. Constitutive expression of pore-forming protein in peripheral blood γ/δ T cells: Implication for their cytotoxic role in vivo. J Exp Med 1990; 172:1877–1880.

24. Koizumi H, Liu CC, Zheng LM, Joag SV, Bayne NK, Holoshitz J, Young JDE. Expression of perforin and serine esterases by human γ/δ T cells. J Exp Med 1991; 173:499–502.

25. Lowin B, Hahne M, Mattmann C, Tschopp J. Cytolytic T-cell cytotoxicity is mediated through perforin and Fas lytic pathways. Nature 1994; 370:650–652.

26. Seko Y, Sato O, Takagi A, Tada Y, Matsuo H, Yagita H, Okumura K, Yazaki Y. Perforin-secreting killer cell infiltration in the aortic tissue of patients with atherosclerotic aortic aneurysm. Jpn Circ J 1997; 61:965–970.

27. Haregewoin A, Soman G, Hom RC, Finberg RW. Human $\gamma\delta^+$ T cells respond to mycobacterial heat-shock protein. Nature 1989; 340:309–312.

28. O'Brien RL, Happ MP, Dallas A, Palmer E, Kubo R, Born WK. Stimulation of a major subset of lymphocytes expressing T cell receptor $\gamma\delta$ by an antigen derived from Mycobacterium tuberculosis. Cell 1989; 57:667–674.

29. Janis EM, Kaufmann HE, Schwartz RH, Pardoll DM. Activation of gd T cells in the primary immune response to Mycobacterium tuberculosis. Science 1989; 244:713–716.

30. Selmaj K, Brosnan CF, Raine CS. Colocalization of lymphocytes bearing $\gamma\delta$ T-cell receptor and heat shock protein hsp65+ oligodendrocytes in multiple sclerosis. Proc Natl Acad Sci USA 1991; 88: 6452–6456.

31. Hohlfeld R, Engel AG, Ii K, Harper MC. Polymyositis mediated by T lymphocytes that express the γ/δ receptor. N Engl J Med 1991; 324:877–881.

32. Xu Q, Dietrich H, Steiner HJ, Gown AM, Schoel B, Mikuz G, Kaufmann SHE, Wick G. Induction of arteriosclerosis in normocholesterolemic rabbits by immunization with heat shock protein 65. Arterioscler Thromb 1992; 12:789–799.

33. Xu Q, Willeit J, Marosi M, Kleidienst R, Oberhollenzer F, Kiechl S, Stulnig T, Luef G, Wick G. Association of serum antibodies to heat-shock protein 65 with carotid atherosclerosis. Lancet 1993; 341:255–259.

34. Aggarwal A, Chag M, Sinha N, Naik S. Takayasu's arteritis: role of Mycobacterium tuberculosis and its 65 kDa heat shock protein. Int J Cardiol 1996; 55:49–55.

35. Moraes MF, Ordway D, Oliveira L, Costa IL, Badura R, Pinheiro MN, da Graca JM, Venture FA. Cellular immune responses to Mycobacterium tuberculosis in a patient with Takayasu's arteritis. Rev Port Cardiol 1999; 18:359–367.

36. Kothari SS. Aetiopathogenesis of Takayasu's arteritis and BCG vaccination: The missing link? Medical Hypotheses 1995; 45:227–230.

37. Marlin SD, Springer TA. Purified intercellular adhesion molecule-1 (ICAM-1) is a ligand for lymphocyte function-associated antigen 1(LFA-1). Cell 1987; 51:813–819.

38. Krensky AM, Robbins E, Springer TA, Burakoff SJ. LFA-1, LFA-2 and LFA-3 antigens are involved in CTL-target conjunction. J Immunol 1984; 132:2180–2182.

39. Dustin ML, Rothlein R, Bhan AK, Dinarello CA, Springer TA. Induction by IL-1 and interferon, tissue distribution, biochemistry, and function of a natural adherence molecule (ICAM-1). J Immunol 1986; 137:245–254.

40. Rothlein R, Czajkowski M, O'Neill MM, Marlin SD, Mainolfi E, Merluzzi VJ. Induction of intercellular adhesion molecule 1 on primary and continuous cell lines by pro-inflammatory cytokines: Regulation by pharmacologic agents and neutralizing antibodies. J Immunol 1988; 141:1665–1669.

41. Dustin ML, Singer KH, Tuck DT, Springer TA. Adhesion of T lymphoblasts to epidermal keratinocytes is regulated by interferon γ and is mediated by intercellular adhesion molecule 1 (ICAM-1). J Exp Med 1988; 167:1323–1340.

42. Acha-Orbea H, Mitchell DJ, Timmermann L, Wraith DC, Tausch GS, Waldor MK, Zamvil SS, McDevitt HO, Steinman L. Limited heterogeneity of T cell receptors from lymphocytes mediating autoimmune encephalomyelitis allows specific immune intervention. Cell 1988; 54:263–273.

43. Urban JL, Kumar V, Kono DH, Gomez C, Horvath SJ, Clayton J, Ando DG, Sercarz EE, Hood L. Restricted use of T cell receptor V genes in murine autoimmune encephalomyelitis raises possibilities for antibody therapy. Cell 1988; 54:577–592.

44. Paliard X, West SG, Lafferty JA, Clements JR, Kappler JW, Marrack P, Kotzin BL. Evidence for the effects of a superantigen in rheumatoid arthritis. Science 1991; 253:325–329.

45. Miceli MC, Finn OJ: T cell receptor β-chain selection in human allograft rejection. J Immunol 1989; 142:81–86.

46. Nitta T, Oksenberg JR, Rao NA, Steinman L. Predominant expression of T-cell receptor Vα7 in tumor-infiltrating lymphocytes of uveal melanoma. Science 1990; 249:672–674.

47. Seko Y, Sato O, Takagi A, Tada Y, Matsuo H, Yagita H, Okumura K, Yazaki Y. Restricted usage of T-cell receptor Vα-Vβ genes in infiltrating cells in aortic tissue of patients with Takayasu's arteritis. Circulation 1996; 93:1788–1790.

48. Swanson SJ, Rosenzweig A, Seidman JG, Libby P. Diversity of T-cell antigen receptor Vβ gene utilization in advanced human atheroma. Arterioscler Thromb 1994; 14:1210–1214.

49. Yokochi T, Holly RD, Clark EA. Lymphoblastoid antigen (BB-1) expressed on Epstein-Barr virus-activated B cell blasts, B lymphoblastoid lines, and Burkitt's lymphomas. J Immunol 1982; 128:823–827.

50. Freeman GJ, Freedman AS, Segil JM, Lee G, Whitman JF, Nadler LM. B7, a new member of the Ig superfamily with unique expression on activated and neoplastic B cells. J Immunol 1989; 143:2714–2722.

51. Azuma M, Ito D, Yagita H, Okumura K, Phillips JH, Lanier LL, Somoza C. B70 antigen is a second ligand for CTLA-4 and CD28. Nature 1993; 366:76–79.

52. Hathcock KS, Laszlo G, Dickler HB, Bradshaw J, Linsley P, Hodes RJ. Identification of an alternative CTLA-4 ligand costimulatory for T cell activation. Science 1993; 262:905–907.

53. Freeman GJ, Gribben JG, Boussiotis VA, Ng JW, Restivo VAJr, Lombard LA, Gray GS, Nadler LM. Cloning of B7-2: A CTLA-4 counter-receptor that costimulates human T cell proliferation. Science 1993; 262:909–911.

54. Smith CA, Farrah T, Goodwin RG. The TNF receptor superfamily of cellular and viral proteins: activation, costimulation, and death. Cell 1994; 76:959–962.

55. Gruss HJ, Dower SK. Tumor necrosis factor ligand superfamily: Involvement in the pathology of malignant lymphomas. Blood 1995; 85:3378–3404.

31

Takayasu's Arteritis: Clinical Aspects

Fujio Numano
Tokyo Medical and Dental University, Tokyo, Japan

I. INTRODUCTION

Takayasu's arteritis (TA) is a chronic idiopathic vasculitis that variably involves the aorta and/or its main branches and the coronary and pulmonary arteries. Inflammation results in stenosis, occlusion, or aneurysm formation. The last may rarely progress to vascular rupture and death (1,2) (Fig. 1).

The first report of TA was in 1830 by R. Yamamoto (3). The first scientific presentation of TA was in 1905 by Mikito Takayasu, at the 12th annual meeting of the Japan Ophthalmology Society. He described a 21-year-old woman who had a peculiar optic fundus abnormality, characterized by coronal anastomoses (4,5) (Fig. 2). At that meeting, K. Ohnishi and T. Kagoshima each presented similar cases and also noted that their patients lacked a palpable radial pulse (5). In 1940, K. Ohta (6) performed the first autopsy of a patient with TA. The patient was a 25-year-old female who had this characteristic optic fundus feature, which was associated with obstruction of cervical vessels. He suggested that the wreath of vessels around the optic disc represented neovascularization and anastomoses secondary to ischemia. In 1951, K. Shimizu and K. Sano (7) summarized the clinical features of the first 25 reported cases, plus their own six cases and pointed out "pulselessness," "coronal anastomosis of retinal vessels," and an "accentuated carotid sinus" as the triad of this condition, which they called "pulseless disease."

Since 1975, in Japan, patients with Takayasu's arteritis have been registered by the Ministry of Health and Welfare as intractable vasculitis of large vessels. Five thousand patients have since been identified (8), and approximately 100 to 200 new patients are recognized every year.

II. CHANGING CLINICAL SPECTRUM OF TAKAYASU'S ARTERITIS

Takayasu's arteritis is known to occur predominantly in women. There are also marked ethnic preferences (1,2,9). High prevalence rates are reported in Asian countries, such as Japan (10), Korea (11), China (12), India (13), Thailand (14), Israel (15), Turkey (16), and certain Central and South American countries such as Peru (17), Columbia (18), Mexico (19), and Brazil (20). Takayasu's arteritis is less common among Caucasian populations (2). A recent international survey among 20 countries revealed some characteristic differences of clinical signs in different ethnic groups (1,8,21,22).

Recent progress in medical technology has made it possible to diagnose TA before pulse-

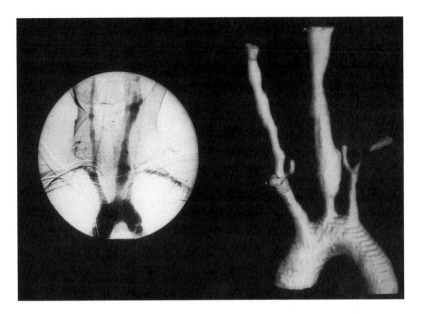

Figure 1   Digital subtraction angiography (DSA) and 3D-CT of a patient with Takayasu's arteritis (24-year-old male).

lessness occurs. Noninvasive angiographic analysis by CT and/or MRA has made it easier to image vessels without risk. Vascular anatomy and qualitative features of the vessel wall can be assessed sequentially over time. Magnetic resonance imaging (MRI) avoids repeated radiation exposure (23–25). Early diagnosis and early treatment are changing clinical features compared with those noted in earlier studies.

In Japan, patients with TA, in general, come to clinics with complaints related to the abnormal cerebral or upper extremity blood flow. Table 1 summarizes the frequencies of complaints in clinic patients. These data are based on the first and second Japanese National Surveys of Takayasu Arteritis (8,10). A high percentage of complaints due to ophthalmic and cerebral ischemic conditions were recorded. The second National Survey of Takayasu Arteritis was carried out 10 years after the first survey. It revealed almost the same clinical manifestations except a reduction of more than 20% of cerebrovascular disorders. It appears that early diagnosis and early treatment may be responsible for this remarkable reduction in severe cerebrovascular disease.

A subcommittee of the American College of Rheumatology recently excluded the rarely encountered ophthalmic findings from the criteria for TA (26). As shown in Figure 3A, although the cases of blindness due to the severe retinal ischemia are decreasing, there are still many patients who develop poor visual acuity or blindness. Ophthalmological follow-up remains an important aspect of care for TA, both because of possible ischemic retinopathy or cataracts (Fig. 3B) or glaucoma.

Cardiac involvement may lead to arrhythmias, ischemic heart disease, and congestive heart failure. Aortic regurgitation may result from aortitis and dilatation of the ascending aorta (Fig. 4). Vasculitis may involve the coronary arteries (1,2,26,28,29). Severe aortic regurgitation may also impair blood flow to patent coronary arteries. Inflammatory lesions of TA have been shown to accelerate the progression of focal atherosclerosis (30–32). Because corticosteroid therapy has further aggravated this complication and patients' life expectancies are now much longer, atherosclerosis is being increasingly recognized. Cardiac complications have become the most common cause of death in patients with TA.

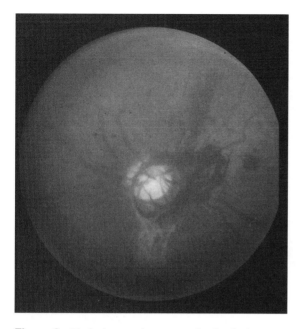

Figure 2   Typical coronal anastomosis of retinal vessels observed in Takayasu's arteritis.

Table 1   Clinical Symptoms of Takayasu's Arteritis

	1973 to 1975 (major complaint at initial consultation) No. Cases (%)	1982 to 1984 (throughout the course of disease) No. Cases (%)
Cerebrovascular disorder[a]	873/1351 (64.6)	551/1302 (42.3)
Ophthalmological symptoms	310/1297 (23.9)	301/1276 (23.6)
Cardiac symptoms	742/1344 (55.2)	536/1296 (41.4)
Hypertension	606/1336 (45.4)	734/1318 (55.7)
Vascular disorder in the extremities[b]	969/1341 (82.3)	930/1261 (73.8)
Acute pain[c]	492/1292 (38.1)	288/1255 (22.9)
Systemic symptoms	885/1324 (66.8)	769/1280 (60.1)

[a]Symptoms/signs of cerebral ischemia.
[b]Extremity ischemia.
[c]Vascular pain.
Source: Ref. 10.

Renal failure associated with nephrotic syndrome has become increasingly recognized in Japan (10).

Figure 5 demonstrates the clinical status of 897 patients with TA surviving through 1998 (unpublished observations). Seventy-one percent of patients were well controlled (Groups I or II) enjoying almost normal healthy lives. Twenty-five percent of patients (Groups IV and V) were suffering from severe complications of TA such as aortic regurgitation, hypertension, ischemic heart disease, congestive heart failure (CHF), poor visual acuity, strokes, or renal failure.

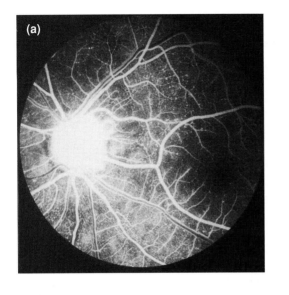
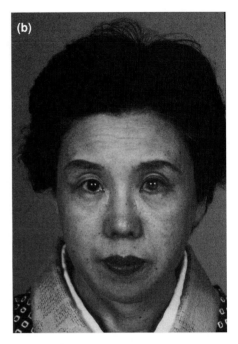

Figure 3   (a) Fluorescent retinal angiography in a 20-year-old woman. Note the many retinal microaneurysms. (b) Forty-five-year-old patient in whom long-standing Takayasu's arteritis and corticosteroid therapy were complicated by monocular blindness due to a left-sided cataract at age 32.

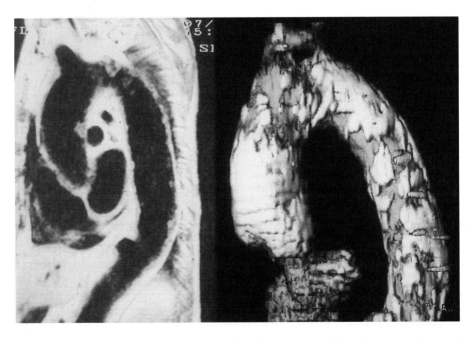

Figure 4   MRI and 3D-CT of a patient with dilated ascending and thoracic aorta causing aortic regurgitation. Thrombus was recognized at aortic arch. White plaques in 3D-CT demonstrate calcified thickened aortic wall.

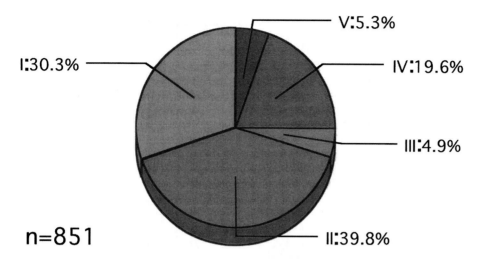

Figure 5 Clinical condition of patients with Takayasu arteritis. Group I: stable clinical condition not requiring steroid therapy. Group II: Stable clinical condition, but medical treatment including corticosteroid therapy needed. Group III: Despite medical and/or surgical treatment, repeated relapses and gradual progression occurred. Groups IV and V: Serious complications of disease and treatment occurred, including aortic regurgitation, ischemic heart disease, dissecting aneurysms, pulmonary infarctions, transient ischemic attacks, strokes, cataracts, psychogenic dysfunction, renal impairment, and renovascular hypertension. (Data from Research Committee for Intractable Vasculitis, Ministry of Health and Welfare, Japan, 1998, unpublished.)

III. DIFFERENT CLINICAL SPECTRUM AMONG ASIAN COUNTRIES

Takayasu's arteritis is more prevalent in Asian and South American countries than elsewhere. A recent international survey revealed that the clinical spectrum of TA may not be the same in other countries as in Japan. Figure 6 shows a comparison of clinical manifestations in Japanese and Indian patients. Many Japanese patients have a weak or absent radial pulse and suffer from aortic regurgitation due to involvement of the ascending aorta and the primary aortic arch branch vessels (1,2,21,22). On the other hand, hypertension is the most characteristic manifestation in Indian patients, suggesting a high frequency of lesions in the abdominal aorta, including the renal arteries, leading to renovascular hypertension (13,34). This is also true for Takayasu's patients in China, Korea, and Thailand (11,12,14). Yajima et al. (21) confirmed these differences in a comparison study of angiographic findings in Korean, Indian, and Japanese patients. Japanese patients frequently showed involvement of the aortic arch and its branches, whereas both Indian and Korean patients more often exhibited involvement of the abdominal aorta (22). Influenced by these findings, in 1994, the XI International Conference on Takayasu Arteritis established a new classification of angiographic findings (Fig. 7) (23). Figure 8 shows a comparison of angiographic findings, based on the new criteria, among 80 Japanese, 102 Indian, and 64 Thai patients. Statistically significant high frequencies of type 1 or type 2 were recorded in Japanese patients compared with both Indian and Thai patients (14,21,23). On the other hand, 28% of Indian and 18% of Thai patients showed type 4, in contrast to only 1.3% of Japanese patients exhibiting limited involvement of the abdominal aorta. These finding support other studies that have noted a differ-

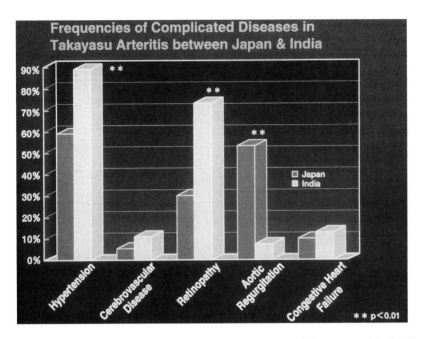

Figure 6 Frequencies of complications in Takayasu arteritis in Japan and India. *Note*: High frequencies of hypertension and retinopathy are recognized in Indian as compared with Japanese patients. On the other hand, Japanese patients more frequently had complicated aortic regurgitation than Indian patients.

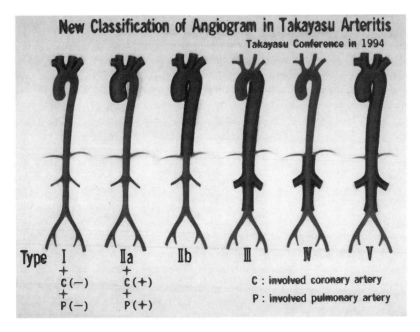

Figure 7 The International Conference on Takayasu Arteritis (1994) revised classification of vessel anatomy. Type I involves branches of the aortic arch. Type IIa involves the ascending aorta and the aortic arch and its branches. Type IIb involves the Type IIa region plus the thoracic descending aorta. Type III involves the thoracic descending aorta, abdominal aorta, and/or renal arteries. Type IV involves only abdominal aorta and/or renal arteries. Type V involves the entire aorta and its branches.

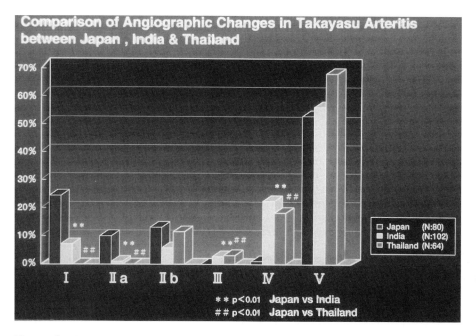

Figure 8 Type I and II changes are more frequently seen in Japanese patients, while type III and IV changes are more frequent in both Indian and Thai patients.

ent clinical spectrum of disease phenotype in Japan and other Asian countries. In contrast, angiographic studies from Columbia (18), Mexico (19), Brazil (20) and the United States (34) have suggested that the pattern of vessel involvement is similar to that noted in Japan.

IV. DIAGNOSIS

The diagnosis of TA is often delayed due to nonspecific symptoms and many physicians not being familiar with this disease. Most patients come to clinics with complaints of cerebral vascular disturbance, such as dizziness, tinnitus, syncope, visual disturbance, and/or headache. Inflammatory signs such as fever, fatigue, swollen cervical lymph nodes or neck pain in young females sometimes tend to be misdiagnosed as tuberculosis, viral infection, rheumatoid arthritis, Behçet's disease, and/or a psychosomatic reaction.

On physical examination, the findings of pulselessness and/or differences in blood pressure between extremities and bruits are helpful in leading to the diagnosis of TA. "Bird-like faces" due to atrophy of facial muscles, intermittent claudication of jaw muscles, perforation of nasal septum due to long-term cervical circulatory disturbances are also helpful signs. Table 2 shows the frequency of abnormal clinical laboratory, chest x-ray, and electrocardiogram (EKG) findings in TA from the first and second Japanese National Surveys. In the Japanese experience, abnormalities of erythrocyte sedimentation rate (ESR) and C-reactive protein (CRP) correlated with clinical features of inflammation and were useful tools to follow disease activity and adjust corticosteroid therapy. The second National Survey in Japan (10) indicated that 88% of patients with active disease had increased ESR values (>20 mm/h) and 69% had a positive CRP (>20). These

Table 2 Findings of Laboratory Examinations in Patients with Takayasu's Arteritis

	1973 to 1975 (at the initial consultation) No. Cases (%)	1982 to 1984 (at deterioration) No. Cases (%)
Enhanced erythrocyte sedimentation	868/1193 (72.8)	997/1130 (88.2)
Increased WBC	437/1249 (35.0)	506/1160 (43.6)
Anemia	563/1175 (47.9)	629/1149 (54.7)
Increase in γ-globulin	483/1008 (47.9)	502/972 (51.6)
Increase in antistreptolysin-O (ASLO)	155/1067 (14.5)	142/920 (15.4)
CRP positive	666/1287 (51.7)	800/1153 (69.4)
RA positive	108/1185 (9.1)	119/1010 (11.8)
Positive Wassermann reaction	23/1105 (2.1)	25/863 (2.9)
Positive tuberculin reaction	366/532 (68.8)	241/342 (70.5)
Increase in cardiothoracic ratio	413/1028 (40.2)	
Aortic calcification	239/1160 (20.6)	251/1142 (22.0)
Abnormal EKG	538/1221 (44.1)	578/1169 (49.4)

Source: Ref. 10.

observations are in contrast to those from the American experience at the National Institutes of Health. In that study, acute phase reactants correlated with clinical, angiographic and biopsy proof of active disease in only about 50% of cases (34). Hypergammaglobulinemia and leukocytosis were noted in 52% and 44%, respectively. Accelerated platelet aggregation, hyperfibrinogenemia, and increased expression of vascular adhesion molecules (35) reflect activation of the coagulation cascade and endothelium, respectively. More than half of Japanese patients are found to carry a haplotype of *HLA A24-B52-DR2,* which may suggest the participation of genetic factors in the pathogenesis of TA (36,37). Patients carrying this haplotype were more prone to having severe, rapidly progressive disease, compared with those without this haplotype (38).

Imaging modalities such as computed tomography (CT), MRI, and/or magnetic resonance angiography (MRA) are very useful noninvasive tools for diagnosis of TA, even in the early stages of illness. Vascular stenoses, dilatation, aneurysm formation, and thrombosis can be demonstrated without serious burden to patients (39,40) (see Fig. 1). These techniques are also very useful to follow the effects of treatment (41). Insofar as aortic regurgitation (AR) due to dilatation of the ascending aorta is a very significant complication of TA and may affect prognosis, follow-up of the aortic root diameter by MR or CT is critically important (29,38,42). Angiography remains an important means of evaluation that allows imaging of the vessel lumen, as well as providing opportunities to record intravascular blood pressures, determine pressure gradients, and perform therapeutic interventions such as angioplasty.

Table 3 lists the guidelines for clinical diagnosis of TA, as proposed by the Committee on Takayasu Arteritis of the Ministry of Health and Welfare in Japan (43). Other criteria, suggested by the American College of Rheumatology (1990), consist of six features (26): age less than 40 years, claudication for an extremity, decreased brachial artery pulse pressure (>10 mm Hg difference in systolic pressure between arms), a bruit over subclavian arteries or aorta, and angiographic evidence of narrowing or occlusion of the aorta or its primary or proximal branches. Presence of three out of six criteria is required for the diagnosis. By those criteria, patients in Asian countries whose abdominal aorta is predominantly involved can be underdiagnosed (23). Furthermore, ophthalmological findings and/or symptoms were not included, perhaps due to their low frequency in American patients.

Table 3 Guidelines for Making a Clinical Diagnosis of Takayasu's Arteritis

1. Symptoms
   (a) Cerebral ischemia: vertigo (especially when looking upward), fainting spells, visual disturbance (especially at direct sunshine)
   (b) Ischemia of the extremities: cold fingers, easy fatigability of the upper extremities
   (c) Stenosis of the aorta or renal arteries: headache, vertigo, shortness of breath, which are considered due to hypertension
   (d) Generalized symptoms: slight fever may be recognized at the onset of the disease
2. Important findings for diagnosis
   (a) Abnormalities of the pulse of the upper extremities (weak or diminution and/or right/left difference of the radial pulse)
   (b) Abnormalities of the pulse of the lower extremities (accentuation or decrease of the pulse)
   (c) Vascular murmur in the arteries of the neck, back, or abdomen
   (d) Ophthalmological abnormalities
3. Abnormalities in laboratory examination
   (a) Increased erythrocyte sedimentation rate
   (b) Positive C-reactive protein
   (c) Increase in γ-globulin levels in the serum
4. Important diagnostic points
   (a) Prevalent in young women
   (b) Final clinical diagnosis can be made by aortography
5. Differential diagnosis: Buerger's disease, arteriosclerosis, collagen disease, congenital vascular abnormalities

V. TREATMENT

Since the etiology of TA is still unknown, treatment is not curative, but rather is primarily medical and symptomatic. Indications for surgical treatment should always be kept in mind. Renovascular hypertension, coarctation of aorta, severe cerebral ischemia, severe aortic regurgitation causing congestive heart failure, or progressive aneurysmal enlargement or dissection may all require prompt surgical treatment. Medical therapy for these conditions is generally inadequate. Ideally, surgical treatment should be provided when inflammatory disease has been adequately suppressed.

A. Medical Treatments

Corticosteroid and antiplatelet therapies are the essential therapies of this morbid condition. Significant improvement can be achieved with corticosteroids, particularly during acutely active disease. Treatment may be initiated with prednisolone, 20–30 mg/day, followed by reduction, after disease is adequately suppressed, by 5 mg/day every 2–3 weeks when clinically feasible, as determined by symptoms, ESR, and CRP (38,44). The target maintenance dose is 5–10 mg/day. Once this maintenance dose is achieved and the patient is stable for some time, later tapering toward discontinuation may be possible. Patients with the *HLA A24-B52-DR2* haplotype may require larger doses (30–40 mg) of corticosteroids for longer periods than patients without this haplotype (38). Some investigators of TA have advocated initial therapy with higher doses (34).

Cytotoxic and other immunosuppressive therapies have been used in Japan for some time, their effects are less than remarkable. Conventionally, 100 mg of cyclosporin has been administered daily or every other day together with 10–20 mg/day of prednisolone. Others have found weekly treatment with methotrexate useful toward achieving better control of active disease and allowing lower maintenance doses of corticosteroids (45).

We believe that antithrombotic therapy is essential in the treatment of TA. Thrombus formation is easily induced on the rough surface of the injured vessel wall. Active inflammation accelerates thrombus formation. When thrombus is forming or established, anticoagulant therapy with or without fibrinolytic treatment may be necessary. Antiplatelet therapy should be considered in all patients for protection from thrombus. In Japan, a small dose (81 mg/day) of acetylsalicylic acid is popular. Other antiplatelet drugs such as dipyridamole, ticlopidin, or cilostazol may also be employed (46).

B. Surgical Treatment

Surgical procedures may be indicated for treatment of TA in the following situations: (1) severe aortic coarctation, (2) severe aortic regurgitation, (3) severe hypertension, (4) congestive heart failure, (5) renovascular hypertension, (6) severe cerebrovascular disease due to stenoses of cervicocranial vessels, (7) progressive aneurysm enlargement, and (8) dissecting aneurysm (47). The Bental operation is a very effective procedure for aortic regurgitation. The timing of surgery must be carefully assessed in regard to achieving disease stability vis-à-vis inflammation, hypertension and hemodynamic status in order to provide optimal results. A variety of grafting and bypass procedures can also be performed (see the following chapter).

VI. PROGNOSIS

Early diagnosis and initiation of treatment leads to improved prognoses. Regardless of disease activity and treatment, it is very important to follow patients carefully at regular intervals. This is particularly relevant to anatomical abnormalities that may be progressive and contribute to hypertension, stroke, heart failure, myocardial infarction, and severe gut or extremity ischemia. Secondary atherosclerosis may cause focal lesions to become progressively worse, even in the absence of inflammation. Congestive heart failure, with or without arrhythmia, is the leading cause of death in Japan, whereas cerebral vascular complications are more common in other Asian countries. It is noteworthy that, in Japan, improved life expectancy for TA has led to increasing awareness of renal dysfunction, associated with nephrotic syndrome.

REFERENCES

1. Numano F. Takayasu arteritis beyond pulselessness. J Int Med 1999; 38:226–232.
2. Numano F, Kobayashi Y. Takayasu arteritis: Clinical characteristics and the role of genetic factors in its pathogenesis. Vascular Med 1996; 1:227–233.
3. Numano F. Kakuta T. Takayasu arteritis: Five doctors in the history of Takayasu arteritis. Int J Cardiol 1996; 54(suppl):1–10.
4. Takayasu M. A case with peculiar changes of the retinal central vessels. Acta Soc Ophthal Japan 1908; 12:554–555.
5. Numano F. Introductory remarks for this special issue of Takayasu arteritis. Heart Vessels 1992; 7(suppl):3–5.
6. Ohta K. Ein seltener Fall on bleiderseitigem Carotis—Subclavia verschluss, Ein Beitrag zur Pathologie der Anastomosis peripapillaris des Auges mit fehlendem Radialpuls. Trans Soc Pathol Jap 1940; 30:680–690.
7. Shimizu K, Sano K. Pulseless disease. J Neuropath Clin Neuro 1951; 1:37–47.

8. Nagasawa T. Current status of large and small vessel vasculitis in Japan. Int J Card 1996; 54(suppl): 75–82.
9. Numano F. Differences in clinical presentation and outcome in different countries for Takayasu arteritis. Curr Opin Rheumatol 1997; 9:12–15.
10. Koide K. Takayasu arteritis in Japan. Heart Vessels 1992; 7(suppl):48–57.
11. Park YB, Hong KJ, Choi DW, Sohn DW, Oh BH, Lee MM, Choi YS, Seo JD, Lee YW, Park JH. Takayasu arteritis in Korea. Clinical and angiographic features. Heart Vessels 1992; 7(suppl):55–59.
12. Zheng D, Fan D, Liu L. Takayasu arteritis in China: A report of 530 cases. Heart Vessels 1992; 7(suppl):32–36.
13. Ganguly NK, Jain S, Kumari S. Current status of Takayasu arteritis in India. Int J Cardiol 1996; 54(suppl):111–116.
14. Suwanwela N, Piyaehon C. Takayasu arteritis in Thailand: Clinical and imaging features. Int J Cardiol 1996; 54(suppl):155–163.
15. Rosenthal T, Morag B, Itzchak Y. Takayasu arteritis in Israel. Heart Vessels 7(suppl):44–47.
16. Turkoglu C, Memis A, Payzing et al. Takayasu arteritis in Turkey. Int J Cardiol 1996; 54:135–136.
17. Lupi-Herrea E, Sanchez-Torres G, Marcushamer J, Horwitz S, Vela JE. Takayasu's arteritis: Clinical study of 107 cases. Am Heart J 93:94–103.
18. Canas CAD, Jimenez CAP, Ramirez LA, Uribe O, Tobon I, Torrenegra A. Takayasu arteritis in Columbia. Int J Cardiol 1998; 66:73–79.
19. Dabague J, Reyes PA. Takayasu arteritis in Mexico. Int J Cardiol 1996; 54:103–109.
20. Sato EI, Hatta FS, Levy-Neto M, Fernandes S. Demographic, clinical and angiographic data of patients with Takayasu arteritis in Brazil. Int J Cardiol 1998; 66:67–70.
21. Yajima M, Numano F, et al. Comparative studies of patients with Takayasu arteritis in Japan, Korea and India. Jpn Circ J 1994; 58:9–14.
22. Moriwaki R, Noda M, Yajima M, Sharma BK, Numano F. Clinical manifestation of Takayasu arteritis in India and Japan. New classification of angiographic findings. Angiology 1997; 48:369–379.
23. Hata A, Noda M, Moriwaki R, Numano F. Angiographic findings of Takayasu arteritis: New classification. Int J Cardiol 1996; 54(suppl):155–163.
24. Yamada I, Numano F, Suzuki S. Takayasu arteritis: Evaluation with MR imaging. Radiology 1993; 188:89–94.
25. Hata A. Numano F. Magnetic resonance imaging of vascular changes in Takayasu arteritis. Int J Cardiol 1995; 52(suppl):45–52.
26. Arend WP, Michael BA, Block DA, et al. The American College of Rheumatology Criteria for the determination of Takayasu arterits. 1990; 33:1129–1134.
27. Kiyosawa M, Baba T. Ophthalmological findings in patients with Takayasu disease. Int J Cardiol 1998; 66(suppl 1):141–147.
28. Yajima M, Namba K, Kakuta T, Nishizaki M, Oniki T, Numano F. Echo cardiographic studies on aortic regurgitation in Takayasu arteritis. J Cardiovascular Technol 1989; 8:223–230.
29. Hashimoto Y, Oniki T, Numano F, et al. Aortic regurgitation in patients with Takayasu arteritis: Assessment by color Doppler echocardiography. Heart Vessels 1992; (suppl 7):111–115.
30. Wissler RW, PDAY Group. Atheroarteritis: a combined immunological and lipid imbalance. Int J Cardiol 1996; 54(suppl 7):11–23.
31. Ross R. Atherosclerosis is the inflammatory disease. N Engl J Med 1999; 340:115–126.
32. Numano F. Inflammation and atherosclerosis. Ann NY Acad Sci. In press.
33. Sharma BK, Sagar S, Singh AP, Suri S. Takayasu arteritis in India. Heart Vessels 1992; (suppl 7): 37–43.
34. Kerr GS, Hallahan CW, Giordano J, Leavitt RY, Fauci AS, Rottem M, Hoffman GS. Takayasu's arteritis. Ann Intern Med 1994; 120:919–929.
35. Noguchi S, Numano F, Gravanis MB, Wilcox JN. Increased levels of soluble form of adhesion molecules in Takayasu arteritis. Int J Cardiol 1998; 66:S23–S33.
36. Numano F, Isohisa I, Maezawa H, Sasazuki T. HLA-B52 in Takayasu disease. Tissue Antigen 1978; 12:246–248.
37. Kimura A, Kitamura H, Date Y, Numano F. Comprehensive analysis of HLA genes in Takayasu arteritis in Japan. Int J Cardiol 1996; 54:61–69.

38. Moriwaki R, Numano F. Takayasu arteritis, follow up studies for 20 years. Heart Vessels 1992; 7(suppl):138–145.

39. Park JH. Conventional and CT, angiographic diagnosis of Takayasu arteritis. Int J Cardiol 1996; 54:S165–S171.

40. Hata A, Numano F. Magnetic resonance imaging of vascular changes in Takayasu arteritis. Int J Cardiol 1995; 52:45–52.

41. Hayashi K, Fukushima T, Matsunaga N. Takayasu arteritis: Decrease in aortic wall thickening following steroid therapy. Br Radiol 1986; 59:281–283.

42. Hashimoto Y, Tanaka M, Hata A, Kakuta T, Maruyama Y, Numano F. Four years follow-up study in patients with Takayasu arteritis and severe aortic regurgitation: assessment by echocardiography. Int J Cardiol 1996; 54:173–176.

43. Sekiguchi M, Suzuki M. An overview on Takayasu arteritis. Heart Vessels 1992; 7(suppl):6–10.

44. Ito S. Medical treatment of Takayasu arteritis. Heart Vessels 1992; 7(suppl):133–137.

45. Hoffman GS, Leavitt RY, Kerr GS, Rottem M, Sneller MC, Fauci AS: Treatment of glucocorticoid-resistent or relapsing Takayasu's arteritis with methotrexate. Arthritis Rheum 1994; 37:578–582.

46. Numano F, Murayama Y, Koyama T, Numano Fe. Antiaggregative aspirin dosage at the affected vessel wall. Angiology 1986; 37:695–701.

47. Tada Y, Sato O, Ohshima A, Miyata T, Shindo S. Surgical treatment of Takayasu arteritis. Heart Vessels 1992; 7(suppl):159–167.

48. Amano J, Suzuki A, Tanaka H, Sunamori M. Surgical treatment for annulo aortic ectasia in Takayasu arteritis. Int J Cardiol 1998; 66:S197–S198.

32

Takayasu's Arteritis: Surgical Treatment

Joseph M. Giordano

George Washington University Medical Center, Washington, D.C.

I. INTRODUCTION

Treatment of Takayasu's arteritis presents unique clinical problems to the surgeon that impact on the outcome of treatment. The disease is infrequent, with an annual incidence in one study of 2.6 cases per one million inhabitants (1,2). Most vascular surgeons rarely, if ever, see a case of Takayasu's arteritis. The ultimate outcome for patients with Takayasu's arteritis depends in part on the appropriate management of ischemia to vital organs. It is tempting and even appropriate to use principles learned in the treatment of elderly patients with advanced atherosclerosis as guidelines in the management of patients with Takayasu's arteritis. The differences, however, between atherosclerosis and Takayasu's arteritis are real and must be considered before surgical treatment of Takayasu's arteritis is undertaken.

II. GENERAL PRINCIPLES OF SURGICAL TREATMENT

1. Patients with Takayasu's arteritis are young, but have significant medical problems that could complicate a surgical procedure. They frequently have hypertension, often unrecognized. Left ventricular hypertrophy and congestive heart failure are common sequelae of unrecognized systemic hypertension (3). Takayasu's arteritis can affect the coronary arteries (3,6). The patients are frequently on steroids and immunosuppressive drugs which may have an impact on the surgical treatment. Therefore, although these patients are young, medical problems require careful coordination of medical and surgical services.
2. Percutaneous transluminal angioplasty is becoming an effective alternative to bypass surgery in certain situations (7,10). Takayasu's arteritis presents the interventionist with a unique set of technical problems. The walls of the arteries are rigid and noncompliant, with the disease affecting all three layers of the artery. At times, the interventionist needs three to five attempts before the "waist" of the narrowing is eliminated. There is a possibility that the impact of trauma from the arterial dilation could rapidly cause restenosis in these clinically inflamed arteries. As in arteries affected with atherosclerosis, dilatation and arterial stenting for patients with Takayasu's arteritis works best in arteries that have short segment stenosis and high flow.
3. The timing of operative procedures is debatable (11,12). Most cases do not require

emergency surgery, but can be done as an elective procedure allowing time for medical evaluation. Performing an operative procedure while the patient still has active disease should be discouraged, but can be done if necessary.

4. In general, bypass of diseased arteries is the procedure of choice. Endarterectomy is difficult because Takayasu's arteritis affects all the layers, making endarterectomy more technically challenging than in patients with atherosclerosis. Note that even though the anastomoses of bypasses are always done in arteries that appear normal on arteriography, 44% of biopsies taken from the arteries show microscopic evidence of active disease (13). This may have long-term impact on the anastomatic sites.

5. Patients with Takayasu's disease are young and have a long life expectancy. Since it is unusual to follow elderly patients with atherosclerosis who have had bypasses for more than 20 years, it is not clear whether bypass grafts or their anastomoses in patients with Takayasu's arteritis will last longer than 20 years.

III. CEREBROVASCULAR DISEASE

Lateralizing cerebrovascular symptoms, including stroke, transient ischemic attacks, and amaurosis fugax, are not uncommon presenting symptoms in patients with Takayasu's arteritis (1,11, 14,6). In elderly patients with atherosclerosis, localized cerebrovascular symptoms occur usually from emboli due to turbulence originating from local plaque formation at the carotid bifurcation. Patients with cerebrovascular involvement from Takayasu's arteritis do not have local plaque formation, but instead have long, smooth, tapered stenoses that can involve the entire length of an artery such as the common carotid artery. It would appear less likely that this type of arterial disease could be a source of emboli.

Stroke in Takayasu's arteritis is most likely to result from occlusion of one or more major arteries of the thoracic aorta (12) (Fig. 1). Knowledge of the blood supply to the brain and the pathology of cerebrovascular involvement in Takayasu's arteritis is important. The brain receives

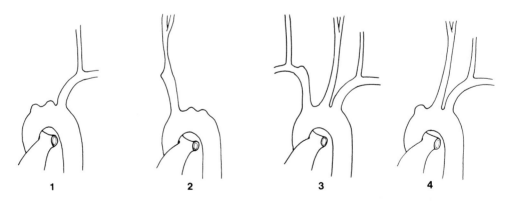

Figure 1 Aortic arch arteriograms in four patients with Takayasu's disease who presented with a stroke. Patient 1: Both the innominate and the left carotid arteries are totally occluded. The left subclavian artery is open with the left vertebral being the only artery to the brain. Patient 2: The left subclavian and the left common carotid arteries are occluded. The patient has an innominate artery but the right subclavian artery is occluded. There is also disease present in the right common carotid artery, the only vessel to the brain. Patient 3: The right common carotid artery is occluded. Patient 4: The innominate artery is totally occluded, which means both the right carotid and the right vertebral arteries are not providing antegrade blood flow to the brain.

its blood supply from four arteries, two carotids and two vertebrals. The two vertebrals originate from the subclavian arteries, the right carotid artery originates from the innominate and the left carotid artery usually comes directly off the aortic arch. Since the right subclavian and the right common carotid are the two branches of the innominate artery, this artery supplies both the right vertebral and the right carotid, in other words, the entire right side of the brain.

The subclavian and carotid arteries are most commonly involved in Takayasu's arteritis, with the innominate slightly less frequently affected. It is common for all the major thoracic arch arteries to be involved with long, tapered stenoses. A sudden occlusion of one of these involved arteries could cause a stroke (12) (Fig. 2). The author has seen asymptomatic patients with left subclavian and, therefore, its left vertebral branch as the only branch of the thoracic aorta not occluded and therefore the sole source of blood supply to the brain. If that artery occludes, a massive stroke could occur.

Since most Takayasu's patients have severe anatomical cerebrovascular involvement without symptoms, there is a question whether these patients should have a prophylactic bypass to preserve or even increase blood flow to the brain in case one of the involved arteries suddenly occludes. There is no large series that proves that prophylactic bypass is indicated. However, the author recommends that if there is significant involvement of more than one of the major branches of the thoracic aorta, then revascularization should be done prophylactically to prevent a major stroke (12). The graft should originate off the ascending aorta, infrequently involved with Takayasu's arteritis and then be anastomosed to the subclavian and/or both carotid arteries. Takayasu's arteritis may affect almost the entire length of the common carotid arteries, but does not usually affect the bifurcation of the carotid artery, so that there usually is an area macroscopically free of disease to serve as the site of the distal anastomosis.

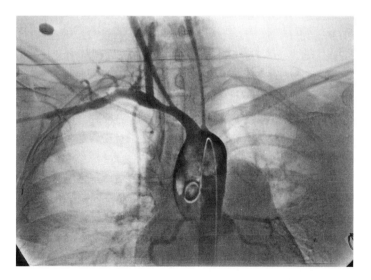

Figure 2   This is a classic arteriogram of a Takayasu's patient with cerebrovascular involvement. The patient is asymptomatic. Note that the left subclavian artery is occluded. The left common carotid and to a lesser extent the right common carotid arteries have significant stenoses. Occlusion of the right or left common carotid artery could cause a significant stroke. This is the type of patient in whom revascularization of the cerebrovascular blood supply may be important to prevent a stroke.

IV. UPPER EXTREMITY

Involvement of the subclavian and axillary arteries frequently causes upper extremity ischemic symptoms. Gangrenous changes in the hands and arms are rare. Upper extremity symptoms of fatigue and pain with exercise are far more common. It is also important to note that since patients with Takayasu's arteritis are young and more active, the arm ischemic symptoms are more likely to interfere with patients' lifestyles. Bilateral involvement of the upper extremities also prevents accurate assessment of arterial blood pressure, which in normal circumstances is measured from the brachial artery. These patients may have undiagnosed systemic hypertension, a serious source of morbidity and mortality. In these patients, revascularization of the upper extremities should be strongly considered as a way to document and treat patients with systemic hypertension.

V. LOWER EXTREMITY

Involvement of arteries to the lower extremities can cause claudication and, in unusual circumstances, rest pain, ulceration, or gangrene (1,11). Claudication occurs from involvement of the terminal aorta and, to a lesser extent, the iliac arteries. The aortic involvement usually begins just below the renal arteries and ends just above the aortic bifurcation often sparing the distal aorta, a peculiar pattern (Fig. 3). It is unusual for Takayasu's arteritis to involve the common femoral artery and its distal branches.

Most patients with leg claudication due to atherosclerosis can be treated conservatively with an exercise program. However, when the arterial disease of Takayasu's arteritis causes stenosis of the abdominal aorta, it is unlikely that an exercise program will be effective. Since these patients are young and more likely to have active lifestyles, indication for surgical treatment of Takayasu's arteritis with severe claudication should be more liberal than in the older patients with claudication due to atherosclerosis. To bypass the affected distal aorta, the graft usually originates in the distal thoracic aorta.

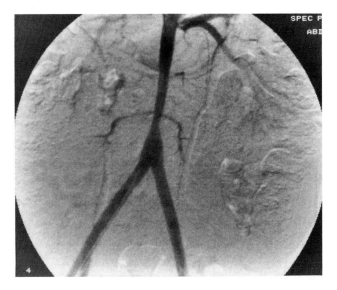

Figure 3 Peculiar involvement of the abdominal aorta in a patient with Takayasu's arteritis. Note that the distal part of the aorta is spared of disease whereas proximal to it there is significant narrowing.

VI. RENAL ARTERY STENOSIS

The incidence of hypertension secondary to renal artery stenosis has been reported in up to 72% of patients (1,15–17). Since the morbidity and mortality of Takayasu's arteritis are frequently due to cardiac decompensation from prolonged systemic hypertension, it is important to diagnose and treat hypertension. Renal artery stenosis, the most common cause of hypertension in patients with Takayasu's arteritis, is easily diagnosed with arteriography and should be treated initially with percutaneous transluminal angioplasty.

Percutaneous transluminal angioplasty is assuming an important role in the management of renal artery stenosis. Since the involvement of the renal artery tends to be a short segment lesion, percutaneous transluminal angioplasty is ideally suited for this type of stenosis. However, the chronic changes in Takayasu's arteritis make the artery more rigid than the arteries affected by atherosclerosis. Therefore, the angiographer may need three to five attempts to dilate the lesion before elimination of the stenosis is achieved. Despite these technical problems, the initial success rate is good with some studies showing patency of 85 to 95% (8,10). Follow-up has been relatively short in most trials. The long-term benefits of stenting to maintain renal artery patency is currently unknown.

If percutaneous transluminal angioplasty is unsuccessful, bypass of stenotic renal arteries is indicated to treat renal artery hypertension or to prevent chronic renal disease. Due to involvement of the abdominal aorta with Takayasu's arteritis, the usual inflow site for bypass of renal arteries presents some technical challenges to surgeons, although, in general, these procedures are successful with good long-term results (1,11,14).

VII. ANEURYSMS

The incidence of aneurysms in patients with Takayasu's arteritis varies in different parts of the world. In the North American experience, aneurysms in major arteries represents one-fourth of all vascular lesions (13), compared with being noted in 22 to 72% of patients reported from India, Japan, and South Africa (1,6,18–20). The incidence of aneurysm rupture is exceptionally low. The author still recommends resection in medically stable patients who have large aneurysms. With good medical care, this young population has a long life expectancy, much longer than patients with aneurysms from atherosclerosis. Although the rupture rate of aneurysms is low, these patients with a relatively long life expectancy ultimately have greater risk of aneurysm rupture.

VIII. CONCLUSIONS

The low incidence of Takayasu's arteritis and unusual patterns of vascular involvement make surgical treatment of this form of vasculitis challenging. However, with careful attention to details, knowledge of what vessels are likely to become involved over time, consultation with the medical service, and, in general, using conservative indications for surgical procedures, patients with Takayasu's arteritis can undergo vascular operations safely and have expectations for good long-term results.

REFERENCES

1. Hall S, Barr W, Lie JT, et al. Takayasu arteritis: A study of 32 North American patients. Medicine 1985; 64:89.

2. Waern AU, Anderson P, Hemmingsson A. Takayasu's arteritis: A hospital-region based study on occurrence, treatment and prognosis. Angiology 1983; 34:311.

3. Panja M, Kar AK, Dutta AL, et al. Cardiac involvement in non-specific aorto-arteritis. Int J Cardiol 1992; 34:289.

4. Numano F, Isohisa I, Maezawa H, et al. HL-A antigens in Takayasu's disease. Am Heart J 1979; 98:153.

5. Amano J, Suzuki A. Coronary artery involvement in Takayasu's arteritis. J Thorac Cardiovasc Surg 1991; 102:554.

6. Talwar KD, Kumar K, Chopra P, et al. Cardiac involvement in non specific aortoarteritis (Takayasu's arteritis). Am Heart J 1991; 122:1666.

7. Sharma S. Rajani M, Kaul U, et al. Initial experience with percutaenous transluminal angioplasty in the management of Takayasu's arteritis. Br J Radiol 1990; 63:517.

8. Park JH, Han MC, Kim SH, et al. Takayasu's arteritis: Angiographic findings and results of angioplasty. Am J Radiol 1989; 153:1069.

9. Sharma S, Thatai D, Saxena A, et al. Renal artery stenosis caused by non-specific arteritis (Takayasu's disease): Results of treatment with percutaneous transluminal angioplasty. Am J Radiol 1982; 158: 417.

10. Sharma S, Thatai D, Saxena A, et al. Renovascular hypertension resulting from non-specific aortoarteritis in children: Midterm results of percutaneous transluminal renal angioplasty and predictors of restenosis. Am J Roentgenol 1966; 166:157.

11. Weaver FA, Yellin AE, Campen DH, et al. Surgical procedures in the management of Takayasu's arteritis. J Vasc Surg 1990; 12:429.

12. Giordano J, Leavitt RY, Hoffman G, et al. Experience with surgical treatment of Takayasu's disease. Surgery 1991; 109:252.

13. Kerr GS, Hallahan CW, Giordano J, et al. Takayasu arteritis. Ann Intern Med 1994; 120:919.

14. Lagneau P, Michel JB, Vuong PN. Surgical treatment of Takayasu's disease. Ann Surg 1987; 205:157.

15. Lupi-Herrera E, Sanchez-Torres G, Marcushamer J, et al. Takayasu's arteritis: Clinical study of 107 cases. Am Heart J 1977; 93:94.

16. Shelhamer JH, Volkman DJ, Parillo JE, et al. Takayasus's arteritis and its therapy. Ann Intern Med 1985; 103:121.

17. Hall S, Buchbinder R. Takayasu's arteritis. Rheum Dis Clin North Am 1990; 16:411.

18. Robbs JV, Abdoll-Carrim A, Kadwa AM. Arterial Reconstruction for nonspecific arteritis (Takayasu's disease). Eur J Vasc Surg 1994; 8:401.

19. Matsumura K. Hirano I, Iakeda K, et al. Incidence of aneurysms in Takayasu's arteritis. Angiology 1991; 42:308.

20. Kumar S, Subramanyan R, Ravi Mandalan K, et al. Aneurysmal form of aortoarteritis (Takayasus's disease): Analysis of thirty cases. Clin Radiol 1990; 42:342.

33
Behçet's Disease

Kenneth T. Calamia
Mayo Clinic Jacksonville, Jacksonville, Florida

J. Desmond O'Duffy
Sarasota, Florida

I. INTRODUCTION

In 1937, the Turkish dermatologist H. Behçet called attention to the association of oral and genital ulceration with hypopyon–uveitis (1). Since then, Behçet's disease has become associated with a number of additional clinical manifestations, each attributed to an underlying vasculitis. Vessels of all sizes may be affected. The most typical clinical lesions are mucocutaneous, reflecting involvement of small vessels, but inflammation of the aorta and its branches and veins of all caliber is also possible. The disease is recognized worldwide, but there are significant differences in the epidemiological, genetic, and clinical characteristics of the disorder among ethnic groups and in different geographical locations. As there are no specific manifestations or specific diagnostic tests, the term "Behçet's syndrome" is preferred by some authors, especially for patients from low-prevalence areas whose disease manifestations are generally less severe and possibly due to other underlying conditions (2). The disease is associated with significant morbidity and mortality. Treatment is dependent on the site and severity of manifestations (3).

II. EPIDEMIOLOGY

The prevalence of Behçet's disease is highest in countries of the eastern Mediterranean, the Middle East and the eastern Asian rim. This geographical distribution coincides with the historic "silk road" of commerce and travel between Europe and the Orient. It is postulated that either agents responsible for the disease or the necessary genetic susceptibility traveled with the ancients along this path. Prevalence rates of up to 300 per 100,000 are reported from Turkey (4) and are in the range of 13–17 per 100,000 in Japan, Korea, and China. In Europe, rates of 0.5–3 per 100,000 are reported (5,6). The prevalence is much higher in Germans who have Turkish origins (6), but is still only about one-fourth of the rate reported in Turkey. Coupled with very low prevalence rates for Behçet's disease in Japanese Americans, a role for environmental contributions to the disease is suggested. Recent data from Olmsted County, Minnesota, reveal a prevalence rate of 6.6 per 100,000 (7), suggesting that the disease may be more common in the United States than previously suspected. Prevalence rates in all areas of the world are increasing, likely due to improved disease recognition and reporting.

The disease occurs primarily in young adults. The mean age of onset is between 25 and 30 years (6,8,9). Less than 10% of cases are reported in juveniles (3,6,10). Earlier reports from Eastern countries have shown a male predominance in patients with Behçet's disease, but recent reports reflect a male/female ratio much closer to 1. In Western countries, females predominate.

In high-prevalence areas, Behçet's disease is associated with the *HLA-B*5101* allele of *HLA-B51,* a split product of *HLA-B5* (11). Clinical features of patients from these areas are more similar than when compared to western patients whose disease has no strong association with HLA antigens (4). Familial Behçet's disease is uncommon, and no clear pattern of inheritance can be determined in most cases, but familial disease was noted in 15% of affected children (10).

III. CLINICAL FEATURES

A. Mucocutaneous Manifestations

The International Study Group (ISG) criteria for the diagnosis of Behçet's disease (Table 1) are weighted heavily in favor of mucocutaneous manifestations (12). The mucocutaneous lesions as well as the pathergy lesion may be varied presentations of the same pathological process (13). Vasculitis is thought to underlie these lesions, and has been demonstrated in a high percentage of ulcers and skin lesions (14). Vasculitis or the perivascular inflammation seen in Behçet's lesions may be either neutrophilic or lymphocytic, and is thought to reflect the age of the lesions (13). The vasculitis seen in some skin biopsy specimens may be secondary to intense perivascular inflammation (15).

Aphthous oral ulcers are usually the first and most persistent clinical feature (Fig. 1). Lesions may be present 50% of the time in some individuals (16). Aphthae occur as 2- to 12-mm discrete, painful, round or oval, red-rimmed lesions. The nonkeratinized mucosa of the cheeks, tongue, palate, and pharynx is mostly affected, whereas the well-keratinized hard palate is less involved. Oral ulcers are identical to the lesions of recurrent aphthous stomatitis, but six or more ulcers, variable in size, with surrounding erythema, and with involvement of the soft palate and oropharynx should increase the suspicion for Behçet's associated lesions. The severity and behavior of the oral ulcers in Behçet's disease often fits the description of "complex aphthosis," in which multiple, recurrent, or persisting lesions result in a severe syndrome that may include perianal or genital ulceration (17,18). Complex aphthosis may be a forme fruste of Behçet's disease when another cause is not found (19). The diagnosis of Behçet's disease in these patients requires

Table 1   International Study Group Criteria for Behçet's Disease

Recurrent oral ulceration	Minor aphthous, major aphthous, or herpetiform ulceration observed by physician or patient, which recurred at least 3 times in one 12-month period[a]
Plus 2 of:	
Recurrent genital ulceration	Aphthous ulceration or scarring, observed by physician or patient[a]
Eye lesions	Anterior uveitis, posterior uveitis, or cells in vitreous on slit lamp examination; or retinal vasculitis observed by ophthalmologist
Skin lesions	Erythema nodosum observed by physician or patient, pseudofolliculitis, or papulopustular lesions; or acneiform nodules observed by physician in postadolescent patients not on corticosteroid treatment[a]
Positive pathergy test	Read by physician at 24–48 h

[a]Findings applicable only in absence of other clinical explanations.
Source: Ref. 12.

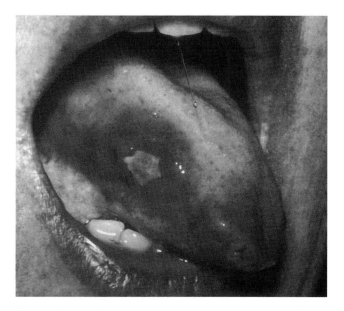

Figure 1 Aphthous ulcer in Behçet's disease.

the presence of other characteristic lesions and exclusion of other systemic disorders (18), most notably sprue, hematological disorders, herpes simplex infection, inflammatory bowel disease, cyclic neutropenia, and acquired immune deficiency syndrome. Other disorders responsible for oral–genital ulcerative syndromes include the hypereosinophilic syndrome and myelodysplasia. Lesions in Stevens–Johnson syndrome, lichen planus, pemphigus, or cicatricial pemphigoid are not aphthous in character (18). The differential diagnosis can be clarified with the aid of an experienced dermatologist and biopsy.

Genital ulcers, resembling oral aphthae, occur on the vulva and vagina in females and on the scrotum or penis in males. Vulvar lesions are painful and may result in scarring, but vaginal ulcers may be asymptomatic or result in a discharge (20). Scrotal lesions may be superficial or deep, and may heal with scarring. Genital ulcers are single or multiple, and typically occur two to four times a year. Perianal ulcers have been found in 7% of children with Behçet's disease (10).

The frequency of skin lesions in Behçet's disease ranges from 41–97% (21). Skin lesions occurred in 64% of Behçet's patients from the United States (22) and are often essential to meet diagnostic disease criteria. The ISG criteria (12) (see Table 1) recognize erythema nodosum, pseudofolliculitis, papulopustular lesions, or acneform nodules for the diagnosis. Histopathological findings in lesions of erythema nodosum are those of a septal and lobular panniculitis and may include a lymphocytic vasculitis (23). These lesions are indistinguishable from erythema nodosum associated with other disorders. Nodose lesions should be distinguished from superficial thrombophlebitis. The distinction between acneform and papulopustular lesions is unclear, but the term "pseudofolliculitis" separates these lesions from follicle-based eruptions. However, distinction of these lesions on clinical examination is not reliable (13), and biopsies are not often performed. A neutrophilic vascular reaction (19) characterizes typical Behçet's lesions, but the pathology is not specific for the disease. Occasionally, intense neutrophilic inflammation results in lesions of Sweet's syndrome. Pyoderma gangrenosum–like lesions or cutaneous aphthosis may also occur (21), and more than one type of skin lesion may occur in the same patient (21,24).

Pathergy, an excessive skin response to trauma, has been considered a unique manifestation of Behçet's disease, reflecting neutrophil hyperreactivity. The phenomenon can also be demonstrated in patients with chronic myelogenous leukemia (25). Pathergy testing is performed by inserting a sterile 20-gauge needle perpendicularly into the skin and subcutaneous tissue of the volar forearm to a depth of 0.5 cm. An erythematous papule or pustule ($\geq$2 mm in diameter) at the puncture site after 48 h constitutes a positive test. Pathergy equivalents in the form of sterile abscesses or pustules after therapeutic injections or skin trauma may occur. The pathergy test is less likely to be positive in Behçet's patients from North America and European countries than in Turkish patients (26). Nonetheless, a positive pathergy test was found in 6 of 18 patients tested from the United States, suggesting that the test may be underutilized in Western countries (22). However, positivity of the test may wax and wane (27), and standardization of the test procedure has been lacking (28,29). The outcome of testing is influenced by the diameter of the needle (30), the use of sharp, disposable needles as compared to blunted reusable needles (31), the number of puncture sites, and the use of cleansing antiseptic (32).

B. Ocular Manifestations

The ocular finding in Behçet's original patients was that of hypopyon–uveitis (1) which may still be found in up to one-third of patients with eye disease (33). While eye disease limited to the anterior chamber does not usually threaten vision (34), hypopyon suggests severe ocular inflammation and a poor visual prognosis. In fully developed Behçet's eye disease, a panuveitis, including posterior uveitis and retinal vasculitis, is usually associated with anterior uveitis and is responsible for the visual loss in these patients. Younger patients and males are at higher risk for ocular involvement (35). Severe eye disease is less common in western countries than in the Middle East or Japan. In Japanese patients, ocular disease is found in about 90% of men, and results in blindness in up to 25% of affected individuals (33). Ocular inflammation in Behçet's disease typically follows mucocutaneous symptoms by a few years and progresses with a chronic, relapsing course affecting both eyes. Vasculitis leads to episodes of retinal occlusion and areas of ischemia, and may be followed by neovascularization, vitreous hemorrhage and contraction, glaucoma, and retinal detachment. The earliest findings of retinal vasculitis may be detected with fluorescein angiography. It is essential for patients with ocular involvement to be monitored very carefully by an experienced ophthalmologist. Isolated optic disc edema in Behçet's disease suggests cerebral venous thrombosis rather than ocular disease (36), but papillitis may occur with ocular inflammation and central nervous system disease. Occasionally, cranial nerve palsies resulting from brain stem lesions are present and visual field defects may occur with intracranial lesions (37). Rarely, conjunctival aphthous lesions are found.

C. Major Vessel Involvement

Large-vessel involvement in Behçet's disease affects about one-fourth to one-third of patients. The types of major vessel lesions seen are shown in Table 2. Sixty-eight percent of patients with vascular disease in one report had involvement of both arterial and venous systems (38). Major vessel problems and their complications are a significant cause of morbidity and mortality in Behçet's disease and are a major determinant of disease prognosis (39–41).

Superficial thrombophlebitis often precedes deep venous disease, and both conditions appear to increase risk for caval thrombosis (38,42,43), as well as for arterial disease (44). Thromboses of superficial veins may occur following venipuncture and have been reported at sites of heparin infusions (45). Deep venous thrombosis is the most common large vascular lesion. It occurs primarily in the lower extremities, but involvement is possible at any site. Vena cava occlu-

Table 2 Vascular Involvement in Behçet's Disease

Systemic arterial vasculitis
   Aneurysms
   Occlusions
Pulmonary arterial vasculitis
   Aneurysms
   Occlusions
Venous occlusions
   Superficial venous thromboses
   Deep venous thromboses
   Vena cava thromboses
   Cerebral venous thromboses
   Budd–Chiari syndrome
   Portal vein thrombosis
   Right ventricular thrombi
   Pulmonary emboli
Varices

sion is a commonly recognized thrombotic complication in Behçet's disease (46), and is associated with a high risk of mortality (46,47). Additional thrombotic complications include Budd–Chiari syndrome (48) and cavernous transformation of the portal vein (49). Chest wall, abdominal, and esophageal varices may occur as a consequence of deep-seated venous thrombosis. Right ventricular thrombi have been reported in Behçet's disease, usually associated with pulmonary vasculitis (50). With cerebral venous thrombosis, patients usually present with symptoms associated with elevated intracranial pressure, including headache and visual obscurations with papilledema. Focal deficits, seizures, and altered consciousness may also occur (51). Magnetic resonance imaging (MRI) may be used to demonstrate acute or recent clots in the larger dural sinuses (Fig. 2a). Magnetic resonance angiography (MRA) provides more reliable imaging of the cerebral venous system, especially of the smaller veins and if thromboses are older. Two-dimensional (see Fig. 2b) and three-dimensional phase contrast MRAs allow imaging of the cerebral veins without administration of contrast.

In spite of the frequency of venous thrombosis, there is a conspicuous rarity of pulmonary emboli in patients within Behçet's disease. This supports histological evidence that the vascular wall itself is a major factor in the process of thrombosis in Behçet's disease, resulting in an adherent thrombus (44). In some cases, however, venous thrombosis may be recurrent and progressive, in spite of treatment with anticoagulants and can result in life-threatening emboli. All of the factors contributing to venous thrombosis in Behçet's disease are not known. Inflammation of the venous endothelium is present. There have been no consistent primary abnormalities of the coagulation, anticoagulation, or fibrinolytic systems yet identified, although some evidence exists for impaired fibrinolysis (52). Thrombophilia has been implicated in some patients with thrombosis (53). Antiphospholipid antibodies have been reported in some patients, but these do not correlate with thrombosis (54).

Arterial complications occur in up to 7% of patients with Behçet's disease (55). Arterial lesions may be seen in the systemic circulation as well as in the pulmonary arterial bed (Fig. 3). In either location, stenoses, occlusions, and aneurysms may result and frequently coexist. Isolated occlusions or stenosis may be asymptomatic or associated with ischemic symptoms, depending upon the adequacy of the collateral circulation (56). Arterial aneurysms, due to vasculitis of the vasa vasorum (57), primarily involve the aorta, but any large vessel may be affected, and the risk

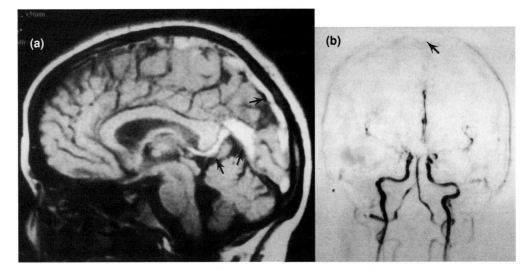

Figure 2 (a) T1-weighted spin echo MRI reveals clot (arrows, high signal intensity) in the sagittal and straight sinuses, the vein of Galen, and an internal cerebral vein. (b) Anterior–posterior view of a 2-D phase contrast MRA demonstrates a flow void in the sagittal sinus (arrow) indicating the presence of thrombosis.

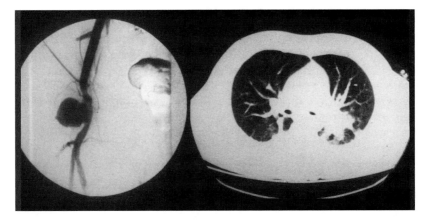

Figure 3 Angiograms showing femoral artery aneurysm and CT scan revealing a pulmonary artery aneurysm in a 37-year-old male with Behçet's disease.

of rupture is high (58). Pulmonary artery vasculitis (Fig. 4) with aneurysm formation was found in about 1% of Behçet patients in Turkey (44). Patients usually present with hemoptysis due to pulmonary artery–bronchial fistula. Hemoptysis may be massive and threaten life. As venous thrombosis often coexists with pulmonary artery–bronchial fistulae, it is extremely important to distinguish these patients from those with hemoptysis due to pulmonary emboli so that anticoagulant treatment is not initiated.

Clinically apparent cardiac vascular involvement is unusual, but may result in myocardial infarction (59). However, subclinical cardiac and vascular abnormalities are common if patients are systematically evaluated (60,61).

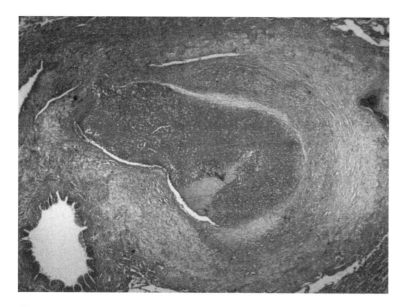

Figure 4   Acute angiitis, thrombosis, and aneurysmal dilatation of a branch pulmonary artery in Behçet's disease.

D.   Central Nervous System Disease

In addition to cerebral venous thrombosis, central nervous system (CNS) symptoms in Behçet's disease may be due to aseptic meningitis or parenchymal lesions, resulting in focal or diffuse brain dysfunction. Aseptic meningitis presents with headache, stiff neck, and fever, and is associated with elevated protein and a lymphocytic pleocytosis in the cerebrospinal fluid (62). Focal or multifocal nervous system involvement reflects the predilection of the disease for brain stem and periventricular white matter involvement (63). Diffuse or recurrent disease may result in dementia. Magnetic resonance imaging is more sensitive than computed tomography in demonstrating focal lesions. Although the findings are nonspecific, the clinical combination of stroke, aseptic meningitis with CSF pleocytosis, and the presence of mucocutaneous lesions can be diagnostic. Cerebral angiography is usually negative because small vessels are involved, but findings consistent with vasculitis can occasionally be seen (64). Magnetic resonance venography is warranted in patients with papilledema or other symptoms suggesting increased intracranial pressure to rule out venous sinus thrombosis.

Central nervous system disease in Behçet's patients may be more common in European and U.S. patients, affecting about 30% (65). Involvement was found in about 5% of patients from Turkey (66), and in 3.2% from Iran (4). Isolated headaches in Behçet's patients are common but may represent secondary migraine or be unrelated to the disease. Follow-up of a group of headache patients, however, revealed neurological abnormalities in one-fourth (67).

E.   Gastrointestinal Lesions

Gastrointestinal disease in Behçet's is much more common in Japanese patients than in patients from other geographical areas (39). Gastrointestinal symptoms include melena or abdominal pain. Lesions consist of single or multiple ulcerative lesions that primarily involve the distal ileum and cecum, but any region can be affected. Gastrointestinal lesions have a tendency to perforate or bleed and may recur after surgery (68,69). Vasculitis has been demonstrated in surgical specimens of operated patients. Lesions should be distinguished from those of Crohn's disease or those due to the use of nonsteroidal antiinflammatory drugs.

F. Arthritis and Spondylitis

An intermittent, symmetrical oligoarthritis of the knees, ankles, hands, and/or wrists, affects 40–70% of patients with Behçet's disease (70–72). Episodes often persist for a few weeks and may not be associated with other clinical manifestations. Synovial fluid analysis reveals inflammatory range white blood cell counts, consisting primarily of polymorphonuclear leukocytes (73). Synovial biopsies reveal superficial neutrophilic infiltration (74), distinct from the lymphocytic synovitis seen in rheumatoid arthritis. A destructive arthropathy is unusual.

Some studies have found an increased frequency of ankylosing spondylitis or radiographic sacroiliitis in patients with Behçet's disease, but others have shown no association (75). *HLA-B27* is present in those Behçet's patients with spondyloarthropathy and patients may have inflammatory bowel disease as well (75). Despite the occasional association with spondylitis, Behçet's disease should not be classified as a seronegative spondyloarthropathy.

G. Miscellaneous Manifestations

There have been sporadic reports of glomerulonephritis in Behçet's disease, but renal involvement is seen much less frequently than one might expect in a systemic vasculitis. Peripheral neuropathy is unusual in Behçet's disease (20). Epididymitis occurs in about 5% of affected patients. Amyloidosis of the AA-type can accompany Behçet's disease, usually presenting as nephrotic syndrome. This complication has occurred primarily in Mediterranean patients (76–78). The MAGIC (mouth and genital ulcers with inflamed cartilage) syndrome is diagnosed in patients who have features of both Behçet's disease and relapsing polychondritis (79). A generalized myositis can rarely be associated with Behçet's disease (80).

IV. LABORATORY FINDINGS

There are no laboratory abnormalities that are diagnostic of Behçet's disease. Acute phase reactants may be elevated, especially in patients with large-vessel vasculitis, but may be normal with active eye disease. Levels of immune complexes may be elevated in Behçet's disease, but measurements of rheumatoid factor, cryoglobulins, and complement components are usually normal or negative. The histocompatibility antigen HLA-B51 is more common in Behçet's disease patients than in control subjects, especially in high-prevalence areas and in patients with ocular disease. The absence of an HLA-B51 association in northern caucasoid patients, 49% of whom were found to have *HLA-DRB1*04* (81), makes HLA testing in these patients unnecessary. Measurement of the T-cell proliferative response to heat shock proteins (HSP) has been proposed for the diagnosis of Behçet's disease (82) as was measurement of impaired fibrinolytic activity (52), but the value of testing has not been confirmed.

V. DIAGNOSIS

The ISG criteria for the diagnosis of Behçet's disease (see Table 1) (12) have been proposed and validated (83), but these criteria were not meant to replace clinical judgment regarding the diagnosis in individual cases. The criteria require the presence of oral ulcerations, which may be absent in about 3% of Behçet's patients. In Japan, Korea, and Iran, alternative criteria are applied concurrently by investigators (21,84). For patients in Western countries, substitution of large-vessel disease or acute central nervous system infarction for missing ISG criteria is acceptable (85). The multiple manifestations of Behçet's disease may not occur simultaneously but may be separated in time, occasionally by several years. For a definitive diagnosis, manifestations must be documented or witnessed by a physician. Acneform lesions should not be attributed to Behçet's disease in an adolescent or in patients taking corticosteriods (12).

The differential diagnosis of Behçet's disease includes those conditions that result in complex aphthosis. The prevalence of recurrent aphthous stomatitis is much greater than Behçet's and the diagnosis of "possible Behçet's" in patients who only have aphthae is inappropriate. In Reiter's disease, mucocutaneous lesions are nonulcerative and painless. The uveitis is usually limited to the anterior chamber. In addition to gastrointestinal lesions, similarities between Behçet's and Crohn's disease include fever, anemia, oral ulcers, uveitis, arthritis, thrombophlebitis, and erythema nodosum (86). However, granuloma formation in intestinal lesions is not typically seen in Behçet's, and in Crohn's the iritis is typically anterior. Genital ulcerations and central nervous system disease are extremely rare in Crohn's disease.

VI. DISEASE ACTIVITY

For mucocutaneous manifestations, disease activity is recognized and monitored by recording the number, size, and location of lesions, and the percentage of time that lesions have been present since the patient's last visit. Frequent ophthalmological examinations are necessary for patients with ocular disease, and periodic monitoring of the eyes is recommended for patients at risk. A careful history and examination with attention to vascular and neurological systems should be part of the physician's assessment. Standardized tools for recording and scoring disease activity have been developed for use in clinical trials as well as for the care of individual patients (87). Validation efforts continue for the Behçet's Disease Current Activity Form (88) and for the Iran Behçet's Disease Dynamic Activity Measure (89), both currently in use. Similar assessment tools for ocular disease activity have been devised (87,90).

For individual patients in whom systemic symptoms or a particular disease manifestation is paralleled by a nonspecific acute phase response, sequential measurements may be of value. A number of cytokines and markers of vascular inflammation are under investigation as tools for monitoring disease activity. Elevated levels of von Willebrand's factor (91) and thrombomodulin in the serum of Behçet's patients reflect vascular cell injury (92,93). As in other vasculitides, levels of soluble intercellular adhesion molecule-1 (sICAM-1), reflecting endothelial activation, were higher in active Behçet patients but were not different in patients with and without clinical vascular disease (94).

VII. MANAGEMENT

Certainty in the treatment of Behçet's disease is limited by the lack of controlled studies. Treatment practices may reflect the experience and biases of clinicians from different geographical areas. Aphthous lesions are treated with topical or intralesional corticosteriods, but results are frequently disappointing. Dapsone can also be used to suppress mucocutaneous lesions. A controlled study, limited to male patients, demonstrated the value of thalidomide for the prevention and treatment of mucosal and follicular lesions (95). Colchicine is widely used in the treatment of mucocutaneous manifestations and as an adjunct in the treatment of more serious manifestations, but proof of its effectiveness in one controlled study was limited to improvement in erythema nodosum

(78). The addition of penicillin to colchicine was found to be beneficial in reducing the number of arthritis attacks (96). Interferon-α (INF-α) has been used in open studies of Behçet's patients and found to be useful in mucocutaneous lesions and arthritis (97,98). Methotrexate has been effective in the treatment of mucocutaneous disease in a small series (99).

In general, younger male patients are at greatest risk for severe disease, especially uveitis, warranting expectant and aggressive treatment. A controlled study has demonstrated the value of azathioprine at a dose of 2.5 mg/kg/day in limiting the progression of ocular disease and preventing new eye disease in male patients (100). Treatment also had benefits on mucosal ulcers, arthritis, deep-vein thrombosis, and on long-term prognosis (101). Cyclosporin A has been recognized as an effective agent for the control of uveitis (102,103), but the long-term benefits of the drug are less certain. Combination treatment with cyclosporin A and azathioprine has been used when single agents fail (104). In an open trial, interferon-α was highly effective in the control of eye disease in seven patients with early ocular disease or with limited damage (105).

Corticosteriods are useful in suppression of inflammation in acute phases of the disease, but these agents do not consistently suppress mucosal ulcers or central nervous system disease, and do not appear to prevent blindness in Behçet's patients with posterior uveitis or retinal vasculitis. Immunosuppression with cyclophosphamide or chlorambucil is used for uncontrolled ocular disease, central nervous system disease, and large-vessel vasculitis including recurrent deep venous thrombosis. The mucocutaneous disease also improves. We favor the use of chlorambucil in these settings based on our positive experience with the use of this agent (62). The toxicity of chlorambucil includes infertility and an increased risk of malignancy (106). Chlorambucil is more lipophilic than cyclophosphamide, giving it a theoretical advantage in the treatment of central nervous system disease.

Surgery is usually indicated for the treatment of systemic arterial aneurysms because of the risk of rupture (58), but isolated arterial occlusions may be asymptomatic and not require surgery. Pulmonary arterial aneurysms with uncontrolled bleeding require surgery. Percutaneous embolization techniques have been reported to thrombose these lesions (107,108). Arterial vasculitis resulting in aneurysms of the systemic or pulmonary circulations should be treated with alkalating agents. If surgery is required, these agents are also necessary to minimize the high risk of anastomotic recurrences or continued disease (55,56).

Cerebral venous thrombosis responds well to treatment with heparin and corticosteroids (51). Venous thrombosis may be progressive or recurrent in spite of warfarin treatment. As inflammation underlies the thrombosis, corticosteroids and immunosuppressive agents should be considered in these cases. The treatment of Budd–Chiari syndrome has included anticoagulants, colchicine, and corticosteriods (109), but others prefer a combination of antiaggregants (48). Portocaval shunting is recommended if the inferior vena cava is patent (109). Successful treatment of right ventricular thrombi has been reported with anticoagulants, corticosteroids, and immunosuppressive agents (110).

VIII. PATHOGENESIS

Clues to the pathogenesis of Behçet's disease come from analysis of the cellular infiltrates from inflammatory lesions as well as from circulating immune cell types and cytokine patterns. While neutrophilic vascular lesions are characteristic on biopsies of established lesions at mucocutaneous sites, perivascular mononuclear cells dominate in early lesions (111,112). In mucocutaneous sites, ocular lesions (113), gastrointestinal lesions (114), and vascular lesions (111), CD4+ T cells are the predominant type. Reversal in the ratio of CD4+/CD8+ cells in the circulation has been found (115). Oligoclonal expansion of T cells with specific Vβ T cell receptors has been found (116). Elevated numbers of $\gamma\delta$ T cells have been found in Behçet's patients (117,118), and are found in mucosal lesions (119). These cells possess activation markers and produce inflammatory cytokines during disease exacerbation, but the exact role of γδ T cells in the pathogenesis of Behçet's disease remains uncertain.

Interleukin-8 (IL-8), a chemokine responsible for neutrophilic activation, is elevated in the serum of Behçet's patients. Elevated levels of other proinflammatory cytokines, including IL-1, IL-6, INF-γ, IL-12, tumor necrosis factor-α (TNF-α), as well as sIL-2R, have been reported in Behçet's patients (120–123), consistent with systemic immune system activation. Mononuclear cells from these patients produce greater amounts of these cytokines ex vivo, when compared with normals (124–127). However, cytokine studies have not yet led to clinically useful measures of disease activity.

Cytokine analysis and cellular characterization suggest a Th1 response by lymphocytes in Behçet's disease (128). Other studies have shown participation of both Th1 and Th2 cells (129). Although circulating immune complexes (130) and antiendothelial antibodies (131,132) have been found in Behçet's patients, there is little evidence for a contribution of B-cell hyperactivity in Behçet's disease.

Extrinsic agents have been suspected to trigger autoimmunity in Behçet's disease. Molecular techniques have identified herpes simplex viral RNA and DNA in cells from Behçet's patients. Streptococcal antigens are suspected to trigger disease activity (133). The use of minocycline reduced symptoms in affected patients (134).

Peptides from mycobacterial heat shock protein (HSP) (135) and homologous human peptides have been found to specifically stimulate γδ T cells from Behçet's patients (82). It is postulated that cross-reactivity and molecular mimicry between peptides from streptococcal and/or viral HSP, homologous human HSP, and mucosal antigens result in selection of autoreactive T cells (136).

Neutrophilic hyperfunction is recognized in Behçet's disease, in normals with *HLA-B51*, and in *HLA-B51* transgenic mice (137). It remains uncertain if this association is due to antigen interaction with HLA, another effect of the molecule, or to genes in linkage disequilibrium with *HLA-B51*. The disease associated *HLA-B*51* and the closely related but disease-unassociated *HLA-B52* molecules differ in two amino acid positions located in an antigen-binding pocket of the HLA groove. This suggests a direct role of the HLA molecule itself in the susceptibility to Behçet's disease, and implies a role for extrinsic agents (138). However, microsatellite data have also suggested a pathogenic role for genes located between the *HLA-B* and tumor-necrosis factor (TNF) regions on chromosome 6 (139). This region contains the MICA gene (major histocompatibility complex class I chain-related gene A), whose cell surface product is preferentially expressed on fibroblasts and endothelial cells. These gene products may have a role in the presentation of antigen to NK cells or to γδ T cells (139). Analysis of triplet repeat polymorphisms of the MICA gene revealed an association of the *A6* allele with Behçet's disease in Japanese patients which is greater than that of *HLA-B5* (11). These findings were also demonstrated in Caucasian patients (140), making MICA, or a closely related gene, a leading candidate gene for the disease.

IX. SUMMARY

The clinical manifestations of Behçet's disease are due to a vasculitis that can involve arteries of all sizes and the venous system as well. The disease has a predilection for the small vessels in mucocutaneous sites and in the eyes, but any organ system may be involved. The diagnosis is made on clinical grounds as there are no specific tests for the disease. Clinical, epidemiological and genetic differences exist between patients of varied ethnic backgrounds and from different geographical areas. The morbidity of Behçet's disease comes primarily from ocular involvement, and mortality relates primarily to large-vessel involvement and central nervous system disease.

In recent years, the development of dedicated Behçet's disease treatment units, collaborative efforts among investigators, biennial international symposia on the disorder, and controlled studies have led to new information on the treatments for the disorder and its pathogenesis. Genetic studies have revealed a strong association with *HLA-B51*, but the role of this gene in the development of the disease remains uncertain. Evidence exists for neutrophil hyperreactivity as well as for antigen-driven immune mechanisms in the pathogenesis of the disease.

ACKNOWLEDGMENT

Thanks to Darlene Gunsolus for assistance in preparation of the manuscript.

REFERENCES

1. Behçet H. Ueber rezidivierende aphthoese, durch ein Virus verursachte Geschwuere am Mund, am Auge und an den Genitalien. Derm Wochenschr 1937; 36:1152–1157.
2. Ehrlich GE. Vasculitis in Behçet's disease. Int Rev Immunol 1997; 14:81–88.
3. Yazici H, Yurdakul S, Hamuryudan V. Behçet's syndrome. Curr Opin Rheumatol 1999; 11:53–57.
4. Gharibdoost F, Davatchi F, Shahram F, et al. Clinical manifestations of Behçet's disease in Iran analysis of 2176 cases. In: Godeau P, Wechsler B, eds. Behçet's Disease. Paris: Elsevier, 1993:153–158.
5. Chamberlain MA. Behçet's syndrome in 32 patients in Yorkshire. Ann Rheum Dis 1977; 36:491–499.
6. Zouboulis CC, Kotter I, Djawari D, et al. Epidemiological features of Adamantiades-Behçet's disease in Germany and in Europe. Yonsei Med J 1997; 38:411–422.
7. O'Duffy JD. Behçet's disease. Curr Opin Rheumatol 1994; 6:39–43.
8. Gurler A, Boyvat A, Tursen U. Clinical manifestations of Behçet's disease: An analysis of 2147 patients. Yonsei Med J 1997; 38:423–427.
9. Davatchi F. Epidemiology of Behçet's disease in Middle East and Asia. (A). Proceedings of the Eighth International Congress on Behçet's disease, Reggio-Emilia, Italy, 1998:36.
10. Kone-Paut I, Yurdakul S, Bahabri SA, et al. Clinical features of Behçet's disease in children: an international collaborative study of 86 cases. J Pediatr 1998; 132:721–725.
11. Mizuki N, Ota M, Kimura M, et al. Triplet repeat polymorphism in the transmembrane region of the MICA gene: A strong association of six GCT repetitions with Behçet disease. Proc Natl Acad Sci USA 1997; 94:1298–1303.
12. International Study Group for Behçet's Disease. Criteria for diagnosis of Behçet's disease. Lancet 1990; 335:1078–1080.
13. Jorizzo JL, Abernethy JL, White WL, et al. Mucocutaneous criteria for the diagnosis of Behçet's disease: An analysis of clinicopathologic data from multiple international centers. J Am Acad Dermatol 1995; 32:968–976.
14. Kienbaum S, Zouboulis CC, Waibel M, et al. Chemotactic neutrophilic vasculitis: A new histopathological pattern of vasculitis found in mucocutaneous lesions of patients with Adamatntiades-Behçet's disease. In: Godeau P, Wechsler B, eds. Behçet's Disease. Paris: Elsevier, 1993:337–341.
15. Chun SI, Su WP, Lee S. Histopathologic study of cutaneous lesions in Behçet's syndrome. J Dermatol 1990; 17:333–341.
16. Lehner T. Oral ulceration and Behçet's syndrome. Gut 1977; 18:491–511.
17. Jorizzo JL, Taylor RS, Schmalstieg FC, et al. Complex aphthosis: A forme fruste of Behçet's syndrome? J Am Acad Dermatol 1985; 13:80–84.
18. Rogers RS, III. Recurrent aphthous stomatitis in the diagnosis of Behçet's disease. Yonsei Med J 1997; 38:370–379.
19. Ghate JV, Jorizzo JL. Behçet's disease and complex aphthosis. J Am Acad Dermatol 1999; 40:1–18; quiz 19–20.
20. O'Duffy JD, Carney JA, Deodhar S. Behçet's disease. Report of 10 cases, 3 with new manifestations. Ann Intern Med 1971; 75:561–570.

21. Lee ES, Bang D, Lee S. Dermatologic manifestation of Behçet's disease. Yonsei Med J 1997; 38:380–389.

22. Balabanova M, Calamia KT, O'Duffy JD. A study of the cutaneous manifestations of Behçet's disease in patients from the United States (A). Proceedings of the 8th International Congress on Behçet's disease, Reggio Emilia, Italy, 1998:118. Accepted for publication.

23. Chun SI, Su WP, Lee S, et al. Erythema nodosum-like lesions in Behçet's syndrome: A histopathologic study of 30 cases. J Cutan Pathol 1989; 16:259–265.

24. Calamia KT, Cohen MD, O'Duffy JD. Large vessel involvement in Behçet's disease (A). Proceedings of the Eighth International Congress on Behçet's disease, Reggio-Emilia, Italy, 1998:70.

25. Budak-Alpdogan T, Demircay Z, Alpdogan O, et al. Behçet's disease in patients with chronic myelogenous leukemia: Possible role of interferon-alpha treatment in the occurrence of Behçet's symptoms. Ann Hematol 1997; 74:45–48.

26. Yazici H, Chamberlain MA, Tuzun Y, et al. A comparative study of the pathergy reaction among Turkish and British patients with Behçet's disease. Ann Rheum Dis 1984; 43:74–75.

27. Chams-Davatchi C, Davatchi F, Shahram F, et al. Longitudinal study of the pathergy phenomenon in Behçet's disease. In: Hamza M, ed. Behçet's Disease. Tunis: Adhoua, 1997:356–358.

28. Dilsen N, Koniçem N, Aral O, et al. Important implications of skin pathergy test in Behçet's disease. In: Godeau P, Wechsler B, eds. Behçet's Disease. Paris: Elsevier, 1993:229–233.

29. Dilsen N. History of pathergy test (A). Proceedings of the Eighth International Congress on Behçet's disease, Reggio-Emilia, Italy. 1998:36.

30. Ozarmagan G, Saylan T, Azizlerli G, et al. Re-evaluation of the pathergy test in Behçet's disease. Acta Derm Venereol 1991; 71:75–76.

31. Samangooei S, Hakim SM, Mohamad Alipour B. The effect of specially blunted needles on the sensitivity of pathergy test in Behçet's disease (A). Proceedings of the Eighth International Congress on Behçet's disease, Reggio-Emilia, Italy, 1998:127.

32. Fresko I, Yazici H, Bayramicli M, et al. Effect of surgical cleaning of the skin on the pathergy phenomenon in Behçet's syndrome. Ann Rheum Dis 1993; 52:619–620.

33. Kim HB. Ophthalmologic manifestation of Behçet's disease. Yonsei Med J 1997; 38:390–394.

34. BenEzra D, Cohen E, Chajek T, et al. Evaluation of conventional therapy versus cyclosporine A in Behçet's syndrome. Transplant Proc 1988; 20:136–143.

35. Demiroglu H, Dündar S. Occular involvement in Behçet's disease. In: Hamza M, ed. Behçet's disease. Tunis: Adhoua, 1997:253–255.

36. Kansu T, Kansu E, Zileli T. Optic nerve involvement in Behçet's disease. In: O'Duffy JD, Kokmen E, eds. Behçet's Disease: Basic and Clinical Aspects. New York: Marcel Dekker, 1991:77–83.

37. Colvard DM, Robertson DM, O'Duffy JD. The ocular manifestations of Behçet's disease. Arch Ophthalmol 1977; 95:1813–1817.

38. Koç Y, Gullu I, Akpek G, et al. Vascular involvement in Behçet's disease. J Rheumatol 1992; 19:402–410.

39. Shimizu T, Ehrlich GE, Inaba G, et al. Behçet's disease (Behçet's syndrome). Semin Arthritis Rheum 1979; 8:223–260.

40. Yazici H, Basaran G, Hamuryudan V, et al. The ten-year mortality in Behçet's syndrome. Br J Rheumatol 1996; 35:139–141.

41. Wong RC, Ellis CN, Diaz LA. Behçet's disease. Int J Dermatol 1984; 23:25–32.

42. Dundar S, Yazici H. Superior vena cava syndrome in Behçet's disease. Vasc Surg 1984; 18:28–33.

43. Kansu E, Özer FL, Akalin E, et al. Behçet's syndrome with obstruction of the venae cavae. A report of seven cases. Q J Med 1972; 41:151–168.

44. Hamuryudan V, Yurdakul S, Moral F, et al. Pulmonary arterial aneurysms in Behçet's syndrome: A report of 24 cases. Br J Rheumatol 1994; 33:48–51.

45. Chajek T, Fainaru M. Behçet's disease. Report of 41 cases and a review of the literature. Medicine (Baltimore) 1975; 54:179–196.

46. Benamour S, Alaoui FZ, Rafik M, et al. Vena cava thrombosis: 31 cases in a series of 601 cases of Behçet's disease. In: Hamza M, ed. Behçet's Disease. Tunis: Adhoua, 1997:290–293.

47. Bang D, Cha MS, Yoo JH, et al. Vena cava syndrome in Behçet's disease. In: Hamza M, ed. Behçet's Disease. Tunis: Adhoua, 1997:286–289.

48. Bayraktar Y, Balkanci F, Kansu E, et al. Budd-Chiari syndrome: Analysis of 30 cases. Angiology 1993; 44:541–551.

49. Bayraktar Y, Balkanci F, Kansu E, et al. Cavernous transformation of the portal vein: A common manifestation of Behçet's disease. Am J Gastroenterol 1995; 90:1476–1479.

50. Le Thi Huong D, Dolmazon C, De Zuttere D, et al. Complete recovery of right intraventricular thrombus and pulmonary arteritis in Behçet's disease. Br J Rheumatol 1997; 36:130–132.

51. Wechsler B, Vidailhet M, Piette JC, et al. Cerebral venous thrombosis in Behçet's disease: Clinical study and long-term follow-up of 25 cases. Neurology 1992; 42:614–618.

52. Haznedaroglu IC, Ozcebe OI, Ozdemir O, et al. Impaired haemostatic kinetics and endothelial function in Behçet's disease. J Intern Med 1996; 240:181–187.

53. Gul A, Ozbek U, Ozturk C, et al. Coagulation factor V gene mutation increases the risk of venous thrombosis in Behçet's disease. Br J Rheumatol 1996; 35:1178–1180.

54. al-Dalaan AN, al-Ballaa SR, al-Janadi MA, et al. Association of anti-cardiolipin antibodies with vascular thrombosis and neurological manifestation of Behçet's disease. Clin Rheumatol 1993; 12:28–30.

55. Le Thi Huong D, Wechsler B, Papo T, et al. Arterial lesions in Behçet's disease. A study in 25 patients. J Rheumatol 1995; 22:2103–2113.

56. Hamza M. Large artery involvement in Behçet's disease. J Rheumatol 1987; 14:554–559.

57. Matsumoto T, Uekusa T, Fukuda Y. Vasculo-Behçet's disease: A pathologic study of eight cases. Hum Pathol 1991; 22:45–51.

58. Urayama A, Sakuragi S, Saki F, et al. Angio Behçet's syndrome. In: Inaba GI, ed. Proceedings of the International Conference on Behçet's Disease, October 23–24, 1981. Tokyo: University of Tokyo Press, 1982:171.

59. Bowles CA, Nelson AM, Hammill SC, et al. Cardiac involvement in Behçet's disease. Arthritis Rheum 1985; 28:345–348.

60. Gullu IH, Benekli M, Muderrisoglu H, et al. Silent myocardial ischemia in Behçet's disease. J Rheumatol 1996; 23:323–327.

61. Assaad-Khalil SH, Rafla SM, Yacout YM, et al. Prevalence of cardiovascular involvement in patients with Behçet's disease using angiography, color duplex sonography, Doppler echocardiography and CATS. Proceedings of the Eighth International Congress on Behçet's disease, Reggio-Emilia, Italy. 1998:187.

62. O'Duffy JD, Robertson DM, Goldstein NP. Chlorambucil in the treatment of uveitis and meningoencephalitis of Behçet's disease. Am J Med 1984; 76:75–84.

63. Willeit J, Schmutzhard E, Aichner F, et al. CT and MR imaging in neuro-Behçet disease. J Comput Assist Tomogr 1986; 10:313–315.

64. Zelenski JD, Capraro JA, Holden D, et al. Central nervous system vasculitis in Behçet's syndrome: angiographic improvement after therapy with cytotoxic agents. Arthritis Rheum 1989; 32:217–220.

65. O'Duffy JD, Goldstein NP. Neurologic involvement in seven patients with Behçet's disease. Am J Med 1976; 61:170–178.

66. Serdaroglu P, Yazici H, Ozdemir C, et al. Neurologic involvement in Behçet's syndrome. A prospective study. Arch Neurol 1989; 46:265–269.

67. Akman-Demir G, Baykan-Kurt B, Serdaroglu P, et al. Seven-year follow-up of neurologic involvement in Behçet syndrome. Arch Neurol 1996; 53:691–694.

68. Lee KS, Kim SJ, Lee BC, et al. Surgical treatment of intestinal Behçet's disease. Yonsei Med J 1997; 38:455–460.

69. Iida M, Kobayashi H, Matsumoto T, et al. Postoperative recurrence in patients with intestinal Behçet's disease. Dis Colon Rectum 1994; 37:16–21.

70. Yurdakul S, Yazici H, Tuzun Y, et al. The arthritis of Behçet's disease: A prospective study. Ann Rheum Dis 1983; 42:505–515.

71. Mason RM, Barnes CG. Behçet's syndrome with arthritis. Ann Rheum Dis 1969; 28:95–103.

72. Kim HA, Choi KW, Song YW. Arthropathy in Behçet's disease. Scand J Rheumatol 1997; 26:125–129.

73. Zizic TM, Stevens MB. The arthropathy of Behçet's disease. Johns Hopkins Med J 1975; 136:243–250.

74. Vernon-Roberts B, Barnes CG, Revell PA. Synovial pathology in Behçet's syndrome. Ann Rheum Dis 1978; 37:139–145.
75. Olivieri I, Salvarani C, Cantini F. Is Behçet's disease part of the spondyloarthritis complex? (editorial). J Rheumatol 1997; 24:1870–1872.
76. Yurdakul S, Tuzuner N, Yurdakul I, et al. Amyloidosis in Behçet's syndrome. Arthritis Rheum 1990; 33:1586–1589.
77. Dilsen N, Konice M, Aral O, et al. Behçet's disease associated with amyloidosis in Turkey and in the world. Ann Rheum Dis 1988; 47:157–163.
78. Akpolat I, Akpolat T, Danaci M, et al. Behçet's disease and amyloidosis. Review of the literature. Scand J Rheumatol 1997; 26:477–479.
79. Firestein GS, Gruber HE, Weisman MH, et al. Mouth and genital ulcers with inflamed cartilage: MAGIC syndrome. Five patients with features of relapsing polychondritis and Behçet's disease. Am J Med 1985; 79:65–72.
80. Lingenfelser T, Duerk H, Stevens A, et al. Generalized myositis in Behçet disease: Treatment with cyclosporine. Ann Intern Med 1992; 116:651–653.
81. O'Duffy JD, Tirzaman O, Weyand CM, et al. HLA-DRB1 alleles in Behçet's disease (A). Proceedings of the Eighth International Congress on Behçet's disease, Reggio-Emilia, Italy, 1998:113.
82. Hasan A, Fortune F, Wilson A, et al. Role of gamma delta T cells in pathogenesis and diagnosis of Behçet's disease. Lancet 1996; 347:789–794.
83. O'Neill TW, Rigby AS, Silman AJ, et al. Validation of the International Study Group criteria for Behçet's disease. Br. J Rheumatol 1994; 33:115–117.
84. Lee S. Diagnostic criteria of Behçet's disease: Problems and suggestions. Yonsei Med J 1997; 38: 365–369.
85. Schirmer M, Calamia KT. Is there a place for large vessel disease in the diagnostic criteria for Behçet's disease? J Rheumatol 1999; 26:2511–2512.
86. Harewood GC, O'Duffy JD. 20-year-old woman with oral and colonic ulcerations. Mayo Clin Proc 1998; 73:773–776.
87. Rigby AS, Chamberlain MA, Bhakta B. Behçet's disease. Baillieres Clin Rheumatol 1995; 9:375–395.
88. Bhakta BB, Chamberlain MA, Brennan P, et al. Interobserver reliability of a new instrument for assessing clinical activity in Behçet's disease. In: Hamza M, ed. Behçet's disease. Tunis: Adhoua, 1997:225–227.
89. Jamshidi A, Shahram F, Davatchi F, et al. The accuracy of IBDDAM (Iran Behçet's disease dynamic activity measure) in the treatment evaluation of Behçet's disease. In: Hamza M, ed. Behçet's Disease. Tunis: Adhoua, 1997:230–233.
90. BenEzra D, Forrester JV, Nussenblatt RB. Uveitis Scoring System. Berlin: Springer-Verlag, 1991.
91. Ozoran K, Dugun N, Gurler A, et al. Plasma von Willebrand factor, tissue plasminogen activator, plasminogen activator inhibitor, and antithrombin III levels in Behçet's disease. Scand J Rheumatol 1995; 24:376–382.
92. Boehme MW, Schmitt WH, Youinou P, et al. Clinical relevance of elevated serum thrombomodulin and soluble E-selectin in patients with Wegener's granulomatosis and other systemic vasculitides. Am J Med 1996; 101:387–394.
93. Haznedaroglu IC, Ozdemir O, Ozcebe O, et al. Circulating thrombomodulin as a clue of endothelial damage in Behçet's disease (letter). Thromb Haemost 1996; 75:974–975.
94. Aydintug AO, Tokgoz G, Ozoran K, et al. Elevated levels of soluble intercellular adhesion molecule-1 correlate with disease activity in Behçet's disease. Rheumatol Int 1995; 15:75–78.
95. Hamuryudan V, Mat C, Saip S, et al. Thalidomide in the treatment of the mucocutaneous lesions of the Behçet syndrome. A randomized, double-blind, placebo-controlled trial. Ann Intern Med 1998; 128:443–450.
96. Calguneri M, Kiraz S, Ertenli I, et al. The effect of prophylactic penicillin treatment on the course of arthritis episodes in patients with Behçet's disease. A randomized clinical trial. Arthritis Rheum 1996; 39:2062–2065.
97. O'Duffy JD, Calamia K, Cohen S, et al. Interferon-alpha treatment of Behçet's disease. J Rheum 1998; 25:10.

98. Dundar S, Demiroglu H, Ozcebe O, et al. Alpha Interferon in Behçet's Disease. Hematol Rev 1996; 9:285–290.

99. Jorizzo JL, White WL, Wise CM, et al. Low-dose weekly methotrexate for unusual neutrophilic vascular reactions: cutaneous polyarteritis nodosa and Behçet's disease. J Am Acad Dermatol 1991; 24:973–978.

100. Yazici H, Pazarli H, Barnes CG, et al. A controlled trial of azathioprine in Behçet's syndrome. N Engl J Med 1990; 322:281–285.

101. Hamuryudan V, Özyazgan Y, Hizli N, et al. Azathioprine in Behçet's syndrome. Arthritis Rheum 1997; 40:769–774.

102. Masuda K, Nakajima A, Urayama A, et al. Double-masked trial of cyclosporin versus colchicine and long-term open study of cyclosporin in Behçet's disease. Lancet 1989; 1:1093–1096.

103. Nussenblatt RB, Palestine AG, Chan CC, et al. Effectiveness of cyclosporin therapy for Behçet's disease. Arthritis Rheum 1985; 28:671–679.

104. Hamuryudan V, Ozdogan H, Yazici H. Other forms of vasculitis and pseudovasculitis. Baillieres Clin Rheumatol 1997; 11:335–355.

105. Kotter I, Eckstein AK, Stubiger N, et al. Treatment of ocular symptoms of Behçet's disease with interferon alpha 2a: A pilot study. Br J Ophthalmol 1998; 82:488–494.

106. Matteson EL, O'Duffy JD. Treatment of Behçet's disease with chlorambucil. In: O'Duffy JD, Kokmen E, eds. Behçet's Disease: Basic and Clinical Aspects. New York: Marcel Dekker, 1991:576–580.

107. Lacombe P, Qanadli SD, Jondeau G, et al. Treatment of hemoptysis in Behçet syndrome with pulmonary and bronchial embolization. J Vasc Interv Radiol 1997; 8:1043–1047.

108. Hamza M, Chaabane MB, Hamza K, et al. Pulmonary artery aneurysm in Behçet's disease: 10 cases. In: Hamza M, ed. Behçet's Disease. Tunis: Adhoua, 1997:294–295.

109. Bismuth E, Hadengue A, Hammel P, et al. Hepatic vein thrombosis in Behçet's disease. Hepatology 1990; 11:969–974.

110. Islim IF, Gill MD, Situnayake D, et al. Successful treatment of right atrial thrombus in a patient with Behçet's disease (letter). Ann Rheum Dis 1994; 53:550–551.

111. Celenligil H, Kansu E, Ruacan S, et al. Characterization of peripheral blood lymphocytes and immunohistological analysis of oral ulcers in Behçet's disease. In: O'Duffy JD, Kokmen E, eds. Behçet's Disease. New York: Marcel Dekker, 1991:487–496.

112. Yamana S, Jones SL, Aoi K, et al. Lymphocyte subsets in erythema nodosum-like lesions from patients with Behçet's disease. In: Lehner T, Barnes CG, eds. Recent Advances in Behçet's Disease. London: Royal Society of Medicine Services, 1986:117–122.

113. Charteris DG, Barton K, McCartney AC, et al. CD4+ lymphocyte involvement in ocular Behçet's disease. Autoimmunity 1992; 12:201–206.

114. Yamana S, Jones SL, Shimamoto T, et al. Immunohistological analysis of lymphocytes infiltrating the terminal ileum in a patient with intestinal Behçet's disease. In: Lehner T, Barnes CG, eds. Recent Advances in Behçet's Disease. London: Royal Society of Medicine Services, 1986:129–130.

115. Kahan A, Hamzaoui K, Ayed K. Abnormalities of T lymphocyte subsets in Behçet's disease demonstrated with anti-CD45RA and anti-CD29 monoclonal antibodies. J Rheumatol 1992; 19:742–746.

116. Direskeneli H, Eksioglu-Demiralp E, Kibaroglu A, et al. Oligoclonal T cell expansions in Behçet's disease (A). Proceedings of the Eighth International Congress on Behçet's disease, Reggio-Emilia, Italy, 1998:36.

117. Suzuki Y, Hoshi K, Matsuda T, et al. Increased peripheral blood gamma delta+ T cells and natural killer cells in Behçet's disease. J Rheumatol 1992; 19:588–592.

118. Yamashita N, Mochizuki M, Mizushima Y, et al. The phenotypic and functional abnormality of gamma delta T lymphocytes in Behçet's disease. In: Godeau P, Wechsler B, eds. Behçet's Disease. Paris: Elsevier, 1993:7–12.

119. Freysdottir J, Lau SH, Hussain L, et al. Activated gamma lambda cells in Behçet's disease (A). Proceedings of the Eighth International Congress on Behçet's disease, Reggio-Emilia, Italy, 1998:36.

120. al-Janadi M, al-Balla S, al-Dalaan A, et al. Cytokine profile in systemic lupus erythematosus, rheumatoid arthritis, and other rheumatic diseases. J Clin Immunol 1993; 13:58–67.

121. Yosipovitch G, Shohat B, Bshara J, et al. Elevated serum interleukin 1 receptors and interleukin 1B in patients with Behçet's disease: correlations with disease activity and severity. Isr J Med Sci 1995; 31:345–348.

122. Turan B, Gallati H, Erdi H, et al. Systemic levels of the T cell regulatory cytokines IL-10 and IL-12 in Bechçet's disease; soluble TNFR-75 as a biological marker of disease activity. J Rheumatol 1997; 24:128–132.

123. Sayinalp N, Ozcebe OI, Ozdemir O, et al. Cytokines in Behçet's disease. J Rheumatol 1996; 23:321–322.

124. Mege JL, Dilsen N, Sanguedolce V, et al. Overproduction of monocyte derived tumor necrosis factor alpha, interleukin (IL) 6, IL-8 and increased neutrophil superoxide generation in Behçet's disease. A comparative study with familial Mediterranean fever and healthy subjects. J Rheumatol 1993; 20: 1544–1549.

125. Yamakawa Y, Sugita Y, Nagatani T, et al. Interleukin-6 (IL-6) in patients with Behçet's disease. J Dermatol Sci 1996; 11:189–195.

126. Ohno S, Ohguchi M, Hirose S, et al. Close association of HLA-Bw51 with Behçet's disease. Arch Ophthalmol 1982; 100:1455–1458.

127. Fujii N, Minagawa T, Nakane A, et al. Spontaneous production of gamma-interferon in cultures of T lymphocytes obtained from patients with Behçet's disease. J Immunol 1983; 130:1683–1686.

128. Frassanito MA, Dammacco R, Silvestris N, et al. Th1 polarization of immune response in Behçet's disease (A). Proceedings of the Eighth International Congress on Behçet's disease, Reggio-Emilia, Italy, 1998:140.

129. Raziuddin S, al-Dalaan A, Bahabri S, et al. Divergent cytokine production profile in Behcet's disease. Altered Th1/Th2 cell cytokine pattern. J Rheumatol 1998; 25:329–333.

130. Korn S, DeHoratius RJ. Immunology: Humoral immunity. In: Plotkin GR, Calabro JJ, O'Duffy JD, eds. Behçet's disease: A contemporary synopsis. Mount Kisco, NY: Futura, 1988:29–50.

131. Cervera R, Navarro M, Lopez-Soto A, et al. Antibodies to endothelial cells in Behçet's disease: Cell-binding heterogeneity and association with clinical activity. Ann Rheum Dis 1994; 53:265–267.

132. Aydintug AO, Tokgoz G, D'Cruz DP, et al. Antibodies to endothelial cells in patients with Behçet's disease. Clin Immunol Immunopathol 1993; 67:157–162.

133. Sohn S. Etiopathology of Behçet's disease: Herpes simplex virus infection and animal model. Yonsei Med J 1997; 38:359–364.

134. Kaneko F, Oyama N, Nishibu A. Streptococcal infection in the pathogenesis of Behçet's disease and clinical effects of minocycline on the disease symptoms. Yonsei Med J 1997; 38:444–454.

135. Pervin K, Childerstone A, Shinnick T, et al. T cell epitope expression of mycobacterial and homologous human 65-kilodalton heat shock protein peptides in short term cell lines from patients with Behçet's disease. J Immunol 1993; 151:2273–2282.

136. Lehner T. The role of heat shock protein, microbial and autoimmune agents in the aetiology of Behçet's disease. Int Rev Immunol 1997; 14:21–32.

137. Takeno M, Kariyone A, Yamashita N, et al. Excessive function of peripheral blood neutrophils from patients with Behçet's disease and from HLA-B51 transgenic mice. Arthritis Rheum 1995; 38:426–433.

138. Mizuki N, Inoko H, Ohno S. Molecular genetics (HLA) of Behçet's disease. Yonsei Med J 1997; 38: 333–349.

139. Mizuki N, Ohno S, Sato T, et al. Microsatellite polymorphism between the tumor necrosis factor and HLA-B genes in Behçet's disease. Hum Immunol 1995; 43:129–135.

140. Amoura Z, Caillat-Zucman S, Wechsler B, et al. Srong association between mica 6 allele and Behçet disease (A). Proceedings of the Eighth International Congress on Behçet's disease, Reggio-Emilia, Italy, 1998:107.

34

Cogan's Syndrome

Rex M. McCallum, E. William St. Clair, and Barton F. Haynes
Duke University Medical Center, Durham, North Carolina

I. INTRODUCTION

The hallmarks of Cogan's syndrome (CS) are interstitial keratitis (IK) and vestibuloauditory dysfunction. The history of CS reflects a growing awareness of its potential for causing not only eye and ear disease, but also complex systemic manifestations. In 1945, David G. Cogan, an ophthalmologist at the Harvard Medical School, reported four cases of recurrent nonsyphilitic IK and vestibuloauditory symptoms (1). These cases were similar to a patient who had been described in 1934 with IK and Ménière's disease (2). Cogan was later credited with the first description of this disorder, which now bears his name (1).

The essence of these new cases portrayed an illness characterized by recurrent bouts of bilateral photophobia, excessive tearing, and eye redness and pain interspersed with attacks of severe vertigo, nausea, tinnitus, and fluctuating hearing loss. Cogan's examination had shown patchy infiltration of the deep corneal stroma with yellowish white granular opacities, little reaction in the anterior chamber, and limited, if any, visual impairment. The vestibuloauditory features had striking similarity to those of Ménière's disease. Two cases had culminated in complete deafness. Cogan stressed the clinical differences between the ocular manifestations in these new cases and syphilitic keratitis, pointing out that the corneal opacities in syphilis were more prominent and typically accompanied by iridocyclitis. Vestibuloauditory involvement in CS also differed from that of syphilis, where hearing loss develops more slowly and without appreciable vertigo.

Serological studies were negative for syphilis in the first reported cases of CS. However, the resemblance of these two disorders stimulated an intense search for an infectious cause of CS. Evaluation in the first four cases showed no consistent pattern of bacterial growth from the conjunctival sac. The appearance of CS following smallpox vaccination led to the suggestion of a possible immunological etiology (3). The next four cases of CS did not provide an answer to this puzzle (4).

Cogan's syndrome was initially believed to be an organ-specific disease confined to the eye and ear. The clinical picture expanded with later case reports of CS characterized by atypical ocular features, including conjunctivitis, uveitis, episcleritis, scleritis, and retinal artery occlusion (5–9). New cases of CS were also described with aortic valvular insufficiency (10,11) and systemic necrotizing vasculitis (6,9,10,12,13). In the 1980s, Haynes et al. (14) from the National Institutes of Health (NIH) and Vollertsen et al. (15) from the Mayo Clinic published two large case series of CS and established a conceptual basis for our current understanding and management of

CS. Additional clinical experience during the past decade has refined our thinking about the clinical spectrum of CS and sharply focused our attention on aggressive treatment (16).

II. EPIDEMIOLOGY

Cogan's syndrome is a rare disease of young adults. The median age of onset for patients in the NIH (14) and Mayo Clinic series (15) was 22 years, with age ranges of 13–31 and 5–63 years, respectively. The disease affects males and females with approximately equal frequency. These demographics are similar to those of 47 patients with CS evaluated more recently at Duke University Medical Center who had a mean age of onset of 29 years, with a range of 5–63 years (17). The 47 patients from the Duke series include the 13 patients from the NIH group. Cogan's syndrome has also been described in children as young as 4 years old (18) and in the elderly (19).

III. CLINICAL FEATURES

Approximately one-half (40–65%) of patients have an antecedent upper respiratory illness in the weeks before the onset of CS (15,20). Fifty percent of patients present with ocular difficulties, 25% present with vestibuloauditory problems, and 25% present with both ocular and vestibuloauditory manifestations within one month of the other (15,17).

Presenting ocular complaints are most commonly pain (90%), redness (79%), and photophobia (68%) (17). Additional symptoms may include tearing, foreign body sensation, alteration in visual acuity, diplopia, and visual field defects (14,15,21). Despite prominent symptoms, the ophthalmological findings may be mild and evanescent. Repeat examinations may be necessary to document ocular inflammation, particularly in the cornea (4,15,21). Ophthalmological examination most frequently shows IK, conjunctivitis, iritis, and scleritis/episcleritis (Table 1) (17) (Fig. 1). Interstitial keratitis may occur in isolation or with other types of ocular problems. Less frequent findings include corneal ulceration, vitritis, choroiditis, subretinal neovascular mem-

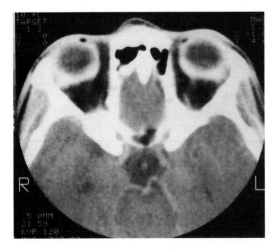

Figure 1   Severe posterior scleritis in a patient with CS. Computerized tomography of the orbits reveals thickened sclera posteriorly, compatible with the clinical picture and examination suggesting posterior scleritis.

Table 1 Major Clinical Features of Cogan's Syndrome[a]

Manifestations	Proportion of cases (%)
Inflammatory eye disease	100
Interstitial keratitis	70
Conjunctivitis	35
Iridocyclitis	30
Episcleritis/scleritis	30
Papillitis	5
Posterior uveitis	5
Retinal vasculitis	5
Exophthalmus	<5
Vestibuloauditory dysfunction	100
Hearing loss	95
Vertigo	90
Tinnitus	75
Nausea and vomiting	65
Ataxia	45
Nystagmus	30
Ocillopsia	15
Systemic vasculitis	15
Aortitis with or without aortic insufficiency	10
Large-sized vessel vasculitis	10
Medium-sized vessel vasculitis	<5

[a]Composite information from Refs. 14–17, 21, 25, 26, and 35.

brane, pars planitis, orbital pseudotumor, cotton wool spots, retinal arterial disease, papillitis, central venous occlusion, conjunctival nodule, vitreous hemorrhage, and posterior uveitis (14,15) (Table 1).

The earliest corneal manifestations of IK are "faint peripheral, subepithelial corneal infiltrates located in the anterior stroma. They measure 0.5 to 1.0 mm in diameter and mimic lesions seen in adenoviral or chlamydial keratitis" (21) (Fig. 2). The corneal infiltrates may evolve to "a granular type of corneal infiltrate, patchy in distribution, situated predominantly in the posterior half of the cornea" (1,4,21). The stromal infiltrates are associated with epithelial erosions in less than 5% of patients (15). The mild and evanescent early findings explain why many patients with CS who present with eye involvement are initially diagnosed with a viral infection. Later, the cornea may become vascularized and opacified. However, corneal opacities occur in less than 5% of patients treated appropriately with topical antiinflammatory therapy (see below) (21,22).

Presenting vestibuloauditory complaints are Ménière's-like with vertigo (85%), sudden decrease in hearing (79%), sudden nausea and vomiting (70%), tinnitus (53%), vertigo (45%), and gradual decrease in hearing (17%) (17). Vestibuloauditory symptoms are often acutely incapacitating and may require hospitalization. Eventually, nearly all patients lose hearing (Table 1). In a significant minority of cases, nystagmus is also present (17). Many patients are ataxic and have absent caloric responses (15,23,24).

Cardiovascular disease of an inflammatory nature develops in 10–15% of patients with CS (14,15,17) (see Table 1). Aortic insufficiency (AI) occurs in 10% of patients with CS and results from aortitis with or without valvulitis (25). Cardiac signs and symptoms of AI range from an asymptomatic diastolic murmur to congestive heart failure to myocardial infarction (10,14, 15,26–32). Aortitis manifests weeks to months after the onset of CS (14,15,26,30). Cardiac

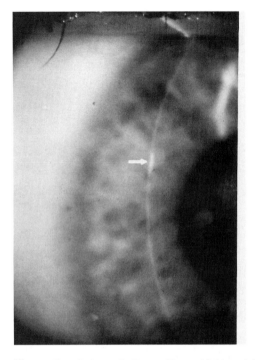

Figure 2   Slit-lamp findings of interstitial keratitis in a patient with CS. Subtle stroma infiltrate (arrow) typical of early interstitial keratitis is demonstrated in the narrow band of light.

catheterization, intraoperative evaluation at the time of aortic valve replacement, electrocardiograms (EKGs), and pathologic material have shown aneurysms of the valve cusps, (10,30) aortic dilatation, (31) arrhythmias, (15) coronary arteritis, (10,26) left ventricular hypertrophy, (15) myocardial infarction, (22) ostial coronary disease, (30–32) pericarditis, (31) torn aortic valve cusp, (32) and valvular fenestrations (10,30).

The most common form of systemic vasculitis associated with CS is a large-sized vessel (Takayasu's disease–like) vasculitis (14,15,17,25,26,33,34) (Fig. 3). It may present with an asymptomatic abdominal bruit (35), an asymptomatic femoral bruit (35), lower extremity claudication (26), symptoms of mesenteric insufficiency (28), hypertension (36), weight loss (37), decreased left brachial artery pulse (38), or abdominal pain from a vasculitic gastric ulcer (26). Cogan's syndrome is less often associated with a medium-sized vessel (polyarteritis nodosa–like) vasculitis (17). Initial symptoms and signs in these cases include claudication, (34) gastrointestinal bleeding, (13) proteinuria and hematuria, (15,34) ischemic loss of limb, (9) and neurological symptoms (15). In CS, vasculitis may involve the coronary artery (10,26) (see Fig. 3B), gastrointestinal tract (26), femoral artery (26), muscle (39), renal artery (26,36) (see Fig. 3A), skin (9,13,40), subclavian artery (26,28,38) (see Fig. 3A,C), or testicle (9).

Other manifestations in CS are relatively non specific (see Table 2) (11,14,15,17). Diverse skin findings, such as cutaneous nodules, rash, cutaneous ulcers, and palpable purpura (15,41), may accompany CS. A minority of patients have developed central nervous system manifestations, which include cavernous sinus thrombosis, encephalitis, localized cerebral infarction, meningismus, seizures, and trigeminal neuralgia (14,15,35,40). In addition, CS has been reported to occur in patients with sarcoidosis, hypothyroidism, inflammatory bowel disease, and interstitial nephritis (15,17,42).

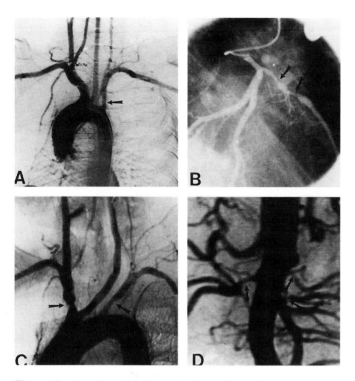

Figure 3 Arteriographic demonstration of large-sized vessel vasculitis in CS. (A) Stenotic lesion in the left subclavian artery (arrow). (B) Stenotic lesions in the left anterior descending coronary artery (arrows) with poststenotic dilatation. (C) Stenotic lesions in the right innominate artery (left arrow) and the subclavian artery (right arrow). (D) Multiple lesions in the single right and duplicated left renal arteries (arrows). (From Ref. 26.)

Table 2 Other Manifestations of Cogan's Syndrome[a]

Manifestations	Proportion of cases (%)
Fever	25
Fatigue	20
Arthralgias/myalgias	15
Arthritis	15
Weight loss	15
Abdominal pain	10
Gastrointestinal bleeding	10
Hepatomegaly	10
Lymphadenopathy	10
Splenomegaly	10
Central nervous system findings	5
Cutaneous nodules	5
Pleuritis	5
Rash	5
Peripheral nervous system findings	<5
Polychondritis	<5

[a]*Source*: Ref. 35.

Table 3 Laboratory Abnormalities in Cogan's Syndrome

Laboratory study	Proportion of abnormal studies (%)	Mean	Range
White blood cell count	75	13,700	1600–47,000
Neutrophilia	50		
Relative lymphopenia	25		
Eosinophilia (mild)	17		
Leukocytosis >24,000 cells/mL	10		
Erythrocyte sedimentation rate		40	3–128
>20 mm/hr	75		
Hemoglobin/hematocrit (anemia)	33		
Platelet count (thrombocytosis)	30		
Cerebrospinal fluid	25		
Cryoglobulins	17–23		
Decreased C_3	21		
Decreased Total hemolytic complement	17		
Decreased C_4	17		
Antinuclear antibodies (low titer)	17		
Rheumatoid factor (low titer)	14		

Source: Compiled from Refs. 14, 15, 17, and 25.

IV. LABORATORY FINDINGS

The laboratory abnormalities in CS are summarized in Table 3 (14,15,17). Hematological findings include leukocytosis and monocytosis (13,15). A few patients with CS have had a false-positive VDRL (14,17). Serum protein electrophoresis may show evidence of chronic inflammation; no monoclonal spikes have been described (14,15,17). Two patients have tested positive for the heterophil antibody (13,45). About one-quarter of patients have abnormalities of the cerebrospinal fluid (CSF) (15), which include pleocytosis, (14,15) elevated protein, and increased γ-globulin fraction (46). Negative or normal findings in CS are tests for anti-DNA, anti-La, anti-Ro, and anti–smooth muscle antibodies, Coomb's test, and hepatitis B antigen (15). Some investigators have noted increased frequencies of *HLA-B17, HLA-A9, HLA-Bw35,* and *HLA-Cw4,* but no conclusions can be drawn from these data because of the small sample sizes (14,43,44).

V. DIAGNOSIS

The diagnosis of CS is based on the presence of both eye inflammation and inner ear dysfunction (see Table 4). In previous studies, CS had been subdivided into "typical" and "atypical" categories depending on the nature of the eye manifestations. Typical CS was the designation when IK was the predominant eye finding. Atypical CS was applied if more than 2 years elapsed between the onset of eye and inner ear disease, or when the ocular component was dominated by conjunctivitis, anterior uveitis, or posterior segment inflammation. The rationale for this distinction came from early observations that systemic necrotizing vasculitis was associated mainly with atypical CS and portended a worse prognosis. This nomenclature has not proven useful because patients initially presenting with typical CS have subsequently developed other types of eye inflammation and systemic necrotizing vasculitis.

Table 4 Differential Diagnosis of Cogan's Syndrome

Disorder	Eye manifestations	Ear manifestations	Other features
Chlamydia infection	Conjunctivitis, IK	Otitis media, CHL	Respiratory tract symptoms
Lyme disease	Conjunctivitis, episcleritis, uveitis, IK, choroiditis, retinitis, optic neuritis		Erythema migrans, meningitis, carditis, arthritis
Congenital syphilis	IK	SNHL	+FTA-ABS
Whipple's disease	Uveitis, vitritis	SNHL	Diarrhea, weight loss, fever, arthritis, skin hyperpigmentation
Sarcoidosis	Conjunctivitis, IK, anterior uveitis, retinitis, keratoconjunctivitis sicca	SNHL	Hilar adenopathy, pulmonary fibrosis, CNS involvement, skin lesions, parotid gland enlargement
Vogt–Koyanagi–Harada	Panuveitis, iridocyclitis	Vertigo, SNHL	Aseptic meningitis, vitiligo, alopecia, poliosis
KID syndrome (congenital)	Keratoconjunctivitis, corneal vascularization	SNHL	Ichthyosis
Sjögren's syndrome	Keratoconjunctivitis sicca	SNHL	Xerostomia, parotid gland enlargement, serum ANA
Rheumatoid arthritis	Episcleritis, scleritis	SNHL	Arthritis, serum rheumatoid factor
SLE	Retinitis, optic atrophy	SNHL (mild)	Skin rash, arthritis, pleurisy, glomerulonephritis, cytopenias, serum ANA
APA syndrome	Retinal vascular occlusion	SNHL	Deep vein thrombosis, pulmonary emboli, arterial thrombosis, thrombocytopenia, serum APA
Polyarteritis nodosa	Retinal vasculitis	SNHL	Renal failure, hypertension, arthritis, skin lesions, neuropathy, CNS involvement, elevated ESR
Wegener's granulomatosis	Conjunctivitis, episcleritis scleritis, uveitis, retinitis	Otitis media (CHL), SNHL	Sinusitis, pulmonary infiltrates, glomerulonephritis, serum ANCA
Relapsing polychondritis	Conjunctivitis, IK, scleritis uveitis	SNHL	Auricular, nasal, and laryngotracheal chondritis, systemic vasculitis
Behçet's syndrome	Anterior uveitis, episcleritis, IK, retinal vasculitis, chorioretinitis	Vertigo, SNHL	Oral and genital ulcers, CNS involvement, arthritis, skin lesions
Ulcerative colitis	Anterior uveitis	SNHL	Colitis
Crohn's disease	Anterior uveitis	SNHL	Enterocolitis
CNS lymphoma	Corneal, anterior chamber and vitreous opacities, sub-RPE infiltrates	SNHL	Cerebellopontine mass
CLL	Optic neuropathy	Otitis media, SNHL	CNS involvement, CSF lymphocytosis
Retinocochleocerebral vasculopathy	Retinal arteriolar occlusions	SNHL	CNS microangiopathy

Abbreviations: CNS, central nervous system; SLE, systemic lupus erythematosus; APA, antiphospholipid antibody; CLL, chronic lymphocytic leukemia; KID, keratitis, ichthyosis, and deafness; IK, interstitial keratitis; RPE, retinal pigment epithelial; SNHL, sensorineural hearing loss; CHL, conductive hearing loss; FTA-ABS, fluorescent treponemal antibody absorption; ANA, antinuclear antibodies; ANCA, antineutrophil cytoplasmic antibodies; CSF, cerebrospinal fluid.

Ocular symptoms such as redness or discomfort, excessive tearing, or impaired vision suggest an ocular process and deserve further evaluation. Interstitial keratitis and other anterior segment disorders are diagnosed by slit-lamp examination, while posterior segment disorders are detected by ophthalmoscopy. Abnormalities of the retinal vasculature may be visualized in more detail using fluorescein angiography. Ophthalmic photography is helpful in documenting and following corneal disease and in monitoring the posterior segment (21). Impaired vision may arise from opacity of the ocular media (e.g., cornea, aqueous humor, vitreous) or a retinal abnormality (e.g., retinal detachment, inflammation, hemorrhage, vessel occlusion). Visual defects may also result from lesions of the optic nerve and chiasm and of the retrochiasmal pathways. Interstitial keratitis, conjunctivitis, anterior uveitis, episcleritis, scleritis, choroiditis, or retinal vasculitis are findings compatible with the diagnosis of CS. Other causes of IK should be considered in the differential diagnosis, including sarcoidosis (47), syphilis (48,49), Lyme borreliosis (50–52), leprosy (53), tuberculosis (54), Chlamydial infection (39,55), and herpes simplex and varicella zoster virus infection (55). However, recurring and bilateral IK suggests an immune-mediated process such as CS.

Vestibuloauditory symptoms may signal either a peripheral (labyrinth, vestibular, or cochlear) or central (brainstem, cerebellum, or cerebral cortex) lesion in the nervous system, or possibly a systemic (cardiovascular or metabolic) disorder. The acute attacks of CS arise from a peripheral lesion and resemble those of Ménière's disease, which are characterized by the sudden onset of severe vertigo, nausea, vomiting, tinnitus, and hearing loss. Important goals of the evaluation are to exclude systemic causes of vestibuloauditory dysfunction and to confirm that the lesion is peripheral rather than central. The examination should initially focus on a careful inspection of the ear canal and tympanic membrane, a hearing check, and a complete neurological evaluation with special attention paid to the cranial nerves, cerebellar function, and the presence of nystagmus. In CS, nystagmus is only seen during an acute attack. Central and peripheral lesions may be distinguished by caloric and rotational testing. In CS, caloric and rotary chair tests between attacks show hypoactive or absent vestibular responses. Electronystagmography (ENG) also reveals abnormal findings indicative of a peripheral lesion.

The hearing loss in CS is sensorineural in origin. Nerve deafness of the type seen in CS results in the finding of air conduction greater than bone conduction (positive Rinne test). Objective assessment of hearing loss by audiometry is an essential part of the evaluation. Pure tone and speech audiometry confirms a sensorineural hearing loss, which preferentially involves the low and high frequencies (Fig. 4) in a pattern similar to that seen in Ménière's syndrome (56). Audi-

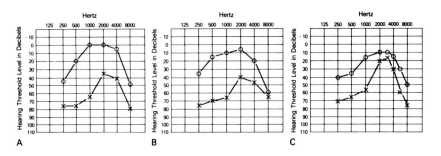

Figure 4 Serial pure tone audiograms over an 8-year period. Note the higher hearing thresholds at the upper and lower frequencies. (A) Two months after onset of CS while on daily corticosteroid therapy. (B) Four and one-half years later on every-other-day corticosteroid therapy. (C) Three years later, demonstrating stable to improved hearing over the period of the tests. (O————O, right ear; X————X, left ear.) (From Ref. 14.)

tory thresholds usually reflect a moderate-to-profound hearing loss. Brain stem auditory evoked potentials may be performed when the lesion cannot be localized with certainty to the peripheral or central nervous system. Peripheral lesions affecting the cochlear nerve demonstrate a delay in the first brain stem wave, but a normal or shortened interpeak latency. The differential diagnosis of vertigo and hearing loss includes Ménière's disease, viral infection, vascular insufficiency, perilymphatic fistulas, drug toxicity, demyelinating disease (e.g., multiple sclerosis) and cerebellopontine angle tumors (which are usually unilateral, but are rarely bilateral). Episodic vertigo without hearing loss or tinnitus is termed vestibular neuronitis. Episodic vertigo and hearing loss without eye disease suggests a diagnosis of Ménière's disease. Demyelinating disease and cerebellopontine angle tumors also cause hearing loss and vertigo and should be excluded by performing a magnetic resonance imaging (MRI) scan of the brain with gadolinium.

Patients with systemic symptoms or findings should be evaluated for possible cardiovascular disease and other sites of organ system involvement. The presence of ischemic chest pain, dyspnea, or a diastolic heart murmur calls for a thorough cardiac evaluation, including chest x-ray, electrocardiogram, echocardiography, and possibly coronary angiography. Echocardiography is important in the evaluation of aortic insufficiency (AI) and may show doppler evidence of regurgitant flow, (15,26) "fluttering" of the anterior mitral leaflet (15), left ventricular enlargement (15,26,31), paradoxical movement of the ascending aorta during systole, (26), or thickening of valve cusps (15,57). In CS, given the association of ostial coronary stenosis with aortitis, the combination of ischemic chest pain and AI demands cardiac catheterization (30,39,57). Patients with severe AI who are surgical candidates should also undergo coronary arteriography. Bruits heard over the large peripheral vessels may indicate a vasculitis of the Takayasu's type and warrant angiographic studies (see Fig. 3). Peripheral vessel angiography can reveal stenosis, dilatations, and aneurysms, such as can be seen in large- and medium-sized vessel vasculitis (14,15,17).

Disorders other than CS may also produce concomitant ocular and vestibuloauditory manifestations. These conditions should be considered in the differential diagnosis of CS and include: viral infection (14,55), Chlamydial infection (39,55), syphilis (48,49,58), Lyme disease (50–52, 59), Whipple's disease (60,61), sarcoidosis (47,62–64), Vogt–Koyanagi–Harada syndrome (65), keratitis, ichthyosis, and deafness (KID) syndrome (66), rheumatoid arthritis (67,68), primary Sjogren's syndrome (69), systemic lupus erythematosus (70), anti-phospholipid antibody syndrome (71–74), Wegener's granulomatosis (75–79), relapsing polychondritis (80–83), Behçet's syndrome (84–86), polyarteritis nodosa (12,87–90), ulcerative colitis (91,92), Crohn's disease (93), primary CNS lymphoma (94–96), chronic lymphocytic leukemia (97), and retinochochleocerebral vasculopathy (Susac syndrome) (98,99). The differentiating features of these conditions are listed in Table 4. Viral infections, sarcoidosis, and systemic vasculitis are the disorders most likely to be confused with CS.

VI. ASCERTAINMENT OF DISEASE ACTIVITY

Collecting information to ascertain disease activity often requires coordination of multiple physicians and providers of care, such as ophthalmologists, audiologists, otolaryngologists, and rheumatologists. The rheumatologist may be best equipped to ascertain inflammatory disease in multiple organ systems, with particular attention focused on the possibility of cardiovascular disease (14,15,17,25).

A complete assessment of ocular disease activity requires a careful ophthalmological examination utilizing a slit lamp and indirect ophthalmoscopy. The slit lamp examination includes a careful evaluation of the cornea with an attentive search for infiltration of the stroma (21,35).

Stromal scars can develop over time and serial evaluations combined with selected corneal photography may be necessary to document these chronic changes (21). Slit lamp examination may also reveal evidence of anterior uveitis (anterior chamber cells) or episcleritis/scleritis (engorged vessels and focal/diffuse redness in the white part of the eye) (14,15,17). Indirect opththalmoscopy may show posterior segment inflammation or central macular edema indicative of intermediate uveitis, retinal vasculitis, retinitis/choroiditis, papillitis, or vitritis (14,15,17,26). Retinal vasculitis, retinochoroiditis, and/or central macular edema may be monitored using fluorescein angiography, which is a useful objective test for judging the response to therapy (26,35).

Vestibuloauditory activity manifests with decreased hearing, vertigo, nausea, emesis, oscillopsia, ear pressure, and tinnitus (14,15,17). Vestibular symptoms are more severe initially than auditory symptoms. Vestibular symptoms decrease in intensity with subsequent flares of CS activity. Loss of hearing, tinnitus, and auricular pressure are more prominent with flares of CS activity after the initial attack. Nystagmus and ataxia can be noted with active vestibular activity. Pure tone audiometry is almost always abnormal and should be followed over time as a measure of disease activity and response to therapy (15,17,20). Since patients with CS often develop cochlear hydrops, (14,100) hearing fluctuations can occur from changes in the amount of cochlear fluid (35,101). Such changes may be brought about by menstrual variation in salt and water metabolism, allergies, upper respiratory infection, barotrauma, or any other cause of salt and water retention. Although it may be difficult to distinguish hearing loss due to cochlear hydrops from that related to active inner ear inflammation, the presence of vestibular symptoms, active eye disease, or an elevated erythrocyte sedimentation rate suggests a recurrent inflammatory process (35,101).

The assessment of cardiovascular manifestations is another major focus. Symptoms of cardiac or limb ischemia should raise suspicion for an inflammatory cardiovascular process (14,15,17,26). The heart examination should be specifically directed toward the recognition of a possible diastolic murmur, arrhythmia, or signs of congestive heart failure. Peripheral vessels should be examined for abnormal pulses or bruits. Arterial vessel abnormalities may be visualized by angiography using radioopaque dye or MRI techniques, which are useful for diagnosis and following the response to therapy. Aortic insufficiency may be evaluated using two-dimensional echocardiography. Rarely, a repeat biopsy of an artery may be utilized to assess disease activity.

VII. MANAGEMENT

Interstitial keratitis and iritis in CS should be treated with topical ocular corticosteroids, such as prednisolone acetate 1% (although lower potency formulations are often adequate), and mydriatics to control inflammation and photophobia, prevent synechiae, and maintain ocular comfort (35,101). Cases in which IK fails to improve with topical therapy should be investigated for other potential causes of corneal inflammation, such as chlamydia (35,39,101). An empirical trial of a tetracycline antibiotic may be considered in such instances (101). Rarely, treatment of IK and iritis may require systemic corticosteroid therapy. Ocular symptoms from IK or iritis in CS usually respond to treatment within 3 to 7 days with concomitant improvement in signs of ocular inflammation (15).

Other forms of anterior segment inflammation, including conjunctivitis, scleritis, and episcleritis, should also be treated with topical corticosteroid therapy. Episcleritis and/or scleritis may also benefit from nonsteroidal antiinflammatory drug (NSAID) therapy. Nodular scleritis or scleritis unresponsive to topical corticosteroids or oral NSAIDs may need treatment with systemic corticosteroids or other immunosuppressive drugs (101).

Progressive corneal opacification sufficient to interfere with visual function may require corneal transplantation. Cataracts may develop and obscure vision, an indication for cataract extraction (22,101). Cataract extraction may be required at an earlier stage than usual in a patient with CS who is also deaf and dependent on lip reading or sign language for communication (35,101).

Posterior-segment inflammation should be treated with systemic corticosteroid therapy if the problem is progressive or persistent and interferes with the patient's function (14,26,101). Patients with continued visual loss despite systemic corticosteroid therapy or the occurrence of significant corticosteroid side effects might require the use of other immunosuppressive drugs. Cyclophosphamide and cyclosporine have each been reported to be effective in patients with CS (26,101).

The presence of compromised auditory acuity and/or vestibular dysfunction in a patient with newly diagnosed CS is an indication for a therapeutic trial of systemic corticosteroid therapy. Treatment should be initiated only after quantifying the degree of abnormality with an audiogram (14,15,17,101). Therapy should be started with 1–2 mg/kg/day of prednisone (or an equivalent dose of another corticosteroid) in divided doses (14,101). After initial signs of improvement are noted, generally 3 to 7 days, the dose should be consolidated to a single morning dose (35,101) (Fig. 5). After 14 days, if a good response is noted subjectively or objectively by examination or audiometry, the decision can be made to continue prednisone for another 1 to 2 weeks with a subsequent gradual reduction in dose. An attempt should be made to taper the corticosteroid dose to an every-other-day regimen within the next 4 weeks, followed by discontinuation of prednisone within the next 1 to 2 months. Tapering of the prednisone dose is contingent on stable auditory acuity and/or vestibular function (101). Certain patients require long-term systemic corticosteroid therapy because of recurrent episodes of hearing loss during attempts to taper the prednisone dose (35). Long-term corticosteroid therapy is not needed to control recurrent vestibular dysfunction.

Down fluctuations in hearing judged to be inflammatory in cause should be documented by audiometry and treated with 0.5 to 2.0 mg/kg/day of prednisone therapy, depending on the severity of change and dose of prednisone at which the hearing loss was noted. If the hearing loss is not believed to be inflammatory, auditory acuity may be monitored without change in prednisone dose. Such patients may benefit from diuretic therapy for presumed cochlear hydrops, which in time may lead to resolution of the hearing deterioration. A trial of increased prednisone therapy

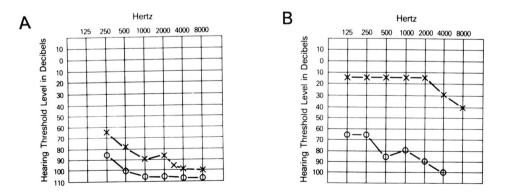

Figure 5 Audiometry demonstrating response to therapy with corticosteroids in patient with CS. (A) Hearing thresholds prior to therapy. (B) Hearing thresholds after therapy for active CS. (O———O, right ear; X———X, left ear.)

may be considered in patients who fail to improve after 4–7 days with this more conservative approach or in the absence of provocative factors (e.g., upper respiratory infection) (35).

If hearing loss occurs during reduction of the prednisone dose, the prednisone dosage may be increased empirically or another immunosuppressive drug can be added to the treatment regimen. Steroid-sparing therapy may be considered for patients in whom excessive corticosteroid doses are required to control the hearing loss or who show signs of corticosteroid intolerance. Other immunosuppressive agents may also be needed in the rare patient with CS whose hearing fails to respond to prednisone therapy within 14 days. Criteria should be established to define the end points for therapy and might include stabilized or improved hearing after 2–3 months, discontinuation or reduction of the prednisone dose, or resolution or improvement of corticosteroid-related side effects (35,101). Cyclophosphamide, methotrexate, azathioprine, and FK-506 have been successfully utilized as adjunctive therapy in anecdotal reports of CS, although their efficacy in controlled trials has not been tested (17,35,102–104). Oral neutral protease therapy has also been reported to be effective in CS (105). Patients have undergone cochlear implants because of severe hearing loss, with improvement in function (106).

Systemic necrotizing vasculitis (SNV) is treated with 1 mg/kg/day of prednisone starting in divided doses with subsequent consolidation. Other immunosuppressive therapies may be added depending on the severity of disease and the nature of organ system involvement (35,101). Cyclosporine at a dose of 5 mg/kg/day or less has been effective for large-vessel vasculitis (26), and cyclophosphamide beginning at 2 mg/kg/day has been effective for medium-sized vessel vasculitis (35,101). After 4 weeks, the prednisone dose is tapered over 4–6 weeks to 0.5 mg/kg/day or less. Subsequently, the prednisone is tapered to every other day therapy and then to zero or the lowest effective dose, which should be <10 mg/day of prednisone (101). The additional immunosuppressive therapy is continued for 9–12 more months beyond the point of disease remission or stabilization and may be discontinued in the case of disease remission (26,101). Response to therapy is monitored by clinical parameters, such as pulses and bruits, the appearance of arterial lesions by doppler ultrasound, standard angiography, or MRI angiography, the sedimentation rate, and appearance of the urinary sediment.

Angina or claudication in a patient with CS should prompt angiography to search for evidence of SNV (35,101). If a surgical procedure is indicated, pathological material should be carefully evaluated for vascular inflammation. As in aortitis, procedures should be avoided, if possible, in the face of active inflammation; however, these can proceed, if clinically necessary, regardless of whether inflammation is present or not (35,101).

VIII. PATHOGENESIS

The cause of CS is still unknown. Since upper respiratory infection precedes the development of CS in up to 40% of cases (15), a microbial etiology with postinfectious immunopathology has long been considered as a possible etiology of CS. Several investigators have attempted to link CS with chlamydial infection based on serological criteria (14,107). In particular, frequent reference has been made to a patient with CS who had a fourfold rise in serum IgG antibodies to *Chlamydia pneumoniae* (39). However, causation cannot be inferred simply from the detection of serum antibodies to chlamydia. Repeated failures to culture chlamydia species from the eyes and ears of CS patients argue persuasively that this organism is not the sole inciting agent in CS.

The histopathology of the eye and inner ear lesions in CS is compatible with immune-mediated mechanisms of disease pathogenesis. Interstitial keratitis is characterized by lymphocytic and plasma cell infiltration in the deeper layers of the cornea (108). Chronic cases may produce neovacularization and scarring. Pathological descriptions of the vestibuloauditory apparatus in

CS have been limited to a few autopsy reports. The autopsy of the patient who was earliest in the disease course showed lymphocytic and plasma cell infiltration of the spiral ligament, endolymphatic hydrops, degenerative changes in the organ of Corti, and demyelination of the vestibular and cochlear branches of the eighth cranial nerve (9). The two cases with more prolonged disease revealed extensive new bone formation, severe hydrops, and degeneration of the sensory receptors and supporting structures (109,110).

Beyond the eye and inner ear, CS may be associated with a medium-sized artery vasculitis in which the histological changes are typical of polyarteritis nodosa (9) (Fig. 6). A minority of patients with CS has been reported with aortitis, narrowing of the major branches of the aortic arch at their origin, dilation of the aortic ring, coronary ostial occlusion, aortic valvulitis, and coronary vasculitis (9,14,26,28,30,31). The pathology of the aortitis resembles that of Takayasu's arteritis (14,30). Aortic valves obtained after valve replacement surgery and at autopsy have grossly shown cusp detachments and outpouchings, fenestrations, thinning, thickening, and retraction (10,28,30,31). Histopathological examination of these specimens has revealed fibrinoid necrosis, lymphocytic infiltration, myxomatous degeneration of the valve leaflets, and irregular thickening of the endocardium (10,28,30,31,111).

A limited body of evidence suggests that the eye and inner ear disease in CS may result from organ-specific autoimmunity. A few cases have been described in which the patients have serum antibodies to undefined corneal antigens (112,113). Peripheral blood from a young woman with CS who had both IK and scleritis was shown to be reactive with retinal S antigen, outer rod segment, and scleroprotein (114). Other case studies have shown peripheral lymphocyte reactivity in vitro to mixtures of inner ear antigens as well as serum antibodies to inner ear proteins

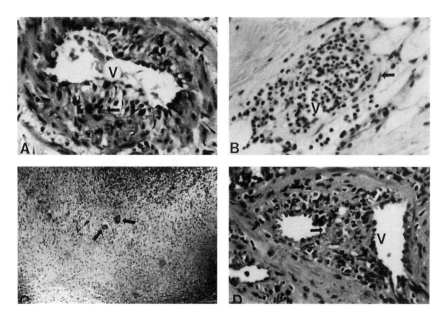

Figure 6 Histology of vascular and splenic inflammation in a patient with CS. (A) Medium-size blood vessel in dermis with inflammatory cells in and around the vessel wall (arrow). V shows the vessel lumen (hemotoxylin and eosin). (B) Inflammatory infiltrate in the lumen (V) and in and around a vessel in the gastric serosa (hematoxylin and eosin). (C) Giant cells (arrows) in splenic granulomatous inflammatory infiltrate (hematoxylin and eosin). (D) A splenic muscular artery with inflammatory cells in a thrombus in the lumen and the vessel wall (arrows) (hematoxylin and eosin). (From Ref. 26.)

(24,115,116). For example, Moscicki et al. (116) found antibodies to a 68-kDa bovine inner ear protein in 8 of 8 patients with CS compared with 42 (58%) of 72 patients with idiopathic, progressive, sensorineural hearing loss and 1 of 53 normal controls. These results are difficult to interpret without a comparison group of patients with other types of immunological disease. However, in another study, serum antibodies to a 68-kDa inner ear protein were detected in only 10 (5%) of 200 patients with rheumatoid arthritis (RA) and systemic lupus erythematosus (SLE) who had no evidence of hearing loss. Interestingly, results from the same study showed that 30% of patients with Ménière's disease also tested positive for serum antibody reactivity with a 68-kDa protein (117). The identity of the 68-kDa antigen is unknown.

The immunopathological mechanisms underlying the chronic inflammatory response in CS are probably similar in the eye and inner ear to those of other tissues, but with some important differences. The cornea and the anterior chamber of the eye are usually considered to be immunologically privileged sites. The anterior chamber and cornea contain transforming growth factor-β, a potent inhibitory cytokine. Other, as yet unidentified, immunosuppressive factors are produced by corneal fibroblasts and epithelial and endothelial cells (118). Corneal injury from infection or other insult may revoke the immune privilege by stimulating corneal vascularization, providing a route for the influx of antigen-presenting cells (APCs) and other immune cells (119). Once immune cells gain access to the eye, interactions between T cells, peptide antigen, and APCs and the production of proinflammatory cytokines likely drive the inflammatory response.

The blood–labyrinthine barrier was initially believed to protect the inner ear from immune attack. However, recent studies show that the inner ear can mount an immunological response. Leukocytes enter the inner ear through the endothelium of the spiral modular vein. Early in the inflammatory process, the endothelial cells undergo morphological transformation to high endothelial venules and are stimulated to express intracellular adhesion molecule (ICAM)-1 and other molecules involved in leukocyte extravasation (120,121). The leukocytes migrate across the endothelium into the cochlear and vestibular labyrinth where they participate in the chronic inflammatory response. The byproduct of chronic inflammation is the accumulation of extracellular matrix and endolymphatic hydrops. Animal studies show that the extracellular matrix is cleared poorly from the inner ear. Ossification is the ultimate outcome regardless of the original insult (121). Histopathological analysis of temporal bone specimens from patients with CS tends to reflect these pathways of inflammation and injury.

IX. SUMMARY

The diagnosis of CS is based on the presence of IK, or other types of ocular inflammation, and vestibuloauditory dysfunction. While initial cases portrayed the ocular and vestibuloauditory components of CS, more recent experience has recognized the association of this disease with aortic insufficiency, coronary arteritis, and SNV. The natural history of IK is relatively benign and does not usually demand aggressive therapy. The ocular outcome in patients with CS is almost always good (14,15,17). However, more serious ocular inflammation, such as scleritis or retinal vasculitis, may cause permanent eye damage and generally warrants the use of corticosteroid plus cytotoxic drugs. Hearing declines in a stepwise progression with repeated attacks of vestibuloauditory dysfunction, and loss of auditory acuity is the major debilitating sequelae for most patients with CS. Progression to deafness is frequent, occurring in 25–50% of patients (15,17). Vestibular symptoms and signs improve with time, but persistent oscillopsia is noted in 15–20% of patients (17). The efficacy of therapy for the auditory manifestations of CS is not well documented. However, auditory thresholds are less than 60 decibels in ~17% of CS patients who had not received oral corticosteroid or cytotoxic therapy, but more than 60 decibels in 81% of CS patients who received oral corticosteroid or oral corticosteroid plus other immunosuppressive therapy (17). Complete deafness may be treated with cochlear implants, which have been shown to improve the hearing and quality of life and provide hope to many patients with this unfortunate outcome.

REFERENCES

1. Cogan DG. Syndrome of nonsyphilitic interstitial keratitis and vestibuloauditory symptoms. Arch Ophthalmol 1945; 33:144–149.
2. Morgan RF, Baumgartner CJ. Ménière's disease complicated by recurrent interstitial keratitis: Excellent results following cervical ganglionectomy. West J Surg 1934; 42:628–631.
3. Rosen E. Interstitial keratitis and vestibuloauditory symptoms following vaccination. Arch Ophthalmol 1949; 41:24–31.
4. Cogan DG. Nonsyphilitic interstitial keratitis with vestibuloauditory symptoms. Arch Ophthalmol 1949; 42:42–49.
5. Lindsay JR, Zuidema JJ. Inner ear deafness of sudden onset. Laryngoscope 1950; 60:238–263.
6. Oliner L, Taubenhaus M, Shapira TM, Leshin N. Nonsyphilitic interstitial keratitis and bilateral deafness (Cogan's syndrome) associated with essential polyangiitis (periarteritis nodosa). N Engl J Med 1953; 248:1001–1008.
7. Quinn FB, Falls HF. Cogan's syndrome. Case report and a review of etiologic concepts. Trans Am Acad Ophthalmol 1958; 62:716–721.
8. Cody DTR, William HL. Cogan's syndrome. Laryngoscope 1960; 70:447–477.
9. Fisher ER, Hellstrom HR. Cogan's syndrome and systemic vascular disease. Arch Pathol 1961; 72:572–592.
10. Eisenstein B, Taubenhaus M. Nonsyphilitic intersitital keratitis and bilateral deafness (Cogan's syndrome) associated with cardiovascular disease. N Engl J Med 1958; 258:1074–1079.
11. Norton EWD, Cogan DG. Syndrome of nonsyphilitic interstitial keratitis and vestibuloauditory symptoms. Arch Ophthalmol 1959; 61:695–697.
12. McNeil NF, Berke M, Reingold IM. Polyarteritis nodosa causing deafness in an adult: Report of a case with special reference to concepts about the disease. Ann Intern Med 1952; 37:1253–1267.
13. Crawford WJ. Cogan's syndrome associated with polyarteritis nodosa. Penn Med J 1957; 60:835–838.
14. Haynes BF, Kaiser-Kupfer MI, Mason P, Fauci AS. Cogan's syndrome. Studies in thirteen patients, long-term follow-up, and a review of the literature. Medicine 1980; 59:426–441.
15. Vollertsen RS, McDonald TJ, Younge BR, Banks PM, Stanson AW, Ilstrup DM. Cogan's syndrome: 18 cases and a review of the literature. Mayo Clin Proc 1986; 61:344–361.
16. St. Clair EW, McCallum RM. Cogan's syndrome. Curr Opin Rheumatol 1999; 11:47–52.
17. McCallum RM, Allen NB, Cobo LM, Weber BA, Haynes BF. Cogan's syndrome: Clinical features and outcomes. Arthritis Rheum 1992; 35(supp 9):S51.
18. Morgan RF, Baumgartner CJ. Mèniére's disease complicated by recurrent interstitial keratitis: Excellent results following cervical ganglionectomy. West J Surg 1934; 42:628–631.
19. Rosen E. Interstitial keratitis and vestibuloauditory symptoms following vaccination. Arch Ophthalmol 1949; 41:24–31.
20. Haynes BF, Pikus A, Kaiser-Kupfer, Fauci AS. Successful treatment of sudden hearing loss in Cogan's syndrome with corticosteroids. Arthritis Rheum 1981; 24:501–503.
21. Cobo LM, Haynes BF. Early corneal findings in Cogan's syndrome. Ophthalmol 1984; 91:903–907.
22. Cogan DG, Kuwabara T: Late corneal opacities in the syndrome of interstitial keratitis and vestibuloauditory symptoms. Acta Ophthalmol 1989; 67:182–187.
23. Benitez JT. Evidence of central vestibulo-auditory dysfunction in atypical Cogan's syndrome: A case report. Am J Otol 1990; 11:131–134.
24. Hughes GB, Kinney SE, Barna BP, Tomsak RL, Calabrese LH. Autoimmune reactivity in Cogan's syndrome: A preliminary report. Otolaryngol Head Neck Surg 1983; 91:24–32.

25. Bielory L, Conti J, Frohman L. Cogan's syndrome. J Allergy Clin Immunol 1990; 85:808–815.
26. Allen NB, Cox CC, Cobo M, Kisslo J, Jacobs MR, McCallum RM, Haynes BF. Use of immunosuppressive agents in the treatment of severe ocular and vascular manifestations of Cogan's syndrome. Am J Med 1990; 88:296–301.
27. Bernhardt O, Veltman R, Dorwald R, Huth F. Cogan Syndrom be Angiitis von Hirnnerven, Aortitis, Endocarditis und Glomerulonephritis. Dtsch Med Worhensche 1967; 101:373–377.
28. Cochrane AD, Tatoulis J. Cogan's syndrome with aortitis, aortic regurgitation, and aortic arch vessel stenoses. Ann Thorac Surg 1991; 52:1166–1167.
29. Cogan DG, Dickerson GR. Nonsyphilitic interstitial keratitis with vestibuloauditory symptoms: A case with fatal aortitis. Arch Ophthal 1964; 71:172–175.
30. Gelfand ML, Kantor T, Gorstein F. Cogan's syndrome with cardiovascular involvement: Aortic insufficiency. Bull NY Acad Med 1972; 48:647–660.
31. Livingston JZ, Casale AS, Hutchins GM, Shapiro EP. Coronary involvement in Cogan's syndrome. Am Heart J 1992; 123:528–530.
32. Hammer M, Witte T, Mugge A, Wollenhaupt J, Laas J, Laszig R, Zeidler H. Complicated Cogan's syndrome with aortic insufficiency and coronary stenosis. J Rheum 1994; 21:552–555.
33. Cheson BD, Bluming AZ, Alroy J. Cogan's syndrome: A systemic vasculitis. Am J Med 1976; 60: 549–555.
34. LaRaja RD. Cogan syndrome associated with mesenteric vascular insufficiency. Arch Surg 1976; 111:1028–1031.
35. McCallum RM, Haynes BF. Cogan's Syndrome. In: Pepose JS, Holland GN, Wilhelmus KR, eds. Ocular Infection and Immunity. St. Louis: Mosby, 1996:446–459.
36. Vella JP, O'Callaghan J, Hickey D, Walshe JJ. Renal artery stenosis complicating Cogan's syndrome. Clin Nephrol 1997; 47:407–408.
37. Thomas HG. Case Report: Clinical and radiological features of Cogan's syndrome—non-syphilitc interstitial keratitis. Audiovascular symptoms and systemic manifestations. Clin Radiol 1992; 45:418–421.
38. Raza K, Karokis D, Kitas GD. Cogan's syndrome with Takayasu's arteritis. Br J Rheumatol 1998; 37: 369–372.
39. Darougar S, John AC, Viswahingam M, Cornell L, Jones BR. Isolation of Chlamydia psittaci from a patient with interstitial keratitis and uveitis associated with otological and cardiovascular lesions. Br J Ophthalmol 1978; 62:709–714.
40. Wohlgethan JR, Stilmant MM, Smith HR. Palpable purpura and uveitis precipitated by splenectomy in an atypical case of Cogan's syndrome. J Rheumatol 1991; 18:1100–1103.
41. Ochonisky S, Chosidow O, Kuentz M, Man N, Fraitag S, Pelisse JM, Revuz J. Cogan's syndrome: An unusual etiology of urticarial vasculitis. Dermatologica 1991; 183:218–220.
42. Jacob A, Ledingham JG, Kerr AIG, Ford MJ. Ulcerative colitis and giant cell arteritis associated with sensorineural deafness. J Laryngol Otol 1990; 104:889–890.
43. Char DH, Cogan DG, Sullivan WR. Immunologic study of nonsyphilitic interstitial keratitis with vestibuloauditory symptoms. Am J Ophthalmol 1975; 80:491–494.
44. Kaiser-Kupfer MI, Mittal KK, Del Valle LA, Haynes BF. The HLA antigens in Cogan's syndrome. Am J Ophthalmol 1978; 86:314–316.
45. Boyd GG: Cogan's syndrome. Report of two cases with signs and symptoms suggesting periarteritis nodosa. Arch Otolaryngol 1957; 65:24–25.
46. Djupesland G, Flottorp G, Hansen E, Sjaastad O. Cogan syndrome: The audiological picture. Arch Otolaryngol 1974; 99:218–225.
47. Lennarson P, Barney NP. Interstitial keratitis as presenting ophthalmic sign of sarcoidosis in a child. J Pediatr Ophthalmol Strabismus 1995; 2:194–196.
48. Brooks AM, Weiner JM, Robertson IF. Interstitial keratitis in untreated (late) syphilis. Aust NZ J Ophthalmol 1986; 14:127–132.
49. Probst LE, Wilkinson J, Nichols BD. Diagnosis of congenital syphilis in adults presenting with interstitial keratitis. Can J Ophthalmol 1994; 29:77–80.
50. Miyashiro MJ, Yee RW, Patel G, Ruiz RS. Lyme disease associated with unilateral interstitial keratitis. Cornea 1999; 18:115–116.

51. Karma A, Seppala I, Mikkila H, Kaakkola S, Viljanen M, Tarkkanen A. Diagnosis and clinical characteristics of ocular Lyme borreliosis. Am J Ophthalmol 1995; 119:127–135.

52. Baum J, Barza M, Weinstein P, Groden J, Aswad M. Bilateral keratitis as a manifestation of Lyme disease. Am J Ophthalmol 1998; 105:75–77.

53. Spaide R, Nattis R, Lipka A, D'Amico R. Ocular findings in leprosy in the United States. Am J Ophthalmol 1985; 100:411–416.

54. Waldman RH. Tuberculosis and the atypical mycobacteria. Otolaryngol Clin North Am 1982; 15: 581–596.

55. Gow JA, Ostler HB, Schachter J. Inclusion conjunctivitis with hearing loss. JAMA 1974; 229:519–520.

56. Meyerhoff WL, Paparella MM, Gudbrandsson FK. Clinical evaluation of Ménière's disease. Laryngoscope 1981; 91:1663–1668.

57. Kundell SP, Ochs HD. Cogan syndrome in childhood. J Pediatr 1980; 97:96–98.

58. Schwartz GS, Harrison AR, Holland EJ. Etiology of immune stromal (interstitial) keratitis. Cornea 1998; 17:278–281.

59. Moscatello AL, Worden DL, Nadelman RB, Wormser G, Lucente F. Otolaryngologic aspects of Lyme disease. Laryngoscope 1991; 101:592–595.

60. Durand DV, Lecomte C, Cathebras P, Rousset H, Godeau P, the SNFMI Research Group on Whipple Disease. Whipple disease: Clinical review of 52 cases. Medicine 1997; 76:170–184.

61. Ramaiah C, Boynton RF. Whipple's disease. Gastroenterol Clin 1998; 27:683–695.

62. Sugaya F, Shijubo N, Takahashi H, Abe S. Sudden hearing loss as the initial manifestation of neurosarcoidosis. Sarcoidosis Vasc Diffuse Lung Dis 1996; 13:54–56.

63. Babin RW, Liu C, Aschenbrener C. Histopathology of neurosensory deafness in sarcoidosis. Ann Otol Rhinol Laryngol 1984; 93:389–393.

64. Sharma OP. Neurosarcoidosis. A personal perspective based on the study of 37 patients. Chest 1997; 112:220–228.

65. Rao NA, Moorthy RS, Inomata H. Vogt-Koyanagi-Harada syndrome. Surv Ophthalmol 1995; 39: 265–292.

66. Alli N, Güngör E. Keratitis, ichthyosis and deafness (KID) syndrome. Int J Dermatol 1997; 36:37–40.

67. Harper SL, Foster CS. The ocular manifestations of rheumatoid disease. Int Ophthalmol Clin 1998; 38:1–19.

68. Kastanioudakis I, Skevas A, Danielidis V, Tsiakou E, Drosos AA, Moutsopoulos MH. Inner ear involvement in rheumatoid arthritis: A prospective study. J Laryngol Otol 1995; 109:713–718.

69. Tumiati B, Casoli P, Parmeggiani A. Hearing loss in the Sjögren syndrome. Ann Intern Med 1997; 126:45–453.

70. Andonopoulos AP, Naxakis S, Goumas P, Lygatsikas C. Sensorineural hearing disorders in systemic lupus erythematosus. A controlled study. Clin Exp Rheumatol 1995; 13:137–141.

71. Naarendorp M, Spiera H. Sudden sensorineural hearing loss in patients with systemic lupus erythematosus or lupus-like syndromes and antiphospholipid antibodies. J Rheumatol 1998; 25:589–592.

72. Hisashi K, Komune S, Taira T, Uemura T, Sadoshima S, Tsuda H. Anticardiolipin antibody-induced sudden profound sensorineural hearing loss. Am J Otolaryngol 1993; 14:275–277.

73. Toubi E, Ben-David J, Kessel A, Podoshin L, Golan TD. Autoimmune aberration in sudden sensorineural hearing loss: association with anti-cardiolipin antibodies. Lupus 1997; 6:540–542.

74. Acheson JF, Gregson RM, Merry P, Schulenburg WE. Vaso-occlusive retinopathy in the primary antiphospholipid antibody syndrome. Eye 1991; 5:48–55.

75. Haynes BF, Fishman ML, Fauci AS, Wolff SM. The ocular manifestations of Wegener's granulomatosis. Fifteen years experience and review of the literature. Am J Med 1977; 63:131141.

76. Luqmani R, Jubb R, Emery P, Reid A, Adu D. Inner ear deafness in Wegener's granulomatosis. J Rheumatol 1991; 18:766–768.

77. Kempf HG. Ear involvement in Wegener's granulomatosis. Clin Otolaryngol 1989; 14:451–456.

78. Abou-Elhmd KA, Hawthorne MR, Flood LM. Cochlear implantation in a case of Wegener's granulomatosis. J Laryngol Otol 1996; 110:958–961.

79. Gran JT, Nordvag BY, Storesund B. An overlap syndrome with features of atypical Cogan's syndrome and Wegener's granulomatosis. Scand J Rheumatol 1999; 28:62–64.

80. Hoshino T, Ishii T, Kodama A, Kato I. Temporal bone findings in a case of sudden deafness and relapsing polychondritis. Acta Otolaryngol 1980; 90:257–261.

81. Clark LJ, Wakeel RA, Ormerod AD. Relapsing polychondritis-two cases with tracheal stenosis and inner ear involvement. J Laryngol Otol 1992; 106:841–844.

82. Kimura Y, Miwa H, Furukawa M, Mizukami Y. Relapsing polychondritis presented as inner ear involvement. J Laryngol Otol 1996; 110:154–157.

83. Albers FWJ, Majoor MHJM, Van der Gaag R. Corneal autoimmunity in a patient with relapsing polychondritis. Eur Arch Otorhinolaryngol 1992; 249:296–299.

84. Bhisitkul RB, Foster CS. Diagnosis and ophthalmological features of Behçet's disease. Int Ophthalmol Clin 1996; 36:127–134.

85. Gemignani G, Berrettini S, Bruschini P, Sellari-Franceschini S, Fusari P, Piragine F, Pasero G, Olivieri I. Hearing and vestibular disturbances in Behçet's syndrome. Ann Otol Rhinol Laryngol 1991; 100:459–463.

86. Brama I, Fainaru M. Inner ear involvement in Behçet's disease. Arch Otolaryngol 1980; 106:215–217.

87. Berrettini S, Ferri C, Ravecca F, LaCivita L, Bruschini L, Riente L, Mosca M, Sellari-Franceschini S. Progressive sensorineural hearing impairment in systemic vasculitides. Semin Arthritis Rheum 1998; 27:301–318.

88. Jenkins HA, Pollack AM, Fisch U. Polyarteritis nodosa as a cause of sudden deafness. A human temporal bone study. Am J Otolaryngol 1981; 2:99–107.

89. Wolf M, Kronenberg J, Engelberg S, Leventon G. Rapidly progressive hearing loss as a symptom of polyarteritis nodosa. Am J Otolaryngol 1987; 8:105–108.

90. Rowe-Jones JM, Macallan DC, Sorooshian M. Polyarteritis nodosa presenting as bilateral sudden onset cochleo-vestibular failure in a young woman. J Laryngol Otol 1990; 104:562–564.

91. Kumar BN, Walsh RM, Wilson PS, Carlin WV. Sensorineural hearing loss and ulcerative colitis. J Laryngol Otol 1997; 111:277–278.

92. Weber RS, Jenkins HA, Coker NJ. Sensorineural hearing loss associated with ulcerative colitis. Arch Otolaryngol 1984; 110:810–812.

93. Bachmeyer C, Leclerc-Landgraf N, Laurette F, Coutarel P, Cadranel J, Médioni J, Dhôte R, Mougeot-Martin M. Acute autoimmune sensorineural hearing loss associated with Crohn's disease. Am J Gastroenterol 1998; 93:2565–2567.

94. Matsuo T, Yamaoka A, Shiraga F, Matsuo N. Two types of initial ocular manifestations in introacular-central nervous system lymphoma. Retina 1998; 18:301–307.

95. Shuangshoti S. Solitary primary lymphoma of the cerebellopontine angle: A case report. Neurosurgery 1995; 36:595–598.

96. Erck S, Ruff T, Lenis A. A rare cause of reversible sensorineural hearing loss. J Otolaryngol 1993; 22:121–124.

97. Cramer SC, Glapsy JA, Efird JT, Louis DN. Chronic lymphocytic leukemia and the central nervous system. A clinical and pathologic study. Neurology 1996; 46:19–25.

98. Petty GW, Engel AG, Younge BR, Duffy J, Yanagihara T, Lucchinetti CF, Bartleson JD, Parisi JE, Kasperbauer JL, Rodriguez M. Retinocochleocerebral vasculopathy. Medicine 1998; 77:12–40.

99. Papo T, Biousse V, Lehoang P, Fardeau C, N'Guyen N, Huong DLT, Aumaitre O, Bousser M, Godeau P, Piette J. Susac syndrome. Medicine 1998; 77:3–11.

100. Beckman H, Trotsky MB. Cogan's syndrome treated with oral glycerine: Report of a case. Arch Otolaryngol 1970; 91:179–182.

101. McCallum RM. Cogan's syndrome. In: Franunfelder FT, Roy FH, eds. Current Ocular Therapy, 4th ed. Philadelphia: Saunders, 1993:410–412.

102. Reiente L, Taglione E, Berrettini S. Efficacy of methotrexate in Cogan's syndrome. J Rheum 1996; 23:1830–1831.

103. Pouchot J, Vinceneux P, Bouccara D, Sterkers O, Bodelet B. Methotrexate as a steroid-sparing agent in Cogan's syndrome: Comment on the concise communication by Richardson. Arthritis Rheum 1994; 38:1348–1349.

104. Roat MI, Thoft RA, Thomson AW, Jain A, Fung JJ, Starzl TE. Treatment of Cogan's syndrome with FK 506: A case report. Transplant Proc 1991; 23:3347.

105. Schedler MGJ, Bartylla M. Retrospektive und prospektive unterscuhungen and patienten mit Cogan-I-syndrom. Laryngo-Rhin-Otol 1994; 73:662–666.

106. Cochlear Implants in Adults and Children. NIH Consens Statement 1995; 13:1–30.

107. Ljungström L, Franzén C, Schlaug M, Elowson S, Vidas U. Reinfection with chlamydia pneumonia may induce isolated and systemic vasculitis in small and large vessels. Scand J Infect Dis 1997; 104(Suppl):37–40.

108. Negroni L, Tiberio G. La sindrome di Cogan. Rev Oto Neuro Oftamol 1969; 44:199–224.

109. Rarey KE, Bicknell JM, Davis LE. Intralabyrinthine osteogenesis in Cogan's syndrome. Am J Otolaryngol 1986; 4:387–390.

110. Schuknecht HF, Nadol JB. Temporal bone pathology in a case of Cogan's syndrome. Laryngoscope 1994; 104:1135–1142.

111. Pinals RS. Cogan's syndrome with arthritis and aortic insufficiency. J Rheumatol 1978; 5:294–298.

112. Arnold W, Gebbers J-O. Serum-antikörper gegen kornea- und innenohrgewebe beim Cogan-syndrom. Laryng Rhinol Otol 1984; 63:428–432.

113. Majoor MHJM, Albers FWJ, van der Gaag R, Gmelig-Meyling F, Huizing EH. Corneal autoimmunity in Cogan's syndrome? Report of two cases. Ann Otol Rhinol Laryngol 1992; 101:679–684.

114. Peeters GJHCM, Cremers CWRJ, Pinckers AJLG, Hoefnagels WHL. Atypical Cogan's syndrome: An autoimmune disease? Ann Oto Rhinol Laryngol 1986; 95:173–175.

115. Arnold W, Pfaltz R, Altermatt H-J. Evidence of serum antibodies against inner ear tissues in the blood of patients with certain sensorineural hearing disorders. Acta Otolaryngol (Stockh) 1985; 99:437–444.

116. Moscicki RA, San Martin JE, Quintero CH, Rauch SD, Nadol JB, Bloch KJ. Serum antibody to inner ear proteins in patients with progressive hearing loss. Correlation with disease activity and response to corticosteroid treatment. JAMA 1994; 272:611–616.

117. Gottschlich S, Billings PB, Keithley EM, Weisman MH, Harris JP. Assessment of serum antibodies in patients with rapidly progressive sensorineural hearing loss and Ménière's disease. Laryngoscope 1995; 105:1347–1352.

118. Jager MJ, Gregerson DS, Streilein JW. Regulators of immunological responses in the cornea and the anterior chamber of the eye. Eye 1995; 9:241–246.

119. Dana MR, Streilein JW. Loss and restoration of immune privilege in eyes with corneal neovascularization. Invest Ophthalmol Vis Sci 1996; 37:2485–2494.

120. Harris JP, Fukuda S, Keithley EM. Spiral modular vein: Its importance in inner ear inflammation. Acta Otolaryngol (Stockh) 1990; 110:357–365.

121. Harris JP, Heydt J, Keithley EM, Chen M. Immunopathology of the inner ear: An update. Ann NY Acad Sci 1997; 830:166.

35

Vasculitis of the Central Nervous System

Leonard H. Calabrese
Cleveland Clinic Foundation, Cleveland, Ohio

George F. Duna
Baylor College of Medicine, Houston, Texas

I. INTRODUCTION

Among the many forms of organ-limited vasculitis, that affecting the central nervous system (CNS) remains one of the most challenging from a clinical and pathophysiological perspective. Reasons for this include (1) lack of specificity of signs and symptoms, (2) limited accessibility of the end-organ for pathological examination, (3) lack of efficient noninvasive diagnostic tests, and (4) the relative rarity of different forms of CNS vasculitis. Despite these limitations, considerable progress has been made over the past decade in our understanding of these conditions.

Vasculitis of the CNS is currently classified as either primary or secondary (1,2). Central nervous system vasculitis that is not associated with a systemic illness or vasculitis outside of the CNS is known as primary angiitis of the CNS (PACNS). Once considered a rare and uniformly fatal disorder, PACNS is now more commonly diagnosed and recognized as a disorder with marked clinical and presumed pathophysiological heterogeneity. Secondary vasculitis of the CNS is found in association with a wide variety of conditions including infections, drugs, malignancies, systemic vasculitides and connective tissue diseases. This chapter focuses on the major forms of CNS vasculitis, with emphasis on their clinical findings, diagnosis, and treatment.

II. EPIDEMIOLOGY OF PACNS

As of 1988 there were only 46 cases of PACNS described in the world literature. At that time, Calabrese and Mallek proposed three criteria for a diagnosis of PACNS (3).

1. A history of a clinical finding of an acquired neurological deficit that remained unexplained after a thorough initial basic evaluation.
2. Either classic (high probability) angiographic evidence or histopathological demonstration of angiitis within the CNS.
3. No evidence of systemic vasculitis or any other condition to which the angiographic or pathological features could be secondary (Table 1).

While these criteria served a useful purpose in providing a basis for analyzing such cases, they did not accommodate the possibility that histologically confirmed cases and those diagnosed

Table 1   Conditions That Resemble PACNS (3,6)

Systemic vasculitides
    Polyarteritis nodosa
    Allergic granulomatosis
    Hypersensitivity vasculitis group disorders
    Vasculitis with connective tissue disease
    Wegener's granulomatosis
    Temporal arteritis
    Takayasu's arteritis
    Behçet's disease
    Lymphomatoid granulomatosis
    Cogan's syndrome
Infections
    Viral, bacterial, fungal, rickettsial
Neoplasm
    Angioimmunoproliferative disorders
    Carcinomatous meningitis
    Infiltrating glioma
    Malignant angioendotheliomatosis
Drug use
    Amphetamines
    Ephedrine
    Phenylpropanolamine
    Cocaine
    Ergotamine
Vasospastic disorders
    Postpartum angiopathy
    Eclampsia
    Pheochromocytoma
    Subarachnoid hemorrhage
    Migraine and exertional headache
Other vasculopathies and mimicking conditions
    Fibromuscular dysplasia
    Moyamoya disease
    Thrombotic thrombocytopenic purpura
    Sickle cell anemia
    Neurofibromatosis
    Cerebrovascular atherosclerosis
    Demyelinating disease
    Sarcoidosis
    Emboli (i.e., SBE, cardiac myxoma, paradoxical emboli)
    Acute posterior placoid pigment epitheliopathy and cerebral vasculitis
    Antiphospholipid antibody syndrome

solely on angiographic grounds may not be clinically equivalent. At the time these criteria were proposed, there was little evidence to suggest that PACNS was other than a homogeneous, highly progressive, and fatal illness. The past decade has witnessed an increasing appreciation that within the spectrum of PACNS, there is considerable clinical heterogeneity including subsets with relatively benign prognosis. In support of this concept are numerous case reports of PACNS with benign outcome and more recently the establishment of criteria to identify such (4–6). In

1983, the importance of this observation became particularly acute after the report of Cupps et al. (7), describing successful therapy of PACNS with a combination of glucocorticoids and cyclophosphamide. Following this, it became common practice for patients diagnosed by either biopsy or solely on angiographic grounds to be treated with such therapy for prolonged periods of time. Based upon these observations, we believe it is imperative to attempt to define subgroups within PACNS, including those cases with relatively benign outcomes that may not require high-intensity immunosuppressive therapy, or at times, any immunosuppressive therapy at all.

III. CLINICAL SUBSETS OF PACNS

A. Granulomatous Angiitis of the Central Nervous System

1. Clinical and Pathological Features

In 1959, Cravioto and Feigin (8) elegantly described a small series of patients with a chronic, progressive, and fatal form of CNS vasculitis with granulomatous pathology limited to the brain and meninges. These original clinical and pathological descriptions have endured as a model of this subset of PACNS that we now refer to as granulomatous angiitis of the CNS or GACNS (8–10). Unfortunately, throughout the last several decades, the term GACNS is often used interchangeably with any form of vasculitis suspected of being confined to the CNS regardless of whether it is diagnosed on pathological grounds or purely through angiographic means, and regardless of whether granulomatous pathology is documented in involved tissue. We believe that GACNS is still a useful diagnostic term, but must be reserved for those cases conforming to the full clinical and pathological features as originally described. The major clinical and pathological features are outlined in Table 2. Using these criteria, there have been approximately 136 cases reported as of 1997 (10).

From a clinical perspective, it is highly useful to categorize PACNS as being either pathologically or angiographically documented (i.e., in the absence of histological confirmation). All patients pathologically documented should further be classified as either having granulomatous or nongranulomatous pathology. Based upon the literature and our own clinical experience, we have estimated that at least half of patients with pathologically defined PACNS have nongranulomatous pathology. The details of this observation are described later in this chapter. The pathology of GACNS is that of a leptomeningeal and cortical vasculitis disease involving the small and

Table 2 Essential Features of GACNS

Clinical
    Variable onset but most frequently a prolonged prodrome of 3–6 or more months
    Mixture of focal and nonfocal neurological signs
    CSF analysis abnormal in 90% (aseptic meningitis formula)
Radiographic
    Neuroimaging reveals signs of multifocal ischemia of varying ages
    Variable presence of leptomeningeal enhancement
    Angiography normal in approximately 40%
Pathological
    Vasculitis of small and medium-sized vessels of leptomeningies and underlying
        cortex with variable degrees of granulomatous changes
    Giant cells may or may not be present.
Exclusions
    Diseases and conditions in Table 1

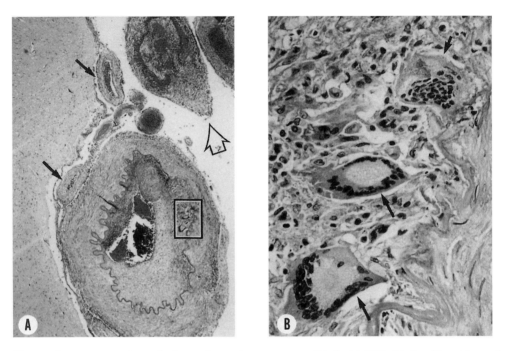

Figure 1 (A) Brain biopsy findings of granulomatous vasculitis in PACNS side-by-side with a poly-arteritis nodosa–type necrotizing vasculitis (open arrow) and two normal arterioles (short arrows). (B) Close-up showing foreign body (short arrows) and Langerhans' (long arrow) giant cells in the granulomatous inflammation. (Hematoxylin and eosin stain, magnification ×64 and ×400.) (From Ref. 1.)

medium-sized cortical arteries, and less commonly, veins (9). The nature and intensity of granuloma formation may markedly vary as evidenced by Figures 1 and 2. At times, well-formed granulomas reminiscent of sarcoidosis may be identified in an angioinvasive pattern, but more frequently, the inflammation merely shows granulomatous features with a mixed infiltrate of mononuclear inflammatory cells, activated histiocytes, and a variable frequency of giant cells. There have been no clinical correlates with any specific pathological feature noted to date.

The clinical manifestations of GACNS are nonspecific (1,2,6,9–11). It may occur at any age and tends to be slightly male predominant. The typical patient is a man or a woman in the fourth or fifth decade of life with the insidious onset of a progressive neurological dysfunction including both focal and nonfocal manifestations. As noted above, the onset is generally insidious with a prodrome that may last several years or more before diagnosis. Rarely, however, the onset may be hyperacute.

The most common symptom is headache, which varies in quality, ranging from mild and chronic to severe and hyperacute. Curiously, the headaches may spontaneously remit for long periods of time. Since virtually any anatomical area of the CNS may be affected by vasculitis, a wide range of focal neurological defects may be seen, including transient ischemic attacks, strokes, paraparesis, quadriparesis, cranial neuropathies, ataxia, and seizures. Retinal vasculitis has occasionally been reported (12,13). The spinal cord may occasionally be involved and may rarely be the exclusive manifestation of the disease. Infrequently, subarachnoid or intracerebral hemorrhage is the initial event.

Nonfocal neurological deficits are characteristic of this disorder and include an acute or subacute encephalopathy (12), which rarely may present as a pure dementia. However, a de-

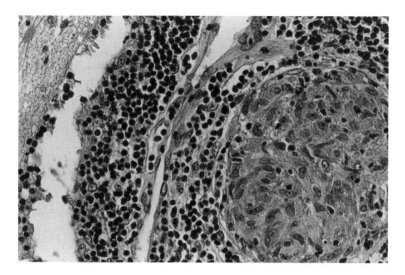

Figure 2   Marked mononuclear inflammatory infiltrate in a cortical vessel with a well-formed paravascular granuloma. (Hematoxylin and eosin stain, magnification ×200.) (From Ref. 2.)

creased or fluctuating level of consciousness is more common. A picture with some similarities to multiple sclerosis has also been described (13). Although there is no clinical presentation specific for GACNS, a chronic, progressive neurological disorder including both focal and nonfocal deficits is most characteristic. Importantly, systemic symptoms such as fever, weight loss, arthralgias, and myalgias, which are typical of systemic vasculitis, are uncommon in PACNS and should suggest a different diagnosis.

2. Laboratory Findings

There are no noninvasive tests or blood studies of sufficient positive predictive value to secure the diagnosis of GACNS. The actual diagnosis relies heavily on several neurologically oriented, diagnostic modalities. These tests include cerebrospinal fluid (CSF) analysis, noninvasive neuroimaging such as computerized tomography (CT) and magnetic resonance imaging (MRI), cerebral angiography, and ultimately biopsy of CNS tissues.

Cerebrospinal fluid analysis is an essential part of the diagnostic process for GACNS. In over 90% of patients with histologically confirmed CNS vasculitis, the CSF is abnormal. However, when angiography is the principal means of diagnosis, CSF is completely normal in over 40% of pathologically documented cases (6). The cause for this discrepancy is unclear, but as detailed in the next section, may indicate that angiography alone may define different subsets of PACNS. Cerebrospinal fluid findings are generally characteristic of an aseptic meningitis, displaying a modest pleocytosis, normal glucose, and an elevated protein. Increased IgG synthesis and the presence of oligoclonal bands are occasionally detected and generally are unhelpful because of their lack of specificity. The most important aspect of CSF analysis is its utility for detection of CNS infection. While the extent of microbial screening should be influenced somewhat by the clinical situation, cultures for bacteria, mycobacteria, and fungi should be routine (14). In addition, we believe all suspected cases should routinely be evaluated for occult viral infections, especially varicella zoster virus, which may mimic GACNS clinically and histopathologically (15).

Angiography is an insensitive tool for the diagnosis of GACNS and probably should be reserved after biopsy of the CNS in the diagnostic algorithm. Despite this, approximately 40% of patients may have high-probability angiograms, which we define as demonstrating multiple areas of stenosis and ectasia in multiple vascular beds (6). Occasionally single or multiple microaneuysms may be noted, but they do not carry the same specificity for arteritis in the CNS as they do in visceral angiography (16). Unfortunately, even a high-probability angiogram lacks specificity and is incapable of securing the diagnosis of GACNS under most circumstances (17). Following successful therapy, regressions of both arterial beading and aneurysms have been documented (16,18).

Noninvasive neuroimaging techniques such as CT and MRI are important in the diagnosis of GACNS as well as other subsets of PACNS. Magnetic resonance imaging is more sensitive than CT and is the preferred diagnostic imaging technique when other than acute cerebral hemorrhage is suspected. Common MRI findings in GACNS, as well as other forms of PACNS, include multiple bilateral supratentorial infarcts, including lesions in the cortex, deep white matter, and/or leptomeninges (19–21). With the use of contrast agents, lesions in both the cortex and leptomeninges may demonstrate enhancement, but this is a nonspecific finding. Enhancement within the leptomeninges is highly predictive of a diagnostic biopsy and should be searched for in all cases (21). Occasionally, PACNS may manifest as diffuse white matter disease mimicking a primary demyelinating disease (22). If one considers only patients with pathologically documented PACNS, the sensitivity of MRI approaches 100% (1,15,23). When combined with the over 90% sensitivity of CSF analysis, the presence of a normal CSF and a normal MRI should strongly dissuade against the diagnosis of GACNS. When considering cases defined solely on the basis of angiography, however, MRI is less sensitive and at times may be completely normal (24).

The gold standard for the diagnosis of all forms of vasculitis is histological confirmation. Biopsy of the CNS is particularly important in the diagnostic process since it is capable of detecting mimicking conditions, such as lymphoproliferative diseases, certain infections, sarcoidosis and other forms of occlusive vascular disease (25). Brain biopsy is unfortunately limited by poor sensitivity. Premortem, biopsies yield false-negative results in an estimated 25% of autopsy-documented cases (7). Reasons belying this low sensitivity include technical factors, such as failing to sample both cortex and leptomeninges, as well as the patchy nature of the disease (24). As noted above, biopsy of a radiographically abnormal area, particularly in the presence of enhancement by MRI, improves the sensitivity of the procedure (25,26).

In the absence of surgically approachable focal lesions, an open biopsy of the temporal tip of the nondominant hemisphere is the preferred procedure (1,25). Sampling of the basilar meninges is important when attempting to exclude certain indolent infections or sarcoidosis (1,25). Steriotactic biopsy is probably not indicated unless approaching a mass lesion (27). Regardless of the technique, tissue samples should be stained and cultured for microorganisms with an effort to preserve frozen tissues for further investigations if found necessary. Although false-positive biopsies are rarely reported, areas of vascular inflammation may be encountered in lymphoproliferative diseases and CNS infections. Even when vasculitis is identified, special stains for microorganisms are essential. In predominantly lymphocytic lesions, immunohistochemistry and/or DNA analysis for clonality may also be needed to help clarify whether one is dealing with a lymphoproliferative process. Since the specificity of a biopsy is not 100%, even a positive biopsy result should be interpreted in light of the entire clinical picture.

B. Benign Angiopathy of the Central Nervous System or Reversible Vasoconstrictive Disorder

The working case definition of PACNS (3) has created a subset of patients in whom the diagnosis has been established solely on angiographic grounds. In this population, an antemortem CNS biopsy may have been nondiagnostic or, more commonly, never performed at all. Such cases represent a sizable subset of the PACNS literature accounting for 44 of 168 recently reviewed (28). Cases diagnosed solely on angiographic grounds have become even more common in recent years with the aggressive application of neuroradiographic techniques in the investigation of unexplained CNS disease.

Given the absence of tissue confirmation in these patients, the reliability of cerebral angiography to secure the diagnosis of CNS angiitis has justifiably come under question. Duna and Calabrese (17) have reported that even a high-probability angiogram, defined as alternating areas of stenosis and ectasia in multiple vascular beds, is likely to represent a false-positive test in the clinical evaluation of suspected vasculitis. In practice, we believe that only rarely can the "classic" angiographic picture of vasculitis be differentiated from the vascular changes resulting from certain infections, degenerative vascular disease, or vasospastic disorders. Based on these data, we and others (1,4,29) believe that within this angiographically defined subset is a group of patients with characteristic features that differentiate them from patients with GACNS.

A careful review of the historical literature on PACNS reveals numerous isolated cases of putative PACNS, diagnosed exclusively on the basis of angiography, with seemingly benign courses that have been labeled isolated benign cerebral vasculitis, isolated benign cerebral arteriopathy, and reversible cerebral segmental vasoconstriction (5). Based upon these reports and a review of all angiographically and pathologically defined cases in the literature, we proposed the diagnostic term "benign angiopathy of the central nervous system," or BACNS. In retrospect, this term appears to be unfortunate since not all patients have a clinically benign outcome, but we still believe that they are generally clinically distinct. The major features of this disorder are summarized in Table 3 and include a female predominance, with acute onset of severe headache or focal neurological event, a normal or nearly normal cerebral spinal fluid analysis, a high-probability angiogram, and a course more often monophasic and benign than that seen in pathologically documented GACNS. It should be emphasized that BACNS has been defined as a clinical and angiographic syndrome and not merely PACNS diagnosed via angiography.

A similar clinical and angiographic picture has been reported in patients exposed to some sympathomimetic drugs (30,31), with pheochromocytoma (32), in the setting of complex headaches such as migraine or exertional headaches (33,34), and in the postpartum period (35–37). The striking similarities between the clinical and angiographic picture of BACNS and these latter conditions suggest that reversible vasoconstriction may belie the underlying angiographic changes. Unfortunately, in the absence of definitive pathophysiological investigations, the underlying pathology responsible for this syndrome remains unknown. We now favor the term, "reversible vasoconstrictive disease," over BACNS since it does not necessarily imply a benign outcome. Cerebral hemorrhage and death can be the sequelae of this presentation, but more often than not, the course is benign.

Table 3   Essential Features of Reversible Vasoconstrictive Disease (BACNS)

Clinical
  Most common in young women
  Acute onset (hours to days)
  Severe headache and or focal neurological event
  Normal or nearly normal CSF analysis
Radiographic
  High-probability angiogram for vasculitis (segmental narrowing, ectasia, or
    beading in multiple vascular beds)
Exclusions
  Diseases and conditions in Table 1

C. Other Forms of PACNS

Reversible cerebral vasoconstrictive disease and GACNS appear to account for no more than 50% of all cases of PACNS fulfilling the working diagnostic criteria (38). The remainder of cases, lacking characteristic features of either subset must at present be defined in descriptive terms based on clinical course, neurological deficits, pathological description, and/or angiographic findings. Within this sizable population of patients are certain recurrent themes that deserve further description.

1. Mass Lesion Presentation

Approximately 15% of PACNS patients present with mass lesions (generally single and occasionally multiple), which should always be considered neoplastic or infective in origin until proven otherwise (1,38). As with all forms of PACNS, the underlying etiology of such cases is unknown. The pathology of such lesions may be granulomatous or nongranulomatous. In our limited experience, the clinical course appears to be relatively benign with treatment generally limited to corticosteroid therapy. Reports of cure by resection have been described. All other patients have required combination immunosuppressive therapy (2) similar to that utilized in GACNS.

2. Spinal Cord Presentation

PACNS can also present with spinal cord involvement and over 75% of these cases appear to have GACNS (38). Such patients most often present with a progressive paraparesis, but acute transverse myelitis and acute spinal subdural hemorrhage have also been reported (39). Differentiation from infective and/or neoplastic forms of spinal cord disease is often difficult and generally requires biopsy confirmation.

3. Amyloid-Associated PACNS

There are approximately 10 patients reported with cerebral amyloid who additionally have features of GACNS (10,40). In these cases, headaches, mental change, gait difficulty, and focal cerebral signs were present in the majority at the onset of their illness. Progressive stupor, coma, and death followed in about half. As expected, these cases have been observed predominantly in older individuals. It has recently been suggested that the inflammatory vascular infiltrates are consistent with a foreign body reaction evoked by amyloid rather than amyloid deposition being secondary to the inflammatory process of arteritis (41). This view is supported by the presence of beta/A4 and cystatin C amyloid within macrophages and giant cells within the lesions, presumably secondary to phagocytosis.

4. CNS Sarcoid Vasculitis

Another interesting subgroup of patients are those with sarcoidosis and a clinical and histological picture virtually indistinguishable from GACNS (10). In several of these cases, including the one illustrated in Figure 2, there was no evidence of any sign of sarcoidosis outside the CNS. How to best classify such patients is currently unsettled.

5. VZV-Associated PACNS

Perhaps the most perplexing subset of patients with PACNS are those with associated varicella zoster virus (VZV) infection. The association of VZV infection with CNS vascular disease has been well described. The most well-known syndrome is that of contralateral hemiplegia in the setting of VZV infection of the trigeminal nerve (42–45). In this syndrome, several weeks to months following VZV infection, the patient suffers an ischemic event secondary to vasculitis of the middle cerebral artery, several of its branches, and occasionally the internal carotid artery. The mechanism appears to be retrograde spread of VZV via anastomotic branches of the gasserian ganglion to the cerebral circulation (44–46). Usually the disease remains anatomically localized and monophasic in course. We do not view such patients with this typical monophasic and focal illness to have true PACNS, since they generally can be readily differentiated on clinical and/or angiographic grounds.

A second VZV-associated syndrome of CNS vascular disease has been described most frequently in patients with altered host defenses, and appears indistinguishable from idiopathic GACNS (14,43). This disease may evolve in the setting of either VZV infection of the trigeminal nerve or infection of other spinal radicular dermatomes, or even in the absence of clinical VZV infection. Gilden et al. (14) have recently described a case of waxing and waning vasculitis originally thought to be idiopathic GACNS and only later demonstrated to be VZV-associated through utilization of molecular techniques demonstrating VZV antigen in cerebral arteries with a patchy or skip distribution. This patient did not have a zosteriform rash preceding the illness. Another recent investigation has demonstrated the frequent subclinical extension of viral infection into the CNS in patients with acute herpes zoster, further supporting the potential role for occult VZV infection in PACNS (47). We believe that all cases of suspected PACNS should have CSF testing for VZV by the polymerase chain reaction.

Lastly, also of note are the sizable number of patients with PACNS with nongranulomatous pathology. Whether these patients represent truly a different disorder or sampling bias of biopsies remains to be determined.

IV. TREATMENT AND OUTCOME OF PACNS

The single most important aspect of successful treatment of any form of PACNS is a secure diagnosis. The diagnoses listed in Table 1 must firmly be excluded even in the presence of a high-probability angiogram or histology demonstrating angiitis within the CNS. In particular, the exclusion of infectious etiologies is of utmost importance. A useful principle for guiding the diagnostic search for PACNS is that the clinician is statistically more likely to encounter other conditions that explain the neurological problem. In a recent study from the Cleveland Clinic Foundation, Duna and Calabrese (17) reviewed the records of 30 patients referred for evaluation of PACNS who ultimately required either cerebral angiography and/or brain biopsy. The final diagnosis revealed that only 7 patients had PACNS while 23 had other disorders including infections, lymphoproliferative disorders, demyelinating disease, vasospastic diseases, and miscellaneous conditions. Careful examination of the CSF is an essential procedure, particularly when suspecting GACNS. A chronic meningitis formula should stimulate further investigations for other possible etiologies including neoplastic, infectious, and other inflammatory diseases (14). If the diagnosis is still in doubt in patients presenting with chronic meningitis, biopsy of the CNS is nearly always indicated. As noted above, the importance of performing a biopsy is as much to rule out mimicking conditions as it is to confirm the suspected diagnosis (48). Performance of a biopsy is particularly important in those patients in whom immunosuppressive therapy with corticosteroids and cytotoxic drugs is being contemplated.

In patients who present with more focal presentation, such as stroke or transient ischemic attacks (TIAs), but who do not display a chronic meningitis formula within the CSF, it is important to perform a detailed search for hypercoagulable states. Transesophageal echocardiography is necessary to search for myxomas and valvular vegetations and to exclude the presence of a patent foramen ovale as a source of paradoxical emboli.

There are no controlled trials of therapy in PACNS diagnosed either by antemortem biopsy or angiography. In general, we believe, based on our limited experience (3,6) and that from the literature (10), that patients with histologically confirmed GACNS should be treated with aggressive combination therapy with corticosteroids and cyclophosphamide. The treatment course is generally 6–12 months with a tapering schedule similar to that used in patients with Wegener's granulomatosis. All patients should receive prophylaxis for *Pneumocystis carinii* pneumonia (49).

Assessment of disease activity in PACNS is problematic. In patients with GACNS variant, serial assessment of MRI looking for decreased enhancement within the leptomeninges (when present) can be helpful. Serial examinations of CSF to demonstrate resolution of inflammatory changes is also helpful in our experience. Unfortunately, neurological deficits, particularly those which are dense, are unlikely to improve and reflect more damage than disease activity.

In patients with the reversible vasoconstrictive variant of PACNS, angiographic improvement or resolution may be documented within 8–12 weeks (2). We believe that this is important to document, since failure to resolve or dramatically improve on therapy is suggestive of alternative diagnoses.

The recommended treatment for the reversible vasoconstrictive syndrome is based solely on our own clinical experience (3,6), with some growing consensus in the literature (50,51). As with GACNS, there are no controlled trials on which to base such recommendations. Given the benefits of high-dose corticosteroids in experimental vasoconstriction secondary to subarachnoid hemorrhage (50), we recommend high-dose corticosteroids (approximately 60–80 mg of prednisone a day) tapered over a 2–4 week period. In addition, we recommend the use of a calcium channel blocker for at least 6–12 months. Avoidance of sympathomimetics and other aggravating factors such as nicotine, caffeine, etc., is also important (53). The role of other experimental agents, such as vasodilators such as papaverin, nonsteroidal antiinflammatory drugs, and biological agents such as monoclonal antibodies directed against ICAM-1, all have a basis in experimental studies, but have not been rigorously clinically tested.

V. SECONDARY FORMS OF CNS VASCULITIS

Cerebral vasculitis may be associated with a variety of conditions, including infections, drugs, lymphoproliferative diseases, systemic vasculitides, and connective tissue diseases (1) (Table 4). Although the evidence for a direct cause and effect mechanism is generally lacking, removal of the exogenous inciting agent or control of the associated systemic disease may result in amelioration of the secondary CNS vasculitis. A diligent search for associated conditions is thus essential in the approach to the patient with suspected cerebral arteritis.

A. Infections

In the evaluation of CNS vasculitis, it is important to search for infection through microbiological analysis of cerebrospinal fluid and biopsy material. This cannot be overemphasized since the clinical and angiographic presentations of infection-related cerebral arteritis mimic those of PACNS (1,54). Furthermore, the underlying infection may be occult when the neurovascular complication occurs. Suspicion of specific pathogens should be guided by epidemiological features and individual risk factors. The possibility of infection with human immunodeficiency virus (HIV-1), VZV, or syphilis should be actively ascertained (see Table 4). Of particular interest, CNS vasculitis has indeed been described in patients infected with hepatitis C virus (HCV) with or without clinical cryoglobulinemia or polyarteritis nodosa (55,56). Furthermore, the hepatitis C

Table 4 Conditions Associated with Secondary CNS Vasculitis and Their Treatment

Condition	Treatment
Infections	Appropriate antimicrobial agent
Viruses (HIV, cytomegalovirus, varicella-zoster, hepatitis C, others)	Adjunctive role of immunosuppressive therapy is unclear
Syphilis	
Neisseria meningitidis and *Neisseria gonorrhoeae*	
Bacterial endocarditis	
Borrelia burgdorferi	
Bartonella	
Tuberculosis	
Fungi (*Aspergillus, Histoplasma, Coccidioides,* chronic mucocutaneous candidiasis, others)	
Rickettsiae (Rocky Mountain spotted fever, typhus, others)	
Neuro-cysticercosis	
Drugs	Withdrawal of the drug
Cocaine	Calcium channel blockers and limited
Heroin	course of steroids
Amphetamines	Cytotoxic drugs in pathological cases
Ephedrine	
Phenylpropanolamine	
Other sympathomimetic drugs	
Lymphoproliferative diseases	Combination chemotherapy ± irradia-
Hodgkin's lymphoma	tion
Non-Hodgkin's lymphoma	
Angioimmunolymphoproliferative lesions (AIL)	
Systemic vasculitides	Steroids ± cytotoxic agents
Polyarteritis nodosa	
Behçet's syndrome	
Wegener's granulomatosis	
Churg–Strauss syndrome	
Others	
Connective tissue diseases	Steroids ± cytotoxic agents
Systemic lupus erythematosus	
Sjögren's syndrome	
Rheumatoid arthritis	
Others	

virus was found in the cerebrospinal fluid of a patient with recurrent papillitis and vasculitis of the anterior spinal artery suggesting a potentially direct pathogenic role for HCV in CNS vasculitis (57). Other organisms of interest include cysticerci. In a recent report from Mexico, angiographic evidence of CNS vasculitis was found in 15 out of 28 patients with subarachnoid cysticercosis (53%); 12 of the 15 presented with a stroke syndrome (58).

Evaluating patients with HIV infection for possible CNS vasculitis is particularly challenging. An array of CNS vascular diseases, both inflammatory and noninflammatory, have been associated with HIV infection. In a pathological analysis of the CNS from 100 cases of acquired immunodeficiency syndrome (AIDS), pathological changes were detected in 87 cases (87%) (59). Encephalitis, leptomeningitis, and/or vasculitis were described in 35 cases (35%) and were typically associated with vacuolar myelopathy and/or leukoencephalopathy. Opportunistic CNS infections, however, accounted for the majority of brain pathology (59 cases; 59%). Lymphoproliferative disease was present in 10 cases (10%). Drug abuse may have contributed to CNS vasculopathy in several cases. Of most interest, the coexistence of multiple pathological processes in the same brain was characteristic in this series. This illustrates the complexity of ascertaining the relationship between HIV infection and CNS vasculitis.

The clinical outcome of infection-associated CNS vasculitis is variable even when appropriate antimicrobial drugs are given. This reflects the diverse pathophysiological mechanisms involved including a direct cytopathic effect of an angioinvasive pathogen, injury to endothelial cells via induction of neoantigen formation or immune complex–mediated damage (60). Adjunctive antiinflammatory or immunosuppressive therapy may be beneficial in patients who do not respond to antimicrobial therapy, although such an approach remains to be tested.

B. Drugs

A variety of drugs, particularly those with sympathomimetic properties, have been associated with a myriad of neurological complications, including cerebral infarcts, intracerebral bleeding, and subarachnoid hemorrhage. Most commonly implicated drugs are oral and intravenous amphetamines, cocaine, heroin, ephedrine, and phenylpropanolamine (see Table 4). Of note, most reported cases of "drug-induced CNS vasculitis" have been diagnosed on the basis of cerebral angiography alone, in the absence of pathological confirmation (1,53). Since the implicated drugs are capable of inducing vasospasm, some of the cases may have represented CNS angiopathy rather than true angiitis. Indeed, CNS vasculitis was absent in a series of 14 autopsy cases of cocaine-related cerebrovascular disease (61). In another series, cocaine administration induced dose-related cerebrovascular vasoconstriction on magnetic resonance angiograms mimicking the appearance of CNS angiitis (60). Ascertaining the relationship between a particular drug exposure and CNS vasculitis is further complicated by numerous other pitfalls (Table 5). Nonetheless, pathologically documented cases of drug-associated CNS vasculitis do exist, with findings ranging from perivascular cuffing to frank vasculitis with or without necrosis (63–65).

Recognizing and withdrawing the offending drug is obviously the cornerstone of treatment. For drugs of abuse, the risk profile dictates the need to also rule out possible associated infections. When present, hypertension should be effectively controlled. For most angiographically defined

Table 5 Pitfalls in the Approach to Drug-Associated CNS Vasculitis

Problems with definition of CNS vasculitis
   Diagnosis made on the basis of angiography alone
   Misinterpretation of pathological findings, i.e., false-positive results
Confounding factors
   Exposure to multiple substances
   Contaminants or impurities in substances used
   Coexisting infections, e.g., HIV, syphilis, tuberculosis, hepatitis B or C, endocarditis
   Other risk factors for CNS events, such as hypertension or trauma
Alternative explanations for angiographic appearance
   Vasospasm due to pharmacological effect of the drug
   Malignant hypertension
   Subarachnoid hemorrhage
   Cerebral emboli
   Vasculitis

cases, we recommend the use of calcium channel blockers and a limited course of corticosteroids. The use of long-term steroid therapy and/or the addition of cytotoxic drugs should be reserved to pathologically documented cases of CNS arteritis.

C. Lymphoproliferative Diseases

Vasculitis of the CNS has been reported in association with Hodgkin's lymphoma, non-Hodgkin's lymphoma, and angioimmunolymphoproliferative lesions (AIL) (1). Of note, the anatomical location of the lymphoproliferative disease may be outside or within the CNS. Although the clinical presentation is generally similar to that of PACNS, mass lesions, spinal cord involvement, and CNS hemorrhage should raise the index of suspicion for an underlying lymphoproliferative disease (1,28). It is important to realize that a biopsy of the CNS lesion(s) and/or mass may only reveal the angiitis without evidence of the malignancy itself. On the other hand, a lymphocytic angiitis may itself be the malignant lesion of AIL, a diagnosis that can be established by detailed immunohistochemistry, T-cell receptor analysis, and B-cell immunoglobulin studies. Finally, one should also ascertain for concomitant infections, particularly with varicella zoster virus.

Treatment is generally directed at the underlying lymphoproliferative disease, be it within or outside the CNS. This generally consists of combination chemotherapy and/or irradiation. Favorable neurological outcomes have been anecdotally reported (66,67).

D. Systemic Vasculitides

Vasculitis of the CNS may occur with any of the systemic vasculitides, but is most commonly reported in polyarteritis nodosa (PAN), microscopic polyangiitis (MPA), Behçet's disease, Wegener's granulomatosis (WG), and Churg–Strauss syndrome (1,68–72). Giant cell arteritis has been associated with cerebral amyloid angiopathy and, on rare occasions, granulomatous CNS arteritis (41,71). The true prevalence of CNS arteritis in systemic vasculitides is difficult to estimate since the diagnosis is most often presumed on clinical grounds when neurological events occur in the setting of systemic disease (i.e., angiographic and/or premortem). Pathological evidence of CNS vasculitis is rarely sought. Alternative explanations for CNS dysfunction should be considered in patients with systemic vasculitis including infections (CNS and systemic), drug toxicities (e.g., steroid-induced CNS effects, cyclophosphamide-induced hyponatremia), metabolic factors (e.g., hypoxic or uremic encephalopathy), and accelerated hypertension (1).

Treatment of CNS disease is generally directed at the underlying systemic vasculitis and generally consists of high-dose corticosteroids. The use of cytotoxic drugs, particularly cyclophosphamide, appears necessary in MPA and WG as well as other systemic vasculitides that threaten life or risk permanent CNS damage (49).

E. Connective Tissue Diseases

Central nervous system involvement is not uncommon in connective tissue diseases, mainly systemic lupus erythematosus (SLE) and Sjögren's syndrome (SS). In SLE, brain pathology most often represents a vasculopathy, with small-vessel hyalinization, thickening, intramural platelet deposition, and thrombus formation (73). Frank CNS vasculitis occurs in less than 7% of cases (73). When SLE patients present with CNS symptoms and signs, it is important to consider mechanisms other than CNS vasculitis. Such mechanisms include antiphospholipid antibody–associated thrombosis, cardiac emboli, thrombotic thrombocytopenic purpura, CNS hemorrhage related to immune thrombocytopenia or acquired coagulation factor deficiency, CNS infections, and side effects of medications. Treatment of CNS vasculitis in SLE generally consists of high-dose intravenous corticosteroids as well as cyclophosphamide in critically ill or progressively deteriorating patients.

In Sjögren's syndrome, CNS manifestations may be caused by a mononuclear inflammatory vasculopathy involving the small vessels of the cortex and meninges (74). Angiographic abnormalities consistent with vasculitis are uncommonly seen. Treatment issues remain unresolved. We would recommend a similar therapeutic approach to patients with CNS disease secondary to SLE.

VI. MISCELLANEOUS CONDITIONS

A variety of other disorders are capable of mimicking the clinical and/or angiographic picture of CNS vasculitis while others are associated with true CNS arteritis (see Table 1) (2). The antiphospholipid antibody (APLA) syndrome is of particular interest since it is clearly associated with CNS ischemic events related to thrombosis. In one study, 74% of patients with the APLA syndrome and ischemic cerebrovascular events had angiographic abnormalities, the majority of which were arterial (75). The abnormalities were solely intracranial in 59%, solely extracranial in 35%, and mixed in 6%. Of patients with intracranial abnormalities, 60% were solitary stem or branch occlusions of the cerebral or basilar arteries while 40% were "suggestive of" vasculitis. This is potentially misleading since the occurrence of true histological vasculitis in the APLA syndrome is distinctly unusual. Treatment consists of anticoagulation rather than immunosuppression.

Radiation and, in particular, excessive irradiation have been associated with CNS vasculitis (76). In one series, in four of eight patients who received excessive irradiation due to a malfunctioning linear electron accelerator, myelopathy due to an obliterative vasculitis was present in all four autopsies performed (76). Of note, MRI of the spine was normal in the acute phase of spinal cord injury in all patients. In a rat pial window model, single high doses of radiation caused an increase in leukocyte/endothelial cell interactions and a decrease or loss of arteriolar flow in the cerebral vasculature, perhaps explaining the radiation vasculitis described in humans (77).

Additional conditions recently reported in association with CNS vasculitis include cerebral amyloid angiopathy (78), Goodpasture's syndrome (79), IgA deficiency (80), and inflammatory bowel disease (81).

REFERENCES

1. Calabrese LH, Duna GF, Lie JT. Vasculitis in the central nervous system. Arthritis Rheum 1997; 40:1189–1201.
2. Calabrese LH. Vasculitis of the central nervous system. Rheum Dis Clin North Am 1995; 21:1059–1076.
3. Calabrese LH, Mallek JA. Primary angiitis of the central nervous system: Report of eight new cases, review of the literature and proposal for diagnostic criteria. Medicine 1988; 67:20–40.
4. Hankey GJ. Isolated angiitis/angiopathy of the central nervous system. Cerebrovasc Dis 1991; 1:2–15.
5. Calabrese L, Gragg LA, Furlan AJ. Benign angiopathy: A distinct subset of angiographically defined primary angiitis of the central nervous system. J Rheumatol 1993; 20:2046–2050.
6. Calabrese LH, Furlan AJ, Gragg LA, et al. Primary angiitis of the central nervous system: Diagnostic criteria and clinical approach. Cleve Clin J Med 1992; 59:293–306.
7. Cupps TR, Moore PM, Fauci AS. Isolated angiitis of the central nervous system. Am J Med 1983; 74: 97–106.

8. Cravioto M, Feigin I. Noninfectious granulomatous angiitis with a predilection for the nervous system. Neurology 1959; 9:599.
9. Younger DS, Hays AP, Burst JCM, et al. Granulomatous angiitis of brain: An inflammatory reaction of diverse etiology. Arch Neurol 1988; 45:514.
10. Younger DS, Calabrese LH, Hays AP. Granulomatous angiitis of the nervous system. Neurol Clin 1997; 15:821–834.
11. Moore PM. Vasculitis of the central nervous system. Semin Neurol 1994; 14:307–312.
12. Rosenbaum JT, Roman-Goldstein S, Lindquist GR, Rosenbaum RB. Uveitis and central nervous system vasculitis. J Rheum 1998; 25:593.
13. Scolding NJ, Jayne DRW, Zajicek JP, Meyer PAR, Wraight EP, Lookwood CM. Cerebral vasculitis: Recognition, diagnosis and management. Q J Med 1997; 90:61.
14. Gripshover BM, Ellner JJ. Chronic meningitis. In: Mandell GL, Bennett JE, Dolin R, eds. Principles and Practice of Infectious Diseases. 4th ed. Philadelphia: Churchill Livingstone, 1998.
15. Gilden DH, Kleinschmidt-DeMasters BK, Wellish M, Headley-Whyte ET, Reintier B, Mahalingam R. Varicella zoster virus: A cause of waning and waning vasculitis. Neurol 1996; 47:1441.
16. Nishikawa M, Sakamoto H, Katsuyama J, Hakuba A, Nishimura S. Multiple appearing and vanishing aneurysms: Primary angiitis of the central nervous system. J Neurosurg 1998; 88:133.
17. Duna G, Calabrese L. Limitations in the diagnostic modalities in the diagnosis of primary angiitis of the central nervous system (PACNS). J Rheumatol 1995; 22:662.
18. Alhalabi M, Moore PM. Serial angiography in isolated angiitis of the central nervous system. Neurology 1994; 44:1221.
19. Greenan TJ, Grossman RI, Goldberg HI. Cerebral vasculitis: MR imaging and angiographic correlation. Radiology 1992; 182:65.
20. Pierot L, Chiras J, Debussche-Depriester C, Dormond D, Bories J. Intracerebral stenosing arteriopathies: Contribution of three radiological techniques to the diagnosis. J Neuroradiol 1991; 18:32.
21. Hurst RW, Grossman RI. Neuroradiology of central nervous system vasculitis. Semin Neurol 1994; 14:320–340.
22. Finelli PF, Onyuike HC, Ophoff DF. Idiopathic granulomatous angiitis of the CNS manifesting as diffuse white matter disease. Neurol 1997; 491:1696.
23. Stone JH, Pomper MG, Roubenoff R, Miller TJ, Hellman DB. Sensitivities of noninvasive tests for central nervous system vasculitis: A comparison of lumbar puncture, computed tomography, and magnetic resonance imaging. J Rheumatol 1994; 21:1277.
24. Cloft HJ, Phillips CD, Dix JE, McNulty BC, Zagardo MT, Kallmes DF. Correlation of angiography and MR imaging in cerebral vasculitis. Acta Radiol 1999; 40:83.
25. Parisi JE, Moore PM. The role of biopsy in vasculitis of the central nervous system. Semin Neurol 1994; 14:341.
26. Cheng TM, O'Neill BP, Schecthauer BW, Piepgras DG. Chronic meningitis: The role of meningeal or cortical biopsy. Neurosurgery 1994; 34:S90.
27. Whiting DM, Barnett GH, Estes ML, Sila CA, Rudick RA, Hassenbusch SJ, Lanzieri. Stereotactic biopsy of non-neoplastic lesions in adults. Cleve Clin J Med 1992; 59:48.
28. Duna GF, George T, Rybicki L, Calabrese LH. Primary angiitis of the central nervous system: An analysis of unusual presentations (abstr). Arthritis Rheum 1995; 38(suppl 9):S340.
29. Rhodes RH, Madelaire C, Petrelli M, Cole M, Karamen BA. Primary angiitis and angiopathy of the central nervous system and their relationship to giant cell arteritis. Arch Pathol Lab Med 1995; 119:334.
30. Fallis RJ, Fischer M. Cerebral vasculitis and hemorrhage associated with phenylpropanolamine. Neurology 1985; 35:405–407.
31. Lake CR, Gallant, Masson E, et al. Adverse drug effects attributed to phenylpropanolamine: A review of 142 cases. Am J Med 1990; 89:195–208.
32. Razavi M, Bendixon B, Maley JE et al. CNS pseudovasculitis in a patient with pheochromocytoma. Neurol 1999; 52:1088.
33. Kapoor R, Kendall, Harrison MJG. Persistent segmental cerebral artery constriction in coital cephalgia. J Neurol Neurosurg Psychiat 1990; 53:266–270.

34. Call GK, Fleming MC, Sealfon S, Levine H, Kistler JP Fisher CM. Reversible cerebral segmental vasoconstriction. Stroke 1988; 19:1159.
35. Bogousslavsky U, Despland PA, Regli F, Dubuis PY. Postpartum cerebral angiopathy: Reversible vasoconstriction assessed by transcranial doppler ultrasounds. Eur Neurol 1989; 29:102.
36. Rascol A, Guitraud B, Manelfe C, et al. Accidents vasculaires cerebraux de a grosses et du post partum. In: La Conference de la Salpetriere sur les Maladies Vasculaires Cerebrales. Balliere, 1980:84.
37. Rass EC, Galetta SL, Broderick M, Atlas SW. Delayed peripartum vasculopathy: Cerebral eclampsia revisited. Ann Neurol 1993; 33:222.
38. Villa Forte A, Vassilopoulos D, Calabrese LH. What is not primary angiitis of the CNS (PACNS) (abstr). 1998; 41:S124.
39. Giovanini MA, Eskin TA, Mukherji SK, Mickle JP. Granulomatous angiitis of the spinal cord: A case report. Neurosugery 1994; 34:540–542.
40. Fountain NB, Eberhard DA. Primary angiitis of the CNS associated with amyloid angiopathy: Report of two cases and review of the literature. Neurology 1996; 46:190.
41. Anders KH, Wang ZZ, Kornfeld M, et al. Giant cell arteritis with cerebral amyloid angiopathy: Immunohistochemical and molecular studies. Hum Pathol 1997; 28:1237.
42. Sigal LH. The neurologic presentation of vasculitis and rheumatologic syndromes. A review. Medicine 1987; 66:157.
43. Martin JR, Mitchell WJ, Henken DB. Neurotropic herpes viruses, neural mechanisms and arteritis. Brain Pathol 1990; 1:6.
44. MacKenzie RA, Forbes GS, Karnes WE. Angiographic findings in herpes zoster arteritis. Ann Neurol 1981; 10:458.
45. Doyle PW, Gibson G, Dolman CL. Herpes zoster ophthalmicus with contralateral hemiplegia: Identification of cause. Ann Neurol 1983; 14:84.
46. Linneman C, Alvira M. Pathogenesis of Varicella-Zoster angiitis of the CNS. Arch Neurol 1980; 37:239.
47. Haaanapa M, Dastidar P, Weinberg A, Levin M, Meittenin A, Lapinlampli A, Laippala P, Nurmikko T. CSF and MRI findings in patients with acute herpes zoster. Neurol 1998; 51:1405.
48. Chu C, Gray L, Goldstein LB, Huylette CM. Diagnosis of intracranial vasculitis: A multidisciplinary approach. J Neuropathol Exp Neurol 1998; 57:30.
49. Calabrese LH. Therapy of systemic vasculitis. Neurol Clin 1997; 15:973.
50. Chyatte O, Sundt TM. Response of chronic experimental vasospasm to methylprednisolone and dexamethasone. J Neurosurg 1984; 60:923.
51. Abu-Shakra M, Kraishi M, Grosman H, et al. Primary angiitis of the CNS diagnosed by angiography. Q J Med 1995; 87:151–158.
52. Crane R, Kerr L, Spura H. Clinical analysis of isolated angiitis of the CNS: Report of 11 cases. Arch Intern Med 1991; 151:2290–2294.
53. Calabrese LH, Duna GT. Drug induced vasculitis. Curr Opin Rheum 1996; 8:34.
54. Grang DW. Central nervous system vasculitis secondary to infections, toxins and neoplasms. Semin Neurol 1994; 14:313.
55. Origgi L, Vanoli M, Carbone A, Grasso M, Scorza R. Central nervous system involvement in patients with HCV-related cryoglobulinemia. Am J Med Sci 1998; 315:208.
56. Petty GW, Duffy J, Houston J III. Cerebral ischemia in patients with hepatitis C virus infection and mixed cryoglobulinemia. Mayo Clin Proc 1996; 71:671.
57. Propst T, Propst A, Nachbauer K, Gradziadei I, Willeit H, Margreiter R, Vogel W. Papillitis and vasculitis of the arteria spinalis anterior as complications of hepatitis C reinfection after liver transplantation. Transplant Int 1997; 10:234–237.
58. Barinagarrementeria F, Cantu C. Frequency of cerebral arteritis in subarachnoid cysticercosis: An angiographic study. Stroke 1998; 29:123–125.
59. Mossakowski MJ, Zelman IB. Neuropathological syndromes in the course of full blown acquired immune deficiency syndrome (AIDS) in adults in Poland (1987–1995). Folia Neuropathol 1997; 35:133.
60. Jenette JP, Falk RJ, Milling DM. Pathogenesis of vasculitis. Semin Neurol 1994; 14:291.
61. Aggarwal SK, Williams V, Levine SR, Cassin BJ, Garcia JH. Cocaine-associated intracranial hemorrhage: Absence of vasculitis in 14 cases. Neurology 1996; 46:1741.

62. Kaufman MJ, Levin JM, Ross MH, Lange N, Rose SL, Kukes TJ, Mendelson JH, Lukas SE, Cohen BM, Renshaw PF. Cocaine-induced cerebral vasoconstriction detected in humans with magnetic resonance angiography. JAMA 1998; 279:376.

63. Citron BP, Halpern M, McCarron M, Lundberg GD, McCormick R, Pincus IJ, Tatter D, Haverback BJ. Necrotizing angiitis associated with drug abuse. N Engl J Med 1970; 283:1003.

64. Fredericks RK, Lefkowitz DS, Challa CR, Troost BT. Cerebral vasculitis associated with cocaine abuse. Stroke 1991; 22:1437.

65. Morrow PL, McQuillen JB. Cerebral vasculitis associated with cocaine abuse. J Forensic Sci 1993; 38:732.

66. Kleinschmidt-DeMasters GK, Filley CM, Bitter MA. Central nervous system angiocentric, angiodestructive T-cell lymphoma. Surg Neurol 1992; 37:130.

67. Greco FA, Kolins J, Rajjoub RK, Brereton HD. Hodgkin's disease and granulomatous angiitis of the central nervous system. Cancer 1976; 38:2027.

68. Moore P, Calabrese LH. Neurologic manifestations of systemic vasculitides. Semin Neurol 1994; 14:300.

69. Nishino H, Rubino FA, DeRemee RA, Swanson JW, Parisi JE. Neurological involvement in Wegener's granulomatosis: An analysis of 324 consecutive patients at the Mayo Clinic. Ann Neurol 1993; 33:4.

70. Tervaert JWC, Kallenberg C. Neurologic manifestations of systemic vasculitides. Rheum Dis Clin North Am 1993; 19:913.

71. Galetta SL, Balcer LJ, Lieberman AP, Syed NA, Lee JM, Oberholtzer JC. Refractory giant cell arteritis with spinal cord infarction. Neurology 1997; 49:1720.

72. Spranger M, Schwab S, Meinck HM, Tischendorf M, Sis J, Breitbart A, Andrassy K. Meningeal involvement in Wegener's granulomatosis cerebrospinal fluid. Neurology 1997; 48:263.

73. Ellis SG, Verity MA. Central nervous system involvement in systemic lupus erythematosus: A review of neuropathologic findings in 57 cases. Semin Arthritis Rheum 1979; 8:212.

74. Alexander EL. Neurologic disease in Sjögren's syndrome: Mononuclear inflammatory vasculopathy affecting the central/peripheral nervous immunopathogenesis. Rheum Dis Clin North Am 1993; 19: 869.

75. Provenzale JM, Barboriak DP, Allen NB, Ortel TL. Antiphospholipid antibodies: Findings at arteriography. Am J Neuroradiol 1998; 19:611.

76. Alfonso ER, De Gregorio MA, Mateo P, Esco R, Bascon N, Morales F, Bellosta R. Radiation myelopathy in over-irradiated patients: MR imaging findings. Eur Radiol 1997; 7:400.

77. Acker JC, Marks LB, Spencer DP, Yang W, Avery MA, Dodge RK, Rosner GL, Dewhirst MW. Serial in vivo observations of cerebral vasculature after treatment with a large single fraction of radiation. Radiat Res 1998; 149:350.

78. Yamada M, Itoh Y, Shintaku M, Kawamura J, Jensson O, Thorsteinsson L, Suematsu N, Matsushita M, Otomo E. Immune reactions associated with cerebral amyloid angiopathy. Stroke 1996; 27:1155.

79. Rydel JJ, Rodby RA. An 18-year-old man with Goodpasture's syndrome and ANCA-negative central nervous system vasculitis. Am J Kidney Dis 1998; 31:345.

80. Liu MF, Li JS, Tsao CJ, Huang JJ, Lee EJ, Tsai YC, Su IJ. Selective IgA deficiency with recurrent vasculitis of the central nervous system. Clin Exp Rheumatol 1998; 16:77.

81. Masaki T, Muto T, Shinozaki M, Kuroda T. Unusual cerebral complication associated with ulcerative colitis. J Gastroenterol 1997; 32:251.

36

Cutaneous Vasculitis and Its Relationship to Systemic Disease

Jeffrey P. Callen
University of Louisville, Louisville, Kentucky

I. INTRODUCTION

The skin is an organ that is well supplied with vasculature and frequently develops manifestations of vasculitis. Often, the skin may be the initial organ affected and, at times, may seem to be the only organ affected (1–3). However, except in some rare disorders, the skin is reflective of a systemic process. The vessels that are affected in the skin are most often small vessels, frequently the postcapillary venule, but vessels of larger size may also be affected. The size of the affected vessel correlates at least in part with the syndrome that affects the patient.

II. DEFINITION

Leukocytoclastic vasculitis (LCV) is a term that refers to the changes observed on light microscopic examination of a biopsy specimen. The features observed include infiltration of the vessel wall by polymorphonuclear neutrophils, deposition of fibrin (fibrinoid necrosis of the vessel wall), fibrin thrombi within the vessels, and disruption of the neutrophils with the presence of nuclear dust in the surrounding tissue (leukocytoclasis). The pathological process is not specific and may be observed in nonvasculitic conditions, including neutrophilic dermatoses such as acute febrile neutrophilic dermatosis (Sweet's syndrome), Behçet's disease, pyoderma gangrenosum, and even insect bites. As lesions age, the histopathological features change from a neutrophil-rich infiltrate to a lymphocyte-rich process (4). Thus, timing of the biopsy is critical in order to appropriately diagnose the process.

III. CLASSIFICATION

The purpose of any system of classification is to be able to predict the prognosis of the patient. From this prediction, the need and aggressiveness of therapy can be assessed. Unfortunately, there is no existing system that functions adequately. The classification of vasculitis is controversial. Zeek (5) suggested a scheme in 1950 that bases its subclasses on size of vessel involved vs. type of infiltrate vs. associated conditions. In 1976, Gilliam and Smiley (6) proposed a revision of this classification scheme by subdividing Zeek's existing categories. Recently, Lotti et al. (2) proposed that vasculitis be classified as either a small-vessel cutaneous vasculitis or as a large-vessel necrotizing vasculitis. The small-vessel category may be subdivided into some of the following: idiopathic hypersensitivity vasculitis, Henoch–Schönlein purpura, essential mixed cryoglobulinemia, Waldenstrom's macroglobulinemia, urticarial vasculitis, vasculitis associated with collagen vascular diseases such as lupus erythematosus or rheumatoid arthritis, and erythema elevatum diutinum. The large-vessel category may be divided into polyarteritis nodosa, granulomatous vasculitis (Wegener's granulomatosis, allergic granulomatosis of Churg–Strauss), vasculitis associated with collagen vascular diseases, and giant cell arteritis. Unfortunately, this proposed system is also problematic because it is well recognized that when vasculitis affects the skin in patients with Wegener's granulomatosis, the vessels involved are usually small. Thus, in the patient who presents with palpable purpura and a biopsy that confirms LCV, the differential diagnosis involves syndromes that may be within either category. Other systems that have recently been proposed by the American College of Rheumatology (ACR) (7) and the Chapel Hill Consensus Conference (8) also have inherent problems.

IV. CUTANEOUS LESIONS OF VASCULITIS

Sams et al. (9) recognized that the lesions of vasculitis are dynamic. Clinically the lesions are often polymorphic, yet at some stage the classic lesions become purpuric and palpable. This dynamic nature of the lesions clinically is also reflected histologically by a shift in the character of the infiltrate as documented by Zax et al. (4). In the early stage of development, the clinical lesions may be urticarial or macular purpura. Later in the process, there may be blistering, necrosis, or ulceration. These types of lesions most often reflect involvement of the small vessels, most often the postcapillary venule. When the larger dermal vessels are involved, the cutaneous manifestation is more likely to be livedo reticularis or nodule formation, and ulceration and necrosis are probably more frequent in these patients than in those with small-vessel involvement.

The characteristic cutaneous lesion observed in patients with leukocytoclastic vasculitis is palpable purpura (Fig. 1). This lesion varies from bright red to purple. The lesions have an in-

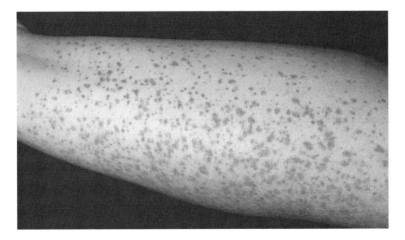

Figure 1   Palpable purpura of hypersensitivity vasculitis.

flammatory component and thus are papular, as opposed to lesions of thrombocytopenia or capillaritis, which are macular. The lesions vary in size from less than a millimeter to several centimeters. The lesions more frequently occur on the dependent surfaces, but may occur anywhere on the body. As the lesions resolve, a residual purpura may be present, but unless ulceration or necrosis occurs, the lesions resolve without scar formation. Piette and Stone (10) have observed that careful analysis of the shape of the purpuric lesions will aid in the differential diagnosis. They have suggested that when there are angulated lesions, so-called retiform purpura, the process is more likely to involve immunoglobulin A (IgA) in its pathogenesis. The lesions of palpable purpura are those that occur in patients with hypersensitivity vasculitis, Henoch-Schönlein purpura, or essential mixed cryoglobulinemia. However, similar lesions may occur in patients with embolic phenomena (such as bacterial endocarditis, left atrial myxoma, or atheromatous emboli) or other neutrophilic dermatoses.

Urticarial lesions (Fig. 2) may be a manifestation of leukocytoclastic vasculitis, and the term urticarial vasculitis (UV) is commonly used (11). The patient with this type of lesion generally has chronic disease. The lesions differ from those observed in "routine" urticaria. They tend to be more long-lasting; often individual lesions are present for over 24 h, whereas in routine urticaria the lesions are transient usually resolving within 2 to 4 h. Urticarial vasculitis lesions also tend to resolve with residual echymosis or dyspigmentation as opposed to routine urticaria in which there is no residual. Patients with UV often complain of burning or pain, rather than pruritus. Patients with UV often have accompanying systemic disease, in particular systemic lupus erythematosus (12). Patients with UV also can be subdivided into those with hypocomplementia and those with normal complement levels. Hypocomplementemic UV is quite rare, and is often complicated by chronic obstructive pulmonary disease (13). There is a middle ground between UV and routine urticaria, which Winkelmann et al. (14) termed neutrophilic urticaria (NU). More persistent lesions characterize NU, but systemic involvement is not present, and although there are neutrophils in and around the vessel walls, they do not cause disruption of the vessels. These patients also have a chronic course.

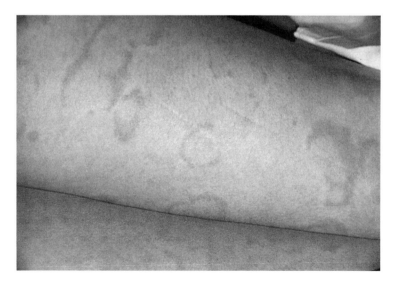

Figure 2 Urticarial lesions of vasculitis. These lesions lasted for over 24 h.

V. WHEN THE DIAGNOSIS OF LCV IS MADE, WHAT IS THE DIFFERENTIAL DIAGNOSIS?

Palpable purpura is the hallmark of cutaneous vasculitis; however, the purpura may not always be clearly palpable. Purpura may also occur as a manifestation of capillaritis, a process of mild inflammation that is rarely associated with internal disorders and does not have associated systemic involvement. Generally, the physical examination and histological evaluation will separate these patients. Purpura may occur with noninflammatory vasculopathy including cryoglobulinemia, antiphospholipid antibody syndrome, or other paraproteins. Cryoglobulinemia may cause both inflammatory and noninflammatory lesions. The clinical lesions may be difficult to separate, but the histopathology will reveal a proteinaceous material within the vessel lumen. Emboli from a left atrial myxoma, bacterial or fungal endocarditis, atheromatous plaques, or the valvular vegetations of patients with the antiphospholipid antibody syndrome may result in lesions that simulate cutaneous vasculitis. Often, these phenomena may be suggested by the presence of symptoms. In addition to palpable purpura, the patients often have reticulated lesions or may have ischemic changes of one or more digits (e.g., a blue toe). Calciphylaxis due to calcium imbalance, most often occurring in patients with renal failure, may present with purpura, but livedo reticularis with or without necrosis is more common.

Leg ulceration is commonly associated with involvement of the cutaneous vasculature. Leg ulceration may occur with palpable purpura and/or livedo reticularis or may be an isolated finding. The patient with purpura or livedo reticularis may have noninflammatory involvement similar to that listed above. Isolated leg ulceration may occur in pyoderma gangrenosum. Biopsy of lesions of pyoderma gangrenosum characteristically lack vessel wall damage; however, some vessel involvement may be present in almost any ulceration regardless of its cause.

Urticarial vasculitis must be differentiated from routine urticaria, erythema multiforme, and insect bites. Clinical examination and historical information are useful, but often a biopsy is necessary. The clinician should communicate with the pathologist and let the pathologist know how strongly vasculitis is being considered, because it appears to me that pathologists often overread biopsies sent to them with the clinical impression "urticarial vasculitis or rule-out urticarial vasculitis." These suggestions often lead to an interpretation that results in the prediction of a poor prognosis, when in fact the patient has chronic urticaria and has no evidence of internal disease.

VI. HYPERSENSITIVITY VASCULITIS

The concept of a separate entity, known as hypersensitivity vasculitis (HSV), dates back to the work of Zeek (5). This concept was furthered by the classification system developed by the American College of Rheumatology (7). Many of these patients develop their disease shortly after the administration or ingestion of a drug or other foreign antigen. Almost any drug can cause a small-vessel vasculitis (HSV), but the more common ones are antibiotics, nonsteroidal antiinflammatory agents, diuretics, and anticonvulsants. Recently, several cases of HSV have been reported with antithyroid drugs, in particular propylthiouracil. These patients are frequently perinuclear antineutrophil cytoplasmic antibody (pANCA)–positive (15). In addition to drugs, foods and food additives may in some individuals be responsible for the reaction (16). Unfortunately, there are patients with small-vessel vasculitis that is not associated with any other condition, in which the causative agent cannot be determined. In addition, small-vessel vasculitis may be part of the process of other vasculitides, such as Wegener's granulomatosis, Henoch–Schönlein purpura, and other processes listed below as associated conditions. It therefore is often difficult, if not impossible, to clearly classify a patient as having HSV without a clear, identifiable causative agent.

Many patients with HSV manifest disease primarily in their skin and do not have identifiable internal organ involvement (17). However, there are individuals who will manifest internal involvement similar to Henoch–Schönlein purpura, with nephritis, arthritis, and bowel disease. Thus, all patients suspected of having HSV should have a careful assessment to exclude other vasculitic syndromes and to document the absence of internal organ involvement.

Hypersensitivity vasculitis is generally manifest by the appearance of palpable purpura, most commonly on the lower extremities below the knees. The disease is usually symmetrically distributed, and may be exacerbated by prolonged dependence of the legs. In patients who are bedridden, the disease frequently is manifest on the back or buttocks. Lesions can be present on any surface, including the mucous membranes. Patients are most often asymptomatic, but occasionally may complain of itching, burning, or pain. The purpuric lesions are usually discrete round papules. Piette and Stone (10) have suggested that the presence of a retiform pattern is predictive of IgA-induced small-vessel vasculitis. Others have not confirmed this observation.

The course of HSV is highly variable. The disease duration may range from several days to a year. In patients in whom the cause is identified and removed, the duration of the process is usually less than a month. When systemic involvement is identified, the course is more prolonged and deaths have been reported.

VII. HENOCH–SCHÖNLEIN PURPURA

Schönlein first described a syndrome manifest by acute purpura and arthritis in 1837. In 1874, Henoch noted a similar syndrome that included nephritis and colicky abdominal pain. Subsequently, this syndrome has become known as Henoch–Schonlein purpura (HSP) (18). Zeek (5) did not separate this syndrome from HSV, while Gilliam and Smiley (6) included it within the category of hypersensitivity vasculitis, and the ACR (7) listed it as a distinct entity.

Henoch–Schönlein purpura was initially described in children, but there are adults who have identical features (19). The syndrome includes purpura, nephritis, arthritis, and gastrointestinal involvement. The disease is usually acute in its onset and often follows an upper respiratory tract infection, particularly ones caused by *Streptococcus*. Children are more frequently affected than adults, and the disease is more common in males. The incidence in the population of 2- to 14-year-olds has been estimated to be 14 per 100,000 per year. Also there appears to be a seasonal variation, with more cases appearing during the winter months.

Skin lesions are one of the defining features of HSP. The rash may begin as a macular erythema or urticaria-like lesions, but within a short time period, the eruption becomes purpuric. The lower extremities and buttocks are the most common sites of involvement. Most often the purpura is present at the onset of the process, but in some patients, abdominal pain, arthritis, or both have preceded the eruption. Other vasculitic syndromes, meningococcemia, and Rocky Mountain spotted fever should be considered in the differential diagnosis.

A detailed description of HSP has been provided in Chapter 22. Therefore the noncutaneous features will only be briefly mentioned at this juncture. The most common features and their frequency of occurrence are arthralgias and/or arthritis in 60–90%, gastrointestinal abnormalities in about 50–70%, and glomerulonephritis in 20–100% of patients.

Henoch–Schönlein purpura is associated with IgA immune complexes. However, its diagnosis is not dependent upon the demonstration of IgA in the vessels or kidneys. The ACR classification basically differentiated HSP from HSV mainly upon the age of the patient (8).

VIII. CUTANEOUS SMALL-VESSEL VASCULITIS AS A MANIFESTATION OF ANOTHER PROCESS

A small-vessel vasculitis with features identical to HSV may occur in relationship to a variety of other processes. The clinical manifestations are identical to HSV, and thus most patients with palpable purpura will need to be assessed to be certain that they do not have one of these associations.

Paraneoplastic vasculitis is the term used when there is clear documentation that a neoplasm has caused the process (20). Small-vessel cutaneous vasculitis has been reported with lymphoproliferative disorders as well as some solid tumors. Often, the vasculitis has been the clinical manifestation that led to the discovery of the neoplasm. The frequency of neoplasm in patients with vasculitis is quite low, representing less than 1% of identified etiologies. Associated neoplasms are often lymphoproliferative.

Vasculitides of small and medium-sized vessels, such as Wegener's granulomatosis and Churg–Strauss syndrome, can affect the skin and produce palpable purpura, which is characterized by a leukocytoclastic vasculitis histopathologically (21). Therefore, in patients who present with small-vessel vasculitis, one must still consider the possibility that it is a manifestation of a more severe syndrome.

Systemic autoimmune disorders, particularly lupus erythematosus, rheumatoid arthritis, and Sjögren's syndrome may be associated with a vasculitis. At times, the vasculitis is a small-vessel vasculitis, although these conditions may also be associated with larger-vessel involvement (see Chapter 44).

Paraproteinemia may be associated with vasculitis. Hepatitis C viral infection is often associated with essential mixed cryoglobulinemia. These patients may present with palpable purpura or with macular purpura. Many of the patients with palpable purpura will have leukocytoclastic vasculitis on biopsy, while some will have proteinaceous intraluminal plugging. The course of the vasculitis may parallel that of the hepatitis. Some studies have demonstrated that the level of cryoglobulinemia decreases with interferon therapy (22), and in addition, some patients treated with ribavirin have achieved control of their cutaneous disease (23). The prevalence of hepatitis C in patients with small-vessel vasculitis may be as high as 20% (24), and thus this simple serological test has become part of the routine evaluation of patients who do not have a readily identifiable cause for their disease.

In addition to hepatitis C–associated cryoglobulinemia, other paraproteinemias may be associated with small-vessel cutaneous vasculitis. Hyperglobulinemic purpura was described by Waldenstrom in 1943, and consisted of recurrent bouts of purpura, hyperglobulinemia, mild anemia, and an elevated sedimentation rate (25). This entity may be a primary process or may be part of another syndrome, particularly systemic lupus erythematosus, Sjögren's syndrome, rheumatoid arthritis, thymoma, thyroiditis, sarcoidosis, or myeloma. The histopathology of this syndrome may be a leukocytoclastic vasculitis or a mononuclear perivascular infiltrate with or without proteinaceous plugging.

Schnitzler et al. described a syndrome characterized by chronic urticaria, fever, an elevated sedimentation rate, a monoclonal IgM paraprotein (usually kappa), and urinary Bence Jones protein (26). These patients may also have bone pain and anemia. The histopathology reveals a leukocytoclastic vasculitis.

Disorders associated with immune complexes, such as inflammatory bowel disease, sarcoidosis, cystic fibrosis, deficiency of the second component of complement, or collagen vascular diseases, may have an accompanying small-vessel vasculitis.

IX. URTICARIAL VASCULITIS

Urticarial vasculitis is characterized clinically by persistent chronic urticarial lesions that often last for more than 24 h and histopathologically by leukocytoclastic vasculitis. McDuffie et al. (27) were the first to describe hypocomplementemic urticarial vasculitis in four patients. The patients had recurrent attacks of erythematous urticarial and hemorrhagic skin lesions with synovitis. Some of the episodes were accompanied by abdominal pain, and two of the patients had glomerulonephritis. Later, Wisnieski et al. (13) recognized that there was a high prevalence of chronic obstructive pulmonary disease among this group of patients. They were able to study only 18 patients among multiple medical centers. In a recent report from the Mayo Clinic, Davis et al. (12) studied 132 patients with urticarial vasculitis, of whom 24 (18%) had hypocomplementemia. Only four of their patients had pulmonary disease. They found a high prevalence of systemic lupus erythematosus in their group (54%).

X. ERYTHEMA ELEVATUM DIUTINUM

Erythema elevatum diutinum is an unusual form of cutaneous vasculitis characterized by persistent erythematous, violaceous, and/or yellow papules, plaques or nodules (28). The lesions tend to occur over bony prominences, are most often on acral or extensor skin surfaces, and are usually symmetrical. Some of these patients will have arthralgias, but other systemic manifestations are absent. Some patients have an IgA paraprotein. Patients with this entity are said to respond well to dapsone.

XI. PATHOGENESIS OF CUTANEOUS VASCULITIS

The pathogenesis of cutaneous vasculitis is more complex than previously suspected. In the mid 1970s it was postulated that the main factor involved was immune complex formation and deposition (9). Different endothelial cell adhesion molecules, including ICAM-1 and -3, VCAM-1, E-selectin, and P-selectin play key roles (2). In addition, inflammatory mediators, neuropeptides, T cells, Langerhans' cells and the fibrinolytic system are all involved in the expression of the disease (29). A full discussion of the proposed mechanisms is beyond the scope of this chapter (see Chapters 1–9).

XII. EVALUATION OF THE PATIENT WITH CUTANEOUS VASCULITIS

The purpose of the evaluation of the patient with cutaneous vasculitis is to identify a cause of the process and assess the presence and severity of systemic involvement. The evaluation begins with a careful history and physical examination, followed by selected testing based upon the acuteness of the process and the findings of the history and physical examination. Blanco et al. (30) have recently proposed an algorithm for evaluation. Their recommended work-up differs for children by not requiring a skin biopsy for "humanitarian" reasons. In adults, they recommend a skin biopsy. For children, the evaluation includes a blood count, sedimentation rate, urinalysis, stool hematest, and biochemistry profile. For adults, they suggest that additional testing include antinuclear antibodies, antineutrophil cytoplasmic antibody, chest x-ray, rheumatoid factor, cryoglobulins, complement levels, hepatitis B surface antigen, and hepatitis C antibody. Subsequent evaluation is directed by additional findings. In children with frequent relapses, suspicion of col-lagen vascular disease, severe vasculitic syndromes, or hepatic involvement, evaluations should be the same as recommended for adults. Adults with persistent fever, abnormal blood smears, risk for HIV infection or severe vasculitis should have cultures, echocardiography, hematological evaluation, human immunodeficiency virus (HIV) testing, and when clinically appropriate, vis-ceral angiography and/or biopsy of involved organs.

XIII. MANAGEMENT OF CUTANEOUS VASCULITIS

Therapy of cutaneous vasculitis depends on whether or not there is clinical or laboratory evidence of internal involvement, the severity of cutaneous disease, and the severity of the systemic dis-ease. Patients with severe systemic necrotizing vasculitis, Wegener's granulomatosis, or poly-arteritis nodosa are generally treated with moderate to high doses of systemic corticosteroids often with addition of a cytotoxic immunosuppressive agent.

Patients with acute cutaneous vasculitis in whom there is an identifiable cause, such as a drug, are treated symptomatically in addition to removing the presumed causative agent. Simi-larly, patients with Henoch–Schönlein purpura usually have self-limiting disease and are often not given specific treatment. Symptomatic measures include rest, elevation, gradient support stockings, and antihistamines.

The challenge is to treat the patient who has chronic cutaneous vasculitis in whom there is no easily identified cause and who does not have significant systemic involvement. There is often a question regarding the need for therapy, since these patients do not have life-threatening dis-ease. However, many of the patients have disease that alters their ability to function normally. Pa-tients may develop small ulcerations that can become secondarily infected or may be painful. Pa-tients may not leave their homes because of psychic distress that the presence of purpura causes. Last, patients with urticarial vasculitis complain of itching and burning of their lesions that may result in sleep disturbance.

Antihistamines have often been suggested as a first line of therapy, based on the observa-tion that histamine may potentiate the deposition of immune complexes in the vessel walls. Pa-tients with palpable purpura rarely benefit from these agents; however, they are the cornerstone of therapy for patients with urticarial vasculitis. I prefer a nonsedating agent in the morning such as loratidine (Claritin) combined with a sedating antihistamine prior to bed such as hydroxizine or doxepin. I will advance the dosage of the evening agent to the maximum tolerated by the pa-tient.

Nonsteroidal antiinflammatory agents have been reported to be beneficial in some patients with vasculitis. Urticarial vasculitis is a subset that may respond to agents such as indomethacin or ibuprofen (12). As yet, there is no information regarding the newer Cox-2 inhibitors.

Pentoxifylline (Trental) has been reported to be useful in some patients. In particular, those patients with evidence of an occlusive vasculopathy, such as livedo vasculitis, may respond.

Dapsone has received some recent attention. It is indicated for the therapy of dermatitis her-petiformis and leprosy. Dermatitis herpetiformis is characterized by a neutrophilic papillitis, and the effect of dapsone is presumably mediated through its effect on the neutrophil. Dapsone is the agent of choice in the rare syndrome of erythema elevatum diutinum (28). In selected patients with cutaneous small-vessel vasculitis, it has been effective in the control of the palpable purpura in doses of 100–200 mg/day. Dapsone may be used with other agents such as pentoxifylline or colchicine (31).

Colchicine has been reported to be effective in open-label trials for cutaneous vasculitis as manifest by palpable purpura or urticarial lesions (32). Its effects in vasculitis may be related to a blockade of disease expression. Colchicine inhibits leukocyte chemotaxis, blocks the release of lysosomal enzymes, inhibits DNA synthesis and cell proliferation, and may inhibit prostaglandins. Of the more than 50 patients that I have treated, colchicine has been effective in about 35, not evaluable in 5, and ineffective in the remaining patients. The only double-blind placebo-controlled trial of colchicine failed to demonstrate a positive benefit; however, the colchicine-treated group included all of the patients who had been previously treated with dapsone and had failed to respond (33). In addition, there were equal numbers of patients with hepatitis C–associated disease in each group. Thus, the study population included patients with more recalcitrant disease and there was an inadvertent bias that occurred during the process of randomization. I continue to utilize colchicine in patients with non–life-threatening disease, beginning with a dose of 0.6 mg twice daily. Effectiveness may be judged within the first 7–14 days of therapy, and if no effect is noted, the therapy may be stopped or dapsone may be added. Long-term therapy is possible without serious toxicity in many patients. In addition to its effect on the skin manifestations, colchicine has been observed to benefit the joint manifestations also. A study of a small number of patients failed to demonstrate any change in the presence of immune complexes following colchicine therapy, suggesting that the mechanism by which it works may be other than by effects on immune complexes. Patients should be monitored with periodic blood counts during long-term therapy. Colchicine probably should not be utilized during pregnancy.

Systemic corticosteroids are effective for leukocytoclastic vasculitis; however, for patients with chronic disease that is localized primarily to the skin, their use should be discouraged and avoided whenever possible. Therefore, I will often utilize a cytotoxic immunosuppressive agent to limit the dosage or eliminate the use of the corticosteroids. Agents such as azathioprine or methotrexate may be utilized in low doses with limited toxicity. Both have been reported to be useful in small open-label case series (34). Other agents such as cyclophosphamide, chlorambucil, or cyclosporin, while they may be useful in systemic vasculitides, have too narrow of a ratio of benefit to toxicity for routine use for patients with cutaneous vasculitis.

REFERENCES

1. Callen JP. Cutaneous vasculitis: Relationship to systemic disease and therapy. Curr Prob Dermatol 1993; 5:45–80.
2. Lotti T, Ghersetich I, Comacchi C, Jorizzo JL. Cutaneous small vessel vasculitis. J Am Acad Dermatol 1998; 39:667–687.
3. Sams WM Jr. Necrotizing vasculitis. J Am Acad Dermatol 1980; 3:1–13.
4. Zax RH, Hodge SJ, Callen JP. Cutaneous leukocytoclastic vasculitis: Serial histopathologic evaluation demonstrates the dynamic nature of the infiltrate. Arch Dermatol 1990; 126:69–72.
5. Zeek PM. Periarteritis nodosa: A critical review. Am J Clin Pathol 1952; 22:777–790.
6. Gilliam JN, Smiley JD. Cutaneous necrotizing vasculitis and related disorders. Ann Allergy 1976; 37:328–339.
7. Hunder GG, Arend WP, Bloch DA, Calabrese LH, Fauci AS, Fries JF, et al. The ACR 1990 criteria for classification of vasculitis. Arthritis Rheum 1990; 33:1065–1136.
8. Jenette JC, Falk RP, Andrassy K, et al. Nomenclature of systemic vasculitides: Proposal of an international consensus conference. Arthritis Rheum 1994; 37:187–192.
9. Sams WM Jr, Thorne EG, Small P, et al. Leukocytoclastic vasculitis. Arch Dermatol 1976; 112:219–226.
10. Piette WW, Stone MS. A cutaneous sign of IgA-associated small dermal vessel leukocytoclastic vasculitis in adults (Henoch-Schönlein purpura). Arch Dermatol 1989; 125:53–56.
11. Soter NA. Chronic urticaria as a manifestation of necrotizing venulitis. N Engl J Med 1977; 296: 1440–1442.

12. Davis MDP, Daoud MS, Kirby B, Gibson LE, Rogers RS III. Clinicopathologic correlation of hypocomplementemic and normocomplementemic urticarial vasculitis. J Am Acad Dermatol 1998; 38:899–905.

13. Wisnieski JJ, Baer AN, Christensen J, Cupps TR, Flagg DN, Jones JV, et al. Hypocomplementemic urticarial vasculitis syndrome: Clinical and serologic findings in 18 patients. Medicine 1995; 74:34–41.

14. Winkelmann RK, Wilson-Jones E, Smith NP, English JSC, Greaves MW. Neutrophilic urticaria. Acta Derm Venereol 1988; 68:129–133.

15. Dolman KM, Gans ROB, Vervaat TJ, et al. Vasculitis and antineutrophil cytoplasmic antibodies associated with propylthiouracil therapy. Lancet 1993; 342:651–652.

16. Lunardi C, Bambarra LM, Biasi D, Zagni P, Caramaschi P, Pacor ML. Elimination diet in the treatment of selected patients with hypersensitivity vasculitis. Clin Exp Rheum 1992; 10:131–135.

17. Ekenstam E, Callen JP. Cutaneous leukocytoclastic vasculitis. Arch Dermatol 1984; 120:484–489.

18. Szer IS. Henoch-Schönlein purpura: When and how to treat. J Rheumatol 1996; 23:1661–1665.

19. Tancrede-Bohin E, Ochonisky S, Vignon-Pennamen M-D, Flageul B, Morel P, Rybojad M. Schönlein-Henoch purpura in adult patients: Predictive factors for IgA glomerulonephritis in a retrospective study of 57 cases. Arch Dermatol 1997; 133:438–442.

20. Sanchez-Guerrero J, Gutiuerrez-Urena S, Vidaller A, Reyes E, Iglesias A, Alarcon-Segovia D. Vasculitis as a paraneoplastic syndrome. Report of 11 cases and review of the literature. J Rheumatol 1990; 17:1458–1462.

21. Barksdale SK, Hallahan CW, Kerr GS, Fauci AS, Stern JB, Travis WD. Cutaneous pathology in Wegener's granulomatosis: A clinicopathologic study of 75 biopsies in 46 patients. Am J Surg Pathol 1995; 19:161–173.

22. Misani R, Bellavita P, Fenili D, et al. Interferon alfa-2a therapy in cryoglobulinemia associated with hepatitis C virus. N Engl J Med 1994; 330:751–756.

23. Durand J-M, Cacoub P, Lunel-Fabiani F, et al. Ribavirin in hepatitis C-related cryoglobulinemia. J Rheumatol 1998; 25:1115–1117.

24. Gungor E, Alli CN, Karakayali G, Gur G, Artuz F. Prevalence of hepatitis C virus antibodies and cryoglobulinemia in patients with leukocytoclastic vasculitis. Dermatology 1999; 198:26–28.

25. Hudson CP, Callen JP. Hyperglobulinemic purpura: A clinical subset of leukocytoclastic vasculitis. Arch Dermatol 1984; 120:1224–1226.

26. Puddu P, Cianchini G, Girardelli CR, Colonna L, Gatti S, dePita O. Schnitzler's syndrome: Report of a new case and a review of the literature. Clin Exp Rheumatol 1997; 15:91–95.

27. McDuffie FC, Sams WM Jr, Maldonado JE, Andreini PH, Conn DL, Samayoa EA. Hypocomplementemia with cutaneous vasculitis and arthritis. Possible immune complex syndrome. Mayo Clin Proc 1973; 48:340–348.

28. Katz SI, Gallin JI, Hertz KC, et al. Skin and systemic manifestations, immunologic studies and successful treatment with dapsone. Medicine 1977; 56:443–455.

29. Kevil CG, Bullard DC. Roles of leukocyte/endothelial cell adhesion molecules in the pathogenesis of vasculitis. Am J Med 1999; 106:677–687.

30. Blanco R, Martinez-Taboada VM, Rodriguez-Valverde V, Garcia-Fuentes M. Cutaneous vasculitis in children and adults: Associated diseases and etiologic factors in 303 patients. Medicine 1998; 77:403–418.

31. Nurenberg W, Grabbe J, Czarnetzic BM. Synergistic effects of pentoxyfylline and dapsone in leukocytoclastic vasculitis. Lancet 1994; 343:491.

32. Callen JP. Colchicine is effective in controlling chronic cutaneous leukocytoclastic vasculitis. J Am Acad Dermatol 1985; 13:193–200.

33. Sais G, Vidaller A, Jucgla A, Gallerdo F, Peyri J. Colchicine in the treatment of cutaneous leukocytoclastic vasculitis: Results of a prospective, randomized controlled trial. Arch Dermatol 1995; 131: 1399–1402.

34. Callen JP, Spencer LV, Burruss JB, Holtman J. Azathioprine: An effective, corticosteroid-sparing therapy for patients with recalcitrant cutaneous lupus erythematosus or with recalcitrant cutaneous leukocytoclastic vasculitis. Arch Dermatol 1991; 127:515–522.

37
Thromboangiitis Obliterans (Buerger's Disease)

Jeffrey W. Olin
The Heart and Vascular Institute, Morristown, New Jersey

Arthur Topoulos
Cleveland Clinic Foundation, Cleveland, Ohio

I. INTRODUCTION

Thromboangiitis obliterans (TAO), or Buerger's disease, is an inflammatory vascular disease affecting small and medium-sized arteries and veins. While Buerger's disease is in the strict sense of the word a vasculitis, it differs pathologically from the most common forms of vasculitis because there is a highly inflammatory thrombus present in the vessel lumen with relatively little inflammation in the vessel wall and the absence of fibrinoid necrosis (1). In addition, autoantibody formation and serological markers of inflammation are absent.

Von Winiwater (2) was the first to describe a patient with thromboangiitis obliterans in 1879. He reported on the pathological findings of a 57-year-old male with a 12-year history of foot pain resulting in gangrene and ultimate amputation. Von Winiwater suggested that the endarteritis and endophlebitis present in the amputated specimen were distinct from atherosclerosis. In 1908, Buerger (3) provided the first detailed and accurate description of the pathology of 11 amputated limbs and based upon his pathological examination called this disease "thromboangiitis obliterans," which later became more commonly known as Buerger's disease. He emphasized that TAO was a distinct clinical pathological entity from atherosclerosis. In 1928, 200 cases of thromboangiitis obliterans were reported from the Mayo Clinic (4). Most of these patients were Jewish and heavy cigarette smokers. They developed foot claudication and trophic changes. The pathology was identical to that in Buerger's original report.

II. EPIDEMIOLOGY

Buerger's disease is most prevalent in the Middle, Near and Far East (5,6). It has been reported less commonly in the United States and Europe, possibly due to the adoption of strict diagnostic criteria and a lower prevalence rate of cigarette smoking. There has been a steady decline in the prevalence of Buerger's disease at the Mayo Clinic from 104 per 100,000 patient registrations in 1947 to 12.6 per 100,000 patient registrations in 1986 (6,7). The proportion of patients from western European countries with peripheral arterial disease who have TAO has been reported to be as low as 0.5–5.6%. These figures stand in dramatic comparison with those from certain other cultures and geographical locations. For example, the proportion of cases of peripheral arterial disease due to TAO in India is 45–63%; in Israel (Ashkenazim), 80%; and in Korea and Japan, 16–66%. The Buerger's Disease Research Committee of the Ministry, Health and Welfare of Japan (8) estimated the incidence of TAO to be 5 per 100,000. In 1986, the Epidemiology of Intractable Disease Research Committee of the Ministry of Health and Welfare of Japan estimated that more than 8000 patients with the disease were being treated at various medical centers (9). According to unofficial estimates, there are 60,000–80,000 patients with Buerger's disease in China (10).

A. Buerger's Disease in Women

Prior to the mid-1980s, Buerger's disease was predominantly encountered in men. In 1987, Lie (7) reported 12 female patients evaluated at the Mayo Clinic. This represented 11% of their entire series from 1981 to 1985. We have demonstrated that 26 (23%) of 112 patients with thromboangiitis obliterans from 1970 to 1987 at the Cleveland Clinic were women (11). In a more recent series, an additional 40 patients with Buerger's disease were studied from 1988 to 1996 at our institution and 30% were women (12). In a study from the University of Oregon, 19% of 26 patients were female. It is unknown why the prevalence of Buerger's disease in women is increasing (13). It may possibly be related to the increased number of women smokers. However, despite an increased prevalence of smoking in women, the prevalence of female Buerger's disease remains low in Japan and Hong Kong (10,14,15).

III. ETIOLOGY AND PATHOGENESIS

The etiology of thromboangiitis obliterans is unknown. Using strict pathological criteria, thromboangiitis obliterans is a vasculitis (5). However, it differs from the more commonly encountered forms of vasculitis in that the thrombus in TAO is highly cellular with considerably less inflammatory cell infiltration in the wall of the blood vessel. In addition, markers of inflammation such as Westergren sedimentation rate and C-reactive protein, and autoantibody formation (antinuclear antibody, rheumatoid factor, complement, circulating immune complexes, etc.) are usually normal or absent.

There are several factors that have been implicated in the etiology of Buerger's disease.

A. Smoking

Heavy tobacco use clearly plays a major role in disease initiation and progression (11,16). There has never been a well-described case of Buerger's disease in a patient who did not use tobacco in some form. While most patients are heavy cigarette smokers, there have been reported cases of Buerger's disease in users of smokeless tobacco or snuff (17–19). Thromboangiitis obliterans is more common in patients from countries where the consumption of tobacco is great. In India, the prevalence of TAO is much higher in individuals of a low socioeconomic class who smoke bidis (homemade cigarettes with raw tobacco) compared with others in the population (20,21).

It is not known if cigarette smoking is causative or contributory to the development of Buerger's disease. Tobacco use is strongly related to the activity of the disease. Progression, continued symptoms, and eventual amputation are closely associated with continued tobacco use (11). There has not been a case of TAO reported in patients exposed to high quantities of environmental tobacco smoke; however, most investigators believe that passive smoking (secondary smoke) may be important in the continuation of symptoms in patients during the acute phase of their illness.

While most investigators believe that tobacco is the most important factor in the development of thromboangiitis obliterans, only a small number of smokers worldwide eventually develop TAO. Therefore, other etiological factors may play a permissive or adjunctive role in the development of TAO.

B. Genetics

While there may be a genetic predisposition to the development of TAO, no gene to date has been identified. There is also no consistent pattern of human leukocyte antigen (HLA) haplotypes in patients with Buerger's disease. The HLA haplotypes appear to be more closely associated with country of origin than presence or absence of TAO (13,16,22–25).

C. Hypercoagulability and Endothelial Function

The presence of hypercoagulable abnormalities is also quite variable among patients with Buerger's disease (26–29). Some investigators (29) have demonstrated increased levels of urokinase-plasminogen activator and decreased levels of free plasminogen activator 1 inhibitor in patients with thromboangiitis obliterans compared with normal healthy controls. Increased platelet response to serotonin has also been demonstrated in Buerger's disease (30). Other investigators have failed to identify clotting abnormalities in these patients.

There have been several studies demonstrating endothelial cell derangement in TAO (31,32). Eikhorn et al. (31) have studied seven patients with active Buerger's disease who had antiendothelial cell antibodies (AECAs) in titers of 1857 ± 450 arbitrary units (AU) compared with titers of 126 ± 15 AU in 30 normal control subjects ($p < 0.001$) and 461 ± 41 AU in 21 TAO patients in remission ($p < 0.01$). Antibodies reacted with both surface epitopes and cytoplasmic antigens of human endothelial cells. If these results can be reproduced, antiendothelial cell antibody titers may be useful in following disease activity in patients with Buerger's disease.

Impairment in endothelium-dependent vasorelaxation has also been demonstrated in patients with Buerger's disease (32). Forearm blood flow (FBF) was measured by plethysmography in the nondiseased limb of patients with active Buerger's disease after the infusion of acetylcholine (an endothelium-dependent vasodilator), sodium nitroprusside (an endothelium-independent vasodilator) and occlusion-induced reactive hyperemia. Patients with active TAO had a smaller increase in FBF compared with healthy controls (14.1 ± 2.8 ml/min/dL of tissue volume vs. 22.9 ± 2.9 ml/min/dL, $p < 0.01$). There was no significant increase in FBF response to sodium nitroprusside and no significant difference between the two groups after reactive hyperemia. These data strongly suggest that endothelium-dependent vasodilatation is impaired even in the nondiseased limb of patients with active TAO.

D. Immunological Markers

Adar et al. (33) demonstrated increased cellular sensitivity to Type I and Type III collagen (normal constituents of human arteries) in patients with TAO compared with patients with arteriosclerosis obliterans or healthy male controls. They also found low but significant levels of anticollagen antibody in 7 of 39 serum samples from patients with TAO, whereas this antibody was not detected in the control group of patients. Some investigators have detected circulating immune complexes in the peripheral arteries of some patients with TAO (20,34–36).

No single abnormality, linked to etiological mechanisms, has been identified in all patients with TAO. It is clear that tobacco plays a central role both in the initiation and continuance of the disease. Other etiological factors, as discussed above, may play an important synergistic role with tobacco to initiate the disease.

IV. PATHOLOGY

The histopathology of the involved blood vessels in Buerger's disease varies according to the chronological age of the lesion. In TAO, there is an inflammatory thrombus that affects both the artery and the veins. The histopathology is most likely to be diagnostic in the acute phase of the disease. In the subacute (intermediate) phase the pathology is suggestive, and in the chronic or end-stage phase all that remains is organized thrombus and fibrosis of the blood vessels. The end-stage lesion is nondescript and can be found in many different types of vascular disease (5,37–41). The histological distinction between Buerger's disease and atherosclerosis is clear-cut and the differentiation can be made with a high degree of accuracy (37). It should also be emphasized that the small blood vessels in the hand and foot are not usually affected by atherosclerosis.

In the acute phase, there is inflammation involving the walls of the blood vessels. This is especially prominent in the veins, and is associated with an occlusive highly cellular inflammatory thrombus. In the periphery of the thrombus, one may encounter polymorphonuclear leukocytes with karyorrhexis, the so-called microabscess, and one or more multinucleated giant cells may be present (Fig. 1). The prominent inflammatory thrombotic lesion occurs more often in veins than in arteries (Fig. 2). If the acute superficial phlebitic lesions of the skin are biopsied at an early stage, one is most likely to see the acute pathological abnormalities of thromboangiitis obliterans.

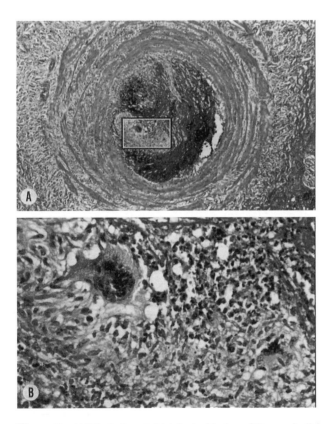

Figure 1   (A) Typical acute histological lesion of Buerger's disease in a vein with intense thromboangiitis (×64). (B) Close-up view of the boxed area in A, showing a microabscess in the thrombus and two multinucleated giant cells (H & E, ×400). (From Ref. 40.)

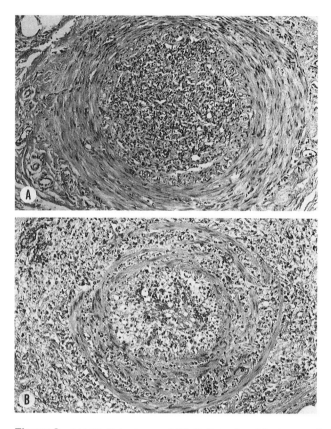

Figure 2 (A) Digital artery and (B) digital vein of the intermediate (subacute) stage of Buerger's disease. Note the prominent inflammatory infiltrates and early organization of the thrombus (H & E, ×64). (From Ref. 40.)

In the intermediate phase, there is progressive organization of the thrombus in the arteries and veins. There are still significant inflammatory cellular infiltrates within the thrombus, but there is much less inflammation in the blood vessel wall. In the chronic or end-stage lesion, there is complete organization of the occlusive thrombus with extensive recanalization, prominent vascularization of the media and adventitia, and perivascular fibrosis. This end-stage lesion can be associated with many different disease entities. "In all three stages the normal architecture of the vessel wall subjacent to the occlusive thrombus and including the internal elastic lamina remains essentially intact. These findings distinguish thromboangiitis obliterans from arteriosclerosis and from other systemic vasculitides in which there is usually more striking disruption of the internal elastic lamina and the media disproportionate to those attributable to aging alone" (1).

Both clinically and pathologically, Buerger's disease is segmental in distribution, and skip areas of normal vessels between diseased ones are commonly encountered. These skip lesions may be observable angiographically and histopathologically.

Pathological studies of Buerger's disease have noted involvement in unusual locations. While the disease most commonly affects the small and medium-sized arteries and veins of the extremities (infrapopliteal and infrabrachial arteries), it has been demonstrated in many other vascular beds. Involvement of the cerebral, coronary, renal, mesenteric, pulmonary, iliac arteries and aorta have been occasionally reported, usually as single cases (42–44). Multiple organ involvement in TAO has also been observed (45,46). There have been reports of Buerger's disease in saphenous vein arterial bypass grafts (47) and in testicular and spermatic arteries and veins (48). When TAO occurs in unusual locations, the diagnosis should only be made when the histopathological findings are "classic" for the acute phase lesion *and* the clinical presentation is consistent for Buerger's disease.

V. CLINICAL FEATURES

Buerger's disease is most commonly encountered in a young male smoker with the onset of symptoms before age 40–45. However, the spectrum of disease appears to be changing, as the prevalence of TAO in women has increased in some reports (7,11,13). Buerger's disease virtually always begins with ischemia of the distal small arteries and veins of the feet and hands. More proximal arteries may become involved as the disease progresses.

From 1970–1996, 152 patients were evaluated at the Cleveland Clinic Foundation (11,49). The demographic characteristics of this group are shown in Table 1. The presenting signs and symptoms of the original 112 patients are demonstrated in Table 2. Early in the course of TAO, patients may present with claudication of the arch of the foot. This is often mistaken for an orthopedic problem, resulting in a significant delay before the patient is referred to the appropriate specialist and the correct diagnosis is made. As the disease progresses, the claudication may move more proximally, and the patient may present with typical calf claudication. A large number of patients present with ischemic ulcerations in the distal toes and fingers at the time of presentation (66% in our series) (1) (Figs. 3 and 4).

Table 1 Demographic Characteristics of Thromboangiitis Obliterans

Variable	Original series[a] (1970–1987)	Present series[b] (1988–1996)
Patients (*n*)	112	40
Mean Age (years)	42	42
Men	86 (77%)	28 (70%)
Women	26 (23%)	12 (30%)

[a]*Source*: Ref. 11.
[b]*Source*: Ref. 12.

Table 2 Presenting Signs and Symptoms of Thromboangiitis Obliterans

	Number (%)
Intermittent claudication	70 (63)
Rest pain	91 (81)
Ischemic ulcers	85 (76)
Upper extremity	24 (28)
Lower extremity	39 (46)
Both	22 (26)
Thrombophlebitis	43 (38)
Raynaud's phenomenon	49 (44)
Sensory findings	77 (69)
Abnormal Allen test	71 (63)

Source: Ref. 11.

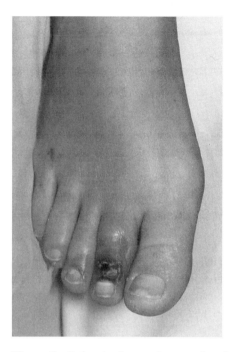

Figure 3 Ischemic ulcer on the second toe in a young woman with TAO. (From Ref. 1.)

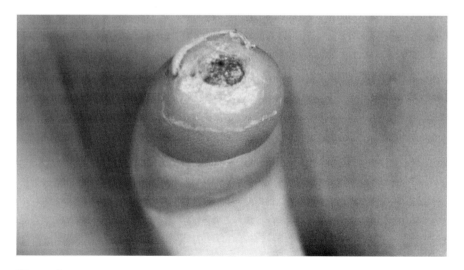

Figure 4 Ischemic ulcer of the index finger in a patient with Buerger's disease. (From Ref. 1.)

It is important to recognize that Buerger's disease almost always involves two or more limbs (10,17). In Shionoya's series, two limbs were involved in 16% of patients, 3 limbs in 41%, and all four limbs in 43% of patients (10). Therefore, it has been our practice to perform an arteriogram of *both* upper extremities and/or *both* lower extremities in patients who clinically present with involvement of only one limb. Angiographic abnormalities are common in limbs that are not yet involved clinically.

If a lower extremity ulceration is present, it is important to perform an Allen's test to assess the circulation in the hands and fingers (50,51). The Allen's test helps to clinically determine if there is occlusion of the radial or ulnar artery distal to the wrist. An abnormal Allen's test in a young smoker with lower extremity ulcerations strongly suggests the presence of TAO, since it signifies that there is small-vessel occlusive disease of both the upper and lower extremities. Thromboangiitis obliterans starts distally and may progress proximally over time. Atherosclerosis is almost always more proximal in its distribution. Atherosclerosis does not usually occur in the hand and rarely is present distal to the subclavian artery except in patients with end-stage renal disease and diabetes. Both superficial thrombophlebitis and Raynaud's phenomenon occur in approximately 40% of patients with TAO (11).

VI. LABORATORY AND ARTERIOGRAPHIC FINDINGS

There are no specific laboratory abnormalities that help to make the diagnosis of TAO. It is important to obtain a complete serological profile so as to exclude other diseases that mimic Buerger's disease. These tests include complete blood count with differential, fasting blood sugar, creatinine, urinalysis, acute phase reactants (Westergren sedimentation rate and C-reactive protein), antinuclear antibody if features of systemic lupus are present, complement measurements if there is evidence of immune complex–mediated disease, and a complete hypercoagulability screen to include antiphospholipid antibodies, factor V Leiden mutation, and the prothrombin gene 20210A. If skin changes suggestive of scleroderma are present, but the diagnosis is uncertain, a biopsy can be very helpful.

Arteriographically, the proximal arteries should be normal and show no evidence of atherosclerosis, aneurysm, or other source of proximal emboli. The disease most often occurs in the infrapopliteal arteries in the lower extremities (Fig. 5) and distal to the brachial artery in the upper extremity (Fig. 6). In some patients, there may be progression to the superficial femoral arteries and even more proximal larger arteries. Isolated disease below the popliteal artery almost never occurs in atherosclerosis. Even patients with diabetes mellitus often have multisegment disease with some evidence of proximal artery involvement. In Buerger's disease, there is involvement of the digital arteries of the fingers and toes as well as the palmar and plantar arteries in the hand and foot. The tibial, peroneal, radial, and ulnar arteries are commonly involved. Buerger's disease is a segmental disorder in which there are areas of diseased blood vessels interspersed with normal blood vessel segments. There may be evidence of multiple vascular occlusions with collateralization around the obstruction (corkscrew collaterals). These collaterals are not pathognomonic of Buerger's disease as they may be present in other small-vessel occlusive diseases such as scleroderma or CREST syndrome. In fact, the arteriographic appearance of Buerger's disease may be identical to many of the connective tissue diseases such as systemic lupus erythematosus (SLE), rheumatoid vasculitis, mixed connective tissue disease, and antiphospholipid antibody syndrome.

It is important to rule out a proximal source of emboli using both arteriography and echocardiography.

The diagnostic algorithm in Figure 7 may help in the diagnosis of TAO. There are also several different proposed diagnostic criteria. Papa et al. (52) use a point scoring system to help make the diagnosis of definite, probable, or unlikely Buerger's disease. Mills and Porter (19) have proposed major and minor diagnostic criteria. We continue to believe that if patients meet the criteria of distal extremity involvement, tobacco use, exclusion of a proximal source of emboli or atherosclerosis, and the absence of hyperlipidemia, diabetes, hypercoagulable states, and systemic antiimmune diseases, one can make the diagnosis of Buerger's disease with a high degree of certainty.

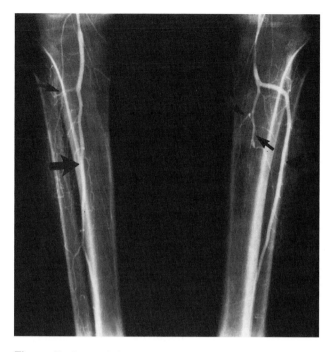

Figure 5 Severe infrapopliteal disease in a patient with TAO. In the right leg, the anterior tibial artery (small arrow) and the posterior tibial artery are occluded at their origin. The peroneal artery is patent (large arrow). In the left leg, the anterior tibial artery is patent (larger arrow), but the posterior tibial and peroneal artery (small arrows) are occluded proximally. (From Ref. 51.)

VII. THERAPY

The most important aspect in the treatment of patients with Buerger's disease is complete abstinence from tobacco. This is the only way to halt the progression of TAO and avoid future amputations (11,26,53). Even modest use of cigarettes or smokeless tobacco (chewing tobacco, snuff) has been reported to trigger or sustain active Buerger's disease (17,18). At the Cleveland Clinic Foundation, 120 patients have been followed long term, and 52 (43%) were able to discontinue cigarette smoking (Fig. 8). If irreversible tissue injury was not present at the time the patient stopped smoking, amputation did not occur. Ninety-four percent of patients avoided amputation in the smoking cessation group. In the 68 patients who continued to smoke, 43% required one or more amputations. There is an extremely strong correlation between smoking cessation and subsidence of disease (ischemic ulcer healing and avoidance of amputation). Therefore, if the patient has stated that they have stopped using tobacco products and the disease remains active, a urine nicotine and cotinine level should be measured to determine if the patient is still smoking or is being exposed to high amounts of environmental (secondary) tobacco smoke (54). Frequent education and counseling is extremely important to encourage discontinuance of tobacco products. The patient should be reassured that if they are able to discontinue tobacco use, the disease will become quiescent and amputation will not occur, assuming critical limb ischemia is not already present. However, patients may continue to experience intermittent claudication or Raynaud's phenomenon since the occluded arterial segments will remain occluded.

Apart from discontinuation of tobacco products, all other forms of therapy are palliative. In a prospective, randomized, double-blind trial comparing a 6 h daily infusion of Iloprost (a prostaglandin analog) to aspirin, Iloprost was superior in providing total relief of pain at rest and

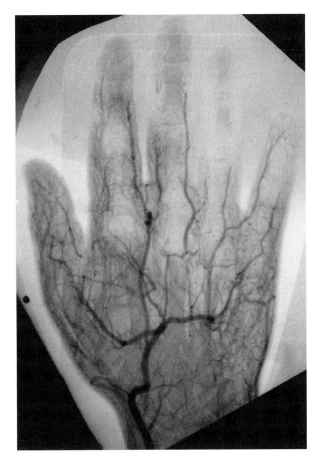

Figure 6 Angiogram demonstrating a normal brachial artery (not shown) with a radial artery that supplies the hand. The interosseous artery ends just above the wrist (not shown). Note the occluded ulnar artery. There are multiple digital artery occlusions. Some digits have multiple "skip" areas with patent arteries interspersed with occluded arteries. (From Ref. 49.)

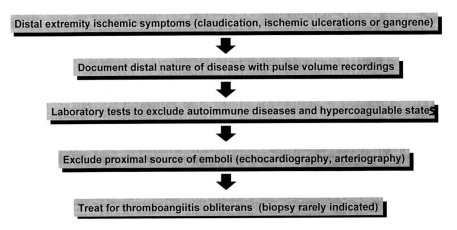

Figure 7 Diagnostic algorithm for the diagnosis of thromboangiitis obliterans. (From Ref. 1.)

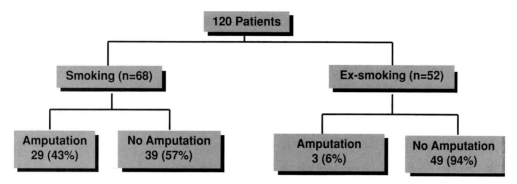

Figure 8 Smoking status related to amputation. (From Ref. 49.)

complete healing of trophic changes. At 6 months, 88% of the patients receiving Iloprost continued to respond to therapy, compared with only 21% of the aspirin group (55). An oral extended-
release preparation of Iloprost has also been studied by the European TAO Study Group (56). Oral
Iloprost was significantly better than placebo in providing total relief of rest pain without the need
of analgesics (57). There was no difference in healing of ischemic lesions. Both sympathectomy
and intraarterial thrombolytic therapy have been used with variable results (11,58). Surgical
revascularization for Buerger's disease is usually not a good alternative because of the distal nature of the disease and the severe segmental involvement. Appropriate distal blood vessels are
generally not available for bypass surgery. In a large series of patients published by Sasajimi et
al. (59), primary patency rate of surgical revascularization was 48.8% and secondary patency rate
was 62.5% at 5 years. These results are better than reported in a number of other series (19,60,61).

Isner and colleagues (62) used intramuscular injection of a plasmid DNA (ph VEGF 165)
that encoded the VEGF 165 (vascular endothelial growth factor 165) gene to treat severe affected
limbs in six patients with TAO. Among nonhealing ulcers present for more than one month, complete healing occurred in three of five limbs after VEGF gene therapy. In the remaining two patients, nocturnal rest pain was relieved. It is too early to tell what role this promising form of gene
therapy will play in patients with TAO in the future.

Good general vascular care is essential in the treatment of patients with severe ischemia
secondary to TAO. A reverse Trendelenburg (vascular) position should be used in patients who
have severe ischemic rest pain. Adequate narcotics should be made available during periods of severe ischemia. Anticoagulation is generally not efficacious in the treatment of Buerger's disease
unless the patient has recurrent episodes of superficial thrombophlebitis. Good foot and hand hygiene and avoidance of injury are obvious important measures. A calcium channel blocking agent
such as nifedipine or amlodipine should be used in patients with vasospasm (51). Pentoxifylline
has not been adequately studied in patients with TAO. Since this drug increases the red blood cell
membrane flexibility and allows red blood cells to fit through a smaller vascular eumen, it is not
unreasonable to try pentoxifylline in the severely ischemic patient. Heel protectors should be used
in patients with severe ischemia to prevent pressure ulcers from developing.

VIII. CONCLUSIONS

Thromboangiitis obliterans (Buerger's disease) is an inflammatory, nonatherosclerotic disease affecting the small and medium-sized arteries and veins in both the upper and lower extremities.
Tobacco plays a central role in both the initiation and the continuance of disease. Discontinuation

of tobacco use, in any form, is the mainstay of treatment. Amputation almost never occurs in patients who are able to discontinue using tobacco.

REFERENCES

1. Olin JW, Lie JT. Thromboangiitis obliterans (Buerger's disease). In: Loscalzo J, Creager MA, Dzau VJ, eds. Vascular Medicine. Boston: Little, Brown, 1996:1033–1049.
2. von Winiwater F. Ueber eine eigenthumliche Form von Endarteritis und Endophlebitis mit Gangran des Fusses. Arch Klin Chir 1879; 23:202–226.
3. Buerger L. Thromboangiitis obliterans: A study of the vascular lesions leading to presenile spontaneous gangrene. Am J Med Sci 1908; 136:567–580.
4. Allen EV, Brown GE. Thrombo-angiitis obliterans: A clinical study of 200 cases. Ann Intern Med 1928; 1:535–549.5.
5. Lie JT. Diagnostic histopathology of major systemic and pulmonary vasculitic syndromes. Rheum Clin North Am 1990; 16:269–292.
6. Lie JT. The rise and fall and resurgence of thromboangiitis obliterans (Buerger's disease). Acta Pathol Jpn 1989; 39:153–158.
7. Lie JT. Thromboangiitis obliterans (Buerger's disease) in women. Medicine 1987; 64:65–72.
8. Ishikawa, ed. Annual Report of the Buerger's Disease Research Committee of Ministry of Health and Welfare of Japan. Tokyo, 1976; 3–15, 86–97.
9. Nishikimi N, Shionoya S, Mizuno S et al. Result of national epidemiological study of Buerger's disease. J Jpn Coll Angiol 1987; 27:1125–1130.
10. Shionoya S. Buerger's disease (thromboangiitis obliterans). In: Rutherford RB, ed. Vascular Surgery. Philadelphia: Saunders, 1989:207–217.
11. Olin JW, Young JR, Graor RA, et al. The changing clinical spectrum of thromboangiitis obliterans (Buerger's disease). Circulation 1990; 82(suppl IV):3–8.
12. Olin JW, Childs MB, Bartholomew JR, Calabrese LH, Young JR. Anticardiolipin antibodies and homocysteine levels in patients with thromboangiitis obliterans. Arthritis Rheum 1996; 39:S–47.
13. Mills JL, Taylor LM, Porter JK. Buerger's disease in the modern era. Am J Surg 1987; 154:123–154.
14. Shionoya S. Buerger's disease. Pathology, diagnosis and treatment. Nagoya: University of Nagoya Press, 1990:261.
15. Lau H, Cheng SWK. Buerger's disease in Hong Kong: A review of 89 cases. Aust NZ J Surg 1997; 67:264–269.
16. Papa MZ and Adar R. A critical look at thromboangiitis obliterans (Buerger's disease). Vasc Surg 1992; 5:1–21.
17. Joyce JW. Buerger's disease (thromboangiitis obliterans). Rheum Dis Clin North Am 1990; 16:463–470.
18. Lie JT. Thromboangiitis obliterans (Buerger's disease) and smokeless tobacco. Arthritis Rheum 1988; 31:812–813.
19. Mills JL, Porter JM. Buerger's disease: A review and update. Semin Vasc Surg 1993; 6:14–23.30.
20. Gulati SM, Madhra K, Thusoo TK, et al. Autoantibodies in thromboangiitis obliterans. Angiology 1982; 33:642–650.
21. Jindal RM, Patel SM. Buerger's disease in cigarette smoking in Bangladesh. Ann R Coll Surg Engl 1992; 74:436–437.
22. McLoughlin GA, Helsby CR, Evans CC, et al. Association of HLA-A9 and HLA-B5 with Buerger's disease. Br Med J 1976; 2:1165–1166.
23. Numano F, Sasazuki T, Koyama T, et al. HLA in Buerger's disease. Exp Clin Immunogenet 1986; 3:195–200.
24. Otawa T, Juji T, Kawano N, et al. HLA antigen in thromboangiitis obliterans. JAMA 1974; 230:1126.
25. Smolen JS, Youngchaiyud U, Weidinger T, et al. Auto immunological aspects of thromboangiitis obliterans (Buerger's diseases). Clin Immunol Immunopathol 1978; 11:168–177.

26. Casellas M, Perez A, Cabero L. Buerger's disease and antiphospholipid antibodies in pregnancy. Ann Rheum Dis 1993; 52:247–248.

27. Craven JL, Cotton RC. Haematological differences between thromboangiitis obliterans and atherosclerosis. Br J Surg 1967; 54:862–867.

28. Siguret V, Alhenc-Gelas M, Aiach M et al. Response to DDAVP stimulation in thirteen patients with Buerger's disease. Thromb Res 1997; 86:85–87.

29. Chaudhury NA, Pietraszek MH, Hachiya T, et al. Plasminogen activators and plasminogen activator inhibitor 1 before and after venous occlusion of the upper limb in thromboangiitis obliterans (Buerger's disease). Thromb Res 1992; 66:321–329.

30. Pietraszek MH, Chaudhury NA, Koyano K, et al. Enhanced platelet response to serotonin in Buerger's disease. Thromb Res 1990; 60:241–246.

31. Eichhorn J, Sima D, Lindschau C, et al. Antiendothelial cell antibodies in thromboangiitis obliterans. Am J Med Sci 1998; 315:17–23.

32. Makita S, Nakamura M, Murakami H, et al. Impaired endothelium dependent vasorelaxation in peripheral vasculature of patients with thromboangiitis obliterans (Buerger's disease). Circulation 1996; 94(suppl II):II-211–II-215.

33. Adar R, Papa MC, Halperin Z, et al. Cellular sensitivity to and thromboangiitis obliterans. N Engl J Med 1983; 308:1113–1116.

34. De Albuquerque RR, Delgado L, Correia P, et al. Circulating immune complexes in Buerger's disease-endarteritis obliterans in young men. J Cardiovasc Surg 1989; 30:821–825.

35. Gulati SM, Saha K, Kant L, et al. Significance of circulating immune complexes in thromboangiitis obliterans (Buerger's disease). Angiology 1984; 35:276–281.

36. Roncon A, Delgado L, Correia P, et al. Circulating immune complexes in Buerger's disease. J Cardiovasc Surg 1989; 30:821–825.

37. Dible JH. The pathology of the limb ischaemia. Edinburgh: Oliver and Boyd, 1966; 79–96.

38. Leu HJ. Early inflammatory changes in thromboangiitis obliterans. Pathol Microbiol 1975; 43:151–156.

39. Leu HJ. Thromboangiitis obliterans Buerger. Schweiz Med Wschr 1985; 115:1080–1086.

40. Lie JT. Thromboangiitis obliterans (Buerger's disease) revisited. Pathol Annu 1988; 23(part 2):257–291.

41. Williams G. Recent view on Buerger's disease. J Clin Pathol 1969; 22:573–578.

42. Deitch EA, Sikkema WW. Intestinal manifestation of Buerger's disease. Am Surg 1981; 47:326–328.

43. Donatelli F, Triggiani M, Nascimbene S, et al. Thromboangiitis obliterans of coronary and internal thoracic arteries in a young woman. J Thorac Cardiovasc Surg 1997; 113:800–802.

44. Rosen N, Sommer I, Knobel B. Intestinal Buerger's disease. Arch Pathol Lab Med 1985; 109:962–963.

45. Harten P, Muller-Huelsbeck S, Regensburger D, Loeffler H. Multiple organ manifestations in thromboangiitis obliterans (Buerger's disease). Angiology 1996; 47:419–425.

46. Cebezas-Moya R, Dragstedt LR III. An extreme example of Buerger's disease. Arch Surg 1970; 101:632–634.

47. Lie JT. Thromboangiitis obliterans (Buerger's disease) in a saphenous vein arterial graft. Hum Pathol 1987;18:402–404.

48. Buerger L. The Circulatory Disturbance of the Extremities: Including Gangrene, Vasomotor and Trophic Disorders. Philadelphia: Saunders, 1924.

49. Olin JW. Thromboangiitis obliterans (Buerger's disease). In: Rutherford RB, ed. Vascular Surgery, 4th ed. Philadelphia: Saunders. In press.

50. Allen EV. Thromboangiitis obliterans. Methods of diagnosis of chronic occlusive arterial lesions distal to the wrist with illustrative cases. Am J Med Sci 1929; 178:237–244.

51. Olin JW, Lie JT. Thromboangiitis obliterans (Buerger's disease). In: Cooke JP, Frohlich ED, eds. Current Management of Hypertension and Vascular Disease. St Louis: Mosby, 1992:265–271.

52. Papa MZ, Rabi I, Adar R. A point scoring system for the clinical diagnosis of Buerger's disease. Eur J Vasc Endovasc Surg 1996; 11:335–339.

53. Corelli F. Buerger's disease: Cigarette smoker disease may always be cured by medical therapy alone. Uselessness of operative treatment. J Cardiovasc Surg 1973; 14:28–36.

54. Matsushita M, Shionoya S, Matsumoto T. Urinary cotinine measurements in patients with Buerger's disease: Effects of active and passive smoking on the disease process. J Vasc Surg 1991; 14:53–58.

55. Fiessinger JN, Schafer M, for the TAO Study. Trial of Iloprost vs. aspirin. Treatment for critical limb ischemia of thromboangiitis obliterans. Lancet 1990; 335:555–557.

56. Hildebrand M. Pharmacokinetics and tolerability of oral Iloprost in thromboangiitis obliterans. Eur J Clin Pharmacol 1997; 53:51–56.

57. The European TAO Study Group. Oral Iloprost in the treatment of thromboangiitis obliterans (Buerger's disease). A double-blind, randomized, placebo-controlled trial. Eur J Vasc Endovasc Surg 1998; 15: 300–307.

58. Hussein EA, Dorri AE. Intra-arterial streptokinase as adjuvant therapy for complicated Buerger's disease: Early trials. Int Surg 1993; 78:54–58.

59. Sasajima T, Kubo Y, Inaba M, et al. Role of infrainguinal bypass in Buerger's disease: An eighteen-year experience. Eur J Vasc Endovasc Surg 1997; 13:186–192.

60. Sayin A, Bozkurt AK, Tuzun H, et al. Surgical treatment of Buerger's disease: Experience with 216 patients. Cardiovasc Surg 1003; 1:377–380.

61. Mills JL, Porter JM. Buerger's disease (thromboangiitis obliterans). Ann Vasc Surg 1991; 5:570–572.

62. Isner JM, Baumgartner I, Rauh G, et al. Treatment of thromboangiitis obliterans (Buerger's disease) by intramuscular gene transfer of vascular endothelial growth factor: Preliminary clinical results. J Vasc Surg 1998; 28:964–75).

38
Virus-Associated Vasculitides: Pathogenesis

Rocco Misiani

Ospedali Riuniti di Bergamo, Bergamo, Italy

I. INTRODUCTION

A wide variety of viral agents have long been associated with different vasculitic processes affecting humans as well as animals (1–10). In recent years, the recognition of vasculitides occurring in patients infected with hepatitis viruses (11–14), human immunodeficiency virus (15), and various agents belonging to the herpes family (16–18), has greatly expanded the interest in this field. The awareness of a causal relationship between specific viruses and some vasculitic syndromes may have important clinical implications. In fact, the recent development of reliable virological tests, along with the availability of effective antiviral drugs may offer the chance of treatment based on etiology, possibly resulting in definitive cure of these often severe diseases. Conversely, treating virus-associated vasculitides with immunosuppressive drugs alone may favor viral replication with potential severe complications (19).

Table 1 is a partial list of viruses that have been found in association with vasculitis in humans. It is noteworthy that many reports in the literature describe isolated cases or small series of patients with vasculitis and simultaneous viral infection, where the responsibility of the virus producing vascular injury remains frequently unproved. In most instances, it is difficult to entirely fulfill the original Koch's postulates that stated: (1) the infectious organism has to be isolated from the appropriate tissue, (2) the same disease has to occur following the inoculation of a suitable animal, and (3) immunity against the agent has to appear as a consequence of the infection. Furthermore, as far as viral infections are concerned, these postulates may not be entirely suitable. As a matter of fact, all studies that prove pathogenicity of hepatitis C virus (HCV) infection have been done without ever isolating the virus. On the other hand, the isolation of any pathogen from a tissue shows that it is present, but not necessarily proves that it induces the disease. Even the appearance of antiviral antibodies in the serum of a patient with vasculitis may become misleading post hoc propter hoc evidence. Definitely more reliable evidence of the causal role of a virus is obtained when the intact virion or its constituents, such as antigens or nucleic acids, are precisely identified in specific tissue lesions, using electron microscopy, immunofluorescence, immunohistochemistry, or in situ hybridization (ISH) techniques. In several cases, improvement following specific antiviral therapy has lent strong, albeit indirect, support to clinical, epidemiological, and serological suspicion of virus-associated vasculitis (12,20).

A number of immunological and nonimmunological pathogenetic mechanisms could be potentially responsible for virus-related inflammatory vascular disease (Table 2). As will be seen, it is possible that in some viral infections more than one mechanism may be operating simulta-

Table 1 Viral Agents Associated with Human Vasculitides

Hepatitis viruses
   Hepatitis A virus (HAV)
   Hepatitis B virus (HBV)
   Hepatitis C virus (HCV)
Retroviruses
   Human immunodeficiency virus (HIV)
   Human T-cell lymphotropic virus type I (HTLV1)
Herpesviruses
   Cytomegalovirus (CMV)
   Epstein–Barr virus (EBV)
   Varicella zoster virus (VZV)
   Herpes simplex virus (HSV)
Enteroviruses
   Echovirus 9
   Poliovirus 1
   Coxsackieviruses B3 and B4
Parvovirus B 19
Rubella virus
Influenza virus

neously or alternatively. It is also important to remember that similar pathological pictures (e.g., cutaneous leukocytoclastic vasculitis) may be caused by different viruses, and the same pathogen may produce various vasculitic syndromes (21). However, viruses are commonly thought to induce vasculitis basically in two ways: (1) direct vessel wall infection and (2) vascular injury mediated by immune complexes (ICs). The direct cytopathogenic effect of viruses or the deposition of immune reactants within the vessel wall should be viewed as initial events that prime and activate endothelium. Subsequently, pathways of inflammation, necrosis, and occlusion are initiated, leading to impairment of blood flow, loss of vascular integrity, and eventually organ dysfunction (Fig. 1).

II. DIRECT VESSEL WALL INFECTION

It has been demonstrated that a number of human and animal viruses can infect endothelial cells (ECs) both in vivo and in vitro (3,5,8–10,16,22,23). In vitro experiments show that viral infec-

Table 2 Possible Mechanisms of Vascular Injury in Viral Diseases[a]

1. Circulating immune complexes of viral antigens and antiviral antibodies
2. In situ formation of immune complexes of viral antigens and antiviral antibodies
3. Circulating immune complexes containing endogenous antigens released by virus-injured cells and host autoantibodies
4. Cell-mediated immunity to viral antigens deposited in the vessel wall
5. Virus-induced autoimmunity against vascular components (e.g., molecular mimicry, induction of self-reactive B or T cells, activation of idiotype–antiidiotype networks)
6. Virus-induced release of cytokines, adhesion molecules, and/or other mediators
7. Direct cytopathogenic effect of the virus on endothelial or other blood vessel cells

[a]Mechanisms may not be mutually exclusive.

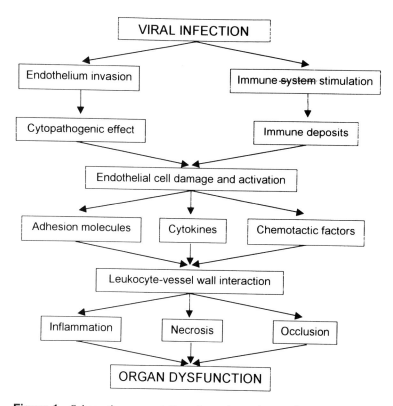

Figure 1 Schematic representation of putative pathogenetic steps in virus-associated vasculitis.

tions may profoundly alter EC function. This functional derangement could stimulate the adhesion of leukocytes to ECs and their migration through the vessel wall, foster the deposition of ICs, and convert the endothelium to a prothrombotic phenotype (22–24). Viruses can also infect other cellular components of the blood vessel wall, particularly smooth muscle cells (SMCs), which then become targets for antiviral immune responses.

A. Animal Models

Among animal models of vasculitis, *equine viral arteritis* has long been recognized as a typical example of virus-induced direct vascular injury (8,10). The disease presents as an acute viral infection of horses associated with a widespread severe vasculitis. A few days after infection, ECs throughout the vasculature show evident microscopic changes that are rapidly followed by leukocyte infiltration and fibrinoid necrosis of the intima and the media. Viral antigen is initially detectable by immunofluorescence in ECs and a few days later in SMCs of the media. Immune mechanisms of vascular injury have not been found in this model of vasculitis.

Infection of genetically susceptible newborn chickens with the *herpesvirus* responsible for *neurolymphomatosis* or *Marek's disease* has been shown to cause a vasculitic process with some similarities to atherosclerosis (25). Some SMCs within atherosclerosis-like proliferative plaques have been found positive for viral antigen or viral DNA by immunofluorescence or ISH, respectively. In contrast, immune deposits were not detectable in the vessel wall by immunohistochemistry. The model of vasculitis induced by Marek's virus brings up the controversial subject of relationship between infectious agents and atherosclerotic vascular disease, which is discussed in other chapters of this book. Other models of inflammatory vascular disease induced by a variety of herpesviruses have been developed in mice (26). Some interesting results of these studies could be helpful in elucidating the pathogenesis of virus-induced human vasculitis: (1) different viruses may cause similar lesions, (2) besides ECs, SMCs, monocytes, and macrophages are targets of viral infection, and (3) interferon-γ and B and T cells play important roles in the generation of vascular inflammation.

B. Human Vasculitides

Similarly to the above-mentioned animal models, various *herpesviruses* have been implicated in many cases of human vasculitis probably due to direct infection of vessel wall (3,5,16–18). Most of these viruses are ubiquitous agents that under conditions of altered host defenses (either acquired or congenital) are capable of inducing inflammatory vascular disease.

Herpes zoster ophthalmicus is occasionally complicated by delayed contralateral hemiparesis owing to cerebral infarction in the internal carotid artery territory. In this condition, the angiographic findings are suggestive of vasculitis in the proximal branches of the anterior or middle cerebral artery (3,27), while pathological studies reveal a necrotizing vasculitis with characteristic granulomatous infiltrates mainly involving the adventitia and intima of small vessels (28,29). This vasculitis could be due to direct invasion of the arteries by *varicella zoster virus* (VZV), but histological evidence has been lacking in most cases. Quite similar vascular lesions have been found in a relatively rare form of vasculitis called primary angiitis of the central nervous system, raising the possibility that at least some cases of this disease may be related to VZV infection. Interestingly, in a patient who was presumed to have primary angiitis of the central nervous system, in the absence of clinical manifestations of VZV infection, a restudy of pathological material demonstrated both VZV DNA and VZV-specific antigen in three of five cerebral arteries (30).

In addition, a recent report on six immunocompromised patients provides radiological, pathological, and virological documentation indicating that VZV encephalitis is predominantly a vasculopathy involving small and large vessels (18). Finally, the relatively frequent association of VZV with cutaneous leukocytoclastic vasculitis demonstrates that the inflammatory vascular disease induced by this pathogen is not confined to the central nervous system or restricted to eliciting only a granulomatous inflammatory response (31).

Cytomegalovirus (CMV) is a member of the herpesvirus family that has been shown to persist in a latent state in the great majority of healthy subjects. However, the virus is a major cause of morbidity and mortality in immunocompromised patients, especially in transplant recipients receiving immunosuppressive therapy and in patients with acquired immunodeficiency syndrome (AIDS). Cytomegalovirus appears to have a specific tropism for vascular endothelium and has been suspected to cause vasculitis predominantly involving small and medium-sized vessels in the gastrointestinal tract, skin, and central nervous system (5,10,16). Cytomegalovirus infection characteristically induces ballooning of ECs with intranuclear or intracytoplasmic inclusions surrounded by a halo (owl eye appearance). In fully expressed CMV vasculitis, EC abnormalities are accompanied by inflammatory infiltrates and necrosis of the vessel wall, along with intraluminal fibrin thrombi. Aiming to study the sequence of histopathological events in CMV vasculitis, a rat model of CMV infection has been developed recently (32). In this experimental model, endothelial ballooning and leukocyte adhesion, interpreted as signs of early activation of ECs, appear prior to detectable infection of these cells. These findings suggest that endothelial activation does not necessarily require direct invasion of ECs. Inflammatory infiltrates of blood vessels consisted mainly of mononuclear cells, many of which were infected with CMV. Since even mononuclear cells in the peripheral blood were infected with CMV, one may postulate that these cells are implicated in both transport of CMV throughout the body and transmission of infection to ECs, as has been suggested by in vitro experiments (33). It is also possible that CMV had infected circulating monocytes and by increasing the production of cytokines, caused extensive activation of ECs. Current evidence points to a direct cytopathogenic effect on ECs as a major pathophysiological mechanism of CMV-associated vasculitis. Nonetheless, the capability of this virus to induce the formation of serum cryoglobulins may occasionally also lead to an IC-mediated vasculitis (34).

III. IMMUNE COMPLEX-MEDIATED VASCULITIS

It is commonly thought that all or nearly all viral infections lead to the formation of circulating ICs. Considering the extremely frequent occurrence of viral infection, the relative rarity of overt vasculitis or other IC-mediated diseases is surprising. Under normal conditions, ICs are rapidly cleared from the circulation by complement-dependent mechanisms. Immune complexes containing IgG or IgM activate complement through the classical pathway and then incorporate C3b, which in turn binds to the complement receptor-1 (CR1) on erythrocytes. The erythrocyte-bound ICs are transported to the liver and spleen where they are eliminated by Kupffer's cells and macrophages. The deposition of virus-induced ICs within the vessel wall may depend on several factors (35,36): (1) persistence of active viral infection, which promotes continuous formation of ICs exceeding the removal capacity by the reticuloendothelial system; (2) characteristics of ICs, such as size, charge, and composition (large-lattice ICs, presence of cationized antibodies, and slight antigen excess facilitate their deposition); (3) increased vascular permeability that is usually mediated by vasoactive amines released from platelets or basophils; (4) presence of virus-induced endothelial receptors for the Fc portion of IgG (Fcγ) and for complement component C3b; and (5) systemic and local hemodynamic factors.

Once the ICs are deposited, vessel injury can be generated by many different mechanisms (37). Among these, the ability of ICs to activate complement seems to be of primary importance. In fact, complement activation is able to damage ECs via formation of the C5b-9 membrane attack complex and to produce chemotactic factors such as C3a and C5a (anaphylatoxins) that attract leukocytes and stimulate the clotting and kinin systems. In addition, ICs deposited within vascular walls can directly bind to Fcγ receptors present on inflammatory cells. Activation of ECs and leukocytes induces increased expression and release of adhesion molecules and cytokines. Subsequently, activated leukocytes adhering to the endothelial surface penetrate the vessel wall where they phagocytose the deposited ICs and release lysosomal enzymes, oxygen radicals, and arachidonic acid metabolites. These and other toxic mediators, as well as the activated components of the extrinsic arm of the coagulation cascade, are likely to lead to the final phase of the vasculitic process.

A. Animal Models

Aleutian disease of mink is a chronic viral infection associated with severe vasculitis and glomerulonephritis (8). In this disease, an IC-mediated pathogenesis is suggested by the presence of virus-induced circulating ICs and, what is more important, by the detection of IgG, C3, and Aleutian disease virus antigen in affected vessels (38). Additional supportive evidence for the role of immune-mediated injury is the observation that immunosuppressive therapy with cyclophosphamide prevents the vasculitis, in spite of persisting viral infection (39).

A systemic vasculitis mainly affecting small blood vessels has been recently described in swine under the name of dermatitis/nephropathy syndrome (40). The disease has been associated with infection by *porcine reproductive and respiratory syndrome virus* (PRRSV), a member of the Arteriviridae. Necrotizing and leukocytoclastic vasculitis accompanied by deposition of immunoglobulins and complement in and around necrotic vessels has been demonstrated in the early stages of the disease, suggesting IC-mediated mechanisms (41). The PRRSV antigens have been detected by immunohistochemistry within macrophages infiltrating perivascular areas, but not in the vessel wall. In pigs experimentally infected with PRRSV, vascular lesions have been found 14 days postinoculation, a time interval consistent with generation and deposition of ICs, but again PRRSV antigen staining was not evident (42). These conflicting results do not exclude that the PRRSV-related vasculitis is IC-mediated. However, a direct cytopathogenic effect of PRRSV on ECs should also be considered since the agent of equine viral arteritis that belongs to the same family of Arteriviridae likely causes vasculitis through this mechanism.

B. Human Vasculitides

A form of necrotizing vasculitis mimicking polyarteritis nodosa (PAN) that usually manifests several weeks to months after *hepatitis B virus* (HBV) infection was recognized almost 30 years ago (1,2,12). The prevalence of this association, accounting for over 30% of all cases of PAN in the early 1980s has been declining to less than 10% in recent years (43), probably due to more effective screening of blood donors and the development of an HBV vaccine. However, following the initial descriptions of HBV-related PAN, it became evident that various vasculitic syndromes may appear in association with HBV infection. The clinical manifestations of acute hepatitis B are frequently preceded by a prodromal syndrome similar to serum sickness, including fever, arthralgia or arthritis, urticaria or purpura, and glomerulonephritis. In some of these cases, the histopathological study of skin lesions revealed small-vessel vasculitis mainly involving postcapillary venules (44,45). In both PAN and small-vessel vasculitis accompanying HBV infection, features suggestive of virus-induced IC disease have been found (1,44,45): (1) circulating complexes of hepatitis B surface antigen (HbsAg), antibody (HbsAb), and complement; (2) serum cryoglobulins containing these ICs; (3) hypocomplementemia due to activation of both classical and alternative pathways; and (4) HbsAg, HbsAb, complement components, immunoglobulins (especially IgM), or viral particles detected by immunofluorescence, immunohistochemistry or electron microscopy in vascular lesions. Moreover, successful treatment of HBV-related PAN with antiviral drugs alone or in combination with plasma exchange has been reported (12,46).

Several lines of evidence indicate a pathogenetic relationship between *hepatitis C virus* (HCV) infection and essential mixed cryoglobulinemia, a systemic vasculitic disorder associated with the presence in the serum of cryoprecipitable ICs consisting of polyclonal IgG bound to either polyclonal or monoclonal IgM with rheumatoid factor activity. The great majority of patients with mixed cryoglobulinemia have antibodies to HCV and have HCV RNA in the serum, while serum cryoglobulins are detectable in a large proportion of patients with chronic hepatitis C (13,14,47). These observations suggest that the production of cryoglobulins is a consequence of HCV infection, probably by an antigen-driven benign proliferation of B cells (48). This hypothesis is indirectly supported by the results of treatment with different antiviral drugs, showing that marked reduction and even disappearance of cryoglobulins regularly follows the clearance of HCV from the serum (20,49,50), as shown in Figure 2. There is also evidence that HCV could be directly or indirectly responsible for the cutaneous vasculitic syndrome of mixed cryoglobuline-

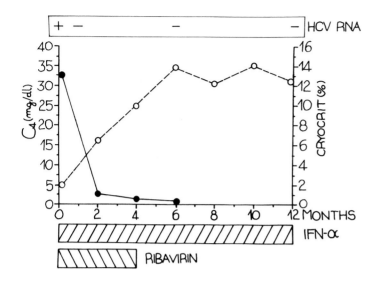

Figure 2 Effects of combined treatment with interferon-α and ribavirin in a patient with HCV-associated mixed cryoglobulinemia. Following the clearance of HCV RNA from the serum, cryoglobulins remarkably decline and become no longer detectable after six months. Simultaneously, the levels of C4 rapidly return to normal. ——— and – – – – indicate cryocrit and serum levels of C4, respectively.

mia. In fact, HCV antigens and HCV RNA have been found in vasculitic skin lesions by immunohistochemistry and ISH, respectively (51,52). The demonstration that HCV RNA is frequently concentrated in cryoprecipitate and that immunoglobulin components of cryoglobulins along with C3 and HCV RNA are detected at the same sites of vessel damage suggests that cutaneous vasculitis could be caused by the deposition of cryoprecipitable HCV-containing ICs. However, this interpretation is in contrast with the lack of direct relationship between the amount of cryoglobulins and clinical manifestations of vasculitis. In addition, cryoglobulins that precipitate in the form of ICs at 4°C usually circulate as monomeric IgG and IgM in the serum at 37°C. On the basis of these findings, it has been suggested that cutaneous vasculitis is mediated by ICs formed in situ from components of the cryoglobulins circulating in a dissociated state (48).

Deposits of IgM and C3 are commonly detected in glomerular lesions of patients with membranoproliferative glomerulonephritis and HCV-associated mixed cryoglobulinemia. However, only one study shows the presence of HCV antigens in glomeruli by immunohistochemistry (53), while ISH failed to detect HCV RNA (54). In an attempt to explain these conflicting results, some authors, on the basis of experimental evidence, suggest that cryoglobulinemic glomerulonephritis could be the consequence of HCV-induced production of monoclonal IgM that forms in situ ICs by binding to mesangial cell fibronectin (55).

Another controversial subject is whether the vasculitis causing peripheral neuropathy in HCV-related mixed cryoglobulinemia is an IC-mediated condition. As a matter of fact, the deposition of immunoglobulins and complement has been infrequently detected in damaged vessels, and in a preliminary study, the search for HCV RNA by ISH assay provided negative results (48). In addition, the inflammatory infiltrate in epineurial vessels has been found to be composed mostly of monocytes and T lymphocytes (56), in contrast with the cutaneous vasculitis where the predominant cells characteristically are polymorphonuclear leukocytes. Thus, the vasculitis of cryoglobulinemic neuropathy is likely to be dependent mainly on cell-mediated immune mechanisms, as described in other vasculitic neuropathies (57). From all these studies, it appears that HCV is capable of triggering different pathophysiological processes leading to multiple pathological and clinical expressions of inflammatory vascular disease.

A variety of vasculitic syndromes have been described in patients with *human immunodeficiency virus* infection. In many of these patients, vasculitis is due to other viral or nonviral infectious agents, including HBV, HCV, CMV, VZV, *Mycobacterium tuberculosis, Aspergillus, Cryptococcus, Candida albicans,* and *Toxoplasma* (15,21,58). Clearly, the identification of one of these pathogens in a patient with AIDS and vasculitis offers the chance of a more specific therapeutic approach. For the same reason, it is important to recognize drug-induced vasculitis or vasculopathy secondary to lymphoma. Even when HIV itself is the likely cause of inflammatory vascular disease, several pathological and clinical expressions may be observed. Indeed, polyarteritis nodosa, leukocytoclastic vasculitis, Henoch–Schönlein purpura, isolated angiitis of the central nervous system, erythema elevatum diutinum, Kawasaki disease, and other forms of vasculitis have been reported. It is possible that different pathogenetic mechanisms underlie all these vasculitic syndromes.

Several features suggestive of IC-mediated disease have been reported in patients with HIV-associated vasculitis: (1) circulating ICs of HIV antigens and antibodies (59), (2) mixed cryoglobulins containing antibodies to HIV and HIV-1 RNA sequences (60), (3) deposits of IgM and complement in vascular lesions of patients with necrotizing and nonnecrotizing vasculitis (15), and (4) vascular deposits of IgA and C3 in skin biopsies of patients with Henoch–Schönlein purpura (61).

The identification of HIV-1 in ECs (62) could suggest a direct cytopathogenic effect of the virus on the vessel wall, a mechanism possibly implicated in the pathogenesis of cerebral aneurysms and arteriopathy occurring in children with longstanding AIDS (63). Experimental evidence supporting an alternative disease mechanism comes from a recently developed model of HIV-associated vasculopathy in transgenic mice (64). The vascular lesions seen in these mice are characterized by marked SMC proliferation involving the media and the intima, along with an infiltrate composed mainly of T cells and localized primarily to the adventitia. Most interestingly, viral transcripts have been identified in SMCs but not in lymphocytes, suggesting that the infiltration of T cells is not the initial event in this condition. Another intriguing observation in this experimental model of HIV-associated vasculopathy is that the endothelium did not appear to express HIV genes or be involved in the pathological process.

REFERENCES

1. Gocke DJ, Hsu K, Morgan C, Bombardieri S, Lockshin M, Christian CL. Association between polyarteritis and Australia antigen. Lancet 1970; ii:1149–1153.
2. Trepo CG, Thivolet J. Hepatitis associated antigen and periarteritis nodosa (PAN). Vox Sanguinis 1970; 19:410–411.
3. Gilbert GJ. Herpes zoster ophthalmicus and delayed contralateral hemiparesis. JAMA 1974; 229: 302–304.
4. Larson A, Forsgren M, Hard AF, Segerstad H, Strauder H, Cantrell K. Administration of interferon to an infant with congenital rubella syndrome involving persistent viremia and cutaneous vasculitis. Acta Ped Scand 1976; 65:105–110.
5. Minars N, Silverman JF, Escobar MR, Martinez AJ. Fatal cytomegalic inclusion disease. Arch Dermatol 1977; 113:1569–1571.
6. Hoffman JS, Franck WA. Infectious mononucleosis, autoimmunity and vasculitis. JAMA 1979; 241: 2735–2736.
7. Oldstone MB, Dixon FJ. Pathogenesis of chronic disease associated with persistent lymphocytic chori-

omeningitis viral infection. II. Relationship of the anti lymphocytic choriomeningitis immune response to tissue injury in chronic lymphocytic choriomeningitis disease. J Exp Med 1970; 131:1–19.

8. Henson JB, Crawford TB. The pathogenesis of virus-induced arterial disease. Aleutian disease and equine viral arteritis. Adv Cardiol 1974; 13:183–191.

9. Wilczynski SP, Cook ML, Stevens JG. Newcastle disease as a model for paramyxovirus induced neurologic syndromes. II. Detailed characterization of encephalitis. Am J Pathol 1977; 89:649–662.

10. Sergent JS. Vasculitides associated with viral infections. Clin Rheum Dis 1980; 6:339–350.

11. Ilan Y, Hillman M, Oren R, Zlotogorski A, Shonval D. Vasculitis and cryoglobulinemia associated with persisting cholestatic hepatitis A virus infection. Am J Gastroenterol 1990; 85:586–587.

12. Guillevin L, Lhote F, Cohen P, Sauvaget F, Jarrousse B, Lortholary O, Noel LH, Trepo C. Polyarteritis nodosa related to hepatitis B virus. A prospective study with long term observation of 41 patients. Medicine 1995; 74:238–253.

13. Misiani R, Bellavita P, Fenili D, Borelli G, Marchesi D, Massazza M, Vendramin G, Comotti B, Tanzi E, Scudeller G, Zanetti A. Hepatitis C virus infection in patients with essential mixed cryoglobulinemia. Ann Intern Med 1992; 119:573–577.

14. Agnello V, Chung RT, Kaplan LM. A role for hepatitis C virus infection in type II cryoglobulinemia. N Engl J Med 1992; 327:1490–1495.

15. Gherardi R, Belec L, Mhiri C, Gray F, Lescs MC, Sobel A, Guillevin L, Wechsler J. The spectrum of vasculitis in human immunodeficiency virus-infected patients. Arthritis Rheum 1993; 36:1164–1174.

16. Golden MP, Scott MH, Wanke CA, Albrecht MA. Cytomegalovirus vasculitis. Case reports and review of the literature. Medicine 1994; 73:246–253.

17. Murakami K, Ohsawa M, Hu SX, Kanno H, Aozasa K, Nose M. Large vessel arteritis associated with chronic active Epstein-Barr virus infection. Arthritis Rheum 1998; 41:369–373.

18. Amlie-Lefond C, Kleinschmidt-Demasters BK, Mahalingam R, Davis LE, Gilden DH. The vasculopathy of varicella-zoster virus encephalitis. Ann Neurol 1995; 37:784–790.

19. Lhote F, Guillevin L. Polyarteritis nodosa, microscopic polyangiitis, and Churg-Strauss syndrome. Clinical aspects and treatment. Rheum Dis Clin North Am 1995; 21:911–947.

20. Misiani R, Bellavita P, Fenili D, Vicari O, Marchesi D, Sironi P, Zilio P, Vernocchi A, Massazza M, Vendramin G, Tanzi E, Zanetti A. Interferon alpha-2a therapy in cryoglobulinemia associated with hepatitis C virus. N Engl J Med 1994; 330:751–756.

21. Somer T, Finegold SM. Vasculitides associated with infections, immunization, and antimicrobial drugs. Clin Infect Dis 1995; 20:1010–1036.

22. Friedman HM. Infection of endothelial cells by common human viruses. Rev Infect Dis 1989; 11(suppl 4):S700–704.

23. Beilke MA. Vascular endothelium in immunology and infectious disease. Rev Infect Dis 1989; 11: 273–283.

24. Vercellotti GM. Effects of viral activation of the vessel wall on inflammation and thrombosis. Blood Coagul Fibrinol 1998; 2(suppl):S3–6.

25. Fabricant CG. Atherosclerosis: The consequence of infection with a herpesvirus. Adv Vet Sci Comp Med 1985; 30:39–66.

26. Dal Canto AJ, Virgin HW. Animal models of infection-mediated vasculitis. Curr Opin Rheumatol 1999; 11:17–23.

27. Walker RJ, Gammal TE, Allen MB. Cranial arteritis associated with herpes zoster. Case report with angiographic findings. Radiology 1975; 107:109–110.

28. Rosenblum WI, Hadfield MG. Granulomatous angiitis of the nervous system in cases of herpes zoster and lymphosarcoma. Neurology 1972; 22:348–354.

29. Kolodny EH, Rebeiz JJ, Caviness VS Jr, Richardson EP. Granulomatous angiitis of the central nervous system. Arch Neurol 1968; 19:510–524.

30. Gilden D, Kleinschmide-Demasters B, Wellish M, Hedley-White E, Rentier B, Mahalingam R. Varicella zoster virus, a cause of waxing and waning vasculitis: The New England Journal of Medicine case 5-1995 revisited. Neurology 1996; 47:1441–1446.

31. Penneys N. Diseases caused by viruses. In: Elder D, Elenitsas R, Jaworsky C, Johnson B Jr. Lever's Hystopathology of the Skin. 8th ed. Philadelphia: Lippincott-Raven, 1997:569–589.

32. Persoons MCJ, Stals FS, Stals FS, Van Dam-Mieras MCE, Bruggeman CA. Multiple organ involve-

ment during experimental cytomegalovirus infection is associated with disseminated vascular pathology. J Pathol 1998; 184:103–109.

33. Waldman WJ, Knight DA, Huang EH, Sedmak DD. Bidirectional transmission of infectious cytomegalovirus between monocytes and vascular endothelial cells: An in vitro model. J Infect Dis 1995; 171:263–272.

34. Wager O, Rasanen JA, Hagman A, Klemola E. Mixed cryoimmunoglobulinemia infectious mononucleosis and cytomegalovirus mononucleosis. Int Arch Allergy Appl Immun 1968; 34:345–361.

35. Moore PM. Immune mechanisms in the primary and secondary vasculitides. J Neurol Sci 1989; 93: 129–145.

36. Mannik M. Experimental models for immune complex-mediated vascular inflammation. Acta Med Scand 1987; 715:145–155.

37. Sneller MC, Fauci AS. Pathogenesis of vasculitis syndromes. Med Clin North Am 1997; 81:221–242.

38. Henson JB, Gorham JR. Animal models of human disease. Am J Pathol 1973; 71:345–348.

39. Cheema A, Henson JB, Gorham JR. Aleutian disease of mink: Prevention of lesions by immunosuppression. Am J Pathol 1972; 66:543–552.

40. Smith WJ, Thomson JR, Done S. Dermatitis/nephropathy syndrome of pigs. Vet Ric 1993; 132:47.

41. Thibault S, Drolet R, Germain MC, D'Allaire S, Larochelle R, Magar R. Cutaneous and systemic necrotizing vasculitis in swine. Vet Pathol 1998; 35:108–116.

42. Cooper VL, Hesse RA, Doster AR. Renal lesions associated with experimental porcine reproductive and respiratory syndrome virus (PRRSV) infection. J Vet Diagn Invest 1997; 9:198–201.

43. Guillevin L, Lhote F, Gerardi R. The spectrum and treatment of virus-associated vasculitides. Curr Opin Rheumatol 1997; 9:31–36.

44. Gower RG, Sausker WF, Cohler PF, Thorne GE, McIntosh RM. Small vessel vasculitis caused by hepatitis B immune complexes. J Allergy Clin Immunol 1978; 62:222–228.

45. Dienstag JL, Rhodes AR, Bhan AK, Dvorak AM, Mihm MC, Wans JR. Urticaria associated with acute viral hepatitis type B. Studies and pathogenesis. Ann Intern Med 1978; 89:34–40.

46. Simsek H, Telatan H. Successful treatment of hepatitis B virus associated polyarteritis nodosa by interferon alpha alone. J Clin Gastroenterol 1995; 20:263–265.

47. Lunel F, Musset L, Cacoub P, Frangeul L, Cresta P, Perrin M, Grippon P, Hoang C, Valla D, Piette JC, Huraux J, Opolon P. Cryoglobulinemia in chronic liver disease: Role of hepatitis C virus and liver damage. Gastroenterology 1994; 106:1291–1300.

48. Agnello V. The etiology and pathophysiology of mixed cryoglobulinemia secondary to hepatitis C virus infection. Springer Semin Immunopathol 1997; 19:111–129.

49. Durand JM, Cacoub P, Lunel-Fabiani F, Cosserat J, Cretel E, Kaplansky G, Frances C, Bletry O, Soubeyrand J, Godeau P. Ribavirin in hepatitis C related cryoglobulinemia. J Rheumatol 1998; 25: 1115–1117.

50. Misiani R, Bellavita P, Baio P, Caldara R, Ferruzzi S, Rossi P, Tengattini F. Successful treatment of HCV-associated cryoglobulinaemic glomerulonephritis with a combination of interferon-α and ribavirin. Nephrol Dial Transplant 1999; 14:1558–1560.

51. Sansonno D, Cornacchiulo V, Lacobelli AR, Di Stefano R, Lospalluti M, Dammacco F. Localization of hepatitis C virus antigens in liver and skin tissues of chronic hepatitis C virus-infected patients with mixed cryoglobulinemia. Hepatology 1995; 21:305–312.

52. Agnello W, Abel G. Localization of hepatitis C virus in cutaneous vasculitic lesions in patients with type II mixed cryoglobulinemia using in situ hybridization. Arthritis Rheum 1997; 40:2007–2015.

53. Sansonno D, Gesualdo L, Manno C, Schena FP, Dammacco F. Hepatitis C virus-related proteins in kidney tissue from hepatitis C virus infected patients with cryoglobulinemic membranoproliferative glomerulonephritis. Hepatology 1997; 25:1237–1244.

54. Agnello W, Abel G, Knight GB, Zhang QX, Elfahal M, Confalonieri R, Montoli A, Muchmore E. The role of hepatitis C virus in the pathogenesis of type II cryoglobulinemia. Keystone Symposia on hepatitis C and Beyond. Burlington, Vermont, 1995; Abstract 7.

55. Fornasieri A, Armelloni S, Bernasconi P, Li M, Pinerolo De Septis C, Sinico RA, D'Amico G. High binding of immunoglobulin MK rheumatoid factor from type II cryoglobulins to cellular fibronectin.

A mechanism for induction of in situ immune complex glomerulonephritis? Am J Kidney Dis 1996; 27:476–483.

56. Bonetti B, Invernizzi F, Rizzuto N, Bonazzi ML, Zanusso GL, Chinaglia G, Monaco S. T-cell mediated epineurial vasculitis and humoral mediated microangiopathy in cryoglobulinemic neuropathy. J Neuroimmunol 1997; 73:145–154.

57. Satoi H, Oka N, Kawasaki T, Miyamoto K, Akiguchi I, Kimura J. Mechanism of tissue injury in vasculitic neuropathies. Neurology 1998; 50:492–496.

58. Mandel BF, Calabrese LH. Infections and systemic vasculitis. Curr Opin Rheumatol 1998; 10:51–57.

59. Morrow WJW, Wharton M, Stricker RB, Levy JA. Circulating immune complexes in patients with acquired immunodeficiency syndrome contain the AIDS-associated retrovirus. Clin Immunol Immunopathol 1986; 40:515–524.

60. Dimitrakopoulos AN, Kordossis T, Hatzakis A, Moutsopoulos HM. Mixed cryoglobulinemia in HIV-1 infection: the role of HIV-1. Ann Intern Med 1999; 130:226–230.

61. Hall TN, Brennan B, Leahy MF, Woodroffe AJ. Henoch-Schönlein purpura associated with immunodeficiency virus infection. Nephrol Dial Transplant 1998; 13:988–990.

62. Bagasra O, Lavi E, Bobroski L, Khalili K, Pestaner JP, Tawadros R, Pomerantz RJ. Cellular reservoirs of HIV-1 in the central nervous system of infected individuals: Identification by the combination of in situ polymerase chain reaction and immunohistochemistry. AIDS 1996; 10:573–585.

63. Dubrovski T, Curless R, Scott G, Chaneless M, Post MJD, Altmann N, Petito CK, Start D, Wood C. Cerebral aneurismal arteriopathy in childhood AIDS. Neurology 1998; 51:560–565.

64. Tinkle BT, Ngo L, Luciw PA, Maciag T, Gilbert J. Human immunodeficiency virus-associated vasculopathy in transgenic mice. J Virol 1997; 71:4809–4814.

39
Virus-Associated Vasculitides: Clinical Aspects

Dimitrios Vassilopoulos and Leonard H. Calabrese
Cleveland Clinic Foundation, Cleveland, Ohio

I. INTRODUCTION

The association between certain viral infections and the development of vascular inflammation involving different size vessels has been well documented in the medical literature over the last 30 years. Since the initial observations of polyarteritis nodosa (PAN) associated with hepatitis B virus (HBV) infection in the early 70's (1,2), an increasing number of vasculitic syndromes developing during the course of an acute or chronic viral infection, have been reported (3–6). The expanding spectrum of viral association with certain vasculitic syndromes that were considered to be "idiopathic" is exemplified by the recent finding of the strong association between hepatitis C virus (HCV) infection and "essential" mixed cryoglobulinemia (EMC) (7).

Typically, virus-associated vasculitides involve small (postcapillary venules, capillaries, arterioles) or medium-sized vessels (Table 1). Rarely, cases of viral infections due to Epstein–Barr virus/human herpesvirus 4 (EBV), parvovirus (B19 virus) or HCV leading to large-vessel involvement have been described (see Table 1). Specific syndromes, such as retinal vasculitis or central nervous system (CNS) vasculitis, have also been related to certain viral infections (see Table 1).

In this chapter we describe the clinical manifestations, laboratory findings, and management of virus-associated vasculitides.

II. HEPATITIS B VIRUS

Two types of vasculitic syndromes can develop during the course of hepatitis B infection. An immune complex–mediated small-vessel vasculitis affecting mainly the skin has been described in the prodromal phase of acute hepatitis B infection ("serum sickness–like syndrome") (8,9) whereas a polyarteritis nodosa–like vasculitis with multisystem involvement is characteristically seen at the early stages of chronic HBV infection (8,10,11).

Table 1 Virus-Associated Vasculitic Syndromes According to Vessel Size and Specific Site of Involvement

Vessel size		
Small vessels	Medium vessels	Large vessels
HBV	HBV	EBV
HCV	HCV	Parvovirus
HIV	HIV	HCV
CMV	CMV	Coxsackie B4 virus (?)
Parvovirus	Parvovirus	
EBV		
HSV-1 or -2		
Rubella virus		
HAV		
Hantavirus		
HTLV-1		
Echovirus		
Coxsackie B1 virus		
Measles		

Specific site of involvement		
Retinal vasculitis	CNS vasculitis	Kawasaki disease
CMV	VZV	EBV
EBV	HSV	Parvovirus
HIV	CMV	Parainfluenza virus
HSV-1 and -2	HIV	Adenovirus
VZV	EBV	
Rubella	HTLV-1	
Coxsackie B virus		
HTLV-1		

[a]Abbreviations: HBV = hepatitis B virus, HCV = hepatitis C virus, HIV = human immunodeficiency virus-1, CMV = cytomegalovirus or human herpesvirus 5, EBV = Epstein-Barr virus or human herpesvirus 4, HSV-1 or -2 = herpes simplex virus type 1 or 2 or human herpesvirus 1 or 2, HAV = hepatitis A virus, HTLV-1 = human T-cell lymphotropic virus 1, VZV = varicella zoster virus or human herpesvirus 3, CNS = central nervous system.

A. Serum Sickness–Like Syndrome

1. Epidemiology

Five to fifteen percent of patients with acute hepatitis B infection develop a transient "serum sickness–like syndrome" consisting of fever, arthralgias, polyarthritis, rash, and occasionally small-vessel vasculitis affecting the skin (9,12). Usually the clinical manifestations appear days to few weeks prior to the onset of jaundice or other typical symptoms of acute hepatitis (Fig. 1).

2. Clinical Findings

The joint manifestations range from arthralgias to a symmetric "rheumatoid arthritis"–like inflammatory polyarthritis. Various forms of rash may accompany the arthritic symptoms, including urticaria, maculopapular rash, palpable purpura, petechial lesions, nodules, or erythematous plaques (9,13). In some cases, the rash may be the only extrahepatic manifestation of acute HBV

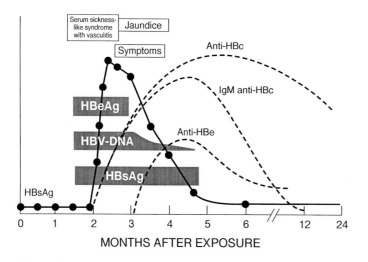

Figure 1 "Serum sickness–like syndrome" with associated vasculitis during acute hepatitis B infection. Abbreviations: HBsAg = hepatitis B surface antigen, HBV = hepatitis B virus, anti-HBe = antibodies against hepatitis B early antigen, anti-HBc = antibodies against hepatitis B core antigen. (Modified from Ref. 17.)

infection. Biopsy of the skin lesions usually reveals a lymphocytic venulitis or neutrophilic vasculitis of small vessels with associated leukocytoclasis or fibrinoid necrosis of the vessel wall (13). Few cases of HBV-associated Henoch-Schönlein purpura have been also reported (14), although their incidence appears to be low (15).

Circulating immune complexes (ICs) play a pivotal role in the pathogenesis of the syndrome. Immune complexes containing hepatitis B surface antigen (HBsAg) and antibodies against HBsAg (anti-HBs) have been demonstrated in the circulation, synovial tissue, and vessel walls (9). High titers of HBsAg and decreased complement levels are frequently detected in the circulation and synovial fluid of these patients. Immunofluorescent (IIF) studies of cutaneous vessels have revealed immunoglobulin G(IgG), IgM, or rarely IgA, complement (C3), and HBsAg, further substantiating the role of ICs in the development of this syndrome (16).

3. Laboratory Findings

Since the majority of the cases occur during the preicteric phase of acute HBV infection, the serological findings are compatible with acute hepatitis B (17). Typically, HBsAg, hepatitis B early antigen (HBeAg), and hepatitis B virus DNA (HBV DNA) are detected in the circulation. Immunoglobulin antibodies against the core antigen (IgM anti-HBc) usually appear with the onset of symptomatic hepatitis and may or may not be present. Complement levels (C3 and/or C4) are usually decreased and ICs can be found in the circulation (8).

Rarely, in cases that exhibit a more chronic course, serological findings suggestive of chronic hepatitis B can be found, including persistence of HBsAg, anti-HBc, and HBV DNA. Bonkovsky et al. (18) recently reported a case of a patient with chronic leukocytoclastic vasculitis associated with chronic HBV infection due to a precore mutant strain of HBV that lacked secretion of HBeAg.

4. Treatment

Typically, the skin and joint manifestations last 2–3 weeks and subside with the appearance of jaundice (12). As the clinical syndrome resolves, complement levels return to normal and HBsAg titers fall (19). Given the transient nature and favorable outcome of this syndrome, no specific therapy is required. Although unusual, cases of chronic leukocytoclastic vasculitis have been described (18,20). In the few cases associated with chronic HBV infection, antiviral therapy with or without immunosuppressive therapy may be warranted.

B.   Hepatitis B Virus–Associated Polyarteritis Nodosa

1.   Epidemiology

Hepatitis B virus–associated PAN is one of the best studied virus-associated vasculitic syndromes. In 1970, two groups of investigators separately reported the development of PAN in patients with hepatitis B infection (1,2). Since then, numerous studies have delineated the possible pathogenetic mechanisms, clinical manifestations, laboratory findings, and treatment options for this systemic vasculitis (8,10,11,21).

Epidemiological data concerning the incidence of HBV-associated PAN are limited. In a retrospective study from 266 HBsAg-positive patients undergoing hemodialysis, Drueke et al. (22) identified HBV-associated PAN in only 1.2% of the cases. In a study of an Alaskan population hyperendemic for HBV infection, the annual incidence of HBV-associated PAN was estimated at 7.7 cases per 100,000 (21). On the other hand, the frequency of HBV infection in patients with PAN varies among different studies from 10–35%. Although studies from France in the early 1980s revealed a 30% frequency of HBV infection in patients with PAN-like syndromes, recent data have shown a decline to 7% (11).

2.   Clinical Findings

(Hepatitis B virus–associated PAN usually develops the first 8–12 months following acute HBV infection (Fig. 2). In a recent large retrospective study from France, Guillevin et al. (11) found that 88% of the cases developed in less than 8 months after viral exposure. Similar findings have been reported by other authors (21,22). The clinical manifestations of HBV-associated PAN reflect the multisystemic nature of the disease (11). These may include constitutional symptoms,

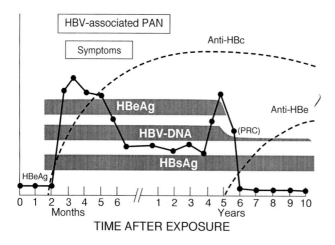

Figure 2   HBV-associated PAN during the course of chronic hepatitis B infection. Abbreviations: HBsAg = hepatitis B surface antigen, HBV = hepatitis B virus, HBeAg = hepatitis B early antigen, anti-Hbe = antibodies against HbeAg, anti-HBc = antibodies against hepatitis B core antigen, PCR = polymerase chain reaction. (Modified from Ref. 17.)

such as weight loss, fever, arthralgias/myalgias, peripheral neuropathy (mainly mononeuritis multiplex), renal insufficiency, ischemic abdominal pain, or hypertension (11).

Despite its initial explosive onset and multisystem involvement, HBV-associated PAN usually lasts only a few months. For patients who achieve remission after treatment, relapses rarely occur. The rate of relapse has been reported to be between 0–9% (10,11,21).

3. Laboratory Findings

Anemia, mild leukocytosis, thrombocytosis, and elevated erythrocyte sedimentation rate (ESR) are common nonspecific laboratory findings in these patients (8,10,11,21) (Table 2). Eosinophilia is present in approximately 19% of cases (8,10,11,21). Taking into account that most cases of HBV-associated PAN occur early in the course of chronic hepatitis (see Fig. 2), serological markers suggestive of early chronic hepatitis B infection are usually present (17). All patients are HBsAg-positive and the majority are HBeAg-positive. In some cases, IgM anti-HBc can be found, whereas moderate to high levels of circulating HBV DNA have been observed in approximately 80% of the cases (11). The presence of HBeAg and increased HBV DNA levels reflect an underlying active viral replication. Recently, a case of PAN associated with a precore mutant of HBV, characterized by the absence of circulating HBeAg and the presence of antibodies against HBeAg (anti-Be), was reported (23). Antineutrophil cytoplasmic antibodies (ANCAs) are rarely present (4%) (11).

Table 2   Clinical and Laboratory Findings in Patients with HBV-Associated PAN-Like Vasculitis[a]

Findings	%
Clinical	
Constitutional symptoms	
Weight loss	80
Fever	66
Arthralgias/arthritis	58
Myalgias	39
Specific organ involvement	
Peripheral neuropathy	66
Abdominal pain	46
Hypertension	46
Orchioepididymitis (males)	26
Renal failure	24
Purpura	22
Laboratory	
Elevated ESR	83
Low C3 or C4	71
Leukocytosis	68
Anemia	49
Eosinophilia	19

[a]Abbreviations: HBV = hepatitis B virus, PAN = polyarteritis nodosa, ESR = erythrocyte sedimentation rate, C3 or C4 = complement 3 or 4.
Source: Data from Refs. 8, 10, 11, and 21.

Abdominal or renal angiograms can reveal the characteristic microaneurysms or stenotic lesions of medium-sized vessels that are frequently seen in patients with classic PAN (11). Biopsies of affected organs usually demonstrate areas of segmental perivascular inflammation of small and medium-sized vessels (mainly arteries and arterioles) accompanied by fibrinoid necrosis alternating with areas of normal or fibrotic appearing vessels (10,11,21). Like the lesions seen in the "serum sickness–like" syndrome, deposition of HBsAg, complement, and immunoglobulins are found by IIF in the vascular wall, suggestive of an IC-mediated process (9). The exact host and/or virus-mediated mechanisms that differentially lead to a small-vessel vasculitis affecting predominantly the skin ("serum sickness–like" syndrome) vs. a multisystemic vasculitis affecting small and medium-sized arteries (PAN) have not been clearly delineated (9,24).

Biopsies of the livers from patients with HBV-associated PAN can display a variety of histological findings but the majority show evidence of chronic hepatitis ($\sim$70%), even though the vasculitis occurs early in the course of chronic HBV infection (9,11).

4. Treatment

Treatment of patients with HBV-associated PAN can be challenging. In patients with life- or major organ–threatening disease, corticosteroids with or without the addition of cytotoxic agents such as cyclophosphamide are needed. Use of these agents can lead to fulminant liver failure or even death, especially after their discontinuation, due to rebound viremia and enhanced host immune response against the virus (25–27). This effect has been mainly observed in HBV-positive patients receiving chemotherapy and attributed to corticosteroids in these regimens (28). Based on these observations, the inclusion of an antiviral agent in the therapeutic regimen would appear to be appropriate (6).

There have been no controlled studies in the treatment of HBV-associated PAN. Although case reports and small uncontrolled studies have suggested a favorable response to antiviral treatment alone (interferon $\pm$ famciclovir) (29–32) or to a combination of antiviral therapy and plasma exchanges (33), the combination of immunosuppressive therapy (corticosteroids and cyclophosphamide), antiviral agents, and plasma exchanges (8,10,11,21) is generally warranted to control this systemic vasculitis. Close monitoring of liver function and markers of viral replication is essential in patients treated in this manner.

The mortality rate of HBV-associated PAN ranges between 20 and 30% in different studies (8,10,11,21). In most cases, death was attributed to complications from the underlying vasculitic process (8,10,11,21), whereas only one patient died from fulminant hepatitis (6%) (11). These findings further emphasize the need for early aggressive immunosuppressive treatment.

III. HEPATITIS C VIRUS

Hepatitis C virus has been particularly associated with small-vessel vasculitis resulting from deposition of ICs containing cryoglobulins in the vessel wall (HCV-associated mixed cryoglobulinemia). Small studies or scattered case reports have indicated the occasional association of HCV with medium- (PAN-like) or large-vessel vasculitides.

A. Hepatitis C Virus–Associated Mixed Cryoglobulinemia

1. Epidemiology

Hepatitis C virus infection is currently one of the most common chronic infections in the United States and worldwide, representing a major public health problem. It has been estimated that approximately 1.8% of the U.S. and 3% of the world population is infected with HCV (34,35). Over the last decade, developments in HCV detection techniques and carefully performed epidemiological studies have identified a continuously expanding number of extrahepatic manifestations associated with this chronic liver infection (36). The association of HCV infection with approximately 80% of cases of mixed cryoglobulinemia (MC), previously referred as EMC, is one of the strongest and best studied (7,37,38). Despite the frequent presence of circulating cryoglobulins in 35–55% of patients with HCV infection (39), the incidence of HCV-associated cryoglobulinemic vasculitis is much lower. Although initial studies suggested a high prevalence of cryoglobulinemic vasculitis in patients with HCV infection (40), several recent studies have estimated this to range between 2–3% (41–45).

2. Clinical Findings

The manifestations of HCV-associated cryoglobulinemic vasculitis can range from leukocytoclastic vasculitis involving only the skin (purpura) to severe membranoproliferative glomerulonephritis (MPGN) leading to renal failure (39) (Table 3).

Purpura is the most common cutaneous finding of HCV-associated MC (82%) and usually represents the presenting feature of the syndrome (41,46). It is usually intermittent, located predominantly in the lower extremities. Other skin findings include leg ulcers, Raynaud's phenomenon, livedo reticularis, urticaria, and nodular lesions (41,42,46,47). Biopsy of the skin typically shows a leukocytoclastic vasculitis of the small vessels. Hepatitis C virus has been demonstrated by in situ hybridization (ISH) in the inflamed areas in the form of ICs with IgM or IgG, suggestive of an immune complex–mediated process (48).

Renal involvement occurs in approximately 34% of patients with HCV-associated MC (39). The majority of patients have circulating type II cryoglobulins (49). Histologically, the most commonly observed lesion is that of a MPGN with subendothelial deposits (49). Indirect immunofluorescence reveals IgG, IgM with rheumatoid factor activity (RF), and C3 deposits, whereas

Table 3 Clinical and Laboratory Findings of HCV-Associated Cryoglobulinemic Vasculitis (Mixed Cryoglobulinemia)[a]

Findings	%
Clinical	
Purpura	82
Weakness	42
Arthralgias	42
Liver involvement	42
Renal involvement	34
Peripheral neuropathy	26
Raynaud's phenomenon	22
Sicca symptoms	6
Laboratory	
Rheumatoid factor	80
Low C4	48–63
Elevated ESR	70
Anemia	70

[a]Abbreviations: ESR = erythrocyte sedimentation rate, C4 = complement 4.
Source: Data from Refs. 39, 50, and 257.

HCV RNA has not been detected (39,49). One-third of the kidney biopsies demonstrate a necrotizing vasculitis of the small and medium-sized renal arteries (even in the absence of glomerular involvement) (49). Hepatitis C virus–associated MPGN presents later than the other typical manifestations of MC (median delay = 4 years) (49,50). Clinically, patients present with hypertension (80%), renal failure (47%), proteinuria (55%), and nephritic (25%) or nephrotic (20%) syndrome. The disease usually follows an indolent course with rare progression to end-stage renal disease (15%) (49,50). By multivariate analysis, older age, low C3, purpura, splenomegaly, cryocrit level of >10%, and elevated serum creatinine (>1.5 mg/dL), were identified as independent predictors of a worse outcome (51).

A distal symmetric sensorimotor polyneuropathy is much more common (39,52–55) than mononeuritis multiplex (56). Electromyography (EMG) shows evidence of multifocal axonal degeneration. Nerve biopsy may show evidence of vasculitis (39,52–55). Immune complex and cell-mediated mechanisms have been implicated in the pathogenesis of the vasculitic lesions (55). Hepatitis C virus has not been identified in the biopsied lesions by ISH (39).

Polyarthralgias, involving mainly the hands and knees, are a common symptom, although inflammatory arthritis or radiographic evidence of erosive changes is rare (50). Whether the severity of liver involvement in patients with HCV-associated MC compared with patients with chronic hepatitis C without cryoglobulinemia differs, remains a controversial issue. The degree of liver inflammation and prevalence of cirrhosis varies significantly among different studies, and may be a function of patient selection bias (57).

3.   Laboratory Findings

The hallmark of HCV-associated MC is the presence of mixed (types II and III) cryoglobulins in the circulation. The majority of circulating cryoglobulins in HCV patients are type II (66%), containing a mixture of polyclonal IgG and monoclonal IgM with RF reactivity (39). Further analysis of the monoclonal RF in these patients revealed a predominance of the WA cross-idiotype (87%) (58). The pathogenesis of cryoglobulin formation is unclear but a direct role for HCV has been proposed through chronic polyclonal activation of B cells (58). Recent data indicating a correlation between disease duration and cryoglobulin formation further support this hypothesis (59). Still, the precise host or viral factors that lead to the development of vasculitis in only a small percentage of patients with HCV-associated cryoglobulinemia remain to be defined.

Other common laboratory findings in patients with HCV-associated MC include anemia (70%), presence of rheumatoid factor (80%), and low complement levels (50–60%) (see Table 3). Typically, the early components of the complement activation cascade are reduced (mainly C4), although C3 levels are frequently low and C3 is present in the glomerular deposits in patients with MPGN (49). The presence of various autoantibodies in patients with chronic hepatitis C infection has been well documented in the literature (36,60,61). However, no difference in the prevalence of autoantibodies between patients with or without mixed cryoglobulinemia has been detected (47,62). Nevertheless, the levels of RF are usually higher in patients with MC, probably reflecting the presence of circulating monoclonal or oligoclonal IgM with RF activity (60,63).

4.   Treatment

Treatment of severe EMC traditionally included a combination of corticosteroids, cytotoxic agents, and plasmapheresis (50,51). Bonomo et al. (65) in 1987 first reported a favorable response of seven patients with type II cryoglobulinemia to interferon-α (IFN-α) treatment (65). The discovery of the strong association between HCV and MC led to further studies that explored the potential therapeutic effect of antiviral agents. Following initial case reports that showed a beneficial effect of IFN-α (66), three controlled trials utilizing IFN-α showed clinical responses ranging from 53–62% in patients with symptomatic HCV-associated MC (67–69). Smaller uncontrolled studies using different IFN-α preparations in various doses and durations showed similar results (40,70–72). The results of these studies should be interpreted with caution since most of the patients had clinically mild disease, especially in regard to renal involvement. Despite these limitations, the results of these studies suggest that IFN-α alone is a moderately effective treatment of HCV-associated MC. Patients who clear HCV viremia during treatment are more likely to achieve a complete remission (69,72). Unfortunately, discontinuation of IFN-α therapy is followed by clinical and virological relapse in the majority of patients (69). In an uncontrolled study, longer duration of treatment and higher doses of IFN-α were associated with long-term responses (72).

Recent multicenter studies have indicated that the addition of ribavirin to IFN-α treatment enhances the rate of virological and biochemical response in patients with chronic hepatitis C. Although it appears logical that the combination of these 2 antiviral agents could be an effective treatment of HCV-associated MC, studies involving large numbers of patients are lacking so far. Interestingly, most of the patients with HCV-associated MC that responded to ribavirin received the agent as monotherapy (73–77).

Concerns regarding the use of immunosuppressive agents such as prednisone and/or cyclophosphamide in patients with MC are focused on their potential effects on liver function, viral replication, and malignant transformation of monoclonal or oligoclonal populations of B cells. D'Amico (49) did not observe any significant deterioration of liver function in over 100 treatment courses of various combinations of prednisone, cyclophosphamide, and plasmapheresis for patients with HCV-associated MPGN (49). In contrast to hepatitis B, case reports of fulminant hepatitis during or after withdrawal of high-dose immunosuppressive therapy have been scarcely reported in HCV infection (78–80).

Prednisone, when given for a short period of time (1–6 months) has been associated with reduction in serum transaminase levels. However, such treatment has been shown to increase viremia in patients with chronic hepatitis C (81–83). Despite these findings, rebound hepatitis has not been observed after completion of therapy. Furthermore, when corticosteroids were combined with IFN-α for 1 year in patients with HCV-associated MC, no elevation of HCV RNA levels or deterioration of liver function was detected (68).

Extrapolating from these limited data, certain recommendations regarding the treatment of HCV-associated MC can be made. For patients with mild disease without major organ involvement, such as skin disease, arthralgias, or GN with stable renal function, a trial of antiviral treatment such as IFN-α at a dose of 3 million units three times a week for 6–12 months is recommended. In patients with IFN-α–resistant manifestations, concomitant short courses of corticosteroids with rapid tapering may be warranted. For severe disease, such as MPGN with worsening renal function or nephrotic syndrome, digital necrotic ulcers, severe neuropathy (peripheral or central nervous system), or other major organ involvement (cardiac, gastrointestinal, etc.), combination therapy with corticosteroids, oral cyclophosphamide (2 mg/kg/day), plasmapheresis (3 times a week for 2–3 weeks), and antiviral treatment is appropriate (49). Close monitoring of liver function, HCV RNA levels and cell counts is essential in these patients. Physicians should also be aware that IFN-α, probably through its immunomodulatory or antiangiogenic properties, may occasionally lead to worsening of the MC manifestations (84–89). The role of other immunosuppressive (cyclosporine) (90,91) or antiviral (ribavirin) therapies remains to be defined.

B. Hepatitis C Virus–Associated Medium- and Large-Vessel Vasculitis

In contrast to the strong association between HCV and cryoglobulinemic vasculitis, HCV has been rarely associated with PAN-like vasculitis (8% in selected HCV-positive populations)

(92–94). A causal relationship cannot be clearly established since some of these patients were co-infected with HBV (92) or had evidence of cryoglobulinemia (94).

Ferracioli et al. (95) recently reported a case of a patient with HCV infection and classic temporal arteritis. Biopsy of the temporal artery revealed infiltration of the media by a mono-clonal B-cell population. A similar oligoclonal B-cell population was found in a salivary gland biopsy. Occasionally, involvement of the vasa vasorum of the temporal arteries in patients with HCV-associated MC can lead to a temporal arteritis-like clinical presentation (96).

IV. RETROVIRAL INFECTIONS

Among human retroviral infections, both the human immunodeficiency virus type 1 (HIV-1) and the human T-cell lymphotropic virus type 1 (HTLV-1) have been associated with vasculitic conditions. Both viral infections share many similar epidemiological and microbiological features but differ significantly in their clinical manifestations.

A. Human Immunodeficiency Virus Type 1

1. Epidemiology

Human immunodeficiency virus type 1 (HIV-1 or HIV) is a common infection worldwide. It has been estimated that since the early 1980s over 40 million individuals have contracted HIV infection. In 1997 alone nearly six million became infected.

The primary clinical manifestations result from opportunistic infections and malignancies, which thrive as a result of a virus-mediated immunosuppressive state. There has also been a wide array of autoimmune and rheumatic complications reported in HIV-infected patients (97). Among these complications are numerous cases of vascular inflammatory disease (98). The frequency of rheumatic complications in general and vasculitis specifically is difficult to ascertain. The only longitudinal study of these complications has suggested that vasculitis is indeed rare in this setting, being observed in less than 2% of infected cases (99). Despite the rarity of vasculitis in HIV-infected patients, its mere presence is important on both clinical and pathophysiological grounds. Clinically, it is challenging to select suitable therapies for an inflammatory/autoimmune disease in the setting of an immunodeficiency state. Pathophysiologically, the presence of vasculitis in patients with a chronic persistent viral infection provides an important opportunity for investigation of mechanisms of disease.

2. Clinical Findings

Numerous forms of vascular inflammatory disease have been reported in HIV-infected patients (Table 4). Unlike other forms of virus-associated vasculitides, such as those observed in the setting of hepatitis B and C, the clinical syndromes associated with HIV are highly heterogeneous. This heterogeneity combined with the fact that most HIV-infected individuals are also coinfected with a variety of other pathogens, including HCV, HBV, cytomegalovirus (CMV), and others, raises questions regarding relative importance of each pathogen, therapeutic agents, and immune dysfunction.

Despite the marked clinical heterogeneity and the limited available pathophysiological data, there are a few clinical themes that stand out. The most frequent vasculitic syndrome encountered in the HIV patient population is that of a PAN-like syndrome (108). Font et al. (108) reported four cases, reviewed an additional 26 from the literature, and compared these cases to previously described non–HIV-infected PAN cases. They pointed out that most cases tended not

Table 4 Vasculitides Associated with HIV Infection

Necrotizing vasculitis (98,100–110)
Leukocytoclastic vasculitis (98,106,111–115)
Cutaneous polyarteritis nodosa (116)
Eosinophilic vasculitis (117,118)
Churg-Strauss vasculitis (119)
Henoch-Schönlein purpura (98,106,120)
Isolated angiitis of the CNS (98,121)
Behcet's syndrome (122–124)
Erythema nodosum (125)
Cryoglobulinemia (126–128)
Zidovudine-induced leukocytoclastic vasculitis (129)
Angiocentric immunoproliferative disorders (98,130,131)
Benign lymphocytic angiitis (98,130)
Lymphomatoid granulomatosis (98,102,130,132,133)
Angiocentric lymphoma (98,130)

---

to become multisystemic or life threatening and tended to resemble PAN limited to muscle and nerve. We would concur with these impressions. A second feature is the frequent presence of digital necrosis (107,108,110,134) associated with vessel narrowing, beading, and occlusion on angiography.

A second propensity for vasculitis in the setting of HIV infection is for CNS involvement, which has been reported with and without systemic disease (98). Similar to the heterogeneity encountered in the systemic vasculitides in the setting of HIV infection, the spectrum of CNS angiitis is heterogeneous as well. One common theme throughout the CNS angiitis and HIV infection literature is that of angiocentric lymphoproliferative lesions. Several cases of angiocentric lymphoproliferative disease reminiscent of lymphomatoid granulomatosis have been reported in HIV-infected patients (132,133). Each case has demonstrated an inflammatory process that is angiocentric and lymphocytic with varying degrees of cellular atypia. Some observers have suggested that these cases merely represent primary CNS lymphomas, with histological variation from one field to another. The clinical manifestations of these cases have reflected multifocal cerebral ischemia and the neuroradiographic findings have ranged from normal to multiple mass lesions. A second theme found throughout the CNS angiitis and HIV infection literature is that of an association with varicella zoster infection (135,136). Similar to varicella zoster infection in the non–HIV-infected individual, this infection can be associated with a spectrum of CNS vascular disease (135). At one extreme are examples of classic, contralateral, delayed hemiplegia following herpes zoster ophthalmicus infection, a disorder overrepresented in the HIV-infected population (135,136). At the other end of the spectrum is a diffuse CNS angiitis occurring in temporal association with systemic varicella zoster infection (135). The pathology of this diffuse arteritis may be granulomatous or nongranulomatous. Attempts to identify varicella zoster virions in the inflammatory infiltrates have generally been unrewarding. This should not be surprising since varicella zoster is difficult to identify in vasculitic lesions in cases of documented infection within the central nervous system (135). As noted above, the precise pathophysiological mechanisms linking varicella zoster to systemic or central nervous system vasculitis are not fully understood.

Aside from these presentations, a variety of other clinical–pathological syndromes have been reported in this setting, including classic granulomatous angiitis of the CNS (121), CNS vasculitis with macroaneurysms (137), and others (98,137).

3. Diagnosis

Given the wide spectrum of vasculitic syndromes reported in association with HIV infection, the ability of HIV disease to remain subclinical for many years and the growing prevalence of the infection, clinicians must have a high index of suspicion to accurately make the diagnosis. Over-reliance upon a history of high-risk behavior, such as male homosexuality and intravenous drug use, will lead to underdiagnosis of the infection. Given the profound ramifications of an underlying HIV infection on both the prognosis and the use of immunosuppressive therapies, a strong argument can be made for a routine screening for HIV as well as other blood-borne pathogens in most patients with suspected systemic or central nervous system vasculitis. Standard testing includes the tandem use of screening by enzyme-linked immunosorbant assay (ELISA) and confirmation by Western blot. False-positive ELISA and indeterminate Western blots have been reported in the setting of systemic vasculitis and other connective tissue diseases. Confirmatory testing by detection of plasma HIV RNA may at times be necessary.

4. Pathophysiology

In a recent report of eight HIV-infected patients by Gisselbrecht et al. (110), a meticulous clinical evaluation strongly ruled out the possibility of the confounding factors (coinfections and multiple therapies) in seven of their cases. Through deductive reasoning, it was suggested that HIV may have served as the major etiological factor in these cases. In a pathophysiological investigation, Gherardi et al. (106) identified HIV virions by immunohistochemistry and electron microscopy in the perivascular infiltrates of two patients with a PAN-like picture involving muscle and nerve. The clinical significance of the detection of the virions in the inflamed tissue could not be directly ascertained. Other cases where HIV has been searched for in vascular inflammatory lesions have not been revealing (109,130). Aside from a direct role for HIV in causing vascular injury and inflammation, another potential but indirect mechanism is HIV-mediated immune activation. It has been postulated that the persistent state of abnormal immune activation that accompanies HIV infection may play a central role in vasculitis as well as other autoimmune manifestations encountered in the HIV-infected population (138). Evidence of such aberrant immune activation includes overexpression of cellular activation markers such as HLA-DR and CD38 on CD4 and CD8 lymphocyte populations as well as the detection of elevated levels of inflammatory cytokines, including TNF-α and interleukin-(IL-1) throughout the natural history of the disease.

5. Treatment

The treatment of HIV-associated vasculitis with immunosuppressive agents must be pursued with caution. Management should include consultation with a physician experienced in the treatment of HIV disease. There are no controlled data on any therapeutic agents in this setting. Anecdotal case reports of successful treatment with corticosteroids, cytotoxic agents including cyclophosphamide, and intravenous immunoglobulin have all been reported. The recent report of Gisselbrecht et al. (110) of eight patients with HIV-associated vasculitis is the largest single published experience. The majority of patients in their series had PAN-like disease with prominent involvement of nerve and muscle. While the treatment protocols were somewhat heterogeneous, the majority were treated with a combination of plasma exchanges and antiretroviral therapy, which was associated with a favorable outcome in most patients. The rationale for this therapy stems from their experience with a similar protocol for treating vasculitis associated with HBV and HCV. These two pathogens, like HIV, and also chronic persistent infections associated with vasculitis. Overall in the setting of HIV infection, it is prudent to avoid high-grade immunosuppressive therapy if at all possible, but in cases of life-threatening vasculitis, such therapy may be necessary for brief periods of time (108,134).

B. Human T Lymphotropic Virus Type 1

Human T lymphotropic virus type 1 (HTLV-1), a human retrovirus that was initially discovered as the causative agent of adult T-cell leukemia, is a member of the oncoretroviridae family (139). Human T lymphotropic virus type 1 infection occurs primarily in endemic areas in southwestern Japan, the Caribbean basin, parts of Africa, and the southeastern United States (139). The virus is transmitted in a similar fashion to HIV-1, but unlike HIV infection, only about 1% of infected patients ever develop clinical disease, most notably adult T-cell leukemia or HTLV-1 associated myelopathy (HAM) (140). Similar to HIV infection, HTLV-1 is also associated with a wide variety of autoimmune and rheumatic disorders. Prominent among these are HTLV-1 arthropathy, which may include marked joint swelling with bone and joint destruction, and Sjögren's syndrome (139,141).

Several inflammatory vascular diseases have also been described in association with HTLV-1 infection, though these appear to be less prevalent than in HIV-1 infection. Both cutaneous and CNS vasculitis have occasionally been reported in the setting of HTLV-1 infection (142,143). The most distinctive vascular inflammatory disease associated with HTLV-1 appears to be one confined to the eye, which includes both uveitis and retinal vasculitis (144,145). In this syndrome, patients present with blurred vision associated with the acute onset of mild inflammation of the vitreous followed by mild iritis and retinal vasculitis. The disease appears to respond well to corticosteroids. Sagawa et al. (144–146) have recently demonstrated the presence of HTLV-1 infected T cells in the ocular lesions. T-cell clones established from these lesions were dually positive for CD4 and CD8 and produced high amounts of TNF-α and IL-6. These investigators have suggested that these activated T cells are responding to yet unrecognized retinal antigens (144–146).

V. VARICELLA ZOSTER VIRUS

Central nervous system vascular disease is the most common form(s) of varicella zoster virus (VZV)–associated vasculitis. Less common patterns of presentation include retinal, localized skin, or hypersensitivity-type vasculitides (Table 5).

A. Central Nervous System Involvement

Martin et al. (147) have proposed a classification of VZV-associated CNS vasculopathies based on pathological findings from autopsy cases (see Table 5).

1. Herpes Zoster Ophthalmicus

Epidemiology. Herpes zoster ophthalmicus (HZO), the most common clinical CNS syndrome associated with VZV, is a unilateral, predominantly large-vessel vasculitis that develops 4–6 weeks after cutaneous VZV infection of the head or neck (usually V_1 distribution) (148,149). Typically, the vascular involvement is ipsilateral to the site of skin involvement. Herpes zoster ophthalmicus has been mainly reported in the elderly, with 65% of the cases involving patients older than 60 (average = 61 years) (150), although there have been scattered cases involving children (151). The exact frequency of the syndrome is unknown, since large prospective studies in elderly patients with herpes zoster infection have not been done. In children, a study from Japan estimated the frequency of HZO after primary VZV infection (varicella) at 1:6500 (152). Clear estimates of its frequency are also complicated by the fact that in some patients, there is no antecedent history of a typical herpes zoster rash (153). The mean delay between skin manifestations and the appearance of the neurological symptoms is approximately 31 days (range 1 week to 2 years) (150). The syndrome has been reported both in immunocompetent and immunosuppressed individuals (135,136,150).

Table 5 VZV-Associated Vasculopathies[a]

Clinical syndrome	Localization of vascular lesions	Vessel involvement
CNS vasculopathy		
Arteritis		
Herpes zoster ophthalmicus (HZO)	Localized involvement contralateral to the VZV skin involvement	Large > small arteries
Disseminated	Disseminated CNS involvement	Small >> large arteries
Angiitis	Disseminated CNS involvement	Small arteries = small veins
Vasculopathy (noninflammatory)	Disseminated CNS involvement	Small >> large arteries
Retinal vasculitis		
Acute retinal necrosis		Retinal arteries
Other forms of vasculitis		
Cutaneous granulomatous vasculitis	Superficial/deep dermis	Small capillaries/venules of the skin
Small-vessel vasculitis (hypersensitivity)	Arms/lower extremities	N/A
Kawasaki disease	Coronary artery aneurysms	Coronary arteries

[a]Abbreviations: CNS = central nervous system, VZV = varicella zoster virus, N/A = not applicable.
Source: Modified from Ref. 147.

Clinical Findings. The typical clinical presentation of patients with HZO consists of the acute onset of contralateral hemiparesis, aphasia, or hemianesthesia, 1 month after the resolution of the cutaneous herpes zoster lesions (148). In approximately 40% of the cases, mental status changes are observed. Headache (14%), fever (6%) or constitutional symptoms are uncommon findings. Involvement of cranial nerves occurs in 45% of the cases, most commonly affecting the VII nerve (150). Usually the disease follows a monophasic course with most patients gradually improving, although recurrent or progressive disease patterns have been described. Mortality rates up to 25% have been reported (148).

Laboratory Findings. Brain imaging studies such as computed tomography (CT) or cerebral angiography are abnormal in the majority of the patients (68 and 95%, respectively) (150). A CT scan of the brain usually reveals infarcts in the deep gray matter or internal capsule, in the distribution of the middle cerebral artery, or its deep penetrating branches, in the hemisphere contralateral to the herpes zoster infection (148). Similar findings have been observed using magnetic resonance imaging (MRI) of the brain (153). Cerebral angiography shows unilateral, segmental circumferentially symmetrical narrowing of the proximal segments of the middle, anterior, and less commonly of the posterior cerebral or internal carotid artery (149,154,155).

Analysis of the cerebrospinal fluid (CSF) is abnormal in almost all cases (96%) (150). The most common finding is a lymphocytic pleocytosis with usually less than 100 white blood cells/mm^3 present (95%) (148,150). Increased protein is detected in two-thirds of the patients (150). Although helpful, these abnormalities are not specific for VZV-related arteritis, since up to 60% of patients with cutaneous herpes zoster infection of the head or neck have similar abnormalities (156).

Similarly, increased titers of antibodies against VZV have been detected in the serum and CSF of patients with HZO (148). Increased intrathecal production of IgG antibodies against VZV has been demonstrated also (151,153). The use of the polymerase chain reaction (PCR) for the detection of viral DNA in CSF has not been extensively studied in patients with HZO. In some cases, VZV DNA was detected (157) in CSF whereas in others the PCR was negative (151,153).

Whether these discrepancies reflect differences in the timing of CSF examination or sensitivity of assays is unclear.

Several histological analyses of vessel specimens obtained from biopsies or autopsies characteristically show segmental infiltration of the vessel by lymphocytes or histiocytes that may be associated with fibrinoid necrosis (148) and/or multinucleated giant cells with granuloma formation. Different size arteries (small/medium/large) can be involved and have fragmentation of the elastic lamina. Electron microscopy studies have identified viral inclusion bodies in infiltrating histiocytes (158) or smooth muscle cells (159) of the arterial wall.

Treatment. Most of the patients who have been reported did not receive therapy (150). Few patients who were treated with acyclovir and/or corticosteroids had stabilization or improvement of their neurological status (150). Considering the monophasic course of illness and its favorable outcome in the majority of cases, it is difficult to make firm recommendations for treatment. In cases with severe or progressive involvement, combination therapy with corticosteroids and acyclovir (orally or intravenously) is warranted.

2. Other Forms of Central Nervous System Involvement

A disseminated CNS arteritis involving mainly small arteries without any particular anatomical location related to a previous herpes zoster infection has been described (160–165). In contrast to HZO, the arteritis occurs predominantly in immunocompromised patients following disseminated herpes zoster infection (147). Patients typically present with mental status changes such as confusion, lethargy, or hallucinations that can be associated with focal neurological deficits. A CT scan of the brain shows evidence of multiple infarcts of different ages, whereas histological findings consist of a disseminated inflammatory CNS arteritis involving predominantly small arteries (147). The prognosis of these patients is poor, mainly due to their underlying systemic illness (Hodgkin's disease, acquired immunodeficiency syndrome [AIDS], etc.).

A similar clinical syndrome, involving predominantly immunocompetent individuals and characterized histologically by a disseminated vasculitis affecting small arteries as well as veins has also been reported (147,160,166–170). A previous history of herpes zoster infection was present in most cases. A granulomatous angiitis with frequent involvement of the leptomeninges was the most common histological finding (147). Immunohistochemical and PCR studies of the involved vessels have revealed the presence of viral proteins and/or in one case DNA (170).

In contrast to these VZV-related inflammatory CNS vasculitides, a noninflammatory vasculopathy involving small and large cerebral arteries has been described predominantly in immunocompromised patients (135,164,171–173). Following herpes zoster infection, patients develop an encephalitis-like picture with mental status changes, seizures, or focal neurological deficits. Multifocal ischemic or hemorrhagic lesions located in the white matter or at the white–gray matter junctions can be seen in CT or MRI scans of the brain (135,164,171–173). Pathologically, "multifocal leukoencephalitis"-like lesions with areas of infarction and demyelination are characteristic. Using immunohistochemistry, VZV antigens can easily be detected in the media of the affected arteries. Occasionally Cowdry type-A inclusions can be found in glial or ependymal cells. These findings suggest a direct effect of VZV in the affected arteries following disseminated viremia and encephalitis in immunocompromised hosts.

Whether the above pathologically defined syndromes actually represent distinct clinical entities with separate pathophysiological mechanisms or just reflect a spectrum of host responses to a disseminated viral insult is unclear.

B. Varicella Zoster Virus–Associated Retinal Vasculitis

Varicella zoster virus is probably the most common etiological agent associated with the development of the acute retinal necrosis (ARN) syndrome (174). The syndrome is characterized by the development of a necrotizing retinitis accompanied by vitreous inflammation, optic neuropathy, and retinal arteritis (174). It initially involves one eye but can subsequently involve the other eye in 35–50% of the cases. Following an initial acute inflammatory phase that lasts 1–3 months, a second phase manifesting by retinal detachment occurs in 75–85% of the cases (174). Arteritis involving the arteries of the retina, iris, choroid, ciliary body, and optic nerve is typically found. Different modes of VZV identification, including direct viral culture, IIF detection of VZV antigens in intraocular fluid specimens or biopsy material, and detection of VZV DNA by PCR, have been employed (174). Most reported cases involve immunocompetent hosts with or without previous history of herpes zoster infection. In AIDS patients, a rapidly progressive form of the disease associated with minimal inflammation has been described (termed progressive outer retinal necrosis syndrome) (175–177).

Therapy with intravenous or intravitreal antiviral agents (acyclovir or gancyclovir) in conjunction with topical and oral steroids is recommended (174).

C.   Other Forms of Varicella Zoster Virus–Associated Vasculitis

A hypersensitivity-type vasculitis manifested by a typical purpuric rash and arthritis has been reported during the incubation period of varicella infection (178). Lesions subsided spontaneously without therapy. Langenberg et al. (179) have described a localized cutaneous granulomatous vasculitis at the areas of previous herpes zoster infection in a patient with HIV infection. Recently, Kuijpers et al. (180) reported the case of a 2-year-old patient who developed a typical presentation of Kawasaki disease following an acute VZV infection (chickenpox).

VI.   PARVOVIRUS

Parvovirus or B19 virus is a small DNA virus, that has been identified as the causative agent of erythema infectiosum or fifth disease and has been increasingly associated with a number of diverse clinical manifestations (181,182). Vasculitides affecting small, medium, and large vessels have been reported. Although there is a definite association with hypersensitivity-type vasculitis, its potential role in other forms of systemic vasculitides is still debated.

A.   Small-Vessel Vasculitis

1.   Epidemiology

Thirteen cases of parvovirus-associated small-vessel vasculitis involving predominantly the skin have been reported in the literature over the last 15 years (183–190). Half of the cases involved children (range 5–11 years). There was no evidence of gender preference. The appearance of the purpuric rash usually coincided with the onset of the second phase of the illness which was characterized by arthralgia, arthritis, or rash, and IgM and later IgG antiviral antibodies (Fig. 3) (191). Given the numerous outbreaks and epidemics of fifth disease worldwide, one can assume that small-vessel vasculitis is an unusual complication of this viral infection. On the other hand, since a search for parvovirus is not commonly performed during the evaluation of patients with hypersensitivity vasculitis, its true incidence remains unknown.

2.   Clinical Findings

Almost all patients presented with purpuric rash involving predominantly the lower extremities (183–190). Polyarthralgias (54%) and fever (61%) were common symptoms, whereas in three

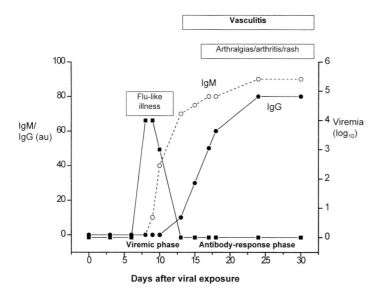

Figure 3 Parvovirus-associated hypersensitivity vasculitis. Abbreviations: au = arbitary units, IgM = immunoglobulin M, IgG = immunoglobulin G. (Modified from Ref. 191.)

cases severe abdominal pain (23%) was present, resembling Henoch-Schönlein purpura (183, 185,188). In most cases, the symptoms were transient and disappeared in few days to weeks. Only in one patient, who was coinfected with HIV, did the disease follow a relapsing course lasting almost 6 months (189).

The timing and pattern of vasculitic involvement observed in these patients suggests an immune complex–mediated process. Parvovirus has been identified by immunohistochemical and electron microscopy studies in the endothelial cells of small skin vessels in patients with various skin manifestations of acute B19 infection (192,193). Furthermore, its putative receptor, globoside or Gb4, has been identified in human endothelial cells (194). These findings imply a direct role for the virus in the vasculitic process.

3. Laboratory Findings

Since most of the vasculitic symptoms appear during the second or antibody-response phase, the majority of the reported cases had IgM antibodies against B19 on presentation whereas in one case the antibodies appeared 1 week later (187). In many cases, IgG antibodies were also detected. Sensitive techniques of viral DNA isolation, such as PCR or dot blot hybridization, were positive in two cases (187,189). Interestingly, in the case of the HIV-coinfected patient, only PCR of material taken from a biopsied vasculitic lesion was positive while serum was negative (189). In two cases, C4 levels were low, further suggesting an immune complex–mediated mechanism (184,188).

4. Treatment

Almost all patients with B19-associated small-vessel vasculitis improved spontaneously without treatment. The patient with concomitant HIV infection, was treated intermittently with oral corticosteroids and, after recurrence of his vasculitic lesions, intravenous immunoglobulin (IVIG) (189).

B.   Medium- and Large-Vessel Vasculitides

Parvovirus has been implicated recently in as a potential etiological agent for medium- and large-vessel vasculitides, such as PAN, Wegener's granulomatosis, Kawasaki disease, and giant cell arteritis.

Four cases of PAN associated with parvovirus have been described (three of them being children) (195–197). In all cases, the diagnosis was established by the presence of IgM antibodies and/or positive PCR for viral DNA. In three of these cases, the disease followed a chronic course lasting several months (196,197). Three patients were initially treated with conventional immunosuppressive therapy, including prednisone and cyclophosphamide, but only one responded. Two of the resistant cases were treated successfully with IVIG (196) whereas the other one responded to intravenous iloprost (197). Following these initial intriguing reports, Leruez-Ville et al. (198) retrospectively analyzed sera from 38 patients with early PAN (55% HBsAg+) but did not find any patient with evidence of recent parvovirus infection.

Similarly, four cases of patients with Wegener's granulomatosis and associated parvovirus infection have been identified (196,199,200). Nikkari et al. (201) utilized a PCR technique to screen a population of 42 adult patients with Wegener's granulomatosis for the presence of parvovirus DNA without success.

Although case reports (202,203) and a small study from Italy (204) suggested parvovirus as a common etiological agent for Kawasaki disease, subsequent reports from different groups including large numbers of patients, did not substantiate these initial findings (205–208). Nevertheless, parvovirus may play a role in some cases of Kawasaki disease.

The recent demonstration of a cyclic pattern of fluctuation in the incidence of giant cell arteritis (GCA) (209), raised reasonable questions about the potential role of infectious agents, particularly viruses, in its pathogenesis. Staud et al. (210) first reported a typical case of GCA developing after posttransfusion infection with parvovirus. Extending their initial epidemiological observations, the group from Mayo Clinic examined temporal artery specimens for the presence of B19 DNA, using PCR (211). Fifty-four percent of the positive specimens for GCA demonstrated evidence of viral DNA. Even though these findings do not prove causality between B19 infection and GCA, they emphasize the need for further studies.

VII.   CYTOMEGALOVIRUS

Cytomegalovirus-associated vasculitis occurs almost exclusively in immunocompromised hosts (212). Usually the vasculitic process is confined to a specific organ, such as skin, CNS, lungs, or gastrointestinal (GI) tract. In severely immunocompromised hosts, disseminated vasculitis may also occur. Case reports of CMV-associated vasculitis in patients with underlying systemic diseases, such as Wegener's granulomatosis (213,214) or systemic lupus erythematosus (SLE) (215), emphasize the need for early diagnosis and aggressive antiviral treatment for this condition.

A.   Epidemiology

Cytomegalovirus is a ubiquitous β-herpesvirus that causes an asymptomatic, latent infection in the majority of immunocompetent hosts. Fifty to 100% of the general population has IgG anti-CMV antibodies, indicating prior exposure to the virus. In contrast to the benign course of primary infection in healthy individuals, primary or reactivation of latent CMV infection is associated with significant morbidity and mortality in immunosuppressed hosts. These include organ transplant recipients, patients with AIDS or various hematological malignancies, and patients receiving chronic immunosuppressive therapy. The characteristic tropism of the virus for the endothelial cells probably accounts for a number of the observed clinical syndromes in these groups of patients (216). So, it is not unusual that a number of cases of CMV vasculitis have been reported in these patient populations (212), although its exact incidence is unknown.

In immunocompetent hosts, there have been only rare case reports of CMV-associated vasculitis affecting the skin or GI tract (212,217–220). Hogarth et al. (220) did not observe the characteristic cytomegalic cells with intranuclear inclusions ("owl's eye") in any of the skin biopsies from 37 consecutive patients with leukocytoclastic vasculitis. The authors acknowledge, though, that serological tests for CMV were performed in only 13% of the cases. Unless prospective studies are performed, utilizing the latest techniques in virus detection, the true incidence of CMV-associated vasculitis in immunocompetent hosts will remain speculative.

B. Clinical Findings

Skin involvement in patients with CMV-associated vasculitis have been reported both in immunocompromised (212) and immunocompetent hosts (217,218,220). A spectrum of skin manifestations has been described ranging from typical purpura to necrotic ulcers. In immunosuppressed patients, skin biopsy reveals the presence of cytomegalic cells (e.g., evidence of active endothelial CMV infection) (212). Interestingly, in "healthy" individuals, changes typical of leucocytoclastic vasculitis with occasional C3 deposits in the absence of direct CMV infection are seen (220).

Gastrointestinal vasculitis due to CMV occurs frequently in patients with advanced AIDS and transplant recipients. Typically, patients present with fever, abdominal pain, and diarrhea, suggestive of underlying colitis (212). Occasionally, the upper GI and the billiary system can be affected. Both small and medium-sized vessels of the bowel wall are involved in the vasculitic process, most likely due to active endothelial infection by the virus. Ailani et al. (219) recently reported a case of a young healthy man who presented with signs of abdominal ischemia and widespread venulitis and thrombophlebitis in the resected bowel wall. Evidence of active CMV infection was established by the presence of CMV-IgM antibodies and positive blood cultures for CMV.

Central nervous system involvement by CMV has been documented in autopsy studies in 2–13% of patients with AIDS. Vasculitis usually occurs in the setting of accompanying encephalitis, demyelinating lesions, or radiculomyelitis (212). Whether vasculitis is the primary process in these conditions is unclear. Koeppen et al. (221) described elegantly the pathological picture of a widespread necrotizing CNS angiitis involving both arteries and veins in a patient with lymphoma and CMV infection. Vasculitic lesions were present even in areas without obvious parenchymal involvement.

Recently, Henry et al. (222) reported five cases of patients with advanced AIDS who presented with alveolar hemorrhage and displayed evidence of pulmonary capillaritis in lung biopsies. Characteristically, giant cytomegalic endothelial cells were present and were associated with microangiopathic hemolytic anemia.

C. Laboratory Findings

Physicians dealing with immunosuppressed patients who present with localized or disseminated vasculitis face the challenging task of trying to identify a causative agent among numerous bacterial, viral, fungal, or parasitic candidates. The development of new methods for CMV isolation and culture from various specimens can be extremely helpful to the clinician (223). In general, isolation of CMV indicates active infection; it does not always prove that the virus is the cause of a specific clinical syndrome. Application of these newer techniques in patients presenting with new onset vasculitides of unknown etiology as well as in those with flares of a known underlying vasculitic process may prove to be of significant clinical importance.

D. Treatment

Once the diagnosis of CMV-associated vasculitis has been made, prompt initiation of treatment with antiviral agents (e.g., gancyclovir or foscarnet) is imperative. In patients who receive immunosuppressive therapy, rapid tapering of these agents is also important. Because of their poor overall status, the prognosis of patients with CMV vasculitis despite antiviral therapy remains poor.

VIII. EPSTEIN–BARR VIRUS

Epstein–Barr virus (EBV) has been recognized as a possible cause of leukocytoclastic vasculitis (224,225), CNS vasculitis (226), Kawasaki disease (227–232), and recently, large-vessel arteritis (233–236). Some authors have also suggested a role for EBV in pulmonary lymphomatoid granulomatosis, a disease that may be a form of T-cell lymphoma (237).

Hoffman and Franck (224) first reported a case of leukocytoclastic vasculitis occurring during the course of acute infectious mononucleosis in an adult. Lande et al. (225) reported a case in a child. C3 and C4 levels were low in both cases, whereas in one case, granular deposition of immunoglobulins were observed in the vessel walls from skin and kidney biopsies (225), suggesting an immune complex–mediated process. Both cases experienced spontaneous improvement.

In contrast to the benign course of leukocytoclastic vasculitis associated with acute EBV infection, chronic EBV infection has been linked to coronary arteritis manifested by coronary aneurysms (Kawasaki disease–like) (229–231), which in some cases was accompanied by arteritis of the large vessels of the thorax and abdomen (233–236). All the cases with large-vessel involvement were from Japan where chronic EBV infection is more common. Affected patients followed a rapidly progressive course leading to death. Autopsy studies revealed dilatation of the coronary arteries and large vessels with prominent lymphocytic infiltrates of the arterial wall. The majority of the infiltrating cells were T cells containing EBV genomic material. It is unclear if this large-vessel arteritis actually represents a form of EBV-associated angiocentric T-cell lymphoma.

IX. HERPES SIMPLEX VIRUS TYPES 1 AND 2

Cutaneous vasculitis (238–240), retinal vasculitis (241,242), and a widespread necrotizing vasculitis of small/medium-sized arteries (243) have been reported in association with herpes simplex virus (HSV) types 1 and 2 infections. Most patients with HSV-associated cutaneous vasculitis presented with localized persistent papular lesions in a zosteriform distribution. Interestingly, a granulomatous vasculitis of small skin vessels was observed in four of six patients (239,240), similar to the one observed in post–herpes zoster cutaneous vasculitis. Polymerase chain reaction of skin biopsy material confirmed the presence of HSV in two cases (240). In the other two cases, a leukocytoclastic vasculitis with evidence of active endothelial infection by HSV was found (238).

Retinal vasculitis in association with HSV-1 and -2 has been reported to occur both in immunocompetent (242) and immunosuppressed (241) individuals. Usually the patients present with a necrotizing retinitis that resembles ARN (241). The application of PCR techniques aids in the early diagnosis and aggressive treatment of these patients.

X. HEPATITIS A VIRUS

Leukocytoclastic vasculitis involving skin vessels and presenting with purpuric rash has been demonstrated in four cases of hepatitis A infection (241,244–247). Cutaneous vasculitis developed either during the acute (two cases) (245,247) or relapsing (two cases) phase (12,246) of hepatitis A infection. Patients with relapsing hepatitis A infection also had evidence of circulating cryoglobulins and/or rheumatoid factor. The possibility of an underlying HCV infection cannot be ruled out entirely in these cases, since testing for HCV was not available at that point. All but one patient, who required a short course of corticosteroids, improved spontaneously in a few weeks.

XI. RUBELLA

Two cases of hypersensitivity vasculitis, one involving a 7-month-old boy and one a 33-year-old man, have been reported in association with rubella infection (248,249). In both cases, an immune complex–mediated mechanism was postulated. Riikonen (250) reported a case of optic neuritis with characteristic findings of retinal vasculitis in a 13-year-old girl following rubella vaccination.

XII. MISCELLANEOUS VIRUSES

Isolated cases of localized or systemic vasculitides have been described in association with certain viruses, mainly based on serological evidence of virus infection. These include cases of Kawasaki disease with parainfluenza (251) or adenovirus (4) infection, leukocytoclastic vasculitis with hantavirus (252) or echovirus-7 (253) infection, Henoch-Schönlein purpura with Coxsackie B1 infection (254), and systemic vasculitis associated with measles (255) or Coxsackie B4 virus infection (256) (see Table 1). Whether these represent meaningful pathogenic associations or coincidental findings is unclear.

XIII. CONCLUSIONS

As the number of techniques that are used for viral isolation expand and new viruses are discovered, one would expect that novel associations between viruses and various localized or systemic vasculitic syndromes will be found. For the time being, physicians evaluating patients with vasculitis must be aware of the characteristic clinical and laboratory findings of the known virus-associated vasculitides. Early and accurate diagnosis of these conditions will facilitate appropriate therapy and may allow avoidance in certain cases of immunosuppressive regimens. Controlled therapeutic trials in conditions such as HCV-associated cryoglobulinemic vasculitis are needed in order to identify more efficacious and less toxic therapies.

REFERENCES

1. Gocke DJ, Hsu K, Morgan C, Bombardieri S, Lockshin M, Christian CL. Association between polyarteritis and Australia antigen. Lancet 1970; 2:1149–1153.
2. Trepo C, Thivolet J. Hepatitis associated antigen and periarteritis nodosa (PAN). Vox Sang 1970; 19:410–411.
3. Sergent JS. Vasculitides associated with viral infections. Clin Rheum Dis 1980; 6:339–350.

4. Somer T, Finegold SM. Vasculitides associated with infections, immunization, and antimicrobial drugs. Clin Infect Dis 1995; 20:1010–1036.
5. Guillevin L, Lhote F, Gherardi R. The spectrum and treatment of virus-associated vasculitides. Curr Opin Rheumatol 1997; 9:31–36.
6. Mandell BF, Calabrese LH. Infections and systemic vasculitis. Curr Opin Rheumatol 1998; 10:51–57.
7. Angello V, Chung RT, Kaplan LM. A role for hepatitis C virus infection in type II cryoglobulinemia. N Engl J Med 1992; 327:1490–1495.
8. Duffy J, Lidsky MD, Sharp JT, Davis JS, Person DA, Hollinger FB, Min KW. Polyarthritis, polyarteritis and hepatitis B. Medicine (Baltimore) 1976; 55:19–37.
9. Dienstag JL. Immunopathogenesis of the extrahepatic manifestations of hepatitis B virus infection. Springer Semin Immunopathol 1981; 3:461–472.
10. Sergent JS, Lockshin MD, Christian CL, Gocke DJ. Vasculitis with hepatitis B antigenemia: long-term observation in nine patients. Medicine (Baltimore) 1976; 55:1–18.
11. Guillevin L, Lhote F, Cohen P, Sauvaget F, Jarrousse B, Lortholary O, Noel LH, Trepo C. Polyarteritis nodosa related to hepatitis B virus: A prospective study with long-term observation of 41 patients. Medicine (Baltimore) 1995; 74:238–253.
12. Inman RD. Rheumatic manifestations of hepatitis B virus infection. Semin Arthritis Rheum 1982; 11:406–420.
13. Popp JW, Jr., Harrist TJ, Dienstag JL, Bhan AK, Wands JR, LaMont JT, Mihm MC, Jr. Cutaneous vasculitis associated with acute and chronic hepatitis. Arch Intern Med 1981; 141:623–629.
14. Maggiore G, Martini A, Grifeo S, De Giacomo C, Scotta MS. Hepatitis B virus infection and Schönlein-Henoch purpura. Am J Dis Child 1984; 138:681–682.
15. Kurokawa M, Hisano S, Ueda K. Hepatitis B virus and Schönlein-Henoch purpura (letter). Am J Dis Child 1985; 139:861–862.
16. Nowoslawski A. Hepatitis B virus-induced immune complex disease. Prog Liver Dis 1979; 6:393–406.
17. Hoofnagle JH, Di Bisceglie AM. Serologic diagnosis of acute and chronic viral hepatitis. Semin Liver Dis 1991; 11:73–83.
18. Bonkovsky HL, Liang TJ, Hasegawa K, Banner B. Chronic leukocytoclastic vasculitis complicating HBV infection: Possible role of mutant forms of HBV in pathogenesis and persistence of disease. J Clin Gastroenterol 1995; 21:42–47.
19. Alpert E, Schur PH, Isselbacher KJ. Sequential changes of serum complement in HAA related arthritis. N Engl J Med 1972; 287:103.
20. Wands JR, Mann E, Alpert E, Isselbacher KJ. The pathogenesis of arthritis associated with acute hepatitis-B surface antigen-positive hepatitis: Complement activation and characterization of circulating immune complexes. J Clin Invest 1975; 55:930–936.
21. McMahon BJ, Heyward WL, Templin DW, Clement D, Lanier AP. Hepatitis B-associated polyarteritis nodosa in Alaskan Eskimos: Clinical and epidemiologic features and long-term follow-up. Hepatology 1989; 9:97–101.
22. Drueke T, Barbanel C, Jungers P, Digeon M, Poisson M, Brivet F, Trecan G, Feldmann G, Crosnier J, Bach JF. Hepatitis B antigen-associated periarteritis nodosa in patients undergoing long-term hemodialysis. Am J Med 1980; 68:86–90.
23. Miguelez M, Bueno J, Laynez P. Polyarteritis nodosa associated with precore mutant hepatitis B virus infection (letter). Ann Rheum Dis 1998; 57:173.
24. Gupta RC, Kohler PF. Identification of HBsAg determinants in immune complexes from hepatitis B virus-associated vasculitis. J Immunol 1984; 132:1223–1228.
25. Hoofnagle JH, Davis GL, Pappas SC, Hanson RG, Peters M, Avigan MI, Waggoner JG, Jones EA, Seeff LB. A short course of prednisolone in chronic type B hepatitis: Report of a randomized, double-blind, placebo-controlled trial. Ann Intern Med 1986; 104:12–17.
26. Hess G, Manns M, Hutteroth TH, Meyer zBK. Discontinuation of immunosuppressive therapy in hepatitis B surface antigen-positive chronic hepatitis: effect on viral replication and on liver cell damage. Digestion 1987; 36:47–54.
27. Anonymous. Chemotherapy and hepatitis B. Lancet 1989; 2:1136–1137.

28. Cheng AL. Steroid-free chemotherapy decreases the risk of hepatitis flare-up in hepatitis B virus carriers with non-Hodgkin's lymphoma (letter). Blood 1996; 87:1202.

29. Simsek H, Telatar H. Successful treatment of hepatitis B virus-associated polyarteritis nodosa by interferon alpha alone. J Clin Gastroenterol 1995; 20:263–265.

30. Sonntag KC, Schwarz-Eywill M, Hunstein W. Is interferon alpha a therapy for hepatitis B-associated polyarteritis nodosa? (letter). Br J Rheumatol 1995; 34:486–487.

31. Kruger M, Boker KH, Zeidler H, Manns MP. Treatment of hepatitis B-related polyarteritis nodosa with famciclovir and interferon alpha-2b. J Hepatol 1997; 26:935–939.

32. Avsar E, Savas B, Tozun N, Ulusoy NB, Kalayci C. Successful treatment of polyarteritis nodosa related to hepatitis B virus with interferon alpha as first-line therapy (letter). J Hepatol 1998; 28:525–526.

33. Guillevin L, Lhote F, Sauvaget F, Deblois P, Rossi F, Levallois D, Pourrat J, Christoforov B, Trepo C. Treatment of polyarteritis nodosa related to hepatitis B virus with interferon-alpha and plasma exchanges. Ann Rheum Dis 1994; 53:334–337.

34. WHO. Hepatitis C: Global prevalence. Wkly Epidemiol Rec 1997; 72:341–344.

35. Centers for Disease Control and Prevention. Recommendations for prevention and control of hepatitis C virus (HCV) infection and HCV-related chronic disease. Centers for Disease Control and Prevention. MMWR 1998; 47:1–39.

36. Hadziyannis SJ. The spectrum of extrahepatic manifestations in hepatitis C virus infection. J Viral Hepat 1997; 4:9–28.

37. Pascual M, Perrin L, Giostra E, Schifferli JA. Hepatitis C virus in patients with cryoglobulinemia type II (letter). J Infect Dis 1990; 162:569–7.

38. Ferri C, Greco F, Longombardo G, Palla P, Marzo E, Moretti A. Hepatitis C virus antibodies in mixed cryoglobulinemia (letter). Clin Exp Rheumatol 1991; 9:95–96.

39. Agnello V. The etiology and pathophysiology of mixed cryoglobulinemia secondary to hepatitis C virus infection. Springer Semin Immunopathol 1997; 19:111–129.

40. Lunel F, Musset L, Cacoub P, Frangeul L, Cresta P, Perrin M, Grippon P, Hoang C, Valla D, Piette JC. Cryoglobulinemia in chronic liver diseases: Role of hepatitis C virus and liver damage [published erratum appears in Gastroenterology 1995 Feb;108(2):620]. Gastroenterology 1994; 106:1291–1300.

41. Karlsberg PL, Lee WM, Casey DL, Cockerell CJ, Cruz PD, Jr. Cutaneous vasculitis and rheumatoid factor positivity as presenting signs of hepatitis C virus-induced mixed cryoglobulinemia. Arch Dermatol 1995; 131:1119–1123.

42. Daoud MS, el-Azhary RA, Gibson LE, Lutz ME, Daoud S. Chronic hepatitis C, cryoglobulinemia, and cutaneous necrotizing vasculitis: Clinical, pathologic, and immunopathologic study of twelve patients. J Am Acad Dermatol 1996; 34:219–223.

43. Wong VS, Egner W, Elsey T, Brown D, Alexander GJ. Incidence, character and clinical relevance of mixed cryoglobulinaemia in patients with chronic hepatitis C virus infection. Clin Exp Immunol 1996; 104:25–31.

44. Buskila D, Shnaider A, Neumann L, Lorber M, Zilberman D, Hilzenrat N, Kuperman OJ, Sikuler E. Musculoskeletal manifestations and autoantibody profile in 90 hepatitis C virus infected Israeli patients. Semin Arthritis Rheum 1998; 28:107–113.

45. Weiner SM, Berg T, Berthold H, Weber S, Peters T, Blum HE, Hopf U, Peter HH. A clinical and virological study of hepatitis C virus-related cryoglobulinemia in Germany. J Hepatol 1998; 29:375–384.

46. Dupin N, Chosidow O, Lunel F, Cacoub P, Musset L, Cresta P, Frangeul L, Piette JC, Godeau P, Opolon P. Essential mixed cryoglobulinemia: A comparative study of dermatologic manifestations in patients infected or noninfected with hepatitis C virus. Arch Dermatol 1995; 131:1124–1127.

47. Pawlotsky JM, Dhumeaux D, Bagot M. Hepatitis C virus in dermatology: A review. Arch Dermatol 1995; 131:1185–1193.

48. Agnello V, Abel G. Localization of hepatitis C virus in cutaneous vasculitic lesions in patients with type II cryoglobulinemia. Arthritis Rheum 1997; 40:2007–2015.

49. D'Amico G. Renal involvement in hepatitis C infection: Cryoglobulinemic glomerulonephritis. Kidney Int 1998; 54:650–671.

50. Gorevic PD, Kassab HJ, Levo Y, Kohn R, Meltzer M, Prose P, Franklin EC. Mixed cryoglobulinemia: Clinical aspects and long-term follow-up of 40 patients. Am J Med 1980; 69:287–308.

51. Tarantino A, Campise M, Banfi G, Confalonieri R, Bucci, Montoli A, Colasanti G, Damilano I, D'Amico G, Minetti L. Long-term predictors of survival in essential mixed cryoglobulinemic glomerulonephritis. Kidney Int 1995; 47:618–623.

52. Nemni R, Corbo M, Fazio R, Quattrini A, Comi G, Canal. Cryoglobulinaemic neuropathy. A clinical, morphological and immunocytochemical study of 8 cases. Brain 1988; 111:541–552.

53. Ferri C, La Civita L, Cirafisi C, Siciliano G, Longombardo G, Bombardieri S, Rossi B. Peripheral neuropathy in mixed cryoglobulinemia: Clinical and electrophysiologic investigations. J Rheumatol 1992; 19:889–895.

54. Apartis E, Leger JM, Musset L, Gugenheim M, Cacoub P, Lyon-Caen O, Pierrot-Deseilligny C, Hauw JJ, Bouche P. Peripheral neuropathy associated with essential mixed cryoglobulinaemia: A role for hepatitis C virus infection? J Neurol Neurosurg Psychiatry 1996; 60:661–666.

55. Bonetti B, Invernizzi F, Rizzuto N, Bonazzi ML, Zanusso, GL, Chinaglia G, Monaco S. T-cell-mediated epineurial vasculitis and humoral-mediated microangiopathy in cryoglobulinemic neuropathy. J Neuroimmunol 1997; 73:145–154.

56. David WS, Peine C, Schlesinger P, Smith SA. Nonsystemic vasculitic mononeuropathy multiplex, cryoglobulinemia, and hepatitis C. Muscle Nerve 1996; 19:1596–1602.

57. Agnello V. Mixed cryoglobulinaemia after hepatitis C virus: More and less ambiguity. Ann Rheum Dis 1998; 57:701–702.

58. Agnello V. Hepatitis C virus infection and type II cryoglobulinemia: An immunological perspective [published erratum appears in Hepatology 1998 Mar; 27(3):889]. Hepatology 1997; 26:1375–1379.

59. Santagostino E, Colombo M, Cultraro D, Muca-Perja M, Gringeri A, Mannucci PM. High prevalence of serum cryoglobulins in multitransfused hemophilic patients with chronic hepatitis C. Blood 1998; 92:516–519.

60. Pawlotsky JM, Ben Yahia M, Andre C, Voisin MC, Intrator L, Roudot-Thoraval F, Deforges L, Duvoux C, Zafrani ES, Duval J. Immunological disorders in C virus chronic active hepatitis: A prospective case-control study. Hepatology 1994; 19:841–848.

61. Clifford BD, Donahue D, Smith L, Cable E, Luttig B, Manns M, Bonkovsky HL. High prevalence of serological markers of autoimmunity in patients with chronic hepatitis C. Hepatology 1995; 21:613–619.

62. Monteverde A, Ballare M, Pileri S. Hepatic lymphoid aggregates in chronic hepatitis C and mixed cryoglobulinemia. Springer Semin Immunopathol 1997; 19:99–110.

63. Polzien F, Schott P, Mihm S, Ramadori G, Hartmann H. Interferon-alpha treatment of hepatitis C virus-associated mixed cryoglobulinemia. J Hepatol 1997; 27:63–71.

64. Zignego AL, Ferri C, Giannini C, Monti M, La Civita L, Careccia G, Longombardo G, Lombardini F, Bombardieri S, Gentilini P. Hepatitis C virus genotype analysis in patients with type II mixed cryoglobulinemia. Ann Intern Med 1996; 124:31–34.

65. Bonomo L, Casato M, Afeltra A, Caccavo D. Treatment of idiopathic mixed cryoglobulinemia with alpha interferon. Am J Med 1987; 83:726–730.

66. Knox TA, Hillyer CD, Kaplan MM, Berkman EM. Mixed cryoglobulinemia responsive to interferon-alpha (letter). Am J Med 1991; 91:554–555.

67. Ferri C, Marzo E, Longombardo G, Lombardini F, La Civita L, Vanacore R, Liberati AM, Gerli R, Greco F, Moretti A. Interferon-alpha in mixed cryoglobulinemia patients: A randomized, crossover-controlled trial. Blood 1993; 81:1132–1136.

68. Dammacco F, Sansonno D, Han JH, Shyamala V, Cornacchiulo V, Iacobelli, AR, Lauletta G, Rizzi R. Natural interferon-alpha versus its combination with 6-methyl-prednisolone in the therapy of type II mixed cryoglobulinemia: A long-term, randomized, controlled study. Blood 1994; 84:3336–3343.

69. Misiani R, Bellavita P, Fenili D, Vicari O, Marchesi D, Sironi PL, Zilio P, Vernocchi A, Massazza M, Vendramin G. Interferon alpha-2a therapy in cryoglobulinemia associated with hepatitis C virus. N Engl J Med 1994; 330:751–756.

70. Mazzaro C, Franzin F, Tulissi P, Pussini E, Crovatto M, Carniello GS, Efremov DG, Burrone O, Santini G, Pozzato G. Regression of monoclonal B-cell expansion in patients affected by mixed cryoglobulinemia responsive to alpha-interferon therapy. Cancer 1996; 77:2604–2613.

71. Akriviadis EA, Xanthakis I, Navrozidou C, Papadopoulos A. Prevalence of cryoglobulinemia in chronic hepatitis C virus infection and response to treatment with interferon-alpha. J Clin Gastroenterol 1997; 25:612–618.

72. Casato M, Agnello V, Pucillo LP, Knight GB, Leoni M, Del Vecchio S, Mazzilli C, Antonelli G, Bonomo L. Predictors of long-term response to high-dose interferon therapy in type II cryoglobulinemia associated with hepatitis C virus infection. Blood 1997; 90:3865–3873.

73. Lopes E, Lopes LV, Silva AE. Mixed cryoglobulinemia and membranoproliferative glomerulonephritis associated with hepatitis C virus infection (letter). Ann Intern Med 1996; 125:781–782.

74. Safadi R, Shouval D, Kaspa RT, Ashur Y, Ilan Y. Beneficial effect of ribavirin on hepatitis C-associated cryoglobulinemia after liver transplantation. Liver Transpl Surg 1996; 2:263–268.

75. Blanche P, Bouscary D. Ribavirin therapy for cryoglobulinemia and thrombocytopenia associated with hepatitis C virus infection. Clin Infect Dis 1997; 25:1472–1473.

76. Durand JM, Cacoub P, Lunel-Fabiani F, Cosserat J, Cretel, Kaplanski G, Frances C, Bletry O, Soubeyrand J, Godeau P. Ribavirin in hepatitis C related cryoglobulinemia. J Rheumatol 1998; 25:1115–1117.

77. Pham HP, Feray C, Samuel D, Gigou M, Azoulay D, Paradis, Ducret F, Charpentier B, Debuire B, Lemoine A. Effects of ribavirin on hepatitis C-associated nephrotic syndrome in four liver transplant recipients. Kidney Int 1998; 54:1311–1319.

78. Kanamori H, Fukawa H, Maruta A, Harano H, Kodama F, Matsuzaki M, Miyashita H, Motomura S, Okubo T, Yoshiba M. Case report: Fulminant hepatitis C viral infection after allogeneic bone marrow transplantation. Am J Med Sci 1992; 303:109–111.

79. Arend SM, Hagen EC, Kroes AC, Bruijn JA, van der Woude FJ. Activation of chronic hepatitis C virus infection by cyclophosphamide in a patient with cANCA-positive vasculitis. Nephrol Dial Transplant 1995; 10:884–887.

80. Funaoka M, Kato K, Komatsu M, Ono T, Hoshino T, Kato J, Kuramitsu T, Ishii T, Toyoshima I, Masamune O. Fulminant hepatitis caused by hepatitis C virus during treatment for multiple sclerosis. J Gastroenterol 1996; 31:119–122.

81. Fong TL, Valinluck B, Govindarajan S, Charboneau F, Adkins RH, Redeker AG. Short-term prednisone therapy affects aminotransferase activity and hepatitis C virus RNA levels in chronic hepatitis C. Gastroenterology 1994; 107:196–199.

82. Magrin S, Craxi A, Fabiano C, Simonetti RG, Fiorentino G, Marino L, Diquattro O, Di M, V, Loiacono O, Volpes R. Hepatitis C viremia in chronic liver disease: Relationship to interferon-alpha or corticosteroid treatment. Hepatology 1994; 19:273–279.

83. Thiele DL, DuCharme L, Cunningham MR, Mimms LT, Cuthbert JA, Lee WM, Combes B. Steroid therapy of chronic hepatitis: Characteristics associated with response in anti-hepatitis C virus-positive and -negative patients. Am J Gastroenterol 1996; 91:300–308.

84. Bojic I, Lilic D, Radojcic C, Mijuskovic P. Deterioration of mixed cryoglobulinemia during treatment with interferon-alpha-2a. J Gastroenterol 1994; 29:369–371.

85. Harle JR, Disdier P, Pelletier J, Azulay JP, Perreard M, Weiller PJ, Jouglard J. Dramatic worsening of hepatitis C virus-related cryoglobulinemia subsequent to treatment with interferon alpha (letter). JAMA 1995; 274:126.

86. Zuber M, Gause A. Peripheral neuropathy during interferon-alpha therapy in patients with cryoglobulinemia and hepatitis virus infection (letter; comment). J Rheumatol 1997; 24:2488–2489.

87. Di Lullo L, De Rosa FG, Coviello R, Sorgi ML, Coen G, Zorzin LR, Casato M. Interferon toxicity in hepatitis C virus-associated type II cryoglobulinemia (letter). Clin Exp Rheumatol 1998; 16:506.

88. Gordon AC, Edgar JD, Finch RG. Acute exacerbation of vasculitis during interferon-alpha therapy for hepatitis C-associated cryoglobulinaemia. J Infect 1998; 36:229–230.

89. Cid MC, Hernandez-Rodriguez J, Robert J, Rio A, Casademont J, Coll-Vinent B, Grau JM, Kleinman HK, Urbano-Marquez A, Cardellach F. Interferon-α may exacerbate cryoglobulinemia-related ischemic manifestations. An adverse effect potentially related to its anti-angiogenic activity. Arthritis Rheum 1999; 42:1051–1055.

90. Ballare M, Bobbio F, Poggi S, Bordin G, Bertoncelli MC, Catania E, Monteverde A. A pilot study on the effectiveness of cyclosporine in type II mixed cryoglobulinemia. Clin Exp Rheumatol 1995; 13 Suppl 13:S201–S203

91. Horsmans Y, Tennstedt D, Cornu C, Geubel AP. Failure of cyclosporin therapy in type II cryo-globulinemia associated with hepatitis C virus infection (letter). Clin Exp Rheumatol 1998; 16:514–515.

92. Quint L, Deny P, Guillevin L, Granger B, Jarrousse B, Lhote F, Scavizzi. Hepatitis C virus in patients with polyarteritis nodosa. Prevalence in 38 patients. Clin Exp Rheumatol 1991; 9:253–257.

93. Cacoub P, Lunel-Fabiani F, Du LT. Polyarteritis nodosa and hepatitis C virus infection (letter). Ann Intern Med 1992; 116:605–606.

94. Carson CW, Conn DL, Czaja AJ, Wright TL, Brecher ME. Frequency and significance of antibodies to hepatitis C virus in polyarteritis nodosa. J Rheumatol 1993; 20:304–309.

95. Ferraccioli GF, Mariuzzi L, Damato R, Rocco M, Pirisi M, Beltrami CA. Jaw and leg claudication in a patient with temporal arteritis, chronic sialoadenitis and previous hepatitis C virus infection. Clin Exp Rheumatol 1998; 16:463–468.

96. Genereau T, Martin A, Lortholary O, Noel V, Guillevin L. Temporal arteritis symptoms in a patient with hepatitis C virus associated type II cryoglobulinemia and small vessel vasculitis. J Rheumatol 1998; 25:183–185.

97. Calabrese LH. The rheumatic manifestations of infection with the human immunodeficiency virus. Semin Arthritis Rheum 1989; 18:225–239.

98. Calabrese LH. Vasculitis and infection with the human immunodeficiency virus. Rheum Dis Clin North Am 1991; 17:131–147.

99. Calabrese LH, Kelley DM, Myers A, O'Connell M, Easley K. Rheumatic symptoms and human im-munodeficiency virus infection. The influence of clinical and laboratory variables in a longitudinal cohort study. Arthritis Rheum 1991; 34:257–263.

100. Said G, Lacroix C, Andrieu JM, Gaudouen C, Leibowitch J. Necrotizing arteritis in patients with in-flammatory neuropathy and human immunodeficiency virus (HIV III) infection (abstr). Neurology 1987; 176.

101. Weber CA, Figueroa JP, Calabro JJ, Marcus EM, Gleckman, RA. Co-occurrence of the Reiter syn-drome and acquired immunodeficiency (letter). Ann Intern Med 1987; 107:112–113.

102. Vinters HV, Guerra WF, Eppolito L, Keith PE. Necrotizing vasculitis of the nervous system in a pa-tient with AIDS-related complex. Neuropathol Appl Neurobiol 1988; 14:417–424.

103. Gherardi R, Lebargy F, Gaulard P, Mhiri C, Bernaudin JF, Gray F. Necrotizing vasculitis and HIV replication in peripheral nerves (letter). N Engl J Med 1989; 321:685–686.

104. Valeriano-Marcet J, Ravichandran L, Kerr LD. HIV associated systemic necrotizing vasculitis. J Rheumatol 1990; 17:1091–1093.

105. Conri C, Mestre C, Constans J, Vital C. [Periarteritis nodosa-type vasculitis and infection with human immunodeficiency virus]. [French]. Rev Med Interne 1991; 12:47–51.

106. Gherardi R, Belec L, Mhiri C, Gray F, Lescs MC, Sobel A, Guillevin L, Wechsler J. The spectrum of vasculitis in human immunodeficiency virus-infected patients: A clinicopathologic evaluation. Arthritis Rheum 1993; 36:1164–1174.

107. Libman BS, Quismorio FPJ, Stimmler MM. Polyarteritis nodosa-like vasculitis in human immuno-deficiency virus infection. J Rheumatol 1995; 22:351–355.

108. Font C, Miro O, Pedrol E, Masanes F, Coll-Vinent B, Casademont J, Cid, MC, Grau JM. Polyarteri-tis nodosa in human immunodeficiency virus infection: Report of four cases and review of the litera-ture. Br J Rheumatol 1996; 35:796–799.

109. Massari M, Salvarani C, Portioli I, Ramazzotti E, Gabbi E, Bonazzi L. Polyarteritis nodosa and HIV infection: No evidence of a direct pathogenic role of HIV. Infection 1996; 24:159–161.

110. Gisselbrecht M, Cohen P, Lortholary O, Jarrousse B, Gayraud M, Lecompte, Ruel M, Gherardi R, Guillevin L. Human immunodeficiency virus-related vasculitis: Clinical presentation of and thera-peutic approach to eight cases. Ann Med Interne 1998; 149:398–405.

111. Velji AM. Leukocytoclastic vasculitis associated with positive HTLV-III serological findings (letter). JAMA 1986; 256:2196–2197.

112. Chren MM, Silverman RA, Sorensen RU, Elmets CA. Leukocytoclastic vasculitis in a patient in-fected with human immunodeficiency virus. J Am Acad Dermatol 1989; 21:1161–1164.

113. Mondain V, Carles M, Bernard E, Dellamonica P, Taillan, Ferrari E, Vinti H. [Leukocytoclasic vas-

culitis and human immunodeficiency virus. 2 new cases (letter)]. [French]. Rev Rhum Mal Osteoartic 1990; 57:367–368.

114. Potashner W, Buskila D, Patterson B, Karasik A, Keystone, EC. Leukocytoclastic vasculitis with HIV infection (letter). J Rheumatol 1990; 17:1104–1107.

115. Weimer CEJ, Sahn EE. Follicular accentuation of leukocytoclastic vasculitis in an HIV-seropositive man: Report of a case and review of the literature. J Am Acad Dermatol 1991; 24:898–902.

116. Peraire J, Vidal F, Mayayo E, Torre L, Richart C. Cutaneous polyarteritis nodosa in human immunodeficiency virus infection (letter). Br J Rheumatol 1993; 32:937–938.

117. Schwartz ND, So YT, Hollander H, Allen S, Fye KH. Eosinophilic vasculitis leading to amaurosis fugax in a patient with acquired immunodeficiency syndrome. Arch Intern Med 1986; 146:2059–2060.

118. Enelow RS, Hussein M, Grant K, Cupps TR, Druckman D, Mortazavi A, Villaflor ST, Glass-Royal M. Vasculitis with eosinophilia and digital gangrene in a patient with acquired immunodeficiency syndrome. J Rheumatol 1992; 19:1813–1816.

119. Cooper LM, Patterson JA. Allergic granulomatosis and angiitis of Churg-Strauss: Case report in a patient with antibodies to human immunodeficiency virus and hepatitis B virus. Int J Dermatol 1989; 28:597–599.

120. Hall TN, Brennan B, Leahy MF, Woodroffe AJ. Henoch-Schönlein purpura associated with human immunodeficiency virus infection. Nephrol Dial Transplant 1998; 13:988–990.

121. Yankner BA, Skolnik PR, Shoukimas GM, Gabuzda DH, Sobel RA, Ho DD. Cerebral granulomatous angiitis associated with isolation of human T-lymphotropic virus type III from the central nervous system. Ann Neurol 1986; 20:362–364.

122. Buskila D, Gladman DD, Gilmore J, Salit IE. Behçet's disease in a patient with immunodeficiency virus infection. Ann Rheum Dis 1991; 50:115–116.

123. Stein CM, Thomas JE. Behcet's disease associated with HIV infection. J Rheumatol 1991; 18:1427–1428.

124. Stein CM, Davis P. Arthritis associated with HIV infection in Zimbabwe. J Rheumatol 1996; 23:506–511.

125. Fegueux S, Maslo C, de Truchis P, Matheron S, Coulaud, JP. Erythema nodosum in HIV-infected patients. J Am Acad Dermatol 1991; 25:113.

126. Taillan B, Garnier G, Pesce A, Ferrari E, Fuzibet JG, Gratecos N, Dujardin P. Cryoglobulinemia related to hepatitis C virus infection in patients with human immunodeficiency virus infection (letter). Clin Exp Rheumatol 11:350.

127. Furie RA. Effects of human immunodeficiency virus infection on the expression of rheumatic illness. Rheum Dis Clin North Am 1991; 17:177–188.

128. Stricker RB, Sanders KA, Owen WF, Kiprov, DD, Miller RG. Mononeuritis multiplex associated with cryoglobulinemia in HIV infection. Neurology 1992; 42:2103–2105.

129. Torres RA, Lin RY, Lee M, Barr MR. Zidovudine-induced leukocytoclastic vasculitis. Arch Intern Med 1992; 152:850–851.

130. Calabrese LH, Estes M, Yen-Lieberman B, Proffitt MR, Tubbs R, Fishleder, AJ, Levin KH. Systemic vasculitis in association with human immunodeficiency virus infection. Arthritis Rheum 1989; 32:569–576.

131. Gold JE, Ghali V, Gold S, Brown JC, Zalusky R. Angiocentric immunoproliferative lesion/T-cell non-Hodgkin's lymphoma and the acquired immune deficiency syndrome: A case report and review of the literature. Cancer 1990; 66:2407–2413.

132. Montilla P, Dronda F, Moreno S, Ezpeleta C, Bellas C, Buzon L. Lymphomatoid granulomatosis and the acquired immunodeficiency syndrome (letter). Ann Intern Med 1987; 106:166–167.

133. Anders KH, Latta H, Chang BS, Tomiyasu U, Quddusi AS, Vinters HV. Lymphomatoid granulomatosis and malignant lymphoma of the central nervous system in the acquired immunodeficiency syndrome. Hum Pathol 1989; 20:326–334.

134. O'Grady NP, Sears CL. Therapeutic dilemmas in the care of a human immunodeficiency virus-infected patient with vasculitis: Case report. Clin Infect Dis 1996; 23:659–661.

135. Gray F, Belec L, Lescs MC, Chretien F, Ciardi A, Hassine D, Flament-Saillour M, de Truchis P, Clair

B, Scaravilli F. Varicella-zoster virus infection of the central nervous system in the acquired immune deficiency syndrome. Brain 1994; 117:987–999.

136. Picard O, Brunereau L, Pelosse B, Kerob D, Cabane J, Imbert JC. Cerebral infarction associated with vasculitis due to varicella zoster virus in patients infected with the human immunodeficiency virus. Biomed Pharmacother 1997; 51:449–454.

137. Dubrovsky T, Curless R, Scott G, Chaneles M, Post MJ, Altman N, Petito, CK, Start D, Wood C. Cerebral aneurysmal arteriopathy in childhood AIDS. Neurology 1998; 51:560–565.

138. Calabrese LH. Vasculitis and chronic persistent viral infections (editorial). Ann Med Interne 1998; 149:395–397.

139. Nishioka K, Sumida T, Hasunuma T. Human T lymphotropic virus type I in arthropathy and autoimmune disorders. Arthritis Rheum 1996; 39:1410–1418.

140. Gessain A, Gout O. Chronic myelopathy associated with human T-lymphotropic virus type I (HTLV-I). Ann Intern Med 1992; 117:933–946.

141. McCallum RM, Patel DD, Moore JO, Haynes BF. Arthritis syndromes associated with human T cell lymphotropic virus type I infection. Med Clin North Am 1997; 81:261–276.

142. Vernant JC, Smadja D, Deforge-Lasseur C, Cabre P, Buisson G, Neisson-Vernant C, Desgranges C. [Vasculitis and neurologic manifestations related to HTLV-1]. [French]. Presse Med 1994; 23:1421–1425.

143. Schwartz J, Gonzalez J, Rosenberg R, Fujihara K, Cottrill CM, Klainer, AS, Bisaccia E. Cutaneous T-cell lymphoma, tropical spastic paraparesis, cerebral vasculitis, and protein S deficiency in a patient with HTLV-I. South Med J 1996; 89:999–1000.

144. Sasaki K, Morooka I, Inomata H, Kashio N, Akamine T, Osame M. Retinal vasculitis in human T-lymphotropic virus type I associated myelopathy. Br J Ophthalmol 1989; 73:812–815.

145. Hayasaka S, Takatori Y, Noda S, Setogawa T, Hayashi H. Retinal vasculitis in a mother and her son with human T-lymphotropic virus type 1 associated myelopathy. Br J Ophthalmol 1991; 75:566–567.

146. Sagawa K, Mochizuki M, Katagirl K, Tsuboi I, Sugita S, Mukaida N, Itoh K. In vitro effects of immunosuppressive agents on cytokine production by HTLV-I-infected T cell clones derived from the ocular fluid of patients with HTLV-I uveitis. Microbiol Immunol 1996; 40:373–379.

147. Martin JR, Mitchell WJ, Henken DB. Neurotropic herpesviruses, neural mechanisms and arteritis. Brain Pathol 1990; 1:6–10.

148. Hilt DC, Buchholz D, Krumholz A, Weiss H, Wolinsky JS. Herpes zoster ophthalmicus and delayed contralateral hemiparesis caused by cerebral angiitis: diagnosis and management approaches. Ann Neurol 1983; 14:543–553.

149. Sigal LH. The neurologic presentation of vasculitic and rheumatologic syndromes. A review. Medicine (Baltimore) 1987; 66:157–180.

150. Sigal LH. Cerebral vasculitis. In: Koopman WJ, ed. Arthritis and Allied Conditions: A Textbook of Rheumatology. 13th ed. Baltimore: Williams & Wilkins, 1997:1547–1559.

151. Hausler MG, Ramaekers VT, Reul J, Meilicke R, Heimann G. Early and late onset manifestations of cerebral vasculitis related to varicella zoster. Neuropediatrics 1998; 29:202–207.

152. Ichiyama T, Houdou S, Kisa T, Ohno K, Takeshita K. Varicella with delayed hemiplegia. Pediatr Neurol 1990; 6:279–281.

153. Nau R, Lantsch M, Stiefel M, Polak T, Reiber H. Varicella zoster virus-associated focal vasculitis without herpes zoster: Recovery after treatment with acyclovir. Neurology 1998; 51:914–915.

154. Mackenzie RA, Forbes GS, Karnes WE. Angiographic findings in herpes zoster arteritis. Ann Neurol 1981; 10:458–464.

155. Hurst RW, Grossman RI. Neuroradiology of central nervous system vasculitis. Semin Neurol 1994; 14:320–340.

156. Haanpaa M, Dastidar P, Weinberg A, Levin M, Miettinen A, Lapinlampi A, Laippala P, Nurmikko T. CSF and MRI findings in patients with acute herpes zoster. Neurology 1998; 51:1405–1411.

157. Koskiniemi M, Mannonen L, Kallio A, Vaheri A. Luminometric microplate hybridization for detection of varicella-zoster virus PCR product from cerebrospinal fluid. J Virol Methods 1997; 63:71–79.

158. Fukumoto S, Kinjo M, Hokamura K, Tanaka K. Subarachnoid hemorrhage and granulomatous angi-

itis of the basilar artery: Demonstration of the varicella-zoster-virus in the basilar artery lesions. Stroke 1986; 17:1024–1028.

159. Doyle PW, Gibson G, Dolman CL. Herpes zoster ophthalmicus with contralateral hemiplegia: identification of cause. Ann Neurol 1983; 14:84–85.

160. Rosenblum WI, Hadfield MG. Granulomatous angiitis of the nervous system in cases of herpes zoster and lymphosarcoma. Neurology 1972; 22:348–354.

161. Linnemann CCJ, Alvira MM. Pathogenesis of varicella-zoster angiitis in the CNS. Arch Neurol 1980; 37:239–240.

162. Jemsek J, Greenberg SB, Taber L, Harvey D, Gershon A, Couch RB. Herpes zoster-associated encephalitis: Clinicopathologic report of 12 cases and review of the literature. Medicine (Baltimore) 1983; 62:81–97.

163. Frank Y, Lim W, Kahn E, Farmer P, Gorey M, Pahwa S. Multiple ischemic infarcts in a child with AIDS, varicella zoster infection, and cerebral vasculitis. Pediatr Neurol 1989; 5:64–67.

164. Kleinschmidt-DeMasters BK, Amlie-Lefond C, Gilden DH. The patterns of varicella zoster virus encephalitis. Hum Pathol 1996; 27:927–938.

165. Kleinschmidt-DeMasters BK, Mahalingam R, Shimek C, Marcoux HL, Wellish M, Tyler KL, Gilden DH. Profound cerebrospinal fluid pleocytosis and Froin's syndrome secondary to widespread necrotizing vasculitis in an HIV-positive patient with varicella zoster virus encephalomyelitis. J Neurol Sci 1998; 159:213–218.

166. Kolodny EH, Rebeiz JJ, Caviness VSJ, Richardson EP, Jr. Granulomatous angiitis of the central nervous system. Arch Neurol 1968; 19:510–524.

167. Ruppenthal M. Changes of the central nervous system in herpes zoster. Acta Neuropathol 1980; 52:59–68.

168. De Reuck J, Crevits L, Sieben G, De Coster W, vander, Eecken H. Granulomatous angiitis of the nervous system: A clinicopathological study of one case. J Neurol 1982; 227:49–53.

169. Blue MC, Rosenblum WI. Granulomatous angiitis of the brain with herpes zoster and varicella encephalitis. Arch Pathol Lab Med 1983; 107:126–128.

170. Gilden DH, Kleinschmidt-DeMasters BK, Wellish M, Hedley-Whyte ET, Rentier, Mahalingam R. Varicella zoster virus, a cause of waxing and waning vasculitis: The New England Journal of Medicine case 5-1995 revisited. Neurology 1996; 47:1441–1446.

171. Eidelberg D, Sotrel A, Horoupian DS, Neumann PE, Pumarola-Sune T, Price, RW. Thrombotic cerebral vasculopathy associated with herpes zoster. Ann Neurol 1986; 19:7–14.

172. Morgello S, Block GA, Price RW, Petito CK. Varicella-zoster virus leukoencephalitis and cerebral vasculopathy. Arch Pathol Lab Med 1988; 112:173–177.

173. Amlie-Lefond C, Kleinschmidt-DeMasters BK, Mahalingam R, Davis LE, Gilden DH. The vasculopathy of varicella-zoster virus encephalitis. Ann Neurol 1995; 37:784–790.

174. Blumenkranz MS, Duker JS, D'Amico DJ. Acute retinal necrosis. In: Albert DM, Jakobiec FA, eds. Principles and Practice of Ophthalmology: Clinical Practice. Philadelphia: Saunders, 1994:945–962.

175. Forster DJ, Dugel PU, Frangieh GT, Liggett PE, Rao NA. Rapidly progressive outer retinal necrosis in the acquired immunodeficiency syndrome. Am J Ophthalmol 1990; 110:341–348.

176. Hellinger WC, Bolling JP, Smith TF, Campbell RJ. Varicella-zoster virus retinitis in a patient with AIDS-related complex: Case report and brief review of the acute retinal necrosis syndrome. Clin Infect Dis 1993; 16:208–212.

177. Rousseau F, Perronne C, Raguin G, Thouvenot D, Vidal A, Leport C, Vilde, JL. Necrotizing retinitis and cerebral vasculitis due to varicella-zoster virus in patients infected with the human immunodeficiency virus (letter; comment). Clin Infect Dis 1993; 17:943–944.

178. Messaritakis J, Psychou F, Dracou C, Nicolaidou P, Kakourou T. Arthritis and vasculitis during the incubation period of varicella. Acta Paediatr 1994; 83:681–683.

179. Langenberg A, Yen TS, LeBoit PE. Granulomatous vasculitis occurring after cutaneous herpes zoster despite absence of viral genome. J Am Acad Dermatol 1991; 24:429–433.

180. Kuijpers TW, Tjia KL, de Jager F, Peters M, Lam J. A boy with chickenpox whose fingers peeled. Lancet 1998; 351:1782.

181. Cherry JD. Parvoviruses. In: Feigin RD, Cherry JD, ed. Textbook of Pediatric Infectious Diseases. 4th ed. Philadelphia: Saunders, 1998:1620–1630.

182. Naides SJ. Rheumatic manifestations of parvovirus B19 infection. Rheum Dis Clin North Am 1998; 24:375–401.

183. Lefrere JJ, Courouce AM, Muller JY, Clark M, Soulier JP. Human parvovirus and purpura. Lancet 1985; 2:730.

184. Mortimer PP, Cohen BJ, Rossiter MA, Fairhead SM, Rahman AFMS. Human parvovirus and purpura. Lancet 1985; 2:730–731.

185. Lefrere JJ, Courouce AM, Soulier JP, Cordier MP, Guesne, Girault MC, Polonovski C, Bensman A. Henoch-Schönlein purpura and human parvovirus infection [letter]. Pediatrics 1986; 78:183–184.

186. Li LT, Coyle PV, Anderson MJ, Allen GE, Connolly JH. Human serum parvovirus associated vasculitis. Postgrad Med J 1986; 62:493–494.

187. Schwarz TF, Bruns R, Schroder C, Wiersbitzky S, Roggendorf M. Human parvovirus B19 infection associated with vascular purpura and vasculitis (letter). Infection 1989; 17:170–171.

188. Veraldi S, Rizzitelli G. Henoch-Schönlein purpura and human parvovirus B19 (letter). Dermatology 1994; 189:213–214.

189. Martinelli C, Azzi A, Buffini G, Comin CE, Leoncini F. Cutaneous vasculitis due to human parvovirus B19 in an HIV-infected patient: Report of a case (letter). AIDS 1997; 11:1891–1893.

190. Cooper CL, Choudhri SH. Photo quiz II. Leukocytoclastic vasculitis secondary to parvovirus B19 infection. Clin Infect Dis 1998; 26:849.

191. Anderson MJ, Higgins PG, Davis LR, Willman JS, Jones SE, Kidd IM, Pattison JR, Tyrrell DA. Experimental parvoviral infection in humans. J Infect Dis 1985; 152:257–265.

192. Takahashi M, Ito M, Sakamoto F, Shimizu N, Furukawa T, Matsunaga Y. Human parvovirus B19 infection: Immunohistochemical and electron microscopic studies of skin lesions. J Cutan Pathol 1995; 22:168–172.

193. Aractingi S, Bakhos D, Flageul B, Verola O, Brunet M, Dubertret L, Morinet F. Immunohistochemical and virological study of skin in the papular-purpuric gloves and socks syndrome. Br J Dermatol 1996; 135:599–602.

194. Cooling LL, Koerner TA, Naides SJ. Multiple glycosphingolipids determine the tissue tropism of parvovirus B19. J Infect Dis 1995; 172:1198–1205.

195. Corman LC, Dolson DJ. Polyarteritis nodosa and parvovirus B19 infection (letter). Lancet 1992; 339:491.

196. Finkel TH, Torok TJ, Ferguson PJ, Durigon EL, Zaki SR, Leung DY, Harbeck RJ, Gelfand EW, Saulsbury FT, Hollister JR. Chronic parvovirus B19 infection and systemic necrotising vasculitis: Opportunistic infection or aetiological agent? Lancet 1994; 343:1255–1258.

197. Zulian F, Costantini C, Montesco MC, Schiavon F, Zacchello F. Successful treatment of gangrene in systemic necrotizing vasculitis with iloprost. Br J Rheumatol 1998; 37:228–230.

198. Leruez-Ville M, Lauge A, Morinet F, Guillevin L, Deny P. Polyarteritis nodosa and parvovirus B19 (letter; comment). Lancet 1994; 344:263–264.

199. Nikkari S, Mertsola J, Korvenranta H, Vainionpaa R, Toivanen P. Wegener's granulomatosis and parvovirus B19 infection. Arthritis Rheum 1994; 37:1707–1708.

200. Corman LC, Staud R. Association of Wegener's granulomatosis with parvovirus B19 infection: Comment on the concise communication by Nikkari et al. (letter; comment). Arthritis Rheum 1995; 38:1174–1175.

201. Nikkari S, Vainionpaa R, Toivanen P, Gross WL, Mistry N, Csernok E, Szpirt W, Baslund B, Wiik A. Association of Wegener's granulomatosis with parvovirus B19 infection: Comment on the concise communication by Nikkari et al. Arthritis Rheum 1997; 38:1175.

202. Nigro G, Pisano P, Krzysztofiak A. Recurrent Kawasaki disease associated with co-infection with parvovirus B19 and HIV-1 (letter). AIDS 1993; 7:288–290.

203. Holm JM, Hansen LK, Oxhoj H. Kawasaki disease associated with parvovirus B19 infection. Eur J Pediatr 1995; 154:633–634.

204. Nigro G, Zerbini M, Krzysztofiak A, Gentilomi G, Porcaro MA, Mango T, Musiani M. Active or recent parvovirus B19 infection in children with Kawasaki disease. Lancet 1994; 343:1260–1261.

205. Cohen BJ. Human parvovirus B19 infection in Kawasaki disease (letter; comment). Lancet 1994; 344:59.
206. Rowley AH, Wolinsky SM, Relman DA, Sambol SP, Sullivan J, Terai M, Shulman ST. Search for highly conserved viral and bacterial nucleic acid sequences corresponding to an etiologic agent of Kawasaki disease. Pediatr Res 1994; 36:567–571.
207. Yoto Y, Kudoh T, Haseyama K, Suzuki N, Chiba S, Matsunaga Y. Human parvovirus B19 infection in Kawasaki disease (letter; comment). Lancet 1994; 344:58–59.
208. Fukushige J, Takahashi N, Ueda K, Okada K, Miyazaki C, Maeda Y. Kawasaki disease and human parvovirus B19 antibody: Role of immunoglobulin therapy. Acta Paediatr Jpn 1995; 37:758–760.
209. Salvarani C, Gabriel SE, O'Fallon WM, Hunder GG. The incidence of giant cell arteritis in Olmsted County, Minnesota: Apparent fluctuations in a cyclic pattern. Ann Intern Med 1995; 123:192–194.
210. Staud R, Corman LC. Association of parvovirus B19 infection with giant cell arteritis. Clin Infect Dis 1996; 22:1123.
211. Gabriel SE, Espy M, Erdman DD, Bjornsson J, Smith TF, Hunder GG. The role of parvovirus B19 in the pathogenesis of giant cell arteritis. Arthritis Rheum 1999; 42:1255–1258.
212. Golden MP, Hammer SM, Wanke CA, Albrecht MA. Cytomegalovirus vasculitis. Case reports and review of the literature. Medicine (Baltimore) 1994; 73:246–255.
213. Sackier JM, Kelly SB, Clarke D, Rees AJ, Wood CB. Small bowel haemorrhage due to cytomegalovirus vasculitis. Gut 1991; 32:1419–1420.
214. Weiss DJ, Greenfield JWJ, O'Rourke KS, McCune WJ. Systemic cytomegalovirus infection mimicking an exacerbation of Wegener's granulomatosis. J Rheumatol 1993; 20:155–157.
215. Bulpitt KJ, Brahn E. Systemic lupus erythematosus and concurrent cytomegalovirus vasculitis: Diagnosis by antemortem skin biopsy. J Rheumatol 1989; 16:677–680.
216. Vossen RC, van Dam-Mieras MC, Bruggeman CA. Cytomegalovirus infection and vessel wall pathology. Intervirology 1996; 39:213–221.
217. Weigand DA, Burgdorf WH, Tarpay MM. Vasculitis in cytomegalovirus infection. Arch Dermatol 1980; 116:1174–1176.
218. Sandler A, Snedeker JD. Cytomegalovirus infection in an infant presenting with cutaneous vasculitis. Pediatr Infect Dis J 1987; 6:422–423.
219. Ailani RK, Simms R, Caracioni AA, West BC. Extensive mesenteric inflammatory veno-occlusive disease of unknown etiology after primary cytomegalovirus infection: first case. Am J Gastroenterol 1997; 92:1216–1218.
220. Hogarth MB, Qureshi T, Lloyd J, Rees RG. A blistering rash and swollen knees. Lancet 1999; 353: 978.
221. Koeppen AH, Lansing LS, Peng SK, Smith RS. Central nervous system vasculitis in cytomegalovirus infection. J Neurol Sci 1981; 51:395–410.
222. Herry I, Cadranel J, Antoine M, Meharzi J, Michelson S, Parrot A, Rozenbaum W, Mayaud C. Cytomegalovirus-induced alveolar hemorrhage in patients with AIDS: A new clinical entity? Clin Infect Dis 1996; 22:616–620.
223. Hodinka RL. Human cytomegalovirus. In: Murray PR, Baron EJ, Pfaller MA, Tenover FC, Yolken RH, eds. Manual of Clinical Microbiology. 7th ed. Washington, DC: American Society for Microbiology, 1999:888–899.
224. Hoffman GS, Franck WA. Infectious mononucleosis, autoimmunity, and vasculitis: A case report. JAMA 1979; 241:2735–2736.
225. Lande MB, Mowry JA, Houghton DC, White CRJ, Borzy MS. Immune complex disease associated with Epstein-Barr virus infectious mononucleosis. Pediatr Nephrol 1998; 12:651–653.
226. Loeffel S, Chang CH, Heyn R, Harada S, Lipscomb H, Sinangil F, Volsky DJ, McClain K, Ochs H, Purtilo DT. Necrotizing lymphoid vasculitis in X-linked lymphoproliferative syndrome. Arch Pathol Lab Med 1985; 109:546–550.
227. Barbour AG, Krueger GG, Feorino PM, Smith CB. Kawasaki-like disease in a young adult. Association with primary Epstein-Barr virus infection. JAMA 1979; 241:397–398.
228. Iwanaga M, Takada K, Osato T, Saeki Y, Noro S, Sakurada. Kawasaki disease and Epstein-Barr virus (letter). Lancet 1981; 1:938–939.

229. Kikuta H, Taguchi Y, Tomizawa K, Kojima K, Kawamura N, Ishizaka A, Sakiyama Y, Matsumoto S, Imai S, Kinoshita T. Epstein-Barr virus genome-positive T lymphocytes in a boy with chronic active EBV infection associated with Kawasaki-like disease. Nature 1988; 333:455–457.

230. Kikuta H, Sakiyama Y, Matsumoto S, Hamada I, Yazaki M, Iwaki T, Nakano. Detection of Epstein-Barr virus DNA in cardiac and aortic tissues from chronic, active Epstein-Barr virus infection associated with Kawasaki disease-like coronary artery aneurysms. J Pediatr 1993; 123:90–92.

231. Muso E, Fujiwara H, Yoshida H, Hosokawa R, Yashiro M, Hongo Y, Matumiya, Yamabe H, Kikuta H, Hironaka T. Epstein-Barr virus genome-positive tubulointerstitial nephritis associated with Kawasaki disease-like coronary aneurysms. Clin Nephrol 1993; 40:7–15.

232. Culora GA, Moore IE. Kawasaki disease, Epstein-Barr virus and coronary artery aneurysms. J Clin Pathol 1997; 50:161–163.

233. Takano Y, Manabe H, Aoyama Y, Nakamichi N, Matsumura T, Kurata T. Measles associated with coronary arteritis. Virchows Arch A Pathol Anat Histopathol 1990; 416:271–276.

234. Nakagawa A, Ito M, Iwaki T, Yatabe Y, Asai J, Hayashi K. Chronic active Epstein-Barr virus infection with giant coronary aneurysms. Am J Clin Pathol 1996; 105:733–736.

235. Murakami K, Ohsawa M, Hu SX, Kanno H, Aozasa K, Nose M. Large-vessel arteritis associated with chronic active Epstein-Barr virus infection. Arthritis Rheum 1998; 41:369–373.

236. Ban S, Goto Y, Kamada K, Takahama M, Watanabe H, Iwahori T, Takeuchi H. Systemic granulomatous arteritis associated with Epstein-Barr virus infection. Virchows Arch 1999; 434:249–254.

237. Guinee DJ, Jaffe E, Kingma D, Fishback N, Wallberg K, Krishnan J, Frizzera G, Travis W, Koss M. Pulmonary lymphomatoid granulomatosis. Evidence for a proliferation of Epstein-Barr virus infected B-lymphocytes with a prominent T-cell component and vasculitis. Am J Surg Pathol 1994; 18:753–764.

238. Cohen C, Trapuckd S. Leukocytoclastic vasculitis associated with cutaneous infection by herpesvirus. Am J Dermatopathol 1984; 6:561–565.

239. Gibson LE, el-Azhary RA, Smith TF, Reda AM. The spectrum of cutaneous granulomatous vasculitis: Histopathologic report of eight cases with clinical correlation. J Cutan Pathol 1994; 21:437–445.

240. Snow JL, el-Azhary RA, Gibson LE, Estes SA, Espy MJ, Smith TF. Granulomatous vasculitis associated with herpes virus: a persistent, painful, postherpetic papular eruption. Mayo Clin Proc 1997; 72:851–853.

241. Cunningham ETJ, Short GA, Irvine AR, Duker JS, Margolis TP. Acquired immunodeficiency syndrome–associated herpes simplex virus retinitis. Clinical description and use of a polymerase chain reaction–based assay as a diagnostic tool [published erratum appears in Arch Ophthalmol 1997 Apr;115(4):559]. Arch Ophthalmol 1996; 114:834–840.

242. Chatzoulis DM, Theodosiadis PG, Apostolopoulos MN, Drakoulis N, Markomichelakis NN. Retinal perivasculitis in an immunocompetent patient with systemic herpes simplex infection. Am J Ophthalmol 1997; 123:699–702.

243. Phinney PR, Fligiel S, Bryson YJ, Porter DD. Necrotizing vasculitis in a case of disseminated neonatal herpes simplex infection. Arch Pathol Lab Med 1982; 106:64–67.

244. Inman RD, Hodge M, Johnston ME, Wright J, Heathcote J. Arthritis, vasculitis, and cryoglobulinemia associated with relapsing hepatitis A virus infection. Ann Intern Med 1986; 105:700–703.

245. Dan M, Yaniv R. Cholestatic hepatitis, cutaneous vasculitis, and vascular deposits of immunoglobulin M and complement associated with hepatitis A virus infection. Am J Med 1990; 89:103–104.

246. Ilan Y, Hillman M, Oren R, Zlotogorski A, Shouval D. Vasculitis and cryoglobulinemia associated with persisting cholestatic hepatitis A virus infection. Am J Gastroenterol 1990; 85:586–587.

247. Press J, Maslovitz S, Avinoach I. Cutaneous necrotizing vasculitis associated with hepatitis A virus infection. J Rheumatol 1997; 24:965–967.

248. Larsson A, Forsgren M, Hard aS, Strander H, Cantell K. Administration of interferon to an infant with congenital rubella syndrome involving persistent viremia and cutaneous vasculitis. Acta Paediatr Scand 1976; 65:105–110.

249. Ohsaki H, Sasaki T, Hatakeyama A, Nose M, Yoshinaga K. Hypersensitivity angiitis in an adult with rubella infection (letter). J Rheumatol 1992; 19:1160–1161.

250. Riikonen RS. Retinal vasculitis caused by rubella. Neuropediatrics 1995; 26:174–176.

251. Johnson D, Azimi P. Kawasaki disease associated with Klebsiella pneumoniae bacteremia and parainfluenza type 3 virus infection. Pediatr Infect Dis 1985; 4:100.
252. Pether JV, Thurlow J, Palferman TG, Lloyd G. Acute hantavirus infection presenting as hypersensitivity vasculitis with arthropathy. J Infect 1993; 26:75–77.
253. Chia JK, Bold EJ. Life-threatening leukocytoclastic vasculitis with pulmonary involvement due to echovirus 7. Clin Infect Dis 1998; 27:1326–1327.
254. Costa MM, Lisboa M, Romeu JC, Caldeira J, De Q, V. Henoch-Schönlein purpura associated with coxsackie-virus B1 infection (letter). Clin Rheumatol 1995; 14:488–490.
255. Bucknall RC, Doshi R. Diffuse vasculitis, eosinophilia, and elevated antibody titre to measles virus. Postgrad Med J 1976; 52:297–303.
256. Corbeel L, Gewillig M, Baeten E, Casteels-Van DM, Eggermont E. Carotid and coronary artery involvement in infantile periarteritis nodosa possibly induced by Coxsackie B4 infection. Favourable course under corticosteroid treatment. Eur J Pediatr 1987; 146:441–442.
257. Monti G, Galli M, Invernizzi F, Pioltelli P, Saccardo F, Monteverde A, Pietrogrande M, Renoldi P, Bombardieri S, Bordin G. Cryoglobulinaemias: A multi-centre study of the early clinical and laboratory manifestations of primary and secondary disease. GISC. Italian Group for the Study of Cryoglobulinaemias. Q J Med 1995; 88:115–126.

40

Vasculitis Secondary to Bacterial, Fungal, and Parasitic Infection

Michael C. Sneller
National Institute of Allergy and Infectious Diseases,
National Institutes of Health, Bethesda, Maryland

I. INTRODUCTION

A wide variety of bacterial and fungal infections may give rise to true vasculitis either by direct extension of a localized focus of infection or hematogenous seeding of normal and abnormal blood vessels. The first section of this chapter summarizes the forms of vasculitis that can be produced by many common bacterial and fungal pathogens. Subsequent sections focus on specific microorganisms that have a predilection to directly infect blood vessels.

II. BACTERIAL AND FUNGAL VASCULITIS

Vasculitis secondary to bacterial or fungal infections is usually the result of direct extension of a localized focus of infection to involve a blood vessel. Certain bacteria and fungi have a propensity to invade the vessel wall from a contiguous focus. The suppurative process initially involves the adventitia and subsequently spreads inward leading to destruction of the vessel wall and thrombosis. Invasion and necrosis of blood vessels is a prominent feature of necrotizing pneumonias due to bacteria such as *Pseudomonas aeruginosa* (1) and *Legionella pneumophila* (2). Vasculitis may also be seen adjacent to areas of necrotizing granulomatous reactions caused by mycobacterial or fungal pathogens and may mimic Wegener's granulomatosis pathologically. Angioinvasion and tissue infarction are characteristic of *Aspergillus* and *Mucor* infections that occur in severely immunocompromised patients (3). Infectious vasculitis may also develop in superficial cerebral vessels in association with bacterial, mycobacterial, or fungal meningitis. Vasculitis can be a particularly prominent feature of meningitis due to *Coccidioides immitis* (and occasionally other fungi) and can mimic primary central nervous system vasculitis (4,5). In patients with active tuberculosis, direct extension from contiguous infected lymph nodes, lung abscess, other viscera, or bone can rarely give rise to tuberculous aortitis (6–8).

Infective vasculitis may also arise from hematogenous dissemination of bacteria or fungi from a clinically obvious focus of infection or from an unidentified portal of microbial entry. This form of infective vasculitis is thought to result from either septic embolization to the vaso vasorum or direct microbial invasion of a normal or previously damaged vessel wall during bacteremia or fungemia. In medium to large arteries, the resulting lesion is often referred to as a "mycotic aneurysm." This term was first used by William Osler to describe the infective arterial lesions seen in subacute bacterial(not fungal) endocarditis. The term "aneurysm" is also a misnomer as many times this infective arterial lesion does not result in true aneurysm formation. Although mycotic aneurysms may occur in any vessel, they most frequently develop in the aorta, intracranial, superior mesenteric, and femoral arteries (9–11). In large arteries such as the aorta, septic emboli may lodge in the relatively large vaso vasorum, leading to suppurative infection and ischemic necrosis of the vessel wall. In smaller vessels, such as intracranial arteries, septic emboli may lodge in the vessel lumen and initiate a similar pathogenic process. Anatomical sites predisposed to mycotic aneurysm formation are arterial bifurcations, arteriovenous fistulae, coarctations, and atherosclerotic vessels.

In the preantibiotic era, most cases of mycotic aneurysms were due to infective endocarditis. With the advent of antibiotics and the decline in rheumatic heart disease, mycotic aneurysms associated with infective endocarditis have become less prevalent. Currently, mycotic aneurysms more commonly arise in older individuals when clinically obvious or occult bacteremia "seeds" a preexisting atherosclerotic lesion. The aorta, which is a frequent site of atherosclerosis, is also the most frequent site of this form of infectious arteritis (12–14). This type of mycotic aneurysm is rare; in one series of 820 consecutive patients who underwent surgery for aortic aneurysm, only five were found to be infected (13). Mycotic aneurysms may also occur in intravenous drug users, especially if they perform arterial injections.

A. Clinical Features

When mycotic aneurysms occur in the setting of infective endocarditis, manifestations of the underlying infection usually dominate the clinical picture. However, it should be noted that many of the nonspecific clinical features of bacterial endocarditis (e.g., fever, myalgias, cutaneous lesions, anemia, and elevated erythrocyte sedimentation rate [ESR]) may mimic polyarteritis nodosa or other systemic vasculitis syndromes. Intracranial mycotic aneurysms due to infective endocarditis are often clinically silent and resolve with appropriate antimicrobial therapy. When rupture occurs, patients usually exhibit severe headache and rapid deterioration in mental status. The time between diagnosis of infective endocarditis and aneurysm rupture in one report was variable (0–35 days) with a mean time of 18 days (11). In some cases, rupture may be preceded by the development of focal neurologic deficits or seizures. The microorganisms most frequently associated with mycotic aneurysms in infective endocarditis are staphylococci and streptococci.

The clinical presentation of mycotic aneurysms not associated with infective endocarditis can be indolent and nonspecific (e.g., unexplained fever, weight loss, and back, abdominal, or chest pain) or acute and catastrophic (aneurysm rupture with hemorrhage). A mycotic aneurysm should be suspected in an elderly patient or intravenous drug user who has no signs of endocarditis, but who nonetheless has persistently positive blood cultures, despite appropriate antibiotic therapy. The etiological agents of primary mycotic aneurysms differ from those secondary to infective endocarditis. *Staphylococcus aureus* or gram-negative bacilli (chiefly *Salmonella* species) are responsible for the majority of primary mycotic aneurysms (14–16). Fungal arterial infections are rare and characteristically occur in chronically immunosuppressed patients or in individuals who inject illicit drugs (17).

Clinically distinct forms of infectious vasculitis involving small cutaneous vessels can be associated with certain types of bacteremia. Ecthyma gangrenosum is a cutaneous lesion commonly associated with *Pseudomonas aeruginosa* bacteremia in neutropenic patients. However, bacteremia with gram-negative organisms other than *P. aeruginosa* can produce this same lesion (18). Ecthyma gangrenosum begins as a 1- to 5-cm macular lesion that rapidly develops a halo of induration and erythema and a central area of necrotic ulceration (see color insert, Fig. 40.1). A biopsy of the lesion reveals direct vascular invasion by bacilli with thrombosis of the vessel. Ecthyma-like lesions can also be seen in immunocompromised patients who develop disseminated infection with *Nocardia*, *Aspergillus*, and *Mucor* species (3). Bacteremia with *Neisseria meningitidis* is often associated with characteristic maculopurpuric skin lesions distinct from ecythyma gangrenosum. Biopsy of this skin lesion demonstrates endothelial necrosis, vasculitis, and thrombosis. Large numbers of *N. meningitidis* organisms are seen both in endothelial cells and being phagocytized by neutrophils.

B. Diagnosis

There are no specific laboratory abnormalities associated with any of the above forms of bacterial or fungal vasculitis. The diagnosis of vasculitis resulting from extension of a localized focus of infection is made by demonstrating organisms within the lesion by histopathological techniques and culture. The diagnosis of small-vessel cutaneous vasculitis associated with certain forms of bacteremia or fungemia is best made by biopsy and demonstration of organisms within the lesion.

When mycotic aneurysms occur in the setting of infective endocarditis, positive blood cultures and findings that indicate an underlying cardiac disease are usually present. In patients with infective endocarditis who develop neurological symptoms, computerized tomography (CT) is useful to rule out intracranial hemorrhage from a ruptured mycotic aneurysm. The diagnosis of intracranial mycotic aneurysms is best made by four-vessel cerebral arteriography (Fig. 2); however, magnetic resonance imaging (MRI) angiography may soon become a safer alternative to standard arteriography.

Patients with infected aortic aneurysms usually have leukocytosis, but this can also be seen with rupture of noninfected aneurysms. Blood cultures are positive in 50–100% of cases (9,14). Evidence of a primary focus of infection (such as pneumonia or osteomyelitis) may be found in up to 46% of cases (19). The CT findings of perianeurysmal fluid collection, enhancing inflammatory mass, or gas in the aortic wall are suggestive features of infection, but CT scanning often cannot distinguish an infected from bland aneurysm. Preoperative angiography is useful to fully delineate the extent of the aneurysm and plan the operative approach.

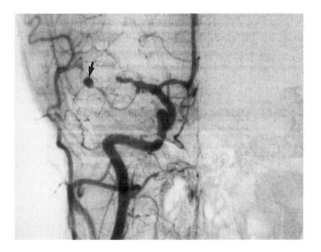

Figure 2 Cerebral arteriogram (AP view) showing a mycotic aneurysm (arrow) of the anterior temporal branch of the middle cereberal artery secondary to *Aspergillus* infection in an immunocompromised patient. (Courtesy of Drs. Holland and Patronas, National Institutes of Health, Bethesda, MD.)

C. Treatment

In the case of vasculitis resulting from extension of a localized focus of infection or cutaneous vasculitis associated with septicemia, the primary mode of treatment is with antimicrobial therapy directed against the specific pathogen.

There is no uniformly acceptable approach to the treatment of mycotic aneurysms that occur in the setting of infective endocarditis. Most of the available studies that address this issue deal with intracranial mycotic aneurysms. One review of 45 patients with infective endocarditis and intracranial mycotic aneurysms found that over 50% of aneurysms resolved with antibiotic therapy (20). In this review, there seemed to be no clear-cut advantage of combined antibiotic and surgical therapy over antibiotic therapy alone. Other series have reported better survival with combined surgical and antibiotic therapy (11,17). Most authorities would agree that serial angiography should be performed every 2 weeks, and surgical therapy is indicated for intracranial aneurysms that increase in size or fail to resolve after 4–6 weeks of appropriate antibiotic therapy. The optimal approach to aneurysms that decrease in size on repeat angiography is unclear.

The mortality rate for patients with infected atherosclerotic aneurysms is high, and successful treatment requires combined surgical and antibiotic therapy. Although organism-specific antibiotic therapy is essential, prompt surgical therapy is critical for survival and should not be delayed in an attempt to "sterilize" the aneurysm before resection and vascular reconstruction. The standard surgical treatment of infected aortic aneurysms includes complete debridement of all infected tissue followed by extraanatomical bypass. However, recent reports suggest that thorough debridement of infected tissue followed by in situ reconstruction can be successful in selected patients (21).

III. SYPHILIS

Syphilis is a complex systemic infection produced by the spirochete *Treponema pallidum*. Syphilis can be acquired by sexual contact, passage through the placenta, direct inoculation, or blood transfusion. The vast majority of cases are transmitted via sexual intercourse. There has been a rise in the number of cases of syphilis in recent years, primarily due to the increasing practice of exchanging sex for drugs and the concomitant epidemic of human immunodeficiency virus (HIV) infection. Pathological findings of endarteritis and periarteritis can be found in all three clinical stages of syphilis. However, aortitis and cerebrovascular disease are the clinically most important forms of syphilitic vasculitis. Although rare today, cardiovascular syphilis was responsible for 10–15% of all cardiovascular disease in the prepenicillin era (22).

A. Clinical Features

Syphilitic aortitis, the classic vascular lesion of tertiary syphilis, usually develops 10–30 years after the initial infection and typically involves the ascending aorta. This lesion is often asymptomatic, but symptoms such as substernal chest pain, congestive heart failure due to concomitant aortic valvular insufficiency, and angina secondary to coronary ostial stenosis occur in 20–25% of patients (22,23). Aneurysm formation in the thoracic aorta occurs in 5–10% of patients (24,25). The histopathological findings of syphilitic aortitis are characterized by adventitial fibrosis, obliterative endarteritis of the vasa vasorum, replacement of the media by vascularized scar tissue, and a lymphoplasmacytic infiltrate throughout the vessel wall (26). Only rarely can *T. pallidum* organisms be detected in this lesion.

Cerebrovascular syphilis is a recognized cause of stroke in young individuals. This form of syphilitic arteritis usually develops 6–10 years after the primary infection and typically involves medium-sized vessels leading to ischemic stroke. There may be a prodromal history of neuro-logical symptoms, such as headache, vertigo, and personality changes, that precedes the stroke by weeks to months. Because there is often diffuse as well as focal endarteritis, patients often present with signs of encephalopathy superimposed on focal neurological deficits (27). Several case reports suggest that concomitant HIV infection may be associated with increased incidence of neurosyphilis syndromes and a decrease in the time from initial infection to presentation of neu-rosyphilis (22).

B. Diagnosis

There are no clinical or radiographic features that reliably distinguish syphilitic aortitis from other causes of aortitis. Thus, the diagnosis of cardiovascular syphilis can only be made serolog-ically. In contrast to primary and secondary syphilis, the nontreponemal reaginic tests (VDRL, RPR) can be negative in late cardiovascular syphilis (28). Specific treponemal tests, such as flu-orescent antibody absorbed test (FTA-abs) or *T. pallidum* hemagglutination assay (TPHA) are positive in the majority (>90%) of cases (28).

The diagnosis of cerebrovascular syphilis should be suspected when stroke occurs in an in-dividual with a prior history of syphilis, in young individuals, and in patients with concomitant HIV infection. Angiographic findings are nonspecific and there is no "gold standard" for the di-agnosis of this form of neurosyphilis. Most patients are diagnosed based on a combination of the reactive serology described above, cerebrospinal fluid (CSF) abnormalities (increased protein, lymphocytic pleocytosis), and a positive CSF VDRL. The CSF VDRL has high diagnostic speci-ficity for neurosyphilis but is only reactive in 30–70% of cases (29). A reactive CSF FTA-abs or TPHA is not specific for neurosyphilis, but negative results may be useful for ruling out neu-rosyphilis. Because reactive CSF FTA-abs or TPHA have been seen in patients with syphilis who have no signs or symptoms of neurological disease, positive tests are not diagnostic of neu-rosyphilis. However, a negative CSF FTA-abs or TPHA may be useful for ruling out neuro-syphilis.

C. Treatment

The effect of antibiotic treatment on syphilitic aortitis is unclear. It is known that aortitis heals with scar formation, and antibiotic treatment may hasten this process (23). The currently recom-mended treatment regimen is three doses of 2.4 million units of benzathine penicillin given at weekly intervals (30). For treatment of cerebrovascular syphilis, the currently recommended reg-imen is intravenous aqueous penicillin G 3–4 million units every 4 h for 10–14 days (30).

IV. LYME DISEASE

A. Clinical Features

Lyme disease is a multisystem, tick-borne disease caused by the spirochete *Borrelia burgdorferi* and is endemic to many parts of the United States and Europe (31). Lyme disease usually begins with a characteristic skin lesion, known as erythema migrans, that occurs at the site of the tick bite. Days to weeks after the appearance of the erythema migrans, the organism hematogenously disseminates to many different sites, particularly the nervous system, heart, and joints. During this phase, patients frequently experience a nonspecific influenza-like illness with fever, myalgia, and headache. Weeks to months later, untreated patients may develop joint, cardiac, or central nervous system (CNS) disease. The most common neurological manifestations of Lyme disease are meningitis, subtle signs of encephalitis, cranial neuritis, motor or sensory radiculopathy, or myelitis. Very rarely, CNS vasculitis has been reported as a neurological manifestation of Lyme disease (32–34).

B. Diagnosis

Lyme disease is usually diagnosed by recognition of the typical clinical picture combined with serological confirmation of infection with *B. burgdorferi.* Serological testing may be negative in the first few weeks of infection, but the majority of patients will have detectable antibody after that time. The major limitations of serological tests are that they cannot reliably distinguish active from inactive infection and there is considerable interlaboratory variation. For a more complete discussion of the diagnostic limitations of serological testing for Lyme disease, the reader is referred elsewhere (31,35). Patients with suspected Lyme disease who develop signs of diffuse CNS disease or stroke should have a lumbar puncture, MRI, and possibly MRI angiography or standard four-vessel cerebral angiography to rule out CNS vasculitis (Fig. 3).

C. Treatment

The treatment of choice for CNS Lyme disease is ceftriaxone 2 g per day or cefotaxime 2 g every 8 h (36). The minimum duration of therapy should be 2–4 weeks.

V. RICKETTSIAL INFECTIONS

Members of the family Rickettsiaceae are fastidious bacterial pathogens that are obligate intracellular parasites. They are maintained in nature through a cycle involving reservoirs in mammals and insect vectors. With the exception of louse-borne typhus, humans are incidental hosts and are not necessary for propagation of the organism in nature. The Rickettsiae can be broadly divided

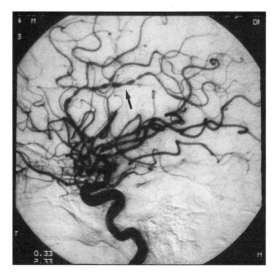

Figure 3   Cerebral arteriogram from a 32-year-old male with CNS vasculitis secondary to Lyme disease. Dramatic beading (arrow) typical of vasculitis is seen. (Courtesy of Dr. Marques, National Institutes of Health, Bethesda, MD.)

into spotted fever and typhus groups based on antigenic and growth characteristics. With the exception of Q fever, the pathogenesis of both the spotted fever and typhus groups is small-vessel vasculitis caused by proliferation of the organisms in endothelial cells. The geographical distribution of selected rickettsial infections are summarized in Table 1.

A. Clinical Features

During the appropriate season, the triad of fever, headache, and rash should alert the physician to the possibility of rickettsial infection. In Rocky Mountain spotted fever (RMSF), fever, headache, malaise, myalgias, nausea, and vomiting are frequent nonspecific manifestations during the first 2–3 days of illness. Rash usually appears during the third to fifth day of fever and is characterized by pink-red macular lesions on the wrist and ankles. These lesions spread centripedially and become maculopapules that blanch with pressure. Up to 10% of patients with RMSF may not develop a rash. If unrecognized and untreated, patients develop widespread microvasculitis with increased vascular permeability, leading to edema, azotemia, and/or pulmonary edema. Significant encephalitis due to cereberal microvasculitis occurs in up to 25% of patients. Lumbar puncture frequently shows CSF pleocytosis and elevated protein but the glucose is usually normal.

Epidemic typhus is characterized by the abrupt onset of fever, prostration, and headache. Maculopapular rash appears by the fifth day of fever, initially involves the axillary folds but later spreads to the trunk and extremities, and can become petechial and confluent. Photophobia and conjunctivitis are frequently seen. Untreated patients frequently develop fatal multisystem involvement with azotemia. Murine typhus resembles epidemic typhus but the clinical course is milder and mortality is less than 1% even without treatment.

Boutonneuse fever and the other spotted fevers are characterized by rash, fever, and, in most cases, the formation of an eshcar at the site of tick bite. These infections generally follow a less severe course than RMSF or epidemic typhus. However, the case fatality rate for Boutonneuse fever ranges from 1–5.6% (37).

B. Diagnosis

Rickettsial illnesses are usually diagnosed on clinical grounds with subsequent serological confirmation. Serological evidence of infection does not occur until at least the second week of illness; thus, therapy must be instituted based on clinical diagnosis. In RMSF, detection of organisms in biopsies of skin lesions by direct immunofluorescence can be used for rapid diagnosis (38).

Table 1 Summary of the Geographic Distribution of Selected Rickettsioses

Disease	Organism	Geographic distribution
Spotted fever group		
RMSF[a]	*R. rickettsii*	Western hemisphere
Boutonneuse fever	*R. conorii*	Africa, Mediterranean, India
Queensland tick typhus	*R. australis*	Australia
Rickettsial pox	*R. akari*	United States, Russia, Korea, Africa
Typhus group		
Epidemic typhus	*R. prowazekii*	South America, Africa, Asia, United States
Murine typhus	*R. typhi*	Worldwide
Scrub typhus	*R. tsutsugamushi*	South pacific, Asia, Australia

[a]Rocky Mountain spotted fever.

C. Treatment

The treatment of choice for RMSF and epidemic typhus is doxycycline 100 mg every 12 h for 7–10 days (RMSF) or until the patient is afebrile (epidemic typhus). For young children or pregnant women, chloramphenicol (50–75 mg/kg every 6 h) can be used, but anecdotal reports suggest this is less effective therapy than doxycycline. The same regimens can be used for other rickettsial infections. Ciprofloxacin (750 mg twice a day for 5 days) is an alternative for the treatment of Boutonneuse fever.

VI. PARASITIC INFECTIONS

Vasculitis has only rarely been reported as a manifestation of parasitic infections and, in most cases, other manifestations of the infection dominated the clinical picture. Localized pulmonary vasculitis has been associated with certain parasitic infections such as *Dirofilaria immitis* and *Wuchereria* species. In dirofilariasis, the adult worm can embolize in a pulmonary artery, occluding the lumen and resulting in localized lung infarction. A granulomatous reaction surrounds the infarcted area and the pulmonary vessel in the center of the infarction may show changes of vasculitis. These lesions usually present as localized pulmonary nodules (with or without respiratory symptoms) and the diagnosis is made following resection and pathological examination (39). Similar forms of localized pulmonary vasculitis have been reported with *Wuchereria* infection (40).

VII. VASCULITIS DUE TO ABERRANT IMMUNOLOGICAL REACTIONS TO BACTERIAL, FUNGAL, AND PARASITIC INFECTIONS

Small-vessel vasculitis with predominantly cutaneous involvement has been indirectly linked to a wide variety of bacterial, fungal, and parasitic infections (41). In the majority of cases, there was a temporal association between infection with a common pathogen and the occurrence of small-vessel vasculitis. However, only rarely is there direct evidence for a casual relationship between the infection and the vasculitis syndrome. In many cases, it is likely that either the temporal relationship of vasculitis and infection was coincidental or due to a hypersensitivity reaction to antimicrobial drugs used to treat the infection. One situation in which an excessive immune response to a bacterial pathogen is likely responsible for vasculitis is erythema nodosum leprosum (ENL). This syndrome affects nearly half of the patients with lepromatous leprosy and occurs following the initiation of antimicrobial therapy. The most frequent clinical manifestations are painful cutaneous nodules that usually ulcerate, neuritis, fever, uveitis, and occasionally glomerulonephritis. Erythema nodosum leprosum may occur any time within the first 2 years of treatment (42). Unlike other forms erythema nodosum, ENL is histologically an acute vasculitis. The vasculitis is thought to be due to immune complex deposition, local increase in T-helper-cell-type-1–mediated immunity, or a combination of these and other factors (43,44). Short courses of corticosteroids effectively treat most cases. Thalidomide (100–300 mg per day) may be used for managing recurrent episodes of ENL.

REFERENCES

1. Soave R, Murray H, Litrenta M. Bacterial invasion of pulmonary vessels: Pseudomonas bacteremia mimicking pulmonary thromboembolism with infarction. Am J Med 1978; 65:864–867.

2. Winn WC Jr, Myerowitz RL. The pathology of the Legionella pneumonias: A review of 74 cases and the literature. Hum Pathol 1981; 12:401–422.

3. Wheat L. Fungal infections in the immunocompromised host. In: Rubin R, Young L, eds. Clinical Approach to Infection in the Compromised Host. 3rd ed. New York: Plenum, 1994:211–237.

4. de Carvalho CA, Allen JN, Zafranis A, Yates AJ. Coccidioidal meningitis complicated by cerebral arteritis and infarction. Hum Pathol 1980; 11:293–296.

5. Kobayashi RM, Coel M, Niwayama G, Trauner D. Cerebral vasculitis in coccidioidal meningitis. Ann Neurol 1977; 1:281–284.

6. Mally A, D'Souza C, Dwivedi S, Shatapathi P. Pulmonary tuberculosis with multiple saccular aneurysms of the aorta: A case report. Angiology 1990; 41:333–336.

7. Goldbaum TS, Lindsay J, Jr., Levy C, Silva CA. Tuberculous aortitis presenting with an aortoduodenal fistula: A case report. Angiology 1986; 37:519–523.

8. Sung CS, Leachman RD, Lufschanowski R, Milam JD, Hougen ML. Tuberculous aneurysms of the aorta. South Med J 1979; 72:750–752.

9. Anderson CB, Butcher HR, Jr., Ballinger WF. Mycotic aneurysms. Arch Surg 1974; 109:712–717.

10. Feigl D, Feigl A, Edwards JE. Mycotic aneurysms of the aortic root: A pathologic study of 20 cases. Chest 1986; 90:553–557.

11. Frazee JG, Cahan LD, Winter J. Bacterial intracranial aneurysms. J Neurosurg 1980; 53:633–641.

12. Reddy DJ, Shepard AD, Evans JR, Wright DJ, Smith RF, Ernst CB. Management of infected aortoiliac aneurysms. Arch Surg 1991; 126:873–878; discussion 878–879.

13. Bitseff EL, Edwards WH, Mulherin JL, Jr, Kaiser AB. Infected abdominal aortic aneurysms. South Med J 1987; 80:309–312.

14. Wang JH, Liu YC, Yen MY, Chen YS, Wann SR, Cheng DL. Mycotic aneurysm due to non-typhi salmonella: report of 16 cases. Clin Infect Dis 1996; 23:743–747.

15. Brown SL, Busuttil RW, Baker JD, Machleder HI, Moore WS, Barker WF. Bacteriologic and surgical determinants of survival in patients with mycotic aneurysms. J Vasc Surg 1984; 1:541–547.

16. Jarrett F, Darling RC, Mundth ED, Austen WG. Experience with infected aneurysms of the abdominal aorta. Arch Surg 1975; 110:1281–1286.

17. Barrow DL, Prats AR. Infectious intracranial aneurysms: Comparison of groups with and without endocarditis. Neurosurgery 1990; 27:562–572; discussion 572–563.

18. Young L. Fever and septicemia. In: Rubin R, Young L, eds. Clinical Approach to Infection in the Compromised Host. 3rd ed. New York: Plenum, 1994:67–104.

19. Bennett D, Cherry J. Bacterial infection of aortic aneurysms: A clinicopathologic study. Am J Surg 1967; 113:321.

20. Bingham WF. Treatment of mycotic intracranial aneurysms. J Neurosurg 1977; 46:428–437.

21. Chiba Y, Muraoka R, Ihaya A, Kimura T, Morioka K, Nara M, Niwa H. Surgical treatment of infected thoracic and abdominal aortic aneurysms. Cardiovasc Surg 1996; 4:476–479.

22. Singh AE, Romanowski B. Syphilis: Review with emphasis on clinical, epidemiologic, and some biologic features. Clin Microbiol Rev 1999; 12:187–209.

23. Kampmeier R. The late manifestations of syphilis: Skeletal, visceral, and cardiovascular. Med Clin North Am 1964; 48:667–697.

24. Heggtveit H. Syphilitic aortitis: A clinicopathologic autopsy study of 100 cases. Circulation 1964; 29:349–355.

25. Kampmeier R. Saccular aneurysm of the thoracic aorta: A clinical study of 633 cases. Ann Intern Med 1938; 12:624–651.

26. Lie JT. Infection related vasculitis. In: Churg A, Churg J, eds. Systemic Vasculitides. Tokyo: Igaku-Shoin, 1991:243–255.

27. Coyle PK, Dattwyler R. Spirochetal infection of the central nervous system. Infect Dis Clin North Am 1990; 4:731–746.

28. Tramont E. Treponema pallidum (syphilis). In: Mandell G, Bennett J, Dolin R, eds. Principles and Practice of Infectious Diseases. New York: Churchill Livingston, 1995:2127–2129.

29. Scheck DN, Hook EW III. Neurosyphilis. Infect Dis Clin North Am 1994; 8:769–795.

30. Centers for Disease Control and Prevention. Guidelines for treatment of sexually transmitted diseases. Morbid Mortal Weekly Rep 1998; 47:28–49.

31. Nadelman RB, Wormser GP. Lyme borreliosis. Lancet 1998; 352:557–565.
32. Brogan GX, Homan CS, Viccellio P. The enlarging clinical spectrum of Lyme disease: Lyme cerebral vasculitis, a new disease entity. Ann Emerg Med 1990; 19:572–576.
33. Veenendaal-Hilbers JA, Perquin WV, Hoogland PH, Doornbos L. Basal meningovasculitis and occlusion of the basilar artery in two cases of Borrelia burgdorferi infection. Neurology 1988; 38:1317–1319.
34. Midgard R, Hofstad H. Unusual manifestations of nervous system Borrelia burgdorferi infection. Arch Neurol 1987; 44:781–783.
35. Tugwell P, Dennis DT, Weinstein A, Wells G, Shea B, Nichol G, Hayward R, Lightfoot R, Baker P, Steere AC. Laboratory evaluation in the diagnosis of Lyme disease. Ann Intern Med 1997; 127:1109–1123.
36. Wormser GP. Treatment and prevention of Lyme disease, with emphasis on antimicrobial therapy for neuroborreliosis and vaccination. Semin Neurol 1997; 17:45–52.
37. Raoult D, Zuchelli P, Weiller PJ, Charrel C, San Marco JL, Gallais H, Casanova P. Incidence, clinical observations and risk factors in the severe form of Mediterranean spotted fever among patients admitted to hospital in Marseilles 1983–1984. J Infect 1986; 12:111–116.
38. Woodward TE, Pedersen CE, Jr., Oster CN, Bagley LR, Romberger J, Snyder MJ. Prompt confirmation of Rocky Mountain spotted fever: Identification of rickettsiae in skin tissues. J Infect Dis 1976; 134:297–301.
39. Ro JY, Tsakalakis PJ, White VA, Luna MA, Chang-Tung EG, Green L, Cribbett L, Ayala AG. Pulmonary dirofilariasis: The great imitator of primary or metastatic lung tumor. A clinicopathologic analysis of seven cases and a review of the literature. Hum Pathol 1989; 20:69–76.
40. Beaver PC, Fallon M, Smith GH. Pulmonary nodule caused by a living Brugia malayi-like filaria in an artery. Am J Trop Med Hyg 1971; 20:661–666.
41. Somer T, Finegold SM. Vasculitides associated with infections, immunization, and antimicrobial drugs. Clin Infect Dis 1995; 20:1010–1036.
42. Gelber R. Leprosy. In: Mandell G, Bennett J, Dolin R, eds. Principles and Practice of Infectious Diseases. New York: Churchill Livingston, 1995:2243–2205.
43. Scollard DM, Bhoopat L, Kestens L, Vanham G, Douglas JT, Moad J. Immune complexes and antibody levels in blisters over human leprosy skin lesions with or without erythema nodosum leprosum. Clin Immunol Immunopathol 1992; 63:230–236.
44. Sreenivasan P, Misra RS, Wilfred D, Nath I. Lepromatous leprosy patients show T helper 1-like cytokine profile with differential expression of interleukin-10 during type 1 and 2 reactions. Immunology 1998; 95:529–536.

41

Vasculitis and Rheumatoid Arthritis

Edward D. Harris, Jr.
Stanford University School of Medicine, Stanford, California

I. INTRODUCTION AND EPIDEMIOLOGY

Systemic vasculitis in rheumatoid arthritis (RA) can be considered, in very simplistic terms, as a "spillover" into extraarticular tissues of very severe synovitis. Fortunately, this complication of rheumatoid arthritis is rare. Some of its forms of presentation are very serious and life threatening; others are more benign. Management of the complication of vasculitis in the context of severe articular disease is often challenging and difficult.

An attempt to estimate the incidence of rheumatoid vasculitis has been made by Watts et al. (1). During a period of 6 years, attempts were made in a relatively closed population of over 400,000 adults to identify all patients with newly diagnosed systemic rheumatoid vasculitis that included nail bed infarcts, usually a benign process. The results showed an overall annual incidence of 12.5 per million (95% CI = 8.5–17.7). The incidence in men exceeded that in women. Despite the fact that RA occurs two to three times more frequently in women than in men, vasculitis occurred approximately four times more often in men. The annual incidence rate for men was 15.8 per million (95% CI = 9.5–24.7) and 9.4 per million (95% CI = 4.8–16.4) for women. In contrast, the annual incidence of RA within a similar population has been estimated to be 140 per million in men and 360 per million in women (2). In practical terms relevant for practioners, the probability of having many patients in a practice who have rheumatoid vasculitis is small. In a survey of 290 rheumatologists practicing in the United States, it was estimated that those physicians who saw 15–50 rheumatoid arthritis patients each week saw fewer than five RA patients with all forms of vasculitis in 1 year (3).

The clinical and laboratory features that predict an increased risk for systemic vasculitis developing in rheumatoid patients are male gender, extraarticular features, a severe course of joint disease, and, most important, high concentrations of rheumatoid factor (4).

The importance of rheumatoid factor as a pathogenic factor in rheumatoid vasculitis is discussed in subsequent sections. The intriguing discordance between the higher incidence of vasculitis in men, when there is a greater frequency of rheumatoid arthritis in women, remains a mystery. Watts et al. (1) have calculated that there is a lifetime risk of developing systemic rheumatoid vasculitis for a patient with RA of 1 in 9 for men and 1 in 38 for women. This may seem to be high numbers, but it must be remembered that when many authors refer to "vasculitis" in RA they include digital infarcts, a complication that is much more common than systemic forms involving internal organs or the nervous system.

What is the incidence of systemic rheumatoid vasculitis compared with other forms of vasculitis? In a study from the United Kingdom, the annual incidence of polyarteritis nodosa has been estimated at 4.6 per million (5), whereas an estimate of annual frequency in the United States, determined at approximately the same time, was 9.0 per million (6). In the Norwich, United Kingdom, population of 414,000 in 1994, it is apparent that Wegener's granulomatosis with an annual incidence of 8.5 per million and systemic rheumatoid vasculitis are the most common of this genre (7).

II. CLINICAL FEATURES

No one knows why rheumatoid arthritis localizes to the joints, but it is very evident that blood vessels are intimately involved in pathogenesis of the disease. It is the microvasculature of synovium that very early in the disease develops activated endothelial cells expressing adhesion molecules enabling lymphocytes, macrophages, and polymorphonuclear (PMN) leukocytes to adhere, bind, and work through the vessel wall into the synovium for perpetuation and amplification of the rheumatoid process (8). Why are vessels not equally involved in other tissues? The answer is unknown, but must relate to an arthritogenic antigen that is, as yet, unknown. In the patients who do develop systemic vasculitis, excluding pulmonary fibrosis and rheumatoid nodules and other manifestations of proliferative granulomata, clinical manifestations may include

> Digital arteritis (splinter hemorrhages to gangrene)
> Cutaneous ulceration (including pyoderma gangrenosum)
> Palpable purpura (i.e., leukocytoclastic vasculitis)
> Peripheral neuropathy
> Myopathy
> Arteritis of viscera (heart, lungs, bowel, kidney, liver, spleen, pancreas, lymph nodes, and
>   testis)
> Central nervous system (CNS) vasculitis

One example of systemic vasculitis in a rheumatoid patient gives a clear picture of the substrate and common findings:

> Picture a 58-year-old man who acutely developed RA associated with low-grade fevers and severe stiffness with abundant synovial proliferation in the PIPJ, MCPJ, wrists, and feet. The laboratory tests revealed a hemoglobin of 10.2 g/dL, mild thrombocytosis, white blood cell count of 10,380/mm^3 with a slight predominance of granulocytes and an excess (7%) of eosinophils, an erythrocyte sedimentation rate of 62 mm/h and C-reactive protein of 3.4 mg/dL (normal <0.6), rheumatoid factor positive at high dilutions, negative FANA, and a normal urinalysis. He was treated first with NSAIDs, then with 10 mg methotrexate each week. The disease was resistant to therapy. Within several months, rheumatoid nodules appeared on both olecranon processes, and prednisone 5 mg/day was added to the therapy. After 2 years of aggressive therapy including methotrexate, 17.5 mg each week, sufasalazine, and hydroxychloroquine, he developed significant joint destruction and was placed on a surgeon's list for a total knee replacement.
>
> He telephoned his primary care physician when he began to notice tingling in the lateral aspects of his right calf and ankle, and a tendency to stub his toe. On examination he was found to have decreased sensation over the right lateral calf and heel. Strength of the extensors of his right forefoot and toes was estimated to be at 2 on a scale of 5. Reflexes were decreased slightly at the right knee and ankle. His joint examination was unchanged and indicative of severe proliferative and destructive synovitis.
>
> Laboratory tests revealed a slight leukocytosis, moderate anemia, normal urinalysis, normal renal and liver function, an erythrocyte sedimentation rate of 84 mm/h and a C-reac-

tive protein of 2.3 mg/dL. Chest radiographs showed mild basilar fibrosis. A sural nerve and adjacent muscle biopsy was performed; the nerve showed fibrosis and atrophy of several fascicles of the nerve, and fibrinoid necrosis in the walls of small arterioles in both the nerve and adjacent muscle.

This example is one of mononeuritis multiplex, and is typical of rheumatoid patients with vasculitis. The evidence for vasculitis gradually appeared, superimposed upon severe joint disease and high titers of rheumatoid factor. This subgroup represents fewer than 1% of patients with RA. The findings on biopsy, usually of skin or muscle, range from mild perivascular infiltration with inflammatory cells to fibrinoid necrosis and immunoglobulin deposits in vessel walls with infarctions within the distal vascular beds. Even in small-vessel involvement (e.g., in obliterative endarteritis of the finger) immune complex deposits have been demonstrated in vessel walls (9). Uninvolved skin from rheumatoid patients is positive for immunoglobulin (Ig) and complement; the presence of IgG correlates directly with circulating immune complexes, vasculitic skin lesions, subcutaneous nodules, and very high titers of rheumatoid factor. Nonspecific findings in patients with RA that should warn the physician about the possibility of a developing vasculitis are weight loss, pleuritis, pericarditis, ocular inflammation, hepatic or splenic enlargement, or Felty's syndrome (10,11). It has been estimated that vasculitis may occur in about 30% of patients with Felty's syndrome (12).

The various forms of vasculitis in rheumatoid disease that are listed above are now described in more detail:

Digital arteritis—This form of rheumatoid vasculitis is more benign than others, and does not presage visceral or more serious cutaneous disease. The lesions can resemble splinter hemorrhages in the nail bed or Osler's nodes in finger pulp (Fig. 1).

Cutaneous ulceration—In Felty's syndrome (neutropenia, frequently with splenomegaly in RA), localized plaques of superficial cutaneous infarction can cause skin breakdown, usually in a circular form ranging from 1–5 cm in diameter. More serious are the lesions of pyoderma gangrenosum. These can be deep, dirty ulcerations that can penetrate through fascia and are marked by heaped up eschar at the edges (Fig. 2). Cytotoxic drugs are often needed for control of this process. Superimposed infection is common.

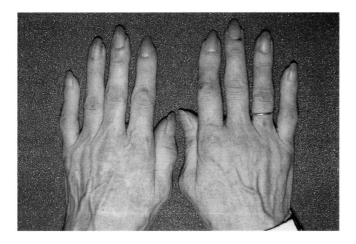

Figure 1 Rheumatoid digital vasculitis. (Courtesy of Dr. Gary S. Hoffman.)

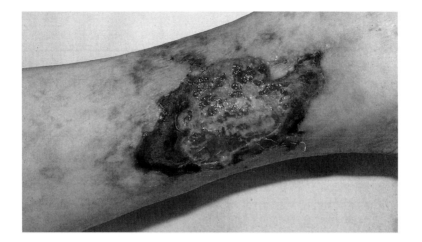

Figure 2 Recurrent vasculitis has occurred about the distal tibia. Tissue destruction has progressed through subcutaneous tissue and fascia, extending to muscle. Gangrenous eschar is present about the periphery. Healed scars indicate the waxing and waning nature of disease at this site. Because of failure of more conservative therapies, treatment was initiated with daily cyclophosphamide, in addition to intensive local care of the wound. Considerable improvement followed within 12 weeks. (Courtesy of Dr. Gary S. Hoffman.)

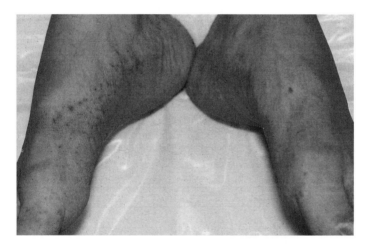

Figure 3 Palpable purpura, affecting the feet of a 55-year-old woman with chronic rheumatoid arthritis. Lesions were nontender and did not proceed to ulceration. Resolution followed the use of prednisone, 20 mg daily, over a period of 2 weeks. Prednisone was gradually discontinued without recurrence of lesions. Whether these lesions would have spontaneously resolved without treatment is uncertain. (Courtesy of Dr. Gary S. Hoffman.)

> *Palpable purpura*—These are the classic lesions of small-vessel (capillary and venule) angiitis. Small purple papules that are neither painful nor pruritic and do not blanch appear in crops, usually on dependent extremities (Fig. 3). At any given time, lesions of varying size and age are present. Over several days after their appearance, the lesions flatten and spread, and the borders of adjacent lesions may coalesce. Ulceration is unusual. Unlike a typical bruise, brown discoloration may persist long after healing. Biopsy reveals lymphocytic infiltrate adjacent to postcapillary venules and abun-

dant nuclear fragments from degraded polymorphonuclear leukocytes. The same lesions can be found in multiple different diseases, including systemic lupus erythematosus (SLE), cryoglobulinemia, allergic reactions to drugs, human immunodeficiency virus (HIV) infection, and other forms of systemic vasculitis. Urinary sediment consistent with a mild glomerulitis occasionally accompanies the skin lesions.

Peripheral neuropathy—A prototype case of this form of vasculitis is given in the case presented above. The typical lesion is unilateral, or one that begins with a staggered start in both legs (legs more common than arms). Sensory and motor nerves are affected in the distribution of a single nerve, although occasionally only a mild distal sensory neuropathy is found (13). This latter group may complain of "burning feet" along with decreased touch and pin sensation distally. Foot drop, paresthesias, and numbness are the most common symptoms.

The sural nerve and adjacent muscle are most often used as biopsy sites; the sural nerve has a relatively small cutaneous sensory distribution and no motor activity.

Myopathy—Active vasculitis in skeletal muscle can produce swollen, tender, and very painful muscles. This is in contrast to the frequently painless weakness that is characteristic of polymyositis, or the deep aching without tenderness found in polymyalgia rheumatica. Muscles on the chest wall can be affected as are those on the arms and legs. When muscle bundles in the paraspinal areas are involved the presenting syndrome is one of a "slipped disk" with occasionally immobilizing back spasm.

Arteritis of viscera—With the exception of isolated cranial arteritis in rheumatoid disease, fibrinoid necrosis of vessel walls within viscera have the most potential for severe morbidity and, rarely, death. The symptoms and signs reflect localized ischemia or infarction. The distribution can resemble that found in polyarteritis. Coronary vasculitis can present as myocardial infarction; intestinal vasculitis can present with symptoms of bowel ischemia. Peritonitis may result from vasculitis of peritoneal vessels or from seepage or perforation of ischemic bowel that gives its contents access to the peritoneum. Exploratory surgery can reveal infarcted loops of bowel (14). A patient has been described who developed abdominal pain, then syncope due to intraabdominal hemorrhage from a ruptured aneurysm of the inferior pancreaticoduodenal artery. This man had prior extraarticular rheumatoid disease, including pulmonary fibrosis and Sjögren's syndrome (15). Testicular vasculitis resembles a cord torsion syndrome. Very rarely, pulmonary hypertension in the absence of interstitial lung disease can be a manifestation of vasculitis in patients with RA (16).

CNS arteritis—Cranial arteritis, indistinguishable from isolated (idiopathic) cranial arteritis that occurs without any accompanying disease, is rare and serious. CNS vasculitis associated with rheumatoid arthritis is exceedingly rare. It was reported to occur in less than 0.1% of admissions to a neurological unit serving 2.5 million people (10). Because these data were not derived from a general population of rheumatoid arthritis patients, they may not be a valid measure of incidence or prevalence. Although there is great heterogeneity in clinical presentations of cerebral vasculitis, there are three more common patterns (17):

1. *Acute or subacute encephalopathy*—Patients presenting in this way may develop headaches, vomiting and lapse into stupor or even coma.
2. *Symptoms and signs resembling multiple sclerosis*—Patients presenting in this fashion may have apparently unrelated events that come and go (e.g., sensory disturbances or small areas of muscle twitching, then visual loss, amnesia, hyperreflexia) and imaging studies that suggest demyelinating diseases. The cerebrospinal fluid (CSF) can reveal oligoclonal bands.

3. *Features simulating a rapidly progressive space-occupying lesion*—These patients can present with global neurological dysfunction. Computed tomography (CT) scans can show an apparent intracranial mass lesion. Biopsy can reveal vasculitis, infarction, or changes consistent with infection. The latter problem is directly proportional to the degree of immunosuppression in individual patients, and thus is very important to rule out by biopsy.

It is important for physicians to be aware that patients can have previously established rheumatoid disease without active arthritis at the time of neurological presentation. In all cases of CNS vasculitis, ophthalmological examination can aid diagnosis. Abnormalities can include marked slowing of flow, multifocal attenuation of arterioles, and aggregates of erythrocytes. Fluorescein studies can confirm these findings and also demonstrate small-vessel infarction and leakage from postcapillary and collecting venules.

III. LABORATORY FINDINGS

Findings from laboratory tests usually help confirm a diagnosis of vasculitis that has been suspected on clinical grounds. As mentioned above, vasculitis appears in rheumatoid patients who often have active disease with extraarticular manifestations. Therefore, it is not unusual for them to have

> *Elevated acute phase reactants (erythrocyte sedimentation rate [ESR] and C-reactive protein [CRP] levels).* Occasionally, because serum gamma globulin and fibrinogen levels are inordinately high, the ESR may be elevated proportionately more than the CRP, which is a protein made by the liver in response to inflammation and is not affected by other acute phase reactants or changes in serum proteins.
> *Anemia.* This is generally characterized as a hypochromic, microcytic anemia that is inversely proportional to the ESR or CRP. Iron stores are usually adequate, but utilization is insufficient to generate adequate red blood cells.
> *Thrombocytosis and leukocytosis.*
> *Hypoalbuminemia.*
> *Rheumatoid factor*—often in high titer.

None of these tests is specific and there is great overlap with patients who have very active joint disease but very few extraarticular manifestations. One test that is of use in systemic vasculitis and crescentic glomerulonephritis is the titer of antibody to neutrophil cytoplasmic antigens (ANCAs). There are two patterns of ANCAs recognized by indirect immunofluorescence: C-ANCA is prominent in Wegener's granulomatosis and indicates the presence of anti–proteinase 3 antibody in the cell cytoplasm; a perinuclear pattern (P-ANCA) is generated often by antibody to myeloperoxidase, although several other target antigens producing a perinuclear pattern have been noted, and include elastase, cathepsin G, and lactoferrrin. In a study of patients with long-standing RA, 48% had significant titers of P-ANCA, although only 29% of RA patients with vasculitis had elevated P-ANCA titers, and the most prevalent antibody in RA was against human elastase (18). Close to half of the patients studied with a diagnosis of SLE also had positive ANCAs. Two other studies, however, have suggested that the presence of ANCAs might be a marker for a more aggressive course of disease in respect to serological variables and extraarticular manifestations, including rheumatoid vasculitis and lung involvement (19). Mulder et al. (19) reported much higher titers of ANCAs in rheumatoid vasculitis compared with uncomplicated RA. These authors found that the dominant antigen in rheumatoid patients for ANCAs was lactoferrin, not proteinase 3, myeloperoxidase, elastase, or cathepsin G. Another series (20) found ANCAs in 16% of patients with RA, all showing a perinuclear pattern. This P-ANCA–positive group had a higher frequency of vasculitis ($p < 0.05$) than did rheumatoid patients who were P-ANCA–negative. Much work is needed to determine whether the ANCA that appears in certain patients with RA is more than an epiphenomenon.

Goronzy and Weyand (21) have set forth the hypothesis that individuals with synovial disease and individuals with synovial plus extraarticular disease, including vasculitis, are parts of two separate groups that can be best defined by immunogenetic analysis. Virtually all patients with extraarticular disease in their clinics carry an HLA-DRB1*04 allele. Of 28 patients who had inherited two disease-linked alleles, all had nodular disease and 61% had other extraarticular manifestations. Fifty percent of the patients with rheumatoid vasculitis were homozygous for *HLA-DRB1*0401*, and an additional 21% were heterozygous for two disease-associated *HLA-DRB1*04* variants (22). In a more recent study, however, no associations were found between rheumatoid vasculitis and any of the *DRB1*04* alleles or with *DQA1* or *DQB1* alleles, although the risk of developing minor skin vasculitis (e.g., palpable purpura) was increased in patients with *DRB1*04* (23).

IV. DIAGNOSIS AND PROGNOSIS

The diagnosis of vasculitis in rheumatoid patients should be primarily a clinical one. To move from a moderate to high degree of suspicion of a diagnosis of rheumatoid vasculitis, histological examination of a biopsy specimen from an affected organ should be obtained (24). Perivascular infiltrates with mononuclear and polymorphonuclear leukocytes are more likely to be found in nonlesional skin biopsies of rheumatoid vasculitis patients than in patients with RA without vasculitis (25). In an attempt to determine whether muscle biopsy might be a more sensitive and specific index of vasculitis, quadriceps (rectus femoris) biopsies were done in patients with RA and vasculitis confirmed by other means, RA patients with no clinical suspicion of vasculitis, and osteoarthritis patients. It was found that the finding in muscle of perivascular infiltrates of > three cell layers of perivascular mono/polymorphonuclear leukocytes was found in 67% of RA patients with vasculitis, and in none of the RA patients without clinical evidence for vasculitis or osteoarthritis patients. Fibrinoid necrosis of vessel walls was found in 33% of the 12 patients with rheumatoid vasculitis, but in none of the other RA patients ($n = 12$) or in muscle from osteoarthritis patients ($n = 11$). The majority of the perivascular infiltrating cells were mononuclear, as opposed to polymorphonuclear. The yield of positive results was increased by examination of multiple sections. Muscle biopsy is appropriate, therefore, when a biopsy of a sural nerve is being taken in cases of clinical mononeuritis multiplex, and when the diagnosis of vasculitis is suspected. Whenever possible, of course, biopsy of tissue from organs suspected of being damaged by vasculitis is preferred.

It would be very useful if blood tests from rheumatoid patients were both sensitive and specific markers of vasculitis. Although several such tests have been evaluated, they remain imperfect tools for the clinician. Plasma levels of circulating cellular fibronectin levels in rheumatoid vasculitis patients have been reported to be significantly ($p = 0.01$) elevated over rheumatoid patients without vasculitis (26). The fibronectin levels correlated with von Willebrand factor antigen levels. In the same group of patients, circulating levels of intercellular adhesion molecules (cICAM-1 and cICAM3) but not cE-selectin were elevated ($p > 0.0001$) compared with patients with RA who did not have evidence of vasculitis (27). The levels appeared to fluctuate directly with clinical activity of the vasculitis.

Prognosis for patients with rheumatoid vasculitis is less good than for those with disease confined to the joints. Indeed, compared with age- and sex-matched control populations, there is an increased risk of death for rheumatoid patients who have cutaneous ulcers, vasculitic rash, or neuropathy (28). Rheumatoid arthritis itself puts patients at significant risk for earlier demise. It is almost an a priori finding that those who are sicker, with extraarticular involvement, and with progressively more vascular involvement (especially in internal organs such as the GI tract, heart and lungs, and CNS) will have a worse prognosis than others. In the survey of 290 North American rheumatologists, the respondents associated the following features most strongly with a poor prognosis in rheumatoid vasculitis: mononeuritis multiplex, digital gangrene, nonhealing leg ulcers, scleromalacia perforans, high titer rheumatoid factor, positive visceral angiography, and necrotizing arteritis on biopsy. From the large Dutch group that has intensively studied rheumatoid vasculitis come data to indicate that the unadjusted relative risk of death in rheumatoid vasculitis patients compared with RA controls was 1.65, and this fell to 1.26 after adjustment for age and sex (29). In this group, infection (probably related to immunosuppressive therapy) was the main cause of death in the rheumatoid vasculitis patients. Cardiovascular disease was the most common cause of mortality in the rheumatoid patients who did not have vasculitis.

V. MANAGEMENT

Therapy depends upon the clinical manifestations of the vasculitis in patients with RA.

Patients with mild cutaneous disease (e.g., fingernail linear hemorrhages, small patches of palpable purpura, asymptomatic digital vasculitis) do not require added therapy to what is appropriate for other aspects of their disease. It is crucial that extra emphasis on smoking cessation be stressed for all patients with vasculitis. Although it has not been rigorously studied, it is logical to assume that the vasoconstrictive and atherogenic influences of tobacco may amplify the pathogenic mechanisms underlying rheumatoid vasculitis. Blood pressure control is recommended for the same reasons. Relatively small, nonprogressive leg ulcers can be managed conservatively with debridement, antimicrobial ointments, and dressing regimens supervised by experienced dermatologists or vascular surgeons. Although rheumatologists make every effort to keep oral prednisone therapy in rheumatoid patients to less than 7.5 mg/day, the appearance of systemic vasculitis other than mild cutaneous forms warrants treatment with higher doses (up to 60 mg daily) until signs or symptoms diminish or are stable, at which time slow tapering can begin. As soon as higher doses of glucocorticoids are prescribed, bone protective regimens (e.g., 1500 mg/day elemental calcium and 400 IU vitamin D, and bisphosphonates or, in postmenopausal women, raloxifine) should be instituted. In general, it is probably inappropriate to risk thrombotic disease by starting estrogen therapy in a woman with RA who has developed vasculitis. D-penicillamine was first used effectively in a group of rheumatoid patients who had cutaneous ulcers associated with high titers of rheumatoid factor (30). In disease that is refractory to moderate doses of glucocorticoids, treatment with cyclophosphamide in doses used for treatment of Wegener's granulomatosis should be considered (31). The usual starting dose is 2 mg/kg/day, orally. Hemorrhagic cysitis and the risk of opportunistic infections and, later, carcinoma of the bladder are major toxicities, but usually the addition of cyclophosphamide enables the prednisone dose to be lowered. Isolated reports of accelerated vasculitis during methotrexate therapy (32) for rheumatoid patients have not been seen with any regularity. If cyclophosphamide is going to be used in patients already taking methotrexate, the latter drug should be stopped. In uncontrolled studies, it has been reported that plasmapheresis combined with prolonged therapy with immunosuppression can reduce the morbidity of cutaneous leg ulcers, but has no effect on long-standing neuropathic manifestations (33). Plasma exchange has been used in severe cutaneous rheumatoid vasculitis. However, these results are not the product of controlled trials and will have to be confirmed by more rigorous study (34).

The pathophysiology of aggressive disease implies processes driven in part by tumor necrosis factor alpha (TNF-α), and it is imperative that well-controlled studies using anti-TNF-α therapy in rheumatoid vasculitis be performed and reported.

REFERENCES

1. Watts RA, Carruthers DM, Symmons DP, et al. The incidence of rheumatoid vasculitis in the Norwich Health Authority. Br J Rheumatol 1994; 33:832–833.
2. Symmons DPM, Barrett EM, Bankhead CR, et al. The incidence of rheumatoid arthritis in the United Kingdom: Results from the Norfolk Arthritis Register. Br J Rheumatol 1994; 33:735–739.
3. Panush RS, Katz P, Longley S, et al. Rheumatoid vasculitis: Diagnostic and therapeutic decisions. Clin Rheumatol 1983; 4:321–330.
4. Voskuyl AE, Zwinderman AH, Westedt ML, et al. Factors associated with the development of vasculitis in rheumatoid arthritis: Results of a case-control study. Ann Rheum Dis 1996; 55:190–192.
5. Scott DGI, Bacon PA, Elliott PJ, et al. Systemic vasculitis in district general hospital 1972–80: Clinical and laboratory features, classification and prognosis of 80 cases. Q J Med 1982; 203:292–311.
6. Kurland LT, Chuang TY, Hunder G. The Epidemiology of the Rheumatic Diseases. New York: Gower, 1984.
7. Watts RA, Carruthers DM, Scott DG. Epidemiology of systemic vasculitis: Changing incidence of definition? Semin Arthritis Rheum 1995; 25:28–34.
8. Harris ED Jr. Rheumatoid Arthritis. Philadelphia: Saunders, 1997.
9. Fischer M, Mielke H, Glafke S, et al. Generalized vasculopathy and finger blood flow abnormalities in rheumatoid arthritis. J Rheumatol 1984; 11:33.
10. Fischer M, Mielke H, Glafke S, et al. Generalized vasculopathy and finger blood flow abnormalities in rheumatoid arthritis. J Rheumatol 1984; 11:33.
11. Vollertsen RS, Conn DL Vasculitis associated with rheumatoid arthritis. Rheum Dis Clin North Am 1990; 16:445–461.
12. Campion G, Maddison PJ, Goulding N, et al. The Felty syndrome: A case-matched study of clinical manifestations and outcome, serologic features and immunogenetic associations. Medicine 1990; 69: 69–80.
13. Schmid FR, Cooper NS, Ziff M, et al. Arteritis in rheumatoid arthritis. Am J Med 1961; 30:56.
14. Babian M, Nasef S, Soloway G. Gastrointestinal infarction as a manifestation of rheumatoid vasculitis. Am J Gastroenterol 1998; 93:119–120.
15. Achkar AA, Stanson AW, Johnson CM, et al. Rheumatoid vasculitis manifesting as intra-abdominal hemorrhage. Mayo Clin Proc 1995; 70:565–569.
16. Balagopal VP da Costa P, Greenstone MA. Fatal pulmonary hypertension and rheumatoid vasculitis. Eur Respir J 1995; 8:331–333.
17. Scolding NJ, Jayne DRW, Zajicek JP. Cerebral vasculitis: Recognition, diagnosis and management. Q J Med 1997; 90:61–73.
18. deBrant M, Meyer O, Haim T et al. Antineutrophil cytoplasmic antibodies in rheumatoid arthritis patients. Br J Rheumatol 1996; 35:38–43.
19. Mulder AHL, Horst G, Van Leewven MA, et al. Antineutrophil cytoplasmic antibodies in rheumatoid arthritis. Characterization and clinical correlations. Arthritis Rheum 1993; 36:1054–1060.
20. Braun MG, Csernok E, Schmitt WH, et al. Incidence, target antigens, and clinical implications of antineutrophil cytoplasmic antibodies in rheumatoid arthritis. J Rheumatol 1996; 23:826–830.
21. Goronzy JJ, Weyand CM. Vasculitis in rheumatoid arthritis. Curr Opin Rheumatol 1994; 6:290–294.
22. Weyand CM, Xie C, Goronzy JJ. Homozygosity for the HLA-DRB1 allele selects for extraarticular manifestations in rheumatoid arthritis. J Clin Invest 1992; 89:2033–2039.
23. Voskuyl AE, Hazes JM, Schreuder GM, et al. HLA-DRB1, DQA1, and DQB1 genotypes and risk of vasculitis in patients with rheumatoid arthritis. J Rheumatol 1997; 5:852–855.
24. Voskuyl AE, Zwinderman AH, Westedt ML, et al. Factors associated with the development of vasculitis in rheumatoid arthritis; results of a case-control study. Ann Rheum Dis 1996; 55:190–192.

25. Westedt ML, Meijer CJLM, Vermeer BJ, et al. Rheumatoid arthritis. The clinical significance of histo- and immunopathological abnormalities in normal skin. J Rheumatol 1984; 11:448–453.

26. Voskuyl AE, Emeis JJ, Hazes JM, et al. Levels of circulating cellular fibronectin are increased in patients with rheumatoid vasculitis. Clin Exp Rheumatol 1998; 16:429–434.

27. Voskuyl AE, Martin S, Melchers L, et al. Levels of circulating intercellular adhesion molecule-1 and -3 but not circulating endothelial leukocyte adhesion molecule are increased in patients with rheumatoid vasculitis. Br J Rheumatol 1995; 34:311–315.

28. Eberhardt CC, Mumford PA, Venables PJW et al. Factors predicting a poor life prognosis in rheumatoid arthritis: An eight year prospective study. Ann Rheum Dis 1989; 48:7–10.

29. Voskuyl AE, Zwinderman AH, Westedt ML, et al. The mortality of rheumatoid vasculitis compared with rheumatoid arthritis. Arthritis Rheum 1996; 39:266–271.

30. Jaffe IA. Penicilamine. In: Kelley WN, Harris EDJr., Ruddy S, Sledge CB, eds. Textbook of Rheumatology. 4th ed. Philadelphia: Saunders, 1993:760–766.

31. Abel T, Andrews BS, Cunningham PH, et al. Rheumatoid vasculitis: Effect of cyclophosphamide on the clinical course and levels of circulating immune complexes. Ann Int Med 1980; 93:407–413.

32. Segal R. Accelerated nodulosis and vasculitis during methotrexate therapy for rheumatoid arthritis. Arthritis Rheum 1988; 31:1182–1184.

33. Winkelstein A, Starz TW, Agarwal A. Efficacy of combined therapy with plasmapheresis and immunosuppressants in rheumatoid vasculitis. J Rheumatol 1984; 11:12–166.

34. Ortonne JP, Cassuto-Viguier E, Quananta JF, et al. Acta Derm Venereol 1983; 63:543–546.

42
Systemic Sclerosis with Vascular Emphasis

M. Bashar Kahaleh
Medical College of Ohio, Toledo, Ohio

E. Carwile LeRoy
Medical University of South Carolina, Charleston, South Carolina

I. INTRODUCTION

Scleroderma (literally "hard skin") is an umbrella term that covers most forms of thickened, sclerotic skin, including both localized (morphea, linear scleroderma, many others) and generalized (limited, diffuse) variants. Generalized scleroderma is synonymous with systemic sclerosis (SSc). Systemic sclerosis, the third most common connective tissue disease and the most lethal, affects the diffuse connective tissues and is associated with immune (autoimmune), vascular, microvascular, and fibrotic manifestations. The diagnosis, when the disease is fully expressed, can be made by visual and certainly by tactile observations alone. In its early prodromal phases, however, SSc usually begins with Raynaud's phenomenon.

> In its aggravated form, diffuse scleroderma is one of the most terrible of all human ills. Like Tithonus, to wither slowly and like him to be beaten down and marred and wasted until one is literally a mummy encased in an evershrinking skin of steel is a fate not pictured in any tragedy ancient or modern. (Osler W. On diffuse scleroderma; with special reference to diagnosis, and the use of thyroid gland extract. J Cutan Genito-urinary Dis 1895; 16: 49.)

II. RAYNAUD'S PHENOMENON

In 1862, Maurice Raynaud described cold-sensitive digital ischemic attacks that are now referred to as Raynaud's phenomenon (RP). Because of recent progress, a clear clinical definition and a precise delineation of associated disorders can be made; the prevalence of RP in the population can be measured. There are now theories of pathogenesis, methods of investigation, and rational approaches to therapy.

A. Clinical Definition

The classical definition, episodic triphasic color changes of pallor, cyanosis, and rubor, is rarely seen sequentially in the same patient, and current definitions do not strictly require all three colors for diagnosis. Biphasic color changes of pallor and cyanosis are commonly reported by patients.

Primary Raynaud's Phenomenon or Raynaud's disease is defined as documented RP, normal peripheral pulse, normal nailfold capillaries, negative antinuclear antibody (ANA) test, and a normal Westergren erythrocyte sedimentation rate. It is a benign condition with negligible consequences. Fibromyalgia, a prolapsed mitral valve, migraine headaches, irritable bowel syndrome, or heightened anxiety may be associated as comorbid, possibly pathogenetically related through sympathetic nervous system interaction.

Secondary Raynaud's Phenomenon or Raynaud's Syndrome signals the presence of an associated disease. The workup of patients with Raynaud's phenomenon without an underlying cause should include a careful history and physical examination, a test for antinuclear antibodies, hands and chest radiographs, and nailfold capillary microscopy. If the results of these evaluations are negative, the diagnosis of primary Raynaud's phenomenon is made. However, if clinical or laboratory abnormalities are detected, then a serial evaluation should be performed periodically to detect transition to a connective tissue disorder, which may take 10 years or more. The vast majority of patients with Raynaud's phenomenon in the general population have the primary, benign form of the disease and do not require extensive evaluation or intensive follow-up.

B. Prevalence

A questionnaire-based study of RP in South Carolina revealed a prevalence of up to 10% in the general population, whereas clinical screening studies reported a prevalence rate of 3–3.5%. The prevalence of RP in established connective tissue diseases is shown in Table 1.

C. Associated Conditions and Methods of Investigation

Conditions most frequently associated with RP are listed in Table 2. A follow-up over several decades of patients with RP who sought medical attention revealed an associated disease in 30–80%. However, local referral patterns significantly affect any clinical series.

Antinuclear antibody testing is positive in 30–50% of patients with RP; accordingly, disease-specific ANA should be evaluated (Table 3). Antibodies to dsDNA, Sm, SSA/SSB, RNP, centromere (ACA) and Scl-70 (see Table 3) are significant for prognosis. Antinuclear antibody has 98% and Scl-70 has 100% specificity for development of scleroderma, comparable to widefield nailfold capillaroscopy.

Table 1 Prevalence of RP in the Rheumatic Diseases

Disease[a]	%
Scleroderma	90
MCTD/UCTS	80
SLE	40
SS	30
PM/DM	20
Rheumatoid arthritis	15

[a]MCTD/UCTS = mixed connective tissue disease/undifferentiated connective tissue syndrome; SLE = systemic lupus erythematosus; SS = Sjögren's syndrome; PM/DM = polymyositis/dermatomyositis.

Table 2 Classification of Raynaud's Phenomenon

Primary Raynaud's disease
Secondary Raynaud's phenomenon
   Chronic occlusive arterial diseases
      Arteriosclerosis obliterans
      Thromboangiitis obliterans
      Embolization
      External compression (carpal tunnel and thoracic outlet syndromes)
   Rheumatic disorders
      Systemic sclerosis
      Rheumatoid arthritis
      Systemic lupus erythematosus
      Vasculitis
      Dermatomyositis–polymyositis
      Sjögren's syndrome
   Occupational trauma
      Pianists, typists, sewing machine operators
      Pneumatic hammer operators, chain-saw operators (manual, vibratory)
      Butchers, mechanics, dairy workers, farmers, miners (silica)
      Solvent exposure (trichloroethylene, toluene, vinyl chloride, epoxy, benzene)
   Chemical and drug exposure

Vinyl chloride	Methysergide	L-Tryptophan
Bleomycin	Pentazocine	L-5-OH-Tryptophan
Cisplatin	Cocaine	
β-Blockers	Ethoxysuximide	
Ergotamines	Amphetamines (and other appetite suppressors)	

   Blood diseases
      Cold agglutinins: primary atypical pneumonia, infectious mononucleosis, lupus erythematosus, lymphoma, and viral infections
      Cryoglobulins and hyperviscosity
      Neoplastic diseases: multiple myeloma, lymphocytic leukemia, polycythemia vera, lymphosarcoma
      Chronic infectious diseases: kala-azar, malaria, and subacute bacterial endocarditis
   Miscellaneous
      Reflex sympathetic dystrophy
      Malignancy
      Hypothyroidism
      Cirrhosis
      Coronary artery disease

Table 3 Serologic Profile in Patients with RP and Connective Tissue Diseases[a]

	RNP	SSA/SSB	Centromere	Scl-70	dsDNA	Sm
UCTS/MCTD	+	+/–	+/–	+/–	+/–	+/–
SSc	+	+/–	+	+	–	–
SLE	+	+	–	–	+	+
SS	+	+	–	–	–	–

[a]Abbreviations: UCTS, undifferentiated connective tissue syndrome; SLE, systemic lupus erythematosus; SSc, systemic sclerosis; SS, Sjögren's syndrome; dsDNA, double-stranded DNA; SSA/SSB, Sjögren's syndrome A and B antigens, same as Ro and La; RNP, RNA protein complex; ACA, anticentromere antibodies; Scl, scleroderma 70 kD, same as topoisomerase.

D. Etiology and Pathogenesis

Considerable evidence indicates that episodes of Raynaud's phenomenon follow closure of the digital arteries. The exact mechanism of arterial closure is not known; however, increased sympathetic tone, local hypersensitivity to cold, increased blood viscosity, occlusive arterial disease, and platelet vessel wall interaction are among the proposed mechanisms. Vascular endothelial injury with associated dysfunction is the principal pathological process in RP. The recent description of decreased tissue levels of the potent vasodilator calcium gene-related peptide and the reported increase in release of the vasospastic mediator endothelin suggest enhanced local vasospasm.

III. SYSTEMIC SCLEROSIS

A. Classification

Taut skin proximal to the metacarpophalangeal joints is the major criterion for diagnosis of scleroderma. Sclerodactyly, digital pitting scars, and bilateral basilar pulmonary fibrosis on chest roentgenogram were identified as the three minor criteria. The presence of the major criterion or two or more minor criteria satisfies the diagnosis of scleroderma.

Patients with systemic sclerosis follow two distinguishable patterns of skin and internal organ involvement. The most prevalent pattern is called limited cutaneous systemic sclerosis (lcSSc); patients with this pattern usually have a long history of Raynaud's phenomenon, skin thickening limited to the fingers and face, and internal organ involvement in the second to fourth decades. Anticentromere antibodies are found mainly in lcSSc, which is associated with an 80% 5-year and 50% 12-year survival. A more serious, but less common, form of systemic sclerosis is diffuse cutaneous systemic sclerosis (dcSSc). These patients may present with the abrupt onset of Raynaud's phenomenon; puffy hands, arms, face, and feet; and the rapid progression of the process to hidebound skin covering both extremities and trunk and the early appearance of internal organ involvement. Antitopoisomerase I (Scl-70) is seen predominately in this group and is associated with more extensive skin and cardiac involvement. Anti-RNA polymerase autoantibodies appear to be associated with skin and renal involvement. Diffuse scleroderma is associated with a 40% 5-year and 15% 12-year survival.

Both limited and diffuse forms of SSc are present within the adult Raynaud's phenomenon population, depending largely on the population sample from which the group was collected, and vary from <10 to >50% in population surveys, depending upon the referral bias. Limited SSc encompasses Raynaud's subjects with the nailfold capillaries and antinuclear antibody profiles characteristic of SSc (usually anticentromere in Caucasians). Years, even decades, of Raynaud's phenomenon may be the sole feature of these most limited of limited SSc patients. Objective skin changes, present eventually in 90–95% of patients, should not be required, especially in the first year of symptoms. In patients with rapidly changing skin puffiness or tautness, where skin changes appear within weeks to months of the onset of Raynaud's symptoms, and when the antinuclear pattern is not anticentromere but may be antitopoisomerase I, the diagnosis of diffuse SSc should be suspected and can be confirmed when skin changes proximal to the elbows and knees are documented, excluding the neck and face which can be affected in limited SSc. Fortunately, there are three to five limited SSc patients for every diffuse patient (1).

Patients who qualify for the strict definition of primary Raynaud's can be reassured that they will not develop connective tissue disease, specifically SSc (2). Those who do not qualify are identified as suspect connective tissue disease, suspect SSc. The classification of suspect, limited, and diffuse SSc is of prognostic significance due to the high mortality and severe morbidity of diffuse, and to a lesser degree, of limited SSc (Table 4). The pace of diagnostic and the risk of

COLOR
PLATES

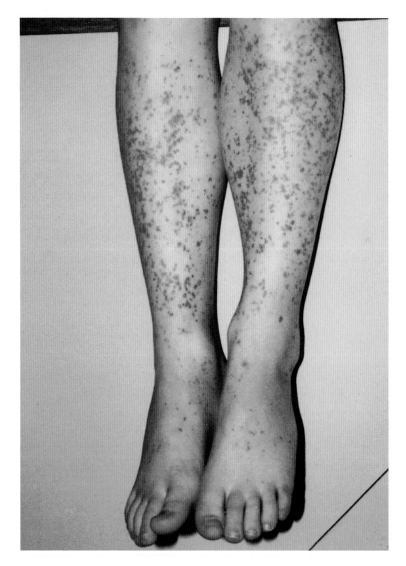

Figure 22.1 Extensive purpuric rash affecting both lower extremities in a 10-year-old girl with HSP.

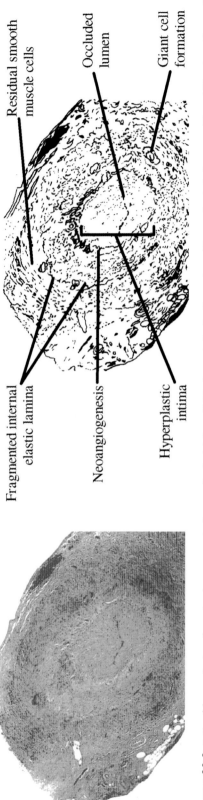

Figure 28.3 *Intimal hyperplasia—the artery's response to immunological injury.* Critical events in the formation of hyperplastic intima are: (1) mobilization of smooth muscle cells and fragmentation of the internal elastic lamina by metalloproteinases; (2) formation of growth factor–secreting giant cells and smooth muscle cell proliferation; and (3) neoangiogenesis in the intima.

Residual smooth muscle cells

Occluded lumen

Giant cell formation

Fragmented internal elastic lamina

Neoangiogenesis

Hyperplastic intima

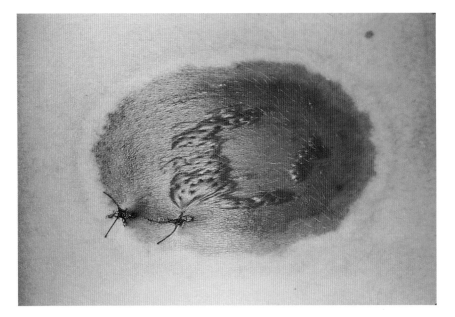

Figure 40.1 Ecthyma gangrenosum secondary to disseminated *Mucor* infection in a neutropenic patient. (Courtesy of Dr. John Bennett, National Institutes of Health, Bethesda, MD.)

Table 4 Scleroderma Deaths

Diagnosis	Mortality ratio
Pulmonary, total	29.4
Hypertension	12.5[a]
Fibrosis	10.1
Failure	5.3
Hemorrhage	1.1
Cancer	0.4
Renal, total	2.7
Heart, total	2.3
Congestive heart failure	1.7
Atherosclerosis	0.6
Sepsis and pneumonia	2.9

[a]The underlined standardized mortality ratios (useful principally for comparison between diagnoses) indicate those diagnoses in SSc death certificates that significantly exceeded those in 29 million non-SSc death certificates.

Source: Adapted from Phillips et al. A Case Study and National Database Report of Progressive Systemic Sclerosis and Associated Conditions. J Women's Health 1998; 7(9):1099–1104.

therapeutic intervention can be focused in the individual patient by this precise subset classification. As an example, limited SSc patients may change little over 5–20 years of visits (the appearance of pulmonary hypertension being the major exception to this rule), whereas diffuse SSc patients may evolve skin changes and develop visceral involvement on a month-to-month basis.

There are many ways to validate the definition of SSc subsets, the most important to the patient being the relative risk of death compared with that of the general population. Limited SSc patients have a twofold increased risk of death; diffuse SSc patients have a 4.5-fold increased risk of death. Only approximately half of SSc deaths are directly attributed to SSc; of these one-third are pulmonary, one-fifth are gastrointestinal, and a decreasing but still significant fraction succumb to scleroderma renal crisis (SRC). There is a twofold increased risk of death in SSc patients from causes that were not directly attributed to SSc, such as cardiovascular disease, cancer, and infection, all of which were probably indirectly associated with the presence of SSc (3).

B. Epidemiology

Using retrospective reviews of patients who attended clinics or who died in hospitals, the incidence of SSc has been estimated to be 1–19 per million. These techniques are inherently insensitive but relatively specific. Prevalence, more difficult to assess due to referral patterns, which instill unmeasurable biases, has been estimated to be 4–290 per million. If one estimates prevalence using 5% for Raynaud's in the general population and 1% for SSc in the Raynaud's population, one obtains 500 SSc per million, consistent with the higher prevalence estimates. The occurrence of SSc is worldwide, in all ethnic groups studied, and females are affected 4–10 times more than males (4). Infant SSc is rare, childhood SSc is uncommon, and there is no age too old to develop the disease. These matters are of less consequence than is subset classification (v.s.) in managing the individual SSc patient.

C. Skin

Each area of skin should be examined separately by an experienced observer and evaluated against the skin of that anatomical area in healthy subjects. These observations can thus be combined into a skin score. Modifications of the original Pittsburgh (Rodnan) skin score technique offer the examiner fewer options where the skin is naturally tight (distal fingers) or thick (back and abdomen) and include fewer examination sites. The Kahaleh or Charleston Skin Score is such a modified technique. The critical feature of taut skin in scleroderma of all types is in fact subcutaneous, where fat and elastic bands are replaced by collagen and the skin feels thickened, unable to be tented, and "hidebound." The skin may also be edematous early, usually developing a "wooden" consistency after edema subsides. The most sensitive areas for detection are the dorsum of the hand and the forearm, where healthy skin is thin and elastic. The patient usually detects changes before the physician does.

   The skin is usually edematous (puffy) early, indurated during the progressive phase, and atrophic late when most disease activity is "burned out." Because visceral involvement is dependent on vascular rather than skin scarring, the phases of skin involvement may not be helpful in the prediction of internal involvement or its severity. The rate of change of skin involvement on repeated examinations is perhaps the most important prognostic tool in predicting future visceral involvement. Prominent cutaneous features in the well-developed SSc patient include flexion contractures of the fingers; hyperpigmentation scattered among depigmented areas ("salt and pepper"); telangiectasia on palms, lips, fingertips and face; and subcutaneous calcifications (5).

   Changes in the epidermis include thinning, loss of rete pegs, loss of subpapillary capillary loops, either increases or decreases of pigmentation (major clinical and cosmetic concerns, especially to persons of increased skin pigment), as well as tautness and a lack of stretchability that inhibits movement and changes appearance. The psychosocial–spiritual effects of a changed appearance should not be underestimated (6).

D. Gastrointestinal System

While all segments of the digestive track can be involved in SSc, esophageal hypomotility is the most common of all organ involvement and the most frequent gastrointestinal (GI) manifestation. Dry eyes and dry mouth (xerostomia) occur in up to one-third of SSc patients but are uncommon early. Virtually every segment of the smooth muscle portions of the gut can be and usually is affected in SSc; secondary and tertiary waves of electrical excitation and consequent smooth muscle propulsion are diminished or absent; sphincters are patulous, atonic, and often atrophic. Symptoms range from dysphagia (with or without odontophagia), to bloating and abdominal distension, and may include fecal and gas incontinence. Reflux leads to esophageal stricture, metaplasia, and neoplasia (Barrett's esophagus), an uncommon but increasing feature as SSc patients live longer. If duodenal and jujunal hypomotility is sufficiently severe to prevent ascending small-bowel bacterial colonization, which consumes bile salts essential for fat absorption, malabsorption can occur with major acute abdominal symptoms and chronic nutritional consequences.

   Many patients with digestive tract SSc are asymptomatic; the first symptoms are usually related to esophageal dysmotility and include fullness and substernal pain on swallowing, especially following the ingestion of large pills or poorly chewed, unusually cold, or unusually spicy food. Lying down soon after eating a large meal can also elicit "heartburn." Esophageal transit time estimates are one of the better screening tests for esophageal dysmotility; if normal, no further testing is indicated and management can be symptomatic. If abnormal, both barium swallow and esophageal manometry are indicated to detect mechanical obstruction and to document hypomotility, respectively. The stomach is often hypomotile if studied dynamically but is seldom symptomatic, has few if any clinical consequences and is not often treated directly. Manometric techniques are usually definitive; laser-based blood flow techniques are experimental but promising.

Dilatation, hypomotility, and inefficient absorption of nutrients in the duodenum and jejunum can lead to a debilitating syndrome characterized by early satiety, abdominal distension, a bloated feeling, and severe, crampy abdominal pains. When acute, these features suggest acute abdominal obstruction and, especially when the diagnosis of SSc is not obvious or has not already been made, can lead to surgical intervention (searching for mechanical obstruction), which is not only not beneficial but can be harmful if unsuspected renal or pulmonary insufficiency is precipitated by surgery. Bowel rest and decompression of dilatation are the management of choice. Chronic management is challenging and includes antibiotics to reduce gut flora, careful dietary management including liquid and partially digested foods, frequent meals, careful upright posture after food ingestion, and, ultimately, complete bowel rest with total parenteral alimentation, a major technique of organ support equivalent to renal hemodialysis and cardiopulmonary life support (7). The use of proton pump inhibitors (omeprazole) and propulsive agents (cisapride, octreotide) has improved the quality of life in many SSc patients.

Stool patterns in SSc usually alternate between constipation and mild to moderate diarrhea. Fiber and stool bulk preparations are helpful. Cathartics and enemata can be dangerous. Major constipating drugs such as codeine should be avoided.

E. Lung

It is appropriate to be especially sensitive to lung involvement in SSc because when fully developed it can be irreversible and lethal, and also because in its early phases it is often clinically silent and a challenge to detect. As an example, up to 75% of diffuse SSc patients with normal chest radiographs and no pulmonary symptoms have abnormal chest computed tomography (CT) scans. Over the last several decades, pulmonary deaths represent a major portion of SSc-related deaths (see Table 4), especially pulmonary hypertension, which remains a major therapeutic challenge, along with end-stage pulmonary fibrosis.

Pleuritis is sufficiently rare that it should be investigated for microbial and other causes, such as rib/chest wall trauma, referred pain, or cardiac/GI causes. Effusions are usually bland with fibrin deposits on the pleural surfaces much as they occur in the synovitis of SSc.

Pulmonary hypertension, heralded by an abrupt reduction in exercise tolerance and occasionally dull chest pains, occurs largely in localized SSc patients often in the absence of interstitial lung disease; it may also occur late in diffuse SSc patients with severe interstitial lung disease, hypoxia, and respiratory insufficiency. Techniques to identify pulmonary hypertension have greatly improved with echocardiography-Doppler as a noninvasive screen and, of course, right heart catheterization when absolute measurements are crucial. The presence of peak pulmonary artery pressures above 60–65 is a very negative prognostic sign, from 40–65 a moderately negative sign, and from 25–40 the prognosis is not entirely clear. Lowering the pressure is the urgent objective. Large doses of several (more than one family) calcium channel blockers can be effective if symptomatic orthostatic hypotension can be managed. Also, hydralazine, isoproterenol, prazosin, and, recently, continuous infusions of epoprostenol (Flolan) have been successful in the individual patient. Flolan may be the most promising of these. Patients with persistent pulmonary hypertension, especially with right heart dilatation and overload, have a 50% 12-month life expectancy. Another study showed a 44% 2-year survival with pulmonary hypertension vs. 88% without.

Interstitial lung disease (ILD) is one of the most subtle and insidious of the manifestations of SSc. Because SSc patients are usually not active aerobically, because ILD is indolent, and because substantial restrictive lung involvement can occur before respiratory symptoms are given priority over skin and musculoskeletal complaints, ILD must be searched for prospectively. The chest film is insensitive; if positive, it usually does not permit the distinction of alveolitis from fibrosis. Pulmonary function tests are useful for management; volume measurements such as vital capacity are reduced late in ILD and are not sensitive early. Diffusion measurements, affected by either ventilation or perfusion, are nonspecific and thus can be sensitive indicators of either ILD or pulmonary hypertension. After several decades of experience with open lung biopsies (invasive, still the gold standard) and with two decades of experience with bronchoalveolar lavage (excellent but invasive), the single best technique to detect ILD early is a high-resolution chest CT scan, which can distinguish alveolitis from fibrosis and both together. The alveolitis-positive group of SSc patients was originally defined by lavage (cellular) criteria and can be currently defined by amorphous alveolar opacities usually at the lung bases on chest CT.

Although the data are not definitive (lacking a large and carefully studied control population unaffected by therapy), the presence of alveolitis is associated with pulmonary functional deterioration of about 5% vital capacity per year and an increased likelihood of future respiratory insufficiency. Aggressive therapeutic measures are indicated to reduce further deterioration and hopefully encourage tissue repair and return of lung function. The two agents of choice for therapeutic intervention are prednisone in moderate doses (20–40 mg PO once daily) and cyclophosphamide (up to 2 mg/kg orally) for a period of 1–3 years, depending on response. Several different groups have had success with this regimen. Others have used monthly pulse cyclophosphamide to reduce bladder toxicity with some success. With increased early detection of ILD it is hoped that fewer and fewer SSc patients will find themselves oxygen dependent and on the list for lung transplantation. More time and experience is needed to determine if this hope will be fulfilled (8).

F. Heart

As a general cadiopulmonary screening procedure, arterial desaturation (O_2) measured by finger oximeter following exercise can, if positive, alert the physician to further study for careful physiological definition of the problem.

There are many ways the heart can be affected in SSc. Pulmonary hypertension can cause the right heart to fail, systemic hypertension can cause the left heart to hypertrophy and fail, and coronary heart disease can damage the myocardium. One common feature of SSc heart disease is a bland pericarditis with pericardial effusion. It is rare for this to become chronic, constricting, or to cause tamponade. Pericardial friction rubs are rare and the only clue may be dependent edema, difficult to distinguish from the puffy phase of scleroderma in the early diffuse SSc patient. Echocardiography is definitive. Gentle decreases in pericardial fluid are in order to avoid renal cortical compromise from hypovolemia. If the pericardial effusion is considered to be potentially significant hemodynamically, a pericardial window should be created surgically.

Cardiopulmonary involvement may be subtle and relatively far advanced before it is detected clinically. Pitting edema of the legs and slight dyspnea should be investigated by physical examination to detect tachypnea, dry rales at the lung bases, and signs of pulmonary hypertension such as increased P2 intensity. Noninvasive cardiac diagnostic techniques have led to more frequent detection of cardiac involvement in scleroderma. Disorders of rhythm and conduction system are the most common abnormalities. Cardiac enlargement may not be impressive, particularly in the presence of restrictive lung disease. Cardiac arrhythmias, including complete heart block and other conduction defects, are common. Echocardiogram and 24-h continuous electrocardiogram (Holter monitor) are helpful for cardiac evaluation. The echocardiogram with Doppler studies is particularly useful to identify pericardial effusion, pulmonary hypertension, and ventricular dysfunction. Thallium perfusion scan is a sensitive tool for the evaluation of perfusion defects in the scleroderma heart. Many cardiac abnormalities have been associated with poor outcome. The combination of left axis deviation in association with moderate pericardial effusion is associated with a particularly poor outcome. One of the more severe acute cardiac features of SSc is diffuse myocarditis. It occurs exclusively in diffuse SSc patients and is usually heralded by malaise, fever, and left ventricular failure. Endocardial biopsy may be indicated. Immunosuppression with both prednisone and cyclophosphamide should be administered aggressively. The outlook is guarded at best.

The indolent, progressive feature of SSc heart development is the obliteration of intramyocardial arterioles and capillaries by the characteristic SSc process of endothelial injury and interstitial fibrosis. This process may be exaggerated by the demands of cardiac perfusion under load conditions; the lesions are characteristic of repeated episodes of ischemia-reperfusion injury with autoimmune systemic vascular wall injury factors added. Chamber dilatation is uncommon. Lack of compliance and diastolic heart failure are the frequent findings and, in a patient with major organ involvement elsewhere, diagnosis and management may be difficult. There are still a number of diffuse SSc patients who die suddenly, diastolic left ventricular failure due to intramyocardial myocardial fibrosis leading to ventricular arrhythmias could be the culprit. Follansbee (9) showed some years ago, in the carefully studied Pittsburgh SSc patient group, that poor thallium myocardial perfusion was a negative prognostic indicator that overrode the limited–diffuse skin subset classification, indicating that an occasional "limited" SSc patient can have myocardial fibrosis with negative prognostic implications. In these patients, angiotensin-converting enzyme (ACE) inhibitors have been shown to improve both systolic and diastolic function. Caution is again urged in the use of diuretics.

Classic coronary heart disease can occur in SSc patients who are often in the fifth to seventh decades of life; whether more or less than would be expected in a control or an autoimmune control population is unknown. When contemplating coronary bypass procedures in SSc patients, intramyocardial disease (microvascular perfusion) should be assessed before bypass is undertaken. If myocardial fibrosis is extensive in SSc patients, technically excellent bypass may not result in adequate myocardial perfusion due to obliterated microvascular beds. This is a difficult situation when angina is debilitating (9).

G. Renal System

At midcentury (1950–1960) as many as half of SSc patients died of the oliguric, hyperreninemic, hypertensive syndrome called scleroderma renal crisis (SRC). Angiotensin-converting enzyme inhibitors have reduced a >90% 1-year mortality rate to <45%. Since early detection of SRC is essential, all diffuse SSc patients should self-determine blood pressures weekly. The patient at risk for SRC is older, often male, may have left ventricular congestive heart failure, and be in the first 3 years of diffuse SSc. Onset of SRC is often abrupt with headache, blurred vision, hypertension with retinopathy and papilledema, microangiopathic hemolytic anemia, oliguria, and sudden death if untreated. These features occur together and represent an acute emergency. Experience has shown that if treatment with ACE inhibitors is begun at serum creatinine levels below 4.0 mg/dL (350 Mm/L), renal function can be stabilized and, over months, returned toward normal. The most likely sequence of events is gradual reduction of renal blood flow from the vascular lesion (intimal proliferation) characteristic of SSc; acute reduction of renal blood flow with reduced glomerular filtration; the appearance of intravascular coagulation; ischemia–reperfusion; microangiopathic hemolytic anemia; renin release; renal cortical vasospasms; cortical ischemia and infarction; underperfusion; proteinuria; renal insufficiency and accelerated hypertension with retinopathy; encephalopathy; myocardial ischemia; and possibly peripheral vasospasm with gangrene. Renin levels in SRC are some of the highest measured in long-term clinical experience with accelerated hypertension. Inhibiting angiotensin production has been very effective in stabilizing these extremely ill patients and resetting the baseline for a return of renal function. Short-term hemodialysis may be needed. Peritoneal dialysis is relatively ineffective because SSc tissues have substantially reduced capillary beds, so that diffusion is slow and inefficient. In most settings, SSc patients on hemodialysis should be given 2 years for endogenous renal function to return before transplantation is considered. Vascular access can be a problem due to widespread vascular and microvascular disease. Arteriovenous (AV) shunts can fail.

We have had modest success reducing microangiopathy and intravascular coagulation with antiplatelet agents such as dipyridamole and aspirin (together). European investigators report some success with the 3- to 5-day protocol of intravenous prostacyclin analogues (IV Iloprost). Unfortunately, oral prostacyclin analogues do not seem to help.

In the initial definition of the renovascular disease in SSc, renal arteriograms were done. Due to the ischemia produced by the dyes injected, especially in settings of low renal blood flow, they are contraindicated. The radioactive differential renal scans carry a lower risk and can be helpful in detecting asymmetry or slight reductions in renal perfusion or urine flow (10).

H. Musculoskeletal System

Symmetrical polyarthralgia with stiffness affecting the hands, wrists, knees, and ankles are frequent initial complaints. The inflammatory features of synovitis are usually minimal to modest, upper extremity joints (wrists, fingers) are usually symmetrically involved, and, except for the occasional patient with an overlap rheumatoid arthritis–SSc pattern of illness, erosive joint disease is very rare. The synovium contains layers of fibrin considered to be due to deficiencies in plasminogen generation and increased concentrations of its inhibitor (PAI-1). In patients whose skin has them "encased in steel," considerable disuse atrophy occurs that may influence joint structure and function. Radiographic evaluation is often complicated by flexion contractures and usually shows bone resorption, soft tissue atrophy, and subcutaneous calcifications.

Skeletal muscles are usually depleted in size and function in SSc. Disuse atrophy is important, loss of microvascular bed is important, and some SSc patients demonstrate an active myositis with elevated enzymes and inflammatory infiltrates. Electrical studies usually indicate neurovascular bundle muscle fiber defects and occasionally severe entrapment syndromes, such as trigiminal neuralgia. About 20% have an active, inflammatory myositis indistinguishable from polymyositis, an overlap syndrome, which usually responds to glucocorticoid therapy. If steroid resistant, azathioprine (2.5 mg/kg daily) or methotrexate (15–25 mg weekly) are used.

IV. LABORATORY DIAGNOSIS

A. Vascular Tests

Occasionally, in the early stages of diagnosis, a confirmation of Raynaud's phenomenon is needed. The literature contains color photographs of hands showing mixtures of pallor, suffusion, cyanosis, and pigmentation; the definitive test is as described by Neilsen in which water of differing temperatures is circulated through cuffs around the middle phalanx of the finger and digital artery pressure is detected by an air cuff around the proximal phalanx of the finger inflated to occlude a distal phalanx pulse plethysmogram. Raynaud's subjects are abnormally sensitive to water temperatures below 25°C. The widefield nailfold capillary examination should be a routine part of the evaluation of all patients suspected of a connective tissue disease (11) (Fig. 1).

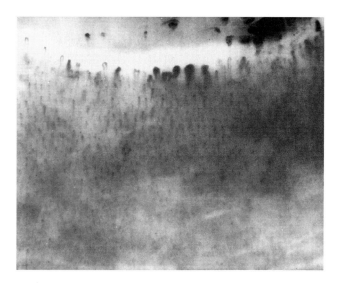

Figure 1 Widefield nailfold capillaroscopy, showing SSc-type nailfold capillary abnormalities, including dilated capillaries and avascular areas. Magnification 15×.

B. Autoantibody Determinations

The type of cell used for the ANA is important. It must be a human cell and it should be a rapidly dividing cell so that mitotic figures are present to bind the anticentromere antibodies of Caucasian females with limited SSc. The preferred cellular substrate is the HEp-2 cell, a human laryngeal carcinoma epithelial cell. When human, rapidly dividing cell substrates were introduced, the proportion of SSc patients who were positive doubled. Associations between autoantibody titers and SSc subset, as well as with specific SSc organ involvement (see Tables 3 and 7), are interesting but may not serve as therapeutic, prognostic, or management beacons in the individual patient (12).

V. PATHOGENESIS

Systemic sclerosis, probably first described in the eighteenth century, has become better understood in the twentieth century but much remains unknown. Paul Klemperer brought SSc together with other systemic autoimmune diseases as a "collagen vascular" or a "diffuse connective tissue" disease in the 1940s. He characterized SSc a progressive systemic disease with skin, gut, lung, heart, and kidney involvement. A generalized vascular hypothesis was proposed in the 1970s (13) initiating the present era of defining immune (including immunogenetic and autoimmune), vascular wall (including endothelial and smooth muscle cell activation/injury), and interstitial (including fibroblast, pericyte, and extracellular matrix) fibrotic mechanisms. This era remains incomplete. Figure 2 indicates only some of the complexities involved. There is a scattering of SSc patients who are genetically deficient in complement components, especially those who carry null alleles for C4a. In general terms, HLA-DR3 tracks with limited, and DR5 with diffuse, SSc; however a much stronger association exists with autoantibody expression and the HLA haplotype. Intriguing as these may be, they do not assist in evaluating the individual patient. Other reported associations include A9, B8, DR1, DR4, DQW7, and DPW5. Most patients express autoantibodies to one of the following: centromere, topoisomerase I (anti-Scl-70), RNA polymerase

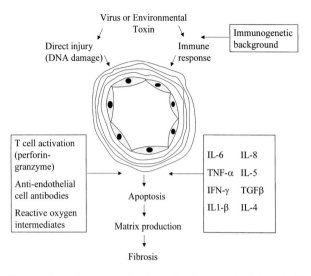

Figure 2   A hypothetical schema for the vascular injury in SSc.

(I, III), and U1 snRNP [formerly ENA, it is the serology purported to characterize mixed, over-lap, or undifferentiated connective tissue disease (UCTD)]. Proportions depend on the sensitivity of the test and the subset of the patients studied (see Table 3). These may or may not be patho-genetically important. Beyond this group of four autoantibody profiles that have been incorporated into subset classification, the list of antibodies found in SSc sera is long and heterogeneous, including cytomegalovirus, fibrillarin, fibrillin, Th (an endoribronuclease), NOR-90 (a nucleolar organizer), PM-Scl (a nucleolar multi-subunit particle), and many overlap patterns.

The fact that nailfold capillary abnormalities and serum markers of endothelial injury (plasma FVIII-vWF levels, serum ACE levels) occur early in SSc indicates that vascular (mi-crovascular) abnormalities are significant in the pathogenesis of the disease. How do these occur? Several different immune-based types of endotheliotoxic agents have been reported. The first was a protease or proteases shown to be endotheliotoxic and later suggested to be a product of acti-vated T cells (granzyme). Antiendothelial antibodies (a term that probably encompasses an-tiphospholipid and antioxidized LDL antibodies) occur in some SSc patients. Antibody-depen-dent cell cytotoxicity (ADCC) mechanisms seem to be operative in some patients. Certain arachidonate products such as thromboxanes and certain leukotrienes are endotheliotoxic, as is the family of endothelin peptides. Angiotensin and norepinephrine can injure a susceptible ves-sel wall. Many of these agents induce vasoconstriction if not balanced by inhibitors or active va-sodilators. Ischemia and subsequent reperfusion is vasculotoxic in its own right as a major setting for the production and release of reactive oxygen species, which may be a common pathway link-ing idiopathic with environmental SSc (Table 5) and the various immune triggers with the vascu-lar lesion of intimal proliferation.

This vascular lesion is similar in autoimmune, rejection, and restenosis vasculopathy, which share a propensity for cytomegalovirus infection. The similarities between SSc and homo-graft rejection, especially chronic graft vs. host reactions (GVHR), has prompted hypotheses that SSc represents an indolent GVHR based on the formation of a microchimeric state between mother and infant in vitro. Whether autoimmunity (and its immunodeficiency) begets mi-crochimerism or vice versa and whether this is unique to SSc remain to be determined.

Unusual circulating T-cell profiles have been reported in SSc. A relative decrease in CD8 T cells in blood may be balanced by a relative increase in CD8 T cells in the fluids of affected or-

Table 5 Environmental Agents Associated with SSc[a]

Drugs: bleomycin, methysergide, pentazocine, cocaine, ethosuximide, amphetamine and other appetite suppressors
Amino acids and derivatives: L-tryptophan, L-5-OH-tryptophan, penicillamine
Occupational exposures:
  Manual and vibrating
  Solvents: epoxy, benzene, toluene, trichloroethylene, vinyl chloride
  Inhalants: silica and related dusts
  Ingestants: adulterated cooking oil (toxic oil)

[a]In vivo feature that many of these agents share is the generation of reactive oxygen species (free radicals, including nitrogen based) with subsequent lipid peroxidation and endothelial activation or injury.
See Nietert PJ, et al. Is Occupational Organic Solvent Exposure a Risk Factor for Scleroderma? Arthritis Rheum 1998; 41:1111–1118.

gans in SSc patients, especially bronchoalveloar lavage fluid (14). Many of these CD8 T cells carry the γ-δ T-cell receptor, which recognizes antigen independent of MHC-restricted antigen-presenting cells (such as dendritic cells), and which seems to have a propensity for recognition of certain heat shock proteins. These γ-δ T cells are oligoclonally expanded and they seem to bind selectively to SSc fibroblasts in vitro (compared with control skin fibroblasts or with autologous α-β T cells). Yet to be determined are which ligands these γ-δ T cells recognize; whether they contain granzyme-perforin (becoming cytolytic T lymphocytes, CTL); whether they recognize cytomegalovirus, a known stimulator of γ-δ T cells; and whether their cytokine profile is more profibrogenic (interleukin-4, IL-4; transforming growth factor-β, TGF-β) than would be expected (15,16).

A. Cellular Immune Reactions

A distinct perivascular lymphocytic infiltrate occurs in involved organs prior to the onset of tissue fibrosis and vascular injury. The cells are composed predominately of the helper-T-cell phenotype and are shown to express mRNA for TGF-β1, IL-2 and IL-4. A variety of circulating cytokines are described including IL-1, IL-2, IL-4, IL-6, IL-8, tumor necrosis factor-α (TNF-α) and TNF-β, and soluble IL-2 receptors.

B. Cellular Interactions in Pathogenesis

The pathogenetic hypothesis for scleroderma indicates the presence of cellular changes that consist of a state of cellular activation in an interactive fashion. Manifestations and consequences of this activated state are fibroblast migration to the perivascular spaces, proliferation, and increase in matrix synthesis. Mast cell migration and degranulation are prominent. Endothelial activation is demonstrated by a change in biological function to a proinflammatory (expression of the adhesion molecules ICAM-1, β1 integrin and ELAM-1), promitogenic (expression of PDGF), and provasospastic (increased endothelin and decreased nitric oxide production) phenotype. Injury to the vascular endothelium, particularly of the microvessels, is the only cellular injury seen in this cellular interactive process, suggesting endothelial cells as the target of the immune reaction.

VI. MANAGEMENT

A. Differential Diagnosis

The differential diagnosis of scleroderma includes a number of fibrotic conditions that will not be described in detail here (Table 6). These conditions may mimic scleroderma skin disease but are

Table 6   Differential Diagnosis of Scleroderma

Eosinophilic fasciitis
Eosinophilia myalgia syndrome
Scleredema
Scleromyxedema
POEMS syndrome
Progeria
Porphyria cutania tarda
Reflex sympathetic dystrophy
Bleomycin and other drug-induced fibrosis
Carcinoid syndrome
Amyloidosis
Phenylketonuria

distinguished by the lack of the classic scleroderma visceral involvement, the absence of RP, and the lack of hand and feet cutaneous involvement; by frequent neuropathy and myalgia; and by characteristic clinical features of their own. An increased incidence of scleroderma has been reported in patients with chronic graft vs. host disease; gold, coal and silica miners; and in those exposed to organic solvent (see Table 5).

B.   Therapy of Raynaud's Phenomenon

The management of Raynaud's phenomenon is aimed at increasing the patient's digital blood flow and at preventing vasospasm. The simplest vasodilatory therapy is protection against cold exposure. Improvement of resting digital skin temperature has been noted after biofeedback training. However, long-term maintenance of the responses is variable.

Several types of drugs have been useful in preventing the ischemic events of Raynaud's (Figs. 3 and 4, Tables 7 and 8). The calcium channel blockers have gained widespread acceptance

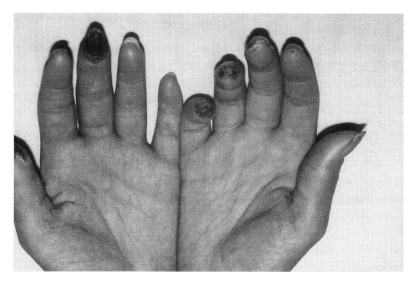

Figure 3   Multiple ischemic digital ulcers in a 33-year-old patient with 3-month history of sclerodactyly and 10-year history of Raynaud's phenomenon. A positive anticentromere antibody of 1:612 was noted.

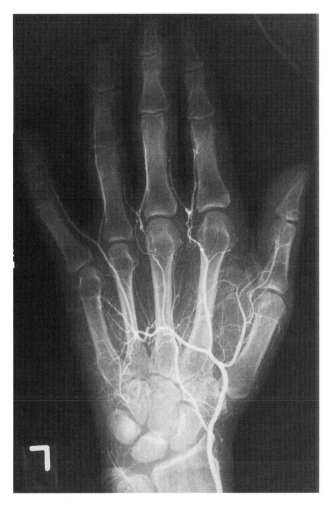

Figure 4 Hand arteriogram of the patient in Figure 1. Note occlusion of the distal ulnar artery approximately 2.0 cm proximal to the articular surface of the distal ulna with collateral vessels at the point of occlusion. The superficial palmer arch is occluded. Diffuse occlusive disease in the digital arteries is prominent.

Table 7 Treatment of Raynaud's Phenomenon

Avoidance of cold
Cessation of cigarette smoking
Biofeedback training
Drug therapy
   Nifedipene-XL 30–60 mg/day
   Diltiazem-cd 120–240 mg/day
   Prazasin 1–2 mg tid
   Tolazoline 80 mg bid
   Phenoxybenzamine 5–80 mg/day
   Alphamethyldopa 250–500 tid
   Ketanserin 20–40 mg tid
   Pentoxifylline 400 mg tid

Table 8   Therapy for RP and Digital Ulcers

Adequate treatment of RP
Topical nitroglycerin
Stanazolol
Tissue plasminogen activator
Prostacyclin, iloprost or PGE1 infusion
Pharmacologic cervical sympathectomy and stellate ganglion blockade
Microsurgical digital sympathectomy
Antibiotics for osteomyelitis

as first choice. Nifedipine-XL, 30–90 mg daily, is the most effective; its use, however, may be associated with orthostatic side effects. Diltiazem-CD, 140–300 mg is less effective but better tolerated. If calcium channel blockers prove to be ineffective, then other agents may be tried, such as prazosin hydrochloride, 1–5 mg daily; α-methyldopa, 1–2 g daily; tolazoline, 80 mg twice daily; reserpine, 0.25–0.5 mg daily; phenoxybenzamine, 5–80 mg daily; and dipyridamole, 200–400 mg daily in combination with 150 mg aspirin daily. Symptomatic improvement has been reported by the use of the angiotensin-converting enzyme inhibitors captopril and enaloapril. Nitroglycerin can be helpful when applied topically 2–3 times daily at the base of the digits. Some improvement has been reported with the oral serotonin antagonist, ketanserin. Beneficial effects have also been reported over several months with drugs that enhance red cell deformability, such as pentoxifyline, 400 mg 3 times daily, and drugs that stimulate fibrinolysis, such as stanozolol, 5 mg daily. Sustained improvement has been reported after 3 days of intravenous infusion of Iloprost (prostacyclin analogue). Persistent digital ulcers can be a difficult management problem (see Tables 7 and 8).

C.   Therapy of Gastrointestinal Systemic Sclerosis

Symptomatic esophageal reflux is best managed by avoidance of recumbent position after meals, elevation of the head of the bed, and regular use of antacids. H_2 antagonists (cimetidine, famotidine, ranitidine) and sucralfate may be effective. The gastric acid pump inhibitor omeprazole is quite effective in the management of reflux; long-term studies document the safety of this agent. Metoclopramide has been shown to have a small beneficial effect in improving esophageal motility. Better results are reported with the use of cisapride, which is shown to increase lower esophageal sphincter pressure and the number of gastric contractions. Octreotide (long-acting somatostatin analogue) and erythromycin can improve GI motility. Malabsorption syndrome is best managed by use of broad spectrum antibiotics to reduce bacterial overgrowth. Cyclic intermittent courses (2 weeks per month) of tetracycline, ampicillin, and erythromycin are effective.

In patients with severe gastrointestinal hypomotility, intermittent ileus, and malnutrition, home hyperalimentation is an effective therapy that restores adequate nutritional status and dramatically improves the quality of life; however, late complications with increased mortality from thrombosis, septicemia, and liver failure have been reported.

D.   Course

The course of scleroderma is extremely variable; early detection of organ involvement and careful therapeutic intervention are essential for optimal patient happiness and survival. Variables that predict poor survival include older age, reduced renal function, anemia, and reduced pulmonary diffusing capacity. These parameters may be useful in predicting individual patients at risk for shortened survival. Scleroderma remains a lethal rheumatic disorder. The cumulative survival rate is 80% at 2 years, 50% at 8 years, and 30% at 12 years of disease onset, with reduced survival predicted by older age, and renal, pulmonary, and cardiac involvement.

E. General

No effective disease-modifying therapy exists to control or cure SSc. Recent controlled trials document the lack of effect of D-penicillamine, methotrexate, antilymphocyte globulin, and α and γ interferons. Organ-specific therapies are the mainstays of management. It is complex to decide how often and how intensively one should search for vascular involvement and functional organ compromise in SSc. Subset classification helps.

In the fully expressed limited SSc patient, who is usually a Caucasian female who has completed her childbearing aspirations and whose disease manifestations include RP with or without evidence of digital ischemia (ulcers, digital pits, paronychia, gangrene, and autoamputation; see Figure 3), sclerodactyly, and/or esophageal dysphagia, monitoring for pulmonary hypertension (by echocardiography with Doppler of the tricuspid valve) every 1–3 years and for interstitial lung disease (alveolitis and fibrosis by chest CT scan) every 3–6 years seems appropriate. In contrast, in the diffuse SSc patient, lung function and CT chest scans should be yearly or, if positive, twice yearly to monitor closely and attempt to find alveolitis, currently detectable by CT and, if equivocal, by lavage. In addition, the diffuse SSc patient should take his or her own blood pressure weekly with a cuff and report increases of 30 mm Hg systolic or 20 mm Hg diastolic immediately.

With the exception of angiotensin-converting enzyme inhibitors to forestall scleroderma renal crisis and with the possible exception of combined therapy with prednisone and cyclophosphamide to inhibit the gradual progression of alveolitis to fibrosis in interstitial lung disease, no therapy has unequivocally been shown to change the natural history of either limited or diffuse SSc. Specifically, D-penicillamine, colchicine, or calcium channel blockers may provide symptomatic relief or reduce changes in one or another target organ but have not as yet been shown to change the pattern or progression of involvement.

It is tempting to use glucocorticoids chronically for the musculoskeletal features of SSc. This powerful antiinflammatory agent should be reserved for acute therapy aimed at specific inflammatory findings. The danger with chronic glucocorticoids is the risk of precipitating scleroderma renal crisis probably via a mineralocorticoid pathway.

Current trials for general SSc therapy in the hope of developing a truly disease-modifying regimen include: relaxin (17), minocycline, the induction of oral tolerance to collagen, extracorporeal photopheresis, high-dose immunosuppression (cyclophosphamide) with or without autologous stem cell rescue, and methotrexate. Trials take long periods, require carefully stratified patients, leave little ethical space for placebo trials, are often unable to obtain financial sponsorship, and are often hammered by regulatory groups because SSc patients die of their disease both in and out of trials.

Just as the tools to monitor therapeutic efficacy are limited, the criteria to ascertain activity are also not well defined. Does one monitor immune (serum IL-2), vascular (plasma vWF levels) or fibrotic (type III collagen propeptide, serum, or urine) parameters? These are only a few of the complicating aspects of determining disease activity, disease severity, or therapeutic efficacy in this variable, episodic disease (4).

REFERENCES

1. LeRoy EC, Black C, Fleischmajer R, Jablonska S, Krieg T, Medsger TA Jr, Rowell N, Wollheim F. Scleroderma (systemic sclerosis): Classification, subsets and pathogenesis. J Rheumatol 1988; 15: 202–205.

2. LeRoy EC, Medsger TA Jr. Raynaud's phenomenon: A proposal for classification. Clin Exp Rheum 1992; 10:485–488.
3. Jacobsen S, Halberg P, Ullman S. Mortality and causes of death of 344 Danish patients with systemic sclerosis (scleroderma). Br J Rheumatol 1998; 37:750–755.
4. Silman AJ, Black CM, Welsh KI. Epidemiology, Demographics, Genetics. In: Clements PJ, Furst DE, eds. Systemic Sclerosis. Philadelphia: Williams & Wilkins, 1996:389–407.
5. Smith EA, LeRoy EC. Scleroderma (systemic sclerosis) and morphea. In: Jameson JL, Collins FS, eds. Principles of Molecular Medicine. Totowa: Humana, 1998: 820–838.
6. Clements PJ, Medsger TA Jr. Organ involvement: Skin. In: Clements PJ, Furst DE, eds. Systemic Sclerosis. Philadelphia: Williams & Wilkins, 1996:23–49.
7. Verne GN, Eaker EY, Hardy E, Sninsky CA. Effect of octreotide and erythromycin on idiopathic and scleroderma-associated intestinal pseudoobstruction. Dig Dis Sci 1995; 40:1892–1901.
8. Silver RM, Miller KS, Kinsella MB, et al. Evaluation and management of scleroderma lung disease using bronchoalveolar lavage. Am J Med 1990; 88:470.
9. Follansbee WP. Organ involvement: Cardiac. In: Clements PJ, Furst DE, eds. Systemic Sclerosis. Philadelphia: Williams & Wilkins, 1996:333–364.
10. Steen VD. Scleroderma renal crisis. In: Steen VD, Rheumatic Disease Clinics of North America. Philadelphia: Saunders, 1996:861–878.
11. Maricq HR, Smith EA. Organ involvement: Peripheral vascular. In: Clements PJ, Furst DE, eds. Systemic Sclerosis. Philadelphia: Williams & Wilkins, 1996:365–385.
12. Bunn CC, Denton CP, Shi-Wen X, Knight C, Black CM. Anti-RNA polymerases and other autoantibody specificities in systemic sclerosis. Br J Rheumatol 1998; 37:15–20.
13. Campbell PM, LeRoy EC. Pathogenesis of systemic sclerosis: a vascular hypothesis. Semin Arthritis Rheum 1975; 4:351–368.
14. Yurovsky VV, Wigley FM, Wise RA, et al. Skewing of the CD8+ T cell repertoire in the lungs of systemic sclerosis patients. Hum Immunol 1996; 48:84.
15. Kahaleh MC, Fan PS, Otsuka T. Gammadelta receptor bearing T cells in scleroderma: Enhanced interaction with vascular endothelial cells in vitro. J Appl Biomaterials 1999; 91:188–195.
16. LeRoy EC. Systemic sclerosis: A vascular perspective. In: Steen VD, ed. Rheumatic Disease Clinics of North America. Philadelphia: Saunders, 1996:675–694.
17. Seibold JR, Clements PJ, Furst DE, Mayes MD, McCloskey DA, Moreland SW, White B, Wigley FM, Rocco S, Erikson M, Hannigan JF, Sanders ME, Amento EP. Safety and pharmacokinetics of recombinant human relaxin in systemic sclerosis. J Rheumatol 1998; 25:302–307.

43
Sjögren's Syndrome

Robert I. Fox and Paul Michelson
Scripps Memorial Hospital and Research Foundation, La Jolla, California

Joichiro Hayashi and Toshiaki Maruyama
The Scripps Research Institute, La Jolla, California

I. INTRODUCTION

Sjögren's syndrome (SS) is a systemic autoimmune disorder characterized by clinical features of severe dry eyes and dry mouth (sicca symptoms) as a result of lymphocytic infiltration of the salivary and lacrimal glands. The patients have clinical and laboratory manifestations of a systemic autoimmune disorder. Vascular involvement in SS takes several forms: (1) inflammatory disease of the blood vessels, including ocular surface, oral surface, skin, lung, heart, kidney and nervous system; (2) noninflammatory disease of blood vessels (Raynaud's phenomena); (3) increased frequency of venous thrombosis as part of the spectrum of anticardiolipin syndrome; and (4) autonomic neuropathy in which local inflammatory response alters vascular permeability and tone.

II. EPIDEMIOLOGY

Sjögren's syndrome is subdivided into primary SS (1° SS) and secondary SS (2° SS), where the sicca symptoms are associated with another well-defined autoimmune disorder such as rheumatoid arthritis (RA), systemic lupus erythematosus (SLE), polymyositis, or progressive systemic sclerosis (scleroderma). Primary SS is predominant in females (9:1), with peak age incidences in the childbearing age (25–35 years) and in the early postmenopausal age (50–55 years). The precise frequency of 1°SS depends on the criteria system used (discussed below). However, the frequency ranges from approximately 0.5% (San Diego criteria) to 3% (original EEC criteria) for primary SS.

In 2°SS associated with SLE, the clinical distinction from 1°SS is often very difficult, since both groups of patients have a positive antinuclear antibody (ANA), anti-SS-A antibody, arthralgias, leukopenia, and increased frequency of HLA-DR3. In considering the differential diagnosis between primary SS and secondary SS with SLE, it is easiest to think of SLE as a group of diseases in which each mutually exclusive subgroup has its own characteristic pattern of autoantibodies (i.e., anti-SS-A, anti-DNA, anti-RNP, etc.). One subset of these SLE patients (HLA-DR3, anti-SS A antibody) shares clinical features, prognosis and therapeutic approach with the primary SS patients. Patients with secondary SS and SLE generally lack renal involvement or anti-DNA, anti-Sm, or anti-RNP antibodies.

The most common disease associated with 2°SS is RA, due to the high frequency of RA in the general population. The onset of sicca symptoms is generally many years after the onset of joint symptoms. Ocular symptoms are more common than oral symptoms in 2°SS plus RA.

Finally, sicca symptoms may be associated with scleroderma. However, the pathogenesis of sicca symptoms in these patients appears different from 1°SS. Minor salivary gland biopsies from 2°SS plus scleroderma patients show a predominant pattern of glandular fibrosis rather than the lymphocytic infiltrates characteristic of 1°SS biopsies. These patients have a different pattern of autoantibodies and different associated HLA-DR alleles. It has been suggested that sicca symptoms in scleroderma are more similar in pathogenesis to those occurring in patients with graft vs. host disease after bone marrow transplantation.

III. DIAGNOSIS

As noted above, there is a current debate over the criteria for diagnosis of primary SS. In 1932, Henrik Sjögren reported the triad of keratoconjunctivitis sicca (KCS), xerostomia, and rheumatoid arthritis. The clinical spectrum of SS as a systemic autoimmune disease was further defined by Bloch et al. (1) in 1956. Although the ocular component of SS was clearly outlined (i.e., keratoconjunctivitis sicca), the criteria for the oral component was not strictly outlined and has led to much of the present confusion in diagnosis. The demonstration of focal lymphocytic infiltrates on minor salivary gland (SG) biopsy has remained the "gold standard" for the oral component of SS. A cluster of 50 or more lymphocytes is called a "focus" and an average focus score of 2 or more per 4 mm^2 fulfills the diagnosis of SS in the San Francisco criteria (2). Multiple studies have shown that a positive SG biopsy is closely correlated with KCS and antinuclear antibodies directed against SS-A (Ro) and SS-B (La) antigens (2).

However, many clinicians are hesitant to perform a minor salivary gland biopsy, due to the risk of numbness of the lip if the biopsy is not performed correctly. Thus, other classification systems have been proposed that do not require a biopsy, including the San Diego criteria where patients have (1) objective KCS and xerostomia, and (2) a characteristic minor SG biopsy *or* evidence of a systemic autoimmune disease as manifested by characteristic autoantibodies (3). Using this criteria, about 0.5% of adult females would be diagnosed as having 1°SS.

The European (EEC) committee for SS proposed a different set of criteria that can be fulfilled without either biopsy or serological abnormality (4). Using this criteria, about 3% of all adults would be classified as 1°SS. Features of each of these classification systems are summarized in Table 1. Also, exclusions to diagnosis of SS differ in the San Diego and EEC criteria. For example, patients with sicca symptoms associated with hepatitis C infection or preexisting lymphoma (5) are excluded from diagnosis as SS in the San Diego criteria (6) but included in the EEC criteria. This is a significant problem, since up to 20% of SS patients fulfilling EEC criteria have hepatitis C (7).

Comparison of SS patients fulfilling different criteria systems indicates that only about 15% of the patients fulfilling the EEC criteria would be diagnosed as SS using the San Diego criteria (4). Therefore, it is difficult to compare studies published from Europe (where EEC criteria are frequently used) to studies published in the United States where other diagnostic criteria are often used. Fortunately, a recent abstract from the EEC study group has suggested modification of the European criteria to require either a positive minor salivary gland biopsy (focus score 1 or greater) or positive antibody against SS-A antigen (8). This revision of the EEC criteria will lead to much closer agreement between the San Diego and EEC criteria. In this chapter, we will use the San Diego criteria for SS (3), since these patients share common features of minor salivary gland biopsy, autoantibodies, and particular HLA-DR/DQ alleles.

Table 1 Comparison of Different Criteria for the Diagnosis of Sjögren's Syndrome

Criteria	Lip biopsy focus score required for diagnosis	Autoantibody (anti–SS-A), % patients	Criteria exclusion: hepatitis C and other diseases[a]	Reference
San Francisco	≥2[b]		yes	2
San Diego	≥2[b]	78	yes	3
European (EEC) original	1[c]	28	no	4
European (EEC) revised	1[d]	74	no	8

[a]Patients with history of preexistent diseases such as hepatitis C, lymphoma, sarcoidosis, or other known causes of lymphocytic infiltrative disease.

[b]A focus refers to a cluster of 50 or more lymphocytes in a minor salivary gland biopsy; the average number of foci in a 4 mm^2 area of salivary gland biopsy is termed the focus score. Lobules with dilated ducts (nonspecific sialadenitis) are excluded from evaluation.

[c]Lip biopsy is not required in EEC criteria, but a focus score of only 1 is described as sufficient to serve as a positive characteristic.

[d]In the proposed revision of the EEC criteria, either a positive minor salivary gland biopsy (focus score 1 or greater) or a positive anti–SS-A antibody is required for diagnosis.

IV. OCULAR SURFACE AND LACRIMAL GLAND ABNORMALITIES

SS provides an opportunity to study the interaction of the neuroimmune and exocrine systems. The regulation of the autonomic nervous system controls the regional blood flow and permeability of blood vessels supplying the salivary and lacrimal glands.

The major component of tears and saliva is water, which is derived from the small postarterial capillaries that supply the glands. Normal lacrimal and salivary flow is regulated through feedback mechanisms shown schematically in Figure 1. The mucosal surfaces of the eye or mouth are heavily innervated by unmyelinated fibers that carry afferent signals to the lacrimatory or salivatory nuclei located in the medulla. These medullary nuclei, which are part of the autonomic nervous system, are influenced by higher cortical inputs, including taste, smell, anxiety, and depression. The efferent neurons innervate both glandular cells and local blood vessels. The blood vessels provide not only water for tears and saliva, but also growth factors including hormones (e.g., insulin) and matrix proteins (e.g., fibronectin and vitronectin) in the perivascular space of the lacrimal and salivary glands. In response to neural stimulation through muscarinic M3 receptors and vasoactive intestinal peptide (VIP) receptors, glandular acinar and ductal cells secrete water, proteins, and mucopolysaccharides (mucins). This complex mixture forms a hydrated gel that lubricates the ocular surface (i.e., tears) and the oral mucosa (i.e., saliva).

A common misconception about SS is that sicca syndrome results from the total immune destruction of the lacrimal or salivary gland. A minor SG biopsy from a SS patient is shown in Figure 2A, which shows lymphocytic infiltrates in the central region of the lobule; in comparison, a histologically normal minor SG biopsy is shown in Figure 2B. Around the periphery of the lobule in Figure 2A, acinar and ductal cells are still present even though this patient has had symptoms of severe sicca syndrome for over 10 years. This retention of almost half of the glandular epithelial cells in SS contrasts with other organ-specific autoimmune disorders such as type I diabetes mellitus, where destruction of insulin producing epithelial cells occurs before clinical symptoms are apparent. Morphometric analysis of SS biopsies shows that almost half of the acinar cells remain histologically intact in patients with long-standing sicca symptoms (9).

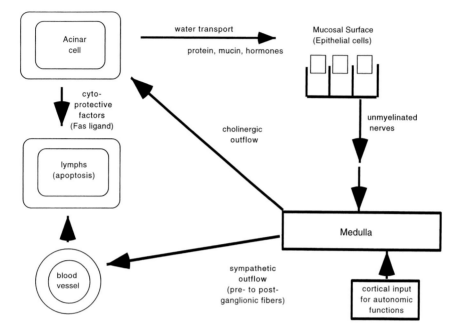

Figure 1   Schematic representation for the regulation of normal lacrimal and salivary secretion. Afferent nerves respond to signals from the mucosal surfaces of the eye and mouth. These unmyelinated nerves travel to areas of the midbrain (lacrimatory and salivatory nuclei), where they are integrated with signals from higher cortical centers. The net signal (i.e., decision for salivation or lacrimation) leads to generation of an efferent nerve signal sent back to blood vessels (sympathetic nerves) and to glands (cholinergic nerves). The blood vessels provide a source of water, proteins, hormones and nutrients that are subsequently pumped onto the mucosal surface as secretions. As part of normal mucosal defense, lymphocytes also routinely traffic through the glands but undergo apoptosis due to constitutive production of Fas by the epithelial cells.

The failure of residual acini in SS glands to function adequately may result partly from the loss of neural innervation, as indicated decreased neural axon specific protein 9.5 and synaptophysin by immunohistological methods (10). Acetylcholine is required for acinar secretion and VIP for glandular homeostasis (11). The release of cytokines, particularly tumor necrosis factor-α (TNF-α) and interleukin-1 (IL-1) may be toxic to local nerves or acini (12,13). Cytokines IL-1 or TNF-α in amounts similar to the levels found in SS glands or saliva are "toxic" to nerve cells grown in vitro (14) or in mice expressing these transgenes (15).

Other factors may be involved in the decreased response of acinar cells to neural stimulation. A recent immunohistological study noted a decrease in the phosphokinase C (PKC) isoform beta pi in acinar epithelial cells and the zeta isoform in myoepithelial cells of minor SG biopsies of SS patients (16). This alteration in PKC isoforms would be predicted to decrease the secretory response to cholinergic stimulation. Further, antibodies against muscarinic M3 receptors have been found in SS patients and may compete with acetylcholine (17).

In the simplest model of SS (Fig. 3), the lacrimal or salivary gland is incapable of adequate response to neural signals as a consequence of local immune infiltrates and their derived cytokines. The actual processes in SS or autonomic neuropathy are more complicated than indicated in these schematic diagrams, which are primarily designed to emphasize that salivation or lacrimation is part of a regulatory circuit involving the central nervous system (18).

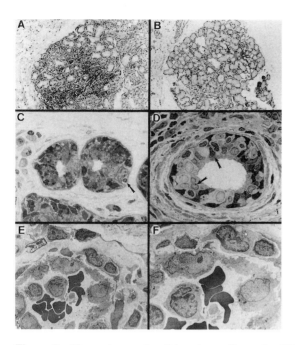

Figure 2   Photomicrographs of the minor salivary gland biopsies. A, C, D, E, and F are from a patient with SS (original magnification 50, 200, and 500 ×). E and F show high endothelial venules containing red blood cells and lymphocytes migrating into the gland. B is a normal salivary gland biopsy (original magnification 50×). Arrows in C and D indicate lymphocytes infiltrating the acinar and ductal structures.

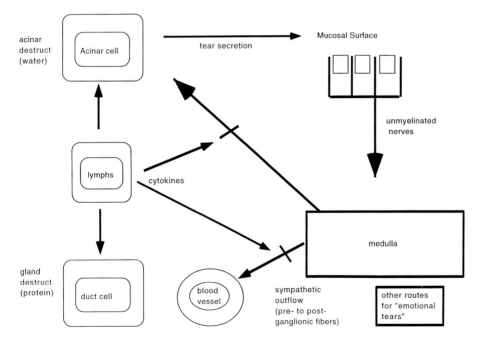

Figure 3   Schematic view of SS where the glandular dysfunction prevents the neural signal from initiating glandular secretion. Lymphocytes in the gland resist apoptosis due to upregulation of bcl-x and release cytokines that impair glandular response to neurotransmitters. Further, antibodies may be secreted to muscarinic M3 receptors that partially block response to acetylcholine.

V. VASCULAR INVOLVEMENT

In addition to ocular manifestations of keratoconjunctivitis sicca discussed above, ocular vas-culitis may be manifest as a "corneal melt" (19). In these unfortunate patients, corneal vasculitis leads to anoxic damage of the cornea and thinning of the cornea with possible rupture of the globe. This occurs most commonly in the presence of nodular scleritis in RA patients with 2° SS (20), but may occur in the absence of nodules in patients with 1° SS (21). Retinal involvement is very uncommon in SS patients (22) and suggests the diagnosis of SLE or uveitis-related diseases such as Reiter's syndrome. Visual loss in SS patients may be due to demyelinating disease or em-bolic disease (21).

In addition to oral problems involving accelerated periodontal disease and increased fre-quency of oral infections (particularly candidiasis) (23), SS patients may rarely develop a necro-tizing vasculitis of the mucus membranes (24). These vasculitic lesions in the nose are clinically and histologically similar to Wegener's granulomatosis (25).

Skin manifestations include leukocytoclastic vasculitis that presents as palpable purpura (26,27). These lesions may have the appearance of erythema multiforme (28,29) or erythema an-nulare (30). These lesions are generally present symmetrically, but an asymmetric distribution should raise a search for possible embolic sources.

Patients with SS develop nonpalpable purpura; symmetric involvement of the lower ex-tremities is much more common than upper extremities (31,32). Hypergammaglobulemic pur-pura is relatively common in SS patients and may lead to sensory peripheral neuropathy (33–35). In a large cohort of patients with hyperglobulinemic purpura, about 50% had coexistent SS (36). The skin lesions are often associated with circulating type II mixed cryoglobulin (polyclonal IgG and monoclonal rheumatoid factor). The rheumatoid factor (RF) is often an IgM-κ monoclonal rheumatoid factor containing the VKIIIb subsubclass of light chains (37). This RF has an idio-type defined by a specific monoclonal antibody called 17-109. The skin biopsies generally show rheumatoid factor containing this idiotype and deposition of complement (38). It has been as-sumed that immune complexes become trapped at the bifurcation of small blood vessels, leading to complement activation by the immune complex. In patients with skin manifestations of mixed cryoglobulinemia and sicca complaints, hepatitis C infection should be excluded (7,39).

Urticarial vasculitis has been reported in SS patients (40) but is relatively uncommon. An unusual skin lesion called "subacute" lupus (with clinical appearance of psoriaform lesions) (41) has been reported in patients with SS (42). These patients often lack an ANA when the mouse kid-ney is used as a substrate but exhibit a positive ANA when Hep 2 cells are used as substrate. Fur-ther, these patients frequently exhibit a positive anti–SS-A antibody.

Patients with SS may develop vascular manifestation of lung disease, including pulmonary hypertension (43,44). Vasculitis involving the lung in SS patients has been reported in association with mixed cryoglobulinemia (38). Interstitial pneumonitis may occur in SS patients (45) with lung biopsies showing features ranging from usual interstitial pneumonitis (46) to lymphocytic interstitial pneumonitis (47).

Gastrointestinal manifestations of SS may include mesenteric vasculitis (48), although this is quite rare (49). Patients with SS with mixed cryoglobulinemia may develop abdominal pain and, rarely, infarcts of the spleen or other abdominal organs. Abnormal liver tests may reflect pri-mary biliary cirrhosis, in which patients frequently exhibit sicca symptoms (49). However, many of the hepatic manifestations initially associated with SS are now recognized as due to hepatitis C and its associated mixed cryoglobulinemia.

Central nervous system involvement in SS covers the same spectrum of disorders as found in SLE patients. This includes small-vessel arteritis causing encephalopathy (50) or thrombotic infarcts of the brain presenting as a stroke (51). The role of vasculitis in neuropsychiatric manifestations in SS patients remains unclear (52) but may involve alterations in regional blood flow within the brain (53). Initial reports suggested an elevated frequency of demyelinating disorders in SS patients that mimicked multiple sclerosis (50,54). However, subsequent studies have not found an increased frequency of demyelinating lesions in SS patients (55,56). Sudden hearing loss in SS patients has been reported and is presumed to result from vasculitic infarct of the acoustic nerve (57).

Similar to SLE, patients may develop pleurisy or pericarditis. However, the incidence of clinically evident pericarditis or pleuritis is probably less than 10% of patients. Coronary arteritis is very rare in SS patients (58). Although cardiomyopathy may be present in SS patients, it is usally due to accelerated atherosclerotic disease (especially in patients on chronic steroids), amyloidosis, or an unrecognized manifestation of as associated polymyositis (58).

Patients with SS have been reported to have increased frequency of interstitial cystitis. Most of the reported studies have not confirmed the clinical diagnosis with bladder biopsies. However, a small proportion of SS patients with a novel autoantibody against a 70-kD protein (59) had biopsy proven interstitial cystitis.

Nephritis is generally interstitial but glomerulonephritis may occur in primary SS patients (60); however, the occurrence of glomerulonephritis should stimulate a search for amyloid or SLE.

Anticardiolipin antibodies are found in a subset of SS patients and are generally IgA isotype, with lower incidence of thrombosis than found in SLE patients (61,62). However, the occurrence of thrombotic events in SS patients should trigger a search for anticardiolipin antibodies, anti-β_2 glycoprotein I antibodies, and elevation of homocysteine levels (63). Of note, the administration of methotrexate in the absence of folic acid (either due to failure to coadminister or noncompliance of patient) may lead to significant elevation of homocysteine levels, a significant cofactor in thrombosis, particularly in the setting of anticardiolipin syndrome.

VI. MANAGEMENT

The treatment of extraglandular symptoms of SS remains similar to treatment of SLE (64). Symptoms of arthralgia may respond to nonsteroidal antiinflammatory agents or antimalarials (65). In the patient with vasculitis, the key question is whether visceral organs are involved.

Initial treatment of systemic vasculitis involving visceral organs (i.e., brain, lung, kidney) remains corticosteroids, usually in doses from 0.5–2 mg/kg. In patients with life-threatening organ involvement, intravenous cyclophosphamide (10–30 mg/kg) is often used at monthly intervals for at least 3 months (66). Although the risk of lymphoma is increased in SS patients (67), the need for immediate therapy with cyclophosphamide takes precedence in the short term (58).

In order to facilitate tapering of corticosteroids, other immune suppressive drugs such as methotrexate (68) and cycloporin A (66) have been used and reported to be useful (68). However cyclosporin A, FK-506, or rapamycin have not been well tolerated in SS due to renal toxicity, increased preexistent interstitial nephritis, and concerns about the tendency toward lymphoma associated with chronic therapy (69). Previous studies with azathioprine have indicated relatively little benefit and limitation due to gastrointestinal and hematologic toxicity (70).

The recent success of "biologic" agents (i.e., anti-TNF antibody and TNF receptors) in RA and IV gammaglobulin in various autoimmune diseases suggests that there may a potential role for these agents.

VII. SUMMARY

The term Sjögren's syndrome (SS) refers to xerophthalmia and xerostomia due to lymphocytic infiltrates of lacrimal and salivary glands. The criteria for diagnosis of primary Sjögren's syndrome has been controversial. The absence of a uniformly accepted criteria has led to confusion in clinical practice and in the research literature. For example, only 15% of patients that fulfill European (EEC) criteria for SS would fulfill the San Diego criteria. This difference in disease classification leads to difficulty in comparing clinical trials and in elucidating pathogenetic mechanisms, since different patient populations are evaluated.

ACKNOWLEDGMENTS

The research of RIF was supported by NIH grant M01-RR000831 and from the Department of Academic Affairs of the Scripps Institute for Research and Medicine. Additional support for postdoctoral fellows (JH and CC) was provided by grants from the Hennings Memorial Trust, the Florence, the Scripps-Stedham, the Kovler, and the Ramsdell Foundations.

REFERENCES

1. Bloch KJ, Buchanan WW, Wohl MJ, Bunim JJ. Sjögren's syndrome: A clinical, pathological and serological study of 62 cases. Medicine (Baltimore) 1956; 44:187–231.
2. Daniels TE, Whitcher JP. Association of patterns of labial salivary gland inflammation with keratoconjunctivitis sicca. Analysis of 618 patients with suspected Sjögren's syndrome. Arthritis Rheum 1994; 37:869–877.
3. Fox RI, Saito I. Criteria for diagnosis of Sjögren's syndrome. Rheum Dis Clin North Am 1994; 20:391–407.
4. Vitali C, Moutsopoulos HM, Bombardieri S. The European Community Study Group on diagnostic criteria for Sjögren's syndrome. Sensitivity and specificity of tests for ocular and oral involvement in Sjögren's syndrome. Ann Rheum Dis 1994; 53:637–647.
5. Haddad J, Deny P, Munz-Gotheil C, Ambrosini JC. Lymphocytic sialadenitis of Sjögren's syndrome associated with chronic hepatitis C virus liver disease. Lancet 1992; 8:321–323.
6. Fox R. Classification Criteria for Sjögren's syndrome. Rheum Dis Clin North Am 1994; 20:391–407.
7. Jorgensen C, Legouffe MC, Perney P, Coste J, Tissot B, Segarra C, Bologna C, Bourrat L, Combe B, Blanc F, Sany J. Sicca syndrome associated with hepatitis C virus infection. Arthritis Rheum 1996; 39:1166–1171.
8. Vitali C, Bombardieri S, European Community Study Group on Diagnostic Criteria. The European classification criteria for Sjögren's syndrome (SS): Proposal for modification of the rules for classification suggested by the analysis of the receiver operating characteristic (ROCS) curve of the criteria performance. J Rheum 1997; 24(suppl):S18.
9. Andoh Y, Shimura S, Sawai T, Sasaki H, Takishima T, Shirato K. Morphometric analysis of secretory glands in Sjögren's syndrome. Am Rev Respir Dis 1993; 148:1358–1362.
10. Konttinen YT, Sorsa T, Hukkanen M, Segerberg M, et al. Topology of innervation of labial salivary glands by protein gene product 9.5 and synaptophysin immunoreactive nerves in patients with Sjögren's syndrome. J Rheumatol 1992; 19:30–37.
11. Ekstrom J. Autonomic control of salivary secretion. Proc Finn Dent Soc 1989; 85:323–331.
12. Main C, Blennerhassett P, Collins SM. Human recombinant interleukin 1 beta suppresses acetylcholine release from rat myenteric plexus. Gastroenterology 1993; 104:1648–1654.
13. Lu G, Beuerman RW, Zhao S, Sun G, Nguyen DH, Ma S, Kline DG. Tumor necrosis factor-alpha and interleukin-1 induce activation of MAP kinase and SAP kinase in human neuroma fibroblasts. Neurochem Int 1997; 30:401–410.

14. Soliven B, Wang N. Tumor necrosis factor-alpha regulates nicotinic responses in mixed cultures of sympathetic neurons and nonneuronal cells. J Neurochem 1995; 64:883–894.

15. Campbell IL. Neuropathogenic actions of cytokines assessed in transgenic mice. Int J Dev Neurosci 1995; 13:275–284.

16. Tornwall J, Konttinen Y, Tuomen R, Tornwall M. Salivary gland acinar epithelial cells are deficient in their protein kinase C expression in Sjögren syndrome. Lancet 1997; 349:1814–1815.

17. Borda E, Camusso JJ, Perez Leiros C, Bacman S, Hubscher O, Arana R, Sterin-Borda L. Circulating antibodies against neonatal cardiac muscarinic acetylcholine receptor in patients with Sjögren's syndrome. Mol Cell Biochem 1996; 163–164:335–341.

18. Stern ME, Beuerman RW, Fox RI, Gao J, Mircheff AK, Pflugfelder SC. The pathology of dry eye: The interaction between the ocular surface and lacrimal glands. Cornea 1998; 17:584–589.

19. Squirrell DM, Winfield J, Amos RS. Peripheral ulcerative keratitis 'corneal melt' and rheumatoid arthritis: A case series. Rheumatol 1999; 38:1245–1248.

20. Hazleman BL. Rheumatic disorders of the eye and the various structures involved. Br J Rheumatol 1996; 35:258–268.

21. Soukiasian SH, Foster CS, Raizman MB. Treatment strategies for scleritis and uveitis associated with inflammatory bowel disease. Am J Ophthalmol 1994; 118:601–611.

22. Rosenbaum JT, Robertson JE Jr. Recognition of posterior scleritis and its treatment with indomethacin. Retina 1993; 13:17–21.

23. Hernandez YL, Daniels TE. Oral candidiasis in Sjögren's syndrome: Prevalence, clinical correlation and treatment. Oral Surg Oral Med Oral Pathol 1989; 68:324–329.

24. Lotti TM, Comacchi C, Ghersetich I. Cutaneous necrotizing vasculitis: Relation to systemic disease. Adv Exp Med Biol 1999; 455:115–125.

25. Daniels TE, Fox PC. Salivary and oral components of Sjögren's syndrome. Rheum Dis Clin North Am 1992; 18:571–589.

26. Alexander EL, Provost TT. Cutaneous manifestations of primary Sjögren's syndrome: A reflection of vasculitis and association with anti-Ro (SSA) antibodies. J Invest Dermatol 1983; 80:386–391.

27. Ramos-Casals M, Cervera R, Yague J, Garcia-Carrasco M, Trejo O, Jimenez S, Morla RM, Font J, Ingelmo M. Cryoglobulinemia in primary Sjögren's syndrome: Prevalence and clinical characteristics in a series of 115 patients. Semin Arthritis Rheum 1998; 28:200–205.

28. Ohosone Y, Ishida M, Takahashi Y, Matsumura M, Hirakata M, Kawahara Y, Nishikawa T, Mimori T. Spectrum and clinical significance of autoantibodies against transfer RNA. Arthritis Rheum 1998; 41:1625–1631.

29. Provost TT, Watson R, Simmons-O'Brien E. Anti-Ro(SS-A) antibody positive Sjögren's/lupus erythematosus overlap syndrome. Lupus 1997; 6:105–111.

30. Ruzicka T, Faes J, Bergner T, Peter RU, Braun-Falco O. Annular erythema associated with Sjögren's syndrome: A variant of systemic lupus erythematosus [see comments]. J Am Acad Dermatol 1991; 25:557–560.

31. Simmonsobrien E, Chen S, Watson RA, Petri CM, Hochberg M, Stevens M, Provost T. One hundred anti-Ro (SS-A) antibody positive patients: A 10-year follow-up. Medicine (Baltimore) 1995; 74:109–130.

32. Provost TT, Watson R, Simmons-O'Brien E. Anti-Ro(SS-A) antibody positive Sjögren's/lupus erythematosus overlap syndrome. Lupus 1997; 6:105–11.

33. Cho CS, Park SH, Min JK, Lee SH, Kim HY. Clinical significances of antibodies to Ro/SS-A autoantigens and its subtypes in primary Sjögren's syndrome. Korean J Intern Med 1997; 12:176–181.

34. Gemignani F, Marbini A, Pavesi G, Di Vittorio S, Manganelli P, Cenacchi G, Mancia D. Peripheral neuropathy associated with primary Sjögren's syndrome. J Neurol Neurosurg Psychiatry 1994; 57:983–986.

35. Hebbar M, Hebbar-Savean K, Hachulla E, Brouillard M, Hatron PY, Devulder B. Participation of cryoglobulinaemia in the severe peripheral neuropathies of primary Sjögren's syndrome. Ann Med Interne 1995; 146:235–238.

36. Kyle R, Gleich G, Baynd E, et al. Benign hyperglobulinemic purpura of Waldenstrom. Medicine (Baltimore) 1971; 50:113–123.

37. Fox RI, Carson DA, Chen P, Fong S. Characterization of a cross reactive idiotype in Sjögren's syndrome. Scand J Rheumatol 1986; 561:83–88.

38. Konishi M, Ohosone Y, Matsumura M, Oyamada Y, Yamaguchi K, Kawahara Y, Mimori T, Ikeda Y. Mixed-cryoglobulinemia associated with cutaneous vasculitis and pulmonary symptoms. Intern Med 1997; 36:62–67.

39. Buezo GF, Garcia-Buey M, Rios-Buceta L, Borque MJ, Aragues M, Dauden E. Cryoglobulinemia and cutaneous leukocytoclastic vasculitis with hepatitis C virus infection. Int J Dermatol 1996; 35:112–115.

40. O'Donnell B, Black AK. Urticarial vasculitis. Int Angiol 1995; 14:166–174.

41. Magro CM, Crowson AN. The cutaneous pathology associated with seropositivity for antibodies to SSA (Ro): A clinicopathologic study of 23 adult patients without subacute cutaneous lupus erythematosus. Am J Dermatopathol 1999; 21:129–137.

42. Sontheimer RD. Subacute cutaneous lupus erythematosus: A decade's perspective. Med Clin North Am 1989; 73:1073–1090.

43. Suzuki M, Hamada M, Sekiya M, Shigematsu Y, Go S, Hiwada K. Fatal pulmonary hypertension in a patient with mixed connective tissue disease: Report of an autopsy case. Intern Med 1992; 31:74–77.

44. Hedgpeth MT, Boulware DW. Pulmonary hypertension in primary Sjögren's syndrome. Ann Rheum Dis 1988; 47:251–253.

45. Franquet T, Gimenez A, Monill JM, Diaz C, Geli C. Primary Sjögren's syndrome and associated lung disease: CT findings in 50 patients. Am J Roentgenol 1997; 169:655–658.

46. Kadota J, Kusano S, Kawakami K, Morikawa T, Kohno S. Usual interstitial pneumonia associated with primary Sjögren's syndrome. Chest 1995; 108:1756–1758.

47. Deheinzelin D, Capelozzi VL, Kairalla RA, Barbas Filho JV, Saldiva PH, de Carvalho CR. Interstitial lung disease in primary Sjögren's syndrome. Clinical-pathological evaluation and response to treatment. Am J Respir Crit Care Med 1996; 154:794–799.

48. Sheikh SH, Shaw-Stiffel TA. The gastrointestinal manifestations of Sjögren's syndrome. Am J Gastroenterol 1995; 90:9–14.

49. Parke AL, Parke DV. Hepatic disease, the gastrointestinal tract, and rheumatic disease. Curr Opin Rheumatol 1994; 6:85–94.

50. Alexander EL, Beall SS, Gordon B, Selnes LA, Yannakakis GD, Patronas N, Provost TT, McFarland HF. Magnetic resonance imaging of cerebral lesions in patients with the Sjögren's syndrome. Ann Intern Med 1988; 108:815–823.

51. Bragoni M, Di Piero V, Priori R, Valesini G, Lenzi GL. Sjögren's syndrome presenting as ischemic stroke. Stroke 1994; 25:2276–2279.

52. Utset TO, Golden M, Siberry G, Kiri N, Crum RM, Petri M. Depressive symptoms in patients with systemic lupus erythematosus: Association with central nervous system lupus and Sjögren's syndrome. J Rheumatol 1994; 21:2039–2045.

53. Spezialetti R, Bluestein HG, Peter JB, Alexander EL. Neuropsychiatric disease in Sjögren's syndrome: Anti-ribosomal P and anti-neuronal antibodies. Am J Med 1993; 95:153–160.

54. Alexander EL, Lijewski JE, Jerdan MS, Alexander GE. Evidence of an immunopathogenic basis for central nervous system disease in primary Sjögren's syndrome. Arthritis Rheum 1986; 29:1223–1231.

55. De Backer H, Dehaene I. Central nervous system disease in primary Sjögren's syndrome. Acta Neurol Belg 1995; 95:142–146.

56. Fox RI. Sjögren's syndrome. Curr Opin Rheumatol 1995; 7:409–416.

57. Tumiati B, Casoli P, Parmeggiani A. Hearing loss in the Sjögren syndrome. Ann Intern Med 1997; 126:450–453.

58. Whaley K, Webb J, McAvoy B, Hughes GR, Lee P, MacSween RN, Buchanan WW. Sjögren's syndrome. 2. Clinical associations and immunological phenomena. Q J Med 1973a; 66:513–548.

59. Ochs RL, Stein TW Jr, Chan EK, Ruutu M, Tan EM. cDNA cloning and characterization of a novel nucleolar protein. Mol Biol Cell 1996; 7:1015–1024.

60. Fox RI, Wilson C. In: Regenbogen LS, Eliahou HE. Sjögren's Syndrome. The Association of Interstitial Nephritis and Keratoconjunctivitis. New York: Karger, 1993:266–293.

61. Asherson RA, Fei HM, Staub HL, Khamashta MA, Hughes GRV, Fox RI. Antiphospholipid antibodies and HLA associations in primary Sjögren's syndrome. Ann Rheum Dis 1992; 51:495–498.

62. Merkel PA, Chang Y, Pierangeli SS, Convery K, Harris EN, Polisson RP. The prevalence and clinical associations of anticardiolipin antibodies in a large inception cohort of patients with connective tissue diseases. Am J Med 1996; 101:576–583.

63. Merkel PA, Chang Y, Pierangeli SS, Harris EN, Polisson RP. Comparison between the standard anti-cardiolipin antibody test and a new phospholipid test in patients with connective tissue diseases [In Process Citation]. J Rheumatol 1999; 26:591–596.

64. Oxholm P, Prause JU, Schiodt M. Rational drug therapy recommendations for the treatment of patients with Sjögren's syndrome. Drugs 1998; 56:345–353.

65. Fox RI, Dixon R, Guarrasi V, Krubel S. Treatment of primary Sjögren's syndrome with hydroxy-chloroquine: A retrospective, open-label study. Lupus 1996; 5(suppl 1):S31–36.

66. Schnabel A, Reuter M, Gross WL. Intravenous pulse cyclophosphamide in the treatment of interstitial lung disease due to collagen vascular diseases. Arthritis Rheum 1998; 41:1215–1220.

67. Kassan SS, Thomas TL, Moutsopoulos HM, Hoover R, Kimberly RP, Budman DR, Costa J, Decker JL, Chused TM. Increased risk of lymphoma in sicca syndrome. Ann Intern Med 1978; 89:888–892.

68. Skopouli FN, Jagiello P, Tsifetaki N, Moutsopoulos HM. Methotrexate in primary Sjögren's syndrome. Clin Exp Rheumatol 1996; 14:555–558.

69. Ferraccioli GF, De Vita S, Casatta L, Damato R, Pegoraro I, Bartoli E. Autoimmune connective tissue disease, chronic polyarthritides and B cell expansion: Risks and perspectives with immunosuppressive drugs. Clin Exp Rheumatol 1996; 14(suppl 14):S71–80.

70. Price EJ, Rigby SP, Clancy U, Venables PJ. A double blind placebo controlled trial of azathioprine in the treatment of primary Sjögren's syndrome. J Rheumatol 1998; 25:896–899.

44
Vasculitis in Systemic Lupus Erythematosus

David P. D'Cruz, Munther A. Khamashta and Graham R.V. Hughes
St. Thomas' Hospital, London, England

I. INTRODUCTION

Systemic lupus erythematosus (SLE) is a multisystem autoimmune connective tissue disease characterized by failure of immune regulation which results in the production of autoantibodies, activation of the complement system, immune complex generation, and abnormalities of cellular immunity. The clinical spectrum of the disease is extremely wide and the disease course and prognosis are variable depending to some extent on the degree of major organ involvement. This chapter briefly reviews the epidemiology, main clinical and serologic features and the manifestations of vascular disease in SLE.

II. EPIDEMIOLOGY

Systemic lupus erythematosus is characteristically seen in young women, with a female to male ratio of 8 or 9:1, a prevalence varying between 12 and 50.8 per 100,000 persons, and an average annual incidence of between 2.0 and 7.6 cases per 100,000 persons. The incidence and prevalence of SLE is higher among women from the Caribbean, the Far East, and Asia (1). For example, the incidence of SLE in black females in Baltimore was 11.4 per 100,000 per year compared with 3.9 per 100,000 per year in white females. Population studies in China suggest a prevalence of between 40 and 70 per 100,000. Mortality rates are 3 times higher for Afro-Caribbeans and twice as high for Asians compared with whites and deaths are mainly attributable to active disease with major organ involvement and infections. The long-term prognosis for Afro-Caribbeans is significantly worse even after adjustment for socioeconomic status (1). In addition, accelerated atheroma may account for increasing numbers of premature deaths (2,3).

In the United Kingdom, SLE is more prevalent among Afro-Caribbeans and Asians from the Indian subcontinent. Johnson et al. (4) found an overall prevalence in Birmingham of 27.7 per 100,000 but 206 per 100,000 in Afro-Caribbean females. Furthermore, the prevalence of undiagnosed SLE was significant (5). Samanta et al. (6) found SLE to be 3 times more common among Indian Asian immigrant females than white females in Leicester and also noted that Asians have more systemic disease and a higher risk of mortality (7).

The overall incidence of SLE is rising concurrent with improvement in survival rates. This was clearly demonstrated in a study of patients over 40 years by Uramoto et al. (8). The reasons for the increased incidence are most likely due to earlier detection of milder cases, and the widespread availability of antinuclear antibody testing. The improved survival rates may be due to a combination of milder disease detected earlier and improved methods of therapy. The long-term prognosis of patients with mild disease is generally excellent with 10-year survival rates of 80–90% (9). However, patients who develop vasculitis, glomerulonephritis, thrombosis, cardiopulmonary or central nervous system disease are at increased risk of morbidity and mortality.

Familial aggregation of SLE is well described and twin studies demonstrate concordance rates from 23–58% of monozygotic twins compared with 9% in dizygotic twins (1). There are HLA associations with SLE and HLA DR-2, DR3 and DQw1 are found in excess in whites with SLE (9). Complement deficiencies are associated with a risk of developing SLE and increased frequencies of the null alleles C4A*Q0 and C4B*Q0 are found in patients with SLE. The extended haplotype HLA-A1, B8 C4A*Q0, C4B1, BfS, C2-1, DR3 is commonly found in whites with SLE and the dominant association with SLE is due to C4A*Q0 (9).

III. CLINICAL FEATURES

Systemic lupus erythematosus is clinically extremely diverse and almost any organ may be involved. Polyarthritis, oral ulcers, and rashes, including photosensitivity, are common early features. Chronic fatigue, a variety of cognitive defects, and mild psychological disturbances such as anxiety and depression are extremely common (10). There is often a delay in diagnosis, especially in patients who have mild disease or in whom only a single manifestation such as arthritis or thrombocytopenia is present.

The diagnosis of SLE is made on clinical grounds, supported by laboratory investigations. Classification criteria may distinguish SLE from other connective tissue diseases; the most widely used are the revised criteria of the American College of Rheumatology (ACR) (11) which have been recently updated (12). These are criteria designed for clinical trials; they are not diagnostic criteria. Thus, in clinical practice, it is possible to make a diagnosis of lupus in patients with mild disease without fulfilling these criteria. Cervera et al. (13) described the clinical and serological features of 1000 SLE patients and Table 1 lists the clinical features at onset and during disease evolution in these patients.

IV. LABORATORY FINDINGS

Systemic lupus erythematosus is characterized by the presence of antinuclear antibodies (ANA), detected by indirect immunofluorescence in 95% or more of patients. The most common pattern is diffuse or homogeneous nuclear staining. Antibodies to native double-stranded DNA (anti-dsDNA) are more specific for SLE, though less sensitive, with 60–80% of patients having this antibody at presentation. Anti-dsDNA antibodies do not predict particular clinical features, though patients with lupus nephritis are much more likely to have high levels (10).

A speckled ANA pattern suggests the presence of antibodies to extractable nuclear antigens and the four most commonly assayed are antibodies to ribonucleoprotein (RNP), Smith (Sm), Ro (SS-A) and La (SS-B). These antibodies are associated with clinical subsets of SLE. Antibodies to SS-A/Ro and SS-B/La, predominantly cytoplasmic antigens, are associated with the photosensitive rash of subacute cutaneous lupus, "ANA-negative lupus" and are found in mothers of newborns suffering from the neonatal lupus syndrome (discoid-like rashes, thrombocytopenia, and cholestatic jaundice) and congenital heart block. These antibodies are also associated with the sicca features of Sjögren's syndrome where anti-Ro have been identified in parotid eluates. Cryoglobulins containing anti-Ro may occur in patients with cutaneous vasculitis and anti-Ro are present in glomerular eluates in lupus nephritis.

Table 1 Clinical Features at Onset and During Evolution of SLE in 1000 Patients

Manifestation	At onset (%)	During evolution (%)
Malar rash	40	58
Discoid lesions	6	10
Subacute cutaneous lesions	3	6
Photosensitivity	29	45
Oral ulcers	11	24
Arthritis	69	84
Serositis	17	36
Nephropathy	16	39
Neurological involvement	12	27
Thrombocytopenia	9	22
Hemolytic anemia	4	8
Fever	36	52
Raynaud's phenomenon	18	34
Livedo reticularis	5	14
Thrombosis	4	14
Myositis	4	9
Lung involvement	3	7
Chorea	1	2
Sicca syndrome	5	16
Lymphadenopathy	7	12

Source: Ref. 13.

Antibodies to uridylic acid–rich small nuclear ribonucleoproteins (anti–U-snRNPs) occur in mixed connective tissue disease (MCTD) and SLE, often with anti-Sm antibodies. Although a great deal is known about the fine specificities of anti–U1-RNP and anti-Sm antibodies (14), they have proved to be somewhat disappointing as clinical tools in delineating subsets of SLE except that they are in general associated with more severe disease (15). By way of illustration, Table 2 shows the prevalence of serological features in the Cervera et al. (13) cohort of patients.

Table 2 Serological Findings in 1000 Patients with SLE

Parameter	Prevalence (%)
ANA	96
High anti-dsDNA	78
Ro (SS-A)	25
La (SS-B)	19
U1-RNP	13
Sm	10
Rheumatoid factor	18
IgG anticardiolipin	24
IgM anticardiolipin	13
Lupus anticoagulant	15

Source: Ref. 13.

V. LUPUS AND VASCULITIS

One of the most characterisitic lesions of SLE is vascular injury, which may manifest as cutaneous vasculitis, cerebrovascular disease, glomerulonephritis, cardiopulmonary, and less commonly, gastrointestinal and ocular damage. The clinical spectrum of these lesions is wide, and endothelial activation and damage are central to the pathogenesis of vascular disease in SLE. Vascular damage may be inflammatory or thrombotic. This chapter focuses mainly on the clinical features and immunopathology of inflammatory vasculitis.

A. Cutaneous Vasculitis

There are surprisingly few data on the prevalence of cutaneous vasculitis in SLE. One reason for this lack of data is that cutaneous lesions are usually diagnosed by clinical examination alone, especially if the lesions are subtle, such as nailfold lesions or splinter hemorrhages. This almost certainly results in an underestimate of the true prevalence of cutaneous vasculitis. Furthermore, reports of clinical manifestations in SLE tend to utilize the ACR classification criteria, which do not include vasculitis.

An early study suggested a prevalence of dermal vasculitis of 21% of 150 patients (16). This was supported by possibly the largest study to date where a point prevalence of 18.7% of vasculitis was observed in 704 European patients with SLE (17). The cutaneous vasculitic lesions included digital infarcts, splinter hemorrhages (Fig. 1), ulcers, purpura, urticaria, and bullous lesions. Livedo reticularis may also be a manifestation of SLE vasculitis. Another large study found a high prevalence of vasculitis (36%, 194/540) over a 10-year follow-up period; the majority (160/194) had cutaneous vasculitis (18).

In severe cases, cutaneous lesions, especially those on the lower limbs and feet, can ulcerate. The majority of these lesions arise from small-vessel vasculitis, but severe ischemic injury and gangrene may result from vasculitis of medium-sized vessels (Fig. 2).

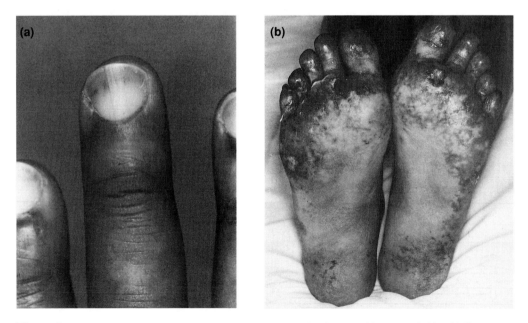

Figure 1 (a) Splinter hemorrhages in a woman with SLE who developed lupus nephritis. (b) Severe cutaneous vasculitis with digital ulcers and pulp infarcts of the toes.

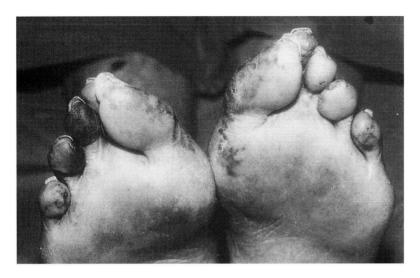

Figure 2   Medium-sized-vessel vasculitis in SLE resulting in digital ischemia and gangrene.

Less commonly, urticarial vasculitis is seen in SLE (19). The term "urticarial vasculitis" (UV) describes recurrent urticarial wheals that show leukocytoclastic vasculitis (rarely lymphocytic vasculitis) on biopsy. The typical cutaneous lesion is a raised erythematous wheal that is visible for 24–72 h, is seldom pruritic, but may be painful, and blanches on pressure. In contrast, true urticaria lasts for less than 24 h and is pruritic. Although vasculitis is usually confined to the skin, some patients with UV subsequently develop angioedema, vasculitis in major organs, and/or experience constitutional symptoms such as fever, malaise, and arthralgia. Serum complement may be decreased in such patients (19).

The diagnosis of cutaneous vasculitis is usually made on clinical grounds but where doubt exists, skin biopsy should be performed. Histologically, the most common lesion is leukocytoclastic vasculitis of arterioles, capillaries, and venules. Polymorphonuclear cells may be seen within the vessel walls and be associated with destruction of the vessel wall, fragmentation of the polymorphonuclear leukocytes, nuclear debris, and extravasation of red cells. Immunofluorescence studies usually demonstrate deposition of immunoglobulin G (IgG), complement, and fibrinogen in and around the cutaneous vessels.

The development of vasculitis is associated with an increase in the risk of morbidity and mortality. Most patients have constitutional symptoms, such as malaise, and other features of active lupus when they develop vasculitis.

B.   Central and Peripheral Nervous System Vasculitis

Central nervous system (CNS) disease is relatively common in SLE. The broad range of CNS clinical features varies from mild cognitive dysfunction to severe psychoses, ischemia, infection, and seizures. One of the problems with CNS lupus is that there have been no standard definitions of these manifestations and this has made the interpretation of studies that attempt to correlate a new imaging or serological investigation with clinical features difficult. The ACR has recently addressed this issue and has suggested revised nomenclature guidelines (20).

The pathophysiology of CNS lupus is poorly understood. Although lupus may be characterized by vasculitis, it seems reasonably clear that true central nervous system vasculitis is uncommon, occurring in 7–12% of patients (21–23). Despite the recognized association between

cutaneous vasculitis and CNS disease (24), the most striking aspect of these postmortem pathological studies is the relatively normal macroscopic appearance of the brain despite significant
neuropsychiatric dysfunction prior to death. Magnetic resonance imaging (MRI) appearances are
usually not diagnostic but may reveal the presence of periventricular white matter lesions, which
are probably vascular in origin. The nature of these lesions remains unknown and they are certainly not specific for neuropsychiatric lupus since they are commonly seen in lupus patients
without any evidence of neurological dysfunction (25) and in older, otherwise healthy individuals. Gadolinium enhancing lesions on MRI may improve with immunosuppressive therapy in a
small number of patients with SLE and this is certainly compatible with an inflammatory abnormality for at least some of these lesions (26). Other forms of imaging such as single photon emission computed tomography frequently show areas of reduced cerebral blood flow but again, these
defects may also seen in asymptomatic lupus patients (27). Subarachnoid hemorrhages have been
reported in association with SLE. While these may be due to rupture of a cerebral artery
aneurysm, vasculitis has been documented in the affected cerebral artery (28). Large-vessel cerebral vasculitis in lupus is extremely rare but is serious: the mortality of 12 reported patients with
documented cerebral large-vessel vasculitis was 67% (29).

Retinal vasculitis is well documented in SLE and, as with cutaneous vasculitis, is commonly associated with more severe disease. Retinal lesions are usually due to retinal infarction
leading to the clinical appearance of so-called cytoid bodies. Other features include retinal hemorrhage and vascular exudation. In a prospective study of 550 patients with SLE, Stafford Brady
et al. (30) found 41 to have retinopathy. In the majority of cases, this consisted of a microangiopathy, which had an excellent prognosis in regard to maintaining vision. Five patients developed other complications that resulted in loss of visual acuity. Lupus retinopathy was associated
with active SLE in 88% of patients, of whom lupus cerebritis was present in 73% of cases.
Retinopathy in this series of patients was a marker of poor prognosis for survival.

Fluorescein angiography may be very useful in diagnosis, assessing the extent of retinal involvement and response to treatment (Fig. 3). Other imaging modalities include magentic resonance imaging. In SLE, Sklar et al. (31) observed orbital MR enhancement within the optic nerve

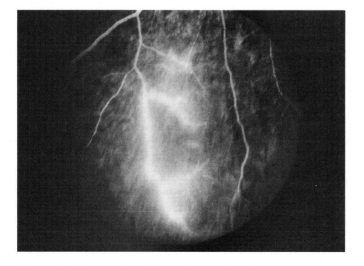

Figure 3 Fluorescein angiogram in a patient with SLE and retinal vasculitis demonstrating extensive
leakage of contrast.

suggesting disruption of the blood–brain barrier within the optic nerve, where optic neuropathy and vasculitis had been documented.

Transverse myelitis is a rare complication of lupus that almost certainly has a vascular basis (Fig. 4). Many of these patients respond rapidly to immunosuppressive therapy with intravenous cyclophosphamide, supporting the idea that transverse myelitis is due to an inflammatory myelopathy (32). Others have suggested a closer association with antiphospholipid antibodies (33).

Peripheral nervous system abnormalities may result from SLE vasculitis. Peripheral neuropathy was seen in 4.8% of patients in one large series (17). Mononeuritis multiplex, which may result from vasculitis of the vasa nervorum and is characterisitic of vasculitic involvement, is uncommon. Cranial nerve lesions may also have a vasculitic basis but are fortunately rare. Sural nerve biopsy may be a useful diagnostic procedure, though in our experience, there is a relatively high complication rate with poor healing following the procedure. Biopsy may show marked vasculitis with inflammatory cell infiltration. Ohkoshi et al. (34) observed occlusions in epineurial arteries greater than 100 μm in diameter, with mild vasculitic changes in arterioles 40–100 μm in diameter.

C. Pulmonary Vasculitis

Microvascular angiitis or capillaritis may occasionally occur in the lungs where the lesion is a necrotizing alveolar capillaritis manifesting as pulmonary hemorrhage. These manifestations are fortunately rare, though when they do occur the appearances are very similar to the alveolar lesions seen in the systemic vasculitides such as Wegener's granulomatosis (WG) or microscopic

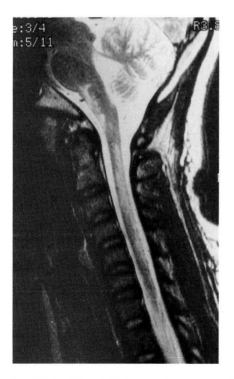

Figure 4   T2-weighted magnetic resonance image of the cervical cord in a patient with SLE and transverse myelitis. There are extensive high-signal abnormalities and edema within the cord.

polyangiitis (MPA). However, unlike WG and MPA, lung tissue from lupus patients with alveolar hemorrhage frequently shows the presence of C3 and/or IgG along the alveolar capillary basement membranes (35).

D. Renal Vasculitis

In any patient with cutaneous vasculitis, the threshold for investigating for glomerulonephritis should be low, since the two problems often coexist. In the kidney, the histological lesion of vasculitis is focal segmental necrotizing glomerulonephritis with fibrinoid necrosis, which may lead to rapidly progressive renal failure. Occasionally, renal and pulmonary vasculitis may coexist. Systemic lupus erythematosus is therefore part of the differential diagnoses of pulmonary–renal syndromes.

The vasculitic renal lesion is quite distinct from the more commonly seen membranous, mesangial, focal or diffuse proliferative glomerulonephritis, though vasculitis may also be seen in these forms of lupus nephritis. Histologically, renal glomerular basement membrane immunofluorescence is almost always positive for immunoglobulins and complement components (36) in necrotizing lupus glomerulonephritis. This is an important distinction compared with the antineutrophil cytoplasmic autoantibody (ANCA)-associated systemic vasculitides, where there is a relative lack of renal immune deposits.

Vasculitic involvement of other parts of the genitourinary system, such as the ureters and bladder, is rare and documented only as case reports.

E. Gastrointestinal Vasculitis

The best-described manifestation of vasculitis of the gastrointestinal (GI) tract in SLE is mesenteric vasculitis, which is uncommon and may occur in 1% of patients (17). Other abdominal organs that may be affected by lupus vasculitis include the pancreas, peritoneum, gallbladder, and the liver, though involvement of these organs, especially the liver, is rare (37).

The clinical presentation of mesenteric vasculitis is similar to that seen in polyarteritis nodosa. The patient may suddenly develop acute severe abdominal pain that leads to laparotomy. Occasionally, the symptoms of intestinal perforation may be masked if the patient is already on high-dose corticosteroid therapy. Severe and extensive bowel vasculitis may result in vigorous GI hemorrhage that is life threatening. On clinical examination, the patient is severely ill, often anemic, and has other evidence of organ involvement (38). Serological abnormalities usually include marked increases in products of the acute phase response, high anti-dsDNA, and low complement levels. Radiological investigations may be helpful: plain abdominal radiographs may show ileus or pseudo-obstruction (39) and chest radiographs may reveal gas under the diaphragm. Imaging with contrast such as barium may be normal or show classical features such as thumb-printing and bowel infarction. When bleeding is severe, angiography may localize the bleeding point and may occasionally reveal visceral artery aneurysms.

Macroscopically, GI vasculitis may lead to mucosal ischemia, infarction, ulceration, perforation, or hemorrhage. Histologically, GI vasculitis is commonly a small-vessel vasculitis, although very rarely, aneurysmal dilation of the mesenteric vessels has been described (40). Other rare manifestations of GI vasculitis are documented as case reports and include pneumatosis cystoides intestinalis and protein-losing enteropathy (37).

F. Cardiac and Large-Vessel Vasculitis

Cardiac involvement in SLE is common. Pericarditis and valvular disease are the most common manifestations. Coronary artery vasculitis is extremely rare and documented only in case reports

(41). Clinically, the patients may give a history of cardiac chest pain, and electrocardiograms may be normal or reveal evidence of ischemia or infarction. The ideal investigation is coronary arteriography, which may reveal aneurysms, tapering stenoses, or abrupt occlusions. If aneurysms are present, they may thrombose, leading to myocardial infarction.

The differential diagnosis of coronary vasculitis includes accelerated coronary atheroma, which may be up to 50 times more likely in women with lupus compared with non-lupus controls (42). The precise reasons for this remain unclear but include the usual cardiovascular risk factors and the additional effects of antiphospholipid antibodies cross-reacting with oxidized low-density lipoproteins (43) and atherogenic drugs such as corticosteroids.

Vasculitic involvement of large vessels such as the aortic arch and its branches resembling Takayasu's arteritis and the distal aorta is exceedingly rare and documented as case reports (44).

G. Evolution of Systemic Lupus Erythematosus into Systemic Vasculitis

There are a few case reports of patients with well-documented SLE evolving over time into a major systemic vasculitis. For example, D'Cruz et al. (45) described five patients in whom long-standing SLE evolved into systemic vasculitis resembling polyarteritis nodosa, Churg–Strauss syndrome, and Wegener's granulomatosis. Vivancos et al. (46) described a similar case. The reasons for this evolution from one disease to another remain obscure but may also reflect limitations in classification of multisystem connective tissue diseases.

H. Other Factors Associated with Vasculitis in Systemic Lupus Erythematosus

There are many other causes of small-vessel vasculitis in SLE. The list of drugs that have been implicated in playing a role is long and includes penicillins, sulfonamides, allopurinol, thiazides, pyrazolones, retinoids, streptokinase, cytokines, monoclonal antibodies, quinolones, hydantoins, carbamazepine, and other anticonvulsants. Patients with SLE have a higher frequency of allergic reactions (47), and the development of a new rash, especially a vasculitic rash, should raise the possibility of a drug-induced process. Viral infections, such as hepatitis C, are associated with the development of cryoglobulinemia (48), and should be considered as possibly complicating lupus and Sjögren's syndrome in patients with vasculitis.

VI. THROMBOSIS IN SYSTEMIC LUPUS ERYTHEMATOSUS

It is well-established that the antiphospholipid antibody (Hughes') syndrome is a major cause of vascular morbidity and mortality in SLE (49). The striking difference between this process and SLE vasculitis is that vascular occlusions are noninflammatory and the result of a markedly increased prothrombotic tendency. There are, however, documented instances where vasculitis and disseminated thrombosis may coexist in the same patient. Lie et al. (50) for example, describe a woman with lupus and antiphospholipid antibodies who had systemic and cerebral vasculitis coexisting with a disseminated coagulopathy, resulting in stroke and myocardial infarction.

VII. MONITORING DISEASE ACTIVITY

There are a number of systems in use for objectively quantifying disease activity in SLE, and active vasculitis is a feature of all these disease activity scores (51). The scoring systems do not include all the serological markers that may be used in the clinic, possibly because of limitations in sensitivity to change in relation to clinical variables. The scoring systems are most useful as research tools and provide some objectivity when interpreting the results of clinical trials in SLE.

VIII. THERAPY

The best strategy for coping with vasculitis in SLE is the prevention of vasculitic episodes in the first place. The most effective agent for this is hydroxychloroquine, and this was clearly demonstrated by the Canadian Hydroxychloroquine Study Group (52). In a randomized prospective double-blind trial, patients on stable doses of hydroxychloroquine were randomized to continue drug therapy or be changed to a placebo. Discontinuation of hydroxychloroquine was associated with a significant increase in clinical flares and severe disease exacerbations complicated in one case each by vasculitis, transverse myelitis, and lupus nephritis. There is, therefore, a compelling case for long-term continuation of hydroxychloroquine in patients even when the disease is stable or in remission, though reduction to alternate-day dosing may be possible.

The development of vasculitis in patients with lupus is frequently associated with an increased risk of morbidity and possibly mortality and justifies intensive immunosuppressive therapy. The most widely used and effective therapy includes corticosteroids and cyclophosphamide, which should be considered in any lupus patient with widespread severe vasculitis. While the dose, route of administration, and length of cyclophosphamide therapy remain controversial, one regimen using intravenous low-dose (500 mg) pulses of cyclophosphamide has been reported to be effective and relatively safe. The regimen uses 3–6 weekly or fortnightly intravenous pulses of cyclophosphamide, and when clear improvement or remission is seen, maintenance therapy with azathioprine or methotrexate is initiated. The main advantage of this therapy is the relative lack of ovarian toxicity when compared with sustained use of high-dose intravenous cyclophosphamide or oral cyclophosphamide (32). Another approach, if the patient is not severely ill, is to consider moderate prednisolone doses (30–40 mg daily) with intravenous pulse methylprednisolone doses followed by azathioprine. It is worth noting that although there are a number of clinical trials in progress assessing therapeutic strategies in lupus nephritis, to our knowledge there are no prospective studies of therapy for lupus vasculitis. The guiding principle in these patients, in the absence of evidence-based data, is to provide close surveillance and careful clinical judgment in balancing the beneficial and toxic effects of intensive immunosuppressive therapy.

In patients with complement deficiencies and vasculitis, infusions with fresh frozen plasma may be of benefit (53).

IX. IMMUNOPATHOLOGY

One commonly accepted hypothesis for vascular damage in SLE is that local deposition of immune complexes, particularly those containing anti–double-stranded DNA antibodies, onto the vascular endothelium triggers an inflammatory response involving activation of the complement cascade, possibly with the eventual formation of the C5b-9 membrane attack complex. There is good evidence that patients with SLE are unable to clear immune complexes efficiently, especially if they have complement deficiencies. For example, Davies et al. (53) showed in a C2-deficient patient that splenic uptake of injected immune complexes was absent despite normal splenic blood flow. Splenic uptake returned to normal following replenishment of complement components with fresh frozen plasma. When erythrocyte binding of immune complexes was measured in their patient, there was minimal binding to red cells, but following replenishment of complement, 72% of protein-bound activity from the labeled immune complexes was seen on the patient's erythrocytes. Thus, patients with lupus, particularly those with congenital hypocomplementemia, have abnormalities of immune complex processing. A further example was reported in a family study of a patient with homozygous C2 deficiency who developed cutaneous vasculitis, mesangial proliferative IgA glomerulonephritis, and polyclonal IgGλ cryoglobulins. The clinical features of the disease responded to immunosuppressive therapy and fresh frozen plasma infusions. The proband's brother had a similar, but much milder, illness that did not require therapy (54).

Antibodies to double-stranded DNA may be relevant to the pathology of vasculitic lesions in SLE, though it is not clear if they are directly pathogenetic. In animal studies, infusion of human monoclonal anti-DNA antibodies may result in the development of glomerulonephritis (55), though these results have not been reproduced (56).

Because endothelium can be a target of immune injury, investigators have sought to identify antibodies directed against vascular endothelium. Antiendothelial cell antibodies (AECAs) have been described in sera from patients with a wide variety of connective tissue diseases. Antiendothelial cell antibodies have been described in SLE in association with nephritis and vasculitis, and appear to correlate with disease activity (57). They may also be associated with digital, cutaneous, nonurticarial, and urticarial vasculitis (58). The hypocomplementemic urticarial vasculitis syndrome is characterized by decreased serum C1q levels, IgG anti-C1q antibodies, and the absence of anti-DNA antibodies. In fact, anti-C1q antibodies appear to be a specific marker for this condition that is clinically characterized by angioedema, arthritis/arthralgia, ocular inflammation, glomerulonephritis, and obstructive lung disease (59). Antiendothelial cell antibodies are seen in the hypocomplementemic urticarial vasculitis syndrome as well as in patients with UV associated with SLE where anti-DNA antibodies and hypocomplementemia were also frequently seen (58). It is possible, therefore, that AECAs may play a role in the pathogenesis of UV in both SLE and hypocomplementemic urticarial vasculitis syndrome.

The antigenic determinants for AECAs are present on the surface of endothelial cells and are independent of HLA class II and blood group antigens. These antigenic epitopes are not specific for endothelial cells since adsorption of AECA-positive sera by other cells, such as fibroblasts and to a lesser extent by leukocytes and monocytes, reduces AECA binding (60). The consensus is that AECAs bind by the F(ab′)2 and not the Fc region. Although this is a heterogeneous group of antibodies, AECA reactivity is unrelated to the presence of antinuclear antibodies, anti-DNA antibodies, or antibodies to extractable nuclear antigens or rheumatoid factor (57). The exact antigenic specificities of AECAs however remain unknown, although Western blot analyses suggest that a large number of different antigens may be recognized (61).

An early study (62) suggested that AECAs from lupus patients may disrupt endothelial monolayers. However, with the exception of a few patients, other groups failed to show direct complement-dependent serum cytotoxicity. Cytotoxic AECAs have been demonstrated in Kawasaki disease, which is characterized by a panvasculitis (63). More recently, Del Papa et al. (64) showed that sera from patients with systemic vasculitis displayed antibody-dependent cellular cytotoxicity in the presence of a mixed lymphocyte population. Thus, the evidence for an endothelial cytotoxic effect of AECAs remains controversial.

An alternative to direct AECA cytotoxicity is that such antibodies may induce functional changes in endothelial cells that promote vasculitis. For example, Carvalho et al. (65) showed that IgG AECAs from SLE and systemic vasculitis patients upregulated adhesion molecule expression and increased leukocyte adhesion. Thus, instead of directly damaging cells, AECAs may contribute to pathogenesis of vasculitis by enhancing leukocyte–endothelial interactions. The possibility remains that AECAs may be a response to vascular damage caused by other mechanisms.

A recent hypothesis suggests that a Shwartzman-like phenomenon may also result in small-vessel vasculitis in SLE (66). The original Shwartzman phenomenon resulted from injection of endotoxin intradermally followed by a further endotoxin injection 4–18 h later. Those manipulations activate complement, which triggers the release of anaphylatoxins (e.g., C3a and C5a). The result is chemotaxis and activation of inflammatory cells that aggregate and adhere to vascular endothelium, occluding small vessels and releasing toxic mediators that damage the vascular wall and the surrounding tissues. This mechanism does not require immune complex deposition and is a departure from the accepted hypotheses of pathogenic mechanisms in SLE.

X. SUMMARY

Vasculitic complications of SLE are relatively common, may affect a variety of organ systems, and vary from being benign to serious and life threatening. Careful regular monitoring for vasculitic complications is essential. Long-term maintenance therapy with hydroxychloroquine has been demonstrated to reduce the risk of vasculitic disease relapses and there is a continuing need for prospective studies.

There have been a number of advances in the understanding of the pathophysiology of lupus vasculitis and further insights will allow new therapies to be developed.

REFERENCES

1. Gladman DD, Hochberg MC. Epidemiology of systemic lupus erythematosus. In: Lahita RG, ed. Systemic Lupus Erythematosus. 3d ed. San Diego: Harcourt Brace, 1999:537–550.
2. Urowitz MB, Bookman AM, Koehler BE, Smythe HA, Ogryzlo MA. The bimodal mortality pattern of systemic lupus erythematosus. Am J Med 1976; 60:221–225.
3. Petri M, Perez-Gutthann S, Spence D, Hochberg MC. Risk factors for coronary artery disease in patients with systemic lupus erythematosus. Am J Med 1992; 93:513–519.
4. Johnson AE, Gordon C, Palmer RG, Bacon PA. The prevalence and incidence of systemic lupus erythematosus in Birmingham, England. Relationship to ethnicity and country of birth. Arthritis Rheum 1995; 38:551–558.
5. Johnson AE, Gordon C, Hobbs FD, Bacon PA. Undiagnosed systemic lupus erythematosus in the community. Lancet 1996; 347(8998):367–369.
6. Samanta A, Roy S, Feehally J, Symmons DP. The prevalence of diagnosed systemic lupus erythematosus in whites and Indian Asian immigrants in Leicester City, UK. Br J Rheumatol 1992; 31:679–682.
7. Samanta A, Feehally J, Roy S, Nichol FE, Sheldon PJ, Walls J. High prevalence of systemic disease and mortality in Asian subjects with systemic lupus erythematosus. Ann Rheum Dis 1991; 50:490–492.
8. Uramoto KM, Michet CJ, Thumboo J, Sunku J, O'Fallon WM, Gabriel SE. Trends in the incidence and mortality of systemic lupus erythematosus 1950–1992. Arthritis Rheum 1999; 42:46–50.
9. Hochberg MC. Epidemiology of the rheumatic diseases: Systemic lupus erythematosus. Rheum Dis Clin North Am 1990; 16:617–639.
10. Mills JA. Systemic lupus erythematosus. N Engl J Med 1994; 330:1871–1879.
11. Tan EM, Cohen AS, Fries JF, Masi AT, McShane DJ, Rothfield NF, et al. The 1982 revised criteria for the classification of systemic lupus erythematosus. Arthritis Rheum 1982; 25:1271–1277.
12. Hochberg MC. Updating the American College of Rheumatology Revised Criteria for the classification of systemic lupus erythematosus. Arthritis Rheum 1997; 40:1725.
13. Cervera R, Khamashta MA, Font J, Sebastiani GD, Gil A, Lavilla P, Domenech I, Aydintug AO, Jedryka-Goral A, De Ramon E, Galeazzi M, Haga HJ, Mathieu A, Houssiau FA, Ingelmo M, Hughes

GRV, and the European Working Party on Systemic Lupus Erythematosus. Systemic Lupus erythematosus: Clinical and immunologic patterns of disease expression in a cohort of 1,000 patients. Medicine (Baltimore) 1993; 72:113–124.

14. Van Venrooij WJ, Sillekens PTG. Review: Small nuclear RNA associated proteins: Autoantigens in connective tissue diseases. Clin Exp Rheumatol 1989; 7:635–645.

15. Montecucco C. Anti-RNP antibodies and their clinical significance (editorial). Br J Rheumatol 1990; 29:322–324.

16. Estes D, Christian CL. The natural history of systemic lupus erythematosus by prospective analysis. Medicine (Baltimore) 1971; 50:85–95.

17. Vitali C, Bencivelli W, Isenberg DA, Smolen JS, Snaith ML, Sciuto M, D'Ascanio, Bombardieri S, and the European Consensus Study Group for Disease Activity in SLE. Disease activity in systemic lupus erythematosus: report of the Consensus Study Group of the European Workshop for Rheumatology Research. I. A descriptive analysis of 704 European lupus patients. Clin Exp Rheumatol 1992; 10:527–539.

18. Drenkard C, Villa AR, Reyes E, Abello M, Alarcon-Segovia D. Vasculitis in systemic lupus erythematosus. Lupus 1997; 6:235–242.

19. Asherson RA, D'Cruz DP, Stephens CJM, McKee PH, Hughes GRV. Urticarial vasculitis in a Connective Tissue Disease Clinic: Patterns, presentations and treatment. Semin Arthritis Rheum 1991; 20:285–296.

20. Ad hoc Committee on neuropsychiatric lupus nomenclature. The American College of Rheumatology nomenclature and case definitions for neuropsychiatric lupus syndromes. Arthritis Rheum 1999; 42: 599–608.

21. Johnson RT, Richardson EP. The neurological manifestations of systemic lupus erythematosus: A clinical pathological study of 24 cases and review of the literature. Medicine (Baltimore) 1968; 47:337–369.

22. Ellis SG, Verity MA. Central nervous system involvement in systemic lupus erythematosus: A review of neuropathological findings in 57 cases 1955–1957. Semin Arthritis Rheum 1979; 8:212–221.

23. Devinsky O, Pettito CK, Alonso DR. Clinical and neuropathological findings in systemic lupus erythematosus: The role of vasculitis, heart emboli and thrombotic thrombocytopenic purpura. Ann Neurol 1988; 23:380–384.

24. Feinglass EJ, Arnett FC, Dorsch CA, Zizic TM, Stevens MB. Neuropsychiatric manifestations of systemic lupus erythematosus: Diagnosis, clinical spectrum and relationship to other features of the disease. Medicine (Baltimore) 1976; 55:323–339.

25. Gonzalez-Crespo MR, Blanco FJ, Ramos A, Ciruelo E, Mateo I, Lopez Pino MA, Gomez-Reino JJ. Magnetic resonance imaging of the brain in systemic lupus erythematosus. Br J Rheumatol 1995; 34: 1055–1060.

26. Miller DH, Buchanan N, Barker G, Morrissey SP, Kendall BE, Rudge P, Khamashta M, Hughes GR, McDonald WI. Gadolinium-enhanced magnetic resonance imaging of the central nervous system in systemic lupus erythematosus. J Neurol 1992; 239:460–464.

27. Kodama K, Okada S, Hino T, Takabayashi K, Nawata Y, Uchida Y, Yamanouchi N, Komatsu N, Ikeda T, Shinoda N, et al. Single photon emission computed tomography in systemic lupus erythematosus with psychiatric symptoms. J Neurol Neurosurg Psychiatry 1995; 58:307–311.

28. Kelley RE, Stokes N, Reyes P, Harik SI. Cerebral transmural angiitis and ruptured aneurysm: A complication of systemic lupus erythematosus. Arch Neurol 1980; 37:526–527.

29. Weiner DK, Allen NB. Large vessel vasculitis of the central nervous system in systemic lupus erythematosus: Report and review of the literature. J Rheumatol 1991; 18:748–751.

30. Stafford Brady FJ, Urowitz MB, Gladman DD, Easterbrook E. Lupus retinopathy: Patterns, associations and prognosis. Arthritis Rheum 1988; 31:1105–1110.

31. Sklar EM, Schatz NJ, Glaser JS, Post MJ, ten Hove M. MR of vasculitis-induced optic neuropathy. Am J Neuroradiol 1996; 17:121–128.

32. Martin-Suarez I, D'Cruz D, Mansoor M, Fernandes AP, Khamashta MA, Hughes GRV. Immunosuppressive therapy in severe connective tissue diseases: effects of low dose intravenous cyclophosphamide. Ann Rheum Dis 1997; 56:481–487.

33. Alarcon-Segovia D, Deleze M, Oria CV, Sanchez-Guerrero J, Gomez-Pacheco L. Antiphospholipid antibodies and the antiphospholipid syndrome in systemic lupus erythematosus: A prospective analysis of 500 consecutive patients. Medicine (Baltimore) 1989; 68:353–356.

34. Ohkoshi N, Mizusawa H, Oguni E, Shoji S. Sural nerve biopsy in vasculitic neuropathies: Morphometric analysis of the caliber of involved vessels. J Med 1996; 27:153–170.

35. Zamora MR, Warner ML, Tuder R, Schwarz MI. Diffuse alveolar hemorrhage and systemic lupus erythematosus. Clinical presentation, histology, survival, and outcome. Medicine (Baltimore). 1997; 76: 192–202.

36. Tsumagari T, Fukumato S, Kinjo M, Tanaka K. Incidence and significance of intrarenal vasculopathies in patients with systemic lupus erythematosus. Hum Pathol 1985; 16:43–49.

37. Fessler BJ, Hoffman GS. SLE and the cardiovascular system: Vasculitis. In: Lahita RG, ed. Systemic lupus erythematosus. 3d ed. San Diego: Harcourt Brace, 1999:707–717.

38. Gladman DD, Ross T, Richardson B, Kulkarni S. Bowel involvement in systemic lupus erythematosus: Crohn's disease or lupus vasculitis? Arthritis Rheum 1985; 28:466–470.

39. Shapeero LG, Myers A, Oberkircher PE, Miller WT. Acute reversible lupus vasculitis of the gastrointestinal tract. Radiology 1974; 112:569–574.

40. Ko SF, Hsien MJ, Ng SH, Wong HF, Lee TY, Lee CM. Superior mesenteric artery aneurysm in systemic lupus erythematosus. Clini Imaging. 1997; 21:13–16.

41. Korbet SM, Schwartz MM, Lewis EJ. Immune complex deposition and coronary vasculitis in systemic lupus erythematosus. Am J Med 1984; 77:141–146.

42. Manzi S, Meilahn EN, Rairie JE, Conte CG, Medsger TA, Jansen-McWilliams L, et al. Age-specific incidence rates of myocardial infarction and angina in women with systemic lupus erythematosus: Comparison with the Framingham study. Am J Epidemiol 1997; 145:408–415.

43. Vaarala O, Alfthan G, Jauhiainen M, Leirisalo-Repo M, Aho K, Palosuo T. Cross-reaction between antibodies to oxidised low-density lipoprotein and to cardiolipin in SLE. Lancet 1993; 341:923–925.

44. Harmon SM, Oltmanns KL, Min K-W. Large vessel occlusion with vasculitis in systemic lupus erythematosus. South Med J 1991; 84:1150–1154.

45. D'Cruz D, Cervera R, Aydintug AO, Ahmed T, Font J, Hughes GRV. Systemic lupus erythematosus evolving into systemic vasculitis: A report of five cases. Br J Rheumatol 1993; 32:154–157.

46. Vivancos J, Soler-Carrillo J, Ara-del Rey J, Font J. Development of polyarteritis nodosa in the course of inactive systemic lupus erythematosus. Lupus 1995; 4:494–495.

47. Sequeira J, Cesic D, Keser G, Bukelica M, Karanagnostis S, Khamashta MA, Hughes GRV. Allergic disorders in systemic lupus erythematosus. Lupus 1993; 2:187–192.

48. Ferri C, La Civita L, Longombardo G, Greco F, Bombardieri S. Hepatitis C virus and mixed cryoglobulinaemia. Eur J Clin Invest 1993; 23:399–405.

49. Hughes GRV. The antiphospholipid syndrome: Ten years on. Lancet 1993; 342:341–344.

50. Lie JT, Kobayashi S, Tokano Y, Hashimoto H. Systemic and cerebral vasculitis coexisting with disseminated coagulopathy in systemic lupus erythematosus associated with antiphospholipid syndrome. J Rheumatol 1995; 22:2173–2176.

51. Gladman DD, Goldsmith CH, Urowitz MB, Bacon P, Bombardier C, Isenberg D, Kalunian K, Liang MH, Maddison P, Nived O, Richter M, Symmons D, Zoma A. Sensitivity to change of 3 systemic lupus erythematosus disease activity indices: International validation. J Rheumatol 1994; 21:1468–1471.

52. Canadian Hydroxychloroquine Study Group. A randomized study of the effect of withdrawing hydroxychloroquine sulfate in systemic lupus erythematosus. N Engl J Med 1991; 324:150–154.

53. Davies KA, Erlendsson K, Beynon HLC, Peters AM, Valdimarsson H, Walport MJ. Splenic uptake of immune complexes in man is complement dependent. J Immunol 1993; 151:3866–3873.

54. D'Cruz D, Taylor J, Ahmed T, Asherson R, Khamashta M, Hughes GRV. Complement factor 2 deficiency: A clinical and serological family study. Ann Rheum Dis 1992; 51:1254–1256.

55. Mendlovic S, Brocke S, Shoenfeld Y, Ben-Bassat M, Meshorer A, Bakimer R, Mozes E. Induction of a systemic lupus erythematosus-like disease in mice by a common human anti-DNA idiotype. Proc Natl Acad Sci 1988; 85:2260–2264.

56. Isenberg DA, Katz D, Knight B, Le Page S, Tucker L, Hutchins P, Watts R, Andre-Schwartz J, Schwartz RS, Cooke A. Independent analysis of the 16/6 idiotype lupus model. A role for an environmental factor? J Immunol 1991; 147:4172–4177.

57. D'Cruz DP, Houssiau FA, Ramirez G, Baguley E, McCutcheon J, Vianna J, Haga H-J, Swana GT, Khamashta MA, Taylor JC, Davies D, Hughes GRV. Antiendothelial cell antibodies in systemic lupus erythematosus: A potential marker for nephritis and vasculitis. Clin Exp Immunol 1991; 85:254–261.
58. D'Cruz D, Wisnieski J, Asherson RA, Khamashta MA, Hughes GRV. Autoantibodies in systemic lupus erythematosus and urticarial vasculitis. J Rheumatol 1995; 22:1669–1673.
59. Wisnieski JJ, Naff GB. Serum IgG antibodies to C1q in hypocomplementemic urticarial vasculitis syndrome. Arthritis Rheum 1989; 32:1119–1127.
60. Meroni PL, D'Cruz DP, Khamashta MA, Youinou P, Hughes GRV. Antiendothelial cell antibodies: Only for scientists or for clinicans too? (editorial) Clin Exp Immunol 1996; 104:199–202.
61. van der Zee JM, Siegert CEH, De Vreede TA, Daha MR, Breedveld FC. Characterisation of anti-endothelial cell antibodies in systemic lupus erythematosus. Clin Exp Immunol 1991; 84:238–244.
62. Cines DB, Lyss AP, Reeber M, Bina M, DeHoratius RJ. Presence of complement fixing anti-endothelial cell antibodies in systemic lupus erythematosus. J Clin Invest 1984; 73:611–625.
63. Tizard J, Baguley E, Hughes GRV, Dillon M. Antiendothelial cell antibodies detected by a cellular based ELISA in Kawasaki's disease. Arch Dis Child 1991; 66:189–192.
64. Del Papa N, Meroni PL, Barcellini W, Sinico A, Radice A, Tincani A, D'Cruz D, Nicoletti F, Borghi MO, Khamashta MA, Hughes GRV, Balestrieri G. Antibodies to endothelial cells in primary vasculitides mediate in vitro endothelial cytotoxicity in the presence of normal peripheral blood mononuclear cells. Clin Immunol Immunopathol 1992; 63:267–274.
65. Carvalho D, Savage COS, Isenberg D, Pearson JD. IgG anti-endothelial cell autoantibodies from patients with systemic lupus erythematosus or systemic vasculitis stimulate the release of two endothelial cell-derived mediators, which enhance adhesion molecule expression and leukocyte adhesion in an autocrine manner. Arthritis Rheum 1999; 42:631–640.
66. Belmont HM, Abramson SB, Lie JT. Pathology and pathogenesis of vascular injury in systemic lupus erythematosus. Arthritis Rheum 1996; 39:9–22.

45

Vasculitis in the Idiopathic Inflammatory Myopathies

Chester V. Oddis

University of Pittsburgh School of Medicine, Pittsburgh, Pennsylvania

I. INTRODUCTION

The idiopathic inflammatory myopathies (IIM) represent a group of diseases of unknown cause in which muscle injury results from inflammation. The major categories of IIM include polymyositis (PM), dermatomyositis (DM), myositis in overlap with malignancy or another connective tissue disease (CTD), childhood myositis (most commonly dermatomyositis), and inclusion body myositis (IBM). Although proximal muscle weakness is the most common symptom of IIM, the clinical features at disease presentation and during the course of the illness vary considerably from patient to patient. The presence of a variety of rashes and cutaneous findings separates the patient with an inflammatory myopathy into the clinical subset of dermatomyositis.

Vasculitis is an uncommon complication of the inflammatory myopathies. It may be seen as a manifestation of the overlap disorder (e.g., systemic lupus erythematosus or Sjögren's syndrome) with which myositis is associated and there are reports of vasculitic muscle involvement in polyarteritis nodosa (1), Churg–Strauss syndrome (2), and inflammatory bowel disease (3) where patients clinically present as PM but evolve into other immunological disorders. However, this chapter discusses vasculitic manifestations of patients with an established diagnosis of IIM. Since vasculitis in IBM is extremely rare, only the five classic subsets (4) of inflammatory myopathy are considered.

II. EPIDEMIOLOGY

It is difficult to determine the prevalence of muscle vasculitis in the inflammatory myopathies due to selection bias and the exclusion of certain IIM subsets in reported series. In one of the largest cohorts of myositis patients, Bohan et al. (4) retrospectively reviewed 153 patients with carefully defined PM and DM and found only 3% (4/135 who had muscle biopsies performed) demonstrating muscle vasculitis. Two had pure adult DM and two had myositis in overlap with another CTD. No other myositis subset, including childhood myositis (11 patients), demonstrated vasculitis.

In a clinicopathological assessment of an Indian population (5), 86 muscle biopsies in as many patients were identified over a 10-year period and 73 of 86 patients met established criteria for myositis (6). Vasculitis was diagnosed when the walls of arterioles and venules were moderate to severely infiltrated by inflammatory cells. Fibrinoid necrosis of the vessel wall, though characteristic, was not essential for the diagnosis of vasculitis. Eight patients (11%) demonstrated muscle vasculitis, four of whom were in the myositis/connective tissue disease overlap category (PM with rheumatoid arthritis, one; PM with systemic sclerosis, one; DM with systemic sclerosis, two). Only one of seven cases of childhood dermatomyositis (CDM) showed acute necrotizing vasculitis. Overall, vasculitis was present in three patients with PM and five with DM. The frequency of vasculitis in DM was double (15.1%) that in PM (7.5%) and women were affected 3 times more commonly than men.

The one feature that has distinguished CDM from the adult variety is the widespread necrotizing vasculitis with small-vessel intimal proliferation, thrombosis, and multiple infarctions first reported many years ago (7). This finding was rarely seen in the CDM patients from studies described above in sharp contrast to series of pure CDM where vasculopathic features are commonly reported (Fig. 1). In one study, 29 patients with childhood poly/dermatomyositis had one or more muscle biopsies performed over a 22-year period (8). Muscle biopsy was performed before corticosteroid treatment in 27 of the 29 patients, while 16 additional posttreatment biopsies were studied in an attempt to correlate tissue manifestations with patient outcome. Vasculitis was identified in 6 of 18 pretreatment muscle biopsies of patients with chronic ulcerative and nonulcerative CDM but none of 9 children with limited DM or chronic PM. These four mutually exclusive clinical course designations were determined retrospectively from analysis of the histopathological data and were determined either by length of patient follow-up or by unequivocal signs of ulcerative disease at any time. Distinctive lesions included nonnecrotizing lymphocytic vasculitis and a spectrum of endovascular injury producing temporary or prominent occlusion of small arteries and capillaries. Only 1 of 16 posttreatment specimens showed vasculitic changes.

III. CLINICAL FEATURES

A. Cutaneous

Patients with IIM with cutaneous vasculitis far outnumber other vasculitic organ manifestations. Cutaneous changes in CDM include telangiectatic involvement of the upper eyelids often associated with periorbital edema and ulceration. More common vasculitis changes affect the nailbeds

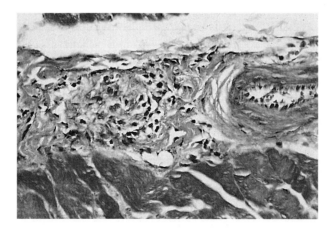

Figure 1   Muscle biopsy of a child with dermatomyositis demonstrating acute necrotizing vasculitis of one vessel (left) adjacent to a normal blood vessel (right) (trichrome, 100×). (Courtesy of A. Vincent Londino, Jr.)

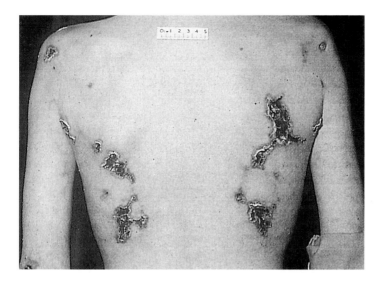

Figure 2 Healing, linear, necrotic lesions on the back of a child with dermatomyositis. Similar lesions may occur in the axillae and groin. (Courtesy of A. Vincent Londino, Jr.)

and digits, and particularly troublesome are the ulcerated and crusting lesions in the skinfolds of the axillae and groin or back (Fig. 2). Infarction of the palate has also been reported (9).

The cutaneous vasculitic features in adult IIM patients have curious clinical associations. In a retrospective study, 7 of 76 (9%) patients with adult-onset PM or DM seen over an 11-year period had cutaneous vasculitis (10). This was manifested by dermal and/or subcutaneous nodules in four, periungual infarcts in three, and digital ulceration in two (Fig. 3). A significant association was noted between cutaneous vasculitis and DM ($p = 0.025$) as only 1 of 31 pure PM and 0 of 18 overlap myositis patients had vasculitis while 6 of the 7 patients with vasculitis had the rash of DM (10). In addition, 2 of the 7 patients (29%) with vasculitis had a malignancy compared

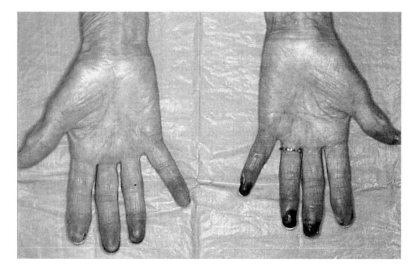

Figure 3 Digital tip infarction in a middle-aged woman with polymyositis and no associated malignancy. (Courtesy of Lawrence M. Mulhern.)

with only 4 of 69 (6%) without vasculitis, suggesting that cutaneous vasculitis may be a marker of underlying malignancy. The absence of vasculitis in muscle biopsy specimens indicated a lack of correlation between dermal and muscle vasculitis. A subsequent report of 32 pure adult DM patients defined predictive signs of cancer and established prognostic factors related to survival (11). Thirteen (41%) of the 32 patients had DM associated with malignancy, and cutaneous necrosis was more commonly found in the cancer patients (31% vs. 5%, $p < 0.05$). Sites of cutaneous necrosis were characterized by eroded or ulcerated necrotic lesions on erythematosus, violaceous indurated plaques (Fig. 4). As opposed to the former study (10), vasculitis on muscle biopsy was frequently (66%) observed (11). Both studies (10,11) suggest that selected DM patients with cutaneous necrosis have a poor prognosis. Other studies have reported cutaneous vasculitis in adult-onset myositis (12,13) but have not confirmed an association with malignancy. Six (24%) of 25 adult PM or DM patients without malignancy had striking skin vasculitis with other classical skin features of DM (12). Similarly, 14 (19%) of 75 adult IIM patients from Singapore had cutaneous vasculitis at presentation (13). Although three of four patients with malignancy at presentation had cutaneous vasculitis, the latter was not more frequent in the myositis/malignancy subset compared with the other groups of myositis patients. Nevertheless, the bulk of the literature does suggest a possible association between cancer and vasculitic skin changes.

Cutaneous vasculitis has been reported in a dermatomyositis patient without overt muscle disease (14), and urticarial skin lesions secondary to lymphocytic vasculitis have been seen in a patient with pure PM (15). Another patient with DM and a remote history of gastric cancer developed multiple punched-out cutaneous ulcers, and a skin biopsy showed vasculitis in the deep dermis with membranocystic changes without panniculitis (16).

B. Gastrointestinal

Gastrointestinal vasculitis often distinguishes childhood from adult DM and it may be extensive in severe cases of CDM. It manifests as hemorrhage, ulceration, perforation, peritonitis, or infarction, and children complain of severe abdominal pain, hematemesis, and melena (9). Its onset is often acute and death may result (7,8). Although there are many reports of gastrointestinal involvement in children, few have documented the histological presence of vasculitis. Early reports of childhood DM have nicely demonstrated the extent and severity of pathological vasculitic in-

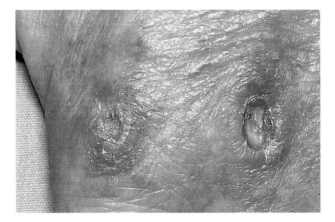

Figure 4   Characteristic, well-demarcated, ulcerative lesions on the dorsum of the hand and wrist in an adult patient with dermatomyositis and cutaneous vasculitis. Note the erythematous, violaceous margin of the ulcer. Similar lesions were noted on the elbows.

volvement in the esophagus, stomach, and small and large bowel (7). In Crowe's series, two of the three fatalities caused by CDM were due to ischemic intestinal ulceration with secondary hemorrhage and perforation, while another patient had necrotizing arteritis typical of polyarteritis nodosa in a large mesenteric artery branch (8).

Two male children with severe DM developed pancreatitis, an unusual complication often associated with multiple organ involvement in patients with diffuse connective tissue diseases. One child had overt duodenal and jejunal vasculitis with multiple perforations, and the other had widespread cutaneous ulcerations and hepatitis with presumptive bowel vasculitis suggesting that pancreatitis was a feature of widespread vasculitic activity due to CDM (17).

In the adult PM and DM series discussed earlier, where 24% of patients had cutaneous vasculitis, one patient developed severe intestinal vasculitis leading to perforation and death, a distinctly unusual complication in adult IIM (12).

C. Pulmonary

In a clinical and autopsy study of 65 patients with PM or DM seen over a 52-year period at the Mayo Clinic, 43 had pulmonary symptoms and 27 had interstitial lung disease (ILD) at autopsy (18). Pulmonary vasculitis (indistinguishable from the vasculitis of other connective tissue diseases and demonstrating either necrotizing or chronic healed proliferative lesions) was seen in five (8%) patients, all with associated ILD. One of the patients with pulmonary vasculopathy presented with rapidly progressive and fatal pulmonary hypertension. Four of the five had PM as well as an inflammatory arthritis raising the possibility that these patients had pulmonary vasculitis in association with the presence of the anti-Jo-1 autoantibody or another of the anti-aminoacyl-tRNA synthetases. The anti-synthetases are known to be associated with the presence of ILD and inflammatory arthritis in the IIM. We have seen muscle vasculitis in a patient with PM, severe ILD and the anti-Jo-1 antibody (Fig. 5).

Pulmonary capillaritis, a distinctive histological lesion with extensive neutrophilic infiltration of the alveolar interstitium, was seen in two patients with the acute onset of PM, respiratory failure and diffuse alveolar hemorrhage (without hemoptysis), and bronchiolitis obliterans–organizing pneumonia (BOOP) (19). One patient had a positive serum anti-Jo-1 autoantibody, and neither had antibodies directed against myeloperoxidase (p-ANCA) or proteinase 3 (c-ANCA).

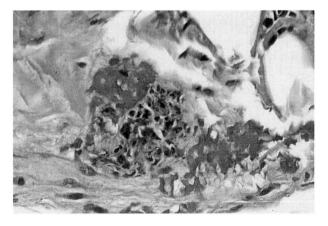

Figure 5   Necrotizing vasculitis in the muscle biopsy of a patient with anti-Jo-1 antibody positive polymyositis with interstitial lung disease (H and E, 60×).

D. Miscellaneous

Retinal vasculitis has been reported in several cases of CDM (20–22). Most often, there are transient retinal and visual changes that respond quite well to treatment. However, retinopathy resulted in permanent and profound central visual loss in one patient with severe bilateral optic neuropathy (22). With retinal vasculitis, the fundus may demonstrate cytoid bodies, cotton wool spots, or hemorrhage, and edema secondary to small-vessel occlusions (9,22). One adult with DM and cutaneous vasculitis also had retinal vasculitis (10), but this is a rare complication in adult IIM.

Central nervous system vasculitis as a feature of severe multisystem disease is an unusual complication of CDM (23–25). Most cases are fatal and patients often have fever, mental status changes, and seizures. Postmortem findings have demonstrated an angiopathy similar to that observed in skeletal muscle, as well as endothelial necrosis, dermal thickening, and parenchymal changes of hypoperfusion (23,24).

Cardiac involvement occurs in the setting of severe DM but may not be vasculitic in etiology. However, myocarditis with vasculitis can lead to atrioventricular heart block or complete heart block (9), hypotension, and left ventricular failure (24). Microscopic findings have revealed ischemic myonecrosis (infarct) secondary to small-vessel lymphocytic vasculitis with superimposed thrombotic luminal occlusion (24).

Other myositis syndromes have been associated with vasculitis. Nodular polymyositis with an acute purpuric rash has been reported (26), and idiopathic eosinophilic myositis with a necrotizing medium-sized-vessel vasculitis and severe symmetric polyneuropathy is described (27). Pseudotumor of muscle associated with necrotizing vasculitis and chronic myositis preceded generalized PM by 7 years in one patient (28).

IV. DIAGNOSIS AND MANAGEMENT

The diagnosis of vasculitic complications in IIM entails various modalities. Cutaneous features are clinically obvious and may require histopathological documentation. Gastrointestinal vasculitis can be diagnosed endoscopically with biopsy, but children often present acutely with abdominal crisis necessitating surgical intervention with bowel resection (8). A white cell scan demonstrating increased small bowel uptake suggestive of vasculitis has been reported (17). Pulmonary capillaritis can be diagnosed thoracoscopically or transbronchially (19). Cardiac and central nervous system vasculitis are difficult to diagnosis and, unfortunately, often substantiated by postmortem analysis (24). Laboratory findings are of little help in establishing vasculitis as a complication of myositis. There are no consistent serological autoantibody correlations, and other indicators of inflammation are much too nonspecific.

Although corticosteroids are the mainstay of treating vasculitis, they can be administered in different ways. In acutely ill children with gastrointestinal vasculitis, intravenous "pulses" of methylprednisolone are the treatment of choice and the dosage is usually 30 mg/kg/body weight up to 1 g daily for 3 consecutive days. However, the most effective frequency and duration of intravenous injections are uncertain. With improvement, children should be converted to oral corticosteroids immediately after pulse treatment, and it may be necessary to administer doses of 2 mg/kg body weight (in divided doses) since gastrointestinal vasculitis may impair drug absorption (9). After at least 1 month of divided dose corticosteroids, a conversion to a single daily dose with sequential tapering is recommended.

Cyclophosphamide (initially intravenous, followed by daily oral therapy in severe cases) should be considered, and has been effective in conjunction with corticosteroids in patients with multisystem disease where corticosteroids are unable to be tapered (17,22). Although both individual and combination therapy (including methotrexate, cyclosporine, cyclophosphamide, intravenous immune globulin) utilizing many immunosuppressive agents have been efficacious, some patients have been unresponsive to multiple modalities (25). Two adults with polymyositis and diffuse alveolar hemorrhage secondary to pulmonary capillaritis responded to a combination of corticosteroids and oral cyclophosphamide (19).

Since gastrointestinal vasculitis with mucosal ulceration can lead to bowel perforation, surgical intervention may be necessary. In addition to the need for concomitant immunosuppressive treatment, it is necessary to meticulously manage sump drains and judiciously administer antibiotics as well as provide parenteral nutrition. In perforations beyond the ligament of Treitz, surgery may include proximal bowel diversion with secondary closure of the colostomy.

V. PATHOGENESIS

There is increasing information on the mechanisms of muscle damage in the inflammatory myopathies (29). It is clear that the process differs among the unique subsets of IIM. Cell-mediated immunity appears to be pathogenetically important in PM and IBM, and investigators have demonstrated CD8+ T lymphocytes surrounding and invading muscle fibers in polymyositis (30,31). The fibers are otherwise normal and intact and the T cell antigen-directed attack on muscle thus seems to be a primary event rather than a secondary response to myofiber necrosis. Although humorally mediated damage to vascular targets is operative in childhood and adult DM, humoral immune mechanisms are involved in both PM and DM as they relate to the formation of distinctive autoantibodies in the myositis syndromes.

The increase of vasculitis-associated clinical complications in adult and childhood DM, as opposed to PM, is borne out histopathologically as well. In most cases of CDM and some adult DM patients, there is early, prominent blood vessel involvement with capillary loss and ischemic muscle damage (8) leading to perifascicular atrophy. The inflammatory infiltrates (CD4+ and B lymphocytes) are interstitial and perivascular (30), and the microvascular injury is complement-mediated with deposition of the membrane attack complex (32). The latter finding is an early feature in DM muscle, occurring prior to other histological changes supporting its primary role in muscle injury (33). The factors that lead to complement activation are unknown and the roles of humoral immunity and complement activation in extramuscular vasculitic disease manifestations remain undefined. However, the role of an obliterative microvasculopathy in the pathogenesis of vasculitic cutaneous lesions in DM is supported by a recent study demonstrating C_{5b-9} deposition and a reduction in the density of the superficial vascular plexus (34). The above observations support the hypothesis that PM is a T cell–mediated myocytotoxic disease, whereas DM is a humorally mediated vasculitis.

VI. SUMMARY

The inflammatory myopathies are a heterogeneous group of systemic autoimmune diseases that can target blood vessels much like any of the diffuse connective tissue diseases. Cutaneous manifestations in the form of nodules, infarcts, or ulcerated lesions are the predominant feature when vasculitic involvement occurs. Childhood dermatomyositis patients most commonly develop vasculitic complications and the effects can be life threatening when gastrointestinal or systemic involvement results. Treatment usually includes the administration of corticosteroids, and other immunosuppressive agents are often necessary for severe or refractory manifestations. The pathogenesis of these interesting diseases reinforces the blood vessel as an immunological target, especially in the case of dermatomyositis.

REFERENCES

1. Fort JG, Griffin R, Tahmoush A, Abruzzo JL. Muscle involvement in polyarteritis nodosa: Report of a patient presenting clinically as polymyositis and review of the literature. J Rheumatol 1994; 21: 945–948.
2. DeVlam K, De Keyser F, Goemaere S, Praet M, Veys EM. Churg-Strauss syndrome presenting as polymyositis. Clin Exp Rheumatol 1995; 13:505–507.
3. Gilliam JH III, Challa VR, Agudelo CA, Albertson DA, Huntley CC. Vasculitis involving muscle associated with Crohn's colitis. Gastroenterology 1981; 81:787–790.
4. Bohan A, Peter JB, Bowman RL, Pearson CM. A computer-assisted analysis of 153 patients with polymyositis and dermatomyositis. Medicine (Baltimore) 1977; 56:255–286.
5. Prasad ML, Sarkar C, Roy S, Bagghi U, Singh RR, Singh YN, Sharma S, Malaviya AN. Idiopathic inflammatory myopathy: Clinicopathological observations in the Indian population. Br J Rheumatol 1992; 31:835–839.
6. Bohan A, Peter JB. Polymyositis and dermatomyositis (I). N Engl J Med 1975; 292:334–347.
7. Banker BQ, Victor M. Dermatomyositis (systemic angiopathy) of childhood. Medicine (Baltimore) 1966; 45:261–289.
8. Crowe WE, Bove KE, Levinson JE, Hilton PK. Clinical and pathogenetic implications of histopathology in childhood polydermatomyositis. Arthritis Rheum 1982; 25:126–139.
9. Ansell BM. Juvenile dermatomyositis. J Rheumatol 1992; 19(33):60–62.
10. Feldman D, Hochberg MC, Zizic TM, Stevens MB. Cutaneous vasculitis in adult polymyositis/dermatomyositis. J Rheumatol 1983; 10:85–89.
11. Basset-Seguin N, Roujeau J-C, Gherardi R, Guillaume J-C, Revuz J, Touraine R. Prognostic factors and predictive signs of malignancy in adult dermatomyositis. Arch Dermatol 1990; 126:633–637.
12. Ramirez G, Asherson RA, Khamashta MA, Cervera R, D'Cruz D, Hughes GRV. Adult-onset polymyositis-dermatomyositis: Description of 25 patients with emphasis on treatment. Semin Arthritis Rheum 1990; 20:114–120.
13. Koh ET, Seow A, Ong B, Ratnagopal P, Tjia H, Chng HH. Adult onset polymyositis/dermatomyositis: clinical and laboratory features and treatment response in 75 patients. Ann Rheum Dis 1993; 52:857–861.
14. Kadoya A, Akahoshi T, Sekiyama N, Hosaka S, Kondo H. Cutaneous vasculitis in a patient with dermatomyositis without muscle involvement. Intern Med 1994; 33:809–812.
15. Kao NL, Zeitz HJ. Urticarial skin lesions and polymyositis due to lymphocytic vasculitis. West J Med 1995; 162:156–158.
16. Yamamoto T, Ohkubo H, Katayama I, Nishioka K. Dermatomyositis with multiple skin ulcers showing vasculitis and membrano-cystic lesion. J Dermatol 1994; 21:687–689.
17. See Y, Martin K, Rooney M, Woo P. Severe juvenile dermatomyositis complicated by pancreatitis. Br J Rheumatol 1997; 36:912–916.
18. Lakhanpal S, Lie JT, Conn DL, Martin WJ II. Pulmonary disease in polymyositis/dermatomyositis: A clinicopathological analysis of 65 autopsy cases. Ann Rheum Dis 1987; 46:23–29.
19. Schwarz MI, Sutarik JM, Nick JA, Leff JA, Emlen W, Tuder RM. Pulmonary capillaritis and diffuse alveolar hemorrhage. Am J Respir Crit Care Med 1995; 151:2037–2040.
20. Fruman LS, Ragsdale CG, Sullivan DB, Petty RE. Retinopathy in juvenile dermatomyositis. J Pediatr 1976; 88:267–269.
21. Brown GC, Brown MM, Hiller T, Fischer D, Benson WE, Magargal LE. Cotton-wool spots. Retina 1985; 5:206–214.
22. Yeo LMW, Swaby DSA, Situnayake RD, Murray PI. Irreversible visual loss in dermatomyositis. Br J Rheumatol 1995; 34:1179–1181.
23. Gotoff SP, Smith RD, Sugar O. Dermatomyositis with cerebral vasculitis in a patient with agammaglobulinemia. Amer J Dis Child 1972; 123:53–56.
24. Jimenez C, Rowe PC, Keene D. Cardiac and central nervous system vasculitis in a child with dermatomyositis. J Child Neurol 1994; 9:297–300.
25. Falcini F, Trapani S, Ermini M, Taccetti G, Bartolozzi G. Systemic vasculitis in juvenile dermatomyositis: A fatal case. Clin Exp Rheumatol 1995; 13(4):531–532.

26. Allen I, Mullally B, Mawhinney H, Sawhney B, McKee P. The nodular form of polymyositis: A possible manifestation of vasculitis. J Pathol 1980; 13:183–191.

27. Espino-Montoro A, Medina M, Marin-Martin J, Jimenez-Gonzalo FJ, Moalla AK, Fernandez-Gonzalez GF, Vahl R. Idiopathic eosinophilic myositis associated with vasculitis and symmetrical polyneuropathy. Br J Rheumatol 1997; 36:276–279.

28. Esteva-Lorenzo FJ, Ferreiro JL, Tardaguila F, de la Fuente A, Falasca G, Reginato AJ. Case report 866: Pseudotumor of the muscle associated with necrotizing vasculitis of medium and small-sized arteries and chronic myositis. Skeletal Radiol 1994; 23:572–576.

29. Targoff IN. Humoral immunity in polymyositis/dermatomyositis. J Invest Dermatol 1993; 100:116S–123S.

30. Arahata K, Engel AG. Monoclonal antibody analysis of mononuclear cells in myopathies. I. Quantitation of subsets according to diagnosis and sites of accumulation and demonstration and counts of muscle fibers invaded by T cells. Ann Neurol 1984; 16:193–208.

31. Engel AG, Arahata K. Monoclonal antibody analysis of mononuclear cells in myopathies. II. Phenotypes of autoinvasive cells in polymyositis and inclusion body myositis. Ann Neurol 1984; 16:209–215.

32. Kissel JT, Mendell JR, Rammohan KW. Microvascular deposition of complement membrane attack complex in dermatomyositis. N Engl J Med 1986; 314:329–334.

33. Emslie-Smith AM, Engel AG. Microvascular changes in early and advanced dermatomyositis: A quantitative study. Ann Neurol 1990; 27:343–356.

34. Crowson AN, Magro CM. The role of microvascular injury in the pathogenesis of cutaneous lesions of dermatomyositis. Hum Pathol 1996; 27:15–19.

46
Relapsing Polychondritis

Sudhakar T. Sridharan
Cleveland Clinic Foundation, Cleveland, Ohio

I. INTRODUCTION

Relapsing polychondritis (RP) is a rare, chronic multisystem disorder of unknown etiology characterized by recurrent episodic inflammation of cartilaginous structures that results in tissue destruction that can be life-threatening (1). All types of cartilage, including the elastic cartilage of the ears and nose, the hyaline cartilage of the tracheobronchial tree and peripheral joints, and the fibrocartilage of the axial skeleton may be involved. Inflammatory injury may also affect the eye, heart, blood vessels, and inner ear. Constitutional symptoms are common. Vasculitis may affect small, medium, or large vessels. There is a paucity of data regarding the epidemiology, incidence, prevalence, and mortality of this rare disease. No specific serological tests for RP have been identified, and the diagnosis is based on the characteristic clinical manifestations. Patients with RP have an increased frequency of HLA-DR4 (2,3), and often have coexistent autoimmune diseases (4). Relapsing polychondritis pursues a fluctuating and often progressive course with bouts of inflammation that may lead to permanent destruction of involved tissues. In a minority of patients, the disease may be self-limited. Glucocorticoids (GCs) are the mainstay of therapy during acute attacks. Cytotoxic agents such as cyclophosphamide (CYC), azathioprine (AZA), and methotrexate (MTX) have been used as additional therapy although no controlled studies have been performed with these agents. Overall, 74% of patients are alive 5 years, and 55% 10 years after disease onset (5).

II. ETIOLOGY AND PATHOGENESIS

The cause of RP is unknown. Cartilage destruction is mediated by release of degradative enzymes, including metalloproteinases and reactive oxygen metabolites from activated chondrocytes and inflammatory cells under the influence of immune-mediated cytokines such as interleukin 1 (IL-1) and tumor necrosis factor (TNF).

The earliest histological abnormality is focal or diffuse loss of basophilic staining, indicating depletion of proteoglycans from the cartilage matrix. Mononuclear cells predominate in established lesions. In the acute stage, polymorphonuclear leukocytes (PMNs) may be seen. Chondrocyte dropout, lacunar breakdown, and centripetal destruction of cartilage are followed by granulomatous changes, fibrosis, and foci of calcification.

Electron microscopic examination of ear cartilage reveals large amounts of electron dense material on the surface of elastic fibers and between collagen fibers (6). Numerous small extracellular matrix granules, thought to be proteoglycans, are also seen. Larger, dense membrane-bound vesicles of variable size are observed budding from the tips of chondrocyte villi into the extracellular space. These may represent chondrocyte-derived lysosomal granules that contribute to the loss of cartilage (7).

Several reports document an immune response against type II collagen in RP and rheumatoid arthritis (RA) (8,9). In addition, antibodies to type II collagen and immune complexes are detected in the sera of some patients (10). Small areas of regenerating cartilage may sometimes be seen. Immunofluorescence techniques have demonstrated deposition of immunoglobulins (IgG, IgA and IgM) and complement (C3) at the chondrofibrous junction extending focally into marginal cartilaginous areas (11). Titers of anticollagen antibodies have been reported to correlate with the activity of the disease (9).

Auricular chondritis occurs in rats immunized with type II collagen (12,13), and fawn-hooded rats develop chondritis spontaneously (12,14). Antibodies to type II collagen are found in the sera of these animals and, as in man, immune deposits (IgG, IgM, IGA, and C3) are detected at sites of ear inflammation. In addition, double transgenic mice for human HLA-DQ6 and HLA-DQ8 develop chondritis and arthritis, which appear similar to human disease (15). Cell-mediated processes appear to also be operative in causing tissue injury. Lymphocyte transformation and macrophage migration inhibition can be demonstrated when patients' lymphocytes (but not controls) are exposed to cartilage extracts (16). Humoral and cellular responses to types IX and XI collagen were found in one patient (17). Thus, it appears that in RP there may be a genetically influenced immune response against type II (and less often other) collagen that causes injury to cartilage or collagen-rich structures via proteolytic destruction.

III. CLINICAL MANIFESTATIONS

In 1923, Jaksch-Wartenhorst (18) reported the first case of RP in a 32-year-old brewer who developed the acute onset of an asymmetric polyarthritis with fever, and bilateral ear inflammation. After auricular inflammation subsided, loss of hearing, dizziness, tinnitus, and deformity of both ears followed, with collapse of the nasal bridge, resulting in a "saddle-nose" deformity. Biopsy of the nasal cartilage revealed loss of cartilage matrix and a hyperplastic mucous membrane. In 1960, Pearson et al. (19) coined the term, "relapsing polychondritis" when they reported two additional cases and reviewed the literature of previously described cases.

Although the disease may develop at any age, the peak period is in the fifth decade, and the mean age is 47 years (5). Cases have been reported at both extremes of life (5). In general, gender preference does not occur, although in one review the female-to-male ratio was found to be 3:1 (1). Caucasians are most commonly affected, and RP is rare in other ethnic groups.

In 40% of patients, the initial manifestation of RP is auricular chondritis (Fig. 1 and 2), affecting one or both ears. Eventually 85% of patients will develop ear involvement (Table 1). Usually both ears are involved. Patients experience the sudden onset of inflammation of the cartilaginous portion of the ear. The noncartilaginous earlobes are spared. The overlying skin is beefy red or violaceous. The episode, which lasts days to weeks, usually resolves spontaneously. Recurrent episodes are also abrupt in nature, unless the patient is receiving GC therapy, in which case episodes can be more insidious. Repeated attacks eventually lead to cartilaginous destruction and a droopy or flabby ear ("cauliflower ear"). Auricular chondritis infrequently develops in other preexisting rheumatic diseases, such as systemic lupus erythematosus (SLE) or Wegener's granulomatosis (WG) (20), causing diagnostic confusion. Similar features may also be seen in lepromatous leprosy (21). Relapsing polychondritis has·also been reported in rheumatoid arthri-

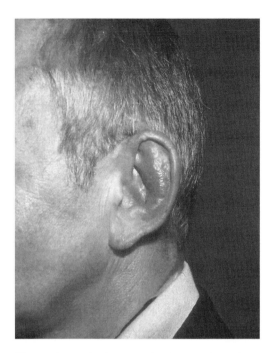

Figure 1 Auricular chondritis in relapsing polychondritis.

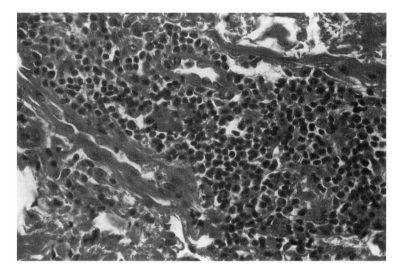

Figure 2 Light microscopy of an ear biopsy specimen from a patient with RP. Infiltrate is primarily mononuclear cells.

Table 1 Clinical Manifestations in 112 Patients with Relapsing Polychondritis

Clinical feature	Frequency (%)	
	At presentation	Cumulative
Ophthalmological disease	21 (19)	57 (51)
Eyelid/periorbital		
Lid edema		9
Tarsitis		2
Orbital inflammation	1	4
Muscle paresis		5
Dacrocystitis		1
Scleral		
Episcleritis	15	39
Scleritis	6	14
Conjunctiva		
Keratitis sicca		10
Nonspecific		6
Cornea		
Peripheral corneal thinning and pannus		4
Peripheral infiltrates		4
Nonspecific		7
Uvea		
Iritis	1	9
Retina		
Retinopathy		9
Retinal vein occlusion		2
Choroiditis		1
Optic nerve		
Optic neuritis	1	5
Ischemic optic neuropathy		2
Papilledema		4
Other visual field defects		3
Lens		
Cataracts		11
Otolaryngological disease		
Auricular chondritis	44 (39)	95 (85)
Nasal chondritis	27 (24)	60 (54)
Saddle-nose deformity	20 (18)	32 (29)
Hearing loss	10 (9)	33 (20)
Vertigo	4 (4)	15 (13)
Respiratory disease		
Laryngotracheal symptoms	29 (26)	54 (48)
Laryngotracheal stricture	17 (15)	26 (23)
Musculoskeletal disorders		
Arthritis	40 (36)	58 (52)
Chest wall tenderness	2 (2)	2 (2)
Renal disease		
Elevated creatinine	8 (7)	15 (13)
Microhematuria	17 (15)	29 (26)
Proteinuria ($\geq$2 on dipstick)	9 (8)	16 (14)

Table 1 (*Continued*)

Clinical feature	Frequency (%)	
	At presentation	Cumulative
Cardiovascular disease		
Aortic regurgitation	0	4 (4)
Mitral regurgitation	0	2 (2)
Aneurysm	3 (3)	11 (10)
Vasculitis	3 (10)	11 (10)
Dermatologic disease		
Skin involvement	8 (7)	32 (28)
Laboratory abnormalities		
Anemia	56 (50)	62 (55)
Elevated sedimentation rate	83 (74)	92 (82)

Source: Modified from Ref. 37.

tis, ankylosing spondylitis (AS), myositis, Behçet's disease, Sjögren's syndrome (SjS), and other vasculitides (Table 2). Hearing loss may occur from blockage of the eustachian tube or the external auditory meatus. Inflammation of the internal auditory artery or its cochlear branch can cause deafness, tinnitus, ataxia, vertigo, nausea, and vomiting (22,23). This may occur in up to 30% of the patients.

The cartilage of the nose becomes inflamed in one quarter of cases during the first attack. Eventually 50% of patients will have nasal involvement (24). Symptoms include nasal stuffiness, rhinorrhea, and epistaxis. Inflammation of the bridge of the nose may lead to collapse, producing a saddle-nose deformity. In some patients, this process may be insidious, without overt inflammation. Saddle nose is more common in younger patients, especially in women.

Arthritis is the presenting manifestation in a third of patients, and may antedate other disease manifestations by several months. The arthritis of RP is typically seronegative, nondeforming, oligoarticular or polyarticular, tends to spare the forefoot, involves both large and peripheral joints (25), and usually resolves spontaneously without residual joint deformity. It has a predilection to involve the central thoracic joints (sternoclavicular, costochondral, and sternomanubrial junctions), which in severe cases can lead to dislocation of the clavicles and ribs, and compromise respiratory function (4). The synovial fluid is usually noninflammatory. Radiographs typically demonstrate joint space narrowing without erosions (26). Rarely, there may be a destructive arthropathy (4,27).

Laryngotracheal involvement, which occurs in 50% of patients, results in hoarseness, nonproductive cough, dyspnea, wheezing, inspiratory stridor, and tenderness over the larynx and proximal trachea (28). Mucosal edema, strictures, and/or collapse of laryngeal or tracheal cartilage may cause life-threatening airway stenosis necessitating tracheostomy (29). Collapse of the bronchial cartilage can lead to pneumonia and death from respiratory insufficiency.

IV. VASCULITIS AND RELAPSING POLYCHONDRITIS

While RP predominantly occurs as a distinct clinical entity, in up to 30% of patients it can be associated with systemic vasculitis, RA, SLE, spondyloarthropathy, or Behçet's syndrome (5). Vasculitis syndromes are the most commonly reported of these disorders, with estimates ranging

Table 2 Systemic Vasculitis in Relapsing Polychondritis

Site	Type of vasculitis/associations
Skin	Leukocytoclastic vasculitis
	Granulomatous vasculitis
	Livedo reticularis
	Erythema nodosum
	Panniculitis
	Subcutaneous nodules
Cardiovascular	Coronary artery vasculitis
	Aortitis
	Aortic regurgitation
	Thoracic and abdominal aortic aneurysms
Renal	Segmental necrotizing crescentic glomerulonephritis
Ocular	Chorioretinitis
	Retinal vasculitis
	Retinal (or branch) vein occlusion
Neurological	Cranial neuropathies
	Encephalopathy
	Stroke
	Ataxia
	Aseptic meningitis
	Transverse myelitis
	Mononeuritis multiplex
Other	Testicular ischemia
	Superficial thrombophlebitis
Association with other systemic vasculitides	Wegener's granulomatosis
	Polyarteritis nodosa
	Takayasu's arteritis
	Giant cell arteritis
	Microscopic polyangiitis
	Churg–Strauss syndrome
	Behçet's disease (MAGIC syndrome)
	Mixed cryoglobulinemia

from 11–56% (4,5). There is a broad range of vasculitis associated with RP (see Table 2). Overlap or undifferentiated vasculitic syndromes can also occur.

A. Cutaneous

Skin lesions, seen in 17–39% of cases, include macules, papules, vesicles, and bullae (5,30,31). Five to 14% of patients have biopsy-proven leukocytoclastic vasculitis (4,5). Necrotizing and granulomatous vasculitis may also occur (32). Occasionally, patients may present with fever and migratory, tender, subcutaneous nodules that histologically resemble erythema nodosum (EN) (33). Other rare cutaneous lesions include urticaria, livedo reticularis, panniculitis, angioedema, erythema elevatum diutinum, and erythema multiforme that may coexist with vasculitis (5,34). In addition, an overlap of RP and Behçet's disease, termed MAGIC syndrome (*mouth and genital ulcers with inflamed cartilage*) may occur (35). This combination is very rare; only eight cases have been reported in the literature (36). Age of onset varied from 10–59 years. Five out of eight patients were women. Two patterns of disease are recognized: (1) Behçet's disease–type, in which oral and genital ulcers are initial signs (6 of 8 patients were in this group) and (2) polychondritis-type, in which oral ulcers and polychondritis were initial signs, with the subsequent appearance of EN or genital ulcers suggesting Behçet's disease.

B. Ocular

Ocular inflammation occurs in about 65% of patients with RP (5). Episcleritis is the most common ocular finding. Conjunctivitis, keratitis, uveitis, chorioretinitis, proptosis, exophthalmos mimicking orbital pseudotumor, and extraocular muscle paralysis can also occur (37,38). In a review of 112 patients, proptosis with chemosis suggesting a pseudotumor was the most common ocular adnexal finding (37). Four patients had proptosis (up to 6 mm), with two having bilateral proptosis simulating orbital pseudotumor. Because imaging studies were not done, proof of pseudotumor is not definitive. There was accompanying extraocular muscle paresis in two patients. Extraocular muscle palsy may occur, which is a known complication of pseudotumor in other diseases (38). Ocular involvement is often episodic. When the manifestations of RP are conjunctivitis, chorioretinitis, or iritis with arthritis, the differential diagnosis includes Reiter's syndrome, sarcoidosis, RA, spondyloarthropathies, reactive arthritis, inflammatory bowel disease, or Behçet's syndrome. Serious ocular sequelae can occur, including severe corneal ulceration and scleromalacia perforans (39). Retinal vasculitis and optic neurits may lead to blindness (37,40). Keratoconjunctivitis sicca is observed in up to 10% of cases. Rarely, a conjunctival mass, a "salmon patch" of lymphoid hyperplasia is observed (41).

C. Cardiovascular

1. Valvular Heart Disease

Cardiovascular involvement is the second leading cause of death in RP (4,5,42), and is seen in 24–52% of patients. Aortic regurgitation (AR), the most common cardiac abnormality in RP, was first described by Yamazaki et al. in 1966 (44). Aortic regurgitation occurs in approximately 10% of patients (43,44). It is usually a late sequel of RP (mean disease duration = 7 years), secondary to aortic root dilatation (78% of cases) (43) or cusp retraction (45). Severe AR complicating cusp rupture can be a rare early manifestation. Microscopically, the valvular cusp shows necrotizing leukocytic inflammation (46). The valve may show cusp thickening, fraying, loss of elastic tissue, and cystic degeneration of cells (47). Cusp rupture with a normal aortic root has been reported (46). Valve replacement is required in more than one-third of patients with AR (48). Surgical repair may be complicated by continued annular inflammation resulting in paravalvular leak, valve dehiscence, and need for further surgical intervention (49). Severe aortic root involvement can sometimes develop in asymptomatic patients despite otherwise apparent remission of RP (50). In either case, this observation underscores the importance of careful cardiac surveillance.

Mitral regurgitation (MR) is less frequent (1.8% of patients) than AR (43,51) and may be caused by annular dilatation (43,49), leaflet thickening (43), anterior leaflet prolapse (43), and, rarely, chordal rupture secondary to endocarditis (43). Histological studies reveal chronic inflammation, fibrosis, and myxomatous degeneration (43,52). In 1.5% of patients, AR and MR lesions coexist (43). Rarely, dilatation of the annulus of both the mitral and tricuspid valves may cause mitral and tricuspid regurgitation (46).

2. Arrhythmias

First- to third-degree atrioventricular conduction blocks occur in about 5% of patients (42). Complete heart block, related to either fibrosis of the conduction system or extension of inflammation and/or fibrosis from the aortic valve, may be the first cardiac manifestation of the disease or may occur later (53,54). Sinus tachycardia, atrial fibrillation, and atrial flutter have been rarely reported (49,55).

3. Pericarditis, Myocardial Infarction

Pericarditis is observed in about 4% of cases of RP. Pericardial effusions usually do not cause tamponade. Diagnosis and severity can be assessed by echocardiography (55). Myocardial infarction can rarely occur as a result of coronary vasculitis or coronary artery aneurysms causing thrombosis or embolism (4,43).

4. Aortic Involvement

Aortic aneurysms (AAs) are observed in 5–7% of patients (43,51). Aortic aneurysms occur most often in the ascending aorta (Fig. 3), but may be multiple and can involve the abdominal aorta (43,56). An aortic arch syndrome, single or multiple thoracic or abdominal aortic aneurysms with rupture, or "pulseless" disease similar to Takayasu's arteritis have been described (see Table 3).

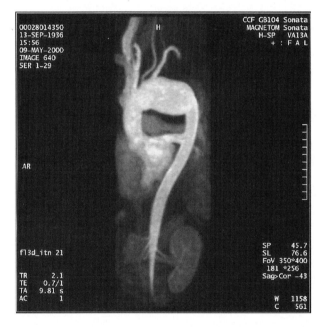

Figure 3   Aneurysm of the aortic arch is visualized using MRI. Progressive dilatation occurred over 1 year. (Courtesy of Chad Deal, Department of Rheumatic and Immunologic Diseases, Cleveland Clinic Foundation.)

Table 3   Aortic Disease in Relapsing Polychondritis

Site	Incidence (%)
Thoracic aortic aneurysm	3.1
Thoracic and abdominal aortic aneurysm	1.1
Abdominal aortic aneurysm	0.9
Aortic dissection	0.9

Source: From Ref. 51.

Aortic root involvement usually results in AR. Grossly, the intimal surface of the affected aorta has a wrinkled appearance that closely resembles syphilis (pseudosyphilis) (57). Histologically, lymphocytic infiltration around the vasa vasorum and fragmentation and loss of elastic tissue eventually leads to fibrosis and hyalinization of the intimal and medial layers of the vessel (58). These lesions are indistinguishable from those seen in Reiter's syndrome and other spondyloarthropathies. Aortic disease may be clinically silent until causing fatality from rupture (56). Large-vessel thrombotic disease has been reported in a patient with antiphospholipid (APL) antibodies (59). Of the remaining seven patients in this study, three had prolonged activated partial thromboplastin times (APTTs) that corrected in mixing studies with controlled plasma. Since this patient was experiencing a flare of RP, the presence of APL antibodies may have been a part of the polyclonal gammopathy that characterizes many inflammatory states. Thrombosis of the aorta and iliac vessels suggests an underlying prothrombotic state, to which APL antibodies may have played a contributing role.

5. Extraaortic Aneurysms and Vasculitis

In RP, asymptomatic aneurysms of the medium-sized vessels may develop and rupture suddenly. Iliac (47,58), femoral (58), subclavian, radial, coronary, and cerebral (60) vessel involvement has been reported. In addition, thrombosis of these vessels secondary to vasculitis can cause catastrophic complications (33).

Apart from aortitis, large-vessel vasculitis is a well-described complication of RP, and occurs in up to 15% of cases (33). The vasculitis may be focal or diffuse, indolent or fulminant, and rapidly fatal. Superficial and deep vein thrombophlebitis occurs in 4% of patients, is frequently relapsing and migratory, can be complicated by pulmonary embolism (47), and may be associated with antiphospholipid antibodies (59).

D. Renal

Glomerulonephritis (GN) occurs in 22% of patients with RP, and is more common than generally recognized (61). The presence of GN imparts a worse prognosis for RP. The 10-year survival rate of RP with GN is only 30%; older age and the presence of vasculitis also impart a worse prognosis (61). The most common renal histopathological finding is mild mesangial proliferation, followed by focal and segmental necrotizing glomerulonephritis with crescents (62). Immunoglobulins (IgG or IgM) and complement components, deposited as granular subendothelial or mesangial deposits, may be observed on electron microscopy (63). Diffuse proliferative glomerulonephritis may be seen if RP is associated with SLE or Sjögren's syndrome (61,64). Other abnormalities include glomerulosclerosis, IgA nephropathy, and tubulointerstitial nephritis. Rheumatoid factor (RF) and cryoglobulins are infrequently present, and C3 and C4 are usually normal. Positive tests for antinuclear antibodies (ANAs), and antineutrophil cytoplasmic antibodies (ANCA) with proteinase 3 (PR3) specificity (2 of 98 patients with biopsy-proven vasculitis) have been reported in RP with renal involvement (65). Therefore, patients with renal involvement should be evaluated for the presence of coexistent diseases, especially SLE, WG, or other systemic vasculitides (66).

E. Neurological

Vasculitis involving the central and peripheral nervous system is a rare complication of RP (4,67). McAdam et al. (4) reported that 2 of 23 patients with RP had cerebral vasculitis, although biopsy confirmation of vasculitis was not sought. Only one biopsy-proven case of central nervous system (CNS) vasculitis has been reported (68). In another case of presumed CNS vasculitis and RP, the patient presented with confusion, nystagmus, facial weakness, and bilateral dysmetria (67). The cerebrospinal fluid (CSF) examination was normal.

The constellation of reported features of CNS involvement in RP includes mononeuritis multiplex, mixed sensorimotor neuropathy, or cranial neuropathies (especially cranial nerves VI and VII, and less often cranial nerves II, III, and XII) (33). These lesions, as well as the typical cochlear or vestibular nerve complications, have been presumed to be vasculitic in etiology (67). Computerized tomography (CT) is often negative in this setting. Aseptic meningitis (69,70), headaches, confusion (71,72), encephalopathy, seizures (4,71), diffuse slowing of the electroencephalogram (72), psychiatric signs (67,72), ataxia (66,71,73), hemiplegia, transverse myelitis, and temporal artery nongranulomatous vasculitis (74) have all been reported.

The pathogenesis of CNS involvement in RP is not understood. Some of the symptoms and signs may be manifestations of small-vessel vasculitis. Since there is a broad overlap with other autoimmune diseases that may involve the CNS (e.g., Behçet's syndrome, polyarteritis nodosa [PAN], giant cell arteritis [GCA], Takayasu's arteritis, WG, and SLE), it is important to consider that some of the findings may be due to coexistent diseases.

V. DIAGNOSIS

McAdam's criteria have been utilized as a guide to diagnosis (4) (Table 4). A definite diagnosis of RP requires three or more clinical features being present. Initial presentation of RP with fewer criteria (66) or the presence of an associated disease may confound the differential diagnosis (75,76). For example, unilateral auricular chondritis may be due to a number of infections that can involve the ear, such as *Pseudomonas aeruginosa* and erysipelas. Chondrodermatitis helicis is characterized by the appearance of a painful, tender, scaling, firm nodule on the helix and can usually be distinguished from auricular chondritis. Rarely, other infiltrating lesions, such as cutaneous lymphoma, may involve the auricle. Biopsy is usually required whenever the diagnosis is uncertain (11,77).

Isolated subglottic involvement may be observed in other inflammatory syndromes, including amyloidois, sarcoidosis, WG, and infectious illnesses such as tuberculosis or atypical mycobacterial diseases (78). Although WG predominantly involves the upper and lower airways and kidneys, in rare cases, the tracheobronchial tree can be the only site of involvement (79). In

Table 4 Diagnostic Criteria for Relapsing Polychondritis

Criterion	Description
1	Recurrent chondritis of both auricles
2	Nonerosive inflammatory polyarthritis
3	Chondritis of nasal cartilage
4	Inflammation of ocular structures, including conjunctivitis, keratitis, scleritis/episcleritis, and/or uveitis
5	Chondritis of the respiratory tract involving laryngeal and/or tracheal cartilages
6	Cochlear and/or vestibular damage manifest by neurosensory hearing loss, tinnitus, and/or vertigo

Source: Modified from Ref. 4.

a series of 51 patients with tracheobronchial WG, half had tracheal abnormalities, and 10% had evidence of subglottic stenosis (80). A rare, inherited, pediatric disorder of hyaline cartilage leading to saddle-nose deformity and degeneration and calcification of subglottic cartilage has been described in an Indian family (81). Other forms of tracheal disease, such as saber-sheath trachea or tracheopathia osteoplastica, can be distinguished by characteristic CT scan appearances and lack of other disease manifestations of RP (82). Tracheopathia osteoplastica is a rare, benign disease of the trachea and major bronchi, characterized by cartilaginous or osseous nodules that project into the tracheobronchial lumen causing considerable deformity (83,84).

The usual findings of RP on CT of the trachea include wall thickening by edema secondary to inflammation and/or granulation tissue. Chronic lesions may become calcified (85). Destruction of tracheal cartilage may lead to softening and dynamic collapse of the airway, best demonstrated by cine CT showing flaccidity of the tracheal wall during inspiration. Laryngotracheal biopsy may be hazardous and lead to acute respiratory distress, especially in cases with stenotic or flaccid airways. Intubation for any reason may be difficult because the glottis may be narrowed due to edema or cartilage destruction (86). In RP patients without laryngotracheal disease, trauma during intubation may induce focal inflammation (87).

Renal status should always be evaluated to exclude the possibility of an accompanying glomerulonephritis (61), and if present, should be carefully screened for coexistent other autoimmune diseases, especially SLE (66). During acute flares of the disease, patients may have elevations of surrogate markers of inflammation.

VI. LABORATORY INVESTIGATION

Mild leukocytosis and normochromic, normocytic anemia are present in approximately 50% of patients (5). If macrocytic anemia is present, the possibility of a rare associated myelodysplastic syndrome should be considered (88). Polyclonal hypergammaglobulinemia, elevated erythrocyte sedimentation rate (ESR), and thrombcytosis reflect nonspecific changes of chronic inflammation. In one study, ESR was elevated in 74% of patients at presentation, and 82% at some point during the disease (5). Low titers of ANA or RF are occasionally seen, and occur more often in patients with other coexistent autoimmune diseases, especially SLE and RA, respectively (66,75). Among 111 patients who met criteria for RP, ANA titers greater than 1:100 were found in 10 patients (9%) (89). Among these patients, five had clinical and/or ophthalmological features suggestive of Sjögren's syndrome, including two with antibodies to both SS-A and SS-B, and two with a myelodysplastic syndrome. None of the 10 patients had antibodies to double-stranded DNA. Antibodies to both native and denatured type II collagen, predominantly of IgG subclass, are found in approximately 50% of patients (8–10). The sensitivity in one study was 33%, with specificity of almost 100%. Data from this study revealed that, during acute attacks of RP, titers of antibody to collagen type II were elevated (9). Antibody titers normalized after treatment with corticosteroids. Circulating immune complexes may be detected, especially in patients with early active disease. In addition, assays for T cell–mediated immune responses to type II collagen may be positive (16,90). Such studies are generally not available in hospital laboratories.

Few studies have included analysis of ANCA by indirect immunofluorescence (IIF) and ELISA techniques, the current standard for diagnosis. In a study of 98 patients who had unequivocal histological proof of RP, cases were stratified according to the ANCA specificity. Anti-PR3 ELISA was positive in only two patients. Previous studies of the relationships between ANCA and RP have relied mainly on IIF titers, which depend on observer interpretation and experience. Current data do not support the notion that the presence of ANCA in RP reflects vascular involvement (91–93).

VII. MANAGEMENT AND TREATMENT

In patients with characteristic presentations, such as bilateral auricular chondritis or multifocal chondritis, biopsy is usually not necessary. Because of the potential for serious airway involvement, all patients with RP regardless of the presence of upper airway symptoms should undergo evaluation for laryngotracheal involvement. Pulmonary function tests, such as flow-volume loops, radiological assessment by tomography or CT scanning, and most importantly, direct visualization of the upper airways by fiberoptic endoscopy are necessary to fully characterize the extent of airway involvement (28,95). A 12-lead electrocardiogram is recommended for all newly diagnosed patients to detect early cardiac involvement. Since cardiac involvement can be asymptomatic, some authors also recommended a baseline echocardiogram to evaluate possible aortic or mitral valve thickening or regurgitation (50). Auscultation over large vessels should be performed to detect bruits. Blood pressure should be measured in all four limbs and periodically repeated. If a significant discrepancy is detected, imaging of the great vessels either by angiography or "edema-weighted" magnetic resonance imaging (MRI) should be performed to delineate vascular anatomy and presence of inflammation. In one study of vascular MRI in Takayasu's arteritis (TA), increased signal density was noted in 94% of patients with unequivocally active disease (96). Comparable data are not available for large vessel involvement in RP.

Distinguishing RP from WG can be difficult because of similarities in clinical phenotypes and, in rare cases, the coexistence of both disorders (97). Saddle-nose deformity, laryngotracheal involvement, arthritis, episcleritis, and vasculitis occur in both disorders (Table 5). Necrotizing GN, otitis, sinusitis, nasal septal perforation, and proptosis, which are more suggestive of WG, may also occur in a minority of patients with RP (61,98). Auricular chondritis, which is considered a hallmark of RP, has been described in several cases of WG (20,99). The presence of cavitary lung lesions and histological evidence of necrotizing granulomas favors a diagnosis of WG.

Table 5   Clinical Features of Relapsing Polychondritis and Wegener's granulomatosis

Clinical feature	Relapsing polychondritis	Wegener's granulomatosis
Auricular chondritis	++++[a]	+
Otitis	++	++
Sinusitis	+	++++
Saddle-nose deformity	+++	+++
Nasal septal perforation	—	++++
Episcleritis	++	++
Pseudotumor	+	++
Laryngotracheal involvement	++++	++
Subglottic stenosis	+++	++
Pulmonary nodules	—	+++
Leukocytoclastic vasculitis	++	++
Glomerulonephritis	++	++++
Mononeuritis multiplex	++	++
Aortitis	+++	—
Aortic aneurysms	++	—
Arthritis	++	++
Myelodysplastic syndrome	++	—
ANCA positivity	++	++++
Necrotizing granuloma	—	++++

[a]Symbols: + rare, ++ occasionally seen, +++ commonly seen, ++++ typically seen.

Tracheobronchial flaccidity and ascending aortic aneurysms favor the diagnosis of RP. In the absence of early discriminating data, a precise diagnosis may not be possible. Because GC therapy alone generally does not lead to remission in WG, critical consideration should be given to the addition of a cytotoxic agent in patients with a WG/RP overlap.

Because RP is a rare disease, treatment recommendations have been derived based on empirical observations. Glucocorticoids are the mainstay of therapy. They have a consistently palliative effect on acute chondritis. Recommended initial doses of prednisone range from 0.5 to 1.0 mg/day. Nonsteroidal antiinflammatory drugs (NSAIDs) can be used to manage mild auricular, nasal, and costochondral chondritis, or synovitis. Anecdotal reports of the use of dapsone (100 mg twice daily), or colchicine (0.6 mg twice daily) have been published as alternatives to GCs in managing auricular or nasal chondritis (100–102). Colchicine (0.6 mg twice daily) has been used with success to abort acute attacks of chondritis (102), and in two patients, therapeutic efficacy was claimed within 96 h, with complete resolution of the auricular inflammation within a week. Because controlled trials have not been performed with colchicine, the efficacy of the agent remains uncertain. Patients with necrotizing scleritis, tracheal involvement, or systemic vasculitis have often experienced progressive disease in spite of GC therapy. In this setting, the most appropriate strategy for a second-line agent remains speculative, but CYC, AZA, and cyclosporin A (CsA) have all been employed (39,103,104). In one report, CsA was reported to induce and maintain remission for 2 years in a patient with progressive tracheal involvement refractory to GCs, dapsone, CYC, and AZA (103). In another series of 11 patients with scleritis and RP, two patients with milder disease were successfully treated with dapsone (39). However, seven patients (63%) required the addition of a cytotoxic agent (CYC, AZA) to systemic GC therapy for optimal control of progressive eye involvement. The authors concluded that ocular manifestations of RP, especially nodular and necrotizing scleritis, are less amenable to either systemic GCs or dapsone therapy and require the addition of a cytotoxic agent. Limited success has been reported with the use of anti-CD4 monoclonal antibodies (Mab) (105,106). In another report, daily infusions of anti-CD4 Mab resulted in regression of symptoms, and allowed reduction of GC doses in a patient with RP that was previously refractory to second-line agents (106).

Acute flares of laryngotracheal disease may be managed with pulse methylprednisolone, and racemic epinephrine, a potent vasoconstrictor, has been reported to be useful to decrease airway inflammation and subglottic edema (107,108). Although reports of its use are also anecdotal, racemic epinephrine may be extremely useful for acute life-threatening airway obstruction because it has a rapid onset of action. Subglottic involvement may require a tracheostomy for relief of upper airway obstruction. Laryngeal stents have not been shown to prolong survival outside the hospital or increase independence from mechanical ventilation (86). However, in a recent study (109), five patients with severe airway disease were managed by the placement of self-expandable metallic stents (SEMSs) and followed prospectively for 20 months. Three patients had previously required ventilator therapy because multiple weaning attempts were unsuccessful prior to stent placement. Seventeen stents were placed, and immediate improvement of symptoms, wheezing, and ventilation was noted in all patients (Fig. 4). Three patients were alive 16 to 18 months after the first stent placement. One patient died after 3 weeks, presumably due to collapse of airways distal to the stents. The other patient survived for 20 months before she died. Advantages of SEMSs include ease of placement, visibility on routine chest radiographs, dynamic expandability, maintenance of ventilation through the stent, conformity of tortuous airways, and ability to intubate through the stent. Complications include migration, granulation tissue formation, retention of secretions, bleeding, ulceration, and, rarely, erosion of the tracheobronchial wall (110,111).

No controlled trials of therapy have been undertaken of cardiovascular complications in RP. Patients with acute conduction abnormalities, presumably due to inflammation affecting the conducting system, may benefit from systemic GC therapy (112). Atrioventricular (AV) blocks may

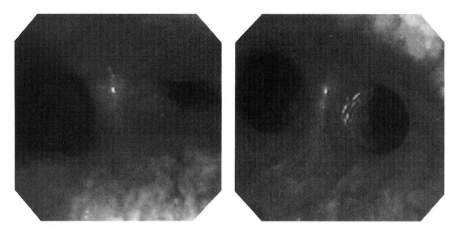

Figure 4 Bronchoscopic view before (right) and after (left) stent placement in a patient with RP. Note near-total collapse of the right mainstem bronchus, and its complete patency following stent placement. The left mainstem bronchus is patent. (Courtesy of Ahtul Mehta, Department of Pulmonary Medicine and Critical Care, Cleveland Clinic Foundation.)

require a permanent pacemaker. Disease progression may occur whether treatment consists of GCs alone or GCs combined with cytotoxic agents (51).

Patients with severe aortic valve involvement should be considered for valve replacement in conjunction with reconstruction or replacement of the aortic root (47). Follow-up of 20 RP patients who underwent valve surgery showed a 1-year mortality of 20% and 2-year rate of 48% (43). The authors contend that early valve replacement is critical to prevent aortic ectasia. If the ascending aorta is contiguously involved, complete replacement using a composite graft with reimplantation of the coronary arteries should be considered, since isolated valve replacement may increase the risk of aortic root aneurysm and secondary prosthesis dehiscence (43). Although there are no controlled studies of the utility of MRI in RP aortitis, we recommend this technique for detection and evaluation of aortic disease (see Fig. 3). Complications following cardiac surgery include the usual limitations of surgical intervention and possible effects of inflammation in producing paravalvular prosthetic leaks and new aneurysms (52).

When RP is associated with vasculitis, the treatment should be tailored to whether critical organs are involved, rate of progression, and prognosis for the specific category of vasculitis. Patients are empirically treated with a combination of a second-line agent and GCs if vasculitis affects major organs such as heart, lungs, gut, kidney, and CNS. Pulse intravenous CYC or oral CYC plus GCs have been successfully employed to treat RP with nephritis (113,114). In reports of individual patients so treated, improvement in creatinine clearance, serum creatinine, and 24-h protein excretion occurred. Similar results were obtained when plasmapheresis was combined to the above regimen in one patient (115). In another report of two patients, one patient had improvement in glomerular filtration rate (GFR) and proteinuria, and another died of uremia when treated with AZA and GCs (116). One cannot make firm recommendations based on these data, but in patients with progressive renal impairment secondary to crescentic GN in RP, we favor the use of a second agent, such as CYC.

VIII. COURSE AND PROGNOSIS

The 5- and 10-year survival from a Mayo Clinic series of 112 patients with RP was 74% and 55%, respectively (5). The median duration of follow-up was 6 years (range, 1 month to 20 years). During the period of observation, 86% of patients had intermittent inflammatory manifestations, the median being five episodes (range, 1–13). Follow-up was available in 90% of patients. The most frequent causes of death, in decreasing order of frequency, were infection, systemic vasculitis, and malignancy. Only 10% of deaths were attributed to acute airway collapse. When multivariate analysis was applied to the group as a whole, age at diagnosis (p <0.0001), anemia (p <0.0016), and laryngotracheal stricture (p <0.0051) best predicted mortality. Other variables imparting high risk included renal involvement (p = 0.04), saddle-nose deformity (p = 0.01), arthritis (p = 0.04), and increased sedimentation rate (p = 0.02). Patients who had RP with systemic vasculitis had a 5-year survival rate of only 45%, and died of causes related to vasculitis.

IX. CONCLUSIONS

Relapsing polychondritis is an uncommon, multisystem disease. The cardinal features include repeated episodes of inflammation involving the ears, nose, or laryngotracheal cartilage. Musculoskeletal, ocular, renal, cardiac, CNS, and vascular involvement can occur at any time during the illness. Vasculitis occurs in about 30% of patients. Relapsing polychondritis can present with organ or life-threatening complications that involve the heart, kidney, CNS, and eyes. It may be associated with various autoimmune disorders, such as SLE, Sjögren's syndrome, RA, myositis, and Behçet's disaease. The diagnosis is based on clinical and, when feasible, histopathological features. There are no specific serological tests for RP. Treatment has been empirically derived. The mainstays of therapy are GCs and NSAIDs. Cytotoxic agents are reserved for more severe features of disease. Newer therapies with monoclonal antibodies to CD4 cells have been explored in a limited number of patients. A role of such interventions has not been defined.

REFERENCES

1. Trentham DE, Le CH. Relapsing polychondritis. Ann Intern Med 1998; 129:114–122.
2. Lang B, Rothenfuser A, Lanchbury JS, et al. Susceptibility to relapsing polychondritis is associated with HLA-DR4. Arthritis Rheum 1993; 36:660–664.
3. Luthra HS, McKenna CH, Terasaki PI. Lack of association of HLA-A and B locus antigens with relapsing polychondritis. Tissue Antigens 1981; 17:442–443.
4. McAdam LP, O'Hanlan MA, Bluestone R, Pearson CM. Relapsing polychondritis: Prospective study of 23 patients and a review of the literature. Medicine 1976; 55:193–215.
5. Michet CJ, McKenna CH, Luthra HS, O'Fallon WM. Relapsing polychondritis: Survival and predictive role of early disease manifestations. Ann Intern Med 1986; 104:74–78.
6. Shaul SR, Schumacher HR. Relapsing polychondritis: Electron microscopic study of ear cartilage. Arthritis Rheum 1975; 18:617–625.
7. Hashimoto K, Arkin CR, Kang AH. Relapsing polychondritis: An ultrastructural study. Arthritis Rheum 1977; 20:91–99.
8. Ebringer R, Rook G, Swana GT, Bottazzo GF, Doniach D. Autoantibodies to cartilage and type II collagen in relapsing polychondritis and other rheumatic diseases. Ann Rheum Dis 1981; 40:473–479.
9. Foidart J, Abe S, Martin GR, et al. Autoantibodies to type II collagen in relapsing polychondritis. N Engl J Med 1978; 299:1203–1207.
10. Yang CL, Brinckmann J, Rui HF, et al. Autoantibodies to cartilage collagens in relapsing polychondritis. Arch Dermatol Res 1993; 285:245–249.
11. Valenzuela R, Cooperrider PA, Gogate P, Deodhar SD, Bergfeld WF. Relapsing polychondritis: Immunomicroscopic findings in cartilage of ear biopsy specimens. Hum Pathol 1980; 11:19–22.
12. Cremer MA, Pitcock JA, Stuart JM, et al. Auricular chondritis in rats: An experimental model of relapsing polychondritis induced with type II collagen. J Exp Med 1981; 154:535–540.

13. McCune WJ, Schiller AL, Dynesius-Trentham RA, et al. Type II collagen-induced auricular chondritis. Arthritis Rheum 1982; 25:266–273.
14. Prieur DJ, Young DM, Counts DF. Auricular chondritis in fawn-hooded rats: A spontaneous disorder resembling that induced by immunization with type II collagen. Am J Pathol 1984; 116:69–76.
15. Bradley DS, Das P, Griffiths MM, Luthra HS, David CS. Double transgenic HLA DQ6/8 mice provide a new model of polychondritis following type II collagen immunization. Arthritis Rheum 1996; 39:S229.
16. Rajapakse DA, Bywaters EGL. Cell-mediated immunity to cartilage proteoglycan in relapsing polychondritis. Clin Exp Immunol 1974; 16:497–502.
17. Alsalameh S, Mollenhauer J, Scheuplein F, et al. Preferential cellular and humoral immune reactivities to native and denatured collagen types IX and XI in a patient with fatal relapsing polychondritis. J Rheumatol 1993; 20:1419–1424.
18. Jaksch-Wartenhorst R. Polychondropathia. Wien Arch J Intern Med 1923; 6:93–100.
19. Pearson CM, Kline HM, Newcomer VD. Relapsing polychondritis. N Engl J Med 1960; 263:51–58.
20. Diaz-Jouanen E, Alarcon-Ségovia D. Chondritis of the ear in Wegener's granulomatosis. Arthritis Rheum 1977; 20:1286–1288.
21. Piepkorn M, Brown C, Zone J. Auricular chondritis as a rheumatologic mainifestation of Lucio's phenomenon: Clinical improvement after plasmapheresis. Ann Intern Med 1983; 98:49–51.
22. Cody DTR, Sones DA. Relapsing polychondritis: Audiovestibular manifestations. Laryngoscope 1971; 81:1208–1222.
23. Moloney JR. Relapsing polychondritis: Its otolaryngological manifestations. J Laryngol Otolaryngol 1978; 92:9–15.
24. McCaffrey TV, McDonald TJ, McCaffrey LA. Head and neck manifestations of relapsing polychondritis: Review of 29 cases. Otolaryngology 1978; 86:473–478.
25. O'Hanlan M, McAdam LP, Bleustone R, et al. The arthropathy of relapsing polychondritis. Arthritis Rheum 1976; 19:191–194.
26. Booth A, Dieppe PA, Goddard PL, et al. The radiological manifestations of relapsing polychondritis. Clin Radiol 1989; 40:147–149.
27. Johnson TH, Mital N, Rodnan GP, Wilson RJ. Relapsing poychondritis. Radiology 1973; 106:313.
28. Eng J, Sabanathan S. Airway complications in relapsing polychondritis. Ann Thorac Surg 91; 51:686–692.
29. Gilliland BC. Relapsing polychondritis and other arthritides. In: Harrison's Principles of Internal Medicine. Vol. 2. 14th ed. New York: McGraw Hall, 1999:1951–1963.
30. West PD. Relapsing polychondritis: An unusual presentation. J Laryngol Otol 1988; 102:254–255.
31. Estes SA. Relapsing polychondritis: A case report and literature review. Cutis 1983; 32:471–476.
32. Mestres CA, Igual A, Botey A, Revert L, Murtra M. Relapsing polychondritis with glomerulonephritis and severe aortic insufficiency surgically treated with success. Thorac Cardiovasc Surg 1983; 31:307–309.
33. Michet CJ. Vasculitis and relapsing polychondritis. Rheum Clin N Amer 1990; 16:441–444.
34. Bernard P, Bedane C, Delrous JL, Catanzano G, Bonnetblanc JM. Erythema elevatum diutinum in a patient with relapsing polychondritis. J Am Acad Dermatol 1992; 26:312–315.
35. Firestein GS, Gruber HE, Weisman MH, Zvaifler NJ, Barber J, O'Duffy JD. Mouth and genital ulcers with inflamed cartilage: MAGIC syndrome. Am J Med 1985; 79:65–72.
36. Imai H, Motegi M, Mizuki N, Ohtani H, Komatsuda A, Hamai K, et al. Mouth and genital ulcers with inflamed cartilage (MAGIC syndrome): A case report and literature review. Am J Med Sci 1997; 314:330–332.
37. Isaak BL, Liesegang TJ, Michet CR Jr. Ocular and systemic findings in relapsing polychondritis. Ophthalmology 1986; 93:681–689.
38. Rucker CW, Ferguson RH. Ocular manifestations of relapsing polychondritis. Arch Ophthalmol 1965; 73:46.
39. Hoang-Xuan T, Foster CS, Rice BA. Scleritis in relapsing polychondritis. Response to therapy. Ophthalmology 1990; 97:892–898.
40. Killiam PJ, Susac J, Lawless OJ. Optic neuropathy in relapsing polychondritis. JAMA 1978; 239:49.

41. Tucker SM, Linberg JV, Doshi HM. Relapsing polychondritis, another cause for a "salmon patch." Ann Ophthalmol 1993; 25:389–391.
42. Godeau P, Bletry O, Guillevin L, Herson S, Piette JC. Le Cöer des collagénoses. Ann Med Interne 1985; 136:496–512.
43. Lang-Lazdunski L, Hvass U, Paillole C, Pansard Y, Langlois J. Cardiac valve replacement in relapsing polychondritis: A review. J Heart Valve Dis 1995; 4:227–235.
44. Yamazaki N, Yawatta K, Hannya H, Kimura E. A case of relapsing polychondritis with aortic insufficiency. Jpn Heart J 1966; 7:188–195.
45. Herman JH. Polychondritis. In Kelley WN, Harris ED Jr, Ruddy S, Sledge CB, eds. Textbook of Rheumatology. Philadelphia: Saunders, 1989:1458–1467.
46. Marshall DAS, Jackson R, Rae AP, Capell HA. Early aortic valve cusp rupture in relapsing polychondritis. Ann Rheum Dis 1992; 51:413–415.
47. Esdaile J, Hawkins D, Gold P, Freedman SD, Duguid WP. Vascular involvement in relapsing polychondritis. Can Med Assoc J 1977; 116:1019–1022.
48. Manna R, Annese V, Ghirlanda G, Pennestri F, Greco AV, Pala MA, et al. Relapsing polychondritis with severe aortic insufficiency. Clin Rheumatol 1985; 4:474–480.
49. Pappas G, Johnson M. Mitral and aortic valvular insufficiency in chronic relapsing polychondritis. Arch Surg 1972; 104:712–714.
50. Buckley LM, Ades PA. Progressive aortic valve inflammation despite apparent remission of relapsing polychondritis. Arthritis Rheum 1992; 35:812–814.
51. Rosso Ad, Petix NR, Pratesi M, Bini A. Cardiovascular involvement in relapsing polychondritis. Semin Arthritis Rheum 1997; 26:840–844.
52. Vandecker W, Panidis IP. Relapsing polychondritis and cardiac valvular involvement. Ann Intern Med 1988; 109:340–431.
53. Bowness P, Hawley IC, Morris T, Dearden A, Walport MJ. Complete heart block and severe aortic incompetence in relapsing polychondritis: Clinicopathologic findings. Arthritis Rheum 1991; 34:97–100.
54. Hughes RAC, Berry CL, Seifert M, Lessoff MH. Relapsing polychondritis: Three cases with a clinico-pathological study and literature review. Q J Med 1972; 41:363–380.
55. Dapogny C, Grollier G, Bertrand JH, et al. Les manifestations cardiaques de la polychondrite atrophiante: A propos d' un cas se manifestant par un épanchement péricardique et un flutter auriculaire. Ann Cardiol Angéiol 1985; 43:621–624.
56. Cipriano PR, Alonso DR, Baltaxe HA, Gay W, Smith J. Multiple aortic aneurysm in relapsing polychondritis. Am J Cardiol 1976; 37:1097–1102.
57. Lande A, Berkmen YM. Aoritis. Pathologic, clinical and arteriographic review. Rad Clin N Am 1976; 2:219–240.
58. Joyeux A, Vavdin F, Caudine M, Thevenet A. L'atteinte artérielle ilio-fémorale dans polychondrite atrophiante. J Mal Vasc 1984; 9:207–210.
59. Balsa-Criado A, Gonzales-Hernandez T, Cuesta MV, et al. Lupus anticoagulant in relapsing polychondritis. J Rheumatol 1990; 17:1426–1627.
60. Strobel ES, Lang B, Schumacher M, Peter HH. Cerebral aneurysm in relapsing polychondritis. J Rheumatol 1992; 19:1482–1483.
61. Chang-Miller A, Okamura M, Torres VE, et al. Renal involvement in relapsing polychondritis. Medicine 1987; 66:202–217.
62. Botey A, Navasa M, del Olmo A, Montoliu J, Ferrer O, Cardesa A, et al. Relapsing polychondritis with segmental necrotizing glomerulonephritis. Am J Nephrol 1984; 4:375–378.
63. Espinoza LR, Richman A, Bocanegra T, Pina I, Vasey FB, Rifkin SI, et al. Immune complex-mediated renal involvement in relapsing polychondritis. Am J Med 1981; 71:181–183.
64. Rodrigues MA, Tapanes FJ, Stekman IL, et al. Auricular chondritis and diffuse proliferative glomerulonephritis in primary Sjögren's syndrome. Ann Rheum Dis 1989; 48:683–685.
65. Geffriaud-Ricourard C, Noel LH, Chauveau D, et al. Clinical spectrum associated with ANCA of defined antigen specificities in 98 selected patients. Clin Nephrol 1993; 39:125–136.
66. Harisdangkul V, Johnson WW. Association between relapsing polychondritis and systemic lupus erythematosus. South Med J 1994; 87:753–757.

67. Sundaram MBM, Rajput AH. Nervous system complications of relapsing polychondritis. Neurology 1983; 33:513–515.

68. Stewart SS, Ashizawa T, Dudley AW, et al. Cerebral vasculitis in relapsing polychondritis. Neurology 1988; 38:150–152.

69. Brod S, Booss J. Idiopathic pleocytosis in relapsing polychondritis. Neurology 1988; 38:322–323.

70. Berg AM, Kasznica J, Hopkins P, Simms RW. Relapsing polychondritis and aseptic meningitis. J Rheumatol 1996; 23(3):567–569.

71. Hull RG, Morgan SH. The nervous system and relapsing polychondritis. Neurology 1984; 34:557.

72. Willis J, Atack EA, Kraag G. Relapsing polychondritis with focal neurologic abnormalities. Can J Neurol Sci 1984; 11:401.

73. Butcher RB, Tahb HG, Dunlap CE. Relapsing polychondritis. South Med J 1974; 67:1443–1449.

74. Luthra HS. Relapsing polychondrtis. In: Klippel and Dieppe, eds. Textbook of Rheumatology. 2d ed. 1998.

75. Franssen MJ, Boerbooms AM, van de Putte LB. Relapsing polychondritis and rheumatoid arthritis: Case report and review of the literature. Clin Rheumatol 1987; 6:453–457.

76. Small P, Black M, Davidman M, de Champlain ML, Kapusta MA, Kreisman H. Wegener's granulomatosis and relapsing polychondritis: A case report. J Rheumatol 1980; 7:915–918.

77. Kindblom LG, Dalen P, Edmar G, et al. Relapsing polychondritis: A clinical, pathologic-anatomic and histochemical study of 2 cases. Acta Pathol Microbiol Scand 1977; 85:656–664.

78. McDonald TJ, Devine KD, Weiland LH. Nontraumatic, non-neoplastic subglottic stenosis. Ann Otol 1975; 84:757–763.

79. Morris CJ, Byrd RP, Roy TM. Wegener's granulomatosis presenting as subglottic stenosis. J Ky Med Assoc 1990; 88:547–550.

80. Daum TE, Specks U, Colby TV, et al. Tracheobronchial involvement in Wegener's granulomatosis. Am J Respir Crit Care Med 1995; 151:522–526.

81. Kurien M, Seshadiri MS, Raman R, Bhanu TS. Inherited nasal and laryngeal degenerative chondopathy. Arch Otolaryngol Head Neck Surg 1989; 115:746–748.

82. Mueller NL, Miller RA, Ostrow DN, Pare PD. Clinico-radiologic conference: Diffuse thickening of the tracheal wall. J Can Assoc Radiol 1989; 40:213–215.

83. Young RH, Sandstorm RE, Mark GJ. Tracheopathia osteoplastica: Clinical, radiologic, and pathologic correlations. J Thorac Cardivasc Surg 1980; 79:537–541.

84. Nienhuis DM, Prakash UBS, Edell ES. Tracheobronchopathia osteochondroplastica. Ann Otol Rhinol Laryngol 1990; 99:689–694.

85. Mendelson DS, Som PM, Crane R, et al. Relapsing polychondritis studies by computerized tomography. Radiology 1988; 157:489–490.

86. Dunne JA, Sabanathan S. Use of metallic stents in relapsing polychondritis. Chest 1994; 105:864–867.

87. Clark J, Wakeel RA, Ormerod AD. Relapsing polychondritis: Two cases with tracheal stenosis and inner ear involvement. J Laryngol Otol 1992; 106:841–844.

88. Diebold J, Rauh G, Jager K, Lohrs U. Bone marrow pathology in relapsing polychondritis: High frequency of myelodysplastic syndromes. Br J Hematol 1995; 89:820–830.

89. Jean-Charles P, El-Rassi R, Zahir A. Antinuclear antibodies in relapsing polychondritis. Ann Rheum Dis 1999; 58:656–657.

90. Herman JH, Dennis MV. Immunopathologic studies in relapsing polychondritis. J Clin Invest 1973; 52:549–558.

91. Papo T, Piette JC, Le Thi Huong Du, et al. Antineutrophil cytoplasmic antibodies in polychondritis. Ann Rheum Dis 1993; 52:384–385.

92. Specks U, Wheatley C, McDonald TJ, Rohrbach MS, De Remee RA. Anticytoplasmic antibodies in the diagnosis and follow-up of Wegener's granulomatosis. Mayo Clin Proc 1989; 64:28–36.

93. Handrock K, Gross WL. Relapsing polychondritis as a secondary phenomenon of primary systemic vasculitis. Ann Rheum Dis 1993; 52:893–895.

94. Crockford MP, Kerr IH. Relapsing polychondritis. Clin Radiol 1988; 39:386–390.

95. Krell WS, Staats BA, Hyatt RE. Pulmonary function in relapsing polychondritis. Am Rev Respir Dis 1986; 133:1120–1123.

96. Flamm SD, White RD, Hoffman GS. The clinical application of "edema-weighted" magnetic resonance imaging in the assessment of Takayasu's arteritis. Int J Cardiol 1998; 66:1(suppl) S151–159.

97. Cauhape PH, Aumaitre O, Papo TH, et al. A diagnostic dilemma: Wegener's garnulomatosis, relapsing polychondritis, or both? Eur J Med 1993; 2:497–498.

98. Vinceneux PH, Pouchot J, Piette JC, Polychondrite atrophiante. In: Kahn MF, Peltier AP, Meyer O, Piette JC, eds. Les Maladies Systémiques. Paris: Flammarion Médecine-Sciences, 1991:735–750.

99. Small P, Black M, Davidman M, Brisson de Champlain ML, Kapusta MA, Kreisman H. Wegener's granulomatosis and relapsing polychondritis: A case report. J Rheumatol 1980; 7:915–918.

100. Barranco VP, Minor DB, Solomon H. Treatment of relapsing polychondritis with dapsone. Arch Dermatol 1976; 112:1286–1288.

101. Martin J, Roenigk HH Jr, Lynch W, Tingwald FR. Relapsing polychondritis with dapsone. Arch Dermatol 1976; 112:1272–1274.

102. Askari AD. Colchine for treatment of relapsing polychondritis. J Am Acad Dermatol 1984; 10:507–510.

103. Svenson KLG, Holmdahl R, Klareskog L, et al. Cyclosporin A treatment in a case of relapsing polychondritis. Scand J Rheumatol 1984; 13:329–333.

104. Anstey A, Mayou S, Morgan K, et al. Relapsing polychondritis: Autoimmunity to type II collagen and treatment with cyclosporin A. Br J Dermatol 1991; 125:588–591.

105. Choy EH, Chikanza IC, Kingsley GH, Panayi GS. Chimeric anti-CD4 monoclonal antibody for relapsing polychondritis. Lancet 1991; 338:450.

106. van der Lubbe PA, Miltenburg AM, Breedveld FO. Anti-CD4 monoclonal antibody for relapsing polychondritis. Lancet 1991; 337:1349.

107. Lipnick RN, Fink CW. Acute airway obstruction in relapsing polychondritis: Treatment with pulse methylprednisolone. J Rheumatol 1991; 18:98–99.

108. Gaffney RJ, Harrison M, Path FRC, Blayney AW. Nebulized racemic ephedrine in the treatment of acute exacerbations of laryngeal relapsing polychondritis. J Laryngol Otol 1992; 106:63–64.

109. Bipin S, Dasgupta A, Mehta C. Management of airway manifestations of relapsing polychondritis: Case reports and review of literature. Chest 1999; 116:1669–1675.

110. Dasgupta A, Dolmatch BL, Abi-Saleh WJ, et al. Self-expandable metallic airway stent insertion employing flexible bronchoscopy: Preliminary results. Chest 1998; 114:106–109.

111. Nesbitt JC, Carrasco H. Expandable stents. Chest Surg Clin N Am 1996; 6:305–328.

112. Routy JP, Pelini RY, Blanc AP, Quittet P, Medvedowsky JL. Les blocs auriculo-ventriculaires dans la polychondrite atrophiante: Cas de blocs complete explorés par voie endocavitare. Presse Méd 1988; 17:36.

113. Stewart AK, Mazanec DJ. Pulse intravenous cyclophosphamide for kidney disease in relapsing polychondritis. J Rheumatol 1992; 19:498–499.

114. Ruhlen JL, Huston KA, Wood WG. Relapsing polychondritis with glomerulonephritis: Improvement with prednisone and cyclophosphamide. JAMA 1981; 245:847–848.

115. Botey A, Navasa M, del Olmo A, et al. Relapsing polychondritis with segmental glomerulonephritis. Am J Nephrol 1984; 4:375–378.

116. Neild CH, Cameron JS, Lessot MIT, Ogg CS, Turner DR. Relapsing polychondritis with crescentic glomerulonephritis. BMJ 1978; 1:743–745.

47
Systemic Vasculitis in Sarcoidosis

Karen E. Rendt and Gary S. Hoffman
Cleveland Clinic Foundation, Cleveland, Ohio

I. INTRODUCTION

Sarcoidosis is a multisystem inflammatory disease of unknown etiology characterized by the formation of noncaseating granulomas in the lungs, lymph nodes, skin, eyes, and other organs (1,2). Since the etiology is not known, sarcoid is described in terms of clinical and histological findings, which are not in actuality specific for the disease. For instance, the characteristic pathological finding is nonnecrotizing granuloma formation, but this may also be seen in berylliosis, primary biliary cirrhosis, Crohn's disease, and infections caused by mycobacteria (tuberculosis [TB], leprosy), fungi, or *Treponema pallidum*. Other clues to the diagnosis include certain systemic features, such as constitutional symptoms, hilar adenopathy, erythema nodosum, uveitis, and splenomegaly. While suggestive of the disease, none of these is pathognomonic. Thus, depending on the presenting manifestations, diagnostic considerations may include infections (fungal, mycobacterial, etc.), other illnesses of unknown etiology (rheumatoid lung, Wegener's granulomatosis, Churg–Strauss granulomatosis), and metastatic cancer.

While the initiating stimulus for the development of sarcoid remains unknown, some details of the immunological response are well established. In involved tissue, increased numbers of CD4+ T helper cells and monocytes/macrophages interact to produce cytokines (tumor necrosis factor [TNF], interferon-γ [IFN-γ], interleukin [IL]-1, IL-6) that stimulate giant cell and granuloma formation. CD8+ T suppressor cells are present in reduced numbers in the affected tissue, yet in the bloodstream the opposite is seen, resulting in suppressed delayed hypersensitivity responses (3). This compartmentalization of immune reactivity, most striking in pulmonary tissues and regional lymph nodes, suggests a host response to an inhaled antigen. Attempts to identify an infectious trigger have thus far been unsuccessful. Earlier theories that mycobacterial infection was responsible are refuted by the stable incidence of new sarcoid cases as the incidence of mycobacterial disease declines, and by the lack of response of sarcoid to antituberculous therapy. To date, sophisticated molecular biological and culture techniques have failed to identify a consistent organism from biopsy specimens (4,5). However, the possibility that an infectious trigger initiates what becomes an autonomous immunologically mediated chronic illness cannot be ruled out at this time.

Sarcoid granulomas may occasionally undergo necrosis, a condition termed necrotizing sarcoid (6,7), and this finding may be associated with small-vessel vasculitis. Vasculitis may also affect medium and large arteries. In this chapter we discuss the clinical spectrum of vasculitis in sarcoidosis, as well as the diagnosis and treatment of this unusual complication.

II. VASCULITIS IN SARCOIDOSIS

Vascular compromise in sarcoidosis may occur by two mechanisms: extrinsic compression of vessels from lymph node enlargement, or by direct extension into a vessel wall from an adjacent focus of inflammation (8–10). While pulmonary vascular involvement is well described (11), extrapulmonary vasculitis due to sarcoid is rare, with fewer than 100 cases reported in the English language. Systemic vasculitis is indeed a heterogeneous complication of sarcoidosis. Small, medium, or large arteries can be involved. Adults and children are equally affected. Vascular disease may occur months to years after an established diagnosis of sarcoid, or vasculitis can herald the onset of the disease. The manifestations range from cutaneous inflammation (leukocytoclastic vasculitis, nodules, papules) (12–20) to life-threatening or major organ system disease (aortitis, stenosis of large arteries, neurovascular disease, glomerulonephritis) (18,21–36). The rarity of sarcoid vasculitis has precluded conducting controlled trials of therapeutic agents. Consequently, recommendations for treatment have been empirically derived. Corticosteroids have been utilized in moderate to high doses when clinically significant vascular disease has been present. In many cases, the dose needed to control disease activity may be unacceptably high, leading to the addition of cytotoxic drugs.

A. Small-Vessel Vasculitis

Cutaneous lesions are the most common manifestation of small-vessel vasculitis in sarcoid. A wide variety of skin lesions occur, including erythema nodosum, scar infiltration, palpable purpura, tender papules and nodules, bullous lesions, leg ulceration, and annular or polycyclic erythematous rashes (Fig. 1). The number of reported cases of cutaneous vasculitis associated with sarcoid is difficult to determine accurately, but is probably around 32 (30 adults, 2 children), with an additional nine possible cases (all children) reported in which typical skin lesions appeared (but were not biopsied) in patients with sarcoid who had histologically or angiographically proven vasculitis in noncutaneous locations. Takemura et al. (19) described the pathological findings of skin biopsies taken from 32 patients with sarcoid and skin abnormalities. Some patients had multiple biopsies. Forty-two biopsies were abnormal. Patients most often had chronic skin lesions, described as being nodular, plaque-like, or subcutaneous. Only one patient had scar infiltration and three had erythema nodosum. The authors point out, however, that erythema nodosum is an uncommon manifestation of sarcoid in the Japanese population. In 39 of 42 speci-

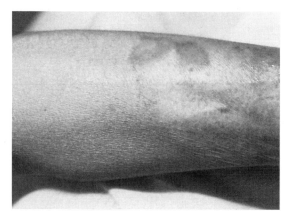

Figure 1   Chronic plaque-like rashes from sarcoid vasculitis.

mens, biopsies revealed granulomas, usually in close proximity to venules. Granulomas were localized to the dermis in 60% of specimens, to the subcutis in 30%, and occupied both regions in 10%. Dermal vessels were obliterated by granulomas in some cases, and 12 specimens (30%) demonstrated granulomatous angiitis. Venous involvement by granulomas was seen in 11 specimens, with one specimen exhibiting both arterial and venous disease. Thus, 22 specimens demonstrated sarcoid-related vascular injury of an arterial or venous type. The report does not indicate the number of unique patients with sarcoid vasculitis (19).

Others have reported the presence of leukocytoclastic vasculitis (LCV) in lesions described as annular or polycyclic erythematous rashes (20) and palpable purpura (16). Leukocytoclastic vasculitis has also been demonstrated in a patient with nodules, purpura, and bullous lesions (17). Cecchi and Giomi (20) found only two other patients in the literature with a similar presentation of annular lesions associated with LCV: both resolved spontaneously and Cecchi's patient improved when glucocorticoids were provided for other manifestations related to sarcoid. As illustrated by these reports, cutaneous vasculitis may be an early or later manifestation of sarcoid, may resolve spontaneously without treatment, or may improve following treatment with nonsteroidal agents or glucocorticoid therapy.

Small-vessel vasculitis may also occur in the lungs. Here, vasculitis has been associated with necrotizing sarcoid granulomatosis (NSG), an unusual variant of sarcoid characterized histologically by necrotizing granulomas with vasculitis of small and larger muscular pulmonary arteries and veins (Fig. 2) (21,37). The vasculitis of NSG may follow three patterns: (1) necrotizing granulomas within the vessel wall, (2) giant cell infiltrates associated with rupture of internal or external elastic lamina (38), or (3) chronic lymphocytic infiltration. Distinguishing NSG from classic sarcoid is the presence of coagulation necrosis, though this may range in severity from being localized within the granulomas, to affecting large areas of the pulmonary parenchyma, creating an infarct-like appearance (37–39). In addition, hilar adenopathy is reported infrequently in NSG as compared with classic sarcoid. Cavitation of parenchymal nodules favors the diagnosis of NSG over sarcoid. Originally regarded as a finding limited to pulmonary sarcoid (6,7,38), NSG has also been documented in the trachea, lymph nodes, liver, and bone (21). Patients with NSG have also exhibited evidence of extrapulmonary disease affecting the central nervous system,

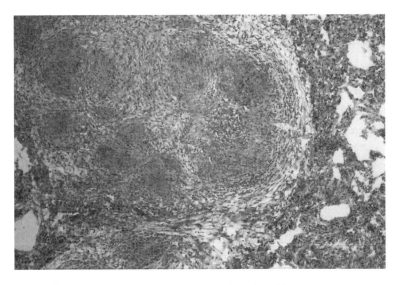

Figure 2 Necrotizing sarcoid granulomata from lung biopsy.

eyes, and spleen (14,21,39–41). Prognosis of NSG is variable: Tauber (42) reported a case of pulmonary NSG which resolved completely without therapy, consistent with early literature that suggested a benign outcome for this condition (6,37). On the other hand, Fernandes et al. (21) described three pediatric patients with NSG and multisystem disease who were treated with glucocorticoids in conjunction with either methotrexate or cyclophosphamide. None achieved complete remission.

Sarcoid synovial involvement may include small vessel vasculitis associated with granulomas or giant cells (21). However, most arthritis associated with sarcoid is not due to underlying vasculitis.

Finally, another manifestation of sarcoid small-vessel vasculitis was found in a 19-year-old male with a 6-year history of sarcoid who developed renal insufficiency due to focal segmental crescentic glomerulonephritis. He is also one of the adults mentioned above who developed synovitis related to small vessel vasculitis (21).

B. Large- and Medium-Vessel Vasculitis

The first report of large-vessel vasculitis complicating sarcoid was in 1959, in an adult female with granulomatous vasculitis involving the pulmonary and mesenteric arteries (22). In subsequent years there have been 18 additional cases in the English literature, including 8 children and 10 adults. An additional case (Table 1, case 6), previously unreported, is included in this chapter. These 20 cases have had involvement of diverse structures, including the aorta, pulmonary, innominate, common and external carotid, subclavian, brachial, radial, ulnar, coronary, renal, mesenteric, splenic, and iliac arteries (21–36) (see Table 1). In the absence of evidence that clearly supports the diagnosis of sarcoidosis, these cases are easily confused with Takayasu's arteritis. In older patients with large-vessel disease, the differential diagnosis includes giant cell (temporal) arteritis.

Aortitis may appear in the form of wall thickening, stenosis, aneurysm formation, and/or dissection (Fig. 3a and b). The ages of nine patients with sarcoid aortitis ranged from 7–56 years. Five of these nine cases were young patients, 7–19 years of age. The racial distribution of aortitis cases was disproportionately skewed toward African-Americans (4 of 9) and Asians (3 of 9). Six deaths due to aortic disease occurred; one survivor underwent aneurysm repair (33), and another had repair of an aortic dissection (21). Aortic disease was associated with inflammation in other large vessels in five of these patients, including involvement of the pulmonary, subclavian, coronary, renal, and/or iliac arteries (Fig. 3c and d). Histologically, the aortic specimens revealed granulomatous arteritis.

In the 11 patients without aortitis, large- or medium-caliber vasculitis developed in branches of the aorta both above and below the diaphragm, as well as in pulmonary, brachial, radial, ulnar, and popliteal arteries (Fig. 4). Mortality rate in these patients was not as high (18%) as in the patients with aortitis (67%). Morbidities included renal failure (34), digital ischemia (29), and bilateral leg amputation and stroke (28). Interestingly, considering this small cohort, a family was identified (30) in which the index case and her maternal aunt both experienced large-vessel vasculitis in the setting of sarcoid. The index case (age 2) experienced malignant hypertension with splenic, renal, and iliac artery stenoses. Her aunt had granulomatous aortitis and died at age 24 of a cardiac arrest.

Among the 20 cases with sarcoid large-vessel disease, claudication in the arms or legs was common and often led to the discovery of vascular disease. Abdominal pain was due to mesenteric arteritis in one case (22) and to dissection of the aorta in a second case (25). Hypertension occurred in seven cases (five children, two adults) and was associated with renal artery stenosis in three instances (see Table 1). Renal arteriography was not performed in three cases. Carotidy-

Table 1 Systemic Vasculitis in Sarcoidosis

		Sarcoidosis			Vascular Disease					
Case	Reference	Age at onset	Sex/race	Clinical features	Age at onset	Clinical features	Vascular histopathology	Arteriography	Treatment/follow-up (yr)	Outcome
1	31	8 mo	F/C	Arthritis, uveitis, erythematous rash, hypertension	4 yr	Hypertension	ND	Renal artery (S), superior mesenteric artery (S)	P, angioplasty/NS	Alive
2	29	5 mo	F/C	Lymph node involvement, fever, rash, foot drop, hepatosplenomegaly, digital ischemia	5 mo	Digital ischemia	LCV (skin)	ND	P, CP, MTX/3.5 yr	Alive, asymptomatic
3	30	8 mo	F/C	Arthritis, iritis, seizures, pericardial effusion, erythematous rash, hypertension	5 yr	Malignant hypertension	ND	Renal arteries (S), iliac arteries (S), splenic artery (S)	P, CP/4 yr	Alive
4	35	9 mo	M/C	Arthritis, deformities, uveitis with blindness, papular rash, seizures, hypertension, pulmonary involvement	10 yr	Hypertension	Aorta (GV)	ND	P, CP, AZA/NS	Died at age 10 yr
5	34	1 yr	F/O	Arthritis, iridocyclitis, papules, hypertension, leg infarction, lymphadenopathy	4 yr	Hypertension		Renal artery (S), popliteal artery (GV)	P/2 yr	Alive at age 24 yrs, with renal failure
6	21	2 yr	F/AA	Fever, erythema nodosum, hilar adenopathy, ILD/pneumonitis, iridocyclitis, periostitis, conjunctival injection, arthralgias	15 yr	New pulmonary infiltrates, R carotid bruit, R femoral bruit, diminished L femoral pulse	Pulmonary vasculitis	Aorta (S), L iliac (S)	P, CP, MTX/4 yr	Alive
7	21	3 yr	F/AA	Cervical adenopathy, fever, maculopapular rash polyarthritis/deformities, anterior bilateral uveitis	12 yr	Carotidynia, ↓ radial and carotid pulses, cardiac murmurs, absent BP L arm	ND	R CCA (A), R ECA(A), innominate artery (A), L SCA (O)	P/5.7 yr	Alive at age 20, arthritis

Table 1 (*Continued*)

Case	Reference	Sarcoidosis			Vascular Disease					
		Age at onset	Sex/race	Clinical features	Age at onset	Clinical features	Vascular histopathology	Arteriography	Treatment/ follow-up (yr)	Outcome
8	32	3.5 yr	F/AA	Arthritis, uveitis, papular rash, carotidynia	11.5 yr	Carotidynia	ND	L carotid artery (S), L SCA (O)	P/12 yr	Alive, asymptomatic
9	33	7 yr	M/AA	Iritis, leg pain, fever	7 yr		ND	Aorta, myxoid degeneration (A)	Surgical repair, P/3 yr	Alive, asymptomatic
10	30	8 yr	F/C	Fever, iritis, hepatomegaly, arthritis, hypertension, blindness, seizure	24 yr	Hypertension	Aorta (GV)	ND	P/NS	Died at age 24 years of cardiac arrest
11	21	13 yr	M/AA	Symmetric polyarthritis, erythema nodosum, Bell's palsy	19 yr	Abdominal bruit, asymmetry of lower extremity pulses and BP at age 19	Synovium: small vessels aortitis FSGN	Aorta (A), bilateral RA(A) and II(A), L SCA(O), R SCA(O)	P, surgical repair for dissection/1.6 yr	Alive at age 22, some improvement
12	26	19 yr	F/O	Fever, cough, proteinuria, pulmonary hemorrhage, lymph node involvement (crescentic GN?)	NS	Pulmonary hemorrhage	Aorta (GV), PA (GV)	ND	None/NS	Died after 2 mo
13	36	29 yr	F/NS	Nodular myositis, weight loss, left arm pain	29 yr	Diminished L radial pulse, L carotid bruit	ND	L SCA(O), L VA(O), L CCA(narrowed), SMA(O)	P, AZA/9 mos	Alive, improved arm pain

#	Ref	Age	Sex/Race	Clinical features		Symptoms	Biopsy/Pathology	Vessels (angiography)	Treatment	Outcome
14	28	31 yr	F/AA	Pulmonary and LN involvement, fever, dyspnea, uveitis, erythema nodosum, stroke, hypertension	NS	Hand and Feet gangrene, Hypertension	ND	Brachial, radial and ulnar arteries(S)	P, CP, IVIg/5 yr	Remission, legs amputated/13 yr
15	21	31 yr	F/AA	Weight loss, hilar adenopathy, bilateral iridocyclitis, leukopenia	31 yr	Claudication of R arm, absent pulse and BP of R arm	ND	R SCA (S), splenic (S)	P/5.5 yrs	Alive at age 36 stable
16	23	51 yr	M/AA	Pulmonary and LN involvement, fever, cough, weight loss, congestive heart failure	NS		Aorta (GV)	Aorta (T)	None/NS	Died, 5 mo
17	24	52 yr	M/O	Pulmonary and LN involvement, palpitation, dyspnea, absent peripheral pulse	NS	Absent peripheral pulse	Aorta, iliac, SCA, PA (GV)	Aorta (A), B SCA(S)	None/NS	Died/6 mo
18	22	55 yr	F/NS	Fever, arthritis, abdominal pain, hypertension, renal impairment, asthma	NS		PA (GV), mesenteric arteries (GV)		None/NS	Died/8 yr
19	25	56 yr	F/O	Pulmonary and LN involvement, abdominal pain	NS		Aorta (GV), coronary and RA (GV)	Aorta (T)(D)	None/NS	Died/NS
20	27	58 yr	F/NS	Pulmonary and LN involvement, pulmonary hypertension	NS	Pulmonary hypertension		PA(A)	None/NS	Died/NS

Abbreviations: ND = not done, NS = not specified, C = Caucasian, AA = African-American, O = Oriental, L = left, R = right, CCA = common carotid artery, ECA = external carotid artery, SCA = subclavian artery, PA = pulmonary artery, RA = renal artery, Il = iliac artery, NSG = necrotizing sarcoid granulomatosis, GV = granulomatous vasculitis, LN = lymph node, FSGN = focal segmental crescentic glomerulonephritis, BP = blood pressure, (A) = aneurysm, (S) = stenosis, (O) = occlusion, (T) = thickening, (D) = dissection, P = prednisone, CP = cyclophosphamide, MTX = methotrexate.

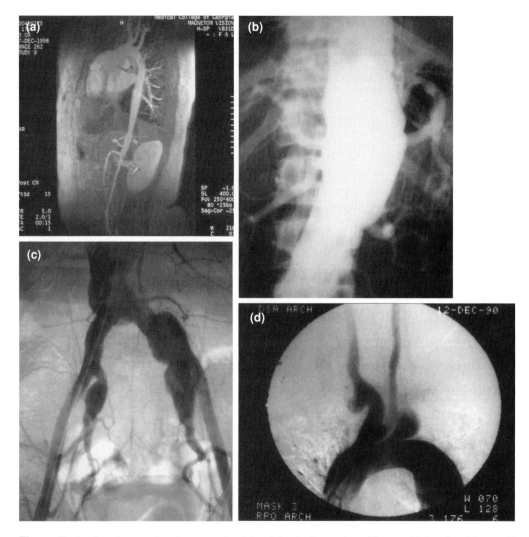

Figure 3 (a) Arteriogram showing stenosis of the abdominal aorta in a 15-year-old female with sarcoid vasculitis (case 6 from Table 1). (b) Arteriogram showing an abdominal aortic aneurysm in a 13-year-old male with sarcoid vasculitis (case 11 from Table 1). (c) Arteriogram showing aneurysms of the distal aorta and iliac arteries (case 11 from Table 1). (d) Arteriogram showing occlusion of the left and right subclavian arteries and thoracic aneurysm of the descending aorta (case 11 from Table 1).

nia occurred in two patients. Constitutional symptoms of fever or weight loss were common, seen in half the patients. The diagnosis of vasculitis in large-vessel disease cases was most often made on the basis of arteriographic findings of stenosis and aneurysm formation. Direct histological evidence was infrequently available in the antemortem state. In recent years, magnetic resonance technology has enabled investigators to identify changes highly suggestive of large-vessel vasculitis in a noninvasive manner (21,43).

Review of the cases of large-vessel vasculitis reveals a very poor prognosis unless aggressive therapy with corticosteroids is employed. Although the small numbers of well-studied cases precludes establishing definitive therapeutic recommendations, certain trends are apparent. Un-

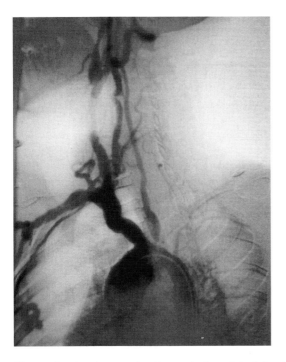

Figure 4 Arteriogram showing occlusion of the left subclavian artery and irregular fusiform aneurysms of the right carotid, innominate and subclavian arteries (case 7 from Table 1).

treated systemic sarcoid vasculitis has a poor prognosis. Six of the eight deaths noted in Table 1 occurred in patients not treated with corticosteroids or cytotoxic agents. Of the 12 patients who received corticosteroids, two died. In some cases, addition of a cytotoxic agent was followed by prolonged remission with a reduced requirement or no need for corticosteroids.

III. CONCLUSION

While vasculitis is an uncommon complication of sarcoid, it is probably more prevalent than reported in the literature. As it may have life-threatening consequences, evaluation of the child or adult with sarcoid should include consideration of this entity. Small-vessel vasculitis presents most commonly as skin lesions, though other vascular beds may be affected. Larger vessel vasculitis may present as limb claudication with physical findings of diminished or absent pulses, asymmetrical blood pressures, bruits over the great vessels, or an aortic regurgitant murmur. Treatment with corticosteroids may be organ- and life-saving.

REFERENCES

1. Neville E, Walker AN, James DG. Prognostic factors predicting the outcome of sarcoidosis: An analysis of 818 patients. Q J Med 1983; 208:525–533.
2. Lynch JP III, Kazerooni EA, Gay SE. Pulmonary sarcoidosis. Clin Chest Med 1997; 18:755–785.
3. Agostini C, Adami F, Semenzato G. New pathogenetic insights into the sarcoid granuloma. Curr Opin Rheumatol 2000; 12:71–76.

4. Moller DR. Systemic sarcoidosis. In: Fishman AP, ed. Fishman's Pulmonary Diseases and Disorders. 3d ed. 1998; 1:1055–1068.
5. Jones RE, Chatham WW. Update on sarcoidosis. Curr Opin Rheumatol 1999; 11:83–87.
6. Liebow AA. The J. Burns Amberson lecture: Pulmonary angiitis and granulomatosis. Am Rev Respir Dis 1973; 108:1–18.
7. Churg A, Carrington CB, Gupta R. Necrotizing sarcoid granulomatosis. Chest 1979; 76:406–413.
8. Hietala SO, Stinnett RG, Faunce HF III, Sharpe AR, Scoggins WG, Smith RH. Pulmonary artery narrowing in sarcoidosis. JAMA 1977; 237:572–573.
9. Cassling RJ, Lois JF, Gomes AS. Unusual pulmonary angiographic findings in suspected pulmonary embolism. Am J Roentgenol 1985; 145:995–999.
10. Fincher RM, Sherman E. Superior vena caval obstruction due to sarcoidosis. South Med J 1986; 79: 1306–1308.
11. Takemura T, Matsui Y, Saiki S, Mikami R. Pulmonary vascular involvement in sarcoidosis: A report of 40 autopsy cases. Hum Pathol 1992; 23:1216–1223.
12. Branford WA, Farr PM, Porter DI. Annular vasculitis of the head and neck in a patient with sarcoidosis. Br J Dermatol 1982; 106:713–716.
13. Johnston C, Kennedy C. Cutaneous leucocytoclastic vasculitis associated with acute sarcoidosis. Postgrad Med J 1984; 60:549–550.
14. Petri M, Barr E, Cho K, Farmer E. Overlap of granulomatous vasculitis and sarcoidosis: Presentation with uveitis, eosinophilia, leg ulcers, sinusitis and past foot drop. J Rheumatol 1998; 15:1171–1173.
15. Gran JT. Multiorgan sarcoidosis presenting with symmetric polyarthralgia, cutaneous vasculitis and sicca symptoms. Scand J Rheumatol 1997; 26:225–256.
16. Garcia-Porrúa C, González-Gay MA, Garcia-País MJ, Blanco R. Cutaneous vasculitis: An unusual presentation of sarcoidosis in adulthood. Scand J Rheumatol 1998; 27:80–82.
17. Aractingi S, Cadranel J, Milleron B, Saiag P, Malepart MJ, Dubertret L. Sarcoidosis associated with leucocytoclastic vasculitis: A case report and review of the literature. Dermatology 1993; 187:50–53.
18. Kennedy C. Sarcoidosis with cutaneous vasculitis. Br J Dermatol 1979; 101(suppl 17):47–49.
19. Takemura T, Shishiba T, Akiyama O, Oritsu M, Matsui Y, Eishi Y. Vascular involvement in cutaneous sarcoidosis. Path Int 1997; 47:84–89.
20. Cecchi R, Giomi A. Annular vasculitis in association with sarcoidosis. J Derm 1999; 26:334–336.
21. Fernandes SRM, Singsen BH, Hoffman GS. Sarcoidosis and systemic vasculitis. Semin Arthritis Rheum 2000; 30:33–46.
22. Bottcher E. Disseminated sarcoidosis with a marked granulomatous arteritis. Arch Pathol 1959; 68: 419–423.
23. Deneberg M. Sarcoidosis of the myocardium and aorta. A case report. Am J Clin Pathol 1965; 43:445–449.
24. Maeda S, Murao S, Sugiyama T, Utaka I, Okamoto R. Generalized sarcoidosis with "sarcoid aortitis." Acta Pathol Jpn 1983; 33:183–188.
25. Murai T, Imai M, Inui M, Watanabe H, Hosoda Y. Generalized granulomatous arteritis with aortic dissection. Zentralbl Allg Pathol 1986; 132:41–47.
26. Shintaku M, Mase K, Ohtsuki H, Yasumizu R, Yasunaga K, Ikehara S. Generalized sarcoidlike granulomas with systemic angiitis, crescentic glomerulonephritis, and pulmonary hemorrhage: Report of an autopsy case. Arch Pathol Lab Med 1989; 113:1295–1298.
27. Barbour DJ, Roberts WC. Aneurysm of the pulmonary trunk unassociated with intracardiac or great vessel left-to-right shunting. Am J Cardiol 1987; 59:192–194.
28. Eid H, O'Connor CR, Catalano E, Reginato AJ. Life-threatening vasculitis associated with sarcoidosis. J Clin Rheumatol 1998; 4:338–344.
29. Kwong T, Valderrama E, Paley C, Ilowite N. Systemic necrotizing vasculitis associated with childhood sarcoidosis. Semin Arthritis Rheum 1994; 23:388–395.
30. Rotenstein D, Gibbas DL, Majmudar B, Chastain EA Familial granulomatous arteritis with polyarthritis of juvenile onset. N Engl J Med 1982; 306:86–90.
31. Gross KR, Malleson PN, Culhan G, Lirenman DS, McCormick AQ, Petty RE. Vasculopathy with renal artery stenosis in a child with sarcoidosis. J Pediatr 1986; 108:724–726.

32. Rose CD, Eichenfield AH, Goldsmith DP, Athreya BH. Early onset sarcoidosis with aortitis: "juvenile systemic granulomatosis"? J Rheumatol 1990; 17:102–106.
33. Gedalia A, Shetty AK, Ward K, Correa H, Venters CL, Loe WA. Abdominal aortic aneurysm associated with childhood sarcoidosis. J Rheumatol 1996; 23:757–759.
34. Umemoto M, Take H, Yamaguchi H, Tokudome T, Tokunaga M. Juvenile systemic granulomatosis manifesting as premature aging syndrome and renal failure. J Rheumatol 1997; 24:393–395.
35. Fink CW, Cimaz R. Early onset sarcoidosis: Not a benign disease. J Rheumatol 1997; 24:174–177.
36. Korkmaz C, Efe B, Tel N, Kabukcuoglu S, Erenoglu E. Sarcoidosis with palpable nodular myositis, periostitis, and large-vessel vasculitis simulating Takayasu's arteritis (letter). Rheumatology (Oxford) 1999; 38(3):287–288.
37. Frazier AA, Rosado-de-Christenson ML, Galvin JR, Fleming MV. Pulmonary angiitis and granulomatosis: Radiologic-pathologic correlation. Radiographics 1998; 18:687–710.
38. Koss MN, Hocholzer L, Feigin DS, Garancis JC, Ward PA. Necrotizing sarcoid-like granulomatosis: Clinical, pathologic and immunopathologic findings. Hum Pathol 1980; 11(suppl 5):510–519.
39. Gibbs AR, Williams WJ, Kelland D. Necrotizing sarcoidal granulomatosis: A problem of identity. A study of seven cases. Sarcoidosis 1987; 4:94–100.
40. Beach RC, Corrin B, Scopes JW, Graham E. Necrotizing sarcoid granulomatosis with neurologic lesions in a child. J Pediatr 1980; 97:950–953.
41. Singh N, Cole S, Krause PJ, Conway M, Garcia L. Necrotizing sarcoid granulomatosis with extrapulmonary involvement: Clinical, pathologic, ultrastructural and immunologic features. Am Rev Respir Dis 1981; 124:189–192.
42. Tauber E, Wojnarowski C, Horcher E, Dekan G, Frischer T. Necrotizing sarcoid granulomatosis in a 14-yr-old female. Eur Respir J 1999; 13:703–705.
43. Rojo-Leyva F, Ratliff NB, Cosgrove DM, Hoffman GS. Study of 52 patients with idiopathic aortitis from a cohort of 1204 surgical cases. Arthritis Rheum 2000; 43(4):901–907.

48

Vasculitis and Malignancy

Paul R. Fortin

University Health Network, University of Toronto, Toronto, Ontario, Canada

I. INTRODUCTION

Although the association between vasculitis and malignancy is rare, a multitude of combinations of vasculitis and malignancies have been reported. Only a few qualify as true paraneoplastic manifestations. In order to be considered as a paraneoplastic syndrome, several criteria should be met. They include: temporal relationship, concordance, consistency, rarity, and unexpected frequency of association between the two conditions (1,2). Temporal relationship is met when both conditions start at about the same time; concordance when both conditions follow a parallel course; and consistency when a defined vasculitis is related to a specific malignancy. These paraneoplastic syndromes are often uncommon but their co-occurrence is unexpectedly frequent. The only associations that satisfy these criteria and that we would recognize as truly paraneoplastic are (1) hairy cell leukemia with small- and medium-sized-vessel systemic necrotizing vasculitis of the polyarteritis nodosa group (3,4), (2) pseudo-Raynaud's phenomenon and solid tumors, and (3) cryoglobulinemia type I or II and hematological malignancies. Table 1 summarizes these paraneoplastic syndromes with their vasculitic component and their concurrent malignancies.

Besides these better-known associations, several anecdotal associations have been reported and are summarized in Tables 2 and 3. They include cutaneous and systemic small-vessel vasculitis with several hematological malignancies and solid tumors (5–8) (see Table 2), and both systemic and limited medium-sized-vessel vasculitis (see Table 3) in association with either hematological or solid tumors. Non–hairy cell leukemias, Hodgkin's and non-Hodgkin's lymphoma, and multiple myeloma have all been reported with systemic necrotizing small- and medium-sized-vessel vasculitis. Solid tumors have very rarely been reported in association with this vasculitis.

Rare case reports of large-vessel vasculitis with hematological malignancies (9–11) or solid tumors (12) have recently been published (Table 4), but this remains controversial since retrospective reviews of large cohorts have not confirmed those results (13,14). This suggests either that the association is indeed quite rare or that the reported cases represents random co-occurrences.

This chapter first reviews the reported associations of vasculitis and malignancies. The next section reviews the capacity for some vasculitides to produce a mass effect that can mislead the best clinician to suspect a malignancy. We review those pseudo-tumors caused by systemic necrotizing medium-sized-vessel vasculitis, such as Wegener's granulomatosis, polyarteritis nodosa, or rheumatoid vasculitis, or by large-vessel vasculitis, such as giant cell arteritis (Table 5). In the

Table 1   Vasculitis as a Paraneoplastic Syndrome

Vasculitis	Malignancy	References
Necrotizing vasculitis of the polyarteritis nodosa group	Hairy cell leukemia	2,4,28,42–64
Pseudo-Raynaud's phenomenon	Hematological malignancies	
	Hodgkin's disease	79
	Solid tumors	
	Adenocarcinoma of lung	78
	Adenocarcinoma of colon	79
	Adenocarcinoma of unknown primary (pancreas or ovary)	79
	Adenopapillary carcinoma of ovary	79
	Hypernephroma	79–81
	Epidermoid carcinoma/cervix	80
	Infiltrating anaplastic carcinoma of breast	80
	Anaplastic carcinoma of maxillary antrum	79
Cryoglobulinemia		
Type I	Lymphoproliferative diseases	82
	Waldenström macroglobulinemia	
	Multiple myeloma	
	Lymphoma	
Type II	Lymphoproliferative diseases	82,84–86
	Waldenström macroglobulinemia	
	Multiple myeloma	
	Chronic lymphocytic leukemia	
	Hodgkin's disease	
	Non-Hodgkin's lymphoma	
	Diffuse "histiocytic" lymphoma	
	Mycosis fungoides	
	Angioimmunoblastic lymphadenopathy	
	Hairy cell leukemia	
	Myeloproliferative diseases	83,87
	Chronic myelocytic leukemia	
	Polycythemia vera	
	Myelofibrosis	
	Solid tumors	
	Breast	83
	Seminoma	165
	Hepatocellular carcinoma	84

next section, we describe the rare malignancies with the capacity to directly invade blood vessels or indirectly injure them, resulting in a pseudo-vasculitis (Table 6).

Two other unusual and nonspecific associations have been reported. They are so rare that they will be mentioned here and not discussed further. They consist of palmar fasciitis and polyarthritis (PFPA) seen rarely as an initial manifestation of a malignancy in the elderly. One case of PFPA with ovarian carcinoma illustrates this syndrome (15). On histopathology, there is diffuse fibrosis with proliferation of the connective tissue and vasculitis. Evidence of deposits of the third component of the complement (C3) and of immunoglobulin M in subcutaneous tissue and in the synovium may support this diagnosis. The other rare syndrome is that of hydroa vacciniforme (HV) described by Ruiz-Maldonado et al. (16). It presents as an edematous, scarring vasculitic

Table 2 Cutaneous, Localized, and Systemic Small-Vessel
Vasculitis with Hematological Malignancies and Solid Tumors

Malignancy	References
Review	2,5–8,166
Hematological malignancies	
Leukemia	24
Acute myelomonocytic leukemia	22,26
Acute myeloid leukemia	25,27
Chronic myelogenous leukemia	31,32
Hairy cell leukemia	28
Myeloproliferative disorders	29
Peripheral T-cell lymphoma	30,33,167,168
Hodgkin's disease	23,33
"Low-grade" lymphoma	24
Multiple myeloma	18,34,169
Solid tumors	
Adenocarcinoma:	
Unknown origin	23,38
Ovary	37
Prostate	33,35
Lung	8,33,40,41
Stomach	36
Liver	39

panniculitis with erythema, vesicles, necrosis, and varicelliform scars on light-exposed skin. This cutaneous vasculitis seen in children is not associated with systemic symptoms. It is most often idiopathic, but severe forms of hydroa vacciniforme have been described to subsequently evolve into aggressive non-Hodgkin's lymphoma.

We do not discuss here the malignancies that may arise as a complication of the treatment of a vasculitis with cytotoxic agents, such as cyclophosphamide (17–20) or azathioprine. Similarly, we do not discuss the vasculitis that may arise as a complication of a treatment for a specific malignancy. This has been described with the use of interleukin-2 (21) or arabinoside-C (22). This chapter does not address either paraneoplastic syndromes related to coagulation abnormalities, such as migratory thrombophlebitis (Trousseau's phenomenon) associated with some adenocarcinoma, disseminated intravascular coagulation seen with some malignancies, or direct vascular infiltration by a solid tumour such as seen with disseminated intravascular carcinomatosis.

II. VASCULITIS AND MALIGNANCY

In the reported associations between vasculitis and malignancy, all three groups of vasculitis as classified by vessel size are described. The group of small-vessel vasculitis is, however, the most frequent and it is associated with several hematological and solid organ malignacies. The medium-sized- and large-vessel vasculitis are not so frequent and are almost entirely restricted to hematological malignancies. In this section, we discuss the associations between vasculitis and malignancy according to the vessel size of the vasculitic component. We discuss pseudo-Raynaud's phenomenon and cryoglobulinemia with the medium-vessel vasculitis section since they

Table 3 Localized and Systemic Small- to Medium-Sized-Vessel Vasculitis with
Hematological Malignancies and Solid Tumors

Malignancy	References
Hairy cell leukemia	Discussed in Table 1
Other hematological malignances	
"Lymphatic leukemia"	88
Monocytic leukemia	89
Chronic myelogenous leukemia	32
Lymphoma	90
Hodgkin's disease	91
Peripheral T-cell lymphoma	168
Lymphosarcoma	91
Multiple myeloma	18,91,92
Lymphoid malignancy and Kawasaki disease	93
Solid tumors and polyarteritis nodosa	
Gastric carcinoma	94,95
Colon	96
Solid tumors and allergic angiitis and granulomatosis	
Melanoma	97
Localized vasculitis and hematological malignancy	
HIV infection, intraocular B-cell lymphoma and retinal vasculitis	109
T-cell lymphoma and renal vasculitis	110
Localized vasculitis and solid tumors	
Choroidal melanoma with retinal vasculitis	111
Localized vasculitis/cerebral granulomatous angiitis	
Chronic myeloid leukemia	46
Hodgkin's disease	102–107
Primary intracerebral lymphoma	108

Table 4 Systemic Large-Vessel Vasculitis with Hematological
Malignancies and Solid Tumors

Malignancy	References
Hematological malignances	
Acute myelogenous leukemia	9
Chronic lymphocytic leukemia	10
B-cell lymphoma	98
Multiple myeloma	11
Not specified	99
Solid tumors	
Lung carcinoma	12
Negative or nonconfirmatory cohort studies	13,14,99

most often involve vessels of that size. Finally, we summarize at the end of this section the rare cases of localized vasculitis associated with a malignancy.

A. Small-Vessel Vasculitis

Small-vessel vasculitis (see Table 2) could be limited to the skin or it could be a more diffuse process. The distinction between the two is often tenuous since most systemic processes present

Table 5 Vasculitis Mimicking Malignancies

Vasculitis	Site misdiagnosed as cancer	References
Wegener's granulomatosis	Breast	112–114
	Subdural, meningeal or base of the skull masses	115
	Eye or orbit	114,116,117
	Lung	118
	Mediastinum	119
	Pituitary/stellar mass	122
	Oropharynx and larynx	123
	Kidney	120,121
Giant cell arteritis	Breast	112,124–129
Polyarteritis nodosa	Testes	131–134
	Breast	128,135
	Uterus and fallopian tubes	136
	Bladder	137
Rheumatoid vasculitis	Soft-tissue tumor	138

Table 6 Tumors Mimicking Vasculitis

Malignancy	Vasculitis	References
Myelomonocytic and monocytic leukemia	Cutaneous leukemic vasculitis	139
Hairy cell leukemia		28
Intravascular lymphoma	Unspecified vasculitis	140
	Cutaneous polyarteritis nodosa	141
	Wegener's granulomatosis	142
	Central nervous system vasculitis	143
	Temporal arteritis	144
	Mononeuritis multiplex	145
Cardiac myxoma	Polyarteritis nodosa	146–156,170–172
Other		
Lymphomatoid granulomatosis	Pulmonary granulomatous vasculitis	161
Mediastinal angiomatoid malignant fibrous histiocytoma	Systemic vasculitis	162
Plasma cell granuloma	Wegener's granulomatosis	163
Malignant glioma	Cerebral vasculitis	164

with palpable purpura and the diagnosis is often be based on a skin biopsy. The systemic component of small-vessel vasculitis may not be apparent at the time of the diagnosis and may resolve with treatment. We therefore discuss below small-vessel vasculitis that often presents as cutaneous vasculitis.

Cutaneous vasculitis may precede the diagnosis of malignancy by weeks to months. It presents usually as palpable purpura. Persistent, unexplained cutaneous vasculitis should raise the possibility of a malignancy, especially in adults over age 50 (5). The vasculitis could be necrotizing (23), leukocytoclastic (5,7), or lymphocytic (6). Schroeter et al. (23) found 4 of 26 cases of biopsy-proven cutaneous necrotizing vasculitis to be associated with an underlying malignancy: two cases of Hodgkin's disease and two cases of adenocarcinoma. A literature review by Naschitz et al. (5) concluded that cutaneous leukocytoclastic vasculitis presenting after the age of 50, compared with before age 50, was more often associated with a malignancy. Similarly, Jessop (7) found 3 of 69 cases of malignancy (one bronchial carcinoma and two lymphoproliferative malignancies) in patients with leukocytoclastic vasculitis. Blanco et al. (8) studied 303 cases of cutaneous vasculitis and reported no association with a malignancy in 131 pediatric cases, while 4 of 172 older adults presented with concomitant neoplasms (one megakaryocytic leukemia, two myelodysplastic syndromes, and one non-Hodgkin's lymphoma).

1. Hematological Malignancies

Several hematological malignancies have been associated with different forms of small-vessel vasculitis. "Chronic leukemias" (24), acute myeloid leukemia (25), Hodgkin's disease (23), non-Hodgkin lymphoma (24), and multiple myeloma have been associated with hypersensitivity lymphocytic or urticarial vasculitis. Leucocytoclastic vasculitis has been described with acute myelomonocytic leukemia (26), acute myeloid leukemia (27), hairy cell leukemia (28), myeloproliferative syndrome (29), and peripheral T-cell lymphoma (30). Henoch–Schönlein purpura is reported more frequently in association with solid tumors and it has only been reported once with a multiple myeloma (18).

Other cutaneous vasculitides without well-described histology are reported with chronic myelogenous leukemia (31,32). Vasculitis of the vasa nervorum resulting in a peripheral neuropathy has been rarely associated with Hodgkin's disease (33).

One case report of an unusual systemic vasculitis in association with multiple myeloma is of interest. This vasculitis presented with gangrene, livedo reticularis, hypertension, renal failure, and small-bowel perforation due to small-vessel necrotizing vasculitis with crystalglobulin deposits observed on the histological examination of the small vessels of the small bowel (34).

2. Solid Tumors

The most common association between a small-vessel vasculitis and a solid tumor appears to be that of Henoch–Schönlein purpura with prostate cancer (35). Henoch–Schönlein purpura has also been reported with a stomach adenoma (36). Other associations include that of leukocytoclastic vasculitis with ovarian (37), colon (38), or liver cancer (39). Clinical diagnosis of cutaneous vasculitis has also been reported with small-cell neuroendocrine carcinoma (40). Necrotizing cutaneous vasculitis with unspecified adenocarcinoma (23) and vasculitis of the vasa nervorum with prostate (33) or lung (33,41) carcinoma have also been rarely reported.

B. Medium-Sized-Vessel Vasculitis

1. Hairy-Cell Leukemia and Systemic Necrotizing Vasculitis

One of the best known paraneoplastic vasculitides is that of necrotizing medium-sized vessel vasculitis seen in association with hairy-cell leukemia (2,4,28,42–64) (see Table 1). This vasculitis is clinically and histopathologically indistinguishable from idiopathic polyarteritis nodosa, although it may present with some unusual features, such as involvement of the temporal (42,52,55) or cerebral (56) arteries, or of the peripheral vessels (4). Two reviews of this topic, one by this author and others (2) in 1991, and one by Hasler et al. (28) in 1995 concur in their conclusions. Forty-two cases of vasculitis have been reported in association with hairy-cell leukemia (28). Of these, 18 would classify as the accepted paraneoplastic vasculitis of the polyarteritis nodosa (PAN) type (see Table 1) initially reported by Hughes et al. (4) in 1979. Twenty-one others are leukocytoclastic vasculitides of the small vessels (28) (see Table 2). Another four demonstrate direct infiltration of the blood vessels by hairy cells and could be considered as direct invasion of the vessel wall by tumor cells (see Table 6).

This leukemia is an unusual chronic leukemia that was first described by Bouroncle et al. (65) in 1958 as a distinct entity and initially referred to as "leukemic reticulo-endotheliosis." Shrek was the first to describe, in 1966, the "hairy" cells that give their name to this leukemia (66). Hairy cell leukemia presents clinically with fatigue, fever, and frequent infections (43,67). Massive splenomegaly, occasional hepatomegaly, and the absence of lymphadenopathy are pathognomonic. The male-to-female ratio is 4:1. Laboratory studies show a moderate pancytopenia with a relative lymphocytosis and the presence of characteristic circulating mononuclear cells with prominent cytoplasmic projections, the so-called "hairy cells" (68). These cells are easily characterized by staining for tartrate-resistant acid phosphatase (69). The diagnosis is confirmed by bone marrow biopsy (70). The majority of patients with this malignancy have leukemic cells of a hairy cell of B-cell lineage, but T-cell types have also been reported (71). Other laboratory abnormalities have not been consistent. Besides the frequent observation of elevated immunoglobulin levels (28), the presence of hepatitis B surface antigen has been found infrequently and there is no clear association with cryoglobulins, serum complement, rheumatoid factor, or antinuclear antibodies.

The polyarteritis nodosa–like vasculitis appears to occur more frequently after the diagnosis of the hairy cell leukemia, splenectomy, and/or infection, while the leukocytoclastic vasculitis tends to develop before the leukemia. Five pathogenetic mechanisms could explain alone, or in combination, the co-occurrence of vasculitis with hairy-cell leukemia: (1) impairment of the clearance of immune complexes by altered monocytes (72,73), (2) the production of antibodies by hairy cells, directed against endothelial cells, (3) increase in antibody production and circulating immune complexes (74,75), (4) autoantibodies against hairy cells may cross-react with antigens on the surface of endothelial cells (55,76), and (5) hairy cells may invade vessel walls. No single theory has been sufficient to explain all reported cases and it is likely that more than one is operative in the development of the vascular inflammation.

The course of the leukemia will more often determine the outcome of these patients. Deaths occur more often due to complications of leukemia, such as infection or exsanguination, rather than from vasculitis. Treatments for hairy cell leukemia include interferon, pentostatin, 2'-deoxycoformycin, or chlorodeoxyadenosine and have been associated with concomitant remission of the leukemia and of the vasculitis (64,77).

2. Pseudo-Raynaud's Syndrome

Atypical Raynaud's phenomenon (see Table 1) has been described in association with solid tumors and lymphoproliferative malignancies (78–81). Raynaud's phenomenon is atypical in this setting because it is accompanied by severe digital ischemia with cyanosis and gangrene rapidly after the onset of cold-induced blanching of the distal phalanges of the fingers. The Raynaud's is not typically triphasic and the blanching phase does not evolve into bluish and reddish phases, but rather into fixed ischemic lesions (78). Symptoms are almost exclusively present in the upper extremities, with only one case having involvement of the feet (80). Ulcerations develop rapidly after the onset of the ischemic symptoms and gangrene may lead to amputation. Half of the patients described are nonsmokers and have no other known risk factors for vaso-occlusive disease. The reported age range is 32–59 with a mean age of 51. In all cases, the pseudo-Raynaud's phenomenon preceded the diagnosis of malignancy.

Malignancies that have been found as presenting with this rare paraneoplastic syndrome include adenocarcinoma of the lung (78), anaplastic carcinoma of the left maxillary antrum (79), hypernephroma (79–81), adenocarcinoma of the colon (79), adenopapillary carcinoma of the ovary (79), metastatic adenocarcinoma (pancreas or ovary as primary) (79), Hodgkin's disease (79), epidermoid carcinoma of the cervix (79), and infiltrating carcinoma of the breast (80).

Arterial angiograms (79,80) have shown patent radial or ulnar arteries with occlusion of the distal digital arteries of the symptomatic fingers (80). This angiographic picture is reminiscent of Buerger's disease but since half of the patients were nonsmokers, it is doubtful that this diagnosis was the explanation for these patients. Furthermore, several of the reported patients (78,80,81) improved following removal of the primary tumor, suggesting a cause-and-effect relationship between the pseudo-Raynaud's and the tumor.

Cryoglobulins were found in two patients. In one patient, the level of cryoglobulins paralleled the course of the vasculopathy. In both cases, removal of the primary tumor was followed by a decline in the cryoglobulin levels and improvement of the ischemic symptoms (78).

3.   Cryoglobulinemia

Types I and II cryoglobulinemia are more often and more specifically associated with malignancies than type III cryoglobulinemia (see Table 1). Type I cryoglobulinemia consists of the production of a monoclonal immunoglobulin that is precipitable in cold (4°C) and produced by a malignant cell line. It is associated with lymphoproliferative diseases such as multiple myeloma, Waldenström's macroglobulinemia, and, rarely, with other lymphomas (82).

Type II cryoglobulinemia, or mixed cryoglobulinemia, results from the production of a monoclonal immunoglobulin with rheumatoid factor activity. This cryoglobulin with rheumatoid factor activity can be produced by lymphoproliferative disorders such as multiple myeloma, Waldenström's macroglobulinemia, chronic lymphocytic leukemia, Hodgkin's and non-Hodgkin's lymphoma, diffuse "histiocytic" lymphoma, mycosis fungoides, angioimmunoblastic lymphadenopathy, and hairy-cell leukemia (82–86). Other myeloproliferative disorders, such as chronic myelocytic leukemia, polycythemia vera, and myelofibrosis, can rarely produce type II cryoglobulins (83,87).

Types II and III cryoglobulinemia are variably present in patients with systemic autoimmune, immune complex–mediated diseases (rheumatoid arthritis, systemic lupus erythematosus, Sjögren's syndrome, primary biliary cirrhosis) and a variety of infectious diseases (viral hepatitis, Epstein–Barr virus, cytomegalovirus, endocarditis, and certain parasitic diseases). Type III cryoglobulins are infrequently found in association with malignancies (less than 10% of cases).

All three types of cryoglobulinemia have been described in patients with solid tumors, but this is extremely rare (82). Since types I and II are the most likely to be associated with a treatable lymphoproliferative disorder, it is important to characterize the clonality of cryoglobulins. In the presence of a monoclonal immunoglobulin, an underlying malignant process should be sought. However, the routine search for a solid tumor in any type of cryoglobulinemia, especially type III, does not appear justified (82).

4.   Other Hematological Malignancies

Medium-sized-vessel vasculitis has been reported in association with the following hematological diagnoses (see Table 3): "lymphatic leukemia" (88), monocytic leukemia (89), chronic myelogenous leukemia (32), lymphomas (90), Hodgkin's disease (91), lymphosarcoma (91), and multiple myeloma (18,91,92). In children, two cases of lymphoid malignancies have been reported with Kawasaki disease (93).

5.   Solid Tumors

Reports of medium-sized-vessel vasculitis with solid tumors (see Table 3) are rare and limited to two cases of gastric tumor (94,95) (one adenoma and one carcinoma) and one case of anaplastic colon carcinoma (96). One unusual case of allergic angiitis and granulomatosis, or Churg–Strauss syndrome, has also been reported in association with malignant melanoma (97).

C. Large-Vessel Vasculitis

1. Hematological Malignancies

Reports of the association between temporal/giant cell arteritis with hematological malignancies (see Table 4) have been increasing in the last decade. Temporal arteritis/giant cell arteritis has been described with acute myelogenous leukemia (9), chronic lymphocytic leukemia (10), multiple myeloma (11), and following chronic lymphocytic leukemia (98). The literature remains equivocal since large retrospective (14,99) and prospective (13) cohort studies have failed to convincingly confirm this association. In retrospective studies, Bahlas et al. (99) found 4 of 149 cases of polymyalgia rheumatica/giant cell arteritis to also have cancer and Mertens et al. (14) found 12 of 111 cases of polymyalgia rheumatica/giant cell arteritis to have cancer, most of which occurred long before or after the diagnosis of polymyalgia rheumatica/giant cell arteritis. Myklebust and Gran (13), in a prospective cohort of 287 cases found only one case of concomitant malignancy. Since giant cell arteritis is not uncommon in this older age group, who are at higher risk for cancer, it remains possible that the reported associations between large-vessel vasculitis and malignancy are fortuitous.

One case of non–giant cell vasculitis of the vasa vasorum of the temporal artery has been reported in association with a malignancy (100).

2. Solid Tumors

Only one concomitant case of adenocarcinoma of the lung has been reported in association with biopsy-proven giant cell/temporal arteritis in a 45-year-old woman (12). She underwent resection of a lung mass and received steroid for the initial 6 months after the diagnosis of her vasculitis. She remained tumor- and vasculitis-free at her 36-month follow-up visit, and 30 months after stopping her steroids.

D. Localized Vasculitis

1. Hematological Malignancies

Cerebral granulomatous angiitis is a rare primary vasculitis of the central nervous system that is characterized by peculiar clinical and histological characteristics first defined by Cravioto and Feigin (101). Localized cerebral granulomatous angiitis has been reported in association with chronic myeloid leukemia (46), Hodgkin's disease (102–107), and primary intracerebral lymphoma (108).

In one case of HIV infection with AIDS, a primary intraocular B-cell lymphoma was described in association with retinal vasculitis (109). Another case of non–HTLV-I T-cell lymphoma in a 6-year-old child was associated with localized bilateral renal vasculitis (110).

2. Solid Tumors

Only one case is reported: choroidal melanoma with retinal vasculitis (111).

III. VASCULITIS MIMICKING TUMORS

Vasculitis of the medium-sized and large vessels can evolve into a conglomerate of inflammatory tissue that may be mistaken for a mass. In atypical presentations such as these, the diagnosis of the malignancy is often made on the pathology specimen obtained from surgical resection of the mass. In some cases, preoperative biopsies could have avoided more radical surgery and/or tissue

716   Fortin

ablation. Wegener's granulomatosis is the single most frequent vasculitis associated with the development of pseudo-tumors. Giant cell arteritis, polyarteritis nodosa, and rheumatoid vasculitis can also present as pseudo-tumors.

In cases of vasculitis presenting as a breast or a testicular mass, the vascular inflammation may be restricted to the area or associated with systemic symptoms and generalized disease. If it is restricted to the area, surgical treatment will often cure the patients. When there is evidence of systemic disease or vasculitis elsewhere, the treatment may include steroids alone if it is a giant cell arteritis, or in combination with a cytotoxic agent if it is Wegener's granulomatosis or polyarteritis nodosa.

A. Wegener's Granulomatosis

This vasculitis has been associated with masses in the breast (112–114), subdural space, meninges and base of the skull (115), eye and its orbit (114,116,117), lung (118), mediastinum (119), kidney (120,121), pituitary gland (122), and oropharynx and larynx (123). In one case, the breast mass presented in a man (113). Another breast mass developed concomitantly with a pseudo-tumor of the orbit (114).

B. Giant Cell Arteritis

Breast masses have been reported infrequently in association with either systemic or localized manifestations of giant cell arteritis (112,124–130). An early diagnosis may prevent an unnecessary mastectomy. The histological material must be examined carefully, however, since carcinoma of the breast has been reported to coexist with necrotizing arteritis of the breast and temporal arteritis (127,129). Management of giant cell arteritis of the breast is the same as that of temporal arteritis. The prognosis is excellent, although exacerbation may be seen with prednisone tapering (130).

C. Polyarteritis Nodosa

The organ most frequently affected by pseudo-tumors due to polyarteritis nodosa has been the testes (131–134). Testicular polyarteritis nodosa may be a localized process without systemic disease. Presurgical biopsies could have prevented unilateral orchiectomy in some patients (133, 134).

Other pseudo-tumors related to polyarteritis nodosa have been reported in the breast (112,135), uterus and fallopian tubes (136), and bladder (137). This last case of bladder vasculitis was associated with HIV disease and hepatitis B infection.

D. Rheumatoid Vasculitis

Rheumatoid vasculitis may resemble polyarteritis nodosa and a rheumatoid arteritis of striated muscles has been described once as mimicking a soft-tissue tumor (138).

In conclusion, pseudo-tumors can be a consequence of small-, medium-sized-, or large-vessel vasculitis. They may be localized or a manifestation of a systemic process. Presurgical biopsies may prevent surgical resection of the organ. In nonsurgical localized processes and in systemic disease, conventional treatment for vasculitis will induce a resorption of the pseudo-tumor.

IV. TUMORS MIMICKING VASCULITIS

Just as vasculitis can masquerade as a neoplasm, some malignancies can initially be misdiagnosed as vasculitis (see Table 6). Specific hematological malignancies and a benign tumor, atrial myxoma, contribute to the large majority of reported cases. This section does not address para-neoplastic syndromes related to coagulation abnormalities, migratory thrombophlebitis (Trousseau's phenomenon), disseminated intravascular coagulation, direct vascular infiltration by a solid tumor, or disseminated intravascular carcinomatosis.

A. Leukemia

The term "leukemic vasculitis" has even been proposed to describe the cutaneous vasculitis seen on occasion with myelomonocytic and monocytic leukemia (139). Six cases of vasculitis accompanying leukemia cutis have been reported. The severity of the vasculitis varies from mild microvascular injury to a necrotizing arteritis. Most often, leukemic infiltration of the dermal blood vessels is observed on histology. The vascular injury, therefore, does not appear to be from reactive inflammation, but is mediated by leukemic blasts.

Similarly, of the 43 cases of hairy cell leukemia discussed above, four have been associated with the infiltration of the vessel wall by hairy cells (28).

B. Lymphoma

Intravascular lymphomas can mimic vasculitis (140) such as cutaneous (141) or systemic poly-arteritis nodosa, Wegener's granulomatosis (142), central nervous system vasculitis (143), temporal arteritis (144), or mononeuritis multiplex (145). The diagnosis of these lymphomas can be challenging, and a definite diagnosis has too often been made at autopsy. Indeed, clinical manifestations of intravascular lymphomas arise from an occlusive angiopathy that may well resemble the clinical manifestations of systemic vasculitis. Treating these lymphomas as systemic vasculitis may slow the course and mask the lymphomatous vascular infiltrates until the malignancy is too far advanced to be effectively treated. Since these lymphomas require treatment that differs from that of vasculitis, one should always keep in mind that a definite diagnosis of vasculitis must be based on obtaining involved tissue and observing vascular wall inflammation. As much as possible, the specimen should be obtained before, or as early as possible after, the introduction of steroids. Even in ideal conditions, the pathologist and the treating physician should keep a very high level of suspicion since the lymphomatous infiltrate can easily be mistaken for the leukocytic infiltrate seen in vasculitis.

C. Cardiac Myxoma

Cardiac myxomas are slow-growing benign intracavitary tumors that may embolize systemically (146,147). Left atrial, or more rarely ventricular, myxomas can cause a syndrome indistinguishable from polyarteritis nodosa (146–156). The clinical and angiographic picture may suggest medium-sized-vessel vasculitis. Although present in the vessel as the cause of the vascular lesion, embolized myxomatous material may be difficult to obtain. A cardiac echocardiogram, since it is an easy noninvasive test with a high yield for myxoma (146–149), should be considered as part of the evaluation of atypical forms of vasculitis that lack characteristic features (e.g., Churg–Strauss, Wegener's granulomatosis, Henoch-Schönlein purpura, Behçet's syndrome, etc.).

The clinical triad that should lead to a high suspicion of myxoma is (1) cardiopulmonary symptoms, (2) constitutional symptoms, and (3) embolic phenomena (148). Cardiac symptoms, however, may be subtle, vary over time, and may be missed clinically (147). Several cases have only been diagnosed at autopsy (149,152). The most common findings on cardiac examination are those of outflow obstruction (mitral valve murmur suggesting mitral stenosis that may change with position) (146,150) and pulmonary hypertension (147).

Nonspecific constitutional symptoms, such as fever, fatigue, and weight loss, are often accompanied by laboratory abnormalities, such as an elevated sedimentation rate, anemia, and serum hypergammaglobulinemia. Their cause in cardiac myxoma is unknown, but they may lead to a premature, incorrect diagnosis of systemic vasculitis (149). In one case, the left atrial myxoma was discovered 31 months after the initial diagnosis of vasculitis (153).

Multiple arterial emboli are frequent in cardiac myxoma. They are seen in up to 45% of myxomas arising from the left atrium (148,150,157–159). The embolized material can be platelet thrombi arising at the surface of the tumor or tumoral myxomatous material itself (149). As often from emboli originating from the left atrium, half of them will localize in the cerebral vessels (153,157) and angiography may confirm the presence of an embolus (150) or multiple cerebral aneurysms (146,148–152,160). More often, the angiographic picture will be nonspecific and may include (1) irregular filling defects in major or minor cerebral arterial branches, (2) fusiform and saccular aneurysms, (3) occlusion of vessels, and (4) delay in the passage of the contrast medium (151).

Since the angiographic picture may be undistinguishable from that of polyarteritis nodosa, it is important to obtain tissue confirmation of diagnosis whenever possible. Myxomatous material has been shown to invade the walls of affected blood vessels at the site of the aneurysms (148,151,152). Histopathological findings include (1) invasion of the endothelium, (2) fragmentation of the elastic lamina with destruction of the normal vascular architecture and dilatation of the arterial lumen, and (3) intimal proliferation within the embolic myxomatous tissue, giving rise to intravascular masses of varying size (148,152).

Differential diagnosis of cardiac myxoma includes bacterial or murantic endocarditis, rheumatic heart disease, coronary artery disease, connective tissue disorders, and occult neoplasm or infection. An early diagnosis is important since it can lead to a curative treatment by surgical excision and the prevention of devastating vascular complications or even death.

D.   Other Tumors

Rare case reports of solid tumors mimicking vasculitis have been published. They include (1) a case of lymphomatoid granulomatosis mimicking a pulmonary granulomatous vasculitis (161), (2) mediastinal angiomatoid malignant fibrous histiocytoma with aberrant production of interleukin-6 (Il-6) and tumor necrosis factor (TNF) causing a clinical syndrome of severe systemic symptoms that was initially mistaken for systemic vasculitis (162), (3) plasma cell granuloma of the maxillary sinus mimicking Wegener's granulomatosis (163), and (4) malignant glioma with leptomeningeal dissemination mimicking cerebral vasculitis (164).

V.   CONCLUSION

True paraneoplastic vasculitides are rare and they include the association of a small- and medium-sized-vessel necrotizing vasculitis with hairy cell leukemia, pseudo-Raynaud's phenomenon and digital gangrene with carcinoma, and type I and II cryoglobulinemia with lymphoproliferative malignancies. With some exceptions, vasculitides thought to be secondary to an antigen–antibody and complement interaction are more often seen with hematological malignancies, while granulomatous vasculitides, thought to be secondary to a cellular immune dysfunction, are more frequently seen with solid tumors. In the workup of these diseases, one has to remain alert to the possibility that vasculitis may mimic a neoplasm, and that, rarely, a malignancy may mimic a vasculitis.

REFERENCES

1. Curth HO. Andrade R, Gumport SL, Popkin GL, eds. Skin lesions and internal carcinoma. In: Cancer of the Skin. Philadelphia: Saunders, 1976:1308–1343.
2. Fortin PR, Esdaile JM. Churg A, Churg J, eds. Vasculitis and malignancy. In: Systemic Vasculitides. New York: Igaku-Shoin, 1991:327–341.
3. Weinstein A. Systemic vasculitis and hairy cell leukemia. J Rheumatol 1982; 9:349–350.
4. Hughes GRV, Elkon KB, Spiller R, Catovsky D, Jamieson I. Poyarteritis nodosa and hairy-cell leukemia (letter). Lancet 1979; 1:678.
5. Naschitz JE, Yeshurun D, Eldar S, Lev LM. Diagnosis of cancer-associated vascular disorders. Cancer 1996; 77:1759–1767.
6. Pavlidis NA, Klouvas G, Tsokos M, Bai M, Moutsopoulos HM. Cutaneous lymphocytic vasculopathy in lymphoproliferative disorders: A paraneoplastic lymphocytic vasculitis of the skin (review). Leukemia Lymphoma 1995; 16:477–482.
7. Jessop SJ. Cutaneous leucocytoclastic vasculitis: A clinical and aetiological study. Br J Rheumatol 1995; 34:942–945.
8. Blanco R, Martinez-Taboada VM, Rodriguez-Valverde V, Garcia-Fuentes M. Cutaneous vasculitis in children and adults: Associated diseases and etiologic factors in 303 patients (review). Medicine (Baltimore) 1998; 77:403–418.
9. Shimamoto Y, Matsunaga C, Suga K, Fukushima N, Nomura K, Yamaguchi M. A human T-cell lymphotropic virus type I carrier with temporal arteritis terminating in acute myelogenous leukemia. Scand J Rheumatol 1994; 23:151–153.
10. Gonzalez-Gay MA, Blanco R, Gonzalez-Lopez MA. Simultaneous presentation of giant cell arteritis and chronic lymphocytic leukemia (letter). J Rheumatol 1997; 24:407–408.
11. Estrada A, Stenzel TT, Burchette JL, Allen NB. Multiple myeloma-associated amyloidosis and giant cell arteritis. Arthritis Rheum 1998; 41:1312–1317.
12. Lie JT. Simultaneous clinical manifestations of malignancy and giant cell temporal arteritis in a young woman. J Rheumatol 1995; 22:367–369.
13. Myklebust G, Gran JT. A prospective study of 287 patients with polymyalgia rheumatica and temporal arteritis: Clinical and laboratory manifestations at onset of disease and at the time of diagnosis. Br J Rheumatol 1996; 35:1161–1168.
14. Mertens JC, Willemsen G, Van Saase JL, Bolk JH, Dijkmans BA. Polymyalgia rheumatica and temporal arteritis: A retrospective study of 111 patients. Clin Rheumatol 1995; 14:650–655.
15. Vinker S, Dgani R, Lifschitz-Mercer B, Sthoeger ZM, Green L. Palmar fasciitis and polyarthritis associated with ovarian carcinoma in a young patient: A case report and review of the literature (review). Clin Rheumatol 1996; 15:495–497.
16. Ruiz-Maldonado R, Parrilla FM, Orozco-Covarrubias ML, Ridaura C, Tamayo SL, Duran MC. Edematous, scarring vasculitic panniculitis: A new multisystemic disease with malignant potential. J Am Acad Dermatol 1995; 32:37–44.
17. Odeh M. Renal cell carcinoma associated with cyclophosphamide therapy for Wegener's granulomatosis. Scand J Rheumatol 1996; 25:391–393.
18. Birchmore D, Sweeney C, Choudhury D, Konwinski MF, Carnevale K, D'Agati V. IgA multiple myeloma presenting as Henoch-Schönlein purpura/polyarteritis nodosa overlap syndrome. Arthritis Rheum 1996; 39:698–703.
19. Wakisaka N, Tanaka S, Nagayama I, Furukawa M. Squamous cell carcinoma of the nasal septum with Wegener's granulomatosis treated with cyclophosphamide and corticosteroids (review). Auris Nasus Larynx 1998; 25:393–396.
20. Westman KW, Bygren PG, Olsson H, Ranstam J, Wieslander J. Relapse rate, renal survival, and cancer morbidity in patients with Wegener's granulomatosis or microscopic polyangiitis with renal involvement. J Am Soc Nephrol 1998; 9:842–852.
21. Michel M, Vincent F, Sigal R, Damaj G, Bensousan TA, Leclercq B, et al. Cerebral vasculitis after interleukin-2 therapy for renal cell carcinoma. J Immunother Emphasis Tumor Immunol 1995; 18:124–126.

22. Ahmed I, Chen KR, Nakayama H, Gibson LE. Cytosine arabinoside-induced vasculitis. Mayo Clinic Proc 1998; 73:239–242.

23. Schroeter AL, Copeman PW, Jordon RE, Sams WMJ, Winkelmann RK. Immunofluorescence of cutaneous vasculitis associated with systemic disease. Arch Dermatol 1971; 104:254–259.

24. McCombs RP. Systemic "allergic" vasculitis: Clinical and pathological relationship. JAMA 1965; 194:1059–1064.

25. Farrell AM, Gooptu C, Woodrow D, Costello C, Bunker CB, Cream JJ. Cutaneous lymphocytic vasculitis in acute myeloid leukaemia. Br J Dermatol 1996; 135:471–474.

26. Bourantas K, Malamou-Mitsi VD, Christou L, Filippidou S, Drosos AA. Cutaneous vasculitis as the initial manifestation in acute myelomonocytic leukemia. Ann Intern Med 1994; 121:942–944.

27. Engelhardt M, Rump JA, Hellerich U, Mertelsmann R, Lindemann A. Leukocytoclastic vasculitis and long-term remission in a patient with secondary AML and post-remission treatment with low-dose interleukin-2. Ann Hematol 1995; 70:227–230.

28. Hasler P, Kistler H, Gerber H. Vasculitides in hairy cell leukemia (review). Semin Arthritis Rheum 1995; 25:134–142.

29. Longley S, Caldwell JR, Panush RS. Paraneoplastic vasculitis. Unique syndrome of cutaneous angiitis and arthritis associated with myeloproliferative disorders. Am J Med 1986; 80:1027–1030.

30. Fernandez AM, Abeles M, Wong RL. Recurrent leukocytoclastic vasculitis as the initial manifestation of acute myelomonocytic leukemia. J Rheumatol 1994; 21:1972–1974.

31. Tomiyama J, Yano K, Uchino S, Ito T, Kudo H, Irimajiri J, et al. Bilateral leg ulcers with pathologic evidence of small vessel vasculitis by skin biopsy during hydroxyurea therapy of chronic myelogenous leukemia. Jpn J Clin Hematol 1997; 38:231–233.

32. Rosen AM, Haines K, Tallman MS, Hakimian D, Ramsey-Goldman R. Rapidly progressive cutaneous vasculitis in a patient with chronic myelomonocytic leukemia. Am J Hematol 1995; 50:310–312.

33. Vincent D, Dubas F, Haun JJ. Nerve and muscle microvasculitis in peripheral neuropathy: A remote effect of cancer? J Neurol Neurosurg Psychiatry 1986; 49:1007–1010.

34. Hasegawa H, Ozawa T, Tada N, Taguchi Y, Ohno K, Chou T, et al. Multiple myeloma-associated systemic vasculopathy due to crystalglobulin or polyarteritis nodosa. Arthritis Rheum 1996; 39:330–334.

35. Garcias VA, Herr H. Henoch-Schönlein purpura associated with cancer of prostate. Urology 1982; 19:155–158.

36. Chong SW, Buckley M. Henoch-Schönlein purpura associated with adenoma of the stomach (letter). Irish Med J 1997; 90:194–195.

37. Stashower ME, Rennie TA, Turiansky GW, Gilliland WR. Ovarian cancer presenting as leukocytoclastic vasculitis. J Am Acad Dermatol 1999; 40:287–289.

38. Callen JP. Cutaneous leukocytoclastic vasculitis in a patient with an adenocarcinoma of the colon. J Rheumatol 1987; 14:386–389.

39. Sanchez-Angulo JI, Benitez-Roldan A, Silgado-Rodriguez G, Ruiz-Campos J. Leukocytoclastic vasculitis as the form of presentation of hepatocarcinoma (review). Gastroenterol Hepatol 1996; 19:255–258.

40. Ponge T, Boutoille D, Moreau A, Germaud P, Dabouis G, Baranger T, et al. Systemic vasculitis in a patient with small-cell neuroendocrine bronchial cancer. Eur Respir J 1998; 12:1228–1229.

41. Blumenthal D, Schochet SJ, Gutmann L, Ellis B, Jaynes M, Dalmau J. Small-cell carcinoma of the lung presenting with paraneoplastic peripheral nerve microvasculitis and optic neuropathy (letter). Muscle Nerve 1998; 21:1358–1359.

42. Elkon KB, Hughes GRV, Catovsky D, Clauvel JP, Dumont J, Seligmann M, et al. Hairy-cell leukemia with polyarteritis nodosa. Lancet 1979; 2:280–282.

43. Rudolph RI. Vasculitis associated with hairy cell leukemia. Arch Dermatol 1980; 116:1077–1078.

44. Pope A, Lazarchik J, Hoyer L, Weinstein A. Hairy cell leukemia and vasculitis. J Rheumatol 1980; 7:895–899.

45. Goedert JJ, Neefe JR, Smith FS, Stahl NI, Jaffe ES, Fauci AS. Polyarteritis nodosa, hairy cell leukemia and splenosis. Am J Med 1980; 71:323–326.

46. LePogamp P, Ghandour C, L Prise PY. Hairy cell leukemia and polyarteritis nodosa. J Rheumatol 1982; 9:441–442.

47. Dorsey JK, Penick GD. The association of hairy cell leukemia with unusual immunologic disorders. Arch Intern Med 1982; 142:902–903.

48. Anuras S, McMahon BJ, Chow KC, Summers RW. Severe abdominal vasculitis with hepatitis B antigenemia. Am J Surg 1980; 140:692–695.

49. Raju SF, Chapman SW, Dreiling B, Tavassoli M. Hairy cell leukemia with the appearance of mixed cryoglobulinemia and vasculitis. Arch Intern Med 1984; 144:1300–1302.

50. Kenny PGW, Shum DT, Smout MS. Leucocytoclastic vasculitis in hairy cell leukemia (leukemic reticuloendotheliosis). Arch Dermatol 1983; 119:1018–1019.

51. Mehta AB, Catovsky D, O'Brien CJ, Lott M, Bowley N, Hemmingway A. Massive retroperitoneal lymphadenopathy as a terminal event in hairy cell leukemia. Clin Lab Hematol 1983; 107:259–263.

52. Krol T, Robinson J, Bekeris L, Messmore H. Hairy cell leukemia and a fatal periarteritis nodosa-like syndrome. Arch Pathol Lab Med 1983; 107:583–585.

53. Thorwarth WT, Jaques PF, Orringer EP. Polyarteritis nodosa in hairy cell leukemia. J Can Assoc Radiol 1983; 34:151–152.

54. Westbrook CA, Golde DW. Autoimmune disease in hairy cell leukemia. Br J Haematol 1985; 61:346–356.

55. Gabriel SE, Conn DL, Phyliky RL, Pittelkow MR, Scott RE. Vasculitis in hairy cell leukemia: Review of literature and consideration of possible pathogenic mechanisms. J Rheumatol 1986; 13:1167–1172.

56. Lowe J, Russell NH. Cerebral vasculitis associated with hairy cell leukemia. Cancer 1987; 60:3025–3028.

57. Lie JT. Isolated polyarteritis of testis in hairy-cell leukemia. Arch Pathol Lab Med 1988; 112:646–647.

58. Komadina KH, Houk RW. Polyarteritis nodosa presenting as recurrent pneumonia following splenectomy for hairy-cell leukemia (review). Semin Arthritis Rheum 1989; 18:252–257.

59. Spann CR, Callen JP, Yam LT, Apgar JT. Cutaneous leukocytoclastic vasculitis complicating hairy cell leukemia (leukemic reticuloendotheliosis). Arch Dermatol 1986; 122:1057–1059.

60. Farcet JP, Weschsler J, Wirquin V, Divine M, Reyes F. Vasculitis in hairy-cell leukemia. Arch Intern Med 1987; 147:660–664.

61. Thorel JB, Grosbois B, Paris G, Schneebeli S, Goasguen J, Leblay R. [Leukocytoclastic vasculitis and hepatic tuberculosis disclosing hairy cell leukemia] [review]. [French]. Rev Med Interne 1988; 9:530–533.

62. Gomez-Almaguer D, Herrera-Garza JL, Garcia-Guajardo BM, Garcia-Taboada BE. Vasculitis in hairy cell leukemia: Rapid response to interferon alpha. Am J Hematol 1989; 30:261–262.

63. Klima M, Waddell CC. Hairy cell leukemia associated with focal vascular damage. Hum Pathol 1984; 15:657–659.

64. Carpenter MT, West SG. Polyarteritis nodosa in hairy cell leukemia: Treatment with interferon-alpha. J Rheumatol 1994; 21:1150–1152.

65. Bouroncle BA, Wiseman BK, Doan CA. Leukemic reticuloendotheliosis. Blood 1958; 13:609–630.

66. Shred R, Donnell WJ. "Hairy" cells in blood in lymphoreticular neoplastic disease and "flagellated" cells of normal lymph nodes. Blood 1966; 27:119–211.

67. Golomb HM, Vardiman J. Hairy cell leukemia: Diagnosis and management. CA 1978; 28:265–277.

68. Turner A, Kjeldsberg CR. Hairy cell leukemia: A review (review). Medicine 1978; 57:477–499.

69. Yam LT, Li CY, Lam KW. Tartrate-resistant acid phosphatase isoenzyme in the reticulum cells of leukemic reticuloendotheliosis. N Engl J Med 1971; 284:357–360.

70. Naeim F, Smith GS. Leukemic reticuloendotheliosis. Cancer 1974; 34:1813–1821.

71. Naeim F, Gatti RA, Johnson CEJ, Gossett T, Walford RL. "Hairy cell" leukemia: A heterogeneous chronic lymphoproliferative disorder. Am J Med 1978; 65:479–487.

72. Hughes GR. Hairy cell leukemia and arteritis. Clin Exp Rheumatol 1983; 1:9.

73. Golomb HM, Catovsky D, Golde DW. Hairy cell leukemia: A clinical review based on 71 cases. Ann Intern Med 1978; 89:t–83.

74. Utsinger PD, Yount WJ, Fuller CR, Logue MJ, Orringer EP. Hairy cell leukemia: B-lymphocyte and phagocytic properties. Blood 1977; 49:19–27.

75. Golde DW, Stevens RH, Quan SG, Saxon A. Immunoglobulin synthesis in hairy cell leukaemia. Br J Haematol 1977; 35:359–365.

76. Posnett DN, Marboe CC, Knowles DM, Jaffe EA, Kunkel HG. A membrane antigen (HCl) selectively present on hairy cell leukemia cells, endothelial cells, and epidermal basal cells. J Immunol 1984; 132:2700–2702.

77. Tallman MS, Peterson LC, Hakimian D, Gillis S, Polliack A. Treatment of hairy-cell leukemia: Current views (review). Semin Hematol 1999; 36:155–163.

78. Domz CA, Chapman CG. Pseudo-Raynaud's: Cryoglobulinemia secondary to occult neoplasm. Calif Med 1961; 95:391–393.

79. Hawley PR, Johnston AW, Rankin JT. Association between digital ischaemia and malignant disease. Br Med J 1967; 3:202–212.

80. Friedman SA, Bienenstock H, Richter IH. Malignancy and arteriopathy: A report of two cases. Angiology 1969; 20:136–143.

81. Andrasch RH, Bardana EJJ, Porter JM, Pirofsky B. Digital ischemia and gangrene preceding renal neoplasm: An association with sarcomatoid adenocarcinoma of the kidney. Arch Intern Med 1976; 136:486–488.

82. Laurance J, Nachman R. Cryoglobulinemia. Disease-A-Month 1981; 27:34–36.

83. Bohrod MG. Plasmacytosis and cryoglobulinemia in cancer. JAMA 1957; 164:18–21.

84. Mody GM, Cassim B. Rheumatologic manifestations of malignancy (review). Curr Opin Rheumatol 1997; 9:75–79.

85. Wooten MD, Jasin HE. Mixed cryoglobulinemia and vasculitis: A novel pathogenic mechanism. J Rheumatol 1996; 23:1278–1281.

86. Ferri C, La Civita L, Longombardo G, Zignego AL, Pasero G. Mixed cryoglobulinaemia: A crossroad between autoimmune and lymphoproliferative disorders (review). Lupus 1998; 7:275–279.

87. Fitzgerald S, Hurst NP, Pannall PR. Sjögren's syndrome, vasculitis, and cryoglobulinaemia associated with a monoclonal IgM (kappa) paraprotein with rheumatoid factor activity. Ann Rheum Dis 1987; 46:485–487.

88. Gerber MA, Brodin A, Steinberg D, Vernace S, Yang CP, Paronetto F. Periarteritis nodosa, Australia antigen and lymphatic leukemia. N Engl J Med 1972; 286:14–17.

89. Leung ACT, McLay A, Boulton-Jones JM. Polyarteritis nodosa and monocytic leukaemia. Postgrad J Med 1986; 62:35–37.

90. Hench PK, Mayne JG, Kiely JM, et al. Clinical study of the rheumatic manifestations of lymphoma. Arthritis Rheum 1962; 5:301.

91. Sams WM, Harvilee DD, Winkelmann RK. Necrotizing vasculitis associated with lethal reticuloendothelial disease. Br J Dermatol 1968; 80:555–560.

92. Seelen MA, de Meijer PH, Arnoldus EP, van Duinen SG, Meinders AE. A patient with multiple myeloma presenting with severe polyneuropathy caused by necrotizing vasculitis. Am J Med 1997; 102:485–486.

93. Murray JC, Bomgaars LR, Carcamo B, Mahoney DHJ. Lymphoid malignancies following Kawasaki disease. Am J Hematol 1995; 50:299–300.

94. Poveda F, Gonzalez-Garcia J, Picazo ML, Gimenez A, Camacho J, Barbado FJ, et al. Systemic polyarteritis nodosa as the initial manifestation of a gastric adenocarcinoma (review). J Intern Med 1994; 236:679–683.

95. Yamada T, Miwa H, Ikeda K, Ohta K, Iwazaki R, Miyazaki A, et al. Polyarteritis nodosa associated with gastric carcinoma and hepatitis B virus infection. J Clin Gastroenterol 1997; 25:535–537.

96. Paajanen H, Heikkinen M, Tarvainen R, Vornanen M, Paakkonen M. Anaplastic colon carcinoma associated with necrotizing vasculitis. J Clin Gastroenterol 1995; 21:168–169.

97. Cupps TR, Fauci AS. Neoplasm and systemic vasculitis: A case report (letter). Arthritis Rheum 1982; 25:475–476.

98. Martinez-Taboada V, Brack A, Hunder GG, Goronzy JJ, Weyand CM. The inflammatory infiltrate in giant cell arteritis selects against B lymphocytes. J Rheumatol 1996; 23:1011–1014.

99. Bahlas S, Ramos-Remus C, Davis P. Clinical outcome of 149 patients with polymyalgia rheumatica and giant cell arteritis. J Rheumatol 1998; 25:99–104.

100. Lesser RS, Aledort D, Lie JT. Non-giant cell arteritis of the temporal artery presenting as the polymyalgia rheumatica-temporal arteritis syndrome. J Rheumatol 1995; 22:2177–2182.

101. Cravioto H, Feigin I. Noninfectious granulomatous angitiis with a prediction for the nervous system. Neurology 1959; 9:599–609.

102. Rewcastle NB, Tom MI. Non-infectious granulomatous angiitis of the nervous system associated with Hodgkin's disease. J Neurol Neurosurg Psychiatry 1962; 25:51–58.

103. Greco FA, Kolins J, Rajjoub RK, Brereton HD. Hodgkin's disease and granulomatous angiitis of the central nervous system. Cancer 1976; 38:2027–2032.

104. Magidson MA, Rajendran MM, Leuthcer WM. Granulomatous angiitis of the central nervous system with an unusual angiographic angiitis of the centreal nervous system. Surg Neurol 1978; 10:355–360.

105. Rajjoub RK, Wood JH, Ommaya AK. Granulomatous angiitis of the brain: A successfully treated case. Neurology 1977; 27:588–591.

106. Rosenblum WI, Hadfield MG. Granulomatous angiitis of the nervous system in cases of herpes zoster and lymphosarcoma. Neurology 1972; 22:348–354.

107. Yuen RW. Primary angiitis of the central nervous system associated with Hodgkin's disease (review). Arch Pathol Lab Med 1996; 120:573–576.

108. Borenstein D, Costa M, Jannotta F, Rizzoli H. Localized isolated angiitis of the central nervous system associated with primary intracerebral lymphoma. Cancer 1988; 62:375–380.

109. Ormerod LD, Puklin JE. AIDS-associated intraocular lymphoma causing primary retinal vasculitis. Ocular Immunol Inflam 1997; 5:271–278.

110. Neuhauser TS, Lancaster K, Haws R, Drehner D, Gulley ML, Lichy JH, et al. Rapidly progressive T cell lymphoma presenting as acute renal failure: Case report and review of the literature (review). Pediatr Pathol Lab Med 1997; 17:449–460.

111. Steel DH, Mahomed I, Sheffield E. Unilateral choroidal melanoma with bilateral retinal vasculitis (letter). Br J Ophthalmol 1996; 80:850–851.

112. Cook DJ, Bensen WG, Carroll JJ, Joshi S. Giant cell arteritis of the breast. Can Med Assoc J 1988; 139:513–515.

113. Trueb RM, Pericin M, Kohler E, Baradun J, Burg G. Necrotizing granulomatosis of the breast. Br J Dermatol 1997; 137:799–803.

114. Gobel U, Kettritz R, Kettritz U, Thieme U, Schneider W, Luft FC. Wegener's granulomatosis masquerading as breast cancer. Arch Intern Med 1995; 155:205–207.

115. Shiotani A, Mukobayashi C, Oohata H, Yamanishi T, Hara T, Itoh H, et al. Wegener's granulomatosis with dural involvement as the initial clinical manifestation. Intern Med 1997; 36:514–518.

116. Agostini HT, Brautigam P, Loffler KU. Subretinal tumour in a patient with a limited form of Wegener's granulomatosis. Acta Ophthalmol Scand 1995; 73:460–463.

117. Janknecht P, Mittelviefhaus H, Loffler KU. Sclerochoroidal granuloma in Wegener's granulomatosis simulating a uveal melanoma. Retina 1995; 15:150–153.

118. Almadori G, Trivelli M, Scarano E, Cadoni G. Misleading clinical features in Wegener's granulomatosis: A case report. J Laryngol Otol 1997; 111:746–748.

119. George TM, Cash JM, Farver C, Sneller M, van Dyke CW, Drus CL, et al. Mediastinal mass and hilar adenopathy: Rare thoracic manifestations of Wegener's granulomatosis. Arthritis Rheum 1997; 40:1992–1997.

120. Villa-Forte A, Hoffman GS. Wegener's granulomatosis presenting with a renal mass. J Rheumatol 1999; 26:457–458.

121. Hoffman GS, Kerr GS, Leavitt RY, Hallahan CW, Lebovics RS, Travis WD, et al. Wegener granulomatosis: An analysis of 158 patients. Ann Intern Med 1992; 116:488–498.

122. Bertken RD, Cooper VR. Wegener's granulomatosis causing sellar mass, hydrocephalus, and global pituitary failure. West J Med 1997; 167:44–47.

123. Wenig BM, Devaney K, Wenig BL. Pseudoneoplastic lesions of the oropharynx and larynx simulating cancer (review). Pathol Annu 1995; 30:143–187.

124. Potter BT, Housley E, Thomson D. Giant-cell arteritis mimicking carcinoma of the breast. Br Med J 1981; 282:1665–1666.

125. Stephenson TJ, Underwood JC. Giant cell arteritis: An unusual cause of palpable masses in the breast. Br J Surg 1986; 73:105.

126. Nirodi NS, Stirling WJ, White MF. Giant cell arteritis presenting as a breast lump. Br J Clini Pract 1985; 39:84–86.

127. Clement PB, Senges H, How AR. Giant cell arteritis of the breast: Case report and literature review (review). Hum Pathol 1987; 18:1186–1189.

128. Waugh TR. Bilateral mammary arteritis-report of a case. J Pathol 1950; 26:851–861.

129. Horne D, Crabtree TS, Lewkonia RM. Breast arteritis in polymyalgia rheumatica. J Rheumatol 1987; 14:613–615.

130. Thaell JF, Saue GL. Giant cell arteritis involving the breasts. J Rheumatol 1983; 10:329–331.

131. Rowling SE, Shapiro ML, Lieberman AP, Coleman BG. Intratesticular vasculitis simulating a testicular neoplasm. J Ultrasound Med 1996; 15:161–163.

132. Levine T. Isolated testicular vasculitis mimicking a testicular neoplasm (letter). J Clin Pathol 1995; 48:496.

133. Mukamel E, Abarbanel J, Savion M, Konichezky M, Yachia D, Auslaender L. Testicular mass as a presenting symptom of isolated polyarteritis nodosa. Am J Clin Pathol 1995; 103:215–217.

134. Warfield AT, Lee SJ, Phillips SM, Pall AA. Isolated testicular vasculitis mimicking a testicular neoplasm. J Clin Pathol 1994; 47:1121–1123.

135. Dega FJ, Hunder GG. Vasculitis of the breast: An unusual manifestation of polyarteritis. Arthritis Rheum 1974; 17:973–976.

136. Grasland A, Pouchot J, Damade R, Vinceneux P. Uterine localization of periarteritis nodosa disclosed by fever of long duration. Rev Med Interne 1996; 17:58–60.

137. Fischer AH, Wallace VL, Keane TE, Clarke HS. Two cases of vasculitis of the urinary bladder: Diagnostic and pathogenetic considerations. Arch Pathol Lab Med 1998; 122:903–906.

138. Andreu JL, Salas C, Mulero J, Martinez-Cal B, Sanz J, Larrea A. Necrotizing arteritis confined to striated muscle mimicking a soft-tissue tumour in a patient with rheumatoid arthritis (letter). Br J Rheumatol 1998; 37:916–917.

139. Jones D, Dorfman DM, Barnhill RL, Granter SR. Leukemic vasculitis: A feature cutis in some patients. Am J Clin Pathol 1997; 107:637–642.

140. al-Chalabi A, Abbott RJ. Angiotropic lymphoma in the differential diagnosis of systemic vasculitis (letter). J Neurol Neurosurg Psychiatry 1995; 59:219.

141. Thomas R, Vuitch F, Lakhanpal S. Angiocentric T cell lymphoma masquerading as cutaneous vasculitis. J Rheumatol 1994; 21:760–762.

142. Walker UA, Herbst EW, Ansorge O, Peter HH. Intravascular lymphoma simulating vasculitis. Rheumatol Int 1994; 14:131–133.

143. Sienknecht CW, Whetsell WOJ, Pollock P. Intravascular malignant lymphoma ("malignant angioendotheliomatosis") mimicking primary angiitis of the central nervous system. J Rheumatol 1995; 22:1769–1770.

144. Tannenbaum CB, Trudel MA, Kapusta MA. Lymphomatous perivascular infiltration involving the temporal artery (letter). J Rheumatol 1996; 23:2009–2010.

145. Roux S, Grossin M, De Bandt M, Palazzo E, Vachon F, Kahn MF. Angiotropic large cell lymphoma with mononeuritis multiplex mimicking systemic vasculitis (review). J Neurol Neurosurg Psychiatry 1995; 58:363–366.

146. Leonhardt ETG, Kullenberg KPG. Bilateral atrial myxomas with multiple arterial aneurysms: A syndrome mimicking polyartertis nodosa. Am J Med 1977; 62:792–794.

147. Huston KA, Combs JJJ, Lie JT, Giuliani ER. Left atrial myxoma simulating peripheral vasculitis. Mayo Clinic Proc 1978; 53:752–756.

148. Price DL, Harris JL, New PFJ, Cantu RC. Cardiac myxoma. Arch Neurol 1970; 23:558–567.

149. Steinmetz EF, Calanchini PR, Aguilar MJ. Left atrial myxoma as a neurological problem: A case report and review. Stroke 1973; 4:451–458.

150. Damasio H, Seabra-Gomes R, da Silva JP, Damasio AR, Antunes JL. Multiple cerebral aneurysms and cardiac myxoma. Arch Neurol 1975; 32:269–270.

151. New PF, Price DL, Carter B. Cerebral angiography in cardiac myxoma: Correlation of angiographic and histopathological findings. Radiology 1970; 96:335–345.

152. Burton C, Johnston J. Multiple cerebral aneurysms and cardiac myxoma. N Engl J Med 1970; 282:35–36.

153. Macedo ME, Reis R, Sottomayor C, Nunes R, Candeias O, Gomez MR, et al. Systemic vasculitis as the initial presentation of a left atrial myxoma (review). Rev Port Cardiol 1997; 16:463–466.

154. Koh WH, Chuah SC, Chng HH. Left ventricular myxoma, adrenal tumour and cutaneous vasculitis: A case report. Singapore Med J 1995; 36:328–330.

155. Gravallese EM, Waksmonski C, Winters GL, Simms RW. Fever, arthralgias, skin lesions, and ischemic digits in a 59-year-old man. Arthritis Rheum 1995; 38:1161–1168.

156. Greeson DM, Wright JE, Zanolli MD. Cutaneous findings associated with cardiac myxomas. Cutis 1998; 62:275–280.

157. Goodwin JF. Diagnosis of left atrial myxoma. Am J Cardiol 1968; 21:464–468.

158. Silverman J, Olwin JS, Graettinger JS. Cardiac myxoma with systemic embolization. Circulation 1962; 26:99–103.

159. Goodwin JF. Symposium on cardiac tumors. Am J Cardiol 1968; 21:307–314.

160. Stoane L, Allen JH, Jr., Collins HA. Radiologic observations in cerebral embolization from left heart myxomas. Radiology 1966; 87:262–266.

161. Hammar SP. Granulomatous vasculitis (review). Semin Respir Infect 1995; 10:107–120.

162. Davies KA, Cope AP, Schofield JB, Chu CQ, Mason JC, Krausz T, et al. A rare mediastinal tumour presenting with systemic effects due to IL-6 and tumour necrosis factor (TNF) production. Clin Exp Immunol 1995; 99:117–123.

163. Ktaili M, Al-Masri N, Williams RC, Jr. Wegener's look-alike. J Rheumatol 1998; 25:180–182.

164. Herman C, Kupsky WJ, Rogers L, Duman R, Moore P. Leptomeningeal dissemination of malignant glioma simulating cerebral vasculitis: Case report with angiographic and pathological studies. Stroke 1995; 26:2366–2370.

165. Lundberg WB, Mitchell MS. Transient warm autoimmune hemolytic anemia associated with seminoma. Yale J Biol Med 1977; 50:419–427.

166. Fortin PR. Vasculitis associated with malignancy Curr Opin Rheumatol 1996; 30–33.

167. O'Shea JJ, Jaffe ES, Lane HC. Peripheral T-cell lymphoma presenting as hypereosinophilia with vasculitis. Am Med J 1987; 82:539–545.

168. Delmer A, Audoin J, Rio B. Peripheral T-cell lymphoma presenting as hypereosinophilia with vasculitis (letter). Am J Med 1988; 84:565–566.

169. Lucas Guillen E, Martinez Ruiz A, Guerao Ramirez MR, Montes Clavero C. Hypersensitivity vasculitis as first manifestation of multiple myeloma (letter). An Med Interna 1997; 14:374–375.

170. Navarro PH, Bravo FP, Berltran GG. Atrial myxoma with livedoid macules as its sole cutaneous manifestations. J Am Acad Dermatol 1995; 32:881–883.

171. Togo T, Hata M, Sai S, Ito T, Sato N, Haneda K, et al. Tricuspid valve myxoma in a child with coronary artery occlusion and aneurysms. Cardiovasc Surg 1994; 2:418–419.

172. Abraham Z, Rozenbaum M, Rosner I, Odeh M, Oliven A. Cutaneous eruption in a patient with cardiac myxoma. J Dermatol 1995; 22:276–278.

49
Drug-Induced Vasculitis

Peter A. Merkel

Boston University School of Medicine, Boston, Massachusetts

I. INTRODUCTION

A wide variety of drugs from many different pharmaceutical classes have been associated with the development of vasculitis (Table 1). These vasculitides range from cases of self-limited leukocytoclastic vasculitis to reports of chronic, life-threatening, systemic necrotizing vasculitis. However, due to problems with classification of drug-induced vasculitis (DIV) and the inherent difficulty in proving causality between particular agents and specific adverse drug reactions, the quality of supporting evidence for drugs that cause vasculitis vary from data from large clinical trials to animal models of disease to individual case reports. This chapter describes the clinical and pathological spectrum of vasculitides putatively ascribed to adverse drug reactions and outlines the evidence supporting these associations.

II. CLASSIFICATION

The nomenclature of DIV is confusing and stems from the proposals of many scientists in the early part of the twentieth century that some forms of vasculitis result from an "allergic" or "hypersensitive" reaction to noninfectious antigens (1). Building upon earlier observations as well as their own large case series, Zeek et al. (1,2) at the University of Cincinnati proposed a classification system for the "necrotizing angiitides." This system describes five types of vasculitis with overlapping clinical and pathological findings. "Hypersensitivity vasculitis" was defined as a response to ". . . serum, sulfonamides, drugs, etc" affecting small vessels and usually lasting less than 1 month.

While Zeek's classification system was a fundamental advance in the study of inflammatory vascular disease, the term "hypersensitivity vasculitis" was broad enough to include such entities as serum sickness, the Arthus reaction, Henoch-Schönlein purpura, post-streptococcal vasculitis, and malignancy-associated vasculitis, as well as DIV. Thus, "hypersensitivity vasculitis" describes a group of vasculitides rather than any one specific entity and is an inappropriate term to apply to all drug-induced vasculitides. While the 1990 American College of Rheumatology (ACR) criteria for the classification of vasculitides included a separate definition for "hypersensitivity vasculitis," these criteria were not exclusive to drug-induced cases of small-vessel disease (3). Furthermore, the ACR criteria were only 71% sensitive and 84% specific for the diagnosis of "hypersensitivity vasculitis." Thus, misclassification is common, even among experts in the di-

Table 1 Drugs Associated with Vasculitis[a]

Antimicrobials	Anticonvulsants/	Antineoplastics/	Psychotropic agents
Antibacterials	Antiarrhythmics	antimetabolites	Amitriptyline
Chloramphenicol	Amiodarone	Allopurinol	Clozapine
Clindamycin	Carbamazepine	Azathioprine	Diazepam
Gentamicin	Phenytoin	Busulfan	Maprotiline
Isoniazid	Procainamide	Chlorambucil	Trazodone
Macrolides[b]	Quinidine	Colchicine	
Penicillins/β-lactams[b]	Trimethadione	Cyclophosphamide	Sympathomimetics
Quinolones[b]	Valproic acid	Levamisole	Ephedrine
Rifampin		Melphalan	Methamphetamine
Sulfonamides[b]	Diuretics	Methotrexate	Phenylpropanolamine
Tetracyclines[b]	Chlorthalidone	Retinoids	
Antivirals	Furosemide	Tamoxifen	Miscellaneous drugs
Acyclovir	Hydrochlorothiazide		Bromide
Zidovudine	Spironolactone	Hematopoietic growth	Cimetidine
Antifungals		factors	Cocaine
Griseofulvin	Other cardiovascular	G-CSF	Chlorpropamide
	agents	GM-CSF	Cromolyn
Vaccines	Acebutolol		Dextran
Hepatitis A	Atenolol	Nonsteroidal antiinflam-	Diphenhydramine
Hepatitis B	Captopril	matories	d-Penicillamine
Influenza	Diltiazem	Acetylsalicylic acid	Gold
Rubella	Guanethidine	Diclofenac	Heroin
Pneumococcal	Hydralazine	Flurbiprofen	Iodinated contrast media
Smallpox	Methyldopa	Ibuprofen	Metformin
	Nifedipine	Indomethacin	Phenacetin
Interferons	Anticoagulants/	Mefenamic acid	Potassium iodide
Alpha, beta, gamma	thrombolytics	Phenylbutazone	Quinine
	Heparin	Piroxicam	Sulfasalazine
Antithyroid agents	Streptokinase		Terbutaline
Carbimazole	Warfarin	Leukotriene inhibitors	
Methimazole		Montelukast	
Propylthiouracil		Pranlukast	
		Zafirlukast	

[a]This list was compiled from multiple sources and is not meant to be comprehensive for all drugs associated with vasculitis. The level of evidence for each agent causing vasculitis varies greatly and readers are advised to investigate any agent individually when making clinical decisions.
[b]More than one agent in this pharmacological class has been reported to cause DIV.

agnosis and management of vasculitides. The recent Chapel Hill Consensus nomenclature does not use the term "hypersensitivity" but rather "cutaneous leukocytoclastic angiitis" (4).

Terms such as "serum sickness–like reactions" or "allergic vasculitis" are also too vague to be useful and imply unproven pathogeneses. Serum sickness is a specific entity that shares features with DIV but the two should not be interchangeable. Serum sickness is only applicable to cases of immune complex reactions to foreign antigens in serum administered for therapeutic purposes.

"Leukocytoclastic vasculitis" (LCV) should not be used to imply a specific disease entity or cause, but rather is one of several histological descriptions of inflammatory blood vessel damage. "Cutaneous vasculitis" is also too vague to be useful since this term incorporates a wide range of disorders and is not exclusive to DIV. Cutaneous LCV most commonly presents as palpable purpura but also presents with urticaria, ulcers, erythematous plaques, or nodules (5–7). While LCV is the major histological finding in most cases of palpable purpura and is a common finding in DIV, it occurs in other settings, including virus-mediated vasculitis, Wegener's granulomatosis and other primary vasculitides, systemic lupus erythematosus, rheumatoid arthritis, and other diseases (5,6). Furthermore, LCV is not the only or even the predominant pathology in DIV. Thus, a finding of LCV does not in itself prove that a patient is suffering from DIV.

For the purposes of this chapter, DIV is defined as any type of inflammatory vascular disorder caused by the administration of a pharmacological agent. This definition includes pathological entities deemed "allergic" or "hypersensitive" as well as other histological types of vasculitis, and excludes other entities that may have similar clinical and pathological findings but different etiologies. As discussed later in this chapter, this differentiation of DIV from other types of vasculitis may have important implications for treatment and clinical management of patients.

III. EPIDEMIOLOGY

Precise and reliable estimates of the frequency of DIV are not established due to the difficulties posed by diagnostic uncertainty, misclassification, underreporting, and methodological problems with research studies. Despite these concerns, it is apparent that DIV is fairly common, especially among patients with disease limited to the skin. In the series of 807 patients with vasculitis collected by the American College of Rheumatology committee on vasculitis classification, 89 (11.0%) were deemed drug induced (3). When limiting cases to cutaneous vasculitis, the prevalence of drug-induced disease is even higher (8).

A number of factors may lead to underestimating the prevalence of DIV. Many cases of self-limited cutaneous vasculitis are not reported to administrative authorities as adverse drug events. Furthermore, unless a skin biopsy is performed, true vasculitis may be underrecognized in many cases of drug eruptions (9). Estimates based on specialty clinic cohorts may underestimate DIV prevalence.

The demographic characteristics, including medical comorbidities, of patients within whom DIV occurs do not seem to be different from those of the overall population of patients receiving pharmacotherapy. There is no age group that is particularly susceptible to DIV, nor is there a different incidence between genders (7).

IV. CLINICAL FEATURES

The clinical presentation of DIV ranges from isolated skin or central nervous system disease to multiorgan involvement (Table 2). Many cases of diffuse, life-threatening disease have been reported. However, the true range of presentations may be milder than reported due to a likely bias toward publishing cases with more severe disease. The literature regarding the clinical features of DIV is of variable quality with individual case reports predominating. Larger case series exist but often involve a mix of drug-induced disease and idiopathic presentations of vasculitis. The evidence of causality for the drugs listed in reports is also highly variable. However, by combining case series and single case reports, a number of reviews of DIV have been compiled allowing reliable patterns of involvement of the clinical manifestations to emerge (6,7,10–16).

Two sources of data on DIV are particularly noteworthy. Haber et al. (7) summarized the clinical manifestations of 100 cases of DIV collected from previously published case series and individual reports, including 30 cases from one source (11). The American College of Rheumatology Subcommittee on Classification of Vasculitis (3) collected 93 cases of "hypersensitivity"

Table 2 Clinical Manifestations of Drug-Induced Vasculitis

Dermatologic manifestations
   *Palpable purpura
   *Petechiae
   Maculopapular lesions
   Ulcers
   Bullae
   Urticaria
   Livedo
   Digital necrosis
Constitutional/miscellaneous symptoms
   *Fever
   *Malaise
   *Arthralgias/arthritis
   Myalgias/myositis
Visceral manifestations
   *Renal: glomerulonephritis, interstitial nephritis
   Lung: alveolar hemorrhage, pleurisy
   Liver: hepatitis, hepatomegaly, hepatic granulomas
   Gastrointestinal: abdominal pain or bleeding, splenomegaly
   Central nervous system: stroke, hemorrhage, seizures
   Peripheral nervous system: mononeuritis multiplex
Laboratory findings
   *Peripheral blood eosinophilia
   *Active urinary sediment
   Elevated acute phase reactants (variable)
   Antineutrophil cytoplasmic autoantibodies

*Denotes relatively common features of drug-induced vasculitis.

vasculitis, of which 89 (96%) were associated with medications felt to be potential "precipitating" factors for the vasculitis. The clinical descriptions of these cases, collected by investigators with particular interests in vasculitis, is valuable.

A. Timing of Clinical Manifestations

The time course of clinical manifestations of DIV is variable. There are three time intervals of interest in studying DIV: (1) the interval between initial drug exposure and onset of vasculitis, (2) the interval between initial clinical manifestation and onset of other features, and (3) the interval between initial clinical feature and resolution of disease (after cessation of drug exposure and/or with treatment). Not all case reports of DIV refer to these time intervals.

The reported interval from drug exposure to first clinical feature of vasculitis ranges from 1 day to many years. Most cases occur within a few weeks of drug exposure. However, a number of cases of drug-associated antineutrophil cytoplasmic antibody (ANCA)-positive vasculitis have been described in which the interval between drug exposure and disease onset was many months (17). Signs and symptoms of disease may progress over days or weeks depending on the extent of disease, timing of drug discontinuation, and initiation of medical therapy. Most patients with isolated dermal vasculitis have abbreviated courses of less than 1 month. Patients with systemic disease are more likely to have manifestations for longer than 1 month (7).

B. Skin Manifestations

Dermatological abnormalities are by far the most common clinical manifestations of DIV. Skin lesions may be the only features of DIV present or they may be found in combination with visceral disease. Two dermatological lesions predominate: palpable purpura and maculopapular rashes. These findings may be seen either alone or in combination in more than 50% of cases (3,7,11). Most cases of maculopapular lesions involve the lower extremities but they may also appear on buttocks, upper extremities, or other areas. When seen in DIV, purpura or petechiae are also almost always found on the lower extremities but can also be seen in other areas. There is usually a symmetrical distribution of purpuric lesions. Other skin findings less commonly occurring in DIV include urticaria, bullae, livedo reticularis, and nonspecific erythema. Edema may be present as well, especially in the lower extremities. Many of these lesions can become confluent or progress to ulceration. Digital necrosis has also been noted in some cases of DIV. One regularly observed skin feature of DIV is that the lesions all appear to be of the same "age" or stage of development.

It is important to realize that while the clinical appearances of the dermatological lesions of DIV differ, the histology of each reveals "vasculitis." These variable skin manifestations of DIV should caution physicians to avoid assuming vasculitis is only present with purpura. Similarly, all that appears to be "purpuric" may not be vasculitis.

C. Extracutaneous Manifestations

Musculoskeletal signs and symptoms are common in cases of DIV. Both diffuse arthralgias and true arthritis (synovitis) occur. The arthritis is usually polyarticular and may be migratory. Myalgias are also common with inflammatory myositis and vasculitis, demonstrated by muscle biopsy, present in some cases.

Central nervous system involvement in DIV has been reported for a number of drugs, both as part of a systemic vasculitis as well as in isolation.

Visceral involvement is common in DIV and can be organ- or life-threatening. Renal disease is the most common visceral manifestation of DIV. Thirty-one of 70 cases (44%) of DIV compiled by Haber et al. (7) and 12 of the 30 (40%) cases from Mullick et al. (11) had some form of renal pathology. Glomerulonephritis frequently occurred with active urinary sediment, elevated serum creatinine, and biopsies demonstrating focal and segmental disease. Patients with DIV and renal manifestations tend to have evidence of other internal organ involvement as well. Hepatic involvement in DIV is also common with 13 of 70 (19%) cases in the Haber et al. series and 15 of Mullick et al.'s 30 (50%) cases having hepatic abnormalities. Frank ascites and jaundice were rare but elevated liver enzymes were common. In the few cases in which hepatic tissue was examined, the findings ranged from inflammatory cell infiltrates to hepatic necrosis.

Other organs are also involved in DIV but with less frequency than skin, joints, kidneys, and liver. The nature of cardiac disease in DIV is not clear from the literature. Cardiac manifestations have been noted in 4–43% of cases (7,11). Other sites of involvement in DIV reported include lungs, pancreas, and spleen, but the number of cases with these manifestations is too small to provide reliable details of pathology.

D. Laboratory Findings

There are no laboratory tests that are diagnostic for DIV. Much of the diagnostic evaluation in patients with suspected DIV is directed at finding causes of the vasculitis other than a drug. To a large extent, the finding of certain markers of disease, such as antinuclear antibodies, cryoglobulins, positive serologies for hepatitis B or C, or hypocomplementemia, all steer clinicians away from a diagnosis of DIV.

Fever and peripheral eosinophilia are common in DIV, especially in cases with internal organ involvement (7,11). In the series from Haber et al. (7), among cases limited to cutaneous disease, fever was present in only 22% and eosinophilia in 22% (only a few patients had both findings). In contrast, 70% of patients with systemic DIV had fever and 79% had eosinophilia. Elevated levels of acute phase reactants or detection of immune complexes may be seen in cases of DIV but are also not universally present. Organ-specific laboratory abnormalities are present in cases of systemic DIV.

V. HISTOPATHOLOGY

The histopathology of DIV is variable, reflecting the multiple clinical manifestations of the disease. The most common site for pathological examination in DIV is the skin since it is frequently involved and easily biopsied. Furthermore, skin biopsies of purpura, macular lesions, or bullae are usually diagnostic for either vasculitis or another specific diagnosis.

The histological findings in skin from patients with DIV include mononuclear (lymphocytic) vasculitis, leukocytoclastic vasculitis, tissue eosinophilia, and various immunofluorescence patterns (5,9,11,12,18–23). Mononuclear vasculitis is the most common histological pattern in DIV. However, leukocytoclastic vasculitis and other pathologies are present in many cases. A "mixed" lymphocytic and leukocytic histology has also been described. It needs to be emphasized that neither mononuclear nor leukocytoclastic vasculitis is specific for DIV and that both can present with identically appearing purpura or other skin lesions. In mononuclear (lymphocytic) vasculitis, mononuclear cells predominate; however, eosinophils and polymorphonuclear cells may also be seen (5,11). Leukocytoclastic vasculitis involves fibrinoid necrosis of small-caliber vessels with infiltration of neutrophils and monocytes, presence of nuclear debris (leukocytoclasia), and extravasation of erythrocytes (5,19).

Immunofluorescence staining of either mononuclear cells or neutrophil-dominant lesions of DIV often, but not always, reveals deposits of IgM and complement but not IgG (5,9,12,19). Some investigators believe that finding IgG deposits in vasculitis is evidence against a drug reaction. Different areas of biopsies are usually all at the same stage or "age" at a given time. However, in a given patient, serial biopsies at different times may yield a spectrum of histological patterns reflecting the evolving nature of the pathology.

VI. DETERMINING CAUSALITY OF SPECIFIC DRUGS FOR VASCULITIS

There are many important reasons to both diagnose cases of DIV and identify the causative agents involved in individual cases. First, the putative agent can and should be discontinued. Second, treatment may differ from that of other types of vasculitis. Glucocorticoids and/or immunosuppressive agents, the mainstays of treatment for idiopathic vasculitis, might not be initiated or only given in short courses in patients with apparent drug-induced disease. Third, for individual patients, prevention of future episodes of vasculitis may be achieved by avoiding use of the previously causative drug and perhaps avoidance of that class of medications. Rechallenge is not advisable. Finally, the medical community and society as a whole also benefit from recognition of potentially serious adverse drug reactions and, when feasible, prophylactic measures can be instituted.

For many reasons, determining that specific drugs cause vasculitis is a difficult and usually imprecise process. Some of these difficulties are common to investigations of any adverse drug reaction (ADR). Drug-induced vasculitis with any particular agent is rare and some of the drugs implicated are not commonly prescribed, making the likelihood of multiple cases available to a single investigator low. Many cases of possible DIV involve patients taking multiple medications or substances, making isolation of the single responsible agent challenging. Precise information regarding time of drug exposure is often surprisingly hard to elicit, especially in cases in which extended drug use occurred prior to the clinical onset of DIV. Accurate data regarding the temporal association between drug exposure, discontinuation, and clinical disease are essential in determining causality for ADRs.

Most of the information on causality and DIV stems from individual case reports. Some data exist from observational cohorts. Cases of rechallenge with recurrent DIV are helpful but unusual. Among the best type of data for documenting ADRs are clinical trials that include both active medication and placebo groups. Adverse drug reactions are carefully documented in clinical trials. However, the number of patients enrolled in premarketing studies of new therapeutic agents is low, resulting in underdetection of less common ADRs such as DIV. Postmarketing studies of new agents are not usually comprehensive.

Guidelines have been developed to help clinicians and researchers faced with diagnosing potential ADRs (24–26). Irey (25) proposed six methods to link specific drugs with ADRs and outlined five categories for evaluating and rating episodes of ADRs (Table 3). Other systems of classifying ADRs have similar approaches (24,26).

Table 3 Linkage of Drugs and Degrees of Certainty for Assigning Causality in Drug-Induced Vasculitis

---

METHODS TO LINK SPECIFIC DRUGS WITH DIV
1. Exclusion of other agents
    Established by either temporal associations of agents to disease or review of medical literature on all agents
2. Dechallenge (withdrawal)
3. Rechallenge
    Generally not performed
4. Singularity of drug
    Exposure to only one drug and no comorbidities explaining clinical findings
5. Pattern
    Clinical or pathological
6. Quantitation of drug level
    Although important in other types of adverse drug reactions, this is usually not pertinent in cases of DIV

DEGREES OF CERTAINTY FOR CAUSALITY IN SINGLE CASES
1. Causative: Certainty of causality established in case. Evidence includes temporal eligibility, drug singularity, and a thorough evaluation excluding other causes of DIV. Ideally, there is an objective and reproducible diagnostic test or procedure that is distinctive and specific for ADR (may not yet exist for DIV)
2. Probable: Category for cases highly consistent with DIV but lack the unique, objective evidence of certainty found in "causative" cases.
3. Possible: Uncertain category where episode can be neither confirmed nor refuted as an ADR. Evidence and factors involved include temporal eligibility and clinicopathological findings that resemble previous reports. However, other causes of DIV are not fully excluded or there are no comparable prior reports. Data may be incomplete or unavailable.
4. Coincidental: DIV is initially diagnosed but subsequent evidence reveals another cause for the vasculitis or no vasculitis at all.
5. Negative: Further evidence reveals DIV was never possible due to factors such as drug mislabeling, drug not actually administered, or temporal eligibility impossible.

Source: Adapted from Ref. 25.

Proposed here is an additional method of evaluating drugs for causality in DIV: "quality of evidence." This term refers to assessing the study design (if any), comprehensiveness, and frequency of reports in the medical literature for specific agents and DIV. This method is outlined in Table 4. While there is considerable overlap in the concepts of degree of certainty and quality of evidence, the two are not fully equivalent but are highly complementary. Readers are encouraged to consider both types of evaluation when reading the medical literature and implicating a specific agent as causing DIV.

VII. CAUSAL AGENTS IN DRUG-INDUCED VASCULITIS

A great number of drugs from almost every pharmaceutical class and category have been cited as causal agents for DIV. Table 1 presented a partial list of those agents reported in the medical literature to cause DIV. This list was compiled from a variety of sources and the degree of evidence for causality ranges form poor to excellent (7,10,12,13,15–17,27–36). The list is organized by medical indication to demonstrate the variety of agents implicated in DIV. That many commonly used drugs are listed may reflect the greater absolute number of patients exposed to these agents rather than an increased incidence of DIV. Furthermore, many cases of DIV likely go unreported in both the medical literature and to regulatory agencies. Evidence of specific drugs causing DIV may reside with the drug's manufacturer or government agencies. Assuming that virtually any drug or therapeutic agent can cause vasculitis is not an unreasonable initial approach for clinicians to take when faced with a possible case of DIV.

Rather than provide details of each drug listed in Table 1, this section highlights several of the broad categories of agents linked to vasculitis that are particularly noteworthy and more re-

Table 4   Quality of Evidence for Assigning Causality in Drug-Induced Vasculitis

---

1. Excellent evidence:
     Prospective, controlled trials *or* properly powered case–control studies
     Animal models
     Details of clinical and pathological evaluations provided, including biopsy material, and temporal
          course
     Exclusion of other diagnoses
     Description of positive rechallenges
     Preponderance of evidence from either
          Large number of cases
          or
          Number of cases that is out of proportion to prevalence of drug's use
2. Good evidence:
     Large case series
     Case reports provide details of clinical and pathological evaluations provided, including biopsy material, and temporal course
     Exclusion of other diagnoses
     Separate case reports are fairly consistent regarding pattern of disease
3. Fair evidence:
     Individual case reports, preferably with clinical details, biopsies, temporal courses, and diagnostic
          evaluations described
     Exclusion of other diagnoses
4. Poor evidence:
     Individual case reports without clear clinical or temporal details
     Other diagnoses *not* excluded

---

cently recognized. Additionally, this section emphasizes the quality of evidence that specific agents are causal for DIV.

A. Antimicrobials

Most classes of antibacterial agents and an increasing number of antiviral agents are linked to DIV (15). It is important in these cases for clinicians to attempt to distinguish between vasculitis as an ADR vs. vasculitis as part of the underlying infection for which the antimicrobial is prescribed. A variety of infections can produce vasculitis or vasculitis-like lesions through either direct infection or immune complex formation and deposition as is seen in cases of subacute bacterial endocarditis (see also Chapters 38–40). Furthermore, the appearance of vasculitis in patients being treated with antimicrobials for organisms not known to cause vasculitis should prompt both consideration of DIV as well as reevaluation of the underlying pathogen.

B. Immunizations

Vasculitis has been reported to follow administration of various vaccines, including those for hepatitis A and B, influenza, rubella, smallpox, tetanus, and tuberculosis (15,37–42). Cases associated with influenza or hepatitis B immunizations were the most common, with fewer than 20 cases reported for each. Many of these cases involved systemic manifestations, including renal, retinal, and cerebral vasculitis. The latency period between vaccine dose and clinical findings of vasculitis ranged from 2 days to several months, with a period of 7–31 days common.

The quality of evidence of causality for these cases is only fair thus far. The temporal relationships, singularity of drugs, evidence of vasculitis, and exclusion of other diagnoses were all documented. However, these are mostly single case reports and the total number of worldwide vaccine recipients is very large. None of the evidence of vaccines causing DIV stems from large vaccine efficacy trials and rechallenges were rarely performed. Nevertheless, the emerging literature on vasculitis following immunizations is particularly fascinating given the growing recognition of the role of various microorganisms in vasculitides.

While programs worldwide to greatly expand the number of people given immunizations will likely prevent far more disease and death than they will induce, the number of DIV cases secondary to vaccination is also likely to increase if these associations are real. Whether administration of specific vaccines could induce "flares" of certain vasculitides is not known. Until new and higher-quality data are available regarding any new risks to vaccination, the standard of care should remain to vaccinate all appropriate people, especially those who are or will become immunocompromised (43). However, in cases of suspected DIV from a vaccine, rechallenge with subsequent doses of the same vaccine should be undertaken with great caution and is probably not advisable.

C. Hematopoietic Growth Factors

Numerous reports have implicated both granulocyte colony-stimulating factor (G-CSF) and granulocyte-macrophage colony-stimulating factor (GM-CSF) as causes of DIV (44–53). In almost all of these cases, vasculitis was present only in the skin and resolved when the drug was discontinued. When patients with neutropenia are given these agents, the neutrophil count seems to be an important predictor of vasculitis: in general, patients who developed DIV did so if the growth factor was continued when their neutrophil count rose above $800/mm^3$. The evidence for causality is good to excellent in these reports with a large total number of cases, many arising from carefully monitored treatment protocols where temporality and drug singularity could be established.

Biopsies were performed and resolution occurred promptly with drug discontinuation. Even more convincing is that drug rechallenge regularly resulted in repeat episodes of vasculitis.

That G-CSF and GM-CSF may cause DIV and other inflammatory conditions might concern clinicians considering using these agents in patients with vasculitides suffering neutropenia secondary to immunosuppressive therapy. There are reports of G-CSF or GM-CSF use inducing flares of psoriasis, rheumatoid arthritis, and lupus (52). Additionally, both of these agents also can cause Sweet's syndrome (54–59) or pyoderma gangrenosum (59,60). However, a recent report by Hellmich et al. (61) described G-CSF administration to six patients with Wegener's granulomatosus and severe neutropenia. Treatment with G-CSF was discontinued prior to the neutrophil count rising above $1000/mm^3$. These six patients did well, with shorter durations of neutropenia compared with controls and no evidence of disease flares.

Only one possible case of vasculitis has been reported in association with erythropoietin (62), a drug in much more widespread use than both G-CSF or GM-CSF combined. No cases of DIV with thrombopoietin have been reported, but this agent is not yet commonly used.

D. Cocaine and Heroin

Both cocaine (63–72) and heroin (10,73–75) have been implicated as causal for DIV. The singularity of a drug in these reports of vasculitis is often difficult to establish because users of these agents often take more than one drug at a time and the drugs are often mixed with other contaminants. These so-called "drugs of abuse" are illegal in most countries and associated with social disapproval, making details of the prevalence of DIV with these agents difficult to determine.

The majority of reports of DIV with cocaine and heroin involve vasculitis of the central nervous system. Because central nervous system vasculitis is so rare, and both drugs have vasoactive properties that could lead to vasospasm and malignant hypertension with hemorrhage, questions about causality remain with these agents with respect to DIV. Users of cocaine and heroin are often at increased risk for infection with human immunodeficiency virus, hepatitis B, and hepatitis C, viruses known to cause vasculitis. Therefore, in any cases of potential DIV with either drug, infections with these viruses need to be to considered.

E. Sympathomimetics

Various sympathomimetics have been associated with DIV including methamphetamine, phenylpropanolamine, and ephedrine (10,73,76–81). Some reports describe a necrotizing vasculitis and include cases of central nervous system vasculitis.

The same questions about causality regarding polysubstance ingestions and vasostimulation as described for cocaine and heroin also apply to the sympathomimetics. In the case of methamphetamine, however, a good animal model of DIV has been described, making the level of evidence of causality of DIV much higher. Sympathomimetics are contained in many over-the-counter decongestants and "diet pills." Patients are often unaware of the active ingredients in these products.

F. Leukotriene Inhibitors

Use of zafirlukast, an oral leukotriene inhibitor used in the treatment of asthma, has been linked to more than 20 cases of Churg–Strauss syndrome (allergic granulomatous vasculitis) (27–32). However, the issue of causality is complicated by both a lack of strong evidence and the unique association between chronic asthma and the development of Churg–Strauss syndrome. Many patients with Churg–Strauss syndrome develop clear manifestations of vasculitis several years after first having symptomatic asthma. Most, but not all, of these cases of DIV occurred during oral glucocorticoid tapering, raising the possibility of that zafirlukast "unmasked" latent vasculitis in susceptible patients (33,34). While patients improved upon drug withdrawal, most were also treated with systemic glucocorticoids. There have also been a few similar cases reported with use of pranlukast and montelukast, implying that DIV may be a class effect for leukotriene inhibitors (35,36).

Because Churg–Strauss syndrome is such a rare form of vasculitis, these reports are being taken quite seriously. It seems prudent to consider avoiding use of leukotriene inhibitors in patients with documented Churg–Strauss syndrome until further information is available. However, at this time, it appears premature to withhold these agents in patients with asthma who have no evidence or history suggestive of vasculitis.

G. Anti–Rheumatic Disease Drugs

Many drugs included in Table 1 as possibly causing DIV are used in the treatment of arthritis and other rheumatic diseases, including vasculitis. These drugs include allopurinol, azathioprine, chlorambucil, colchicine, cyclophosphamide, gold, interferons, methotrexate, nonsteroidal anti-inflammatory agents, penicillamine, sulfasalazine, and tetracyclines. When patients with underlying rheumatic diseases manifest signs or symptoms of vasculitis, both expressions of the primary syndrome as well as DIV should be considered. Differentiating an ADR from worsening primary disease may be difficult, but important treatment decisions will be based on such evaluations.

H. Drug-Induced ANCA-Positive Vasculitis

An increasing number of drugs have been reported to cause vasculitis associated with positive tests for antineutrophil cytoplasmic antibodies (ANCAs). This topic has been reviewed recently (16). The traditional association with ANCAs has been with Wegener's granulomatosis, microscopic polyangiitis, necrotizing and crescentic glomerulonephritis, and Churg–Strauss syndrome (82–84). Antineutrophil cytoplasmic antibody testing by immunofluorescence and ELISA is highly specific for this spectrum of vasculitis and has become an important diagnostic and classification tool.

The drugs thus far reported to cause ANCA-positive DIV include hydralazine (17,85–91), propylthiouracil (and related thionamide antithyroid drugs) (92–101), penicillamine (17,90,102–106), minocycline (107,108), clozapine (109), ciprofloxacin (110), sulfasalazine (17,111), allopurinol (17,112), and phenytoin (113). Of these agents, the best evidence for true causality exists for hydralazine and propylthiouracil. The large number of cases, the detailed documentation of the clinical manifestations including biopsies, the exclusion of other diagnoses, the temporal associations, and singularity of the drugs used all make the evidence good to excellent for these two drugs. A fall in titer or complete disappearance of ANCAs after drug withdrawal in some of the cases is further evidence of causality. The evidence of causality of the other agents, some of which are commonly prescribed medicines, is of lower quality.

The clinical manifestations in ANCA-positive DIV range from mild cutaneous lesions to severe, life-threatening glomerulonephritis, pulmonary hemorrhage, and necrotizing vasculitis. Even drug discontinuation does not always prevent disease progression. Most of the reported patients were treated with glucocorticoids and a second immunosuppressive agent. The time course from the introduction of the putative causal agent to disease presentation ranged from weeks to many months. Most patients were positive for antimyeloperoxidase ANCA and not anti–proteinase 3 ANCA. One case of DIV was reported in a patient with established Wegener's granulomatosis who was positive for anti–proteinase 3 antibodies and then developed a transient DIV from propylthiouracil and was temporarily positive for antimyeloperoxidase antibodies (99).

It is important to differentiate cases of ANCA-positive DIV from drug-induced systemic lupus erythematosus (DILE). While there is some clinical overlap between these two entities, many of the cases of ANCA-positive DIV included features not found in DILE, such as upper respiratory disease and pulmonary hemorrhage. It is quite likely that some previously published cases of DILE, especially in association with hydralazine, would now be classified as ANCA-positive DIV (85,89,90).

Because investigations into possible drug-induced ANCA-positive vasculitis began relatively recently, other drugs will likely be found to cause this subset of DIV. Further understanding the role of ANCA testing in the evaluation of possible ADRs could be an important advance in methods to determine causality of some cases of DIV.

VIII. DIAGNOSIS

Clinicians faced with a potential case of vasculitis should have a high index of suspicion for the possibility of DIV and then work simultaneously on three fronts: (1) firmly establish the diagnosis, whether vasculitis or another condition; (2) determine the extent of disease; and (3) establish an accurate and complete drug exposure history (Table 5).

A. Tissue Biopsy

Unless a nonvasculitis diagnosis is made or highly specific testing such as a positive ANCA, an active urinary sediment with red blood cell casts, or a characteristic angiogram are found, tissue diagnosis is usually required for DIV. Since skin lesions are common and easily biopsied, this is usually the first tissue sampled. Skin pathology can not only document active vasculitis, but also can identify other considered diagnoses, including cutaneous polyarteritis nodosa, Sweet's syndrome, pyoderma gangrenosum, calciphylaxis, cholesterol emboli, various infections, thrombosis, and other entities. In addition to routine histological stains, skin tissue should be sent for immunofluorescence, microbial stains and cultures, and occasionally for electron microscopy. Other tissues may need to be biopsied to establish a diagnosis of vasculitis, depending on the clinical situation.

B. Laboratory Testing

Although there are no pathognomic laboratory findings of DIV, many test results help establish an alternative diagnosis and guide therapy. Drug-induced vasculitis is usually a diagnosis of ex-

Table 5 Guidelines for Obtaining Comprehensive Drug Exposures Histories on Patients with Possible Drug-Induced Vasculitis

---

Pursue drug histories immediately as the "trail" gets "cold" quickly as patients forget key details.

Request assistance from family, friends, other clinicians, and pharmacists associated with the patient.

Inquire about details on drug histories for at least the preceding 6 months, perhaps more.

Ask about exact drug start and stop dates and their temporal relation to the onset or resolution of key signs and symptoms of disease.

Attempt to determine both exposure and drug singularity.

Seek details of:
  Prescription medications
  Over-the-counter preparations (listing each ingredient)
  Herbs, supplements, and vitamins
  "Natural" or "alternative" products
  Illegal drugs and diluents/contaminants.

---

clusion in the setting of proper timing of a candidate drug. Thus, a series of tests for vasculitis are usually performed prior to establishing this diagnosis. These tests should include complete blood counts with lymphocyte differential, liver and renal function tests, urinalysis, quantitative C3 and C4 complement measures, serum and urine protein electrophoreses, and tests for the presence of cryoglobulins. Serological studies for antinuclear antibodies, rheumatoid factor, hepatitis B and C antigens, syphilis, and antibodies to human immunodeficiency viruses should be considered in the appropriate clinical settings. Blood cultures should be obtained, especially if endocarditis is being considered. Antineutrophil cytoplasmic antibodies (ANCAs) should be tested for by both immunofluorescence and antigen-specific ELISAs for antibodies to myeloperoxidase and proteinase 3.

Clinicians should also consider ordering a blood and/or urine toxicology screen for illegal drugs and controlled substances. These screens often also include over-the-counter sympathomimetics and other agents. Toxicology screens may reveal drug use not otherwise suspected or acknowledged.

Acute phase reactants should not be used as screening tests for vasculitis, including drug-associated cases. In a series of patients with cutaneous vasculitis of various causes, including drug-induced disease, Ekenstam and Callen (6) noted elevated erythrocyte sedimentation rates in only 60% of patients. Additionally, most of the diseases in the differential diagnosis of DIV, especially infections, are generally associated with elevated acute phase reactants, further indicating the lack of diagnostic utility of these tests in this setting.

C. Reporting Adverse Drug Reactions

Clinicians and pharmacists are strongly encouraged to report all cases of possible, probable, or certain DIV to the United States Food and Drug Administration (FDA) or the equivalent monitoring agency in their country. The FDA maintains "MedWatch," a large program for reporting all types of ADRs on old and new drugs, biologicals, supplements, and medical devices (http://www.fda.gov/medwatch/; 800-FDA-1088). Other countries and many hospitals and clinics also have their own ADR reporting systems to aid clinicians. Methods specifically addressing causality assessment in ADRs have also been published (114). Only through comprehensive postmarketing surveillance will more accurate and useful data on ADRs, including DIV, be available to clinicians and their patients.

IX. MANAGEMENT

The precise management of DIV is not clear, but general guidelines can be offered based on the literature. Drug manufacturers may also have unpublished information available to aid clinicians, especially for newly released drugs. Treatment decisions in cases of DIV should be made only after considering the extent of disease, rate of progression or remission, the risks of treatment for an individual patient, and the reported experience with DIV from the specific causative agent.

A. Management of Causative Agents

The first step in treatment of DIV is withdrawal of the putative causative agent. If DIV is suspected but drug singularity can not be established, then it is prudent to discontinue multiple drugs simultaneously. The action of most medications can be duplicated by substitute agents. The rate of drug elimination after the last dose varies widely among different drugs and also depends on patients' renal and hepatic functions. It seems reasonable to make efforts at increasing the elimination and metabolism of putative causative agents in cases of DIV. However, given that DIV may be the result of an already established immune activation, such efforts may be less imperative than in cases of overdose with a drug that has direct toxic effects.

Withdrawal of causative agents in cases of DIV may result in full clinical resolution without any other interventions. This may be especially true in cases of DIV limited to the skin. The resolution of vasculitis after such dechallenges provides additional evidence for causality.

Reintroduction of causative agents after resolution is not recommended. There are many documented cases of recurrent vasculitis upon drug rechallenge. Whether patients who have had DIV need to avoid other drugs from the same or a similar pharmaceutical class as the causative agent is not known, but such action should be avoided if feasible. The dangers of drug desensitization are not clear, but this practice certainly entails risk and should only be attempted when substitute medications are not available for serious clinical problems. In cases where multiple drugs where discontinued simultaneously, further data often become available either favoring causality of one agent or eliminating other agents as possible candidates. Such information may allow physicians to comfortably represcribe some of the agents previously discontinued.

B. Immunosuppressive Therapy

While drug withdrawal alone may be sufficient in some cases, it is important to remember that DIV can result in widespread disease and lead to significant morbidity and death. Glucocorticoids and immunosuppressive/cytotoxic therapy are often prescribed in cases of DIV, especially for patients with systemic involvement and in refractory cases. Glucocorticoids alone may be appropriate for cases limited to skin, although it is uncertain whether this approach actually changes the long-term outcome of patients. Treatment is often begun prior to firm establishment of the diagnosis of systemic DIV when other forms of vasculitis are considered possible. Once begun, glucocorticoids or cytotoxic agents may not need to be given as long for DIV as for other forms of vasculitis.

The subset of patients with ANCA-positive DIV may have some unique features that affect treatment decisions. These patients may have major organ system disease, including renal or respiratory failure, and many often have been treated with both glucocorticoids and cyclophosphamide. Furthermore, the possibility of drug-induced disease may not be considered because the clinical picture fits well with idiopathic Wegener's granulomatosis or microscopic polyangiitis (17).

It is important to maintain quite close clinical surveillance of patients with DIV, even after treatment cessation. Not only might recurrent flares of DIV occur, but withdrawal of therapy might also reveal an underlying chronic vasculitis that was misdiagnosed as DIV at first.

X. PATHOGENESIS

The exact pathogenesis of DIV is not yet known, but there is some evidence suggesting these ADRs occur through a combination of alterations in humoral and/or cellular immunity in the context of drug-specific and patient-related factors. It is also possible that different drugs result in DIV through different mechanisms.

Actual evidence of a precise immunological basis for DIV is lacking (7,12,23,115). While immune complexes are found in some cases with DIV, the more commonly seen lymphocytic infiltrates suggest that cellular immunity may also play an important role. Various drugs may provoke different mechanisms and, in many cases, multiple immunological pathways may be involved. Histological findings are also likely to differ based on the timing of biopsies.

Individual patient-related factors may also play a role in the development of DIV from specific drugs. Different genetic predispositions leading to variations in the pharmacokinetics of drug metabolism, distribution, and elimination may exist among people exposed to the same drug. Comorbidities and coingestion of other drugs may contribute to an individual's susceptibility to various ADRs including DIV.

XI. SUMMARY

Drug-induced vasculitis occurs as an adverse drug reaction to multiple different agents from almost every pharmacological class. The timing of DIV ranges from a few days to months or more. Clinical manifestations range from cutaneous-only presentations to multiorgan system involvement and death. The clinical spectrum of DIV encompasses those manifestations seen among the various primary inflammatory vasculitides. No tests are specific for the diagnosis of DIV, and proving causality in a single case or for a specific medication requires a vigilant evaluation process. The number of new pharmaceutical agents introduced to clinical practice is rapidly increasing and is far more than the number of drugs withdrawn from use. Therefore, it is reasonable to assume the spectrum of DIV will only expand in the coming years. Further identification of markers of disease will help both diagnostically and therapeutically. Treatment is based on drug withdrawal and selective use of glucocorticoids and cytotoxic agents. The best protection patients have from suffering morbidity due to DIV is an increased awareness of the varied presentations of DIV among treating physicians and a low threshold to consider the diagnosis in patients presenting with signs or symptoms of vasculitis. Prompt diagnosis should lead to improved clinical outcome.

REFERENCES

1. Zeek PM. Periarteritis nodosa: A critical review. Am J Clin Pathol 1952; 22:777–790.
2. Zeek PM, Smith CC, Weeter JC. Studies on periarteritis nodosa III. The differentiation between the vascular lesions of periarteritis nodosa and of hypersensitivity. Am J Pathol 1948; 24:889–917.
3. Calabrese LH, Michel BA, Bloch DA, Arend WP, Edworthy SM, Fauci AS, Fries JF, Hunder GG, Leavitt RY, Lie JT, Lightfoot RW, Jr., Masi AT, McShane DJ, Mills JA, Stevens MB, Wallace SL, Zvaifler NJ. The American College of Rheumatology 1990 criteria for the classification of hypersensitivity vasculitis. Arthritis Rheum 1990; 33:1108–1113.
4. Jennette JC, Falk RJ, Andrassy K, Bacon PA, Churg J, Gross WL, Hagen EC, Hoffman GS, Hunder GG, Kallenberg CGM, McCluskey RT, Sinco RA, Rees AJ, van ES LA, Waldherr R, Wiik A. Nomenclature of systemic vasculitis: Proposal of an international conference. Arthritis Rheum 1994; 37: 187–192.
5. Winkelmann RK. The spectrum of cutaneous vasculitis. Clin Rheum Dis 1980; 6:413–452.
6. Ekenstam E, Callen JP. Cutaneous leukocytoclastic vasculitis. Clinical and laboratory features of 82 patients seen in private practice. Arch Dermatol 1984; 120:484–489.
7. Haber MM, Marboe CC, Fenoglio JJ. Vasculitis in drug reactions and serum sickness. In: Churg A, Churg J, eds. Systemic Vasculitides. New York: Igaku-Shoin, 1991:305–313.
8. Garcia-Porrua C, Gonzalez-Gay MA, Lopez-Lazaro L. Drug associated cutaneous vasculitis in adults in northwestern Spain. J Rheumatol 1999; 26:1942–1944.
9. Gibson LE, van Hale HM, Schroeter AL. Direct immunofluorescence for the study of cutaneous drug eruptions. Acta Derm Venereol 1986; 66:39–44.
10. Citron BP, Halpern M, McCarron M, Lundberg GD, McCormick R, Pincus IJ, Tatter D, Haverback BJ. Necrotizing angiitis associated with drug abuse. N Engl J Med 1970; 283:1003–1011.
11. Mullick-FG, McAllister HA Jr, Wagner BM, Fenoglio JJ Jr. Drug related vasculitis: Clinicopathologic correlations in 30 patients. Hum Pathol 1979; 10:313–325.
12. Dubost JJ, Souteyrand P, Sauvezie B. Drug-induced vasculitides. Baillieres Clin Rheumatol 1991; 5:119–138.

13. Jain KK. Drug-induced cutaneous vasculitis. Adverse Drug React Toxicol Rev 1993; 12:263–276.
14. Roujeau JC, Stern RS. Severe adverse cutaneous reactions to drugs. N Engl J Med 1994; 331:1272–1285.
15. Somer T, Finegold SM. Vasculitides associated with infections, immunization, and antimicrobial drugs. Clin Infect Dis 1995; 20:1010–1036.
16. Merkel P. Drugs Associated with Vasculitis. Curr Opin Rheumatol 1998; 10:45–50.
17. Choi HK, Merkel PA, Walker AM, Niles JL. Drug-associated ANCA-positive vasculitis: Prevalence among patients with high titers of anti-myeloperoxidase antibodies. Arthritis Rheum 2000; 43:405–413.
18. Winkelmann RK, Ditto WB. Cutaneous and visceral syndromes of necrotizing or "allergic" angiitis: A study of 38 cases. Medicine 1964; 43:59–89.
19. Gower RG, Sams WM, Jr., Thorne EG, Kohler PF, Claman HN. Leukocytoclastic vasculitis: Sequential appearance of immunoreactants and cellular changes in serial biopsies. J Invest Dermatol 1977; 69:477–484.
20. Zeek PM. Periarteritis nodosa and other forms of necrotizing angiitis. N Engl J Med 1953; 248:764–772.
21. Massa MC, Su WP. Lymphocytic vasculitis: Is it a specific clinicopathologic entity? J Cutan Pathol 1984; 11:132–139.
22. Soter NA, Mihm MC, Jr., Gigli I, Dvorak HF, Austen KF. Two distinct cellular patterns in cutaneous necrotizing angiitis. J Invest Dermatol 1976; 66:344–350.
23. McAllister HA, Jr. An overview of human arterial pathology. Toxicol Pathol 1989; 17:219–231.
24. Seidl LG, Thornton GF, Cluff LE. Epidemiological studies of adverse drug reactions. Am J Pub Health 1965; 55:1170–1175.
25. Irey NS. Teaching monograph. Tissue reactions to drugs. Am J Pathol 1976; 82:613–647.
26. Venulet J, Ciucci A, Berneker GC. Standardized assessment of drug-adverse reaction associations: Rationale and experience. Int J Clin Pharmacol Ther Toxicol 1980; 18:381–388.
27. Josefson D. Asthma drug linked with Churg-Strauss syndrome. Br Med J 1997; 315:330.
28. Holloway J, Ferriss J, Groff J, Craig TJ, Klinek M, Klinik M. Churg-Strauss syndrome associated with zafirlukast. J Am Osteopath Assoc 1998; 98:275–278.
29. Wechsler ME, Garpestad E, Flier SR, Kocher O, Weiland DA, Polito AJ, Klinek MM, Bigby TD, Wong GA, Helmers RA, Drazen JM. Pulmonary infiltrates, eosinophilia, and cardiomyopathy following corticosteroid withdrawal in patients with asthma receiving zafirlukast. JAMA 1998; 279:455–457.
30. Katz RS, Papernik M. Zafirlukast and Churg-Strauss syndrome [letter]. JAMA 1998; 279:1949.
31. Knoell DL, Lucas J, Allen JN. Churg-Strauss syndrome associated with zafirlukast. Chest 1998; 114:332–334.
32. Green RL, Vayonis AG. Churg-Strauss syndrome after zafirlukast in two patients not receiving systemic steroid treatment [letter]. Lancet 1999; 353:725–726.
33. Churg J, Churg A. Zafirlukast and Churg-Strauss syndrome [letter]. JAMA 1998; 279:1949–1950.
34. Wechsler ME, Drazen JM. Zafirlukast and Churg-Strauss syndrome [letter]. JAMA 1998; 279:1950.
35. Kinoshita M, Shiraishi T, Koga T, Ayabe M, Rikimaru T, Oizumi K. Churg-Strauss syndrome after corticosteroid withdrawal in an asthmatic patient treated with pranlukast. J Allergy Clin Immunol 1999; 103:534–535.
36. Wechsler ME, Pauwels R, Drazen JM. Leukotriene modifiers and Churg-Strauss syndrome: Adverse effect or response to corticosteroid withdrawal? Drug Saf 1999; 21:241–251.
37. Blumberg S, Bienfang D, Kantrowitz FG. A possible association between influenza vaccination and small-vessel vasculitis. Arch Intern Med 1980; 140:847–848.
38. Mader R, Narendran A, Lewtas J, Bykerk V, Goodman RC, Dickson JR, Keystone EC. Systemic vasculitis following influenza vaccination: Report of 3 cases and literature review. J Rheumatol 1993; 20:1429–1431.
39. Allen MB, Cockwell P, Page RL. Pulmonary and cutaneous vasculitis following hepatitis B vaccination. Thorax 1993; 48:580–581.
40. Kelsall JT, Chalmers A, Sherlock CH, Tron VA, Kelsall AC. Microscopic polyangiitis after influenza vaccination. J Rheumatol 1997; 24:1198–1202.

41. Guillevin L, Cohen P, Gayraud M, Lhote F, Jarrousse B, Casassus P. Churg-Strauss syndrome. Clinical study and long-term follow-up of 96 patients. Medicine 1999; 78:26–37.

42. Le Hello C, Cohen P, Bousser MG, Letellier P, Guillevin L. Suspected hepatitis B vaccination related vasculitis. J Rheumatol 1999; 26:191–194.

43. Avery RK. Vaccination of the immunosuppressed adult patient with rheumatologic disease. Rheum Dis Clin North Am 1999; 25:567–584.

44. Kluin-Nelemans JC, Hollander AA, Fibbe WE, Heinhuis RJ, Brand A. Leucocytoclastic vasculitis during GM-CSF therapy. Br J Haematol 1989; 73:419–420.

45. Dreicer R, Schiller JH, Carbone PP. Granulocyte-macrophage colony-stimulating factor and vasculitis [letter]. Ann Intern Med 1989; 111:91–92.

46. Welte K, Zeidler C, Reiter A, Muller W, Odenwald E, Souza L, Riehm H. Differential effects of granulocyte-macrophage colony-stimulating factor and granulocyte colony-stimulating factor in children with severe congenital neutropenia. Blood 1990; 75:1056–1063.

47. Yang YM, Mankad VN, Manci E. Granulocyte colony-stimulating factor associated leukocytoclastic vasculitis mimicking Henoch-Schönlein purpura [letter]. Pediatr Hematol Oncol 1993; 10:193–195.

48. Jain KK. Cutaneous vasculitis associated with granulocyte colony-stimulating factor. J Am Acad Derm 1994; 31:213–215.

49. Bonilla MA, Dale D, Zeidler C, Last L, Reiter A, Ruggeiro M, Davis M, Koci B, Hammond W, Gillio A, Welte K. Long-term safety of treatment with recombinant human granulocyte colony-stimulating factor (r-metHuG-CSF) in patients with severe congenital neutropenias. Br J Haematol 1994; 88:723–730.

50. Farhey YD, Herman JH. Vasculitis complicating granulocyte colony stimulating factor treatment of leukopenia and infection in Felty's syndrome. J Rheumatol 1995; 22:1179–1182.

51. Couderc LJ, Philippe B, Franck N, Balloul-Delclaux E, Lessana-Leibowitch M. Necrotizing vasculitis and exacerbation of psoriasis after granulocyte colony-stimulating factor for small cell lung carcinoma [letter]. Respir Med 1995; 89:237–238.

52. Euler HH, Harten P, Zeuner RA, Schwab UM. Recombinant human granulocyte colony stimulating factor in patients with systemic lupus erythematosus associated neutropenia and refractory infections. J Rheumatol 1997; 24:2153–2157.

53. Stanworth SJ, Bhavnani M, Chattopadhya C, Miller H, Swinson DR. Treatment of Felty's syndrome with the haemopoietic growth factor granulocyte colony-stimulating factor (G-CSF). Q J Med 1998; 91:49–56.

54. Glaspy JA, Baldwin GC, Robertson PA, Souza L, Vincent M, Ambersley J, Golde DW. Therapy for neutropenia in hairy cell leukemia with recombinant human granulocyte colony-stimulating factor. Ann Intern Med 1988; 109:789–795.

55. Park JW, Mehrotra B, Barnett BO, Baron AD, Venook AP. The Sweet syndrome during therapy with granulocyte colony-stimulating factor. Ann Intern Med 1992; 116:996–998.

56. Paydas S, Sahin B, Seyrek E, Soylu M, Gonlusen G, Acar A, Tuncer I. Sweet's syndrome associated with G-CSF. Br J Haematol 1993; 85:191–192.

57. van Kamp H, van den Berg E, Timens W, Kraaijenbrink RA, Halie MR, Daenen SM. Sweet's syndrome in myeloid malignancy: a report of two cases. Br J Haematol 1994; 86:415–417.

58. Fukutoku M, Shimizu S, Ogawa Y, Takeshita S, Masaki Y, Arai T, Hirose Y, Sugai S, Konda S, Takiguchi T. Sweet's syndrome during therapy with granulocyte colony-stimulating factor in a patient with aplastic anaemia. Br J Haematol 1994; 86:645–648.

59. Johnson ML, Grimwood RE. Leukocyte colony-stimulating factors: A review of associated neutrophilic dermatoses and vasculitides. Arch Dermatol 1994; 130:77–81.

60. Ross HJ, Moy LA, Kaplan R, Figlin RA. Bullous pyoderma gangrenosum after granulocyte colony-stimulating factor treatment. Cancer 1991; 68:441–443.

61. Hellmich B, Schnabel A, Gross WL. Granulocyte colony-stimulating factor treatment for cyclophosphamide- induced severe neutropenia in Wegener's granulomatosis. Arthritis Rheum 1999; 42:1752–1756.

62. Buchbinder A, Adler H, Ballard H. An unusual and unreported toxicity to erythropoietin [letter]. Am J Hematol 1993; 42:412–413.

63. Kaye BR, Fainstat M. Cerebral vasculitis associated with cocaine abuse. JAMA 1987; 258:2104–2106.
64. Klonoff DC, Andrews BT, Obana WG. Stroke associated with cocaine use. Arch Neurol 1989; 46:989–993.
65. Krendel DA, Ditter SM, Frankel MR, Ross WK. Biopsy-proven cerebral vasculitis associated with cocaine abuse. Neurology 1990; 40:1092–1094.
66. Fredericks RK, Lefkowitz DS, Challa VR, Troost BT. Cerebral vasculitis associated with cocaine abuse. Stroke 1991; 22:1437–1439.
67. Enriquez R, Palacios FO, Gonzalez CM, Amoros FA, Cabezuelo JB, Hernandez F. Skin vasculitis, hypokalemia and acute renal failure in rhabdomyolysis associated with cocaine [letter]. Nephron 1991; 59:336–337.
68. Morrow PL, McQuillen JB. Cerebral vasculitis associated with cocaine abuse. J Forensic Sci 1993; 38:732–738.
69. Merkel PA, Koroshetz WJ, Irizarry MC, Cudkowicz ME. Cocaine-associated cerebral vasculitis. Semin Arthritis Rheum 1995; 25:172–183.
70. Gradon JD, Wityk R. Diagnosis of probable cocaine-induced cerebral vasculitis by magnetic resonance angiography. South Med J 1995; 88:1264–1266.
71. Chevalier X, Rostoker G, Larget-Piet B, Gherardi R. Schoenlein-Henoch purpura with necrotizing vasculitis after cocaine snorting [letter]. Clin Nephrol 1995; 43:348–349.
72. Orriols R, Munoz X, Ferrer J, Huget P, Morell F. Cocaine-induced Churg-Strauss vasculitis. Eur Respir J 1996; 9:175–177.
73. Kessler JT, Jortner BS, Adapon BD. Cerebral vasculitis in a drug abuser. J Clin Psychiatry 1978; 39:559–564.
74. Gendelman H, Linzer M, Barland P, Bezahler GH. Leukocytoclastic vasculitis in an intravenous heroin abuser. NY State J Med 1983; 83:984–986.
75. Montoliu J, Miro JM, Campistol JM, Trilla A, Mensa J, Torras A, Revert L. Henoch-Schönlein purpura complicating staphylococcal endocarditis in a heroin addict. Am J Nephrol 1987; 7:137–139.
76. Weiss SR, Raskind R, Morganstern NL, Pytlyk PJ, Baiz TC. Intracerebral and subarachnoid hemorrhage following use of methamphetamine ("speed"). Int Surg 1970; 53:123–127.
77. Stafford CR, Bogdanoff BM, Green L, Spector HB. Mononeuropathy multiplex as a complication of amphetamine angiitis. Neurology 1975; 25:570–572.
78. Wooten MR, Khangure MS, Murphy MJ. Intracerebral hemorrhage and vasculitis related to ephedrine abuse. Ann Neurol 1983; 13:337–340.
79. Glick R, Hoying J, Cerullo L, Perlman S. Phenylpropanolamine: An over-the-counter drug causing central nervous system vasculitis and intracerebral hemorrhage. Case report and review. Neurosurgery 1987; 20:969–974.
80. Forman HP, Levin S, Stewart B, Patel M, Feinstein S. Cerebral vasculitis and hemorrhage in an adolescent taking diet pills containing phenylpropanolamine: Case report and review of literature. Pediatrics 1989; 83:737–741.
81. Yin PA. Ephedrine-induced intracerebral hemorrhage and central nervous system vasculitis [letter]. Stroke 1990; 21:1641.
82. Gross WL. Antineutrophil cytoplasmic autoantibody testing in vasculitis. Rheum Dis Clin North Am 1995; 21:987–1011.
83. Niles JL. Antineutrophil cytoplasmic autoantibodies in the classification of vasculitis. Annu Rev Med 1996; 47:303–313.
84. Falk RJ, Jennette JC. ANCA small-vessel vasculitis. J Am Soc Nephrol 1997; 8:314–322.
85. Nassberger L, Sjoholm AG, Jonsson H, Sturfelt G, Akesson A. Autoantibodies against neutrophil cytoplasm components in systemic lupus erythematosus and in hydralazine-induced lupus. Clin Exp Immunol 1990; 81:380–383.
86. Nassberger L, Sjoholm AG, Thysell H. Antimyeloperoxidase antibodies in patients with extracapillary glomerulonephritis. Nephron 1990; 56:152–156.
87. Nassberger L, Johansson AC, Bjorck S, Sjoholm AG. Antibodies to neutrophil granulocyte myeloperoxidase and elastase: Autoimmune responses in glomerulonephritis due to hydralazine treatment. J Intern Med 1991; 229:261–265.

88. Almroth G, Enestrom S, Hed J, Samuelsson I, Sjostrom P. Autoantibodies to leucocyte antigens in hydralazine-associated nephritis. J Internal Med 1992; 231:37–42.

89. Pedrollo E, Bleil L, Bautz FA, Kalden JR, Bautz EK. Antineutrophil cytoplasmic autoantibodies (ANCA) recognizing a recombinant myeloperoxidase subunit. Adv Exp Med Biol 1993; 336: 87–92.

90. Cambridge G, Wallace H, Bernstein RM, Leaker B. Autoantibodies to myeloperoxidase in idiopathic and drug-induced systemic lupus erythematosus and vasculitis. Br J Rheumatol 1994; 33:109–114.

91. Short AK, Lockwood CM. Antigen specificity in hydralazine associated ANCA positive systemic vasculitis. Q J Med 1995; 88:775–783.

92. Dolman KM, Gans RO, Vervaat TJ, Zevenbergen G, Maingay D, Nikkels RE, Donker AJ, von dem Borne AE, Goldschmeding R. Vasculitis and antineutrophil cytoplasmic autoantibodies associated with propylthiouracil therapy. Lancet 1993; 342:651–652.

93. Vogt BA, Kim Y, Jennette JC, Falk RJ, Burke BA, Sinaiko A. Antineutrophil cytoplasmic autoantibody-positive crescentic glomerulonephritis as a complication of treatment with propylthiouracil in children. J Pediatr 1994; 124:986–988.

94. D'Cruz D, Chesser AM, Lightowler C, Comer M, Hurst MJ, Baker LR, Raine AE. Antineutrophil cytoplasmic antibody-positive crescentic glomerulonephritis associated with anti-thyroid drug treatment. Br J Rheumatol 1995; 34:1090–1091.

95. Tanemoto M, Miyakawa H, Hanai J, Yago M, Kitaoka M, Uchida S. Myeloperoxidase-antineutrophil cytoplasmic antibody-positive crescentic glomerulonephritis complicating the course of Graves' disease: Report of three adult cases. Am J Kidney Dis 1995; 26:774–780.

96. Yuasa S, Hashimoto M, Yura T, Sumikura T, Takahashi N, Shoji T, Uchida K, Fujioka H, Kihara M, Matsuo H. Antineutrophil cytoplasmic antibodies (ANCA)-associated crescentic glomerulonephritis and propylthiouracil therapy. Nephron 1996; 73:701–703.

97. Kitahara T, Hiromura K, Maezawa A, Ono K, Narabara N, Yano S, Naruse T, Takenouchi K, Yasumoto Y. Case of propylthiouracil-induced vasculitis associated with anti-neutrophil cytoplasmic antibody (ANCA): Review of literature. Clin Nephrol 1997; 47:336–340.

98. Pillinger M, Staud R. Wegener's granulomatosis in a patient receiving propylthiouracil for Graves' disease. Semin Arthritis Rheum 1998; 28:124–129.

99. Choi HK, Merkel PA, Tervaert JW, Black RM, McCluskey RT, Niles JL. Alternating antineutrophil cytoplasmic antibody specificity: Drug-induced vasculitis in a patient with Wegener's granulomatosis. Arthritis Rheum 1999; 42:384–388.

100. Kawachi Y, Nukaga H, Hoshino M, Iwata M, Otsuka F. ANCA-associated vasculitis and lupus-like syndrome caused by methimazole. Clin Exp Dermatol 1995; 20:345–347.

101. Hori Y, Arizono K, Hara S, Kawai R, Hara M, Yamada A. Antineutrophil cytoplasmic autoantibody-positive crescentic glomerulonephritis associated with thiamazole therapy [letter]. Nephron 1996; 74:734–735.

102. Jones BF, Major GA. Crescentic glomerulonephritis in a patient taking penicillamine associated with antineutrophil cytoplasmic antibody [letter]. Clin Nephrol 1992; 38:293.

103. Endo H, Hosono T, Kondo H. Antineutrophil cytoplasmic autoantibodies in 6 patients with renal failure and systemic sclerosis. J Rheumatol 1994; 21:864–870.

104. Gaskin G, Thompson EM, Pusey CD. Goodpasture-like syndrome associated with anti-myeloperoxidase antibodies following penicillamine treatment. Nephrol Dial Transplant 1995; 10:1925–1928.

105. Mathieson PW, Peat DS, Short A, Watts RA. Coexistent membranous nephropathy and ANCA-positive crescentic glomerulonephritis in association with penicillamine. Nephrol Dial Transplant 1996; 11:863–866.

106. Locke IC, Worrall JG, Leaker B, Black CM, Cambridge G. Autoantibodies to myeloperoxidase in systemic sclerosis. J Rheumatol 1997; 24:86–89.

107. Elkayam O, Yaron M, Caspi D. Minocycline induced arthritis associated with fever, livedo reticularis, and pANCA. Ann Rheum Dis 1996; 55:769–771.

108. Gaffney K, Merry P. Antineutrophil cytoplasmic antibody-positive polyarthritis associated with minocycline therapy [letter]. Br J Rheumatol 1996; 35:1327.

109. Jaunkalns R, Shear NH, Sokoluk B, Gardner D, Claas F, Uetrecht JP. Antimyeloperoxidase antibodies and adverse reactions to clozapine [letter]. Lancet 1992; 339:1611–1612.

110. Shih DJ, Korbet SM, Rydel JJ, Schwartz MM. Renal vasculitis associated with ciprofloxacin. Am J Kidney Dis 1995; 26:516–519.

111. Caulier M, Dromer C, Andrieu V, Le Guennec P, Fournie B. Sulfasalazine induced lupus in rheumatoid arthritis. J Rheumatol 1994; 21:750–751.

112. Choi HK, Merkel PA, Niles JL. ANCA-positive vasculitis associated with allopurinol therapy. Clin Exp Rheumatol 1998; 16:743–744.

113. Parry RG, Gordon P, Mason JC, Marley NJ. Phenytoin-associated vasculitis and ANCA positivity: A case report. Nephrol Dial Transplant 1996; 11:357–359.

114. Venulet J, Ciucci AG, Berneker GC. Updating of a method for causality assessment of adverse drug reactions. Int J Clin Pharmacol Ther Toxicol 1986; 24:559–568.

115. Fauci AS, Haynes B, Katz P. The spectrum of vasculitis: Clinical, pathologic, immunologic and therapeutic considerations. Ann Intern Med 1978; 89:660–676.

50
Inflammatory Aspects of Acute Coronary Syndromes

Giovanna Liuzzo, Luigi M. Biasucci, and Attilio Maseri
Catholic University of Sacred Heart, Rome, Italy

I. INTRODUCTION

Growing evidence indicates that atherosclerosis is a dynamic process, with an important inflammatory component. In patients, quantitative differences in the inflammatory component have been observed in acute coronary syndromes compared with stable atherosclerosis, suggesting that the inflammation plays a role in the pathogenesis of atherosclerosis. The process of atherosclerosis as proposed by Ross (1) is a "response to injury." In this theory, atherosclerosis is the result of an excessive inflammatory–fibroproliferative response to different forms of injury to the arterial wall. The process, once initiated, is regulated and sustained by a number of inflammatory mediators, such as cytokines, adhesion molecules, and growth factors, and involves all the cellular elements with inflammatory properties, such as T lymphocytes, macrophages, neutrophils, and mast cells, as well as activated endothelial cells and smooth muscle cells. Cytokines, adhesion molecules, and other inflammatory mediators typical of immune interactions, have also been found to be increased in the peripheral circulation of patients with atherosclerosis, suggesting that at least some of the mechanisms are not confined to the arterial wall, but may have a systemic "reverberation."

II. INFLAMMATION AND ATHEROGENESIS

In patients with acute coronary syndromes, coronary atherosclerotic plaques include the presence of activated macrophages, lymphocytes, and mast cells (2–13). Quantitative, rather than qualitative, differences in inflammatory components were observed in patients with acute coronary syndromes compared with stable patients (14) and unselected patients with aortic and coronary atherosclerotic lesions of variable severity (15), suggesting that the inflammatory infiltrates are largely related to the underlying pathogenesis of atherosclerosis.

Different causes of arterial injury include hypercholesterolemia with oxidized low-density lipoproteins (LDLs), hyperhomocysteinemia, hypertension, cigarette smoking, diabetes, viral and bacterial infections, and immune complex deposition. In hypercholesterolemic animal models, the first morphological evidence of disease is the attachment of monocytes to endothelium (1) via specific adhesive glycoproteins (VCAM-1, ELAM-1) on endothelial cells. These adhesive molecules play a pivotal role in attachment and migration of monocytes and T lymphocytes across the endothelial barrier. The process is under the influence of growth-regulatory molecules and chemoattractants released by altered endothelium, adherent leukocytes, and possibly underlying smooth muscle cells. Recent studies have raised the intriguing question of whether infectious agents, such as *Chlamydia pneumoniae*, *Helicobacter pylori* and cytomegalovirus may be responsible for the initiation and progression of atherosclerotic disease (16–21).

The fate of the initial atherosclerotic plaque is largely influenced by the local and systemic inflammatory response. Mature atherosclerotic plaques develop from proliferation of smooth muscle cells, macrophages, and possibly lymphocytes (1). In many mature plaques, there are two different but not independent regions: the "fibrous cap," rich in collagen fibers and smooth muscle cells, and the "core," which is rich in foam cells, macrophages, and cellular necrotic debris. There is evidence that macrophages and lymphocytes infiltrating the plaque are activated (6,15). T lymphocytes have been show to be CD4+ helper and CD8+ cytotoxic cells, present in approximately equal numbers, and activated as memory CD45RO+ cells expressing HLA-DR antigen (6,15,22). Lymphocytes in plaque produce interferon-γ (IFN-γ), a pleiotropic cytokine that activates macrophages that produce matrix-degrading proteases and inhibits collagen secretion by smooth muscle cells (23–27). Protease-producing macrophages and mast cells are particularly abundant in the shoulder regions of the plaque, where their enzymes may contribute to plaque rupture (8–13). Macrophages, as well as circulating monocytes, also produce proinflammatory cytokines, such as interleukin (IL)-1, IL-6 and tumor necrosis factor-α (TNF-α), which activate the endothelium, have procoagulant properties, and may activate neutrophils (Fig. 1) (28–31).

Although the processes involved in plaque formation and growth have received great attention, the triggers that shift the chronic stable phase of atherosclerotic disease to an acute coronary syndrome remain elusive.

III. TRANSITION FROM STABLE PLAQUE
TO UNSTABLE CORONARY SYNDROMES

When examining the relation between coronary atherosclerosis and ischemic syndromes, a major discrepancy emerges. Many patients with very severe atherosclerosis remain stable for years without developing myocardial infarction or unstable angina. Other patients develop myocardial infarction or unstable angina as the very first manifestation of ischemic heart disease, and they may have less extensive and severe coronary atherosclerosis (32). Local and systemic markers of inflammation appear to correlate better with acute coronary syndromes than with the severity of coronary atherosclerosis (33).

Unstable coronary syndromes are clinically characterized by sudden onset or stuttering recurrence of ischemic episodes over a period of weeks or even months. This may evolve to either myocardial infarction or, conversely, a stable or even quiescent phase of ischemic heart disease. In acute coronary syndromes, thrombosis has become the fundamental target for therapy. Understanding why coronary thrombosis becomes a mechanism of disease, instead of remaining a self-limiting step in vascular repair, would open the way to additional novel forms of therapy. In principle, thrombosis can develop in response to two types of stimuli: (1) a fissure of an atherosclerotic plaque caused by purely mechanical forces (in this case the size of thrombus is determined by the thrombogenicity of the fissure), and (2) inflammatory activation of the vessel wall (in this case, the growth of thrombus is proportional to the intensity and duration of inflammation). The two causes are not mutually exclusive and, in both cases, the final acute occlusion of the vessel is also determined by the hemostatic and by the local vasoconstrictor response (32).

Inflammatory cytokines can cause a persistent waxing and waning activation of endothelium, abolishing its antithrombotic and vasodilator properties. They can also directly promote

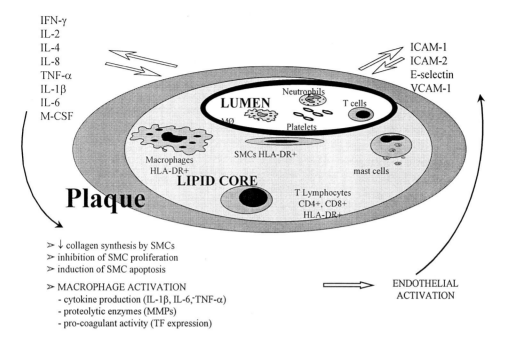

IFN-γ
IL-2
IL-4
IL-8
TNF-α
IL-1β
IL-6
M-CSF

ICAM-1
ICAM-2
E-selectin
VCAM-1

LUMEN   Neutrophils   T cells

MΦ   Platelets

Macrophages
HLA-DR+

SMCs HLA-DR+

mast cells

LIPID CORE

Plaque

T Lymphocytes
CD4+, CD8+
HLA-DR+

➢ ↓ collagen synthesis by SMCs
➢ inhibition of SMC proliferation
➢ induction of SMC apoptosis

➢ MACROPHAGE ACTIVATION
  - cytokine production (IL-1β, IL-6, TNF-α)
  - proteolytic enzymes (MMPs)
  - pro-coagulant activity (TF expression)

ENDOTHELIAL
ACTIVATION

Figure 1 Atherosclerotic plaque contains inflammatory cells. Activated macrophages and lymphocytes have been found in the atherosclerotic plaque. T lymphocytes have been shown to be CD4+ helper and CD8+ cytotoxic cells, which are present in similar proportions and are memory (CD45RO+) cells, expressing HLA-DR antigen (sign of recent activation). Plaque-related lymphocytes mainly produce interferon-γ (IFN-γ), a pleiotropic cytokine that activates macrophages, which synthesize matrix-degrading proteases and inhibit collagen secretion by smooth muscle cells. Macrophages and mast cells are particularly abundant in the shoulder regions of the plaque, which are more prone to rupture. It is through the synthesis of macrophage and mast cell proteases that these cells may contribute to plaque rupture. Macrophages, as well as circulating monocytes, also produce proinflammatory cytokines, such as interleukin (IL)-1, IL-6, and tumor necrosis factor (TNF)-α, which activate the endothelium and have procoagulant properties.

thrombosis, vasoconstriction, and activation of metalloproteases, which digest intercellular matrix, increase vascular permeability, and cause detachment of endothelial cells and lysis of the cap of vulnerable plaques at their thinnest site (34).

Only a minority of acute coronary thrombi are composed of red cells and fibrin, which would be indicative of their development in the presence of blood flow stasis or intense thrombogenic stimuli. The majority of thrombi are largely composed of platelets, which implies their gradual formation in flowing blood in response to weak, but persistent thrombogenic stimuli. In acute coronary syndromes, such thrombi are often multiple and sometimes multilayered, suggesting multiple recurrent thrombogenic stimuli. Recurring, multiple platelet thrombi could be due to diffuse and recurring inflammatory reactions. This would be more plausible than purely mechanical injury. It would also more easily explain the common fluctuations in instability over a period of days and weeks (33).

Several histological studies have shown that inflammatory cells infiltrate acute coronary thrombi, which may lead to plaque fissure (Table 1) (2–13). However, coronary plaques with inflammatory cell infiltrates are also found in stable angina patients (14) and in accident victims

Table 1 Local and Systemic Signs of Inflammation in Acute Coronary Syndromes

---

INFLAMMATORY INFILTRATES OF ATHEROSCLEROTIC PLAQUES
Activated lymphocytes (CD4+ and CD8+ T cells, CD45RO+, HLA-DR+) and macrophages (HLA-DR+)
  Localized to the culprit lesion
  Spread to multiple coronary sites
ACTIVATED CIRCULATING LEUKOCYTES
  Lymphocytes: HLA-DR+, CD25+, IFN-+, IL-2 soluble receptor
  Monocytes: integrin up-regulation, tissue factor expression
  Neutrophils: integrin up-regulation, elastase, neutrophil degranulation, reduced intracellular myeloper-
    oxidase content
ELEVATED LEVELS OF SOLUBLE INFLAMMATORY MARKERS
  Acute phase proteins: fibrinogen, CRP, SAA
  Cytokines: IL-6, TNF-, IL-1Ra
  Adhesion molecules: soluble VCAM-1, soluble ICAM-1, soluble E-selectin
  Others: ceruloplasmin, neopterin, heat shock proteins
POSSIBLE SYSTEMIC SIGNS OF INFLAMMATION IN ACUTE CORONARY SYNDROMES
  Part of the inflammatory response to atherosclerosis
  A consequence of acute ischemia
  A pathogenetic component associated with prognosis

---

without ischemic symptoms (7,15,35). Thus, inflammation, under some conditions, may contribute to the development of atherosclerosis; in other circumstances it may cause acute activation of the vascular wall with consequent local thrombosis and vasoconstriction, with or without plaque fissure. The incomplete specificity of stenosis severity, plaque fissure, the histological features, and the cellular alterations for acute ischemic syndromes suggest that the development of instability and the progression toward infarction may require the simultaneous presence of multiple pathogenetic components, one of which is represented by an inflammatory reaction (33).

An intriguing observation made at the time of bypass surgery is the finding of red streaks with perivascular inflammatory infiltrates along one or more coronary artery branches. This was noted in 21 of 200 patients with unstable angina (3). Patients with red streaks were indistinguishable clinically from those without red streaks. In some patients, the involvement of long segments of one or more coronary arteries, including those that were angiographically normal, suggests a diffuse process rather than localization to the site of a single coronary plaque.

IV. SYSTEMIC MARKERS OF INFLAMMATION IN UNSTABLE ANGINA AND ACUTE MYOCARDIAL INFARCTION

In many patients with unstable angina and acute myocardial infarction, systemic signs of inflammation are detectable (see Table 1). Thus, in acute coronary syndromes, the inflammatory process is not confined to the coronary plaque, but is systemic or at least has a systemic component. Moreover, systemic inflammatory markers, such as C-reactive protein, have an independent prognostic value, thus supporting the pathogenetic role of inflammation.

The existence of an acute inflammatory state in unstable angina and myocardial infarction is supported by clinical studies demonstrating increased urinary excretion of leukotrienes (36), activation of circulating neutrophils (37–40), lymphocytes (41,42), and monocytes (39,43), and elevated levels of acute-phase proteins in serum (44,45).

Mehta et al. (37) and Dinerman et al. (38) demonstrated 15-fold higher levels of a neutrophil elastase–derived fibrinopeptide B-beta in patients with unstable angina compared to controls and stable angina patients. Mazzone et al. (39) observed increased expression of neutrophil

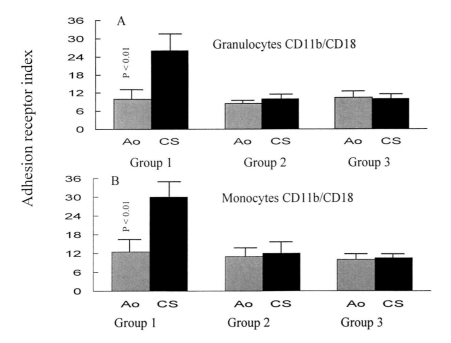

Figure 2 Expression of adhesion receptors in granulocytes and monocytes during their passage through the coronary circulation. CD11b/CD18 adhesion receptor expression is higher in granulocytes (A) and monocytes (B) sampled from the coronary sinus (CS) than in those sampled from the aorta (Ao) in unstable angina patients (Group 1), but not in stable angina patients (Group 2) or controls (Group 3). Thus, in unstable angina patients, leukocyte activation occurs during their passage through the coronary circulation. (Modified from Ref. 39.)

and monocyte adhesion molecules during the passage of these cells through the coronary circulation. This may have been due to endothelial activation (Fig. 2). Circulating neutrophils in patients with acute myocardial infarction and unstable angina were found to have evidence suggestive of activation (e.g., reduced myeloperoxidase content, indicative of a significant release of myeloperoxidase) (40).

Neri Serneri et al. (41) reported activation of monocytes by lymphocytes in unstable vs. stable patients. They proposed that unstable angina is associated with an acute transient inflammatory event with lymphocyte activation. These findings are supported by increased procoagulant activity in circulating monocytes (43), increases in circulating monocytes/macrophages and T lymphocytes with HLA-DR expression (42) and expression of HLA-DR antigens on adjacent smooth muscle cells in plaques beneath thrombi (8,9).

Vejar et al. (46) found that in patients with unstable angina, in whom platelet production of thromboxane A_2 was blocked by low-dose aspirin, urinary excretion of a thromboxane A_2 metabolite (11-dehydrothromboxane B_2) was often much higher than in stable patients undergoing coronary angioplasty, who were on a similar dose of aspirin (47). This observation suggests the possible origin of this metabolite from inflammatory cells in which thromboxane A_2 production is not inhibited by low-dose aspirin (48). Recently, thromboxane A_2 biosynthesis in unstable angina was examined as modified by two cyclooxygenase inhibitors differentially affecting cyclooxygenase 2, despite comparable impact on platelet cyclooxygenase 1 (49). Indobufen, which largely suppresses monocyte cyclooxygenase 2 activity at therapeutic plasma concentration, is more efficient in reducing urinary excretion of 11-dehydrothromboxane B_2 than aspirin in unstable angina (49).

V.   PROGNOSTIC VALUE OF ACUTE-PHASE PROTEINS

Increased concentrations of the highly sensitive acute-phase proteins, C-reactive protein (CRP) and serum amyloid A protein (SAA) (44,45), and of IL-6 and IL-1 receptor antagonist (IL-1Ra, a member of the IL-1 gene family) (50,51) were reported in patients with unstable angina. More interestingly, the intensity of the acute-phase response was shown to be closely related to the in-hospital outcome (45,50,51).

Several studies have reported elevated levels of acute-phase proteins in patients with un-stable angina (45,52,53) or myocardial infarction (54). We have examined whether CRP and SAA have prognostic value in severe unstable angina patients with normal troponin levels (45). On ad-mission, a value of CRP >0.3 mg/dL in patients with unstable angina had a sensitivity of 90% and a specificity of 82% for predicting subsequent in-hospital cardiac events such as cardiac death, myocardial infarction, or the urgent need for coronary revascularization. The sensitivity increased to 100% in patients with a value for CRP >1.0 mg/dL on admission and in those who had any in-crease in the CRP level during the study. In the same study, patients who presented with an acute myocardial infarction, with symptoms of <3 h duration, and a history of preceding unstable angina also had elevated levels of CRP (Fig. 3) (45). These data suggest that two different patient populations can be defined: one with high CRP and high risk, and one with low CRP and low risk. In the first population, an inflammatory reaction is likely to play an important role in altering the stable course of disease. A third population also exists, in which a severe course of disease is to-tally unrelated to inflammation, as in the majority of patients with unheralded myocardial infarc-tion (54); in these patients, other factors, such as mechanical plaque rupture, hypercoagulable state, or vasospasm, can trigger plaque instability (33). Similar data have been reported also by other groups (52,53), and it has been shown that the prognostic value of CRP is also maintained in the presence of elevated plasma levels of troponins, the major prognostic indicator for unsta-ble coronary syndromes (55,56).

Elevated levels of CRP imply an increased synthesis of these proteins, mainly in the liver, stimulated by proinflammatory cytokines (Fig. 4) (57). A recent study has demonstrated that ele-vated serum levels of IL-6 and IL-1Ra are common in unstable angina, correlate with CRP, and are related with prognosis, thus strengthening the importance of inflammation in unstable angina (Figs. 5 and 6) (50,51).

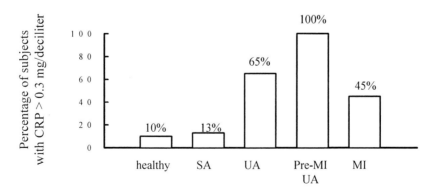

Figure 3   Systemic inflammation in acute coronary syndromes indicated by elevation of acute phase pro-teins. About 65% of patients with Braunwald class IIIB unstable angina (UA) have C-reactive protein (CRP) levels higher than 0.3 mg/dL (90th percentile of normal distribution). The percentage of patients with ele-vated CRP on admission increases to 100% in patients in whom myocardial infarction was preceded by un-stable angina (Pre-MI UA), but decrease to 45% in patients in whom myocardial infarction was totally un-heralded (MI). Stable angina (SA) patients do not significantly differ from healthy subjects. (Modified from Ref. 45.)

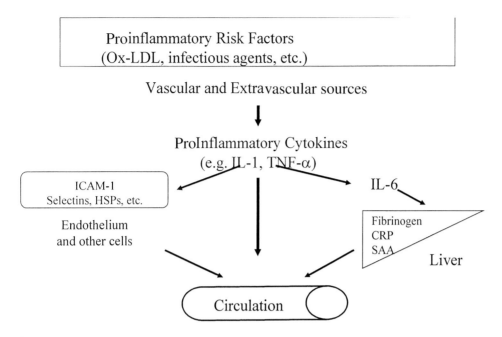

Figure 4 Circulating levels of serum inflammatory markers reflect the underlying inflammatory response. Inflammation, systemic or local, either in the blood vessel itself or elsewhere, triggers the production of proinflammatory cytokines (e.g., IL-1 or TNF-α). These cytokines can directly elicit production by endothelial cells, leukocytes, and other cells of adhesion molecules, procoagulants, and other mediators. Interleukin-1 or TNF-α can also stimulate the production of IL-6, which induces expression of hepatic genes encoding acute-phase reactants found in blood, including C-reactive protein (CRP), serum amyloid A protein (SAA), and fibrinogen. (Modified from Ref. 57.)

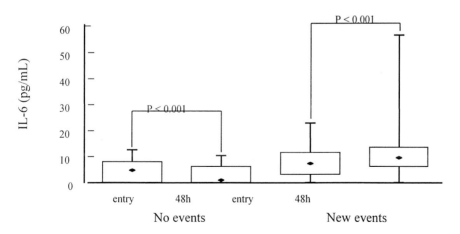

Figure 5 Increasing serum levels of IL-6 during hospitalization in unstable angina are associated with increased risk of coronary events. Elevated serum levels of IL-6 are common in patients with unstable angina, correlate with C-reactive protein levels, and are related to prognosis. Levels of IL-6 are higher at admission than after 48 h, although not significantly, in patients event-free during hospitalization. Conversely, patients with a complicated in-hospital course (death, myocardial infarction, refractory angina) have an increase of IL-6 after 48 h, despite the same medical therapy. Interleukin-6 levels are displayed as boxes and whiskers with median levels (•), 25% to 75% percentiles, and range. (Modified from Ref. 51.)

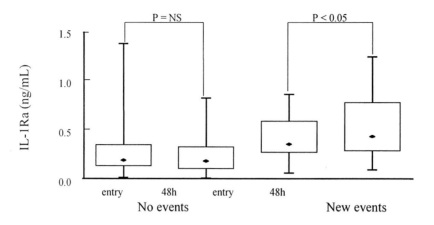

Figure 6 Increasing serum levels of IL-1 receptor antagonist (IL-1Ra) during hospitalization in unstable angina are associated with increased risk of coronary events. IL-1Ra is a member of the IL-1 gene family that can block IL-1 cell-surface receptors. As a member of the IL-1 gene family, its production increases under the same inflammatory conditions that stimulate IL-1 and IL-1. As IL-1Ra has a signal peptide and is readily secreted from cells into the circulation, measurement of this cytokine rather than IL-1 or IL-1 is a more reliable assessment of increased production of IL-1 family members. Patients with unstable angina and with worsening disease exhibit higher IL-1Ra levels than patients who do not experience an in-hospital event, despite the same medical therapy. In addition, a fall in IL-1Ra after 48 h is associated with a good outcome, and conversely, an additional increase is associated with a complicated in hospital-course (death, myocardial infarction, refractory angina). IL-1Ra levels are displayed as boxes and whiskers with median levels (•), 25% to 75% percentiles, and range. (Modified from Ref. 51.)

VI. INFLAMMATION IN ACUTE CORONARY SYNDROMES: A PRIMARY OR SECONDARY PHENOMENON?

An important issue to be investigated is the relevance of the acute inflammatory reaction that seems to differentiate unstable angina from stable angina. It needs to be determined if it is only a marker of instability and represents a response to endothelial disruption and thrombus formation, or if it is a primary pathological process in which lymphocyte and monocyte/macrophage activation cause myocardial ischemia and the occurrence of unstable angina via the formation of a variety of inflammatory mediators (see Table 1). Recently, data have given strong support to the notion that the inflammatory response in unstable angina is not an epiphenomenon. It cannot be attributed to minor degrees of myocardial cell necrosis, a potent stimulus of acute-phase reactants. No evidence of myocardial cell damage, as assessed by troponin-T, was found in hospital patients with raised concentrations of CRP and severe unstable angina (45). It also cannot be attributed to the severity of atherosclerosis, as there is no correlation between the degree of atherosclerosis and the acute-phase response in patients with chronic stable angina or peripheral vascular disease, in spite of much more extensive atherosclerotic and thrombotic involvement (45, 58). It cannot be attributed to episodic activation of the hemostatic system because the systemic elevation of markers of thrombin production is not followed by further elevation of acute phase proteins (59). Nor can increased CRP be attributed to ischemia–reperfusion injury, as circulating neutrophils were not activated and CRP levels were not increased in patients with variant angina, which is a "human model" of transmural myocardial ischemia not associated with plaque instability or thrombus formation. Variant angina is caused by occlusive epicardial coronary artery spasm. Normal CRP was observed despite a significantly larger number of ischemic episodes and a greater total ischemic burden during Holter monitoring (40,60).

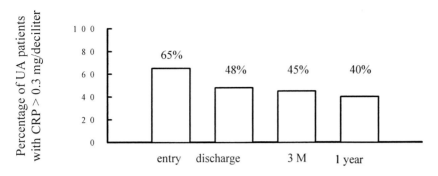

Figure 7 Persistence of elevated levels of C-reactive protein after the waning of symptoms in patients with unstable angina. C-reactive protein (CRP) levels may remain elevated (>0.3 mg/dL, which represents the 90th percentile of normal distribution) for months after an index acute event in almost one-half of patients admitted to the hospital with a diagnosis of Braunwald class IIIB unstable angina. Such an elevation is associated with a significantly higher incidence of new phases of instability within 1 year. (Modified from Ref. 61.)

Indeed, most patients with unstable angina have concentrations of CRP above the normal range at hospital discharge and at 3-month follow-up (Fig. 7). These elevated concentrations carry a greatly increased risk of new episodes of instability and of myocardial infarction and cardiac death at 1 year (Fig. 8) (61). Thus, recurrent instability may be associated with persisting inflammatory stimuli, the cause of which is still unknown. This observation has important implications for clinical practice and research. It provides a new way of identifying patients at risk of recurrent instability, who may benefit from more careful clinical monitoring and more aggressive preventive management. This observation is in line with the long-term prognostic value of mildly elevated concentrations of CRP observed in the ECAT study in a large group of outpatients, including patients with stable and unstable angina (Fig. 9) (52). It is in line with the long-term prognostic value of very high levels of CRP observed in the FRISC study in patients with unstable angina and non–Q-wave myocardial infarction (53). It is also in agreement with the recent observation that the baseline plasma concentration of CRP in apparently healthy men can predict

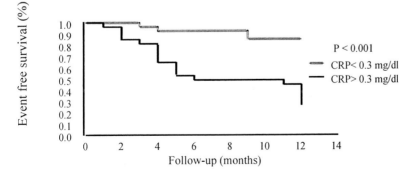

Figure 8 One-year survival free from readmission for unstable angina, myocardial infarction, and death according to C-reactive protein (CRP) levels at hospital discharge in patients with unstable angina. The 1-year survival free from readmission, myocardial infarction, and death was significantly higher in patients with normal CRP levels at discharge (<0.3 mg/dL) than in patients with CRP levels >0.3 mg/dL as assessed by the long-rank test ($p < 0.001$) and was independent of treatment, including coronary revascularization procedures, performed during the initial hospitalization. (Modified from Ref. 61.)

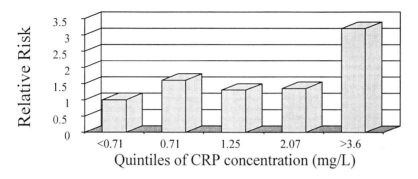

Figure 9   Relative risk of coronary events by quintiles of distribution of C-reactive protein (CRP) concentration in patients with angina. Slightly increased production of CRP is common in patients with angina and is significantly associated with increased risk of myocardial infarction and sudden cardiac death. In a large group of 2121 outpatients from 15 European centers, including patients with stable and unstable angina, the relative risk of a coronary event was about 2 times greater in the fifth quintile of CRP concentration than in the first four quintiles, irrespective of adjustment for other coronary risk factors. Approximately one-third of the coronary events that occurred during the 2-year follow-up were among the fifth quintile of CRP concentration. (Modified from Ref. 52.)

the risk of first myocardial infarction independently of other risk factors, even for events occurring 6 or more years later (Fig. 10) (62). Thus, available data converge to suggest that the effects of inflammation are likely mediated by a chronic process, not confined to the plaque, and disfavor that acute ischemia, thrombosis, or undetected acute illness are solely responsible for the acute-phase response in unstable angina.

VII.   MECHANISMS OF THE ACUTE-PHASE RESPONSE IN ACUTE CORONARY SYNDROMES

The mechanisms that relate the level of acute-phase proteins to short- and long-term prognosis in ischemic heart disease are unclear. Atherosclerosis by itself shares many characteristics of a chronic inflammatory process. Many stimuli may incite the ongoing reaction found in atherosclerosis, including chronic infection of the vessels with microorganisms such as *Cytomegalovirus* and *Chlamydia pneumoniae* (see below), but the cause(s) of the acute exacerbation or activation of an until-then chronic, quiet inflammatory process resulting in the formation of adhesion molecules, inflammatory cytokines, lytic proteases, and leading to endothelial dysfunction and platelet aggregation with subsequent thrombosis are incompletely understood (Table 2). Although the acute-phase response is universal, there can be substantial differences among individuals in the magnitude of their responses to similar stimuli.

Interleukin-1, TNF-α, and in particular IL-6, produced by activated circulating monocytes, resident macrophages, and activated endothelium, are the major inducers of acute-phase protein production by the liver. C-reactive protein is the prototypical acute-phase reactant, as it may increase several hundredfold after an inflammatory stimulus, its level in the circulating blood is dependent only on its rate of production and excretion, and it is not consumed. Because its half-life is 19 h and it is relatively easy and not expensive to measure, CRP is an ideal marker of inflammation. For these reasons, CRP is used as a marker of disease activity in infectious and inflammatory diseases. However, in conditions such as sepsis or rheumathoid arthritis, the inflammatory response is strong, and therefore CRP levels are markedly increased. Conversely, in atheroscle-

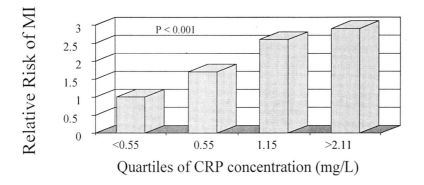

Figure 10 Relative risk of future myocardial infarction by quartiles of distribution of C-reactive protein (CRP) concentration in apparently healthy men. Among apparently healthy men participating in the Physicians' Health Study, the baseline levels of inflammation as assessed by the plasma concentration of CRP can predict the risk of first myocardial infarction (MI), independently of other risk factors, even for events occurring 6 or more years later. In this population of low-risk individuals, CRP concentration was only mildly increased. Nevertheless, the relative risk of first MI increased significantly with each increasing quartile of baseline concentration of CRP. Individuals in the highest quartile had a risk of future MI almost 3 times that among those in the lowest quartile. Finally, the effect of aspirin in preventing a first myocardial infarction was greatest among the men with the highest baseline CRP concentrations and the benefit diminished significantly with decreasing concentration of this inflammatory marker. (Modified from Ref. 62.)

rosis, the inflammatory response is mild, and ultrasensitive methods that allow measurement of low levels of CRP are required (57).

Using these methods, CRP has been shown to be a reliable marker of disease activity in acute coronary syndromes, where up to 60% of unstable patients and 90% of those with unfavorable outcomes have elevated levels of CRP (45,53,54). More recently, CRP has been shown to be related to long-term prognosis in other forms of atherosclerotic disease. Levels of CRP in the top quartile were associated with increased risk of myocardial infarction, stroke (62), and peripheral vascular disease (63) in apparently healthy subjects with a low risk-factor profile, and CRP levels in the top quintile were associated with increased risk of infarction in high-risk subjects (64–66). In particular, the observation that mildly elevated levels of CRP are associated with events occurring 8 or more years later (62,65), together with the finding that CRP levels may remain elevated for months after an index acute event (61), suggest that CRP levels are associated with the activity of atherosclerotic disease. Whether CRP is only a marker of the underlying inflammatory process or has specific properties relevant to plaque instability is still unclear. However, CRP may induce the expression of procoagulant tissue factor on human monocytes and has numerous modulatory affects on inflammation, inducing proinflammatory cytokine production by monocytes and reducing free oxygen radicals by neutrophils, which suggests that CRP may be more than a marker (67).

Table 2 Possible Causes of Inflammation in Acute Coronary Syndromes

Oxidized LDL
Infections: Cytomegalovirus
    Chlamydia pneumoniae
    Helicobacter pylori
Altered immune and/or inflammatory response

The response of patients with coronary artery disease to stress was directly investigated by exploring whether "active" coronary plaque disruption could alter circulating markers of inflammation in unstable angina (68). Percutaneous transluminal coronary angioplasty (PTCA) was followed by an increase of IL-6 levels, and subsequently of CRP and SAA, only in those unstable angina patients with detectable levels of this cytokine prior to the procedure. This acute phase reaction could not be attributed simply to the disruption of particularly "active" coronary plaques because it was also observed in the absence of PTCA following diagnostic cardiac catheterization and coronary angiography.

Moreover, the acute-phase response to myocardial cell necrosis is greatly enhanced in patients with preinfarction unstable angina as compared with those presenting with a totally unheralded myocardial infarction (54). As the two groups did not differ significantly in estimated infarct size and clinical signs of reperfusion, it could be hypothesized that the nature and intensity of the stimuli provoked by myocardial cell necrosis and by reperfusion were similar in the two groups of patients. Thus, patients with preinfarction unstable angina may be more responsive than patients with unheralded myocardial infarction to the inflammatory stimuli caused by myocardial necrosis and reperfusion. These findings suggest that the magnitude of the acute-phase response is determined to a greater extent by individual responsiveness than by the type of provocative stimuli.

These findings are in agreement with the recent observation that the monocytes of patients with recurrent unstable angina and persistent elevation of acute phase reactants exhibit greatly enhanced production of IL-6 in response to LPS challenge 6 months after the last acute event (69). The magnitude of this response is linearly related to baseline levels of acute-phase reactants. These in vitro findings confirm the hypothesis that the individual response to stimuli of different types, including possibly infectious agents, may be responsible for instability. The causes of such hyperresponsiveness are largely unknown and are probably multiple. It is possible that genetic factors or the presence of a recently described population of unusual proinflammatory T lymphocytes play an important role.

If this hypothesis is confirmed, "acute-phase hyperresponsiveness" may contribute to the marked elevation of acute-phase proteins observed in patients with persistent severe unstable angina associated with unfavorable in-hospital outcomes (45). It might also explain the strong positive correlation between baseline CRP values within the normal range and the incidence of myocardial infarction over an 8-year follow-up in the Physicians' Health Study (62) and the long-term prognostic implications of elevated CRP levels in patients with known ischemic heart disease (52,53,61) and high frequencies of risk factors (65,66). Thus, individuals with a high acute-phase response of CRP to low-grade stimulation by chronic infection, oxidized LDL, or other factors, may be at increased risk of acute thrombotic complications.

VIII. ROLE OF IMMUNE SYSTEM AS DETERMINANT OF INFLAMMATORY RESPONSE

Neri Serneri et al. (41) reported that monocyte activation in patients with unstable angina is lymphocyte dependent. More recently, the same group provided direct evidence that circulating T lymphocytes from patients with unstable angina, but not from patients with stable angina, are activated and that enhanced lymphocyte activation is associated with a unfavorable prognosis (42). At variance with Neri Serneri et al. is the work of Caligiuri et al. (70), who found that in unstable angina lymphocyte activation was inversely related to the intensity of inflammation as indicated by plasma CRP. They noted that lymphocyte activation increased 2 weeks after angina, with waning of symptoms (70). These findings may be in keeping with reported elevations of IL-2 soluble receptor in patients with stable angina and a lower restenosis rate after PTCA (71). These data suggest that lymphocyte activation may be protective, possibly by secretion of antiinflammatory cytokines such as IL-4 and IL-10.

The presence of activated T lymphocytes in unstable angina implies antigenic stimulation. The identity of possibly important antigens has only been partially investigated. Several autoantigens expressed in the atherosclerotic plaque are able to elicit an immune response, including oxidized LDLs (72) and heat shock proteins (20,73,74). Infectious agents like *Chlamydia pneumoniae* (16,18), cytomegalovirus (75), and *Helicobacter pylori* (17,18,21) have been associated to ischemic heart disease in several epidemiological studies. Cytomegalovirus (76,77) and *Chlamydia pneumoniae* (19,20) have been frequently detected in advanced coronary atherosclerotic lesions and could be the target for activated lymphocytes within the plaques (Fig. 11) (78). Yet, Kol et al. (79) failed to find evidence of active cytomegalovirus replication in atherectomy specimens from unstable coronary plaques. More promising are the results of studies testing the possibility of a pathogenetic role of *Chlamydia pneumoniae* and its sensitivity to antibiotic treatment. Gurfinkel et al. (80) found a beneficial effect of roxithromycin on the combined end points of death, myocardial infarction, and severe recurrent ischemia at 30 days in patients with non–Q-wave coronary syndromes. Gupta et al. (81) found a persistent beneficial effect of azithromycin at 1 year follow-up in patients with recent myocardial infarction and high levels of antibodies to *Chlamydia pneumoniae*. However, these encouraging results have not been confirmed by more recent trials using antibiotic therapy to reduce the risk of acute coronary events (82).

Recently, Liuzzo et al. (83) have found that unstable angina patients have expansion of an unusual subset of T cells, expressing the CD4+ CD28^{null} phenotype (Fig. 12). These unusual T

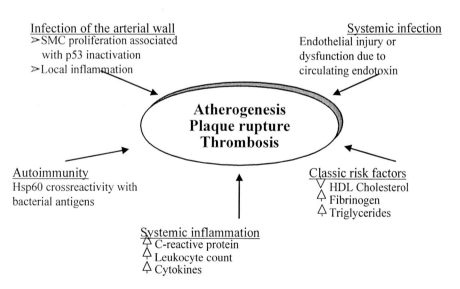

Figure 11 Postulated mechanisms to link infections and ischemic heart disease. Various potential causative mechanisms that may act either acutely (precipitating plaque rupture) or chronically (promoting plaque growth) have been proposed for the reported association between infections and ischemic heart disease. Some involve possible direct effects of infectious agents on the arterial wall, including endothelial injury or dysfunction, smooth muscle proliferation, and local inflammation. But most involve possible indirect effects mediated in the circulation through chronic inflammation, cross-reactive antibodies, or changes in known or suspected cardiovascular risk factors (such as lipids, coagulation proteins, oxidative metabolites, or homocysteine). (Modified from Ref. 78.)

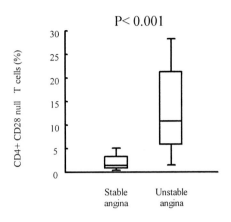

Figure 12 Increased frequencies of CD4+ $CD28^{null}$ T lymphocytes in patients with unstable angina. The frequency of $CD28^{null}$ cells within the CD4+ compartment was compared in stable and unstable angina patients. Data are presented as box plots displaying medians, 25th and 75th percentiles (as boxes), and 10th and 90th percentiles (as whiskers). CD4+ $CD28^{null}$ T cells were significantly expanded in unstable angina patients ($p < 0.001$). Patients with stable angina did not differ from age-matched normal controls. CD4+ $CD28^{null}$ T cells have functional activities that predispose for vascular injury, possibly directly contributing to plaque instability. CD4+ $CD28^{null}$ T cells are characterized by their ability to produce high amounts of IFN-γ, which is a potent stimulator of macrophages and, if present in the local microenvironment of the plaque, could stimulate the production of tissue-destructive metalloproteinases. CD4+ $CD28^{null}$ T cells are cytotoxic effector cells, possibly attacking smooth muscle cells and endothelial cells. (Modified from Ref. 83.)

cells are committed to the production of IFN-γ. The chronic upregulation of IFN-γ in unstable angina patients could lead to subsequent activation of monocytes/macrophages in the circulation as well as in tissue lesions (Fig. 13). In addition, the finding that CD28-deficient T cells have cytolytic capability suggests that immune reactions in individuals with such T cells are deviated toward a high risk for tissue damage. Environmental as well as genetic mechanisms could underlie the perturbation of the T-cell repertoire. In particular, because the defect in CD28 cell surface ex-

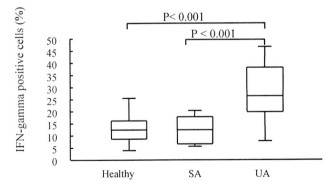

Figure 13 Stable angina and unstable angina patients differ in their repertoire of cytokine-producing T lymphocytes. The frequencies of CD4+ T lymphocytes producing IFN-γ after in vitro activation were determined by three-color flow cytometry. Data are presented as box plots displaying medians, 25th and 75th percentiles (as boxes), and 10th and 90th percentiles (as whiskers). The numbers of CD4+ T cells producing IFN-γ was increased in unstable angina patients compared with patients with stable angina and healthy individuals.

pression may result from chronic exposure to antigen, the expansion of CD4+ CD28^{null} T cells may reflect a persistent immune response to microorganisms or autoantigens contained in atherosclerotic plaques.

IX. CONCLUSIONS

Inflammation plays a pivotal role in both the development of atherosclerosis and the acute activation of the vascular wall with consequent local thrombosis and vasocostriction (with or without plaque fissure) (Fig. 14).

In many patients with unstable angina and acute myocardial infarction, systemic signs of inflammation are detectable. Thus, in acute coronary syndromes, the inflammatory process is not confined to the coronary plaque, but is systemic or at least has a systemic component. Moreover, systemic inflammatory markers, such as CRP, have an independent prognostic value, thus supporting their pathogenetic role of inflammation. The use of CRP as a marker of disease activity and short- and long-term prognosis seems to be of clinical value (Table 3).

However, only about 50–70% of patients with Braunwald class IIIB unstable angina have systemic markers of inflammation. In about 40–50% of these patients, the elevation of CRP and IL-6 persists at discharge and at 3 months and is associated with recurrent instability and myocardial infarction at 1 year follow-up. The percentage of patients with elevated CRP and IL-6 on admission increases to 90–100% in patients in whom myocardial infarction was preceded by unstable angina, but is noted in only 40% of patients in whom myocardial infarction was totally unheralded. Thus, markers of an acute systemic inflammatory reaction appear to be an independent

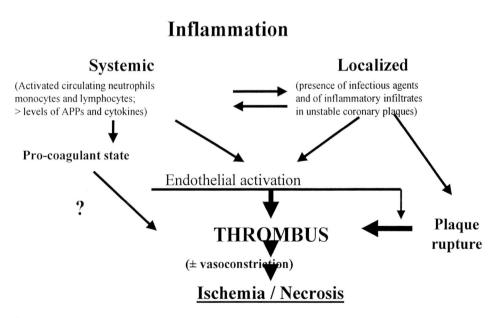

Figure 14 Role of inflammation in the pathogenesis of acute coronary syndromes. Inflammation may cause local endothelial activation and plaque fissure, leading to episodic thrombogenic and vasoconstrictor stimuli, which could be important components of the onset, waxing, and waning of unstable angina and of its evolution toward infarction.

Table 3 Conditions Required to Determine Clinical Utility of Inflammatory Markers in Acute Coronary Syndromes

---

For a novel inflammatory marker to have a clinical role there must be:
  a widely available diagnostic test with high reproducibility
  (this is the case for CRP as measured by highly sensitive assays)
  prospective prognostic studies
  (several studies are available for CRP and fibrinogen)
  additive information to traditional prognostic indicators and risk factors
  (no conclusive data; some studies suggest an incremental prognostic value of CRP)
  treatments able to modify the inflammatory marker alone
  (no conclusive data; statins?, antibiotics?)

---

determinant of prognosis in some patients with acute ischemic syndromes. However, signs of inflammation are not detectable in all such cases (54). Inflammatory events may reflect the impact of a variety of infectious and noninfectious stimuli and also may be an indication of the individual's unique ability to respond to such stimuli.

REFERENCES

1. Ross R. The pathogenesis of atherosclerosis: A prospective for the 1990s. Nature 1993; 362:801–808.
2. Kohchi R, Takebayashi S, Hiroki T, Nobuyoshi M. Significance of adventitial inflammation of the coronary artery in patients with unstable angina: Results at autopsy. Circulation 1985; 71:709–716.
3. Wallsh E, Weinstein GS, Franzone A, et al. Inflammation of the coronary arteries in patients with unstable angina. Tex Heart Inst J 1986; 16:105–113.
4. Sato T. Increased subendothelial infiltration of the coronary arteries with monocytes-macrophages in patients with unstable angina: Histological data on 14 autopsy patients. Atherosclerosis 1987; 68:191–197.
5. Baroldi G, Silver MD, Mariani F, Giuliano G. Correlation of morphological variable in the coronary atherosclerotic plaque with clinical patterns of ischemic heart disease. Am J Cardiovasc Pathol 1988; 2:159–172.
6. Hansson GK, Holm J, Jonasson L. Detection of activated T lymphocytes in the human atherosclerotic plaque. Am J Pathol 1989; 135:169–175.
7. Kragel AH, Reddy SG, Wittes JT, Roberts WC. Morphometric analysis of the composition of coronary arterial plaques in isolated unstable angina pectoris with pain at rest. Am J Cardiol 1990; 66:562–567.
8. van der Wal AC, Becker AE, van der Loos CM, Das PK. Site of intimal rupture or erosion of thrombosed coronary atherosclerotic plaques is characterized by an inflammatory process irrespective of the dominant plaque morphology. Circulation 1994; 89:36–44.
9. van der Wal AC, Piek JJ, de Boer OJ, Koch KT, Teeling P, van der Loos CM, Becker AE. Recent activation of the plaque immune response in coronary lesions underlying acute coronary syndromes. Heart 1998; 80:14–18.
10. Moreno PR, Falk E, Palacios IF, et al. Macrophage infiltration in acute coronary syndromes: implications for plaque rupture. Circulation 1994; 90:775–778.
11. Moreno PR, Bernardi VH, López-Cuéllar J, et al. Macrophages, smooth muscle cells, and tissue factor in unstable angina: Implications for cell-mediated thrombogenicity in acute coronary syndromes. Circulation 1996; 94:3090–3097.
12. Kaartinen M, Penttilä A, Kovanen PT. Accumulation of activated mast cells in the shoulder region of human coronary atheroma, the predilection site of atheromatous rupture. Circulation 1994; 90:1669–1678.

13. Kovanen PT, Kaartinen M, Paavonen T. Infiltrates of activated mast cells at the site of coronary athero-matous erosion or rupture in myocardial infarction. Circulation 1995; 92:1084–1088.

14. van der Wal AC, Becker AE, Koch KT, Piek JJ, Teeling P, van der Loos CM, David GK. Clinically sta-ble angina pectoris is not necessarily associated with histologically stable atherosclerotic plaques. Heart 1996; 76:312–316.

15. van der Wal AC, Das PK, van de Berg DB, et al. Atherosclerotic lesions in humans: In situ immuno-phenotypic analysis suggesting an immune mediated response. Lab Invest 1989; 61:166–170.

16. Saikku P, Leinonen M, Mattila KJ, Ekman MR, Nieminen MS, Makela PH, Huttunen JK, Valtonen V. Serological evidence of an association of a novel Chlamydia TWAR with chronic coronary artery dis-ease and acute myocardial infarction. Lancet 1988; 2:983–986.

17. Mendall MA, Goggin P, Levy J, Molineaux N, Strachan D, Camm A, et al. Relation of Helicobacter pylori infection and coronary hearth disease. Br Health J 1994; 71:437–439.

18. Patel P, Mendall MA, Carrington D, Strachan D, Leatham E, Molineaux N, Levy J, Blakeston C, Sey-mour CA, Camm AJ, Northfield TC. Association of Helicobacter pylori and Chlamydia pneumoniae infections with coronary hearth disease and cardiovascular risk factor. Br Med J 1995; 311:711–714.

19. Muhlestein JB, Hammond EH, Carlquist JF, et al. Increased incidence of Chlamydia species within the coronary arteries of patients with symptomatic atherosclerosis versus other forms of cardiovascular disease. J Am Coll Cardiol 1996; 27:1555–61.

20. Kol A, Sukhova GK, Lichtman AH, Libby P. Chlamydial heat shock protein 60 localizes in human atheroma and regulates macrophage tumor necrosis factor-α and matrix metalloproteinase expression. Circulation 1998; 98:300–307.

21. Pasceri V, Cammarota G, Patti G, Cuoco L, Gasbarrini A, Grillo RL, Fedeli G, Gasbarrini G, Maseri A. Association of virulent Helicobacter pylori strains with ischemic heart disease. Circulation 1998; 97:1675–1679.

22. Stemme S, Holm J, Hansson GK. T lymphocytes in human atherosclerotic plaques are memory cells expressing CD45RO and the integrin VLA-1. Arter Thromb 1992, 12:206–11.

23. Libby P, Hansson GK. Biology of Disease. Involvement of the immune system in human atheroscle-rosis: Current knowledge and unanswered questions. Lab Invest 1991; 64:5–15.

24. Henney AM, Wakeley PR, Davies MJ, et al. Localization of stromelysin gene expression in athero-sclerotic plaques by in situ hybridization. Proc Natl Acad Sci USA 1991; 88:8154–8158.

25. Gallis Z., Sukhova G, Lark M, Libby P. Increased expression of matrix metalloproteinases and matrix degrading activity in vulnerable regions of human atherosclerotic plaques. J Clin Invest 1994; 94:2493–2503.

26. Shah PK, Falk E, Badimon JJ, et al. Human monocyte-derived macrophages induce collagen break-down in fibrous caps of atherosclerotic plaques. Potential role of matrix-degrading metalloproteinases and implication for plaque rupture. Circulation 1995; 92:1565–1569.

27. Brown DL, Hibbs MS, Kearney M, et al. Identification of 92-kD gelatinase in human coronary athero-sclerotic lesions. Association of active enzyme synthesis with unstable angina. Circulation 1995; 91:2125–2131.

28. Wilcoxon JN, Smith KM, Schwartz SM, Gordon D. Localization of tissue factor in the normal vessel wall and in the atherosclerotic plaque. Proc Natl Acad Sci USA 1989; 86:2839–2843.

29. Leatham EW, Bath PMW, Tooze JA, Camm AJ. Increased monocyte tissue factor expression in coro-nary disease. Br Heart J 1995; 73:10–13.

30. Peng J, Friese P, George J, Dale G, Burstein SA. Alteration of platelet function mediated by inter-leukin-6. Blood 1994; 83:398–403.

31. Bevilacqua MP, Gimbrone MA. Inducible endothelial functions in inflammation and coagulation. Semin Thromb Hemost 1987; 13:425–433.

32. Cianflone D, Ciccirillo F, Buffon A, Trani C, Scabbia EV, Finocchiaro ML, Crea F. Comparison of coronary angiographic narrowing in stable angina pectoris, unstable angina pectoris, and in acute myo-cardial infarction. Am J Cardiol 1995; 76:215–219.

33. Maseri A. Ischemic Heart Disease: A Rational Basis for Clinical Practice and Clinical Research. New York: Churchill Livingstone, 1995:237–301.

34. Libby P. Molecular bases of the acute coronary syndromes. Circulation 1995; 91:2844–2850.

35. Arbustini E, Grasso M, Diegoli M, et al. Coronary atherosclerosis plaques with and without thrombus in ischemic heart syndromes: A morphologic immunohistochemical and biochemical study. Am J Cardiol 1991; 68:36B–50B.

36. Carry M, Korley V, Willerson JT Weigekt L, Ford-Hutchinson AW, Tagari P. Increased urinary leukotriene excretion in patients with cardiac ischemia: In vivo evidence for 5-lipoxygenase activation. Circulation 1992; 85:230–236.

37. Mehta J, Dinerman J, Mehta P, et al. Neutrophil function in ischemic heart disease. Circulation 1989; 79:549–556.

38. Dinerman JL, Mehta JL, Saldeen TGP, et al. Increased neutrophil elastase release in unstable angina pectoris and acute myocardial infarction. J Am Coll Cardiol 1990; 15:1559–1563.

39. Mazzone A, De Servi S, Ricevuti G, et al. Increased expression of neutrophil and monocyte adhesion molecules in unstable coronary artery disease. Circulation 1993; 88:358–363.

40. Biasucci LM, D'Onofrio G, Liuzzo G, et al. Intracellular neutrophil myeloperoxidase is reduced in unstable angina and myocardial infarction, but its reduction is not related to ischemia. J Am Coll Cardiol 1996; 27; 3:611–616.

41. Neri Serneri GG, Abbate R, Gori AM, et al. Transient intermittent lymphocyte activation is responsible for the instability of angina. Circulation 1992; 86:790–797.

42. Neri Serneri GG, Prisco D, Martini F, Gori AM, Brunelli T, Poggesi L, Rostagno C, Giensini GF, Abbate R. Acute T-cell activation is detectable in unstable angina. Circulation 1997; 95:1806–1812.

43. Jude B, Agraou B, McFadden EP, et al. Evidence for time-dependent activation of monocytes in the systemic circulation in unstable angina but not in acute myocardial infarction or in stable angina. Circulation 1994; 90:1662–1668.

44. Berk BC, Weintraub WS, Alexander RW. Elevation of C-reactive protein in active coronary disease. Am J Cardiol 1990; 65:168–172.

45. Liuzzo G, Biasucci LM, Gallimore JR, Grillo RL, Rebuzzi AG, Pepys MB, Maseri A. The prognostic value of C-reactive protein and serum amyloid A protein in severe unstable angina. N Engl J Med 1994; 331:417–424.

46. Vejar M, Fragasso G, Hackett D, et al. Dissociation of platelet activation and spontaneous myocardial ischemia in unstable angina. Thromb Haemost 1990; 63:163–168.

47. Ciabattoni G, Ujang S, Sritara P, et al. Aspirin, but not heparin, suppresses the transient increase in thromboxane biosynthesis associated with cardiac catheterization or coronary angioplasty. J Am Coll Cardiol 1993; 21:1377.

48. Neri Serneri GG, Gensini GF, Modesti PA, et al. The role of extraplatelet thromboxane A2 in unstable angina investigated with a dual thromboxane A2 inhibitor: Importance of activated monocytes. Coron Artery Dis 1994; 5:137–145.

49. Cipollone E, Patrignani P, Greco A, Panara MR, Padovano R, Cuccurullo F, Patrono C, Rebuzzi AG, Liuzzo G, Quaranta G, Maseri A. Differential suppression of thromboxane biosynthesis by indobufen and aspirin in patients with unstable angina. Circulation 1997; 96:1109–1116.

50. Biasucci LM, Vitelli A, Liuzzo G, Altamura S, Caligiuri G, Monaco C, Rebuzzi AG, Ciliberto G, Maseri A. Elevated Levels of IL-6 in Unstable Angina. Circulation 1996; 94:874–877.

51. Biasucci LM, Liuzzo G, Fantuzzi G, Caligiuri G, Rebuzzi AG, Ginnetti F, Dinarello CA, Maseri A. Increasing levels of IL-1Ra and of IL-6 during the first two days of hospitalization in unstable angina are associated with increased risk of in-hospital coronary events. Circulation 1999; 99:2079–2084.

52. Haverkate F, Thompson SG, Pyke DM, Gallimore JR, Pepys MB. Production of C-reactive protein and risk of coronary events in stable and unstable angina. Lancet; 1997; 349:462–466.

53. Toss H, Lindahl B, Siegbahn A, Wallentin L. Prognostic influence of increased fibrinogen and C-reactive protein levels in unstable coronary artery disease. FRISC Study Group. Fragmin during Instability in Coronary Artery Disease. Circulation 1997; 96:4204–4210.

54. Liuzzo G, Biasucci LM, Gallimore JR, Caligiuri G, Buffon A, Rebuzzi AG, Pepys MB, Maseri A. Enhanced inflammatory response in patients with pre-infarction unstable angina. J Am Coll Cardiol 1999; 34:1696–1703.

55. Morrow DA, Rifai N, Antman EM, Weiner DL, McCabe CH, Cannon CP, Braunwald E. C-reactive protein is a potent predictor of mortality independently of and in combination with troponin T in acute

coronary syndromes: A TIMI 11A substudy. Thrombolysis in Myocardial Infarction. J Am Coll Cardiol 1998; 31:1460–1465.

56. Rebuzzi AG, Quaranta G, Liuzzo G, et al. Incremental prognostic value of serum levels of troponin T and C-reactive protein on admission in patients with unstable angina. Am J Cardiol 1998; 82:715–719.

57. Libby P, Ridker PM. Novel inflammatory markers of coronary risk. Theory versus practice. Circulation 1999; 100:1148–1150.

58. Monaco C, D'Onofrio G, Rossi E, Milazzo D, Citterio F, Zini G, Biasucci LM, Maseri A. Neutrophil are activated in acute coronary syndromes but not in severe peripheral vascular disease: A clue for different pathogenetic mechanisms? Circulation 1994; 8:1–732, 1996.

59. Biasucci LM, Liuzzo G, Caligiuri G, van de Greef W, Quaranta G, Monaco C, Rebuzzi AG, Kluft C, Maseri A. Activation of the coagulation system doesn't elicit a detectable acute phase reaction in unstable angina. Am J Cardiol 1996; 77:85–87.

60. Liuzzo G, Biasucci LM, Rebuzzi AG, Gallimore JR, Caligiuri G, Lanza GA, Quaranta G, Monaco C, Pepys MB, Maseri A. The plasma protein acute phase response in unstable angina is not induced by ischemic injury. Circulation 1996, 94:874–877.

61. Biasucci LM, Liuzzo G, Grillo RL, Caligiuri G, Rebuzzi AG, Buffon A, Summaria F, Ginnetti F, Fadda, G, Maseri A. Elevated levels of C-reactive protein at discharge in patients with unstable angina predict recurrent instability. Circulation 1999; 99:855–860.

62. Ridker PM, Cushman M, Stamper MJ, Tracy RP, Hennekens CH. Inflammation, aspirin, and the risk of cardiovascular disease in apparently healthy men. N Engl J Med 1997; 336:973–979.

63. Ridker PM, Cushman M, Stampfer MJ, Tracy RP, Hennekens CH. Plasma Concentration of C-reactive protein and risk of developing peripheral vascular disease. Circulation 1998, 97:425–428.

64. Mendall MA, Patel P, Ballam L, Strachan D, Northfield TC. C-reactive protein and its relation to cardiovascular risk factors: A population based cross sectional study. Br Med J 1996; 312:1061–1065.

65. Kuller LH, Tracy RP, Shaten J, Meilahn for the MRFIT Research Group. Relation of C-reactive protein and coronary heart disease in the MRFIT nested case-control study. Am J Epidemiol 1996; 144: 537–547.

66. Koenig W, et al. C-Reactive protein, a sensitive marker of inflammation, predicts future risk of coronary heart disease in initially healthy middle-aged men: Results from the MONICA (Monitoring Trends and Determinants in Cardiovascular disease) Augsburg Cohort Study, 1984 to 1992. Circulation 1999; 99:237–242.

67. Lagrand WK, Visser CA, et al. C-reactive protein as a cardiovascular risk factor. More than an epiphenomenon? Circulation 1999, 100:96–102.

68. Liuzzo G, Buffon A, Biasucci LM, Gallimore JR, Caligiuri G, Vitelli A, Altamura S, Ciliberto G, Rebuzzi AG, Crea F, Pepys MB, Maseri A. Enhanced inflammatory response to coronary angioplasty in patients with severe unstable angina. Circulation 1998; 98:2370–2376.

69. Liuzzo G, Angiolillo DJ, Ginnetti F, et al. Monocytes of patients with recurrent unstable angina are hyper-responsive to LPS-challenge (abstr). J Am Coll Cardiol 1998; March, Special Issue: 272A.

70. Caligiuri G, Liuzzo G, Biasucci LM, Maseri A. Immune system activation follows inflammation in unstable angina: Pathogenetic implications. J Am Coll Cardiol 1998; 32:1295–1304.

71. Blum A, Sclarovsky S, Shohat B. T lymphocyte activation in stable angina pectoris and after percutaneous transluminal coronary angioplasty. Circulation 1995; 91:20–22.

72. Stemme S, Faber B, Holm J, Wiklund O, Witztum JL, Hansson GK. T lymphocytes from human atherosclerotic plaques recognize oxidized low density lipoprotein. Proc Natl Acad Sci USA 1995; 92:3893–3897.

73. Berberian PA, Myers W, Tytell M, Challa V, Bond MG. Immunohistochemical localization of heat shock protein-70 in normal-appearing and atherosclerotic specimens of human arteries. Am J Pathol 1990; 136:71–80.

74. Xu Q, Willeit J, Marosi M, et al. Association of serum antibodies to heat-shock protein 65 with carotid atherosclerosis. Lancet 1993; 341:255–259.

75. Zhou YF, Martin BL, Waclawiw MA, Popma JJ, Yu ZX, Finkel T, Epstein S. Association betwwen prior cytomegalovirus infection and the risk of restenosis after coronary atherectomy. N Engl J Med 1996; 335:624–630.

76. Hendrix MGR, Daemen, Bruggeman CA. Cytomegalovirus nucleic acid distribution within the human vascular tree. Am J Pathol, 1991; 138:563–567.

77. Speir E, Modali R, Huang E-S, et al. Potential role of human cytomegalovirus and p53 interaction in coronary stenosis. Science 1994; 265:391–394.

78. Danesh J, Collins R, Peto R. Chronic infections and coronary artery disease: Is there a link? Lancet 1997; 350:430–436.

79. Kol A, Sperti G, Shani J, et al. Cytomegalovirus replication is not a cause of instability in unstable angina. Circulation 1995; 91:1910–1913.

80. Gurfinkel E, Bozovich G, Daroca A, Beck E, Mautner B. Randomised trial of roxithromycin in non-Q-wave coronary syndromes: ROXIS Pilot Study. ROXIS Study Group. Lancet 1997; 350:404–407.

81. Gupta S, Leatham EW, Carrington D, Mendall MA, Kaski JC, Camm AJ. Elevated Chlamydia pneumoniae antibodies, cardiovascular events, and azithromycin in male survivors of myocardial infarction. Circulation 1997; 96:404–407.

82. Anderson JL, Muhlestein JB, Carlquist J, Allen A, Trehan S, Nielson C, Hall S, Brady J, Egger M, Horne B, Lim T. Randomized secondary prevention trial of azithromycin in patients with coronary artery disease and serological evidence for Chlamydia pneumoniae infection. The Azithromycin in Coronary Artery Disease: Elimination of Myocardial Infection with Chlamydia (ACADEMIC) Study. Circulation 1999; 99:1540–1547.

83. Liuzzo G, Kopecky SL, O'Fallon MW, Frye RL, Maseri A, Goronzy JJ, Weyand CM. Perturbation of the T cell repertoire in patients with unstable angina. Circulation 1999; 100:2135–2139.

51
Dyslipidemia in Rheumatic Disorders

Byron J. Hoogwerf, Rossana Danese, and Alexandra Villa-Forte
Cleveland Clinic Foundation Cleveland, Ohio

I. INTRODUCTION

An important relationship exists between certain rheumatic disorders, dyslipidemia, and increased frequency of atherosclerotic vascular disease, especially coronary heart disease (CHD) (1,3,8,27,36,38,43,54,59,60,63,65,67,75,79,86,88). Systemic lupus erythematosus (SLE) and rheumatoid arthritis (RA) are the most widely studied disorders in regard to CHD. Increased CHD risk is related to associated hypertension, dyslipidemia, renal disease/nephrotic syndrome, vascular inflammation, presence of procoagulant proteins, and use of proatherogenic therapies. Treatment of rheumatic diseases often includes medications that cause alterations and lipids and lipoproteins. To what degree the increased risk of CHD is related to the disease process itself or its treatment is uncertain. However, adverse changes in lipids contribute substantially to CHD risk in general. Therefore, benefits of aggressive lipid lowering in these high-risk groups may be applicable to patients with rheumatic disorders who are at increased risk for CHD.

II. ATHEROSCLEROTIC VASCULAR DISEASE IN PATIENTS WITH RHEUMATIC DISORDERS

A. Systemic Lupus Erythematosus

1. Coronary Heart Disease Prevalence

Premature CHD is a significant cause of morbidity and mortality in patients with SLE. A bimodal mortality pattern of SLE has been reported in a series of patients followed for 5 years. Early deaths occurring in patients with active disease receiving large doses of corticosteroids are often due to infection. Late deaths occurring in patients with inactive disease who have had a long duration of corticosteroid therapy are often due to CHD (67,79). In a prospective survey of 75 SLE patients, 46% of the deaths were caused by myocardial infarction (75). In the Hopkins Lupus Cohort there was an 8% cumulative incidence of coronary artery disease, defined as angina or myocardial infarction (58). This is likely to underestimate the true frequency of atherosclerosis, insofar as autopsy series reported a greater incidence of coronary artery disease in SLE patients (27).

2. Dyslipidemia

Leong et al. (49) reported that 73 of 100 consecutive patients with SLE had dyslipoproteinemia. Fifty-six percent of participants in the Hopkins Lupus Cohort Study had hypercholesterolemia, defined as at least one total cholesterol level ≥200 mg/dL (60). Multivariate analysis in the Hopkins Lupus Cohort Study identified several factors predictive of serum cholesterol. Renal involvement and antihypertensive and anti-inflammatory medications were associated with increased cholesterol. Increasing proteinuria from 0 to 2+ was associated with increasing serum cholesterol by 14 mg/dL and from 0 to 3–4+ by 21 mg/dL (59) (Table 1). Other studies report that SLE is associated with low high-density lipoprotein (HDL)-C and elevated triglyceride/very low-density lipoprotein (TG/VLDL) levels (7,14,22,32,50). Ettinger and Hazzard (15) compared HDL-C levels in 14 untreated adult females with SLE to controls (49.7 ± 3.2 vs. 59 ± 2.3 mg/dL); TG values were not statistically different but tended to be higher in the SLE patients (87.0 ± 8.8 vs. 73.0 ± 6.9 mg/dL). Total cholesterol (TC) and LDL values were similar in patients and controls. Furthermore, SLE disease activity scores have shown significant negative correlation with TC, LDL, and HDL, and a significant positive correlation with TG and VLDL. Borba and Bonfa (7) reported that 29% of patients with inactive disease and 79% of patients with active disease had HDL-C <36 mg/dL.

B. Rheumatoid Arthritis

Patients with RA have significantly increased risk of mortality with a 2.4 times higher incidence of cardiovascular death compared with an age- and sex-matched population (63). Variable concentrations of serum and synovial fluid lipids and lipoproteins have been described in RA (47). There appears to be a relationship between disease activity and dyslipidemia; however, the abnormalities of lipoproteins are not consistent (33,35,47,50,56,76). In juvenile RA, low HDL-C and elevated TG are reported with active disease compared with inactive disease (33). In adult RA, hypocholesterolemia (TC, HDL-C, LDL-C) without an increase in TG has been reported (47,76). These patients may have mean cholesterol levels 20% less than controls. In one study, 69 (predominantly female) patients with RA had significantly lower mean total cholesterol and LDL-C levels (187 and 117 mg/dL, respectively) compared with normal subjects (231 and 142 mg/dL, respectively) and patients with osteoarthritis (222 and 138 mg/dL, respectively). Further analysis of the data showed a statistically significant decrease in total cholesterol, LDL-C, and HDL-C in patients with severe disease activity compared with minimal disease activity (45).

Table 1 Estimated Effect of Various Factors on Serum Cholesterol (mg%): Multivariate Analysis

Factor	Effect on cholesterol (mg%)	Standard error	Z-test	p Value
Sex (women vs. men)	23.49	7.79	3.02	0.001
Race (black vs. white)	−11.59	5.46	−2.12	NS
Age (yr)	0.83	0.21	4.02	0.001
Smoking status (yes vs. no)	−5.39	5.53	−0.97	NS
Weight (lb)	0.10	0.07	1.40	NS
Prednisone dosage (mg/day)	0.75	0.15	5.16	<0.001
Hydroxychloroquine	−8.94	3.44	−2.60	0.009
Diuretic use	8.54	4.88	1.75	0.040
β-Blocker use	6.58	7.37	0.89	NS
Urine protein, trace to 1+	1.06	2.58	0.41	NS
Urine protein 2+	14.88	6.60	2.25	0.12
Urine protein 3–4+	21.26	6.36	3.34	<0.001

Source: Adapted from Ref. 57.

In summary, RA is associated with increased risk for CHD and CHD mortality; RA is associated with a variety of lipid abnormalities. No clear data exist on the contribution of lipid abnormalities to CHD risk in RA.

C. Other Putative Coronary Heart Disease Risk Factors in Rheumatic Disorders

Other mechanisms may contribute to CHD risk. Immune complex–mediated endothelial cell damage appears to be involved in the initiation of the atherosclerotic process in the arterial intima. Lupus sera contains factors that stimulate the accumulation of cholesterol in the cultured smooth muscle cells of the aorta. These may be the LDL-circulating immune complex bonds formed with the ability to promote cholesterol incorporation into the cells (38). Wick et al. (86) suggested that an undefined autoimmune reaction against heat shock protein 60, a mitochondrial protein, expressed by stressed endothelial cells may be an initiating event in atherogenesis. The role of antiphospholipid antibodies in the production of coronary thrombosis has been suggested as another pathogenic mechanism that may enhance atherogenesis, but this is yet to be confirmed. Some studies have not shown any difference in frequency or titer of these antibodies between SLE patients with and without coronary artery disease (2).

Lipoprotein(a), or Lp(a), consists of a particle of LDL-C linked by a disulfide bond to a large hepatically derived glycoprotein, apolipoprotein(a). Lp(a) has structural similarities to plasminogen and has been identified as a strong independent risk factor for CAD (9,43,53,66,71,74,80,83). Lp(a) has been shown to be increased in patients with SLE compared with controls (7) and in SLE patients with myocardial or cerebral infarction compared with patients without infarction (43). No significant relationship between disease activity and Lp(a) was observed.

III. MEDICATIONS USED IN RHEUMATIC DISEASES THAT MAY AFFECT LIPID PROFILES

A. Antihypertensive Agents

Drugs causing dyslipoproteinemia were recently reviewed by Donahoo et al (11). Many antihypertensive agents alter lipid and lipoprotein levels (Table 2). β-Blockers (including β-selective and non–β-selective agents) raise TG and lower HDL-C levels. Triglyceride levels have been reported to increase by 16–46%. The LDL and total cholesterol levels are more variably affected. β-Blockers with intrinsic sympathomimetic activity and those with combined α- and β-blockade generally are lipid neutral. Thiazide diuretics may also adversely affect lipid levels. Triglyceride levels are most adversely affected, increasing by approximately 15%. The LDL-C and total cholesterol levels increase 5–8%; HDL-C is not consistently affected. α-Blockers are reported to have a beneficial effect on lipids. Generally, total cholesterol, LDL-C, and TG levels decrease while the HDL-C level increases. Calcium channel blockers, angiotensin-converting enzyme (ACE) inhibitors, angiotensin II antagonists, and centrally acting agents are reported to be lipid neutral.

B. Immunosuppressive Agents

Among the immunosuppressive agents, glucocorticoids have the greatest effect on lipids and lipoproteins (see Table 2). Observations from studies of patients with rheumatic disorders on glucocorticoids show generally consistent increases in total cholesterol, LDL-C, and HDL-C levels with variable TG responses (5,15,16,33–35,49,50,56,58,59,78,89). In the Hopkins Lupus Cohort

Table 2 Dyslipidemia Associated with Rheumatic Disease and Its Treatment

Dyslipidemia in rheumatic disease	TC	TG	HDL	LDL
Rheumatic disorder				
SLE	⇑	⇑	⇓	⇑
RA	⇓	⇓	⇓	⇓
Complications of rheumatic disease				
Nephrosis	⇑	⇑	V[a]	⇑
Treatment regimens				
Thiazide diuretics	⇑	⇑	⇔	⇑
β-blockers	V	⇑	⇓	V
Alpha blockers	⇓	⇓	⇑	⇓
ACE inhibitors	⇔	⇔	⇔	⇔
Calcium channel blockers	⇔	⇔	⇔	⇔
Angiotensin II receptor blockers	⇔	⇔	⇔	⇔
Glucocorticoids	⇑	V	⇑	⇑
Cyclosporine	⇑	V	⇑	V
Hydroxychloroquine	⇓	⇓	⇓	⇓
Gold	⇔	⇔	⇔	⇔
Azathioprine	⇔	⇔	⇔	⇔

[a]V = Variable responses.

Study, a 10-mg increase in prednisone dose was associated with a change in serum cholesterol of 7.5 mg/dL (59). Furthermore, with increasing prednisone dose a continuous increase in the cholesterol level was reported. Similarly, 23 patients with rheumatic disease (mostly RA) treated with prednisone for 1 month showed statistically significant increases in mean HDL (~34%) and mean total cholesterol (12%) levels, while LDL and TG levels did not change significantly (16). Likewise, 10 pediatric patients followed 4–8 weeks on prednisone showed statistically significant increases in total cholesterol, HDL, LDL and VLDL levels; the most dramatic increase was in HDL (100%, 26 ± 6 vs. 52 ± 13 mg/dL) (22). Ettinger et al. (14), in a study of 32 adult patients with SLE treated with prednisone showed a trend to higher mean HDL (53.5 ± 3.6 mg/dL) compared with untreated patients (49.7 ± 3.2 mg/dL) as well as increased total cholesterol (214 ± 9.2 vs. 170 ± 6.9 mg/dL), LDL-C (130 ± 8.2 vs. 103 ± 7.8 mg/dL), and TG (158 ± 11.0 vs. 87 ± 8.8 mg/dL). Increased HDL-C has also been reported in glucocorticoid-treated patients with localized inflammatory reactions (89) and normal healthy men (78). Limited data exist on other lipoprotein changes, but glucocorticoid therapy in rheumatic disease has been shown to decrease lipoprotein(a) (5).

Cyclosporine has been shown to cause dyslipidemia in many transplant studies. Generally, increases in total cholesterol and LDL levels have been seen with variable responses in TG level (11). Similarly, in patients with amyotrophic lateral sclerosis (6) and psoriasis (13), increases in LDL (30%), total cholesterol (20%), and TG (18%) levels were noted; HDL levels decreased approximately 5%.

Hydroxychloroquine has been shown to decrease cholesterol levels. In the Hopkins Lupus Cohort Study (58,61) hydroxychloroquine was associated with approximately a 9% decline in total cholesterol levels. Hydroxychloroquine ameliorates the increase in cholesterol seen with glucocorticoids. Wallace et al. (82) studied women with RA or SLE and reported that women treated with hydroxychloroquine and glucocorticoid had lipid levels resembling those of patients treated with hydroxychloroquine alone. Much of the effect may be in the TG-containing moieties as Hodis (29) reported a 46% decrease in TG levels. In fact, Munro et al. (56) has suggested hydroxychloroquine as treatment for rheumatic disease in patients with increased coronary artery disease risk factors.

Azathioprine has not been studied in rheumatic disease, but in renal transplantation has been shown to be lipid neutral (28,30,81). In a limited number of studies, gold is likewise thought to be lipid neutral or may show a trend to dyslipoproteinemia (56). Nonsteroidal anti-inflammatory drugs (NSAIDs) do not appear to affect lipid levels. No data exist regarding the effects of chlorambucil or colchicine on lipoproteins in rheumatic patients.

IV. INSIGHTS FROM OTHER DISEASES

Proteinuria is a well-known risk factor for CHD, and rheumatic diseases may be associated with renal disease causing proteinuria. Few data on this risk in rheumatic disorders are available. However, information from other studies may be applicable. Renal disease, in particular the nephrotic syndrome, can cause hyperlipidemia (21,37,42,55,84,85). In the combined results of 16 studies, Kasiske (42) found that 90% of nephrotic patients had total cholesterol levels greater than 240 mg/dL, compared with 30% of participants with nonnephrotic chronic renal insufficiency and 20–25% of end-stage renal disease patients. The degree of lipid abnormality is most commonly a mixed dyslipidemia that correlates with disease severity. Other authors (21,37,55) have corroborated these observations.

V. LIPID ABNORMALITIES AND RELATIONSHIP TO CORONARY HEART DISEASE RISK

A. Epidemiological Studies

Both observational studies and randomized controlled trials have looked at the relationship of lipid abnormalities and coronary heart disease risk. The Framingham Study demonstrated that coronary heart disease risk increases with increased total cholesterol, LDL-C, and TG levels. Framingham data have demonstrated that low levels of HDL-C amplify the adverse effects of elevated LDL-C, and high levels of HDL-C (e.g., >65 mg/dL) abrogate the adverse effects of elevated LDL-C. Framingham investigators have looked at the impact of multiple risk factors on CHD risk. Adding diabetes, hypertension, smoking, and left ventricular hypertrophy to lipid abnormalities progressively increases the observed CHD risk (39,40,87). Such a clustering of risk factors has been reported in a number of observational studies (10,41,72).

The Multiple Risk Factor Intervention Trial (MRFIT) screenees cohort has been followed for more than a decade (73). These data demonstrated that the relationship between total (and LDL) cholesterol and coronary heart disease events and mortality was continuous and graded across the range of lipid values. Overall risk increases with the addition of other CHD risk factors. For example, presence of diabetes nearly tripled the risk of CHD across the total range of cholesterol values.

B. Intervention Trials: Lipid Lowering

1. Primary Prevention Trials

Primary prevention, randomized double-blind clinical trials in general populations have demonstrated reductions in CHD events as a result of lipid lowering (12,19,51,70) using different lipid strategies, including gemfibrozil, bile acid sequestrants, and statins across a wide range of lipid levels at study entry. Although early studies were done in middle-aged men, more recent studies have included women and older subjects. Hence, the results of these trials, which generally show a 2% reduction in CHD risk for each 1% reduction in cholesterol should be applicable to those patients with rheumatic disorders and no evidence of CHD.

2. Secondary Prevention Trials

Five major randomized clinical trials evaluated secondary prevention of CHD risk (52,57,62, 68,69). Four of these trials have looked at LDL-C lowering in patients with documented CHD (52,62,68,69) while one recent trial assessed the effects of raising HDL-C (57). These trials have used statins (sometimes with a bile acid sequestrant) or a fibric acid derivative. The results of these trials show that LDL-C lowering reduced CHD events, coronary revascularization procedures, strokes, and, in fact, all causes of mortality.

3. Intervention Trial Results in High-Risk Patients

Several of these studies have demonstrated that benefits of aggressive cholesterol lowering can be demonstrated in high-risk subgroups, such as patients with diabetes mellitus. Data from diabetic patients in these trials show the benefits of cholesterol lowering in this high-risk group. In the Helsinki Heart Study and AFCAPS/TexCAPS, diabetic patients in the placebo groups had approximately twice the CHD risk compared with nondiabetic patients on placebo. However, diabetic patients achieved greater incremental reduction in CHD risk compared with nondiabetic patients (12,46). In the secondary prevention trials, diabetic patients also had comparable or greater incremental CHD risk reduction with cholesterol-lowering therapy (23,31,52,64).

VI. LIPID-LOWERING STRATEGIES

A. Dietary Therapy

Dietary therapy recommended for CHD risk reduction has focused on reduction of LDL-C. This is largely because intervention trials have supported the benefits of such LDL-C reduction. The current National Cholesterol Education Program (NCEP) (17,18) and American Diabetes Association (ADA) (4) dietary guidelines recommend as a first step total fat intake of <30% of total calories with <10% from saturated fat and total daily cholesterol intake <300 mg. Step II is total fat intake <20% of total calories with <7% from saturated fat and total daily cholesterol intake <200 mg. There is still uncertainty about whether this same dietary modification should be recommended in populations who are at risk for elevations for TG. This is certainly the case in people who have diabetes that is either genetically determined or unmasked by glucocorticoids. Some data suggest that a "Mediterranean" diet with decreased carbohydrate and increased monounsaturated fat intake may have better efficacy in such patients (4). Alcohol intake has also been an unresolved issue. There are data that indicate that alcohol increases TG concentrations in persons with a familial predisposition to hypertriglyceridemia. Therefore, avoidance of excess alcohol has been recommended for patients with high plasma TG levels. The epidemiological data to suggest that there may be benefits in this reduction for coronary heart disease have not (and likely never will be) corroborated by intervention trials. Therefore, fewer than two drinks daily are likely safe in patients without hypertriglyceridemia, hypertension, or other risks associated with alcohol use. However, the data are too limited to recommend alcohol intake as a dietary prescription.

B. Secondary Dyslipidemia

Dyslipidemia is associated with other disease processes—some of which may also be associated with rheumatic disorders. Hypothyroidism elevates both LDL-C and TG levels. If a screening thyroid-stimulating hormone (TSH) level is high, treatment with thyroid hormone replacement prior to other lipid-lowering pharmacotherapy is advisable. Diabetes mellitus, especially Type I diabetes, may be associated with other autoimmune syndromes. Insulin-resistant diabetes may be associated with glucocorticoid and cyclosporin use. When dyslipidemia is associated with suboptimal glycemic control, management of the glucose may be associated with improvement and TG and HDL-C levels. Reduction in dose of other medications contributing to the lipid abnormalities may also result in an improvement in the lipid profile. Therefore, intervention strategies with medications need to take into account the effect of dosage adjustment in the therapies for the rheumatic disorder.

C. Medications (17,18,20,26,45)

Four major classes of medications for lipid lowering currently exist, including niacin/nicotinic acid, fibric acid derivatives, bile acid sequestrants, and statins/HMG CoA reductase inhibitors (Table 3). Efficacy and common side effects of each class are discussed below.

1. Niacin

Niacin lowers TG concentrations by 30–40%. When used for isolated elevation of LDL-C (normal TG), 15% reduction of LDL-C levels may be achieved. Niacin has the greatest efficacy of all the medication classes in raising HDL-C levels. Currently, the recommended doses are in the range of 1–3 g per day. Regular-release niacin is preferred over sustained-release niacin because the efficacy is slightly greater than with the sustained-release form, and the risk for severe hepatotoxicity is less. Flushing may be worse with regular-release preparations. Other adverse effects, including gastrointestinal (GI) disturbances, increase in uric acid and, modest effects on raising blood glucose, are comparable for both preparations. The usual strategy is to start with a 100-mg dose twice a day with meals (often preceded by aspirin), with progressively increasing doses over a period of days to weeks to 1 to 1.5 g per day in divided doses. If desired lipid/lipoprotein targets have not been achieved, then combination therapy is a consideration (see below).

Niaspan (KOS, Miami, FL), a controlled-release form of niacin, is an acceptable alternative to regular-release preparations. Niaspan is given at bedtime, is associated with less flushing than regular-release niacin, and its use has not been associated with serious hepatotoxicity.

2. Fibrates

The commonly used fibric acid derivatives in the United States include gemfibrozil and fenofibrate. (Bezafibrate is widely used in many other parts of the world.) Fibrates have their major effect on lowering TG concentrations. When markedly elevated TG levels are reduced, there is a

Table 3 Lipid-Lowering Medications: Effects on Lipid and Lipoproteins and Common Side Effects

Medication	Total cholesterol	Triglycerides	HDL cholesterol	LDL cholesterol	Side effects
Niacin/nicotinic acid	⇓	⇓⇓⇓	⇑⇑⇑	⇓	Flushing, pruritis, increased glucose, acanthosis, hepatotoxicity
Fibrates/fibric acid derivatives	⇓	⇓⇓	⇑⇑	Variable Effects	GI disturbances, hepatotoxicity, myositis, myalgias
Bile acid sequestrants	⇓⇓	⇑	⇔	⇓⇓	Constipation, bloating
Statins/HMG CoA reductase inhibitors	⇓⇓⇓	⇔⇓	⇔⇑	⇓⇓⇓	Hepatotoxicity, myositis, myalgias

corresponding increase in HDL-C concentration. Fibrate effect on LDL-C levels is variable. When TG levels are high before treatment, then reduction of TG will be associated with increasing LDL-C levels. When TG levels are only mildly elevated prior to treatment, then fibrates may have no effect on LDL-C levels or even cause a modest LDL-C reduction. Adverse effects of fibrates are uncommon and include mild abdominal discomfort, occasional liver enzyme abnormalities, and, rarely, myositis.

3. Bile Acid Sequestrants

The common bile acid sequestrants include cholestyramine and colestid. Both are available in powder form and colestid is available in tablet form. The major effect is on LDL-C reduction. Their use is associated with a mild increase in TG levels and a neutral effect on HDL-C levels. Adverse effects include constipation and bloating. These symptoms tend to improve over time and can be reduced if a powder (which is usually mixed with water or some other liquid) is sipped rather than gulped. Because the resins bind not only bile acids (and the associated cholesterol), but also other medications, resin ingestion must occur at a separate time than ingestion of other medications. Ideally, this separation should be several hours. This is a limiting factor for patients with complex medical problems in whom several medications may be used in therapeutic regimens.

4. Statins/HMG CoA Reductase Inhibitors

Statins have their major effect on LDL-C reduction. At higher doses, statins are associated with reduction in TG levels as well. Low doses of the oldest available statin (lovastatin) may be associated with 10% reduction in LDL-C levels. There is a log linear dose–response curve for most of the statins. There is variation in potency, with atorvastatin and rosuvastatin having the greatest potency, which may achieve LDL-C reductions of 50% or greater. The adverse effects of statins are infrequent and include liver enzyme abnormalities. At low doses, less than 1% of patients will have an abnormal increase in serum liver enzymes. At higher doses, such signs of hepatotoxicity occur in ≤2% of cases. Myalgias and myositis are rare. Of interest is the fact that in double-blind clinical trials, patients rarely discontinued medications because of myalgias. This is in contrast to clinical experience where patients more commonly discontinue medication for muscle aches. In addition to myositis, periarticular pain may occur in patients who are physically active. Involved sites include joints used in physical exercise, e.g., shoulders for swimmers, or hips, knees, and ankles for runners. Routine screening with creatine kinase (CK) is rarely indicated. A reasonable approach to determine if myalgias are related to medication is to discontinue medication and assess the effect on joint pain, and then rechallenge (often starting at a lower dose or with a different statin). In patients with rheumatic disorders, this may be a particularly difficult situation. However, in general, joint and muscle pain is more likely to be related to their rheumatic condition than to the use of the statin.

5. Combination Therapy

For patients who have mixed dyslipidemias, i.e., elevations of both TG and LDL-C levels, several medication combinations may be effective. These include niacin and bile acid sequestrants (a common approach prior to the availability of the statins), fibric acid derivatives plus bile acid sequestrants, niacin plus statins, or fibric acid derivatives plus statins. Each of these combinations will have efficacy that is additive in lipid lowering. Adverse effects are related to the individual medications being used. The combinations of niacin plus the statins or fibric acid derivatives plus the statins are more likely to be associated with liver enzyme abnormalities or myositis. Patients need to be warned about these adverse effects even though they occur in less than 10% patients, and probably closer to 2–5%. For patients with pure LDL-C abnormalities, niacin combined with a bile acid sequestrants or statin, or a statin plus a bile acid sequestrant are very potent in lowering LDL-C levels. Adverse effects are related to the individual medications. Dosing of the bile acid sequestrants needs to be separated temporally from the associated lipid-lowering therapy.

6. Other Considerations in Dyslipidemia

There are a number of other disorders and medications that may have effects on lipid lowering. As noted previously, hypothyroid patients should have thyroid hormone (most commonly levothyroxine) administered to achieve a euthyroid state before other lipid-lowering therapy is initiated. In patients with diabetes mellitus (either primary or as a result of glucocorticoid use), glycemic control is often associated with improvement in TG concentrations. Improvement in hypertriglyceridemia has been associated with every class of glucose-lowering medication, including sulfonylureas, biguanides, thiazolidinediones, carbohydrase inhibitors, metiglinides, and insulin. For postmenopausal women, estrogen therapy is associated with increasing HDL-C and lowering LDL-C levels. Estrogen use may be associated with a modest increase in TG (although this may be part of a larger VLDL moiety that is less atherogenic). Psyllium as a soluble fiber when taken in high quantities is associated with modest LDL-C lowering. Fish oil capsules containing omega-3 polyunsaturated fatty acids are useful in selected patients with hypertriglyceridemia—usually refractory to other diet and medication treatment. Palatability limits fish oil use in routine clinical practice.

VII. TREATMENT OF PATIENTS WITH RHEUMATIC DISEASE AND LIPID ABNORMALITIES

Cumulative data indicate that high-risk patients for CHD accrue greater benefit from aggressive cholesterol lowering. Hence, the National Cholesterol Educational Program Adult Treatment Panel guidelines have recommended lower LDL-C targets (less than 100 mg/dL) for patients with CHD compared with those with two or more risk factors but without coronary artery disease (less than 130 mg/dL) (Table 4). Ongoing investigations are addressing whether patients with coronary artery disease should actually have an LDL target of less than 75 mg/dL. Furthermore, the American Diabetes Association has recommended that diabetic patients (even without known CHD) have LDL-C targets of less than 100 mg/dL. This is based on the observation that diabetic patients without known CHD have the same risk for a coronary event as nondiabetic patients with established CHD. It has become common clinical practice to use the same strategy in other very-high-risk patients without CHD, e.g., familial dyslipidemias, family history of very early coronary heart disease, or very high levels of Lp(a). Models for CHD risk assessment have been developed.

Table 4 LDL Cholesterol Targets in Patients Based on CHD Risk Factors and Presence of CHD

Risk Factors[a]	NCEP guidelines, mg/dL (17,18)	Alternative approach, mg/dL
≤1	<160	<160
≥2	<130	<130
CHD	<100	<100
High-risk[b] patients without known CHD		<100
High-risk[b] patients with CHD		<75 mg/dl

[a]Risk factors include male gender, hypertension, diabetes mellitus, family history of CHD, and obesity (17,18).
[b]High risk includes patients with diabetes mellitus (4,26), elevated Lp(a) (51), very strong family history of premature CHD, and selected rheumatic disorders (SLE, RA)

More aggressive lipid-lowering therapy for patients at high risk has been proposed (1,4,17,18, 24,25,26,53). Although rheumatic diseases such as SLE and RA have not been included in these models, the concept of aggressive LDL-C lowering seems applicable to these high-risk groups.

The benefits of lipid lowering (in randomized clinical trials) are usually evident within 2 years of therapy. More aggressive cholesterol lowering may accrue benefit within 6–12 months. Investigations are underway to determine whether there may be acute benefits to cholesterol lowering that are mediated through atheromatous plaque stabilization. Patients who are at high risk for coronary disease, such as those with SLE, should be approached with a similar aggressive strategy. If lipid abnormalities are associated with glucocorticoid or cyclosporine therapy, and if chronic use (≥ 1 year) is anticipated, then lipid-altering strategies should be implemented. The rationale for this approach is based on benefits of lipid lowering seen in other high-risk populations.

A. General Therapeutic Strategies

Most patients with rheumatic disorders are likely to have a mixed dyslipidemia. Dietary strategies, evaluation for secondary conditions that alter the lipid profiles, and treatment with lipid-lowering medication should be based on the nature of the primary lipid disorder. If LDL concentrations are clearly elevated and TG levels are normal or mildly elevated (≤ 300 mg/dL), then a strategy addressed at lowering LDL-C levels (such as the statins) should be the first choice. If the LDL concentrations remain high with maximally tolerated doses of statins, then fibric acid derivatives or niacin may be added to lower LDL-C and any residual elevation of TG levels. As noted above, these combinations may be more difficult to use in patients with rheumatic problems because of the uncertainty about muscle and joint aches, which may be associated with these combinations of medications. If the major abnormality is an elevation of TG, the fibric acid derivatives are the therapeutic medication of choice. Rarely will there be any confounding interaction with the underlying rheumatic disorder or associated therapeutic strategies. Niacin is difficult to use in rheumatic disorders. Associated GI side effects (especially in patients taking nonsteroidal anti-inflammatory agents), elevations of uric acid (which may precipitate gout), elevations of glucose (which may be additive to effects of glucocorticoids), and systemic symptoms of flushing and muscle aches may confound the clinical picture of the underlying rheumatic disorder.

Bile acid sequestrants are rarely the drug of choice for patients with rheumatic disorders because of limited efficacy and interference with the absorption of medications. Statins are well tolerated, have greater potency at lowering LDL-C levels and have an excellent safety profile. Drug interactions with statins are less of a consideration. Bile acid sequestrants may be necessary as additive therapy with the statins to lower LDL-C levels when statins alone are insufficient to reach LDL-C targets. Bile acid sequestrants are useful when statins are not tolerated. It is important to recall that bile acid sequestrants must be taken at times separate from those medications used for antirheumatic therapies.

VIII. SUMMARY

Selected patients with rheumatic disorders may be at increased risk for coronary artery disease. Dyslipidemia may occur as a result of the underlying disorder, associated diseases, and therapeutic interventions. The nature of the lipid abnormality determines appropriate therapy that may include diet, treatment of associated disorders, and primary lipid-lowering therapy. Aggressive lipid lowering for both LDL-C and TG is justified in patients at high risk of coronary disease. This includes patients with rheumatic disorders.

REFERENCES

1. Anderson, KM, Wilson PWF, Odell PM, Kannel WB. An updated coronary risk profile: A statement for health professionals. Circulation 1991; 83:356–362.
2. Asherson RA, Khamashta MA, Baguley E, Oakley CM, Rowell NR, Hughes GRV. Myocardial infarction and antiphospholipid antibodies in SLE and related disorders. Q J Med 1989; 73(272):1103–1115.
3. Alverson D, Chase P. Systemic lupus erythematosus in childhood presenting as hyperlipoproteinemia. J Pediatr 1988; 91:72–75.
4. American Diabetes Association. Management of dyslipidemia in adults with diabetes. American Diabetes Association: Clinical Practice Recommendations 1999. Diabetes Care 1999; 22:556–559.
5. Aoki K, Kawai S. Glucocorticoid therapy decreases serum lipoprotein(a) concentration in rheumatic diseases. Int Med 1993; 32:382–386.
6. Ballantyne C, Podet E, Patsch W, Harati Y, Appel V, Gotto A, Young J. Effects of cyclosporine therapy on plasma lipoprotein levels. JAMA 1989; 262:53–56.
7. Borba E, Bonfa E. Dyslipoproteinemias in systemic lupus erythematosus: Influence of disease, activity, and anticardiolipin antibodies. Lupus 1997; 6:533–539.
8. Bulkley BH, Roberts WC. A study of 36 necropsy patients. The heart in systemic lupus erythematosus and the changes induced in it by corticosteroid therapy. Am J Med 1975; 58:243–264.
9. Cressman MD, Heyka RJ, Paganini EP, et al. Lipoprotein(a) is an independent risk factor for cardiovascular disease in hemodialysis patients. Circulation 1992; 86:475–482.
10. DeFronzo RA, Ferrannini E. A multifaceted syndrome responsible for NIDDM obesity, hypertension, dyslipidemia, and atherosclerotic cardiovascular disease. Insulin resistance. Diabetes Care 1991; 14:173–194.
11. Donahoo WT. Kosmiski LA. Eckel RH. Drugs causing dyslipoproteinemia. Endocrin Metab Clin North Am 1998; 27:677–697.
12. Downs JR, Clearfield M, Weis S, Whitney E, Shapiro DR, Beere PA, et al. Primary prevention of acute coronary events with lovastatin in men and women with average cholesterol levels: Results of AFCAPS/TexCAPS.Air Force/Texas Coronary Atherosclerosis Prevention Study. JAMA 1998; 279:1615–1622.
13. Ellis C, Gorsulowsky D, Hamilton T, Billings J, et al. Cyclosporine improves psoriasis in a double-blind study. JAMA 1986; 256:3110–3116.
14. Ettinger W, Goldberg A, Applebaum-Bowden D, Hazzard W. Dyslipoproteinemia in systemic lupus erythematosus. Am J Med 1987; 83:503–508.
15. Ettinger W, Hazzard W. Elevated apolipoprotein-B levels in corticosteroid treated patients with systemic lupus erythematosus. J Clin Endocrin Metab 1988; 67:425–428.
16. Ettinger W, Klinefelter H, Kwiterovitch P. Effect of short-term low-dose corticosteroids on plasma lipoprotein lipids. Atherosclerosis 1987; 63:167–172.
17. Expert Panel of Detection, Evaluation, and Treatment of High Blood Cholesterol in Adults. National Cholesterol Education Program. Second report of the expert panel on detection, evaluation and treatment of high blood cholesterol in adults (Adult Treatment Panel II). Circulation 1994; 89:1333–1345.
18. Expert Panel of Detection, Evaluation, and Treatment of High Blood Cholesterol in Adults. National Cholesterol Education Program. National Cholesterol Education Program. Summary of the second report of the National Cholesterol Education Program expert panel on detection, evaluation and treatment of high blood cholesterol in adults (Adult Treatment Panel II). JAMA 1993; 269:3002–3008.
19. Frick MH, Elo O, Haapa K, Heinonen OP, Heinsalmi P, Helo P, et al. Helsinki Heart Study: Primary-prevention trial with gemfibrozil in middle-aged men with dyslipidemia. Safety of treatment, changes in risk factors, and incidence of coronary heart disease. N Engl J Med 1987; 317:1237–1245.
20. Friedrich CA, Rader DJ. Management of lipid disorders. Rheum Clin North Am 1999; 25:507–520.
21. Gherardi E, Rota E, Calandra S, Genova S, Tamborino A. Relationship among the concentrations of serum lipoproteins and changes in their chemical composition in patients with untreated nephrotic syndrome. Eur J Clin Invest 1977; 7:563–570.
22. Glueck C, Levy R, Glueck H, Gralnick H, Greten H, Frederickson D. Acquired Type I hyperlipopro-

teinemia with systemic lupus erythematosus, dysglobulinemia and heparin resistance. Am J Med 1969; 47:318–324.

23. Goldberg RB, Mellies MJ, Sacks FM, Moye LA, Howard BV, Howard WJ, et al. The Care Investigators. Cardiovascular events and their reduction with pravastatin in diabetic and glucose intolerant myocardial infarction survivors with average cholesterol levels: Subgroup analyses in the cholesterol and recurrent events (CARE) trial. Circulation 1998; 98:2513–2419.

24. Grundy SM, Balady GJ, Criqui MH, Fletcher G, Greenland P, Hiratzka LF, Houston-Miller N, Kris-Ehterton P, Krumholz HM, LaRosa J, Ockene IS, Pearson TA, Reed J, Washington R, Smith SC Jr. Primary prevention of coronary heart disease: Guidelines from Framingham. A statement for healthcare professionals from the American Heart Association's Task Force on Risk Reduction. Circulation 1998; 97:1876–1887.

25. Grundy, SM Integrating risk assessment with intervention. Primary Prevention of Coronary Heart Disease. Circ 1999; 100:988–998.

26. Haffner SM. Management of dyslipidemia in adults with diabetes: Technical review. Diabetes Care 1998; 21:160–178.

27. Haider Y, Roberts W. Coronary arterial disease in systemic lupus erythematosus: Quantification of degrees of narrowing in 22 necropsy patients (21 women) aged 16 to 37 years. Am J Med 1981; 70:775–781.

28. Harris KP, Russell GI, Parvin SD, Veitch PS, Walls J. Alterations in lipid-CHO metabolism attributable to cyclosporin A in renal transplant recipients. Br Med J 1986; 292:16.

29. Hodis H, Quismorio F, Wickham E, Blankenhorn D. The lipid, lipoprotein, and apolipoprotein effects of hydroxychloroquine in patients with systemic lupus erythematosus. J Rheumatol 1993; 20:661–665.

30. Hollander AA, van Saase JL, Kootte AM, van Dorp WT, van Bockel HJ, van Es LA, van der Woude FJ. Beneficial effects of conversion from cyclsporin to azathioprine after kidney transplantation. Lancet 1995; 345:610–614.

31. Hoogwerf, BJ, A Waness, M Cressman, et al. for the Post CABG Trial Investigators. Effects of aggressive cholesterol lowering on clinical and angiographic outcomes in patients with diabetes mellitus: Post CABG trial. Diabetes 1999; 48:1289–1294.

32. Hricik DE, Mayes JT, Schulak JA. Independent effects of cyclosporine and prednisone on posttransplant hypercholesterolemia. Am J Kidney Dis 1991; 28:353–358.

33. Ilowite N, Samuel P, Beseler L, Jacobson. Dyslipoproteinemia in juvenile rheumatoid arthritis. Med J Pediatr 1989; 114:823–826.

34. Ilowite N, Samuel P, Ginzler E, Jacobson M. Dyslipoproteinemia in pediatric systemic lupus erythematosus. Arthritis Rheum 1988; 31:859–863.

35. Ilowite N. Hyperlipidemia and the rheumatic diseases. Curr Opin Rheumatol 1996; 8:455–458.

36. Jonsson H, Nived O, Sturfelt G. Outcome in systemic lupus erythematosus: A prospective study of patients from a defined population. Medicine (Baltimore) 1989; 68(3):141–150.

37. Joren J, Villabona C, Vilella E, Masana L, Alberti R, Valles M. Abnormalities of lipoprotein metabolism in patients with the nephrotic syndrome. N Engl J Med 1990; 323:579–584.

38. Kabakov AE, Tertov VV, Saenko VA, Poverenny AM, Orekhov AN. The atherogenic effect of lupus sera: Systemic lupus erythematosus-derived immune complexes stimulate the accumulation of cholesterol in cultured smooth muscle cells from human aorta.

39. Kannel WB, D'Agostino RB, Wilson PW, Belanger AG, Gagnon DR. Diabetes, fibrinogen, and risk of cardiovascular disease: The Framingham experience. Am Heart J 1990; 120:672–676.

40. Kannel WB. Lipids, diabetes, and coronary artery disease: Insights from the Framingham Study. Am Heart J 1985; 110:1100–1107.

41. Kaplan NM. Upper-body obesity, glucose intolerance, hypertriglyceridemia, and hypertension: The deadly quartet. Arch Intern Med 1989; 149:1514–1520.

42. Kasiske B. Hyperlipidemia in patients with chronic renal disease. Am J Kid Dis 1998; 32:S142–S156.

43. Kawai S, Mizushima Y, Kaburaki J. Increased serum lipoprotein(a) levels in systemic lupus erythematosus with myocardial and cerebral infarctions. J Rheumatol 1995; 22:6, 1210–1211.

44. Khachadurian AK. Migratory polyarthritis in familial hypercholesterolemia (Type II hyperlipoproteinemia). Arthritis Rheum 1968; 11:385–393.

45. Knopp RH. Drug Treatment of lipid disorders. N Engl J Med 1999; 341:498–511.

46. Koskinen P, Manttari M, Manninen V, Huttunen JK, Heinonen OP, Frick MH. Coronary heart disease incidence in NIDDM patients in the Helsinki Heart Study. Diabetes Care 1992; 15:820–825.

47. Lazarevic M, Vitic J, Mladenovic V, Myones B, Skosey J, Swedler W. Dyslipoproteinemia in the course of active rheumatoid arthritis. Sem Arthritis Rheum 1992; 22:172–180.

48. Lehto S, Ronnemaa T, Haffner SM, Pyorala K, Kallio V, Laakso M. Dyslipidemia and hyperglycemia predict coronary heart disease events in middle-aged patients with NIDDM. Diabetes 1997; 46:1354–1359.

49. Leong KH, Koh E, Feng P, Boey Lipid profiles in patients with systemic lupus erythematosus. Med J Rheum 1994; 21:1264–1267.

50. Leong KH. Lipid disorders and rheumatic diseases. Ann Acad Med 1988; 27:8992.

51. LIPID Research Study Group. The relationship of reduction in incidence of coronary heart disease to cholesterol lowering. The Lipid Research Clinics Coronary Primary Prevention Trial results. II. JAMA 1984; 251:365–374.

52. MacMahon S, Sharpe N, Gamble G, Hart H, Scott J, Simes J, et al. Effects of lowering average of below average cholesterol levels on the progression of carotid atherosclerosis: Results of the LIPID Atherosclerosis Substudy. LIPID Trial Research Group [published erratum appears in Circulation 1996; 97:2479]. Circulation 1998; 97:1784–1790.

53. Maher VM, Brown BG, Marcovina SM, et al. Effects of lowering elevated LDL-C on the cardiovascular risk of lipoprotein(a). JAMA 1995; 274:1771–1774.

54. Mandell B. Cardiovascular involvement in systemic lupus erythematosus. Semin Arthritis Rheum 1987; 17:126–141.

55. Muls E, Rosseneu M, Daneels R, Schurgers M, Boelaert J. Lipoprotein distribution and composition in the human nephrotic syndrome. Atherosclerosis 1985; 54:225–237.

56. Munro R, Morrison E, McDonald AG, Hunter J, Madhok R, Capell H. Effect of disease modifying agents on the lipid profiles of patients with rheumatoid arthritis. Ann Rheum Dis 1997; 56:374–377.

57. Bloomfield H, Robins SJ, Collins D, et al. for the Veterans Affairs High-Density Lipoprotein Cholesterol Intervention Trial Study Group. Gemfibrozil for the secondary prevention of coronary heart disease in men with low levels of high-density lipoprotein cholesterol. N Engl J Med 1999; 341:410–418.

58. Petri M, Lakatta C, Magder L, Goldman D. Effect of prednisone and hydroxychloroquine on coronary artery disease risk factors in systemic lupus erythematosus: A longitudinal data analysis. Am J Med 1994; 96:254–259.

59. Petri M, Perez-Gutthann S, Spence D, Hochberg M. Risk factors for coronary artery disease in patients with systemic lupus erythematosus. Am J Med 1992, 93:513–519.

60. Petri M, Spence D, Bone L, Hochberg M. Coronary artery disease risk factors in the Johns Hopkins Lupus Cohort: Prevalence, recognition by patients, and preventive practices. Medicine (Baltimore) 1992; 71:291–302.

61. Petri M. Hydroxychloroquine use in the Baltimore Lupus Cohort: Effects on lipids, glucose and thrombosis. Lupus 1996; 5:S16–S22.

62. Post Coronary Artery Bypass Graft Trial Investigators. The effect of aggressive lowering of low density lipoprotein cholesterol levels and low dose anticoagulation on obstructive changes in saphenous-vein coronary-artery bypass grafts. [published erratum appears in N Engl J Med 1997; 337:1859]. N Engl J Med 1997; 336:153–162.

63. Prior P, Symmons DPM, Scott DL, Brown R, Hawkins CF. Cause of death in rheumatoid arthritis. Br J Rheumatol 1984; 23:92–99.

64. Pyorala K, Pedersen TR, Kjekshus J, Faergeman O, Olsson AG, Thorgeirsson G. Cholesterol lowering with simvastatin improves prognosis of diabetic patients with coronary heart disease. A subgroup analysis of the Scandinavian Simvastatin Survival Study (4S) [published erratum appears in Diabetes Care 1997; 20:1048]. Diabetes Care 1997; 20:614–620.

65. Reveille JD, Bartolucci A, Alarcon G. Prognosis in systemic lupus erythematosus. Arthritis Rheum 1990; 33:37–48.

66. Ridker PM, Hennekens CH, Stampfer MJ. A prospective study of lipoprotein(a) and the risk of myocardial infarction. JAMA 1993; 270:2195–2199.

67. Rubin LA, Urowitz MB, Gladman DD. Mortality in systemic lupus erythematosus: The bimodal pattern revisited. Q J Med 1985, 55:87–98.

68. Sacks FM, Pfeffer MA, Moye LA, Rouleau JL, Rutherford JD, Cole TG, et al. The effect of pravastatin on coronary events after myocardial infarction in patients with average cholesterol levels. Cholesterol and Recurrent Events Trial Investigators. N Engl J Med 1996; 335:1001–1009.

69. Scandinavian Simvastatin Survival Study (4S). Randomized trial of cholesterol lowering in 4444 patients with coronary heart disease: The Scandinavian Simvastatin Survival Study (4S). Lancet 1994; 344:1383–1389.

70. Shepherd J, Cobbe M, Ford I, et al. for the West of Scotland Coronary Prevention Study Group. Prevention of coronary heart disease with pravastatin in men with hypercholesterolemia. N Engl J Med 1995; 333:1301–1307.

71. Situnayake RD, Kitas G. Dyslipidemia and rheumatoid arthritis (comment). Ann Rheum Dis 1997; 56:341–342.

72. Sowers JR. Insulin resistance, hyperinsulinemia, dyslipidemia, hypertension, and accelerated atherosclerosis. J Clin Pharmacol 1992; 32:529–535.

73. Stamler J, Vaccaro I, Neaton JD, Wentworth D. Diabetes, other risk factors, and 12-yr cardiovascular mortality for men screened in the Multiple Risk Factor Intervention Trial. Diabetes Care 1993; 16: 434–444.

74. Stein JH, Rosenson RS. Lipoprotein Lp(a) excess and coronary heart disease. Arch Intern Med 1997; 157:1170–1176.

75. Sturfelt G, Eskilsson J, Nived O, Truedsson L, Valind S. Cardiovascular disease in systemic lupus erythematosus: A study of 75 patients from a defined population. Medicine 1992 71:216–223.

76. Svenson K, Lothell H, Hallgren R, Selinus I, Vessby B. Serum lipoprotein in active rheumatoid arthritis and other chronic inflammatory arthritides. Arch Intern Med 1987; 147:1912–1916.

77. Symmons DPM, Jones MA, Scott DL, Prior P. Long-term mortality outcome in patients with rheumatoid arthritis: Early presenters continue to do well. J Rheumatol 1998, 25:1072–1077.

78. Taskinen M, Kuusi T, Yki-Jarvinen H, Nikkala E. Short-term effects of prednisone on serum lipids and high density lipoprotein subfractions in normolipidemic healthy men. J Clin Endocrinol Metab 1988; 67:291–299.

79. Urowitz MB, Bookman AM, Koehler BE, Gordon DA, Smythe HA, Ogryzlo MA. The bimodal mortality pattern of systemic lupus erythematosus. Am J Med 1976; 60:221–225.

80. Utermann G. Lipoprotein(a). In: Scriver CR, Beaudet AL, Sly WS, Valle D, eds. The Metabolic and Molecular Bases of Inherited Disease. New York: McGraw-Hill, 1995:1887–1912.

81. Versluis DJ, Wenting GJ, Derkx FH, Schalekamp MA, Jeekel J, Weimar W. Who should be converted from cyclosporine to conventional immunosuppression in kidney transplantation and why. Transplantation 1987; 44:387–389.

82. Wallace D, Metzger A, Stecher V. Cholesterol lowering effect of hydroxychloroquine in patients with rheumatic disease: Reversal of deleterious effects of steroids on lipids. Am J Med 1990; 89:322–326.

83. Wanner C, Rader D, Bartens W, et al. Elevated plasma lipoprotein(a) in patients with nephrotic syndrome. Ann Intern Med 1993; 119:263–269.

84. Warwick G, Packard C. Lipoprotein metabolism in the nephrotic syndrome. Nephrol Dial Transplant 1993; 8:385–396.

85. Wheeler D, Bernard D. Lipid abnormalities in the nephrotic syndrome: Causes, consequences, and treatment. Am J Kidney Dis 1994; 23:331–346.

86. Wick G, Schett G, Amberger A, Kleindienst R, Xu Q. Is atherosclerosis an immunologically mediated disease? Immunol Today 1995; 16:27–33.

87. Wilson PWF, D'Agostino RB, Levy D, Belanger AM, Silbershatz H, Kannel WB. Prediction of coronary heart disease using risk factor categories. Circulation 1998; 97:1837–1847.

88. Wolfe F, Mitchell DM, Sibley JT, Fries JF, Bloch DA, Williams CA, Spitz PW, Haga M, Kleinheksel SM, Cathey MA. The mortality of rheumatoid arthritis. Arthritis Rheum 1994, 37:481–494.

89. Zimmerman J, Fainaru M, Eisenberg S. The effects of prednisone therapy on plasma lipoproteins and apolipoproteins: A prospective study. Metabolism 1984; 33:521–526.

52
Considerations for Novel Therapies in the Future

David Jayne
Addenbrooke's Hospital, Cambridge, England

I. INTRODUCTION

The small-vessel vasculitides are suitable paradigms for new forms of therapy in autoimmune disease. They are treatment-responsive and many components of the immune and inflammatory systems are involved in their pathogenesis. In particular, there is convincing evidence of T-cell and autoantibody contributions to injury. Today's drugs are usually effective—a remission rate of 93% was achieved in a recent study of generalized systemic vasculitis—but concern to avoid relapse necessitates prolonged therapy, and drug toxicity is almost universal (1,2). Even in "expert" centers, severe adverse effects of therapy in systemic vasculitis occur in one-quarter of patients, and there is an appreciable treatment-related mortality, especially in the elderly (2,3). Current therapy rests on the combination of steroids with cytotoxic drugs and regimens continue to be refined in order to maintain efficacy and minimize adverse effects (4,5). Newer approaches to treatment have arisen from a growing understanding of the pathogenesis of vasculitis and from the development of immunotherapeutic drugs with specificity for circulating agents or membrane receptors. The use of synergistic combinations of existing and newer immunosuppressive drugs allows improved efficacy with reduced toxicity. Finally, more sophisticated subgrouping at diagnosis according to prognostic markers and risk for drug toxicity will facilitate "tailored" protocols (5).

The goal of treatment for an immune-mediated disease is an intervention that has specificity for the deregulated processes that are causing injury, "specific immunotherapy," and the ability to prevent recurrence by induction of tolerance to the provoking factors. Specificity implies that physiological mechanisms, such as the ability to fight infection, are unaffected and the treatment will have low associated toxicity.

II. SPECIFIC IMMUNOTHERAPY: T CELL

Current hypotheses for the pathogenesis of vasculitis in autoimmunity give a central role to the T cell. The B-cell response has the characteristics of T-cell control with affinity maturation and isotype switching; activated T-cells are present at sites of injury and there are restrictions in the T-cell receptor (TCR) repertoire; also, T-cells from patients demonstrate proliferation to antineutrophil cytoplasmic antibody (ANCA) antigens (6–14). T cells have been identified in giant cell arteritis that infiltrate and damage vascular structures in response to vascular antigens (15). Further evidence for the primacy of the T cell comes from treatment: cyclosporin, antithymocyte globulin, and T cell–depleting monoclonal antibodies, which have led to remission in vasculitis (16–19). Strategies for controlling autoreactive T cells can be classified according to their mechanism of action (Table 1).

A. Antigen Presentation

Direction of T-cell immunotherapy toward the trimolecular complex, comprised of the TCR, major histocompatibility complex (MHC), and autoantigens, could confer specificity for the autoreactive response: of these three molecular structures, the MHC appears least useful because MHC restrictions, at least in small-vessel vasculitis, are weak or not present at all, implying presentation of antigen by multiple MHC alleles (20–22). Restrictions of both Vα and Vβ TCR gene usage have been demonstrated in circulating T cells from patients with active disease but not from bronchoalveolar lavage (8–10,23). A common TCR-Vβ complementarity-determining region (CDR)3 sequence has been identified in T cells from vasculitis patients; the CDR3 region is the major peptide antigen binding site and is highly polymorphic. This restriction implies a common vasculitis T-cell antigen response and potential new target for therapy (9). Although several groups have identified T-cell proliferative responses to the ANCA antigens, proteinase 3 (PR3), and myeloperoxidase (MPO), the antigenic peptides participating in pathogenic responses have not been identified (13,14). Where antigenic peptides have been identified in other autoimmune processes, immune manipulation with artificial peptide antigens can suppress the pathogenic response and tolerize the host to the autoantigen (24,25).

There is evidence for T-cell stimulation by microbial antigens in the etiology of Kawasaki disease, a systemic vasculitis of young children (26). This results in expansion of T-cell families bearing the BV segments recognized by the superantigen. Binding of superantigen to the BV regions on the TCR can be inhibited by pooled intravenous immunoglobulin (IgIV), which contains antibodies that compete for the same sequences resulting in abrogation of T-cell activation (27,28). Superantigens have been proposed to play a role in Wegener's granulomatosis where infection of the upper respiratory tract is a frequent occurrence (29). Nasal colonization with *Staphylococcus aureus* is associated with disease relapse, and this organism produces several superantigens capable of activating human T cells (30–32). It is unclear whether this mechanism pertains to clinical improvements seen in Wegener's patients after IgIV or sulfamethoxazole/

Table 1 T-Cell Targets for Immunotherapy in Vasculitis and Potential New Interventions

Mechanism	Target	Agent
Antigen presentation	T-cell receptor	Blocking peptides
	Superantigen	IgIV
Costimulation	CD4	Anti-CD4 (nondepleting)
	CD40:CD40L	Anti-CD40L
	CD28/CTLA4:CD80186	CTLA4Ig
T-cell proliferation	IL-2	Anti-IL-2 receptor
Cytokine regulation	Th1:Th2 counterregulation	IL-10Fc
T-cell depletion	CD52	Anti-CD52
	CD4	Anti-CD4 (depleting)
		Immunoablation

trimethoprim (33–35). Control of staphylococcal infection is a likely explanation for success with antibiotics in Wegener's granulomatosis and has prompted investigation of long-term topical antiseptics to prevent bacterial colonization (33,36).

B. T-Cell Proliferation

Activated T cells release interleukin-2 (IL-2) and express the IL-2 receptor (IL-2r), and proliferation is dependent on IL-2:IL-2r interaction. Soluble IL-2r (sIL-2r) levels correlate with disease activity in Wegener's granulomatosis and remain elevated during remission, pointing to continued T-cell dysregulation despite clinical inactivity (37,38). Preliminary evidence from the use of cyclosporin in vasculitis points to the value of suppressing IL-2–mediated T-cell proliferation and suggests that more-specific agents could also be successful (16,17). Monoclonal anti–IL-2r has suppressed the induction of experimental autoimmunity and has recently been licensed for use in human solid organ allografting (39). In combination with conventional immunosuppressive therapy, anti–IL-2r antibodies further reduce allograft rejection rates without adding to the risk of opportunistic infection, and short-term use leads to suppression of IL-2r expression for several months (40). Such therapy may contribute to T-cell control in vasculitis but so far has only been explored in animal models.

C. T-Cell Costimulation

An alternative approach to the T cell is by inhibition of costimulatory mechanisms required to produce a proliferative response, which include CD4, CD28/CTLA4:CD80186, and CD40:CD40 ligand (CD40L, CD152) (41). Use of a nondepleting anti-CD4 antibody has led to allograft tolerance in animal models and has contributed to sustained remissions in human vasculitis (19). An immunoglobulin antigen conjugate, CTLA4Ig, effectively inhibits CD28/CTLA4: CD80186 interactions and prevents allograft rejection and experimental nephritis. Interestingly, T-cell CD28 expression is inversely correlated with disease activity in Wegener's granulomatosis, and patient-derived T-cell lines do not express CD28, suggesting that the CD28:CD80186 interaction is less significant to this subgroup of vasculitis (42–44). The CD40:CD40L interaction has various roles including T-cell costimulation and T cell–dependent B-cell activation, and antibodies to CD40L block allograft rejection, a T cell–mediated process (45). Marked upregulation of CD40 and CD40L on T and B cells in human systemic lupus erythematosus has prompted studies with anti-CD40L antibodies previously shown to reverse disease and reduce autoantibody levels in animal models (46–48). Inflamed tissues also express CD40L, for example, in the gut in Crohn's disease and in the kidney in inflammatory renal disease; this upregulation of CD40L is likely to contribute to local augmentation of inflammation and cytotoxic T-cell injury (49,50). Blockade of multiple costimulatory interactions can act synergistically, potentiating the therapeutic effect (42). However, costimulation is a fundamental principle of adaptive immune responses and its blockade could have profound immunosuppressive effects.

D. T-Cell Depletion

Monoclonal anti–T-cell depletion with anti-CD52 (CAMPATH-1H) has led to remissions in Wegener's granulomatosis, ANCA-positive and -negative polyarteritis, and rheumatoid vasculitis (19,51). Cytototoxics were withheld prior to antibody therapy and the remissions allowed the subsequent programmed removal of corticosteroids. Transient improvement to CAMPATH-1H has been observed in other autoimmune conditions, including rheumatoid arthritis and multiple sclerosis (52,53). The CD52 antigen is abundantly expressed on T cells and is not subject to downregulation, as occurs with CD4, and total lymphopenia is rapidly obtained (51). Lymphopenia after a single course is usually prolonged but serious opportunistic infection and lymphoma have been rare. Return of CD4+ T cells often presages relapse, indicating the lack of specificity of this treatment for autoreactive T cells, but disease relapses have responded to repeated dosing (51). Antithymocyte globulin (ATG) has induced sustained remissions of refractory Wegener's granulomatosis for over 1 year in a small number of patients without prolonged lymphopenia (18).

A more radical approach to T-cell depletion for severe autoimmunity has been immunoablation with stem cell rescue (54). In theory, this technique destroys all autoreactive T cells with the hope that the immune system regenerates from previously isolated CD34+ stem cells in a more tolerant form (54). Clearly, it does not reverse genetic factors relevant to disease etiology and total T-cell removal appears difficult to achieve, with some T cells surviving immunoablation and others contaminating the graft. The European Bone Marrow Transplant Registry has reported an overall 1-year patient survival of 9% from a population of 74 patients with various autoimmune diseases, including three with vasculitis (55). Allogeneic transplantation currently carries too high a morbidity to be considered for treating human autoimmune disease, but has prevented spontaneous vasculitis in a genetically prone animal model (56).

E. T-Cell Regulation by Cytokines

Controversy exists as to the importance of T-cell counterregulatory networks in vasculitis: experimental models with Th-2 dominant responses are associated with ANCA production and vasculitis; conversely, human vasculitis is often associated with granulomata, a Th-1 phenomenon, and T-cell lines derived from biopsies of vasculitic inflammation in Wegener's granulomatosis have all had a Th-1 phenotype (57,58). It has been postulated that this bias results from excess macrophage IL-12 release that can be reversed in vitro by interleukin 10 (IL-10) (58). Fusion of IL-10 with an immunoglobulin fragment has produced a stable compound capable of suppressing Th-1 responses and Th-1–mediated autoimmunity in experimental animals; clinical studies in vasculitis are awaited (58,59). However, the relevance of Th-1:Th-2 balance to human vasculitis is unlikely to be simple; in Kawasaki disease IL-10 levels are associated with inflammatory activity, and human IgG ANCA induces a Th-2 immune response and vasculitis in experimental animals (60,61). Other interventions that have selectively biased Th-1:Th-2 regulation toward a Th-2 phenotype include thalidomide, pentoxifylline, and CTLA4Ig (62–64).

F. The Antiglobulin Response

A potential problem with biological agents is the development of antibodies in the patients that neutralize the effect of subsequent treatments and can lead to serum sickness reactions, observed, for example, with antithymocyte globulin. Recombinant technology has allowed the generation of "humanized" and chimeric antibodies in which this difficulty is greatly reduced (65). However, an antiglobulin response is still detectable in a proportion of patients that has stimulated strategies, including concurrent immunosuppression, to prevent formation of, and plasma exchange to remove, antiglobulin antibodies (51,66).

III. SPECIFIC IMMUNOTHERAPY: B CELL AND AUTOANTIBODY

A. B Cells

Autoantibody-producing B cells can be targeted by the B-cell receptor, surface-bound immunoglobulin defined by its antigenic specificity or idiotype. Were a dominant idiotype to be demonstrated for ANCA antibodies, monoclonal antiidiotype antibodies might become a realistic treatment. Monoclonal anti-idiotype (anti-id) antibodies have been produced that have the potential to interact with ANCA-secreting B cells; the 5/7 anti-id reacts with an idiotype present on PR3-ANCA from 50% of Wegener's granulomatosis patients, which inhibited the PR3-ANCA binding of 11/19, 5/7 Id–positive sera, and the 7F2C11 anti-id detected a cross-reactive idiotype in four MPO-ANCA–positive sera not present in controls (67,68). Idiotypic network theory proposes that autoimmunity results from a failure of physiological suppression mediated in health by naturally occurring anti-idiotype antibodies (69). Circulating anti-idiotype antibodies reactive with PR3-ANCA and MPO-ANCA occur in both patients and normal individuals, which lends support to this theory (70–72). Idiotypic suppression of autoreactive B-cell activity has been proposed as a mechanism for IgIV and has been found in other autoimmune conditions, such as anti–factor VIII disease (73). IgIV also contains ANCA antiidiotype activity, and falls in ANCAs have been observed in certain, but not all, patients after IgIV. It is unclear whether this is a direct effect on ANCA production or mediated via cytokines or an influence on autoreactive T cells (70–74).

Depletion of B cells, analogous to T-cell depletion above, has been performed by anti-CD20 monoclonal antibodies in B-cell lymphoma patients and might have a role in vasculitic scenarios where autoantibodies predominate (75).

B. Autoantibodies

There is evidence that ANCAs contribute to the pathogenicity of those vasculitides where they are present, through neutrophil activation, blocking protease inhibitors and promoting endothelial injury (76–81). Experimental models have also demonstrated a role for ANCAs in crescentic nephritis and pulmonary capillaritis; both presentations are closely associated with ANCAs in human disease (82,83). Physical removal of ANCAs by plasma exchange might explain the improvement reported in earlier studies of crescentic nephritis not associated with antibodies to glomerular basement membrane, and this forms the subject of an ongoing trial (5,84). Plasma exchange also removes coagulation factors and cytokines, and nonspecific immunoglobulin depletion provokes a rebound in antibody synthesis, including autoantibodies. Selective immunoabsorption is a logical development of plasma exchange that aims to remove the circulating component alone without depleting other plasma proteins and avoiding the need for their replacement. Semiselective removal of immunoglobulins by adsorption against protein-A, heterologous anti-human IgG antibodies, or the charged amino acids tryptophan and phenylalanine has been applied to limited numbers of patients with vasculitis receiving concurrent immunosuppression (85–89). A randomized–controlled trial of 44 patients with renal vasculitis found similar efficacy between plasma exchange and protein A immunoadsorption; both treatments reduced ANCA levels (89). Allergic adverse effects to protein A occur, with skin vasculitis being reported (90). The availability of recombinant ANCA antigens recognized by the majority of ANCA-positive sera has raised the possibility of autoantibody-specific immunoabsorption (91). In vitro study has confirmed the practicability of this treatment in terms of the affinity of MPO-ANCA binding to the recombinant proteins and the capacity of columns containing relatively small quantities of protein (50 mg) to deplete circulating ANCAs (92). Theoretical advantages of this approach are the preferential removal of high-affinity autoantibodies, which have been associated with disease activity in vasculitis, the removal of other isotypes in addition to IgG, and the avoidance of hypogammaglobulinemia (6,7,93).

The antigenic targets for ANCAs are proteolytic enzymes, capable of organ damage in the absence of an immune response, whose activity is normally controlled by protease inhibitors, specifically, 1-antitrypsin for PR3 and ceruloplasmin for MPO (94–96). Binding of ANCAs to PR3 or MPO impairs protease inhibition, prolonging enzymatic activity, and this mechanism has been proposed to explain the increased severity of PR3-ANCA–associated vasculitis in patients with l-antitrypsin deficiency (80,81,94). Pharmacological supplementation of protease inhibitors is feasible but has not been explored in vasculitis.

IV. SPECIFIC IMMUNOTHERAPY: CYTOKINES AND LEUKOCYTE–ENDOTHELIUM INTERACTIONS

The endothelium can be regarded as one target tissue in vasculitis; injury is dependent on interaction between the endothelium and circulating leukocytes, and a pathological hallmark of vasculitis is the infiltration throughout vessel walls of neutrophil and mononuclear leukocytes. Several stages in this process are amenable to therapeutic intervention, including leukocyte migration, endothelial cell activation, and leukocyte adhesion.

A. Leukocyte Attraction

The neutrophil chemoattractants C5a, interleukin-8 (IL-8) and transforming growth factor-β (TGF-β) are present at increased levels in vasculitic sera, and as ANCAs stimulate monocyte IL-8 release and TGF-β activation, these factors serve to amplify inflammation through a positive feedback loop (97–99). Two potential treatments have been explored in experimental models: antibodies to C5a reduce deposition of the membrane terminal attack complex (C5-9) and inhibit endothelial NF-κB translocation and adhesion molecule expression in models of complement-mediated endothelial cell injury, while anti–IL-8 monoclonal antibodies reduced neutrophil migration into sites of vasculitis and consequent injury (57,100,101).

B. Leukocyte Adhesion

The interaction between leukocytes and the endothelium is mediated by receptor–counterreceptor pairs on inflammatory and endothelial cells that govern not only cellular adhesion and traffic but also cellular activation, and play a role in many autoimmune processes (102). Antiadhesion therapy has been shown to abrogate inflammation in models of human inflammatory disease, including antigen-induced arthritis, ischemia–reperfusion injury, and renal allograft rejection, and in patients with rheumatoid arthritis treated with anti-intercellular adhesion molecule 1 (ICAM-1) (103). Upregulation of the neutrophil integrin CD18 and endothelial adhesion molecules, including E-selectin and vascular cell adhesion molecule (VCAM), is induced by ANCAs, and neutrophils from patients with active vasculitis have increased neutrophil CD18 expression (79,105). CD18 also plays a crucial role in transendothelial migration of T cells as well as being an accessory molecule for T-cell activation, and CD18 blockade induces tolerance in a cardiac allograft model (106). A humanized anti-CD18 monoclonal antibody has been given to five patients with refractory vasculitis with apparent clinical benefit in four (107).

C. Endothelial Activation

Cytokines, in particular TNF and IL-1, and ANCAs participate in activation of the endothelium in vasculitis; this is reflected by surface expression and an increase in plasma levels of adhesion molecules (104,108). Tumor necrosis factor has other actions of potential importance in vasculitis, increasing the release of IL-6, IL-8, and IL-12 and supporting a Th-1 T-cell phenotype (58,109,110). The success and safety of TNF inhibitors in rheumatoid arthritis and Crohn's disease has prompted their study in vasculitis (66,111). Other techniques to manipulate leukocyte–endothelium interactions include inhibitors of angiogenesis, which reverse endothelial activation and have minimized coronary vasculitis in an animal model, and antibodies to VCAM-1 and IL-6 (112–114).

V. POOLED INTRAVENOUS IMMUNOGLOBULIN: SPECIFIC IMMUNOTHERAPY?

Multiple mechanisms have been proposed to explain the immunotherapeutic effects of IgIV, which can be divided simply into antiimmune and antiinflammatory. Interactions between the variable regions of IgG in IgIV with autoantibodies, B-cell receptors, and surface antigens on T-cells have the potential to influence antigen-driven immune responses (28,70). Anti-inflammatory effects of IgIV include reversal of lymphocyte activation, increased immunoglobulin clearance, and modulation of cytokine release as well as neutralization of circulating cytokines and activated complement (115–120). IgIV suppresses ANCA-induced neutrophil IL-1 secretion, and anti-idiotypic antibodies in IgIV inhibit ANCA binding; less specific effects of IgIV are inhibition of macrophage TNF release and reduction of complement-mediated endothelial cell injury (70,74,121–123). Clinical study of IgIV has been complicated by, apparently, dramatic improvements in certain cases and more modest or no effects in others (34,74,124–128). In a placebo-controlled trial involving patients with persistent or relapsing diseases, a reduction in disease activity with IgIV was demonstrated with concurrent falls in C-reactive protein, which were maintained for up to 3 months (35). There was no effect of IgIV on ANCA levels or reduction in the subsequent relapse rate, thus the mechanism appeared more likely to be anti-inflammatory than anti-immune (35). This suggests that repeated IgIV dosing, at 1- to 3-month intervals merits further study. If the major mechanism of action of IgIV in vasculitis could be determined, IgIV could be purified or enriched for this activity. For example, anti-idiotype antibodies have been purified from IgIV and are increased in concentration in its dimeric fraction and in normal IgM preparations (129–131).

Sequential antibody depletion with plasma exchange or immunoadsorption followed by IgIV has shown promise in single cases (132). In addition to correcting hypogammaglobulinemia, this strategy suppresses autoantibody rebound and may potentiate the immunomodulatory effects of IgIV.

VI. EXPERIMENTAL IMMUNOSUPPRESSIVES

Two small studies have indicated a role for cyclosporin as a remission-maintaining agent for systemic vasculitis, but its use in vasculitis has been limited by concern over its toxicity, particularly to the kidney and endothelium (16,17,133). Tacrolimus has a similar mode of action to cyclosporin with a different toxicity profile and has proved superior to cyclosporin in autoimmune eye disease (134). Interleukin-2–dependent T-cell proliferation is also suppressed by rapamycin and SDZ-RAD, drugs that are not nephrotoxic and exhibit synergy with cyclosporin and tacrolimus in transplantation (135–137) (Table 2).

The antiproliferative drug mycophenolate mofetil has a selective effect on lymphocytes that lack a salvage pathway for purine metabolism and has additional actions of interest in vasculitis, such as reduction of adhesion molecule expression, antifibrotic effects, and preservation of renal function in partial nephrectomy models (138). A pilot study in small-vessel vasculitis used mycophenolate to prevent relapse after remission induction with cyclophosphamide; only 1 of 12 patients relapsed during the 18-month study (139). Other, anecdotal, reports in vasculitis and accumulating data from systemic lupus erythematosus and primary glomerulonephritis argue for larger studies in vasculitis (139,138). Other immunosuppressives attracting interest in vasculitis

Table 2 Newer Immunosuppressive Drugs for Treatment of Vasculitis and Their Modes of Action

Drug	Target	References
Cyclosporin, tacrolimus	T cell, IL-2 production	16,17
Rapamycin, SDZ-RAD	IL-2–dependent T-cell proliferation	
Mycophenolate mofetil	T-cell and B-cell proliferation	139,138
	Adhesion molecule expression	
	Antifibrotic	
Leflunomide	T cell	140
Deoxyspergualin	T cell, monocyte	142

are leflunomide, a pyrimidine antagonist, and deoxyspergualin (140–142). Deoxyspergualin and its analogues have a novel mechanism of action that is incompletely understood but includes binding to heat shock proteins, suppression of NF-κB–mediated cytokine release and antiproliferative effects (143). Synergy has been shown between deoxyspergualin and rapamycin and between deoxyspergualin and T-cell depletion in transplant models (144,145).

VII. A RATIONAL APPROACH TO NEW THERAPIES

A. Combination Therapy

There have been several examples above of synergy between treatments resulting in improved efficacy or reduced toxicity. The length of remission in Wegener's granulomatosis following T-cell depletion with anti-CD52 has been improved by its combination with a nonlytic anti-CD4 antibody; and it has been proposed that reducing T-cell numbers with anti-CD52, and thereby T-cell interactions, increases the effect of blocking accessory molecules with anti-CD4 (19). The combination of cyclosporin or tacrolimus with rapamycin has allowed reduced cyclosporin dosing, avoiding nephrotoxicity, while improving efficacy in transplantation and experimental autoimmunity (135,137,146). In rheumatoid arthritis, low-dose methotrexate has both improved the outcome with TNF blockade and reduced the frequency of an antiglobulin response (66). For the purposes of designing newer therapies, the vasculitic process may be conveniently divided into autoimmune, inflammatory, and autoantibody effects, and future combination therapy constructed to address each compartment (Table 3).

B. Evaluation of New Therapy

Specific immunotherapy provides the opportunity to explore pathogenesis as well as to develop new treatments, and precise monitoring of the effect of immunotherapy on the pathogenetic process is likely to be informative. It is also necessary to confirm that a drug is operating through its intended mechanisms; an example is the application of anti-CD18 antibodies, which was monitored by measuring neutrophil expression of CD18, in vitro neutrophil activity, and in vivo trafficking of neutrophils to sites of vasculitis (107). The methodology for performing therapeutic trials in vasculitis has been developed over the last decade with the organization of collaborative research networks and design of scoring tools to assess disease activity and damage (5,147–149). Comparative studies remain expensive and are prolonged over several years; the identification of surrogate markers to substitute for current end points and more efficient tools to assess vasculitic activity are therefore desirable. Steps toward the objective assessment of vasculitis activity include white cell scanning using [111]Indium, particularly useful for Wegener's granulomatosis, and

Table 3 Simplified Overview of Sequence of Pathogenesis in Vasculitis with Targets for Immunotherapy and Therapeutic Agents Either Available Now (Bold) or Potentially Available in the Future

Etiology		Autoimmunity			Inflammation and leukocyte–endo-thelium interaction
Genetic sus-ceptibility	Environmental agents	T cell	B cell	Autoanti-body	Cytokines, chemo-kines Leukocytes, en-dothelial cells
					INJURY
	Antibiotics	Anti-IL2r anti-thymocyte globulin	IgIV	Plasma exchange	Anti-TNF IgIV
Gene therapy	Identification and avoidance	Anti-CD52 IL-10Fc Anti-CD4 Anti-CD40L Immunoablation	Anti-CD40L Anti-idiotype Anti-CD20	Immunoad-sorption	Anti-CD18 Anti-VCAM Anti-IL-6 Anti-IL-8 Anti-C5a

targeting isotopes to endothelial adhesion molecules (150,151). The expense of newer agents will require cost–benefit analyses, and detailed economic assessment of vasculitis has not yet been performed (152).

VIII. CONCLUSIONS

Improved therapy would make an important contribution to better outcome in vasculitis but other major factors include avoidance of diagnostic delay, a comprehensive and accessible system of classification, and organization of health care to deliver specialized, multidisciplinary advice. The twin aims of novel therapies are to replace existing drugs, in particular cyclophosphamide and high-dose steroids, and at an immunological level, to induce sustained tolerance against pathogenic autoantigens. From the wide range of potential agents above, a logical strategy can be assembled combining anti–T-cell and anti-inflammatory agents at disease onset and selecting single or multiple agents with low cumulative toxicity for the longer-term prevention of relapse. At present, patients are treated on an empirical basis at diagnosis according to disease severity; with better definition of prognostic factors, subgroupings are likely to be redefined (5,153). Furthermore, the immunogenetic composition of the patient will influence response to immunotherapy, as has been observed in transplantation, and will influence choice of therapy (154).

Identification of genetic and environmental factors relevant to the etiology, presentation, and persistence of vasculitis will also offer new opportunities for disease control. Meanwhile, the accessibility of one of the target organs in vasculitis, the endothelium, from the vascular compartment makes it a suitable target for gene therapy, and techniques to direct genetic vectors to activated endothelial cells have been developed (155). Finally, there is a danger that increasing the complexity of treatment will conflict with the need for simple, comprehensible guidelines that are required to permit improvements in treatment to be spread beyond specialist centers.

REFERENCES

1. Hoffman GS, Kerr GS, Leavitt RY, et al. Wegener granulomatosis: An analysis of 158 patients. Ann Intern Med 1992; 116:488–498.
2. Jayne DRW, Gaskin G, (EUVAS). Randomized trial of cyclophosphamide versus azathioprine during remission in ANCA-associated vasculitis (CYCAZAREM). J Am Soc Nephrol 1999; 10:105A.
3. Krafcik SS, Covin RB, Lynch JPr, Sitrin RG. Wegener's granulomatosis in the elderly. Chest 1996; 109:430–437.
4. Fauci AS, Katz P, Haynes BF, Wolff SM. Cyclophosphamide therapy of severe systemic necrotizing vasculitis. N Engl J Med 1979; 301:235–238.
5. Rasmussen N, Jayne D, Abramowicz D, Andrassy K, Bacon PA, Cohen Tervaert JW, Dadoniené J, Feighery C, van Es LA, Ferrario F, Gregorini G, de Groot K, Gross WL, Grönhagen-Riska C, Guillevin L, Hagen C, Heigl Z, J.H, Kallenberg CGM, Landais P, Lesavre P, Lockwood CM, Luqmani R. European therapeutic trials in ANCA-associated systemic vasculitis: Disease scoring, consensus regimens and proposed clinical trials. Clin Exp Immunol 1995; 101(suppl 1):29–34.
6. Jayne DR, Weetman AP, Lockwood CM. IgG subclass distribution of autoantibodies to neutrophil cytoplasmic antigens in systemic vasculitis. Clin Exp Immunol 1991; 84:476–481.
7. Esnault VL, Jayne DR, Weetman AP, Lockwood CM. IgG subclass distribution and relative functional affinity of anti-myeloperoxidase antibodies in systemic vasculitis at presentation and during follow-up. Immunology 1991; 74:714–718.
8. Giscombe R, Grunewald J, Nityanand S, Lefvert AK. T cell receptor (TCR) V gene usage in patients with systemic necrotizing vasculitis. Clin Exp Immunol 1995; 101:213–219.
9. Grunewald J, Halapi E, Wahlstrom J, et al. T-cell expansions with conserved T-cell receptor beta chain motifs in the peripheral blood of HLA-DRB1*0401 positive patients with necrotizing vasculitis. Blood 1998; 92:3737–3744.
10. Simpson IJ, Skinner MA, Geursen A, et al. Peripheral blood T lymphocytes in systemic vasculitis: Increased T cell receptor V beta 2 gene usage in microscopic polyarteritis. Clin Exp Immunol 1995; 101:220–226.
11. Muschen M, Warskulat U, Perniok A, et al. Involvement of soluble CD95 in Churg-Strauss syndrome. Am J Pathol 1999; 155:915–925.
12. Ballieux BE, van der Burg SH, Hagen EC, van der Woude FJ, Melief CJ, Daha MR. Cell-mediated autoimmunity in patients with Wegener's granulomatosis (WG). Clin Exp Immunol 1995; 100:186–193.
13. King WJ, Brooks CJ, Holder R, Hughes P, Adu D, Savage CO. T lymphocyte responses to anti-neutrophil cytoplasmic autoantibody (ANCA) antigens are present in patients with ANCA-associated systemic vasculitis and persist during disease remission. Clin Exp Immunol 1998; 112:539–546.
14. Brouwer E, Stegeman CA, Huitema MG, Limburg PC, Kallenberg CG. T cell reactivity to proteinase 3 and myeloperoxidase in patients with Wegener's granulomatosis (WG). Clin Exp Immunol 1994; 98:448–453.
15. Brack A, Geisler A, Martinez-Taboada VM, Younge BR, Goronzy JJ, Weyand CM. Giant cell vasculitis is a T cell-dependent disease. Mol Med 1997; 3:530–543.
16. Haubitz M, Koch KM, Brunkhorst R. Cyclosporin for the prevention of disease reactivation in relapsing ANCA-associated vasculitis. Nephrol Dial Transplant 1998; 13:2074–2076.
17. Szpirt WM, Rasmussen N, Pedersen J. Plasma exchange and cyclosporin A in Wegener's granulomatosis: A controlled study. Int J Artif Organs 1996; 10:501.
18. Hagen EC, de Keizer RJ, Andrassy K, et al. Compassionate treatment of Wegener's granulomatosis with rabbit anti-thymocyte globulin. Clin Nephrol 1995; 43:351–359.
19. Lockwood CM. Refractory Wegener's granulomatosis: A model for shorter immunotherapy of autoimmune diseases. J R Coll Physicians Lond 1998; 32:473–478.

20. Zhang L, Jayne DR, Zhao MH, Lockwood CM, Oliveira DB. Distribution of MHC class II alleles in primary systemic vasculitis. Kidney Int 1995; 47:294–298.

21. Hagen EC, Stegeman CA, D'Amaro J, et al. Decreased frequency of HLA-DR13DR6 in Wegener's granulomatosis. Kidney Int 1995; 48:801–805.

22. Spencer SJ, Burns A, Gaskin G, Pusey CD, Rees AJ. HLA class II specificities in vasculitis with antibodies to neutrophil cytoplasmic antigens. Kidney Int 1992; 41:1059–1063.

23. Schnabel A, Renz H, Petermann R, Csernok E, Gross WL. T cell receptor vbeta repertoire in bronchoalveolar lavage in Wegener's granulomatosis and sarcoidosis. Int Arch Allergy Immunol 1999; 119:223–230.

24. Kaye JF, Kerlero de Rosbo N, Mendel I, et al. The central nervous system-specific myelin oligodendrocytic basic protein (MOBP) is encephalitogenic and a potential target antigen in multiple sclerosis (MS). J Neuroimmunol 2000; 102:189–198.

25. Burkhart C, Liu GY, Anderton SM, Metzler B, Wraith DC. Peptide-induced T cell regulation of experimental autoimmune encephalomyelitis: A role for IL-10. Int Immunol 1999; 11:1625–1634.

26. Kotzin BL, Leung DY, Kappler J, Marrack P. Superantigens and their potential role in human disease. Adv Immunol 1993; 54:99–166.

27. Takei S, Arora YK, Walker SM. Intravenous immunoglobulin contains specific antibodies inhibitory to activation of T cells by staphylococcal toxin superantigens. J Clin Invest 1993; 91:602–607.

28. Baudet V, Hurez V, Lapeyre C, Kaveri SV, Kazatchkine MD. Intravenous immunoglobulin (IVIg) modulates the expansion of V beta 3+ and V beta 17+ T cells induced by staphylococcal enterotoxin B superantigen in vitro. Scand J Immunol 1996; 43:277–282.

29. Cohen Tervaert JW, Popa ER, Bos NA. The role of superantigens in vasculitis. Curr Opin Rheumatol 1999; 11:24–33.

30. Stegeman CA, Tervaert JW, Sluiter WJ, Manson WL, de Jong PE, Kallenberg CG. Association of chronic nasal carriage of Staphylococcus aureus and higher relapse rates in Wegener granulomatosis. Ann Intern Med 1994; 120:12–17.

31. Abe Y, Nakano S, Aita K, Sagishima M. Streptococcal and staphylococcal superantigen-induced lymphocytic arteritis in a local type experimental model: Comparison with acute vasculitis in the Arthus reaction. J Lab Clin Med 1998; 131:93–102.

32. Darville T, Milligan LB, Laffoon KK. Intravenous immunoglobulin inhibits staphylococcal toxin-induced human mononuclear phagocyte tumor necrosis factor alpha production. Infect Immun 1997; 65:366–372.

33. Stegeman CA, Cohen Tervaert JW, de Jong PE, Kallenberg CG. Trimethoprim-sulfamethoxazole (cotrimoxazole) for the prevention of relapses of Wegener's granulomatosis. Dutch Co-Trimoxazole Wegener Study Group. N Engl J Med 1996; 335:16–20.

34. Richter C, Schnabel A, Csernok E, De Groot K, Reinhold-Keller E, Gross WL. Treatment of anti-neutrophil cytoplasmic antibody (ANCA)-associated systemic vasculitis with high-dose intravenous immunoglobulin. Clin Exp Immunol 1995; 101:2–7.

35. Jayne DRW, Chapel H, Adu D, et al. Intravenous immunoglobulin for ANCA-associated systemic vasculitis with persistent disease activity. Q J Med 2000; 93:433–439.

36. Jayne DRW, Rasmussen N. Treatment of antineutrophil cytoplasm autoantibody-associated systemic vasculitis: Initiatives of the European Community Systemic Vasculitis Clinical Trials Study Group. Mayo Clin Proc 1997; 72:737–747.

37. Schmitt WH, Heesen C, Csernok E, Rautmann A, Gross WL. Elevated serum levels of soluble interleukin-2 receptor in patients with Wegener's granulomatosis. Association with disease activity. Arthritis Rheum 1992; 35:1088–1096.

38. Stegeman CA, Cohen Tervaert JW, Huitema MG, Kallenberg CG. Serum markers of T cell activation in relapses of Wegener's granulomatosis. Clin Exp Immunol 1993; 91:415–420.

39. Guex-Crosier Y, Raber J, Chan CC, et al. Humanized antibodies against the alpha-chain of the IL-2 receptor and against the beta-chain shared by the IL-2 and IL-15 receptors in a monkey uveitis model of autoimmune diseases. J Immunol 1997; 158:452–458.

40. Maes BD, Vanrenterghem YF. Anti-interleukin-2 receptor monoclonal antibodies in renal transplantation. Nephrol Dial Transplant 1999; 14:2824–2826.

41. Datta SK, Kalled SL. CD40-CD40 ligand interaction in autoimmune disease. Arthritis Rheum 1997; 40:1735–1745.

42. Daikh DI, Finck BK, Linsley PS, Hollenbaugh D, Wofsy D. Long-term inhibition of murine lupus by brief simultaneous blockade of the B7/CD28 and CD40/gp39 costimulation pathways. J Immunol 1997; 159:3104–3108.

43. Moosig F, Csernok E, Wang G, Gross WL. Costimulatory molecules in Wegener's granulomatosis (WG): Lack of expression of CD28 and preferential up-regulation of its ligands B7-1 (CD80) and B7-2 (CD86) on T cells. Clin Exp Immunol 1998; 114:113–118.

44. Giscombe R, Nityanand S, Lewin N, Grunewald J, Lefvert AK. Expanded T cell populations in patients with Wegener's granulomatosis: characteristics and correlates with disease activity. J Clin Immunol 1998; 18:404–413.

45. Pierson RN III, Chang AC, Blum MG, et al. Prolongation of primate cardiac allograft survival by treatment with ANTI-CD40 ligand (CD154) antibody. Transplantation 1999; 68:1800–1805.

46. Vakkalanka RK, Woo C, Kirou KA, Koshy M, Berger D, Crow MK. Elevated levels and functional capacity of soluble CD40 ligand in systemic lupus erythematosus sera. Arthritis Rheum 1999; 42: 871–881.

47. Devi BS, Van Noordin S, Krausz T, Davies KA. Peripheral blood lymphocytes in SLE: Hyperexpression of CD154 on T and B lymphocytes and increased number of double negative T cells. J Autoimmun 1998; 11:471–475.

48. Kalled SL, Cutler AH, Datta SK, Thomas DW. Anti-CD40 ligand antibody treatment of SNF1 mice with established nephritis: Preservation of kidney function. J Immunol 1998; 160:2158–2165.

49. Yellin MJ, D'Agati V, Parkinson G, et al. Immunohistologic analysis of renal CD40 and CD40L expression in lupus nephritis and other glomerulonephritides. Arthritis Rheum 1997; 40:124–134.

50. Battaglia E, Biancone L, Resegotti A, Emanuelli G, Fronda GR, Camussi G. Expression of CD40 and its ligand, CD40L, in intestinal lesions of Crohn's disease. Am J Gastroenterol 1999; 94:3279–3284.

51. Lockwood CM, Thiru S, Isaacs JD, Hale G, Waldmann H. Long-term remission of intractable systemic vasculitis with monoclonal antibody therapy. Lancet 1993; 341:1620–1622.

52. Paolillo A, Coles AJ, Molyneux PD, et al. Quantitative MRI in patients with secondary progressive MS treated with monoclonal antibody Campath 1H. Neurology 1999; 53:751–757.

53. Isaacs JD, Manna VK, Rapson N, et al. CAMPATH-1H in rheumatoid arthritis: An intravenous dose-ranging study. Br J Rheumatol 1996; 35:231–240.

54. Passweg J, Gratwohl A, Tyndall A. Hematopoietic stem cell transplantation for autoimmune disorders. Curr Opin Hematol 1999; 6:400–405.

55. Tyndall A, Fassas A, Passweg J, et al. Autologous haematopoietic stem cell transplants for autoimmune disease-feasibility and transplant-related mortality. Bone Marrow Transplant 1999; 24:729–734.

56. Cherry, Engelman RW, Wang BY, Kinjoh K, El-Badri NS, Good RA. Prevention of crescentic glomerulonephritis in SCG/Kj mice by bone marrow transplantation. Proc Soc Exp Biol Med 1998; 218:223–228.

57. Qasim FJ, Mathieson PW, Sendo F, Thiru S, Oliveira DB. Role of neutrophils in the pathogenesis of experimental vasculitis. Am J Pathol 1996; 149:81–89.

58. Ludviksson BR, Sneller MC, Chua KS, et al. Active Wegener's granulomatosis is associated with HLA-DR+ CD4+ T cells exhibiting an unbalanced Th1-type T cell cytokine pattern: reversal with IL-10. J Immunol 1998; 160:3602–3609.

59. Zheng XX, Steele AW, Hancock WW, et al. A noncytolytic IL-10/Fc fusion protein prevents diabetes, blocks autoimmunity, and promotes suppressor phenomena in NOD mice. J Immunol 1997; 158: 4507–4513.

60. Noh GW, Lee WG, Lee W, Lee K. Effects of intravenous immunoglobulin on plasma interleukin-10 levels in Kawasaki disease. Immunol Lett 1998; 62:19–24.

61. Tomer Y, Barak V, Gilburd B, Shoenfeld Y. Cytokines in experimental autoimmune vasculitis: Evidence for a Th2 type response. Clin Exp Rheumatol 1999; 17:521–526.

62. Sayegh MH, Akalin E, Hancock WW, et al. CD28-B7 blockade after alloantigenic challenge in vivo inhibits Th1 cytokines but spares Th2. J Exp Med 1995; 181:1869–1874.

63. McHugh SM, Rifkin IR, Deighton J, et al. The immunosuppressive drug thalidomide induces T helper

cell type 2 (Th2) and concomitantly inhibits Th1 cytokine production in mitogen- and antigen-stimulated human peripheral blood mononuclear cell cultures. Clin Exp Immunol 1995; 99:160–167.

64. Calderon MJ, Landa N, Aguirre A, Diaz-Perez JL. Successful treatment of cutaneous PAN with pentoxifylline. Br J Dermatol 1993; 128:706–708.

65. Riechmann L, Clark M, Waldmann H, Winter G. Reshaping human antibodies for therapy. Nature 1988; 332:323–327.

66. Maini R, St Clair EW, Breedveld F, et al. Infliximab (chimeric anti-tumour necrosis factor alpha monoclonal antibody) versus placebo in rheumatoid arthritis patients receiving concomitant methotrexate: A randomised phase III trial. ATTRACT Study Group [In Process Citation]. Lancet 1999; 354:1932–1939.

67. Nachman PH, Reisner HM, Yang JJ, Jennette JC, Falk RJ. Shared idiotypy among patients with myeloperoxidase-anti-neutrophil cytoplasmic autoantibody associated glomerulonephritis and vasculitis. Lab Invest 1996; 74:519–27.

68. Strunz HP, Csernok E, Gross WL. Incidence and disease associations of a proteinase 3-antineutrophil cytoplasmic antibody idiotype (5/7 Id) whose antiidiotype inhibits proteinase 3-antineutrophil cytoplasmic antibody antigen binding activity. Arthritis Rheum 1997; 40:135–142.

69. Coutinho A. The network theory: 21 years later. Scand J Immunol 1995; 42:3–8.

70. Rossi F, Jayne DR, Lockwood CM, Kazatchkine MD. Anti-idiotypes against anti-neutrophil cytoplasmic antigen autoantibodies in normal human polyspecific IgG for therapeutic use and in the remission sera of patients with systemic vasculitis. Clin Exp Immunol 1991; 83:298–303.

71. Jayne DR, Esnault VL, Lockwood CM. ANCA anti-idiotype antibodies and the treatment of systemic vasculitis with intravenous immunoglobulin. J Autoimmun 1993; 6:207–219.

72. Jayne DR, Esnault VL, Lockwood CM. Anti-idiotype antibodies to anti-myeloperoxidase autoantibodies in patients with systemic vasculitis. J Autoimmun 1993; 6:221–226.

73. Sultan Y, Kazatchkine MD, Maisonneuve P, Nydegger UE. Anti-idiotypic suppression of autoantibodies to factor VIII (antihaemophilic factor) by high-dose intravenous gammaglobulin. Lancet 1984; 2:765–768.

74. Jayne DR, Davies MJ, Fox CJ, Black CM, Lockwood CM. Treatment of systemic vasculitis with pooled intravenous immunoglobulin. Lancet 1991; 337:1137–1139.

75. Cook RC, Connors JM, Gascoyne RD, Fradet G, Levy RD. Treatment of post-transplant lymphoproliferative disease with rituximab monoclonal antibody after lung transplantation [letter]. Lancet 1999; 354:1698–1699.

76. Falk RJ, Terrell RS, Charles LA, Jennette JC. Anti-neutrophil cytoplasmic autoantibodies induce neutrophils to degranulate and produce oxygen radicals in vitro. Proc Natl Acad Sci USA 1990; 87:4115–4119.

77. Ewert BH, Jennette JC, Falk RJ. Anti-myeloperoxidase antibodies stimulate neutrophils to damage human endothelial cells. Kidney Int 1992; 41:375–383.

78. Kettritz R, Jennette JC, Falk RJ. Crosslinking of ANCA-antigens stimulates superoxide release by human neutrophils. J Am Soc Nephrol 1997; 8:386–394.

79. Mayet WJ, Schwarting A, Orth T, Duchmann R, Meyer zum Buschenfelde KH. Antibodies to proteinase 3 mediate expression of vascular cell adhesion molecule-1 (VCAM-1). Clin Exp Immunol 1996; 103:259–267.

80. Griffin SV, Chapman PT, Lianos EA, Lockwood CM. The inhibition of myeloperoxidase by ceruloplasmin can be reversed by anti-myeloperoxidase antibodies. Kidney Int 1999; 55:917–925.

81. Dolman KM, Stegeman CA, van de Wiel BA, et al. Relevance of classic anti-neutrophil cytoplasmic autoantibody (C-ANCA)-mediated inhibition of proteinase 3-alpha 1-antitrypsin complexation to disease activity in Wegener's granulomatosis. Clin Exp Immunol 1993; 93:405–410.

82. Foucher P, Heeringa P, Petersen AH, et al. Antimyeloperoxidase-associated lung disease: An experimental model. Am J Respir Crit Care Med 1999; 160:987–994.

83. Brouwer E, Huitema MG, Klok PA, et al. Antimyeloperoxidase-associated proliferative glomerulonephritis: An animal model. J Exp Med 1993; 177:905–914.

84. Pusey CD, Rees AJ, Evans DJ, Peters DK, Lockwood CM. Plasma exchange in focal necrotizing glomerulonephritis without anti-GBM antibodies. Kidney Int 1991; 40:757–763.

85. Esnault VL, Testa A, Jayne DR, Soulillou JP, Guenel J. Influence of immunoadsorption on the re-

moval of immunoglobulin G autoantibodies in crescentic glomerulonephritis. Nephron 1993; 65: 180–184.

86. Elliott JD, Lockwood CM, Hale G, Waldmann H. Semi-specific immune-absorption and monoclonal antibody therapy in ANCA positive vasculitis: Experience in four cases. Autoimmunity 1998; 28: 163–171.

87. Haas A, Langmann A, Pizzera B, Winkler J, Zach G. Immunoadsorption as alternative treatment in a case of Wegener's granulomatosis with orbital apex syndrome. Spektrum der Augenheilkunde 1992; 6:240–243.

88. Palmer A, Cairns T, Dische F, et al. Treatment of rapidly progressive glomerulonephritis by extracorporeal immunoadsorption, prednisolone and cyclophosphamide. Nephrol Dial Transplant 1991; 6: 536–542.

89. Stegmayr BG, Almroth G, Berlin G, et al. Plasma exchange or immunoadsorption in patients with rapidly progressive crescentic glomerulonephritis. A Swedish multi-center study. Int J Artif Organs 1999; 22:81–87.

90. Arbiser JL, Dzieczkowski JS, Harmon JV, Duncan LM. Leukocytoclastic vasculitis following staphylococcal protein A column immunoadsorption therapy: Two cases and a review of the literature. Arch Dermatol 1995; 131:707–709.

91. Short AK, Lockwood CM, Bollen A, Moguilevsky N. Neutrophil and recombinant myeloperoxidase as antigens in ANCA positive systemic vasculitis. Clin Exp Immunol 1995; 102:106–111.

92. Griffin S CP, Elliott J, Brownlee A, Short A, Barclay A, Moguilevsky N, Bollen A, Lockwood CM. Recombinant human autoantigens as an extracorporeal immunoadsorbent in therapeutic apheresis. Jpn J Apheresis 1997; 16:17–22.

93. Mulder AH, Heeringa P, Brouwer E, Limburg PC, Kallenberg CG. Activation of granulocytes by antineutrophil cytoplasmic antibodies (ANCA): A Fc gamma RII-dependent process. Clin Exp Immunol 1994; 98:270–278.

94. Esnault VL, Audrain MA, Sesboue R. Alpha-1-antitrypsin phenotyping in ANCA-associated diseases: one of several arguments for protease/antiprotease imbalance in systemic vasculitis. Exp Clin Immunogenet 1997; 14:206–213.

95. Kao RC, Wehner NG, Skubitz KM, Gray BH, Hoidal JR. Proteinase 3: A distinct human polymorphonuclear leukocyte proteinase that produces emphysema in hamsters. J Clin Invest 1988; 82: 1963–1973.

96. Segelmark M, Persson B, Hellmark T, Wieslander J. Binding and inhibition of myeloperoxidase (MPO): A major function of ceruloplasmin? Clin Exp Immunol 1997; 108:167–174.

97. Ralston DR, Marsh CB, Lowe MP, Wewers MD. Antineutrophil cytoplasmic antibodies induce monocyte IL-8 release: Role of surface proteinase-3, alpha1-antitrypsin, and Fcgamma receptors. J Clin Invest 1997; 100:1416–1424.

98. Tesar V, Masek Z, Rychlik I, et al. Cytokines and adhesion molecules in renal vasculitis and lupus nephritis. Nephrol Dial Transplant 1998; 13:1662–1667.

99. Csernok E, Szymkowiak CH, Mistry N, Daha MR, Gross WL, Kekow J. Transforming growth factor-beta (TGF-beta) expression and interaction with proteinase 3 (PR3) in anti-neutrophil cytoplasmic antibody (ANCA)-associated vasculitis. Clin Exp Immunol 1996; 105:104–111.

100. Tanaka T, Abe M, Mitsuyama T, Fukuoka Y, Sakurada T, Hara N. Hyperresponsiveness of granulocytes to anaphylatoxins, C5a and C3a, in Churg-Strauss syndrome. Intern Med 1995; 34:1005–1008.

101. Collard CD, Agah A, Reenstra W, Buras J, Stahl GL. Endothelial nuclear factor-kappaB translocation and vascular cell adhesion molecule-1 induction by complement: inhibition with anti-human C5 therapy or cGMP analogues. Arterioscler Thromb Vasc Biol 1999; 19:2623–2629.

102. Oppenheimer-Marks N, Lipsky PE. Adhesion molecules as targets for the treatment of autoimmune diseases. Clin Immunol Immunopathol 1996; 79:203–210.

103. Kavanaugh AF, Davis LS, Jain RI, Nichols LA, Norris SH, Lipsky PE. A phase I/II open label study of the safety and efficacy of an anti-ICAM-1 (intercellular adhesion molecule-1; CD54) monoclonal antibody in early rheumatoid arthritis. J Rheumatol 1996; 23:1338–1344.

104. Coll-Vinent B, Vilardell C, Font C, et al. Circulating soluble adhesion molecules in patients with giant cell arteritis. Ann Rheum Dis 1999; 58:189–192.

105. Haller H, Eichhorn J, Pieper K, Gobel U, Luft FC. Circulating leukocyte integrin expression in Wegener's granulomatosis. J Am Soc Nephrol 1996; 7:40–48.

106. Isobe M, Yagita H, Okumura K, Ihara A. Specific acceptance of cardiac allograft after treatment with antibodies to ICAM-1 and LFA-1. Science 1992; 255:1125–1127.

107. Lockwood CM, Elliott JD, Brettman L, et al. Anti-adhesion molecule therapy as an interventional strategy for autoimmune inflammation. Clin Immunol 1999; 93:93–106.

108. Muller Kobold AC, van Wijk RT, Franssen CF, Molema G, Kallenberg CG, Tervaert JW. In vitro up-regulation of E-selectin and induction of interleukin-6 in endothelial cells by autoantibodies in Wegener's granulomatosis and microscopic polyangiitis. Clin Exp Rheumatol 1999; 17:433–440.

109. Bengtsson A, Redl H, Schlag G, Hogasen K, Gotze O, Mollnes TE. Anti-TNF treatment of baboons with sepsis reduces TNF-alpha, IL-6 and IL-8, but not the degree of complement activation. Scand J Immunol 1998; 48:509–514.

110. Kitagawa M, Mitsui H, Nakamura H, et al. Differential regulation of rheumatoid synovial cell inter-leukin-12 production by tumor necrosis factor alpha and CD40 signals. Arthritis Rheum 1999; 42:1917–1926.

111. Targan SR, Hanauer SB, van Deventer SJ, et al. A short-term study of chimeric monoclonal antibody cA2 to tumor necrosis factor alpha for Crohn's disease. Crohn's Disease cA2 Study Group. N Engl J Med 1997; 337:1029–1035.

112. Brahn E, Lehman TJA, Peacock DJ, Tang C, Banquerigo ML. Suppression of coronary vasculitis in a murine model of Kawasaki disease using an angiogenesis inhibitor. Clin Immunol 1999; 90:147–151.

113. Nishimoto N, Sasai M, Shima Y, et al. Improvement in Castleman's disease by humanized anti-inter-leukin-6 receptor antibody therapy. Blood 2000; 95:56–61.

114. Yoshizaki K, Nishimoto N, Mihara M, Kishimoto T. Therapy of rheumatoid arthritis by blocking IL-6 signal transduction with a humanized anti-IL-6 receptor antibody. Semin Immunopathol 1998; 20:247–259.

115. Okitsu-Negishi S, Furusawa S, Kawa Y, et al. Suppressive effect of intravenous immunoglobulins on the activity of interleukin-1. Immunol Res 1994; 13:49–55.

116. Sharief MK, Ingram DA, Swash M, Thompson EJ. I.v. immunoglobulin reduces circulating proin-flammatory cytokines in Guillain-Barré syndrome. Neurology 1999; 52:1833–1838.

117. Ito Y, Lukita-Atmadja W, Machen NW, Baker GL, McCuskey RS. Effect of intravenous immuno-globulin G on the TNF-alpha-mediated hepatic microvascular inflammatory response. Shock 1999; 11:291–295.

118. Aukrust P, Muller F, Svenson M, Nordoy I, Bendtzen K, Froland SS. Administration of intravenous immunoglobulin (IVIG) in vivo: Down-regulatory effects on the IL-1 system. Clin Exp Immunol 1999; 115:136–143.

119. Menezes MC, Benard G, Sato MN, Hong MA, Duarte AJ. In vitro inhibitory activity of tumor necro-sis factor alpha and interleukin-2 of human immunoglobulin preparations. Int Arch Allergy Immunol 1997; 114:323–328.

120. Stangel M, Schumacher HC, Ruprecht K, Boegner F, Marx P. Immunoglobulins for intravenous use inhibit TNF alpha cytotoxicity in vitro. Immunol Invest 1997; 26:569–578.

121. Levy Y, Sherer Y, George J, et al. Serologic and clinical response to treatment of systemic vasculitis and associated autoimmune disease with intravenous immunoglobulin. Int Arch Allergy Immunol 1999; 119:231–238.

122. Suzuki H, Uemura S, Tone S, et al. Effects of immunoglobulin and gamma-interferon on the produc-tion of tumour necrosis factor-alpha and interleukin-1 beta by peripheral blood monocytes in the acute phase of Kawasaki disease. Eur J Pediatr 1996; 155:291–296.

123. Brooks CJ, King WJ, Radford DJ, Adu D, McGrath M, Savage CO. IL-1 beta production by human polymorphonuclear leucocytes stimulated by anti-neutrophil cytoplasmic autoantibodies: Relevance to systemic vasculitis. Clin Exp Immunol 1996; 106:273–279.

124. Antonelli A, Agostini G, Agostini S. Preliminary results of intravenous immunoglobulins in treating patients with vasculitis. Clin Ter 1992; 141:33–36.

125. Boman S, Ballen JL, Seggev JS. Dramatic responses to intravenous immunoglobulin in vasculitis. J Intern Med 1995; 238:375–377.

126. Jayne DR, Lockwood CM. Intravenous immunoglobulin as sole therapy for systemic vasculitis. Br J Rheumatol 1996; 35:1150–1153.

127. Levy Y, George J, Fabbrizzi F, Rotman P, Paz Y, Shoenfeld Y. Marked improvement of Churg-Strauss vasculitis with intravenous gammaglobulins. South Med J 1999; 92:412–414.

128. Tuso P, Moudgil A, Hay J, et al. Treatment of antineutrophil cytoplasmic autoantibody-positive systemic vasculitis and glomerulonephritis with pooled intravenous gammaglobulin. Am J Kidney Dis 1992; 20:504–508.

129. Nachbaur D, Herold M, Gachter A, Niederwieser D. Modulation of alloimmune response in vitro by an IgM-enriched immunoglobulin preparation (Pentaglobin). Immunology 1998; 94:279–283.

130. Vassilev TL, Bineva IL, Dietrich G, Kaveri SV, Kazatchkine MD. Variable region-connected, dimeric fraction of intravenous immunoglobulin enriched in natural autoantibodies. J Autoimmun 1995; 8: 405–413.

131. Silvestris F, Cafforio P, Dammacco F. Pathogenic anti-DNA idiotype-reactive IgG in intravenous immunoglobulin preparations. Clin Exp Immunol 1994; 97:19–25.

132. Welcker M, Helmke K. Therapy of autoimmune nephrotic glomerulopathies by combined immunoadsorption and IVIG therapy. Immun Infekt 1995; 23:140–141.

133. Qasim FJ, Mathieson PW, Thiru S, Oliveira DB. Cyclosporin A exacerbates mercuric chloride-induced vasculitis in the brown Norway rat. Lab Invest 1995; 72:183–190.

134. Sloper CM, Powell RJ, Dua HS. Tacrolimus (FK506) in the treatment of posterior uveitis refractory to cyclosporine. Ophthalmology 1999; 106:723–728.

135. Martin DF, DeBarge LR, Nussenblatt RB, Chan CC, Roberge FG. Synergistic effect of rapamycin and cyclosporin A in the treatment of experimental autoimmune uveoretinitis. J Immunol 1995; 154: 922–927.

136. Schuler W, Sedrani R, Cottens S, et al. SDZ RAD, a new rapamycin derivative: Pharmacological properties in vitro and in vivo. Transplantation 1997; 64:36–42.

137. Ikeda E, Hikita N, Eto K, Mochizuki M. Tacrolimus-rapamycin combination therapy for experimental autoimmune uveoretinitis. Jpn J Ophthalmol 1997; 41:396–402.

138. Jayne D. Non-transplant uses of mycophenolate mofetil. Curr Opin Nephrol Hypertens 1999; 8:563–567.

139. Nowack R, Gobel U, Klooker P, Hergesell O, Andrassy K, van der Woude FJ. Mycophenolate mofetil for maintenance therapy of Wegener's granulomatosis and microscopic polyangiitis: A pilot study in 11 patients with renal involvement. J Am Soc Nephrol 1999; 10:1965–1971.

140. Metzler IL-F, E Reinhold-Keller, C Fink, W L Gross. Maintenace of remission with leflunomide in Wegener's granulomatois. Arthritis Rheum 1999; 42.

141. Hotta O, Furuta T, Chiba S, Yusa N, Taguma Y. Immunosuppressive effect of deoxyspergualin in proliferative glomerulonephritis. Am J Kidney Dis 1999; 34:894–901.

142. Birck R NR, Gobel U, Drexler JM, Hotta O, van der Woude FJ. 15-deoxyspergualin induces remission in Wegener's granulomatosis: Report of three cases. J Am Soc Nephrol 1999; 10:154A.

143. Lebreton L, Annat J, Derrepas P, Dutartre P, Renaut P. Structure-immunosuppressive activity relationships of new analogues of 15-deoxyspergualin. 1. Structural modifications of the hydroxyglycine moiety. J Med Chem 1999; 42:277–290.

144. Thomas JM, Contreras JL, Jiang XL, et al. Peritransplant tolerance induction in macaques: early events reflecting the unique synergy between immunotoxin and deoxyspergualin. Transplantation 1999; 68:1660–1673.

145. Muramatsu K, Doi K, Kawai S. Limb allotransplantation in rats: Combined immunosuppression by FK-506 and 15-deoxyspergualin. J Hand Surg [Am] 1999; 24:586–593.

146. Kahan BD, Julian BA, Pescovitz MD, Vanrenterghem Y, Neylan J. Sirolimus reduces the incidence of acute rejection episodes despite lower cyclosporine doses in caucasian recipients of mismatched primary renal allografts: A phase II trial. Rapamune Study Group. Transplantation 1999; 68:1526–1532.

147. Luqmani RA, Bacon PA, Moots RJ, et al. Birmingham Vasculitis Activity Score (BVAS) in systemic necrotizing vasculitis. Q J Med 1994; 87:671–678.

148. Exley AR, Bacon PA, Luqmani RA, et al. Development and initial validation of the Vasculitis Dam-

age Index for the standardized clinical assessment of damage in the systemic vasculitides. Arthritis Rheum 1997; 40:371–380.

149. Hoffman GS, Ahmed AE. Surrogate markers of disease activity in patients with Takayasu arteritis: A preliminary report from The International Network for the Study of the Systemic Vasculitides (IN-SSYS). Int J Cardiol 1998; 66(suppl 1):S191–194; discussion S195.

150. Jamar F, Chapman PT, Harrison AA, Binns RM, Haskard DO, Peters AM. Inflammatory arthritis: Imaging of endothelial cell activation with an indium-111-labeled F(ab′)2 fragment of anti-E-selectin monoclonal antibody. Radiology 1995; 194:843–850.

151. Reuter H, Wraight EP, Qasim FJ, Lockwood CM. Management of systemic vasculitis: Contribution of scintigraphic imaging to evaluation of disease activity and classification. Q J Med 1995; 88:509–516.

152. Hoffman GS, Drucker Y, Cotch MF, Locker GA, Easley K, Kwoh K. Wegener's granulomatosis: Patient-reported effects of disease on health, function, and income. Arthritis Rheum 1998; 41:2257–2262.

153. Hogan SL, Nachman PH, Wilkman AS, Jennette JC, Falk RJ. Prognostic markers in patients with antineutrophil cytoplasmic autoantibody-associated microscopic polyangiitis and glomerulonephritis. J Am Soc Nephrol 1996; 7:23–32.

154. Sankaran D, Asderakis A, Ashraf S, et al. Cytokine gene polymorphisms predict acute graft rejection following renal transplantation. Kidney Int 1999; 56:281–288.

155. Harari OA, Wickham TJ, Stocker CJ, et al. Targeting an adenoviral gene vector to cytokine-activated vascular endothelium via E-selectin. Gene Ther 1999; 6:801–807.

Index